CU01011314

SPECT in Neurology and Psychiatry

A Textbook of:
SPECT in Neurology and Psychiatry

Edited by
P.P. De Deyn
R.A. Dierckx
A. Alavi
B.A. Pickut

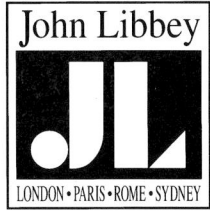

John Libbey

LONDON • PARIS • ROME • SYDNEY

British Library Cataloguing in Publication Data

A textbook of SPECT in neurology and psychiatry
   1. Tomography, Emission   2. Brain-Imaging
   3. Nervous system - Diseases - Diagnosis
   I. De Deyn, P.P. *et al.*
   616.8'047575

ISBN: 0 86196 542 6

Published by

**John Libbey & Company Ltd, 13 Smiths Yard, Summerley Street, London
SW18 4HR, England**
Telephone: 0181 947 2777   Fax: 0181 947 2664
John Libbey & Company Pty Ltd, Level 10, 15/17 Young Street, Sydney,
NSW, 2000, Australia
John Libbey Eurotext Ltd, 127 Avenue de la République, 92120 Montrouge,
France

Printed in Great Britain by WBC Bookbinders Ltd, Bridgend, Unit 5, Waterton
Industrial Estate, Bridgend, Mid Glamorgan, CF13 3YN, U.K.

Contents

Foreword

The neurologist of the nineties disposes of an extensive armamentarium for neuroimaging, including techniques such as CT scan, MRI, angiography, echo-doppler sonography, brainmapping, SPECT and PET scan. In particular, the introduction of computerised tomography in the seventies had a dramatic impact on clinical neurology, enabling direct non-invasive evaluation of central nervous system involvement obtained with high spatial resolution. In practice, for most neurological disorders associated with structural lesions, imaging may be limited to this technique. While magnetic resonance imaging (MRI) has already added sensitivity and spatial resolution to morphological imaging, the application of its principle is further explored in areas, such as spectroscopy, magnetic resonance angiography and functional MRI.

Meanwhile, the parallel growth of positron emission tomography (PET) in the area of functional neuroimaging provided better insights into physiopathological processes such as crossed cerebellar diaschisis. PET may be considered the parade horse of nuclear medicine, offering a considerable degree of freedom in the choice of tracers. In addition to neuroreceptor binding studies, PET explorations involve neuropsychological activation studies. In the latter area, the emerging functional MRI may prove to be a competitive alternative because of a higher spatial resolution and better temporal resolution, in the absence of radiodosimetric limitations.

Moreover, the tendency to implement PET in a hospital environment may be restricted by cost and practical feasibility. The clinical limitations of PET have stimulated the development of neuroSPECT in most nuclear medicine departments. Application of the tomographic principle to the conventional gamma camera, resulting in single photon emission computerised tomography (SPECT), together with the development of adequate radiopharmaceuticals, allowed functional information at a reasonable price in a wide range of neurological and psychiatric disorders.

Although Professor P. Ell, D.C. Costa and the late N.A. Lassen had already edited and written neuropsychiatric imaging works, based on their own wide experience, and not forgetting an illustrative compilation of case reports edited by Van Heertum *et al.*, we felt that a detailed textbook presenting an up-to-date and systematic approach of SPECT in the major neurological and psychiatric disorders, would serve as reference and base line work.

This comprehensive and colour-illustrated textbook in atlas format provides a 'state-of-the-art' view of SPECT in relation to its application in the fields of neurology and psychiatry. While most of the chapters contain the latest reviews from experts in the respective fields, some chapters are shorter and deal with more limited sets of original research and/or clinical experience data. The broad range of topics covered by specialists in the fields of nuclear medicine, neurology and psychiatry from all over the world, reflects the most recent evolution in functional neuroimaging within clinical neuropsychiatric sciences. The book is written in such a way that it remains stimulating throughout for both clinicians and nuclear physicians. Chapters deal with the clinical problems, providing sufficient clinical information and defining questions related to diagnosis, pathophysiology and evaluation of therapy. Each chapter illustrates the contribution of SPECT to the respective neurological and psychiatric fields.

The editors have organised the book with respect to clinical indication, which implies that whenever possible, methodological problems related to clinical indication are categorised under the relevant clinical topic. The textbook contains eleven sections devoted to: dementia; neuropsychology; psychiatric syndromes such as schizophrenia, obsessive-compulsive disorders, depression; movement disorders; epilepsy; paediatric neuropsychiatry; cerebrovascular disorders; neuro-oncology; trauma capitis; headache; infectious disorders and chronic fatigue syndrome. SPECT techniques that are presented involve perfusion as well as receptor-binding studies regarding basal and neuroprovocation paradigms. Special attention is also given to methodological issues and SPECT technology.

We gratefully thank all contributing scientists to this comprehensive work and especially acknowledge the skilful and diligent effort of Ms S. Van den Broeck, who provided secretarial assistance in this endeavour.

With the preparation of the textbook we hope to have provided an important tool for all nuclear physicians, neurologists, psychiatrists, neuropsychologists and neuropaediatricians. May this book serve as a guide towards the optimal application of SPECT in diagnosis, study of pathophysiology and therapeutic follow-up in neuropsychiatric illnesses.

Co-ordinating Editor: **P.P. De Deyn,** Department of Neurology, Middelheim Hospital, University of Antwerp, Belgium
Co-Editors: **R.A. Dierckx,** Division of Nuclear Medicine, University Hospital Ghent, Belgium
A. Alavi, Department of Radiology, Hospital of the University of Pennsylvania, USA
B.A. Pickut, Department of Neurology, Middelheim Hospital, University of Antwerp, Belgium

Dementia

SPECT in Neurology and Psychiatry, edited by P.P. De Deyn, R.A. Dierckx, A. Alavi and B.A. Pickut
© 1997 John Libbey & Company Ltd, pp. 3–9

SPECT in the Differential Diagnosis of Frontal Lobe Type Dementia and Dementia of the Alzheimer Type

Chapter

1

B.A. Pickut[*], J. Saerens[*], P. Mariën[*], J. Goeman[*], F. Borggreve[*],
J. Vandevivere[*], A. Vervaet[*], R. Dierckx[**] and P.P. De Deyn[*†]

Introduction

Neurodegenerative diseases of the brain are complex and interrelated illnesses which may share important behavioural and pathological characteristics. The differential diagnosis may present difficulties in some cases and therefore research continues into seeking new diagnostic tools. Current knowledge of these diseases is based largely on post mortem studies, mostly from the final stages of the diseases. Functional imaging provides a measure of the vital functions of the brain such as microperfusion and, by inference, local metabolism during life, and may help assist clinicians.

The focus of this paper is on the SPECT differentiation of two important forms of neurodegenerative dementia, the most frequent form being senile dementia of the Alzheimer type, and the less predominant form being dementia with frontal lobe features (FLD).

FLD has been recognised as a variant of progressive non-Alzheimer dementia and is a relatively new concept. Clinical, regional cerebral blood flow and neuropathological data suggest that this disease, once thought to be synonymous with Pick's dementia, is a member of a larger clinico-pathological syndrome related to the site of cortical involvement. The aetiology of FLD is still unknown, but a positive family history for the disease was reported in 60% of a group of 30 Swedish patients[1]. Frontal lobe degeneration of the non-Alzheimer's type follows (S)DAT as the second most common primary degenerative dementia, and it has been suggested that 8%[1] to 20%[2] of early-onset dementia may be attributed to this variant.

The term FLD was launched in 1987 to describe a disease characterised by a neuropsychiatric syndrome[3], a non-specific type of histo-pathological picture[4,5] and a typical pattern of reduced regional cerebral blood flow[6], in patients who generally begin to exhibit symptoms in middle age[7].

The neuropsychiatric syndrome of FLD has been described as follows. The progression of a variety of neurobehavioural changes is highly characteristic. At the early onset of the disorder, disturbances of social skills, apathy, depressed mood, hypomania, sloppiness, inadequate behaviour at social gatherings and impaired judgement constitute the most frequently reported behavioural anomalies. Impulsiveness, disinhibition, emotional restlessness, hyperorality

*Memory Clinic, Departments of Neurology and Nuclear Medicine, General Hospital Middelheim
†Department of Neurology, Laboratory of Neurochemistry and Behavior, Born-Bunge Foundation, University of Antwerp
**University Hospital of Ghent, Belgium

and psychotic changes usually appear in a somewhat later stage of the disease, while rigid behaviour, a tendency to simplicity in activities, oral dietary changes and repetitive habits reflect marked character alterations. Besides prominent personality changes, the disorder is typically characterised by a progressive loss of expressive speech initiation (verbal inhibition, adynamia) with verbal stereotypes often evolving into echolalia and a frontal mutism syndrome. In contrast to (S)DAT, in which behavioural changes mostly occur either only at a late stage or as a secondary reaction to cognitive failure, the neurocognitive dysfunction of memory, praxis, gnosis, temporal and spatial orientation are preserved for comparatively longer in FLD. The neuropathological presentation of FLD involves no distinctive subcellular dysmorphic features such as neurofibrillary tangles, Pick bodies, Lewy bodies or ballooned cells[8]. FLD is a primary cortical disorder with degeneration of the superficial layers of the frontal and anterior temporal cortex (lamina I-III) with mild gliosis and microvacuolation.

Finally, it has been suggested that a typical pattern of frontally reduced regional cerebral blood flow might further characterise FLD. SPECT is reported, in early studies using xenon, to give highly characteristic results in patients suspected to have FLD[9-12]. Patients with FLD were found to have focal frontal or frontotemporal blood flow reductions involving both hemispheres. This pattern of reduced flow in the frontal lobes is, however, not specific. Such an abnormality can be found in Pick's disease, Creutzfeldt-Jakob's disease, and in some cases of Alzheimer's disease[4,13]. Low frontal flow has also been described in schizophrenia and in toxic encephalopathy (alcohol, organic solvents)[14] as well as in depression[15]. Moreover, HIV infected demented patients are also reported to have frontal hypoperfusion [16,17]. Dementias associated with motor neuron disease and primary progressive aphasia yield SPECT scans with fronto-temporal hypoperfusion, possibly related to regional atrophies[18]. Moretti *et al.*[19] assessed cortical perfusion in patients with normal pressure hydrocephalus (NPH) and found a frontal hypoactive pattern that was not attributable to focal anatomical changes.

This paper reports the findings of a study of brain perfusion in two clinically defined populations, one consisting of 21 patients suffering from FLD and another group consisting of 19 age- and severity matched (S)DAT patients, to ascertain whether there were characteristics which could support the clinical diagnosis and further demonstrate pathological differences.

Materials and methods

Patients

All 40 patients selected for this study underwent a general internal examination, routine blood screening, neuroimaging consisting of CT and/or MRI to exclude intercurrent pathology (vascular dementia, atrophy, tumours, focal or more than age-associated atrophy), BEAM and EEG. The age of the patients in both groups was 70 ± 9 (M ± s.d.) years; the MMSE score in the FLD group was 16 ± 5.8 (M ± s.d.) and 15 ± 5.2 (M ± s.d.) in the (S)DAT group.

Twenty-one patients clinically diagnosed with FLD were selected from the records at the Memory Clinic, amounting to 7.3% of the newly investigated patients for cognitive deterioration between 1992 and 1995. Selection was based on the clinical presentation and neuropsychological diagnosis of FLD. The histories of the patients' families were also obtained, along with extensive neuropsychological assessments, revealing a characteristic neurocognitive profile that clearly indicated frontal lobe involvement and the degenerative course of the disease during follow-up. All 21 FLD patients underwent an initial battery of tests consisting of the MMSE, the hierarchic dementia scale[20] and Raven's coloured or progressive matrices. The patients with a presenile onset underwent additional tests: the Wechsler Adult Intelligence Scale; the Wechsler Memory Scale; Rey's 15 word list of auditory learning; the Rey-Osterrieth figure; Benton's visual form discrimination; Benton's judgement of line orientation; the Boston Naming Test; the Wisconsin Card Sorting Test; a verbal fluency task consisting of a one minute semantic category generation (animals, transportation, vegetables, clothing) and a two minute phonemic word generation task starting with the phonemes F, A and S. In addition, the MFS (Middelheim Frontality Score) was determined for all patients. This score is indicative of frontal lobe features and was obtained by adding the scores obtained on ten items. Each item was scored either 0 (=absent) or 1 (=present) based on (hetero)anamnesis and/or clinical observation yielding a total maximal score of 10. The ten items scored were: initially comparatively spared memory and spatial abilities (1); personality and behavioural changes: loss of insight and judgement (2), disinhibition (3), dietary hyperactivity (4), changes in sexual behaviour (5), stereotyped behaviour (6), impaired control of emotions (7), aspontaneity (8); speech disturbances such as stereotyped phrases, logorrhea, echolalia, mutism, amimia (9) and restlessness (10).

For the aim of the present study, age- and severity-matched FLD (n=21) and (S)DAT (n=19) groups were considered. The diagnosis of probable SDAT was based on National Institute of Neurological and Communicative Disorders and Stroke/Alzheimer's Disease and Related Disorders Association criteria (NINCDS/ADRDA)[21]. The patients also fulfilled the DSM IV-criteria. In matching both groups, the global MMSE score was used to determine severity levels.

SPECT acquisition and analysis

All 40 patients underwent a ^{99m}Tc-HMPAO SPECT using a previously inserted and fixed butterfly needle, administering 20 mCi (740 MBq) [99m]HMPAO (Ceretec, Amersham International plc, UK) to the patient, who was lying down in a quiet room with indirect neon lighting, eyes open and ears unplugged. Four point sources were fixed along the orbitomeatal axis as reference for later reorientation of the transverse slices. The manufacturer's instructions were followed for the preparation of ^{99m}Tc-HMPAO using one vial.

Data acquisition was started 20 minutes after radiopharmaceutical injection, using a three-detector system (Triad 88, Trionix Research Laboratory, USA) equipped with lead high-resolution fan-beam collimators. Data were collected for 40 projections per camera head (3° steps, 40 s per projection, 128x64 matrix, pixel size 3.6 mm). Projection images were smoothed and reconstructed in a 64x64 matrix, using a Butterworth filter with a high cut-off frequency and roll-off of 5. The slices were reoriented parallel to the orbitomeatal axis.

The SPECT images were all read by two physicians (BP and RD), experienced in nuclear medicine and neurology. The physicians were unaware of the type and severity of cognitive impairment of the patient studied. The images were assessed qualitatively by visual interpretation of colour shades in the cortical regions. The monitor display format had a 10 component colour scale with cerebellum, visual cortex and basal ganglia representing the maximum of reconstructed activity. Each patient data set was normalised individually to the mean cerebellar pixel values. Brain SPECT perfusion deficits were scored by visual qualitative analysis with respect to location: frontal, parietal, temporal and occipital; lateralisation, left and/or right; and severity score:

> 0 = normal (no perfusion deficit)
> 1 = slight (13-30%)
> 2 = moderate (30-50%)
> 3 = severe (>50%, including
>   breaching of the cortex).

In the case of bilateral lesions, the adjacent cortex was used as a guideline.

A total severity score was calculated by adding all the severity scores for right and left frontal, parietal and temporal lobes, yielding a theoretical maximum value of 18 (6x3). In addition, a severity score of bifrontal hypoperfusion (Fs) was calculated. Fs was obtained by adding the severity scores (minimal 0 to maximal 3) of both frontal lobes, yielding a minimal value of 0 in the case of normal bifrontal perfusion and a maximal score of 6 in the case of severe bifrontal hypoperfusion. In cases in which there was a bilateral anterior-posterior gradient, the cerebellum was used as a reference with a minimal index of 65%. The images were interpreted, according to Holman's method[22], into the following perfusion patterns:

A: normal
B: bilateral posterior temporal and/or parietal cortex defects
C: bilateral posterior temporal and/or parietal cortex defects with additional defects
D: unilateral posterior temporal and/or parietal cortex defects with or without aditional defects
E: frontal cortex defects only
F: other large (>7cm) defects
G: multiple small (≤7cm) cortical defects

Results

The MMSE score, MFS, classification according to Holman, temporal, parietal and frontal hypoperfusion on the right and on the left side, as well as the clinical diagnosis of all patients involved, are listed in Table 1. There were no regions of occipital hypoperfusion with more than 13% asymmetry. Figures 1 and 2 illustrate the perfusional differences between (S)DAT and FLD.

No significant correlation was found between MMSE score and total severity SPECT score. When temporal lobe hypoperfusion was examined uni- and bi-laterally, no significant difference was found between FLD and (S)DAT. However, analysis of parietal and frontal lobe hypoperfusion yielded significant results. Biparietal hypoperfusion was found to be greater in (S)DAT (Whitney-Mann p = 0.016) and bifrontal hypoperfusion was significantly higher in clinical FLD (Whitney-Mann p = 0.0054). A logistic regression model predicting FLD versus (S)DAT based on SPECT was developed. This stepwise test allowed significant discrimination between FLD and (S)DAT. The probability of predicting a (S)DAT based on the SPECT scan is calculated as follows:

$$p\ (DAT) = 1\ /\ [1 + e - (1.1 - 6.661 \times Fs\ )]$$

Table 1 MMSE, MFS and SPECT findings in dementia

Patient number	MMSE	MFS	Holman score[a]	Temporal hypoperfusion[b]		Parietal hypoperfusion[b]		Frontal hypoperfusion[b]		Clinical diagnosis
				Left	Right	Left	Right	Left	Right	
1	20	7	D	1	0	1	0	2	1	FLD
2	14	7	C	2	3	2	3	1	2	FLD
3	5	5	D	0	1	0	1	0	0	DAT
4	16	2	G	1	0	1	1	1	0	DAT
5	14	7	D	0	0	0	1	0	0	FLD
6	16	0	C	2	0	2	0	2	2	DAT
7	16	8	C	2	1	2	0	2	1	FLD
8	18	5	D	0	2	0	0	1	2	FLD
9	10	4	C	3	2	2	1	2	2	DAT
10	12	5	E	0	0	0	0	2	1	FLD
11	5	5	C	2	1	1	0	2	1	FLD
12	15	1	C	2	2	2	2	1	1	DAT
13	8	3	D	1	0	2	0	0	0	FLD
14	7	2	B	2	3	1	2	0	0	DAT
15	7	2	C	1	2	1	2	0	1	DAT
16	20	6	E	0	0	0	0	1	1	FLD
17	21	0	C	2	3	1	2	1	0	DAT
18	21	1	C	2	3	1	2	2	2	DAT
19	26	3	B	0	2	1	2	0	0	FLD
20	12	4	C	2	1	1	1	1	1	FLD
21	10	0	B	2	1	1	1	0	0	DAT
22	18	5	D	2	0	1	0	2	1	FLD
23	14	3	D	2	0	1	0	0	0	DAT
24	20	7	D	2	0	1	0	2	1	FLD
25	15	4	C	2	1	2	1	1	0	DAT
26	24	3	C	1	2	1	0	0	1	DAT
27	13	6	D	2	0	1	0	2	2	FLD
28	20	6	C	3	2	2	1	2	1	FLD
29	18	4	C	1	2	1	2	0	1	DAT
30	13	2	D	0	1	0	2	1	2	FLD
31	16	3	C	2	0	1	1	0	0	DAT
32	21	1	C	0	0	1	1	1	0	DAT
33	20	1	D	0	0	2	0	1	2	FLD
34	16	6	C	1	2	1	2	0	2	FLD
35	17	7	C	1	0	1	1	1	1	FLD
36	19	0	C	0	1	1	2	0	0	DAT
37	12	7	D	0	2	1	1	2	2	FLD
38	10	7	D	0	2	0	1	0	1	FLD
39	11	4	D	0	0	1	0	1	1	DAT
40	16	0	D	2	0	1	0	0	1	DAT

[a], A: normal, B: bilateral posterior temporal and/or parietal cortex defects, C: bilateral posterior temporal and/or parietal cortex defects with additional defects, D: unilateral posterior temporal and/or parietal cortex defects with or without additional defects, E: frontal cortex defects only, F: other large (>7cm) defects, G: multiple small (<7cm) cortical defects
[b], severity score: 0, normal; 1, slight (13-30%); 2, moderate (30-50%); 3, severe (>50%)

in which Fs is the severity score of bifrontal hypoperfusion. Using this equation, a value above 0.5 was indicative of (S)DAT and 74% of the SPECT studies of (S)DAT were correctly classified. A calculated value below 0.5 was indicative of FLD and 81% of the SPECT studies of FLD were correctly classified.

Following the Holman criteria, 34 of the 40 patients in our study were classified into categories C and D. There were 19 patients in category C, which amounted to 63% (S)DAT and 37% FLD. Category D included 15 patients of which 27% were (S)DAT and 73% were FLD. Category E included 2 patients, both of which were FLDs.

Discussion

MMSE scores do not correlate with SPECT severity in either group. The MMSE is perhaps not the best measure of cognitive decline for the patients suffering from FLD since the MMSE emphasises orientation and memory, functions located in the parietal and temporal lobes rather than executive or frontal lobe functions. Performance on the MMSE was not correlated with the frontal rCBF in a group of FLD patients studied by Miller et al.[10].

In our group of 19 (S)DAT patients we found no correlation with hypoperfusion patterns and MMSE scores. This is in contrast to the literature where rCBF was found to correlate with severity of dementia[23,24]. The population studied was not graded with respect to severity and MMSE scores as our aim was not to look for such a correlation, but rather at differential diagnosis. The MMSE may have more significance as a measure in combination with SPECT as a predictive or longitudinal tool when taking the temporal perfusion into account[25].

With respect to the perfusion itself, significantly more frontal deficits were found in the patients with a clinical diagnosis of FLD and significantly more parietal deficits were found in (S)DAT. The correlation between parietal and or temporo-parietal hypoperfusion patterns and (S)DAT dates back to the late 1980s[26,27], and has been further validated using post mortem studies[28]. While early studies carried out on patients with frontal type dementia used xenon, Neary et al.[11] described 7 patients with dementia of the frontal type who underwent ^{99m}Tc-HMPAO SPECT scans which yielded higher resolution images. All of these patients exhibited selective reductions in uptake of tracer in the anterior cerebral hemispheres, whereas patients with proven Alzheimer's disease showed reduced uptake in the posterior cerebral hemispheres. Miller et al.[10] reported on 8 patients with frontal lobe dementia characteristics, showed a selective frontal hypoperfusion on SPECT and found SPECT extremely useful in separating these patients from Alzheimer's disease patients.

Some findings indicate that patients clinically corresponding to FLD may not demonstrate the typical cerebral perfusion pattern described above. Launes[29] reported on a group of 160 patients in which only 2 out of 5 clinically defined patients with frontal lobe dementia could be separated from other forms of dementia by SPECT. Our study is the first to report on a substantial group (n=21) of patients with the clinical diagnosis of FLD undergoing brain SPECT using ^{99m}Tc-HMPAO.

Our logistic regression model, based on SPECT, allows discrimination between (S)DAT and FLD. The percentage classified correctly (81% of the FLD group

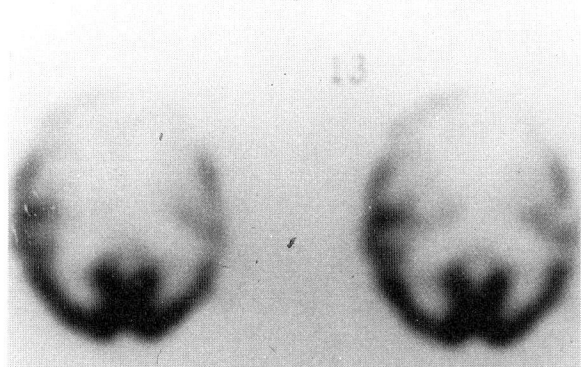

Figure 1 SPECT image of patient number 37 suffering from dementia of the frontal type showing bifrontal hypoperfusion with total frontal severity score (Fs) of 4

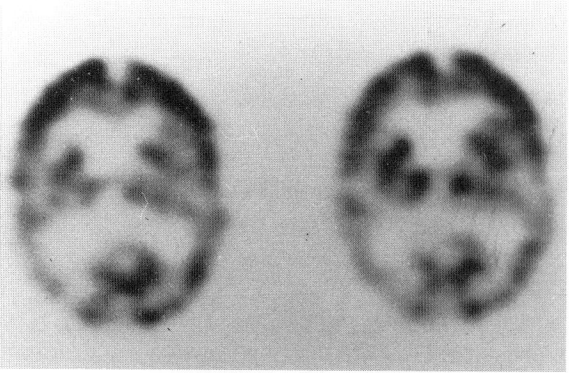

Figure 2 SPECT image of patient number 17 suffering from dementia of the Alzheimer type showing hypoperfusion in the parieto-temporal regions more pronounced on the right

and 74% of the (S)DAT group) might be an overestimation since it is based upon the same data that were used for the formulation of the model. The model requires further validation with independent data in order to investigate whether it is still applicable to new groups of patients suffering from FLD and (S)DAT. In order to achieve this, the percentage classified correctly in the new group will be calculated, based upon application of the old model. Nevertheless, the use of a logistic regression model for successful differential diagnosis between FLD and (S)DAT seems promising.

Using the Holman criteria category E (frontal cortex defects only), only 2 of the 21 (9.5%) patients with clinical FLD were selected. However, by making use of the severity of bifrontal hypoperfusion, or the frontal severity score, rather than by simply scoring presence or absence of hypoperfusion, the diagnostic yield was increased to 81%. The Holman criteria do not take severity of hypoperfusion into account and may not be applicable for a broad dementia population.

According to these results, SPECT yields an important clinical tool in that it may give an additional biological parameter. The tomographic information may furthermore allow the clinician to estimate the extent and severity of disease as well as providing an important means for follow-up in cases in which quantified SPECTs could be performed. In helping to understand dementia, SPECT, compared with PET, gives an affordable method for cumulative diagnostic yield. In the search for new treatment strategies within sub-populations of dementia such as (S)DAT and FLD, which might respond differently to therapy, SPECT allows us to view the functional repercussions on the brain. Moreover, early diagnosis is of particular importance in socio-psychological guidance and counselling given the different clinical presentation and prognosis of FLD and (S)DAT[3].

In conclusion, SPECT seems to be an important functional neuroimaging tool for discrimination of FLD versus (S)DAT. Further validation of the presented logistic regression model is ongoing.

Acknowledgements

This work was supported by: the Flemish Ministry of Education; the Baron Bogaert-Scheid Fund; Born-Bunge Foundation; Medical Research Foundation OCMW Antwerp; University of Antwerp; the United Fund of Belgium; and NFWO grants 3.0044.92 and 3.0064.93.

References

1 Gustafson, L. Clinical picture of frontal lobe degeneration of the non-Alzheimer type. *Dementia* 1993, 4, 143

2 Neary, D. Dementia of frontal lobe type. *J. Am. Ger. Soc.* 1990, 38, 71

3 Gustafson, L. Frontal lobe degeneration of non-Alzheimer type.II Clinical picture and differential diagnosis. *Arch. Gerontol. Geriatr.* 1987, 6, 209

4 Brun, A. Frontal lobe degeneration of non-Alzheimer type: *Neuropathology. Arch. Gerontol. Geriatr.* 1987, 6, 193

5 Englund, E. and Brun, A. Frontal lobe degeneration of non-Alzheimer type.IV White matter changes. *Arch. Gerontol. Geriatr.* 1987, 6, 235

6 Risberg, J. Frontal lobe degeneration of non-Alzheimer type.III Regional cerebral blood flow. *Arch. Gerontol. Geriatr.* 1987, 6, 225

7 Brun, A. Dementia of frontal type. *Dementia* 1993, 4, 125

8 Knopman, DS. Overview of dementia lacking distinctive histology: pathological designation of a progressive dementia. *Dementia* 1993, 4,132

9 Goulding, P., Burjan, A., Smith, R. *et al.* Semi-automatic quantification of regional cerebral perfusion in primary degenerative dementia using ^{99m}technetium-hexamethylpropylene amine oxime and single photon emission tomography. *Eur. J. Nuc. Med.* 1990, 17, 77

10 Miller, B.L., Cummings, J.L., Villanueva-Meyer, J. *et al.* Frontal lobe degeneration: clincial, neuropsychological, and SPECT characteristics. *Neurology* 1991, 41, 1347

11 Neary, D., Snowden, J.S., Northen, B. and Goulding, P. Dementia of the frontal lobe type. *J. Neurol. Neurosurg. Psych.* 1988, 51, 353

12 Ohnishi, T., Hoshi, H., Jinnouchi, S., Nagamachi, S. *et al.* The utility of cerebral blood flow imaging in patients with unique syndrome of progressive dementia with motor neuron disease. *J. Nucl. Med.* 1990, 31, 688

13 Brun, A. Frontal lobe degeneration of non-Alzheimer type.I *Neuropathology. Arch. Gerontol. Geriatr.* 1987, 6, 193

14 Risberg, J., Passant, U., Warkentin, S. and Gustafson, L. Regional blood flow in frontal lobe dementia of non-Alzheimer type. *Dementia* 1993, 4, 186

15 Van Heertum, R.L. in 'Clinical diagnosis: major depressive disorder in Cerebral SPECT Imaging', (Eds. R.L. Heertum and R.S. Tikofsky), Raven Press, USA, 1995, p. 194

16 Costa, D.C., Ell, P., Burns, A. *et al.* CBF tomograms with ^{99m}Tc-HMPAO in patients with dementia (Alzheimer type and HIV) and Parkinson's disease - initial results. *J. Cereb. Blood Flow Metab.* 1988, 8, S109

17 Pohl, P., Vogel, G., Fill, H. *et al.* Single photon emission computed tomography in AIDS dementia complex. *J. Nucl. Med.* 1988, 29, 1382

18 Neary, D., Snowden, J.S. and Mann, D.M.A. The clinical pathological correlates of lobar atrophy. *Dementia* 1993, 4, 143

19 Moretti, J.L., Sergent, A., Louarn, F. *et al.* Cortical perfusion assessment with 123I-isopropyl amphetamine (I-123-AMP) in normal pressure hydrocephalus (NPH). *Eur. J. Nucl. Med.* 1988, 14, 73

20 Cole, M.G., and Dastoor, D. A new hierarchic approach to the measurement of dementia. *Psychosomatics* 1987, 28, 298

21 McKhann, G., Drachman, D., Folstein, M. *et al.* Clinical diagnosis of Alzheimer's disease: report of the NINCDS-ADRDA work group under the auspices of Department of Health and Juman services task force on Alzheimer's disease. *Neurol.* 1984, 34, 939

22 Holman, B.L., Johnson, K.A., Greada, B. *et al.* The scintigraphic appearance of Alzheimer's disease: a prospective study using technetium-99m-HMPAO SPECT. *J. Nucl. Med.* 1992, 33, 1941

23 Eagger, S., Syed, G.M.S., Burns, A. *et al.* Morphologic (CT) and functional (rCBF SPECT) correlates in Alzheimer's disease. *Nucl. Med. Comm.* 1992, 13, 644

24 Johnson, K.A., Holman, B.L., Mueller, S.P. *et al.* Single photon emission computed tomography in Alzheimer's disease. Abnormal iofetamine I-123 uptake reflects dementia severity. *Arch. Neurol.* 1988, 45, 392

25 Wolfe, N., Reed, B.R., Eberling, J.L. and Jagust, W.J. Temporal lobe perfusion on single photon emission computed tomography predicts rate of cognitive decline in Alzheimer's disease. *Arch. Neurol.* 1995, 52, 257

26 McGeer, P.L., Kamo, H., Harrop, R. *et al.* Comparison of PET, MRI and CT with pathology in a proven case of Alzheimer's disease. *Neurol.* 1986, 36, 1569

27 Perani, D., DiPiero, V., Vallar, G. *et al.* Technetium-99m HMPAO-SPECT study of regional cerebral perfusion in early Alzheimer's disease. *J. Nucl. Med.* 1988, 29, 1507

28 Jobst, K.A., Smith, A.D., Barker, C.S. *et al.* Association of atrophy of the medial temporal lobe with reduced blood flow in the posterior parietotemporal cortex in patients with a clinical and pathological diagnosis of Alzheimer's disease. *J. Neurol. Neurosurg. Psych.* 1992, 55, 190

29 Launes, J., Sulkava, R., Erkinjuntti, T. *et al.* Technetium-99m HMPAO SPECT in suspected dementia. *Nucl. Med. Comm.* 1991, 12, 757

SPECT in Neurology and Psychiatry, edited by P.P. De Deyn, R.A. Dierckx, A. Alavi and B.A. Pickut
© 1997 John Libbey & Company Ltd, pp. 11–17

SPECT Findings in Vascular Dementia and Alzheimer's Disease

Chapter

2

S.E. Starkstein and S. Vázquez

Introduction

Vascular disease is a major cause of dementia, and may account for about 15% of all dementia cases[1]. The prevalence of vascular dementia increases with age and is higher in men[1]. While formal criteria for the diagnosis of ischaemic vascular dementia (IVD) have been proposed recently[1,2] (Tables 1 and 2), whether these criteria reliably separate IVD from other dementias such as Alzheimer's disease (AD) has only recently been addressed.

SPECT studies in IVD

Several studies examined the presence of cerebral blood flow (CBF) differences between patients with IVD or AD using photon emission tomography (SPECT). Jagust *et al.*[3] examined 9 patients with AD, 2 patients with multi infarct dementia (MID), and 5 normal controls using SPECT with N-isopropyl-p-iodoamphetamine (IMP) labelled with [123] I. They found that all 9 patients with AD had bilateral diminished radionuclide uptake in the temporo-parietal cortex, while patients with MID showed less activity in the frontal cortex.

In a study that included a larger sample, Gemmell *et al.*[5] assessed 17 patients with AD and 10 patients with IVD using HMPAO SPECT. They found that perfusion deficits were significantly more frequent in AD patients as compared with IVD patients. Bilateral temporo-parieto-occipital perfusion deficits were found in 76% of the AD patients but in only 20% of the IVD patients (p<0.05). The limitations of this study were that the SPECT findings were not quantitated, patients were not matched for demographic variables, and it was not stated whether AD and IVD groups had a comparable severity of dementia.

Deutsch and Tweedy[5] examined 15 patients with AD and 15 patients with IVD, matched for age and severity of dementia using the ^{133}Xe inhalation technique. They found that 13 of the 15 AD patients showed lower blood flow in the left parietal lobe, while MID patients showed frequent regional anomalies in CBF, but without a consistent pattern. This finding may be explained partially by the limited localising value of the xenon technique.

Mc Keith *et al.*[6] carried out HMPAO SPECT studies in 20 patients with IVD, 20 patients with AD, and 20 normal controls. While they found lower bilateral fronto-parietal perfusion in the AD as compared with the IVD group, IVD patients were significantly younger than AD patients, and there were also significant between-group differences in gender distribution.

Raúl Carrea Institute of Neurological Research, Montañeses 2325, 1428 Buenos Aires, Argentina

Table 1 Diagnosis of probable ischaemic vascular dementia (criteria of the State of California Alzheimer's Disease Diagnostic and Treatment Centers)

Dementia

Dementia is a deterioration from a known or estimated prior level of intellectual function sufficient to interfere broadly with the conduct of the patient's customary affairs of life, which is not isolated to a single narrow category of intellectual performance, and which is independent of level of consciousness.

Evidence of two or more ischaemic strokes by history, neurological signs, and/or neuroimaging studies (CT or T_1-weighed MR imaging), or the occurrence of a single stroke with clearly documented temporal relationship to the onset of dementia.

Evidence of a least one infarct outside the cerebellum by CT or T_1-weighted MR imaging.

Table 2 Diagnosis of probable vascular dementia (criteria of the NINDS-ARIEN International Work Group)

Dementia

Defined by cognitive decline from a previously higher level of functioning and manifested by impairment of memory and of two or more cognitive domains (orientation, attention, language, visuospatial functions, executive functions, motor control, and praxis) preferably established by clinical examination and documented by neuropsychological testing; deficits should be severe enough to interfere with activities of daily living, with the impairment not being due to physical effects of stroke alone.

Cerebrovascular disease

Defined by the presence of focal signs on neurological examination, such as hemiparesis, lower facial weakness, Babinski sign, sensory deficit, hemianopsia, dysarthria, etc. consistent with stroke (with or without history of stroke), and evidence of relevant cerebrovascular disease by brain imaging (CT or MR imaging) including multiple large-vessel stokes or a single multiple basal ganglia and white matter lacunes or extensive periventricular white matter lesions, or combination thereof.

A relationship between the above two disorders

Onset of dementia within 3 months following a recognised stroke

Abrupt deterioration in cognitive functions; or fluctuating, stepwise progression of cognitive deficits.

In a recent study, Mielke *et al.*[7] assessed 20 AD patients, 12 IVD patients, and 13 normal controls using HMPAO SPECT. While the AD patients had significantly lower perfusion in the temporo-parietal association cortex, no significant between-group differences were found in the remaining brain areas. However, one important limitation of this study was that IVD patients had higher mini-mental scores than AD patients (i.e. they were less demented).

While all the above studies have certainly advanced our understanding of the CBF correlates of IVD, several methodological limitations should be briefly addressed. First, in several SPECT studies, IVD and AD groups were not comparable in relevant demographic variables such as age and gender, and there were important between-group differences in the severity of the cognitive impairment. Another limitation was that since formal criteria for IVD have been proposed only recently, most SPECT studies have used different criteria for the diagnosis of dementia (e.g., a cut-off score on the Hachinski ischaemic scale[8] or the DSM-III9 criteria for vascular dementia).

We have recently assessed a consecutive series of 10 patients with IVD and 20 patients with AD using HMPAO SPECT. Patients with IVD met the State of California AD Diagnostic and Treatment Centers criteria[1] for probable IVD, while patients included in the AD group met the NINCDS-ADRDA[10] criteria for probable AD. IVD and AD patients were matched for age (± 2 years), gender, and mini-mental score (± 2 points).

Regional cerebral blood flow images were obtained by SPECT one week after the neuro-psychological examination. We used ^{99m}Tc-HMPAO (740 MBq) (Ceretec, hexamethyl-propylene amineoxime, exam-etazime, Amersham International) which was injected intravenously in an ante-cubital vein. Patients sat with eyes closed and ears unplugged in a quiet room with dim lights. Fifteen minutes after the injection patients were positioned supine and with the orbitomeatal line positioned vertically. The alignment was carried out using vertical and horizontal laser beams, and the head was held still by an ad-hoc head-holder. SPECT was carried out with a General Electric 400 AC/T rotating gamma camera attached to a Starcam 3200 computer. The resolution of the system has been measured to be 12 mm full-width at half-maximum in the plane of reconstructed transverse sections.

SPECT studies were carried out using a low energy high resolution collimator and a 64 x 64 matrix. There were 64 images obtained over 360° degrees, with an acquisition time of 30 s, and a zoom of 1.6. Processing was carried out by filtered back-projection using

Butterworth filtering, a critical frequency of 0.44, a slice-width of 1 pixel, and ramp filter. A coefficient of 0.12 was used for attenuation correction. Reconstructed brain slices were then reorientated in the orbitomeatal line using the sagittal and axial views, and a set of 30 axial, sagittal, and coronal sections at 6.4 mm increments were obtained. This procedure was carried out using Starcam software (General Electric, Wisconsin). Following the procedure of Burns et al.[11] square regions of interest (ROI) consisting of 3 x 3 pixels (voxel (3x3x1 pixels)= 2.35 cm^3) were used to obtain activity ratios in axial slices, taking the cerebellum as reference. Specific ROIs were identified using the Matsui and Hirano Atlas[12], and defined using each patient's CT scan. Three measurements (anterior, medial, and posterior) were carried out for each of the following cortical areas: frontal inferior (orbital), frontal superior (dorsal), temporal inferior, temporal superior, and parietal. These measurements were averaged for each cortical region on the right and left hemispheres. ROIs were also placed in the basal ganglia, thalamus, and cerebellum. To determine the activity ratio (brain region/cerebellum), the counts per ROI of each cortical area were divided by the average counts per ROI found in each cerebellar hemisphere in the region with the highest average count. This ratio was used as a measure of rCBF. All SPECT measurements were carried out by a neuroradiologist blind to the clinical data. A CT scan was carried out in every patient, and 5 mm thick slices were obtained parallel to the orbitomeatal line using a General Electric 8800 CT scanner.

A 2-way ANOVA with repeated measures showed a significant group x region interaction ($F(6,168)=2.29$, $p<0.05$). Patients with IVD showed significantly lower blood flow in frontal regions (both inferior ($p<0.001$) and superior ($p<0.01$)) and basal ganglia ($p<0.01$) as compared with AD patients (Figures 1 to 4). All 10 IVD patients had at least one ischaemic lesion on the CT scan, which involved the putamen (5 patients), internal capsule (3 patients), corona radiata (2 patients), thalamus (1 patient) , parietal white matter (1 patient), and the occipital lobe (1 patient).

Thus, while we could not find significant differences in temporo-parietal perfusion between AD and IVD patients, the latter had significantly lower CBF in the frontal lobes and basal ganglia. The presence of basal ganglia hypoperfusion in IVD may be related to the fact that 8 of the 10 IVD patients had ischaemic lesions involving the basal ganglia and/or the internal capsule. On the other hand, our finding of frontal hypoperfusion was not related to structural damage since none of the 10 IVD patients had frontal lobe lesions, but may be secondary to the anterior subcortical lesions.

In conclusion, while some studies showed frontal perfusion deficits in patients with IVD, others demonstrated a more severe bilateral temporo-parietal hypoperfusion among patients with AD. Frontal hypoperfusion in IVD may result from subcortical ischaemic lesions involving the basal ganglia and the internal capsule.

IVD vs. AD - SPECT FINDINGS

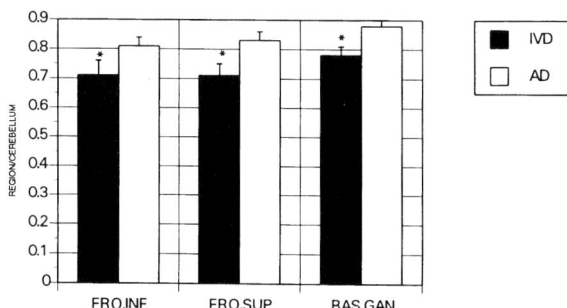

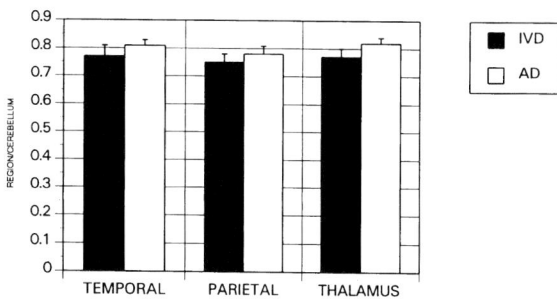

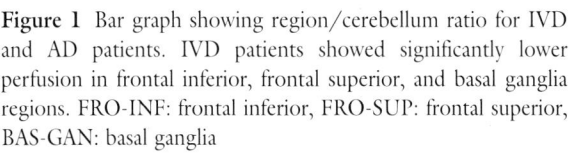

Figure 1 Bar graph showing region/cerebellum ratio for IVD and AD patients. IVD patients showed significantly lower perfusion in frontal inferior, frontal superior, and basal ganglia regions. FRO-INF: frontal inferior, FRO-SUP: frontal superior, BAS-GAN: basal ganglia

Figure 2 Bar graph showing region/cerebellum ratio for IVD and AD patients. No significant between-group differences were found in temporal, parietal, and thalamic regions

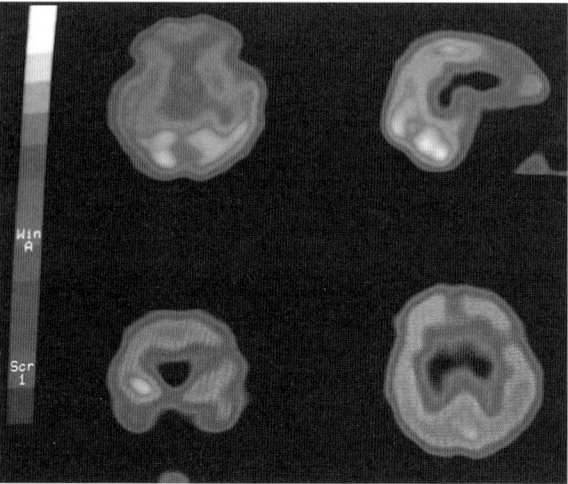

Figure 3 SPECT scan of a patient with IVD showing relatively more severe frontal perfusion deficits

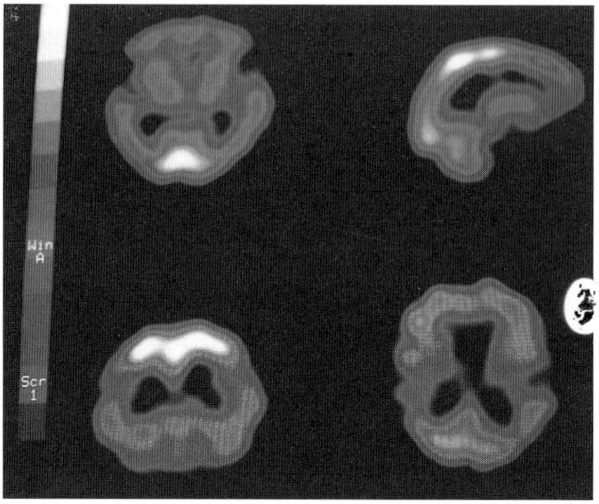

Figure 4 SPECT scan of a patient with AD showing relatively more severe temporo-parietal deficits

Neuropsychological differences between IVD and AD

Most SPECT studies in IVD only included a brief neuropsychological evaluation, and none of them assessed patients with a structured psychiatric interview. Thus, whether AD and IVD patients have a different profile of cognitive and psychiatric impairments has been rarely examined.

Powel *et al.*[13] assessed speech and language deficits in 18 patients with IVD and 14 patients with AD. While IVD patients showed significantly more impairments than AD patients in pitch, melody, articulation, and rate of speech, IVD patients showed significantly more deficits on information content and confrontation naming. These results suggest that the mechanical aspects of speech are more abnormal in IVD, whereas linguistic deficits are more prevalent in AD.

Villardita[14] assessed 30 patients with IVD, 48 patients with AD and 48 normal controls with a neuropsychological battery that included tests of spatial and temporal orientation, memory, visual-perceptual and constructional skills, language, conceptualisation, attention, and executive functions. He found that AD patients had significantly more severe deficits on tasks of orientation, verbal memory, and naming, whereas IVD patients showed significantly more severe deficits in tasks assessing attention, fine motor coordination, and executive functions. Villardita suggested that neuropsychological deficits found in IVD are similar to cognitive deficits characteristic of patients with frontal lobe damage.

Almkvist *et al.*[15] examined the presence of neuropsychological differences between patients with AD (n=83) and patients with IVD (n=42). Based on mini-mental state examination (MMSE) scores, they classified patients into groups with very mild, moderate, and severe dementia. While both groups showed a similar cognitive deterioration along the different stages of the illness, IVD patients had significantly more severe deficits on tasks assessing motor and cognitive speech.

Kertesz *et al.*[16] assessed 35 patients with AD and 11 patients with IVD using a neuropsychological battery that included tests of language, memory, and executive functions. They found that while patients with AD performed worse on memory and language tasks, IVD patients had significantly more deficits on tests 'that are influenced by frontal and subcortical mechanisms'.

In a recent study, we assessed 20 patients with IVD and 40 patients with AD matched for age, gender, and MMSE scores. All patients were examined with a neuropsychological battery that included tests of visual and abstract reasoning (the Raven's progressive matrices[17], and similarities from the Wechsler adult intelligence scale[18]), visual and verbal memory (the Benton visual retention test[19] and the Buschke selective reminding test[20]), attention (the digit span[18]), language (Token test[9] and Boston naming test[21], constructional praxis (block design[18]), and frontal lobe-related functions (verbal fluency[22], Wisconsin card sorting test[23], and trail making test[24]). We found that IVD patients had significantly lower scores than the AD

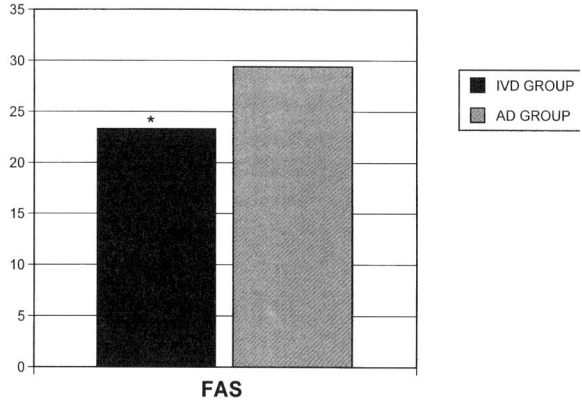

Figure 5 Patients with IVD showed significantly more severe deficits on verbal fluency than AD patients

TRAIL MAKING TEST - TIME B - A

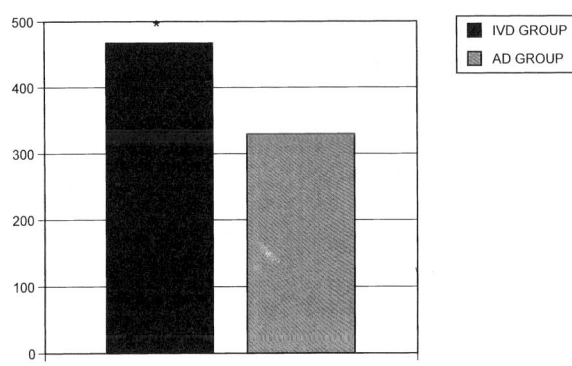

Figure 6 Patient with IVD showed significantly more severe deficits on the trail making test than AD patients

patients on the trail making test (F(1,58)=4.72, p<0.05) and the verbal fluency test (F(1,58)=4.71, p<0.05) (Figures 5 and 6), while no significant between-group differences were found on the remaining neuropsychological variables.

In conclusion, several studies compared groups of patients with IVD or AD and a similar severity of dementia, assessing the presence of different neuropsychological deficits. While some studies reported more severe language deficits in AD patients, most studies have reported selective deficits on frontal lobe-related functions in patients with IVD.

PATHOLOGICAL CRYING IN IVD AND AD

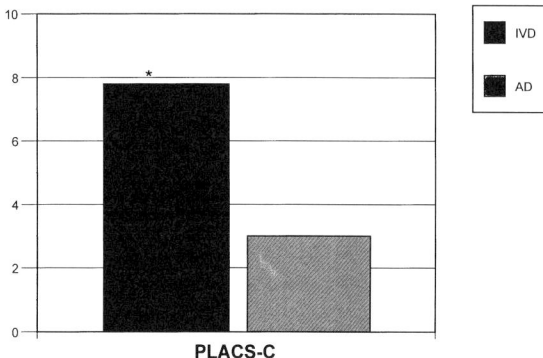

Figure 7 Patients with IVD showed significantly more severe pathological crying than AD patients

Psychiatric differences between IVD and AD

Few studies have examined the presence of differences in the prevalence of psychiatric disorders such as depression, emotional lability, and anosognosia (i.e., denial of intellectual deficits) between patients with AD and IVD. Cummings *et al.*[25] examined the prevalence of delusions, hallucinations, and depression in 30 patients with AD and 15 patients with IVD. They found depression to be significantly more frequent in IVD patients, while the prevalence of delusions and hallucinations was similar in both groups.

In our study of psychiatric disorders among patients with either AD (n=40) or IVD (n=20) we could not find significant between-group differences in the prevalence of major depression, dysthymia, anxiety, or delusions. On the other hand, 55% of patients with IVD showed pathological crying as compared with 15% of patients with AD (X^2 Yates=8.63, df=1, p<0.01) (Figure 7). Another important finding was that patients with IVD showed significantly more severe anosognosia than AD patients. These findings confirm the report of Ishii *et al.*[26] on frequent 'frontal lobe symptoms' (such as emotional lability, apathy, and urinary incontinence) among IVD patients with frontal white matter and internal capsule ischaemic lesions.

Conclusions

SPECT studies in IVD patients produced somewhat inconsistent results. While some studies showed that AD patients had significantly lower temporo-parietal perfusion than IVD patients, other studies demonstrated significantly lower frontal lobe perfusion in IVD. Several methodological limitations may account for these discrepancies. Some studies included IVD and AD groups that were not comparable in demographic variables or the severity of cognitive impairment. Moreover, few of the SPECT studies reported the prevalence and location of ischaemic lesions in patients with IVD, and studies may differ in the number, location, and cortical extension of those lesions. Thus, future studies should match IVD and AD patients for demographic variables and severity of dementia, and report the characteristics of ischaemic lesions.

Neuropsychological studies have consistently demonstrated that patients with IVD have significantly more deficits on tasks assessing frontal lobe-related functions (such as set alternation, planning, sequencing, and verbal fluency) than AD patients with a similar severity of cognitive decline. On the other hand, AD patients showed deficits on tasks usually associated with temporo-parietal functions, such as verbal and visuo-spatial memory. Neuropsychiatric findings in patients with IVD further support the association with frontal lobe dysfunction, since they showed significantly more severe anosognosia than AD patients, and we have recently demonstrated in a HMPAO SPECT study that demented patients with anosognosia had significantly lower right frontal perfusion than demented patients without anosognosia[27].

References

1　Chui, H.C., Mortimer, J.A., Slager, U. *et al.* Pathologic correlates of dementia in Parkinson's disease. *Arch. Neurol.* 1986, 43, 991

2　Roman, G.C., Tatemichi, T.K., Erkinjuntti, T. *et al.* Vascular dementia: diagnostic criteria for research studies. Report of the NINDS-ARIEN International Workshop. *Neurol.* 1993, 43, 250

3　Jagust, W.J., Budinger, T.F. and Reed, B.R. The diagnosis of dementia with single photon emission computed tomography. *Arch. Neurol.* 1987, 44, 258

4　Gemmel, H.G., Sharp, P.F., Besson, J.A.O. *et al.* Differential diagnosis in dementia using the cerebral blood flow agent ^{99m}Tc-HMPA: a SPECT study. *J. Comp. Assist. Tomography* 1987, 11, 398

5　Deutsch, G. and Tweedy, J.R. Cerebral blood flow in severity matched Alzheimer and multi-infarct patients. *Neurol* 1987, 37, 431

6　McKeith, I.G., Bartholomew, P.H., Irvine, E.M. *et al.* Single photon emission computerised tomography in elderly patients with Alzheimer's disease and multi-infarct dementia. *Brit. J. Psychiatry* 1993, 163, 597

7　Mielke, R., Pietrzyk, U., Jacobs, A. *et al.* HMPAO SPET and FDG PET in Alzheimer's disease and vascular dementia: comparison of perfusion and metabolic pattern. *Eur. J. Nucl. Med.* 1994, 21, 1052

8　Hachinski, V., Iliff, L.D., Zilhka, L. *et al.* Cerebral blood flow in dementia. *Arch. Neurol.* 1975, 40, 103

9　De Renzi and Faglioni, P. Development of a shortened version of the Token test. *Cortex* 1978, 14, 41

10　McKhann, G., Drachman, D., Folstein, M.F. *et al.* Clinical diagnosis of Alheimer's disease: report of the NINCDS-ADRDA Work Group under the auspices of the Department of Health and Human Services Task Force on Alzheimer's disease. *Neurol.* 1984, 34, 939

11　Burns, A., Philpot, M.P., Costa, D.C. *et al.* The investigation of Alzheimer's disease with single photon emission tomography. *J. Neurol. Neurosurg. Psychiatry* 1989, 12, 248

12　Matsui, T. and Hirano, H. in ' An atlas for the human brain for computerized tomography', Igaku-Shoin, New York, USA, 1978

13　Powell, A.L., Cummings, J.L., Hill, M.A. and Raven, J. in 'Manual for Raven's progressive matrices and vocabulary scales', H.K. Lewis & Co. Ltd, London, UK, 1986

14　Villardita, C. Alzheimer's disease compared with cerebrovascular dementia. Neuropsychological similarities and differences. *Acta Neurol. Scand.* 1993, 87, 299

15　Imkvist, O., Backman, L., Basun, H. and Wahlund, L.O. Patterns of neuropsychological performance in Alzheimer's disease and vascular dementia *Cortex* 1993, 29, 661

16　Kertesz, A. and Clydesdale, S. Neuropsychological deficits in vascular dementia vs Alzheimer's disease *Arch. Neurol.* 1994, 51, 1226

17　Raven, J.C., Court, J.H. and Raven, J. in 'Manual for Raven's progressive matrices and vocabulary scales', H.K. Lewis & Co. Ltd, London, UK

18　Wechsler, D. in 'Wechsler adult intelligence scale manual', The Psychological Corp., New York, USA, 1955

19　Benton, A.L. in 'The revised visual retention test', 4th Ed., The Psychological Corp., New York, USA, 1974

20　Buschke, H. and Fuld, P.A. Evaluating storage, retention, and retrieval in disordered memory and learning. *Neurol.* 1974, 24, 1019

21　Kaplan, E.F., Goodglass, H. and Weintraub, S. in 'The Boston naming test', Lea & Feibiger, Philadelphia, USA, 1983

22　Benton, A.L. Differential behavioral effects in frontal lobe disease. *Neuropsychol.* 1968, 6, 53

23　Nelson, H.E. A modified card sorting test sensitive to frontal lobe defects. *Cortex* 1976, 12, 313

24　Reitan, R.M. Validity of the trail making test as an incubator of organic brain damage. *Perc. Mot. Skills* 1958, 8, 271

25　Cummings, J., Miller, B. and Hill, M.A. Neuropsychiatric aspects of multi-infarct dementia and dementia of the Alzheimer type. *Arch. Neurol.* 1987, 44, 389

26 Ishii, N., Nishihara, Y. and Imamura, T. Why do frontal lobe symptoms predominate in vascular dementia with lacunes? *Neurol.* 1986, 36, 340

27 Starkstein, S.E., Migliorelli, R., Sabe, L.R. *et al.* A SPECT study of anosognosia in Alzheimer's disease. *Arch. Neurol.* 1995, 52, 41

SPECT in Neurology and Psychiatry, edited by P.P. De Deyn, R.A. Dierckx, A. Alavi and B.A. Pickut
© 1997 John Libbey & Company Ltd, pp. 19-25

Comparison of Cholinergic Neuroreceptor SPECT with ^{123}I- Iododexetimide and ^{99m}Tc-HMPAO in the Early Diagnosis of Alzheimer's Disease

Chapter

3

K.L. Boundy, C.C. Rowe, M. Reid, M. Kitchener,
L. Barnden, M. Kassiou*, A. Katsifis* and R. Lambrecht**

Introduction

The prevalence of dementia is increasing as the elderly proportion of the population increases. In Australia there is a predicted 120% increase[1] by the year 2025. Despite recent major genetic advances[2] in the aetiology and predisposition to Alzheimer's disease (AD), no reliable biological marker has been identified. The histopathological changes in this heterogeneous disease are said to occur earliest in the basal forebrain nuclei, the posterior parietal and temporal cerebral cortex [3]. Volumetric studies of the post mortem brain have shown that the most marked loss of volume is in the temporal lobes, especially the hippocampus [4]. Unfortunately, many forms of dementia can affect the temporal lobes causing hippocampal volume loss, making these changes non-specific. MRI of this region shows maintenance of the internal structures of CA1 and endofolium[5] and early magnetic resonance spectroscopic studies in AD show tissue characteristics similar to those found in elderly normals[6].

The central cholinergic deficit in AD as identified by researchers in the 1970s showed reduction in presynaptic cholinergic markers (ChAT, choline acetyl-transferase; AChE, acetyl cholinesterase) in post mortem Alzheimer's disease brain, consistent with degeneration of the presynaptic projection neurons to the cerebral cortex[7]. A lesser degree of degeneration occurs in the dopaminergic and serotonergic neuronal systems[7].

The well described neurofibrillary changes (neuritic plaques, neurofibrillary tangles, neurophil threads) exhibit a distinct but varying distribution in different cortical areas, particularly involving the cortical association areas, the entorhinal cortex of the temporal lobes. The density of plaques is inversely proportional to the density of cholinergic markers[8]. This clearer understanding of the neurochemical basis of AD prompted the application of modern cellular and molecular biological techniques to the study of AD.

Cholinergic neurons exert their effect through mediation of muscarinic and nicotinic cholinergic neurons. These receptors are classified by their

The Queen Elizabeth Hospital, (TQEH), 28 Woodville Rd, Woodville, Adelaide, South Australia, Australia 5011
*Australian Nuclear Science & Technology Organisation, Private Mail Bag 1 Menai, Sydney, NSW, Australia
**Eberhard-Karls-Universitat, Universitatsklink PET-Zentrum, Tubingen 15 Rontgenway, D-72076, Tubingen, Germany

pharmocological response, for example, the M1 receptor has a low affinity for carbachol and high affinity for pirenzipine, while the M2 receptor has reverse affinities. The M1 receptor is both pre- and post-synaptic and present throughout the grey matter of the brain, while the M2 receptor is predominantly presynaptic[8].

Conflicting reports of muscarinic receptor levels in AD (*in vitro* studies and post mortem brain) being reduced[9] or unchanged[10,11] have been published. Subsequent studies have indicated that a reduction in M2 receptor number or affinity in the cortical association areas in AD may be responsible for these discrepancies[12].

Because of these conflicting results regarding the muscarinic receptor status in AD and the paucity of neuroreceptor mapping of the muscarinic receptor *in vivo*, we assessed whether reductions in these receptors occurred in persons with Alzheimer's disease compared with elderly normals and whether these changes altered with increasing disease severity. We also evaluated the utility of an *in vivo* cholinergic neuroreceptor scan in early diagnosis of AD, and compared this with currently available cerebral blood flow SPECT.

Cholinergic antagonists scopolamine, dexetimide and 3-quinuclidinylbenzilate (QNB), and benztropine exhibit a high affinity for the mAChR, and have all been labelled with C-11 for investigation with PET[13,14]. Only QNB and dexetimide have been successfully labelled for SPECT[15,16]. After radio-iodination, both maintained their high affinity and selectivity for mChR *in vivo* and *in vitro*. A small study with [124]I-QNB, showed reductions of mChR in the frontal and parietal regions in persons with dementia[17]. We have recently evaluated the clinical utility of ^{123}I-iododexetimide (IDEX) in AD.

[123]I-iododexetimide is a muscarinic neuroreceptor ligand that can be imaged *in vivo* with SPECT[18,19] (Figure 1). Dexetimide, an anti-cholinergic drug was used for many years in Europe for the treatment of extrapyramidal disorders[18]. It has a high affinity for all subtypes of muscarinic receptor[20] and a long duration of action (> 72 h). Laduron[21] showed that the 3-hydrogen labelled D-isomer (D-benzetimide) was preferentially taken up in the striatum, nucleus accumbens and olfactory tubercle, frontal cortex and hippocampus in rats, and had very little activity in the medulla and cerebellum. ^{3}H-dexetimide was displaced at low concentrations in rat striatal homogenates by low concentration of 'cold' dexetimide, in contrast to L-benzetimide which required 2000 times more concentration to displace the ^{3}H-dexetimide. They concluded that greater than 95% of ^{3}H-dexetimide binding was stereospecific, with very low non-specific binding[22]. The L isomer, levitimide (L-benzetimide) whose action is on peripheral cholinergic receptors showed no preferential uptake in any particular brain area, and has subsequently been used to assess the effect of non-specific binding[22]. The preparation and evaluation of iododexetimide and its radioiodination was first described by Wilson and Dannals[16]. A small study of 4 normals and 4 persons with temporal lobe epilepsy was performed[23]. SPECT cerebral blood flow[24-28] and PET[29] metabolic studies are widely used in the assessment of persons with dementia. The typical findings are of hypometabolism and hypoperfusion in the temporo-parietal regions, with relative preservation of the primary motor and sensory cortex[25-28]. These changes frequently involve both cerebral hemispheres, but may be asymmetrical and less frequently show hypometabolism of the frontal association cortex[29]. In the earliest stages of Alzheimer's disease these cerebral blood flow studies may not show any of these typical abnormalities.

The aim of our study was to assess the usefulness of cholinergic neuroreceptor SPECT in the diagnosis of Alzheimer's disease, with particular emphasis on the earliest phases of the disorder in which novel treatments may be beneficial.

Methods

Ten elderly normal persons over the age of 60 (average age = 67 years) were recruited by local advertisement and underwent clinical and neurological examination, neuropsychological testing, (MMSE, ADAS-COG)

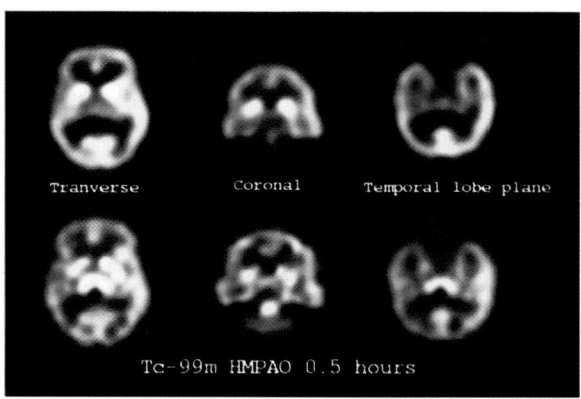

Figure 1 Cerebral distribution of IDEX in a normal male age 65 in comparision with HMPAO cerebral blood flow imaging. Note high IDEX uptake in the striatum and low activity in the thalamus and cerebellum, both areas of high blood flow but low muscarinic receptor concentration

prior to inclusion in this study. Brain SPECT scans were acquired after HMPAO and [123]I -iododexetimide SPECT[19](see methods below).

Recruitment of AD patients (n=30) was through local neurologists, and by advertisement through the Alzheimer's Association. The patients were assessed by a neurologist, a neuropsychologist and underwent a clinical examination and blood screens to exclude others causes of dementia. The average ages were: 64 years in the mild group; 75 years in the moderate group; and 68 years in the severe group. There was a family history in one third of all AD subjects. The duration from onset of symptoms of dementia was: 1.75 years in the mild; 3 years in the moderate group; and 4 years in those cases rated as severe.

All AD subjects had a CT brain scan. Those with evidence of previous cerebrovascular disease or a Hachinski ischaemic score of 4 or greater were excluded [30]. In our normal and AD group the Hachinski score was 2 or less.

Neuropsychological assessment included the MMSE[31] and ADAS-COG[32] test. All persons included in this study were required to fit the DSM III-R criteria for dementia[33] and the NINCDS-ADRAS for Alzheimer's disease [34]. The average MMSE in the normal group was 29.5/30, with the results in the mild = 25, moderate = 20 and severe = 8/30.

The severity of the dementia was graded using the clinical dementia rating scale[35] dividing the AD group into mild (n=12), moderate (n=11) and severe (n=7). Evidence of cognitive deficit in language (dysphasia),

motor skills (apraxia), and spatial skills (agnosia) in addition to memory impairment was required to fit the criteria above and those with very mild (MMSE >27) or isolated memory impairment were not included. Other systemic or neurological conditions, and frontal lobe dementia were excluded as well.

Single photon emission computerised tomography was performed on all normal subjects and persons with probable Alzheimer's disease. The cerebral blood flow study with 600 MBq HMPAO (Amersham) (injected in a resting position with the subjects' eyes closed for two minutes) followed by SPECT 30 min later. A standard solution of 1.5g KI was taken orally 30 min before injection of 185 MBq of IDEX. The neuroreceptor SPECT was performed 6 h after injection. The timing of scan acquisiton was assessed in our previous study and the radiation dosimetry was determined to be safe for human use[19].

The [123]I- iododexetimide was prepared at the Australian Nuclear Science and Technology Organisation. The technique of radio-iodination has been described elsewhere[16]. The radioligand was prepared on the day prior to use and was shipped overnight by air 1000 km from Sydney to Adelaide. The dose was administered at 9 am, and the patient returned for a brain SPECT scan at 3 pm that day.

SPECT was performed with ultra high resolution fan-beam collimators on a triple headed gamma camera (TRIAD 88, Trionix Research Laboratories, Ohio). SPECT acquisiton was of 72 angles, into a 128 x 64 matrix (3.56 pixel size) for 30 s per view. There was a simultaneous acquisition technique for ^{99m}Tc and

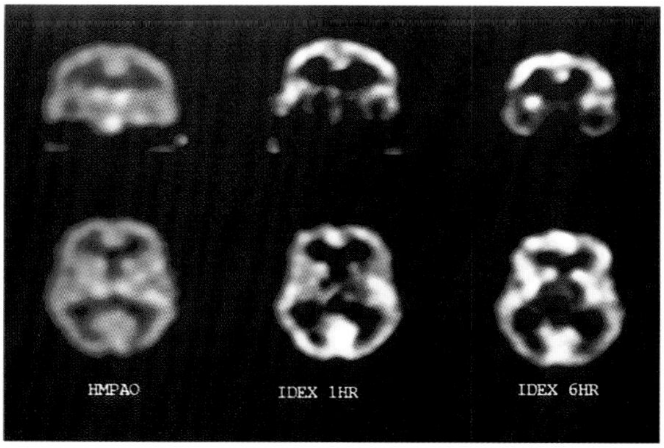

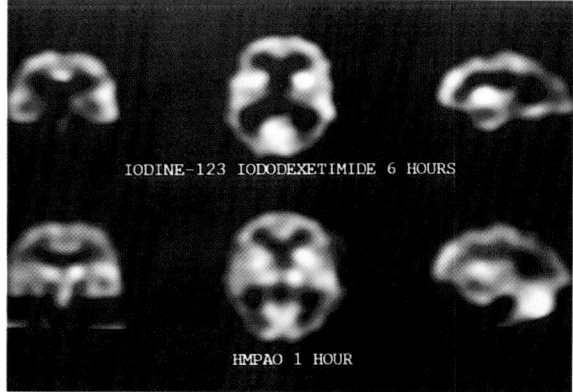

Figure 2 Comparative views of HMPAO SPECT versus IDEX SPECT at 1 and 6 h, in a 64 year old woman with mild Alzheimer's disease. The cerebral blood flow SPECT at 1 and 6 h and IDEX scan at 1 h do not show any deficits. However at 6 h there is clear reduction in IDEX activity in the temporoparietal cerebral cortex

Figure 3 IDEX SPECT scans at 6 h and HMPAO SPECT at 1 h in a 70 year old with moderately severe AD. There is a reduction in IDEX binding and in CBF in the temporal and parietal regions on both scans; both regions where AD neuropathology is prominent

[123]I, with a 10% window for ^{99m}Tc, in conjunction with a 10% asymmetric ^{123}I window (upper peak) [36]. Dual acquisition of the two isotopes was performed in 50% of the normals and all moderate and severe Alzheimer's sufferers, who were unable to lie still for two 30 min scans. Previous analysis of the dual acquisition technique via assessment of cerebellar ratios indicated that there was no significant 'cross contamination'.

The projection data were prefiltered in two dimensions with a Metz filter. The images were reconstructed to produce transverse slices (with the inferior surface of the frontal and occipital lobes aligned horizontally) and coronal slices in the temporal lobe plane.

Visual interpretation of all SPECT scans was carried out by three blinded observers and distribution of abnormalities identified and an overall assessment of whether the scan was normal, had non-specific or focal changes seen in only one plane. Possible AD scans were those with unilateral temporal or parietal, bilateral temporal deficits or global change in activity in two planes. Scan changes due to Alzheimer's disease were designated as those with the typical changes in the temporo-parietal cortical regions bilaterally. These scores were recorded for all HMPAO and IDEX scans and any disagreements were resolved by consensus.

Semi-quantitative analysis of the images was by a standard tranverse template with regions of interest over the striatum, frontal, temporo-parietal, occipital cortex and cerebellum. A further template was applied to the coronal temporal lobe slices with small regions placed over the medial and lateral temporal lobe. A 30% threshold was applied to these regions. Particular interest was paid to regions placed over the frontal association cortex, the posterior parietal association cortex, the temporal lobes and hippocampi. Two slices at the level of greatest activity through the basal ganglia were added together for analysis with the transverse template. Using the coronal temporal views, two slices each through the anterior, mid and posterior temporal lobes were analysed with small square regions placed over the medial and lateral cortex.

This semi-quantitative analysis has been validated for use in SPECT[37]. The striatum was chosen as a reference region, since it has the highest concentration of muscarinic receptors in the brain, and the cerebellar counts for IDEX were extremely low at 6 h as there are very few muscarinic receptors in the cerebellum. Statistical analysis was performed using non-parametric methods, between the normal elderly group and AD of different severity, for each ratio of cortical region to striatum.

Table 1 Semiquantitative analysis shows the ratio to striatum of the parietal and frontal cortical regions for IDEX and HMPAO. The reduction between the normal and mild AD group in the temporoparietal region with IDEX is statistically significant $p=0.02$

Disease	Frontal IDEX	Frontal HMPAO	T/Parietal IDEX	T/Parietal HMPAO
Normal	0.69	0.72	0.701	0.68
	s.d. 0.05	s.d. 0.06	s.d. 0.04	s.d. 0.05
Mild	0.65	0.71	0.595	0.6
	s.d. 0.04	s.d. 0.12	s.d. 0.07	s.d. 0.09
Moderate	0.63	0.69	0.602	0.58
	s.d. 0.08	s.d. 0.08	s.d. 0.07	s.d. 0.06
Severe	0.69	0.71	0.58	0.54
	s.d. 0.04	s.d. 0.06	s.d. 0.09	s.d. 0.07

Results

Blinded visual interpretation of HMPAO scans revealed temporal and posterior parietal cortical deficits in persons with clinical AD, as has been described clinically[24]. The blinded visual interpretation of the HMPAO scans for probable AD scan changes revealed a sensitivity of 70% and specificity of 81%. Adding the possible scan category increased this to 85% sensitivity, but 69% specificity. The negative predictive value of a normal scan was 88%. There were several HMPAO scans of the elderly normals that were labelled as abnormal with non-specific deficit, which was interpreted as possible AD scan abnormalities. There were also several IDEX scans that revealed abnormalities when the corresponding HMPAO was normal, or non-specific (Figure 2).

The IDEX brain SPECT scans were abnormal in all persons with the clinical picture of AD, but there were three normal subjects that showed non-specific abnormalities and two with possible AD changes. All normals are unchanged over two years. The areas of deficit in IDEX binding were in the temporal lobes, hippocampus, posterior parietal and frontal association areas with some appearance suggesting a global cortical reduction in receptor binding. Blinded visual review of IDEX SPECT showed a sensitivity of 83 % with a specificity of scan abnormalities of 80%.

This gives a positive predictive value of 90% for an abnormal IDEX brain SPECT (compared with 62% for HMPAO). The predictive value of a negative scan was only 62%. The accuracy of the IDEX scan was 83%.

Semi-quantitative analysis using ratios of cortical regions to the striatal reference region showed that there was a statistically significant reduction in the binding of IDEX in the posterior temporo-parietal cerebral cortex between the normal and mild AD group (p=0.02) (Table 1). There appeared to be further reductions in the IDEX binding in the temporo-parietal regions with increasing severity of AD. An example of moderately severe AD is given in Figure 3. These further reductions in IDEX binding did not however reach statistical significance. There were also significant reductions of IDEX binding in the frontal association cortex (p=0.01) in the mild AD sufferers, but no significant reductions in the sensorimotor or occipital cortex between normals and mild and moderate AD.

The frequent visual reductions in IDEX binding in the hippocampal region and temporal lobes (where there is the highest cortical density of cholinergic receptors) in mild AD compared with elderly normals, was confirmed by our semiquantitative analysis particularly in the medial temporal regions (p=0.0089). Semi-quantitative methods, which have been validated with PET, are sensitive to small reductions in activity[37].

Discussion

The results of this study, showing a significant reduction in muscarinic receptors in mild AD compared with normal elderly, are in contrast with post mortem studies in late stage AD which suggest that muscarinic receptor concentration is unaltered[11]. The limitation of this method of semiquantitative analysis is that it cannot separate an alteration in receptor affinity from a reduction in receptor concentration. PET studies with tropanyl benzilate of 10 persons with AD suggested that there was no alteration in mChR in AD compared with elderly controls, but did demonstrate a reduction in receptor density with ageing[38]. There was no significant difference in the age groups between

our mild and normal elderly group. This is the first large *in vivo* study of this condition and these results are consistent with a small study with ^{123}I QNB where there was reduced uptake in focal areas in the parietal and frontal cortices in AD[15]. [123]I QNB has a slow brain uptake with images obtained after 15 h with the four diastereoisomers with different affinities for muscarinic receptors making interpretation

complex. The use of the R-R isomer of QNB may enable assessment of the M2 receptor loss[15].

Although the delivery of ligand is necessarily related to local cerebral blood flow, IDEX is stereo-selective for cerebral muscarinic receptors and has very low non-specific binding[21]. Binding of [123]I- iododexetimide can be displaced by muscarinic agents from the receptor, even at the time of delayed imaging[15]. Other researchers have used the L-isomer levitimide to assess non-specific binding in the brain. They found that there was very little binding of levitimide in the brain and after an initial peak of activity. This agent showed a slow washout over several hours[21].

The sensitivity of visual analysis of IDEX scans was high with a number of false positives, but no false negatives. The positive predictive value of a normal IDEX scan was 90%, with an accuracy of 83%. The regional alterations in IDEX binding match the described areas of greatest histopathological abnormality in AD. The reduction in IDEX binding in the temporoparietal region was more significant (p = 0.01) than the reduction in cerebral blood flow with HMPAO on quantitative analysis between the normal elderly and the mild Alzheimer's disease group.

IDEX is a specific muscarinic neuroimaging ligand that is suitable for widespread use. It can be produced in high specific activity (<2000 mCi) with high yield (>70%) which would permit cost effective production. This compares well with the low yields of ^{123}I QNB (<20%), which also has the problem of delayed imaging at over 15 hours and subsequent low counts[15]. The chemical stability of IDEX and the 13 h half-life of ^{123}I enables IDEX to be transported long distances, (over 1000 km for the present study), from the production cyclotron prior to use. The degree of brain uptake is sufficient for SPECT imaging to be performed with widely available rotating gamma cameras with safe radiation dosimetry[19]. The counts at 6 h are sufficient to produce good quality images for analysis.

This is the first large study of muscarinic receptors in Alzheimer's disease *in vivo* and it has extended the work of early researchers[15-18].

We hope that further studies with this agent, particularly in the early phases of dementia, will enable more specific identification of Alzheimer's disease. This will be useful in the assessment of the success of the large number of ongoing drug trials for possible treatment for AD, and allow diagnosis and treatment at a time when least memory loss has occurred and greatest benefit would be obtained.

Acknowledgements

The authors are grateful to the following organisations for financial support for this research: University of Adelaide; Australian Nuclear Science and Technology Organisation; Australian Institute Nuclear Science and Engineering; and Australian Brain Foundation Grant.

References

1   Jorm, A.F., Korten A.E. and Henderson A.S. The prevalence of dementia: A quantitative integration of the literature. *Acta. Scand. Psychiatr.* 1987, 76, 465

2   Saunders A., Strittmatter W.J., Schmechel S., St George-Hyslop P. *et al.* Association of apolipoprotein E4 with late-onset familial and sporadic Alzheimer's disease. *Neurology* 1993, 43, 1467

3   Terry, D. *et al.* Structural basis of cognitive alterations in Alzheimer's disease in 'Alzheimer's Disease', (Eds. R.D. Terry, R. Katzman, K.L. Blick), Raven Press, New York, 1994, p.181

4   Double, K.I., Halliday, G.M., Kril I.J., Harasty J.A., Cullen, K. *et al.* Topography of brain atrophy in Alzheimer's disease. *Neurobiology of Ageing* (in press)

5   Desmond, P.M., Tress, P.M. *et al.* Volumetric and visual assessment of the mesial temporal structures in Alzheimer's disease . *Aust. NZ J. Med.* 1994, 24, 547

6   Murphy, D.G.M., Bottomley P.A., Salerno J.A. *et al.* An in vivo study of phosphorus and glucose in Alzheimer's disease using Magnetic Resonance Spectroscopy and PET. *Arch. Gen. Psychiatry* 1993, 50, 341

7   Davies, P. and Maloney A.J.F. Selective loss of central cholinergic systems and related neuropathological patterns in Alzheimer's disease. *Lancet*, 1976, 2, 1403

8   Guela, C. and Mesulam, M.-M. Cholinergic systems and related neuropathological patterns receptor classification in 'Alzheimer's Disease', (Eds. R.D. Terry, R. Katzman, K.L. Blick), Raven Press, New York, 1994, p.264

9   Davies, P. and Verth, A.H. Regional distribution of muscarinic acetylcholinergic receptors in normal and Alzheimer's type dementia brains. *Brain Res.* 1979, 1387, 389

10   Araujo, D.M., Lapchak, P.A., Robitaille, Y. *et al.* Differential alteration of various cholinergic markers in cortical and subcortical regions of human brain in Alzheimer's disease. *J. Neurochem.* 1988, 50, 1914

11   Keller, K.J., Whitehouse, P.J. *et al.* Muscarinic and nicotinic binding sites in AD cerebral cortex. *Brain Res.* 1987, 436, 62

12   Mash, D., Flynn, D.D. and Potter L.T. Loss of muscarinic receptors in the cerebral cortex in Alzheimer's disease and experimental cholinergic denervation. *Science* 1985, 228, 1115

13   Maziere, B. and Maziere, M. Where have we got to with neuroreceptor mapping of the human brain? *Eur. J. Nucl. Med.* 1990, 16, 817

14   Wilson, A.A., Scheffel, U.A., Dannals, R.F. *et al. In vivo* biodistribution of two (18F)- labelled muscarinic cholinergic receptor ligands: 2-(18F)- and 4-(18F)-fluoro-3-dexetimide. *Life Sciences* 1991, 48, 1385

15   Eckelman, W.C., Eng, R., Rzeszitarski, W.J. *et al.* Use of 3-quinuclidyl 4-iodobenzilate as a receptor binding tracer. *J. Nucl. Med.* 1985, 26, 637

16   Wilson, A.A., Dannals, R. and Ravert, J. Synthesis and biological evaluation of I-123 and I-124 iododexetimide, a potent muscarinic cholinergic receptor antagonist. *J. Med. Chem.* 1989, 32, 1057

17   Weinberger, D.R., Gibson, R.E. *et al.* Distribution of muscarinic receptors in patients with dementia. A controlled study of ^{123}I QNB and SPECT. *J. Cereb. Blood Flow* 1989, 9, S537

18   Muller-Gartner, H.W., Wilson, A.A., Dannals, R.F. *et al.* Imaging muscarinic cholinergic receptors in the human brain *in vivo* with SPECT, ^{123}I-4-iododexetimide. *J. Cereb. Blood Flow Metab.* 1992, 12, 562

19   Boundy, K.L., Barnden, L.R., Rowe, C.C. *et al.* Human dosimetry and normal brain distribution of iodine-123 iododexetimide: A SPECT imaging agent for cholinergic muscarinic neuroreceptors. *J. Nucl. Med.* 1995, 36, 1332

20   De Smedt, R., Rodrigus, E., Debandt, R. and Brugman, J. Dexbenzetimide in neuroleptic-induced parkinsonism. *J. Clin. Pharmacology* 1970, 207

21   Laduron, P.M. and Janssen, P.F.M. Characterisation and subcellular localisation of brain muscarinic receptors labelled in vivo by H-3-dexetimide. *J. Neurochem.* 1979, 32, 421

22   Laduron, P.M., Verwimp, M. and Leyson, J.E. Stereospecific *in vitro* binding of H-3 dexetimide to brain muscarinic receptors. *J. Neurochem.* 1978, 33, 1223

23   Muller-Gartner, H.W., Mayberg, H.S., Fisher, R.S. *et al.* Decreased hippocampal muscarinic cholinergic receptor binding measured by I-123-iododextimide and single photon emission computed tomography in epilepsy. *Ann. Neurol.* 1993, 34, 235

24   Burns, A.P.M., Costa, D.C., Ell, P.J. and Levy, R. The investigation of Alzheimer's disease with single photon emission tomography. *J. Neurol. Neurosurg. Psych.* 1989, 52, 248

25   Waldemar, G., Bruhn, P., Kristensen, A. *et al.* Heterogeniety of neocortical cerebral blood flow deficits in dementia of the Alzheimer type: a [99m-Tc]-d,l-HMPAO SPECT study. *J. Neurol. Neurosurg. Psychiatry* 1994, 57, 285

26   Johnson, K.A., Holman, L., Rosen, J. *et al.* Iofetamine ^{123}I SPECT is accurate in the diagnosis of Alzheimer's disease. *Arch. Int. Med.* 1990, 150, 752

27   Claus, J.J., Breteler, M.M.B., Krenning, E.P. *et al.* The diagnostic value of SPECT with Tc-99m HMPAO in Alzheimer's disease. *Neurology* 1994, 44, 454

28   Dierckx, R.A., Vanderwoude, M., Saerens, J. *et al.* Sensitivity and specificity of Tc-99m HMPAO single headed SPECT in dementia. *Nuclear Medicine Communications* 1993, 14, 792

29 Hodge, M, Souder, E and Chawiak, J. Is there a typical FDG-PET scan pattern for Alzheimer's disease? *J. Nucl. Med.* 1991, 33, 181

30 Hachinsli, V.C., Lassen, N.A. and Marshall, J. Multiinfarct dementia: a cause of mental deterioration in the elderly. *Lancet* 1974, 2, 207

31 Folstein, M.F., Folstein, S.E. and McHugh, P.R. "Mini-mental state": a practical method for grading the cognitive state of patients for the clinician. *J. Psychiatr. Res.* 1975, 12, 189

32 Rosen, W.G., Mohs, R.C. and Davis, K.L. A new rating scale for Alzheimer's disease. *Am. J. Psychiatry* 1984, 141, 1356

33 American Psychiatric Association, Committee on Nomenclature and Statistics in 'Diagnostic and Statistical Manual of Mental Disorders', (3rd edition), American Psychiatric Association, Washington DC, USA, 1980

34 McKhann, G., Drachmann, D., Folstein, M. *et al.* Clinical diagnosis of Alzheimer's disease: report of the NINCDS-ADRAS Work Group under the auspices of the Department of Health and Human Services Task Force on Alzheimer's disease. *Neurology* 1984, 34, 939

35 Hughes, C., Berg, L., Danziger, W.L. *et al.* A new clinical scale for staging dementia. *Brit. J. Psychiatry* 1988, 140, S66

36 Madsen, M.T., O'Leary, D.S., Andreason, N.C. and Kirchner, P.T. Dual isotope brain SPECT imaging for monitoring cognitive activation and physical considerations. *Nucl. Med. Comm.* 1993, 14, 391

37 Costa, D.C., Morgan, G.F. and Lassen, NA. in 'New Trends in Nuclear Neurology and Psychiatry', John Libbey & Co. Ltd, London, 1993, p.25 and p.85

SPECT in Neurology and Psychiatry, edited by P.P. De Deyn, R.A. Dierckx, A. Alavi and B.A. Pickut
© 1997 John Libbey & Company Ltd, pp. 27–32

Can SPECT Distinguish Lewy Body Dementia from Alzheimer's Disease During Life?

Chapter

4

Z. Walker, D.C. Costa[*], A. Janssen[**] and C. Katona

Introduction

Lewy body dementia (LBD), a recently delineated entity, is emerging as the second most common cause of degenerative dementia[1-3]. Other names currently used for this condition are diffuse Lewy body disease (DLBD)[2,4-8], Lewy body variant of Alzheimer's Disease (LBV)[9,10] and senile dementia of the Lewy body type (SDLT)[11,12].

The development of new techniques, particularly anti-ubiquitin immuno-histochemistry [3], which is more sensitive than conventional techniques in the detection of Lewy bodies in the cortex, has led to the increased recognition of LBD. Lewy body dementia is neuropathologically defined by the presence of rounded eosinophilic inclusion bodies (Lewy bodies) within the cytoplasm of neurones in certain brainstem, subcortical and cortical regions. These invariably include the locus coeruleus and substantia nigra, which also show evidence of cell loss and gliosis[13]. This pathology closely resembles that of Parkinson's disease, with the important exception that there are much larger numbers of Lewy bodies throughout the cortex in LBD.

There continues to be controversy about the classification of LBD. Some regard it as a variant of Alzheimer's disease[10], and others as part of the Lewy body brain syndrome, where at one end of a spectrum patients are presenting with Parkinson's disease and at the other end patients have predominantly dementia with mild extrapyramidal features[1,3,7,11,14-16].

As more cases are identified from post mortem studies, retrospective analysis of these cases has helped in defining a clinical picture which comprises progressive dementia with fluctuating cognitive performance, frequent psychiatric symptoms (mainly visual and auditory hallucinations, delusions) and Parkinsonism. Other common features are recurrent falls, autonomic failure and hypersensitivity to neuroleptic medication.

At present LBD can only be diagnosed with certainty by neuropathological examination. Diagnosis during life remains at best probable, based on the presence of symptoms known from autopsy studies to be frequently associated with LBD. Sets of clinical diagnostic criteria have been proposed by Byrne[4] and McKeith[11], but as yet neither has been validated in a prospective study. Apart from distinguishing LBD from other Parkinsonism-dementia syndromes (e.g. Steele-Richardson-Olszewski syndrome, corticobasal degeneration) the greatest problem arises in distinguishing LBD from multi-infarct dementia (MID) and Alzheimer's disease (AD). In MID, the presence of cerebrovascular risk factors, a fluctuating course with stepwise deterioration and periods of stable cognitive

University College Medical School, London and Princess Alexandra Hospital, Harlow, UK
[*]Institute of Nuclear Medicine and University College Medical School, London, UK
[**]Eindhoven University of Technology and Amsterdam Cygne b.v., Netherlands

function, and neuroimaging (CT and MRI scan) are usually of help in making the diagnosis. However this is not the case with AD. All the clinical features described in LBD have been encountered in patients with AD, albeit not as frequently and usually in later stages[17]. Routine neuroimaging has not been shown to be of much value in distinguishing the two conditions. Both are associated with cerebral atrophy. Forstl[9] reported that patients with Lewy body pathology had more marked frontal cerebral atrophy than patients with AD, but the numbers were small and this feature cannot be used to distinguish the conditions.

Measures of dopamine neurotransmission may be a useful way of differentiating LBD from AD. It is estimated that in clinically manifest Parkinson's disease (PD) 60-70% of nigral neurones have de-generated with 80-90% depletion of striatal dopamine by the time that symptoms first appear[18-20]. In LBD the depletion of dopamine is not as severe (40-60%) and in AD there are no significant changes in dopamine metabolism[21].

In autopsy studies, Perry[21] and Langlais[22] showed that dopamine and its metabolite homovanillic acid were significantly reduced in the basal ganglia in LBD and PD but not in AD. The dopamine levels of the LBD group were not as low as in the PD group, but were significantly below the AD group. In both the PD and LBD groups the dopamine levels in basal ganglia correlated with the number of melanin neurones in substantia nigra. There was an inverse association between extrapyramidal features on the one hand, and basal ganglia dopamine concentration and the number of substantia nigra neurones on the other. Although eight out of the 14 AD cases had extra-pyramidal features, there was no significant reduction in dopamine levels and the pathological basis of their movement disorder was not determined.

Functional neuroimaging has not as yet been applied as a diagnostic tool in LBD, although it has been used to study changes in neurotransmitter systems in patients with Parkinson's disease and in individuals at risk of PD[23-25].

Both positron emission tomography (PET) and single photon emission computerised tomography (SPECT) scanning can assess the functional integrity of the nigrostriatal dopaminergic projections26. SPECT is a relatively less expensive technique than PET and is available in most departments of nuclear medicine. The ligand 123I-iodobenzamide has been developed recently. It enables post-synaptic dopaminergic receptors to be studied with a reconstructed resolution of about 7-9 mm.

In contrast to other studies, we decided not to use the basal ganglia density (BG) : frontal cortex density (FC) ratio, since we knew from CT/MRI brain scans that most of our patients had a degree of cerebral atrophy which would have led to reduced cortical IBZM signals and inflated the uptake ratios. We had no means of correcting for decrease of radioactivity uptake due to cerebral atrophy and felt that the caudate:putamen ratio would be a more appropriate measure of the changes in post-synaptic dopamine receptors. We therefore chose the caudate:putamen ratio as our primary measure, hypothesising that in LBD, as in PD, post-synaptic putamen D_2 binding capacity is up-regulated and caudate capacity unaltered resulting in a reduced caudate:putamen ratio compared with both AD and control subjects.

Methods

Approval for the study was obtained from West Essex Health Authority Ethics Committee and the Administration of Radioactive Substances Advisory Committee of UK prior to starting the project. All controls, patients and, if available, their relatives gave written consent.

Patients

Twenty-six patients were recruited for the study from the memory clinic, the old age psychiatry out-patients clinic and hospital wards at Princess Alexandra Hospital, Harlow. Of the 26 patients recruited, 11 patients were diagnosed as having LBD using clinical criteria developed by McKeith[11]. Out of the 15 patients with Alzheimer's disease according to NINCDS ADRDA criteria[27], four were excluded after having CT/MRI scan which showed prominent periventricular lucencies and/or infarcts. Healthy elderly controls were recruited from relatives and friends of patients.

Assessment

Each patient and informant gave a detailed history of memory impairment. This was followed by a full psychiatric history, mental state examination and physical examination. A number of tests were per-formed: the mini-mental state examination (MMSE), adapted from Folstein[29]; the Clifton assessment procedure for the elderly (behaviour part only)[29]; the geriatric depression scale (GDS)[30]; the Clinical Dementia rating (CDR)[31]; and the Cambridge Cognitive Examination (CAMCOG)[13].

Investigations

The following investigations were arranged for all patients if not already performed by a referring doctor: FBC, ESR, U and Es, glucose, LFTs, Ca^{2+}, TFTs, VDRL, B_{12}, folate and CT/MRI brain scan.

^{123}I IBZM SPECT scan

^{123}I-iodobenzamide(IBZM) was supplied by Eindhoven University of Technology and Cygne b.v. All studies were carried out at The Institute of Nuclear Medicine, University College London Medical School, where a high resolution SPECT scanner is available which is able to distinguish between caudate nucleus and putamen radioactivity distribution. All subjects underwent scanning with the SME 810 brain scanner 1.5 to 2 h post-injection (i.v.) of approximately 185 MBq of IBZM. Regular circular regions of interest were employed to calculate average caudate nucleus:lentiform nucleus (mainly putamen) radio-activity ratios for both hemispheres, Figures 1 and 2. All scans were analysed by DC, who was blind to the diagnostic status of the subjects.

Statistics

Data were analysed using SPSS/PC+ version 3.1 (Statistical Package for Social Sciences). Analysis of variance (ANOVA) was used to assess differences between the three groups (LBD, AD and controls) and their basic indices (age, MMSE, CAMCOG, CDR, GDS and CAPE) and the right caudate:putamen (R Cd/Pt) and the left caudate:putamen (L Cd/Pt) tracer concentration ratios. The same data (the tracer concentration ratios in the three groups) were then reanalysed with the non-parametric Kruskal-Wallis (K-W) test.

Results

The means of age at time of the IBZM SPECT scan, age at onset of disease, MMSE, CAMCOG, CDR, CAPE and GDS for LBD and AD group are shown in Table 1. The mean age of the controls (69.4 years), was lower compared with AD patients (73.8 years) and of patients with LBD (76.1 years), but the differences were not statistically significant. There was no significant difference between AD group and LBD group on MMSE, CDR, CAPE or GDS, but LBD patients performed significantly better on CAMCOG than AD patients (p< 0.03, 95% confidence interval [CI] 65.3-82.4, 38.8- 70.3).

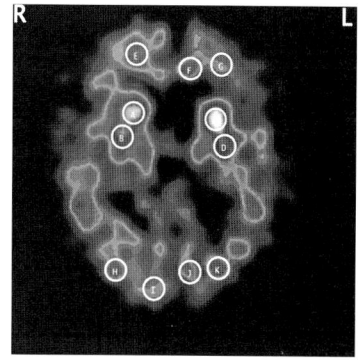

A, B, C, D - Basal ganglia

E, F, G - Frontal cortex

H, I, J, K - Occipital cortex

Figure 1 Data Analysis - ROIs

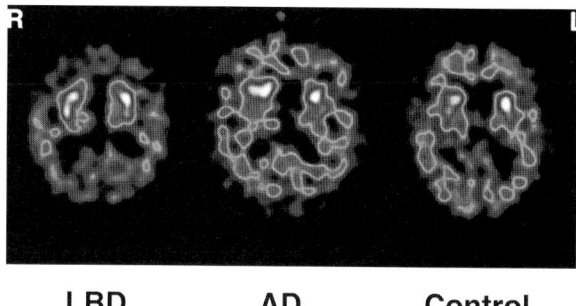

LBD   AD   Control

Figure 2 Dopamine D_2 receptors - ^{123}I-IBZM/SPECT

Table 1

Means (range)	LBD	AD
Age at onset (years)	71.4 (56-85)	70.0 (59-80)
Age at scan (years)	76.1 (58-88)	73.8 (62-87)
MMSE	21.4 (15-29)	16.5 (5-26)
CAMCOG (p<0.03)	73.8 (51-91)	54.5 (17-92)
CDR	1.0 (0.5-2.0)	1.3 (0.5-2.0)
CAPE	11.0 (0-21)	3.4 (2-16)
GDS	3.6 (1-8)	9.4 (0-8)
Male : Female ratio	10 : 1	3 : 8

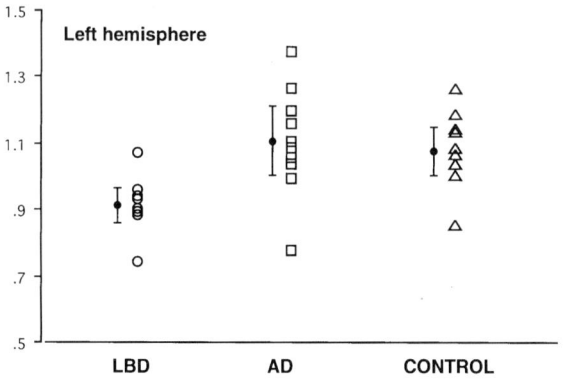

Figure 3 Caudate:putamen (radioactivity ratios)

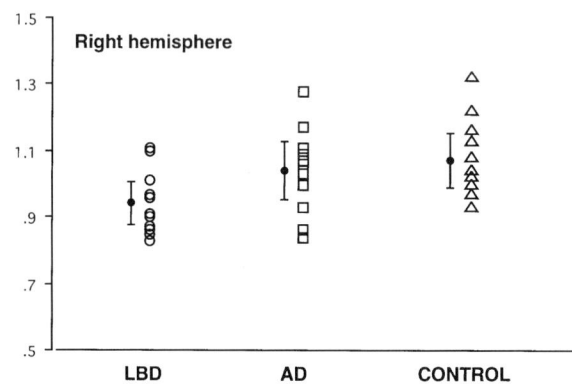

Figure 4 Caudate:putamen (radioactivity ratios)

Radioactivity ratios are shown in Figures 3 and 4. The LBD group had significantly lower L Cd/Pt ratio than controls and AD group (ANOVA overall: F = 8.54, p<0.002; CI: LBD 0.863-0.968, AD 1.005-1.212, controls 1.005-1.152). There was a highly significant difference between L Cd/Pt ratio of LBD and AD group (p<0.0006) and between LBD group and controls (p<0.003), but no difference between AD group and controls. Using the K-W test, the results continued to be highly significant (K-W overall: p<0.002, LBD v AD p<0.006, LBD v controls p<0.03).

The LBD group also had a significantly lower R Cd/Pt ratio than the AD group and the controls (ANOVA overall: F = 4.04, p<0.03), but there was an overlap of the CI, which was 0.877-1.01 for the LBD group, 0.953-1.127 for the AD group, and 1.000-1.158 for the controls. When comparing individual groups, although there was a significant difference between LBD group and controls (p<0.01), the difference between LBD and AD group did not reach statistical significance (p<0.06).

Discussion

This is the first study to examine the changes in post-synaptic D_2 receptors in patients with a clinical diagnosis of LBD. Although there are no studies of patients with LBD, there are a number of studies examining post-synaptic dopaminergic system in patients with Parkinson's disease[32-34]. Brooks[26] summarised the findings of seven studies and concluded that the putamen D_2 binding potential ranges from normal to upregulated but that the caudate D_2 binding potential is low or normal. This means that there are a number of possible explanations for the decreased caudate:putamen radioactivity ratios in patients with LBD. The putamen D_2 binding potential

could be raised (upregulated) and this would represent an adaptive response to loss of nigro-putamen dopaminergic afferents, or, alternatively, there could be a loss of caudate D_2 receptors with the putamen binding capacity staying unchanged. McKeith[35,36] suggests that only some patients with LBD upregulate post-synaptic D_2 receptors in the striatum and that neuroleptic sensitivity in LBD is a result of a critical reduction in nigral dopaminergic output in conjunction with failure to upregulate post-synaptic D_2 receptors in the striatum either in response to the dopaminergic deficit or to D_2 blocking drugs.

In our study the post-synaptic dopaminergic dysfunction in LBD was more pronounced on the left. Where side to side striatal uptake has been compared in patients with Parkinson's disease, tracer uptake was greater in the putamen contralateral to the more affected limbs[3,26,37]. In most patients with LBD, the extrapyramidal symptoms are fairly mild or even absent and it is not always possible to decide which side is more severely affected.

A shortcoming of our study is that the three groups were poorly matched for gender, the male : female ratio being 10 : 1 for LBD group, 3 : 8 for AD group and 7 : 4 for controls. This discrepancy most probably mirrors the unequal prevalence of AD in both genders, females being more commonly affected than males. Moreover McKeith,[11] reported a higher male : female ratio in LBD patients compared with AD patients, although this has not been observed in the majority of other studies[13]. In our study, LBD patients also tended to be older, but less cognitively impaired as measured on MMSE and CAMCOG.

In summary, these preliminary data suggest that patients with LBD have clear changes of striatal D_2 receptors. This observation could be of clinical value in distinguishing LBD patients during life from patients with AD. Further studies with larger numbers of patients, a further control group of patients with untreated PD and post mortem confirmed that diagnoses need to be undertaken to replicate our preliminary findings. In our series the IBZM SPECT results correctly predicted the pathology of the first two patients who came to autopsy (1 LBD, 1 AD; unpublished).

References

1 Byrne, E.J., Lennox, G., Lowe, J. and Godwin-Austen, R.B. Diffuse Lewy body disease: clinical features in 15 cases. *J. Neurol. Neurosurg. Psychiatry* 1989, 52, 709

2 Dickson, D.W., Crystal, H.A., Mattiace, L.A. *et al.* Diffuse Lewy body disease: light and electron microscopic immunocytochemistry of senile plaques. *Acta Neuropathologica* 1989, 78, 572

3 Lennox, G., Lowe, J., Landon, M. *et al.* Diffuse Lewy body disease: correlative neuropathology using anti-ubiquitin immunocytochemistry. *J. Neurol. Neurosurg. Psychiatry* 1989, 52, 1236

4 Byrne, E.J. Diffuse Lewy body disease. *Rec. Adv. Geriatr.* 1991, 33

5 Crystal, H.A., Dickson, D.W., Lizardi, J.E. *et al.* Antemortem diagnosis of diffuse Lewy body disease. *Neurology* 1990, 40, 1523

6 Dickson, D.W., Davies, O., Mayeux, R. *et al.* Diffuse Lewy body disease (neuropathological and biochemical studies of six patients). *Acta Neuropathologica* 1987, 75, 8

7 Dickson, D.W., Ruan, D., Crystal, H.A. *et al.* Hippocampal degeneration differentiates diffuse Lewy body disease (DLBD) from Alzheimer's disease: light and electron macroscopic immunocytochemistry of CA2-3 neurites specific to DLBD. *Neurology* 1991, 41, 1402

8 Fearnley, J.M., Daniel, S.E. and Lees, A.J. Lewy body variant. *Neurology* 1990, 40, 1149

9 Forstl, H., Burns, A., Luthert, P. *et al.* The Lewy body variant of Alzheimer's disease (clinical and pathological findings). *Br. J. Psychiatry* 1988, 162, 385

10 Hansen, L., Salmin, D., Galasko, D. *et al.* The Lewy body variant of Alzheimer's disease: a clinical and pathologic entity. *Neurology*, 1990, 40, 1

11 McKeith, I.G., Perry, R.H., Fairbairn, A.F. *et al.* Operational criteria for senile dementia of Lewy body type (SDLT). *Pathological Medicine* 1992, 22, 911

12 Perry, R.H., Irving, D., Blessed, G. *et al.* Senile dementia of Lewy body type. *J. Neurol. Sci.* 1990, 95, 119

13 Lennox, G. Lewy body dementia. *Balliere's Clinical Neurology* 1992, 1(3), 653

14 Dickson, D.W. Lewy body variant. *Neurology* 1990, 40, 1147

15 Fearnley, J.M., Daniel, S.E. and Lees, A.J. Lewy body variant. *Neurology* 1990, 40, 1149

16 Kosaka, K., Yoshimura, M., Ikeda, K. and Budka, H. Diffuse type of Lewy body disease: progressive dementia with abundant corical Lewy bodies and senile changes of varying degree–a new disease? *Clin. Neuropathol.* 1984, 3, 185

17 Forstl, H., Sattel, H. and Bahro, M. Alzheimer's disease: clinical features. *Int. Rev. Psychiatry* 1993, 5, 327

18 Fearnley, J.M. and Lees, A.J. Ageing and Parkinson's disease: substantia nigra regional selectivity. *Brain* 1991, 114, 2283

19 Jenner, P., Schapira, A.H.V. and Marsden, C.D. New insight into the cause of Parkinson's disease. *Neurology* 1992, 42, 2241

20 Koller, W.C. When does Parkinson's disease begin? *Neurology* 1992, 42, 27

21 Perry, E.K., Marshall, E., Perry, R.H. *et al.* Cholinergic and dopaminergic activities in senile dementia of Lewy body type. *Alzheimer's disease and associated disorders* 1990, 4, 87

22 Langlais, P.J., Thal, L., Hansen, L. *et al.* Neurotransmitters in basal ganglia and cortex of Alzheimer's disease with and without Lewy bodies. *Neurology* 1993, 43, 1927

23 Burn, D.J., Mark, M.H., Playford, E.D. *et al.* Parkinson's disease in twins studies with 18F-Dopa and positron emission tomography. *Neurology* 1992, 42, 1894

24 Sawle, G.V., Wroe, S.J., Lees, A.J. *et al.* The identification of presymptomatic parkinsonism: clinical and 18F Dopa positron emission tomography studies in an Irish kindred. *Ann. Neurol.* 1992, 32, 609

25 Sawle, G.V. The detection of preclinical Parkinson's disease: what is the role of positron emission tomography? *Movement Disorders* 1993, 8, 271

26 Brooks, D.J. Functional imaging in relation to Parkinsonian syndromes. *J. Neurolog. Sci.* 1993, 115, 1

27 McKhann, G., Drachman, D., Folstein, M. *et al.* Clinical diagnosis of Alzheimer's disease: report of the NINCDS-ADRDA Work Group under the auspices of the Department of Health and Human Sevices Task Force on Alzheimer's disease. *Neurology* 1984, 34, 939

28 Folstein, M.F., Folstein, S.E. and McHugh, P.R. 'Mini-mental state': a practical menthod for grading the cognitive state of patients for the clinician. *J. Psychiatr. Res.* 1975, 12, 189

29 Pattie, A.H. and Gilleard, C.J. in 'Clifton assessment procedures for the elderly (CAPE): behaviour rating scale', Hodder and Stoughton Educational, UK, 1979

30 Yesavage, J.A. Geriatric depression scale. *Psychopharmacol. Bull.* 1988, 24, 709

31 Berl, L. Clinical dementia rating (CDR). *Psychopharmacol. Bull.* 1988, 24, 637

32 Brooks, D.J., Ibanez, V., Sawle, G.V. *et al.* Striatal D_2 receptor status in patients with Parkinson's disease, striatonigral degeneration, and progressive supranuclear palsy, measured with 11C-racloprode and poitron emission tomography. *Ann. Neurol.* 1992, 31, 184

33 Brucke, T., Podreka, I., Angelberger, P. *et al.* Dopamine D2 receptor imaging with SPECT: studies in different neuropsychiatric disorders. *J. Cereb. Blood Flow Metab.* 1991, 11, 220

34 Laulumaa, V., Kuikka, J.T., Soininen, H. *et al.* Imaging of D_2 dopamine receptors of patients with Parkinson's disease using single photon emission computed tomography and iodobenzamide I-123. *Arch. Neurol.* 1993, 50, 509

35 McKeith, I.G., Ballard, C.G. and Harrison, R.W.S. Neuroleptic sensitivity to risperidone in Lewy body dementia. *The Lancet* 1995, 346, 699

36 McKeith, I.G. Cortical Lewy body disease: the view from Newcastle in 'Developments in dementia and functional disorders in the elderly', (Eds. R. Levy and R. Howard), Wrightson Biomedical Publishing Ltd, 1995, p.9

SPECT in Neurology and Psychiatry, edited by P.P. De Deyn, R.A. Dierckx, A. Alavi and B.A. Pickut
© 1997 John Libbey & Company Ltd, pp. 33–38

Huntington's Chorea: IBZM SPECT Role in Preclinical Diagnosis

Chapter

5

D. Giobbe, F. Squitieri[*] and G.C. Castellano[**]

Introduction

Huntington's disease (HD) is a devastating progressive neurodegenerative disease characterised by movement disturbances, cognitive abnormalities and psychiatric disorders (Table 1). It is inherited in an autosomal dominant fashion and affects about 1 in 10,000 in most populations of European origin[1]. The disorder typically has an insidious onset in middle age (fourth or fifth decade), worsening gradually over the course of 10 to 20 years until death. Gross wasting of the head of the caudate nucleus and putamen bilaterally is the characteristic neuropathological abnormality, and is usually associated with moderate cortical atrophy in the frontal and temporal lobes. At present, there is no effective treatment. Chorea can, however, be reduced by neuroleptic drugs.

The features of the illness explain the interest of investigations that may allow a preclinical diagnosis. A very important step in this direction was made in 1993 when the gene responsible for HD was identified in the short arm of chromosome 4. Near the 5' end of the gene there is a CAG repeat that is expanded and unstable in HD patients. Thus HD constitutes the fifth example of trinucleotide repeat expansion in neurological diseases after fragile X syndrome, myotonic dystrophy, spino-bulbar muscular atrophy (SBMA) and spinocerebellar ataxia type[1] (SCA 1). The repeat number associated with the normal phenotype is under 35 CAGs, while the pathological number is > 36[2]. However, the molecular analysis of the specific CAG repeat sequence has not solved all the problems. DNA tests cannot predict the age of onset in presymptomatic at risk individuals. This is particularly important in asymptomatic at risk people with a CAG repeat number at the low border of the pathological range (36-39), who may manifest the disease either very late or never[3]. Furthermore, the first stage of HD is often difficult to identify. A major concern arises for at risk HD individuals who receive a result showing that they present a mutation carrier at the genetic analysis, and manifest minor aspecific psychiatric symptoms, frequently observed in the general population. Positive mutation analysis, in these cases, may erroneously let clinicians suspect a disease onset with obvious dramatic implications for patients and their families. Cases involving phenocopies, which are clinically symptomatic but without evidence of CAG expansion, have been described[4-6]. Finally, alleles in the intermediate range of CAGs, with a repeat number of between 29 and 35 inclusive, may be unstable when transmitted through the male germline and may expand in the pathological range in offspring[7,8]. They constitute the pool that new HD mutations come from, and seem to be more unstable when originating from HD families compared with those in the general population[9].

Department of Neurology Osp. Maria Vittoria, Turin, Italy
[*] Ist. Neurologico Mediterraneo Neuromed, Isernia, Italy
[**] Serv. Di Medicina Nucleare, University of Turin Italy

Table 1 Symptoms most frequently observed in Huntington's chorea

Movement disorders	Psychiatric disorders	Cognitive disorders
Chorea	Character abnormalities	Attentiveness decline
Athetosis	Poor self-control	Memory impairment
Tardive dystonia	Depression	Intellectual deterioration
Dysarthria	Delusions	Agnosia
Dysphagia	Suicide	Apraxia
Ataxia	Hypomania	

Among other preclinical diagnostic investigations, the L-DOPA test, performed with the administration of 3.0 g of L-DOPA daily for a period of a month, is based on the hypothesis that the disease is related to an enhanced sensitivity of striatal neurons to dopamine. However, the predictive value of this test is not clearly established and until information becomes available it should be better not to administer L-DOPA to patients at risk of developing the disease. Besides neuropsychological and electrodiagnostic tests (thresholds for a foveal blue test, long latency EMG responses, the masseter inhibitory reflex), functional neuroimaging techniques may offer further important information on this pathology. This view is supported, for example, by the observation that HD patients studied with PET show a characteristic decrease in glucose utilisation, which appears early in the disease and precedes the loss of tissue[2,10-13]. Nevertheless, PET is a very expensive technique and is available only in a few centres. The recent introduction of 3-iodo-6-methoxybenzamide ^{123}I-IBZM, a new dopamine D_2 receptor ligand, allows the study of this receptor by SPECT. As the D_2 receptor is mainly concentrated in the areas of the central nervous system (CNS) involved by HD, IBZM SPECT seems a promising technique to provide more data on this type of pathology.

Methods

We studied an HD family, formed from 16 live members (seven male and nine female), subdivided into three generations (Figure 1). The members of the first (four people, two affected and two healthy) and of the second generation (seven individuals, all healthy) were subjected to IBZM SPECT, neuropsychological

evaluation and MRI. DNA testing was perfomed in the two affected patients.

The first patient was a 65 year old man. The disease had begun 10 years before with choreic movements involving the hands and the face and had slightly worsened in the past 2 years, with extension to the feet and initial impairment of gait. He had been treated for the chorea with neuroleptic drugs (haloperidol). During the course of the illness neither psychiatric nor cognitive abnormalities were observed.

The second patient was a 51 year old woman. The onset of the disease dated back ten years, when she was admitted to a psychiatric hospital due to a severe depressive syndrome. Afterwards she was hospitalised many more times for the same reason, and she was chronically assisted by the local psychiatric service. Choreic movements had begun only recently in the previous months, but had worsened quickly with extension from the hands and face to the feet and legs. At the moment of the neurological examination, dysarthria, dysphagia and gait abnormalities were evident. She had been treated for depression with tryciclic compounds (amitriptyline, clomipramine) and more recently with serotonin reuptake inhibitors (fluoxetine, fluvoxamine and paroxetine).

The neuropsychological assessment was performed employing the mini mental state examination (MMSE) and the Sandoz clinical assessment geriatrics (SCAG) scale. For DNA analysis, a polymerase chain reaction (PCR) amplification of the HD CAG repeat was carried out. The genomic DNA was isolated from leukocytes. For MRI we employed an ESATOM MR 5000 0.5 Tesla unit; 8 mm axial sections and 5 mm coronal sections were performed.

Single photon emission tomography (SPECT) studies were carried out using about 370 MBq ^{123}I-IBZM (10 mCi) intravenously. Acquisition started 2 h after

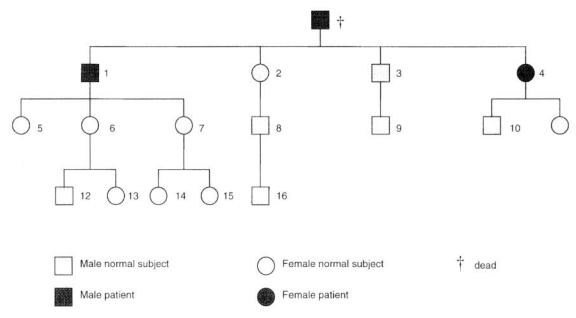

Figure 1 The genealogical tree of HD family living in Piemonte, Northern Italy (provinces of Turin and Cuneo)

injection. Patients were positioned supine with an immobilised head and with the orbito-meatal line perpendicular to the collimator. Acquisitions were performed by means of a single head rotating gamma-camera (GE 400T), equipped with a general purpose collimator (GP), on line with a dedicated computer (GE STAR II); sixty-four views (each over 25 s) were acquired on 360° into 64x64 pixels matrix, setting a 159 Kev 20% window, recording at least 3000 Kcounts. Raw data were filtered with a Butterworth filter (cut-off frequency = 0.5 cycles/cm, slope = 15), then two pixels 1.2 cm thick transaxial slices were reconstructed by filtered back projection algorithm using a Ramp filter. Images were corrected for attenuation (coefficient = 0.12^{-1}). Transaxial images were evaluated both qualitatively and semi-quantitatively. Semiquantitative analysis was performed on the significant sections by putting four, two by two symmetric, equal (8 pixel diameter) circular regions of interest (ROIs) on basal ganglia (BG) and two, equal to the preceeding ones, on the cerebellar lobes (Figure 2). Percentage activity ratios were then calculated between symmetric BG ROI counts (normal range 90-110) and between each BG ROI count and mid-cerebellar ROI count (S/C ratio). Asymmetries >10% were considered significant. The statistical significance was evaluated by Student's t test for unpaired groups. The two patients interrupted their treatment 24 h before the examination.

Results

The MMSE proved normal in all the cases, while the SCAG scale showed high values (76) in the patient with predominant psychiatric disorders. The DNA testing confirmed the clinical diagnosis in both the patients, showing 52 CAG repeats in the first patient and 42 in the second one. With MRI, a moderate hypotrophy of the head of the caudate nucleus was observed in both the patients, resulting in an obliteration of the bulge in the inferolateral border of the lateral ventricle, normally created by this structure. Moreover a slight cortical, mainly temporal, atrophy was present in both the patients. On the contrary MRI was absolutely normal in all the relatives examined.

IBZM SPECT performed with semiquantitative analysis and calculation of the S/C ratio detected very low values in both the patients and normal values in all the relatives but one (Table 2). Interestingly, statistical analysis showed significant differences in S/C between normals and patients and between normals and a healthy relative, no differences between this healthy relative and patients and between the other relatives and normals (Table 3).

No significant asymmetries were detected using IBZM SPECT with semiquantitative analysis and calculation of the uptake ratio between homologous areas of the basal ganglia. Finally, IBZM SPECT with qualitative analysis (Figures 3-6), provided results similar to the semiquantitative one but proved much less accurate in the evaluation of the data.

Discussion

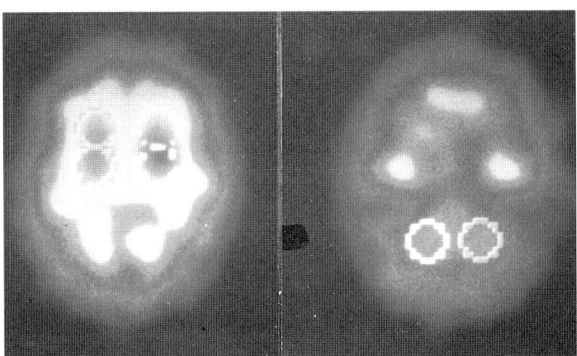

Figure 2 Exemplification of ROI positioning for semi-(quantitative analysis. Basal ganglia are shown on the left) and cerebellum on the right

Table 2 Values of striatocerebellar ratio in patients and relatives. All the patients show striatocerebellar ratios much lower than normals (171 ± 15). Among the clinically healthy relatives one subject ([a]) has values similar to the patients

	Anterior ROIs		Posterior ROIs	
	Dx	Sn	Dx	Sn
I Generation				
I Pt	115	124	119	110
II Pt	130	129	129	127
I Rel	156	157	158	175
II Rel	198	193	197	190
II Generation				
I Rel[a]	132	138	130	123
II Rel	181	180	173	174
III Rel	178	175	164	165
IV Rel	198	195	175	191
V Rel	163	165	162	166
VI Rel	183	176	180	197
VII Rel	185	188	169	166

Table 3 Striatal cerebellar ratio: statistical data. Student's t test for unpaired groups was employed. [a]Significant difference from normals p <0.000001; [b]significant difference from normals p <0.00001

Normals	171 ± 15
Patients	123 ± 7[a]
Healthy relative	131 ± 6[b]
Other relatives	177 ± 14

Our data show that, similarly to what was observed in previous PET and SPECT studies[10,11,13,14-17], IBZM SPECT can easily identify patients affected by HD. The very low uptake values detected in the basal ganglia in the two patients seem to indicate an involvement of striatal dopaminergic system in the disease. Moreover the biochemical abnormality, as outlined by the case of the clinically healthy relative

with significantly decreased S/C ratio and normal MRI, appears to precede the anatomical damage, and so it seems unlikely that it can be a simple epiphenomenon of atrophy. More unclear is why we could not find significant differences in S/C ratio among the patient with pure motor symptomatology, the patient with predominant psychiatric abnormalities and the clinically healthy relative. For both patients, it may be hypothesised that two different neuronal striatal pools are involved: a pool with prevalent connections with the limbic system[18] in the psychiatric one, and a pool with prevalent connections with the pallidum in the purely choreic one[19]. Similarly in the HD patients with predominant cognitive disturbances the disease could mainly involve a third pool connected with the prefrontal[12] and temporal cortical areas. The case of the clinically healthy relative with abnormal S/C values could be explained by the intervention, in the early phase, of counterbalancing pathways, which in the course of the disease become exhausted. Furthermore,

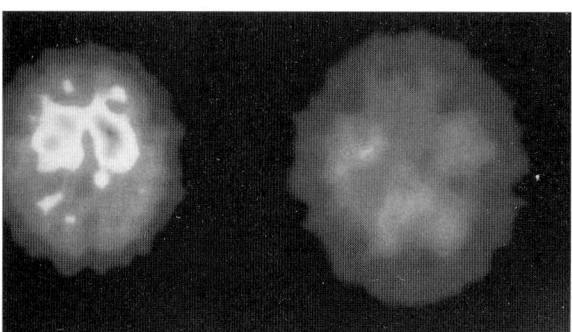

Figure 3 Normal subject: high striatal uptake if compared with cerebellum

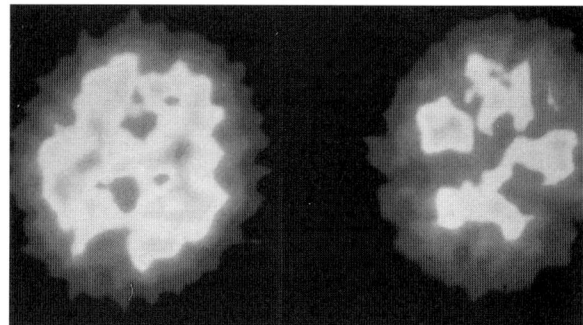

Figure 5 Patient affected by Huntington's chorea: slight difference between striatal and cerebellar uptake

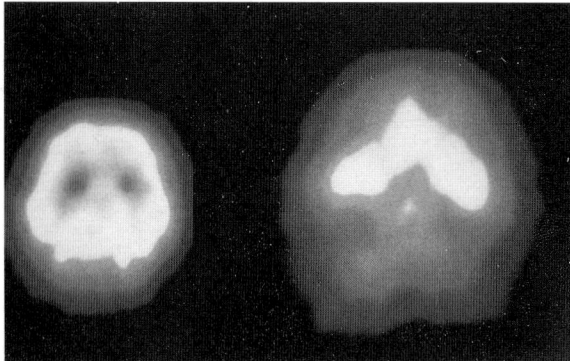

Figure 4 Clinically healthy relative with normal S/C ratio: high striatal uptake if compared with cerebellum, as in normals

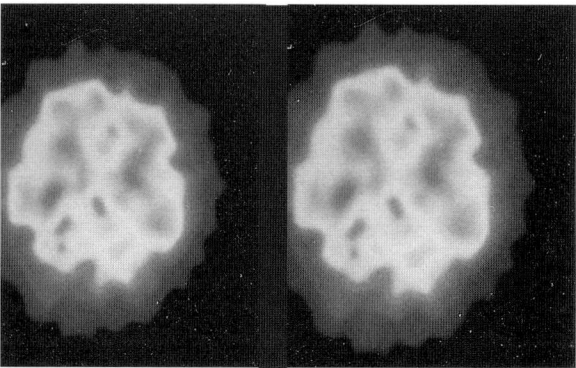

Figure 6 Clinically healthy relative with low S/C ratio: slight difference between striatal and cerebellar uptake, as in patients

chorea is thought to be the opposite of parkinsonian symptomatology and high doses of L-DOPA or dopamine agonists induce chorea in PD patients. However IBZM SPECT data show that the postsynaptic dopaminergic uptake is decreased both in PD and HD. So it appears likely that two different striatal neuronal pools are involved in the two diseases, and the same is probably true for striatonigral degeneration, a form of multisystem atrophy. Finally, the data agree with the pathophysiological mechanism proposed for chorea by Crossman et al.[20]. According to this theory, the injured striatal neurons could no longer inhibit the lateral pallidal neurons. As these lateral pallidal neurons inhibit the subthalamic nucleus (STN), the neurons of this nucleus would become less active, mimicking the STN lesions which induce hemiballism. Nevertheless, in our opinion at present the SPECT abnormalities observed must be considered only as an early marker of the disease. However, this role may be important as a source of further information in the situations in which DNA testing is not completely exhaustive, such as prediction of the age of onset in asymptomatic people with 36 to 39 CAG repeats, identification of the first stage of the disease in doubtful cases, study of phenocopies and detection of the alleles in the intermediate range, which may expand in the pathological range in offspring.

In conclusion, IBZM SPECT proved a useful technique to identify HD patients. Its use in preclinical diagnosis must be better evaluated with the study of other families and in association with DNA analysis. Due to the very large genetic differences between normals and patients SPECT investigations seem to be promising. Moreover, this technique appears to provide new data for better evaluation of the pathophysiology of the basal ganglia and to monitor the effects of therapies, when they become available.

References

1 The Huntington's Disease Collaborative Research Group. A novel gene containing a trinucleotide repeat that is expanded and unstable on Huntington's disease chromosomes. *Cell* 1993, 72, 971

2 Kremer, B., Goldberg, Y.P., Andrew, S.E. *et al.* Worldwide study of the Huntington disease mutation: the sensitivity and specificity of CAG expansion. *New Eng. Med. J.* 1994, 330, 1401

3 Rubinsztein, C.D., Leggo, J., Coles, R. *et al.* Phenotypic characterization of individuals with 30-40 CAG repeats in the Huntington disease (HD) gene reveals HD cases with 36 repeats and apparently normal elderly individuals with 36-39 repeats. *Am J. Hum. Genet.* 1996, 59, 16

4 Andrew, S.E., Goldberg, Y.P., Kremer, B. *et al.* Huntington disease without CAG expansion: phenocopies or errors in assignment? *Am. I. Hum.Genet.* 1994, 54, 852

5 Duyao, M., Ambrose, C., Myers, R. *et al.* Trinucleotide repeat length instability and age on onset in Huntington's disease. *Nat.Genet.* 1993, 4, 387

6 Snell, R.G., MacMillan, J.C., Cheadle, J.P. *et al.* Relationship between trinucleotide repeat expansion and phenotypic variation in Huntington's disease. *Nature Genetics* 1993, 4, 393

7 Goldberg, Y.P., Andrew, S.E., Theilmann, I. *et al.* Familial predisposition to recurrent mutations causing Huntington's disease: genetic risk to sibs of sporadic cases. *J. Med. Genet.* 1993, 30, 987

8 Goldberg, Y.P., Kremer, B., Andrew, S.E. *et al.* Molecular analysis of new mutations for Huntington's disease: intermediate alleles and sex of origin effects. *Nat. Genet.* 1993, 5, 174

9 Goldberg, Y.P., McMurray, C.T., Zeisler, J. *et al.* Increased instability of intermediate alleles in families with sporadic Huntington's disease compared to similar sized intermediate alleles in the general population. *Hum. Mol. Gent.* 1995, 4, 1911

10 Hayden, M.R., Martin, W.R.W. and Stoessl, A.J. PET in the early diagnosis of Huntington's disease. *Neurology* 1986, 36, 888

11 Ichise, M., Toyama, H., Fomazzari, L. *et al.* Iodine-[123]-IBZM dopamine D2 receptor and technetium-[99m]-HMPAO brain perfusion SPECT in the evaluation of patients with and subjects at risk for Huntington's disease. *J. Nucl. Med.* 1993, 34(8), 1274

12 Kemp, J.M. and Powell, T.P.S. The cortico striate projection in the monkey. *Brain* 1970, 93, 525

13 Kuhl, B., Phelps, M.E., Markham, C.H. *et al.* Cerebral metabolism and atrophy in HD determined by FDG and computed tomographic scan. *Ann. Neurol.* 1982, 12, 425

14 Boecker, H., Kuwert, T., Langen, K.J. *et al.* SPECT with HMPAO compared to PET with FDG in Huntington's Disease. *J. Comput. Assist. Tomogr.* 1994, 18(4), 542

15 Brucke, T., Podreka, I., Angelberger, P. *et al.* Dopamine receptor imaging with SPECT: studies in different neuropsychiatric disorders. *J. Cereb. Blood Flow Metab.* 1991, 11(2), 220

16 Brucke, T., Wenger, S., Asenbaum, S. *et al.* Dopamine D2 receptor imaging and measurement with SPECT. *Adv. Neurol.* 1993, 60, 494

17 Bruyn, R.P., Hageman, G., Geelen, J.A. *et al.* SPECT, CT and MRI in a Turkish family with Huntington's disease. *Neuroradiology* 1993, 35(7), 526

18 Selemon, L.D. and Goldman-Rakic, P.S. Longitudinal topography and interdigitation of corticostriatal projections in the rhesus monkey. *J. Neurosci.* 1985, 5, 776

19 Percheron, G., Yelnik, J. and Francois, C.A. A Golgi analysis of the primate globus pallidus.III. Spatial organization of the striato-pallidal complex. *J. Comp. Neurol.* 1984, 227, 21

20 Crossman, A.R., Mitchell, I.J. and Sambrook, M.A. Chorea and myoclonus in the monkey induced by GABA antagonism in the lentiform complex. *Brain* 1988, 111, 1211

T in Neurology and Psychiatry, edited by P.P. De Deyn, R.A. Dierckx, A. Alavi and B.A. Pickut
7 John Libbey & Company Ltd, pp. 39–43

ssessment by ^{99m}Tc-HMPAO SPECT in atients with Normal Pressure ydrocephalus Treated by Acetazolamide

. Moretti, G. Baillet, C. Szekely[*], B. Roualdès[**],
Vanhove[***], G. Demonceau[***], J.M. Rocchisani and
alama

:roduction

mal Pressure Hydrocephalus (NPH) is interesting to the clinician since associated dementia can more or less be reversed by ventriculoatrial shunting[1]. cause of the disease is unknown, but probably results from a low-grade defect cerebrospinal fluid (CSF) resorption. Meningitis, trauma, or subarachnoid morrhage are also possible causes.

clinical syndrome is characterised by a triade consisting of progressive mentia, gait disorder and urinary incontinence. CT shows ventricular enlargement radionuclide injection into the cerebrospinal fluid (lumbar injection) has been d to study the pattern of CSF flow. These tests, however, do not predict which ents are going to benefit from surgical shunting since the response to ventricular nting varies[2].

SF tap of 40 to 50 ml that is accompanied by an improvement in psychomotor onse is said to be a good predictor of improvement after ventricular shunting[3]. similar way, long standing preoperative symptoms yield the worst results, while I resulting from subarachnoid haemorrhage has a good response to surgery[4].

ents with enlargement of the third ventricle and temporal horns improve after gery[5]. There is a high incidence of postoperative complications such as infection, ke, subdural haematoma and valve dysfunction, with as much as 31% shunt function[5].

nough the mechanism of the NPH is not well understood, it is now believed that arachnoidal granulations display decreased CSF resorption. Pressure in brain ues increases and compression of small vessels leads to cerebral blood flow iction. Furthermore, stretching of anterior cerebral arteries over the corpus osum caused by hydrocephalus can induce a decrease in frontal lobe cerebral d flow (CBF), resulting in cognitive disorders. Stretching of middle cerebral ries over the lateral walls of dilated ventricles can induce a reduction in cerebral d flow in parietal regions with walking and gait disorders. Oedema present nd the third ventricle is assumed to cause urinary incontinence.

ventricular tissue changes develop slowly and gradually become irreversible axonal destruction and demyelinisation of the periventricular white matter. ue pressure increases in the periventricular structures, and this affects the rogenic mechanism of CBF regulation including loss of autoregulation and her decreasing CBF. It is tempting then to assume that lowering CSF pressure restore CBF autoregulation.

tazolamide (ACZ) has been proposed as an alternative treatment to surgical nting[6]. ACZ is a carboxic anhydrase inhibitor and its major local effect is to raise

Service Central de Médecine Nucléaire et Service de Neurologie, Hôpital Avicenne, 125 rue de Stalingrad - 93009 Bobigny Cedex, France
[*]Hôpital René Muret, Avenue du Docteur Schaeffner - 93270 Sevran, Belgium
[**]Centre Hospitalier Intercommunal, 40 Avenue de Verdun - 94010, Creteil, Belgium
[***]Hôpital Sainte Elisabeth, Zottegem, Belgium

intravascular CO_2 tension, and increase CBF via flow autoregulation[7]. ACZ also reduces CSF production by the choroid plexus and lowers CSF pressure in hydrocephalic patients.

This effect takes 24 to 48 h to become manifest and continues as long as the drug is given. Lowering CSF pressure may restore CBF autoregulation, and this can be assessed by studying CBF with [99m]Tc- HMPAO SPECT.

We studied patients with NPH treated with ACZ and compared clinical improvement with changes in regional cerebral blood flow (rCBF) assessed by HMPAO SPECT.

Patients and methods

We studied 20 patients that had the clinical diagnosis of normal pressure hydrocephalus. Each of them had the classical triade of clinical symptoms of NPH described by Hakim and Adams[8], dementia, gait disorder and urinary incontinence. There were 8 males and 12 females with a mean age of 81.3 ± 5.6 yrs (range 73-92 yrs). The patients were evaluated clinically in the following manner.

Cognitive functions were evaluated using the mini mental state examination (MMSE), which assesses whether the patient is fully orientated, can repeat words, calculate, memorise, speak and draw clearly. The resulting score varies between 0 (severe impairment) and 30 (normal).

Walking ability was scored as follows:

- normal — 20
- gait ataxia, walking possible — 15
- walking with cane — 10
- walking with human support — 5
- walking impossible — 0

Sphincter control:

- continence — 20
- urination — 10
- complete incontinence — 0

Thus a patient could obtain a total score of between 0 and 70.

This evaluation was performed initially and after six weeks of treatment, and repeated after six months of treatment.

All patients had ventricular dilation on CT. They underwent initial HMPAO SPECT before treatment and then after 6 weeks of treatment (Table 1). Treatment consisted of 500 mg ACZ per day, orally. HMPAO (740 MBq) was injected at rest, without any visual or acoustic stimulation, within 10 min of HMPAO labelling. Heart rate and blood pressure were measured at the time of injection.

SPECT acquisition was performed 15 min later, wit images 64 x 64 over 360° on a General Electric 40 gamma camera. Reconstruction was performed Shepp and Logan prefiltering and an attenua correction was used (Bartec Medical System Ltd, U Transverse slices were reorientated parallel to orbitomeatal line. Coronal and sagittal cuts were obta as well, with a slice thickness of 6.25 mm.

Quantitation was obtained after transformation Talairach space and comparison with a normal data derived from 120 normal patients (Vanhove Demonceau, unpublished data). Accordingly a 3D orientation of the data was performed, followed l normalisation using the histogram mode of the voxe voxel ratio. Significant areas in size and signal ampli were identified, and a slice by slice axial display dep changes in rCBF before and after treatment. Furtherr a global regional cerebral blood flow index was der as the total uptake in the whole brain calibrated by injected dose. This index was used to assess CBF or SPECT image before and after treatment and to tes improvement.

Results

After six week of treatment, the results were as follo

1. In 20/20 patients, the average clinical score improved under treatment, from 40.3 ± 9. 47.7 ± 14.8 with a mean increase of $7.4 \pm$ (p <0.05). The average CBF increased by 17.7% in 20/20 patients (p < 0.02).

2. In 13/20 patients, there was both a cli improvement and an increase in cerebral blood There was a satisfying correlation between increase in the two scores

$$(r = 0.51, p < 0.01).$$

3. In 5/20 patients, there was no improvement ir clinical score and no improvement in the reg cerebral blood flow either.

4. Disagreement between clinical score and I perfusion was present in 2/20 patients :

- 1/20 showed no rCBF improvement on SPE but improved clinically (from 33/70 to 47/7

- 1/20 had rCBF improvement of 31%, but d not improve clinically (54/70 to 52/70).

Improvement of clinical score in 14 patients with improvement was 39.1 ± 8.6 before ACZ versus 5 8.6 after ACZ. There was a good agreement bet clinical improvement and CBF changes (Table 2), an kappa value was high, equal to 0.76.

le 1 Cerebral blood flow change between initial SPECT and SPECT after 6 weeks of treatment with acetazolamide. Clinical score
ge = clinical score after six weeks of acetazolamide minus clinical score before treatment

nt	CBF change %	Clinical score change	CBF improvement after ACZ[a]	Clinical improvement[b]	Agreement[c]
	-13	14	-	Y	0
	-11	-9	-	N	1
	-21	-1	-	N	1
	13	13	+	Y	1
	-13	-27	-	N	1
	50	17	+	Y	1
	65	10	+	Y	1
	34	11	+	Y	1
	31	-2	+	N	0
	15	14	+	Y	1
	0	-19	-	N	1
	17	16	+	Y	1
	15	18	+	Y	1
	44	13	+	Y	1
	10	5	+	Y	1
	55	18	+	Y	1
	16	17	+	Y	1
	57	15	+	Y	1
	-15	2	-	N	1
	5	17	+	Y	1

+ = rCBF has increased; - = rCBF has decreased. [b], Y = yes; N = no. [c], 0 = No agreement; 1 = clinical score and CBF did not improve under
atment. Otherwise CBF and clinical score improved

ble 2 Comparison of HMPAO SPECT changes versus clinical
atus improvement under acetazolamide treatment. There was a
ry good agreement between SPECT and clinical improvement
d the Kappa value was high, equal to 0.76

MPAO SPECT	Clinical grading	
	Improvement	No improvement
BF improvement	13	1
o CBF improvement	1	5

Changes were sometimes quite significant, as in the
following example: patient number 6, aged 80 years old,
presented with some walking impediment and marked
anterograde amnesia. CT was suggestive of NPH. SPECT
showed decreased rCBF bilaterally in the frontal and
parietal cortex in the vicinity of the anterior and posterior
ventricular horns. After six weeks of treatment, the
patient was markedly improved clinically especially as
far as walking was concerned. The overall clinical score
increased from 40 to 57. Regional cerebral blood flow
increased by 50% in the frontal regions. The rCBF and
clinical score remained increased at 6 months (close to
the values obtained at 6 weeks).

Discussion

NPH can improve with surgical or medical treatment. However, the response to treatment is difficult to predict. The response to surgery is less satisfactory when Evan's ratio on CT or MRI is more than 0.3 (this is the ventricular to brain broadness ratio), or when dementia has been present long before surgery or if gait impairment has started before dementia[9]. It has been shown that improvement in the psychomotor functions and gait pattern after lumbar puncture correlated with improvement after shunt operation[3].

Cerebral perfusion itself cannot predict response to surgical shunting since Tamaki *et al.*[10] found no difference in CBF patterns between patients with good or poor outcome. They found that an increase in CBF after surgery correlated with clinical improvement.

Moretti *et al.*[11,12] measured CBF after lumbar puncture and found that an increase in CBF after CSF tap correlated with clinical improvement after shunting. Furthermore, Kamiya *et al.*[13], reported that frontal blood flow increased in comparison with temporal flow after CSF tap in cases who benefitted most from shunting.

The frontal cortex is certainly a critical region in NPH, since Ishikawa *et al.*[14], using positron emission tomography, found that NPH involves impairment of cerebral oxygen metabolism in the lower regions of the cerebral cortex, particularly in the lower frontal region. Meyer *et al.*[15] also found a reduction in CBF throughout frontal and temporal lobes in NPH patients.

These results were confirmed by Larsson *et al.*[16], who found that CBF changes in the frontal and hippocampal regions have pathophysiological and prognostic value in NPH. Accordingly, when posterior cortical CBF is more decreased than the anterior frontal cortical CBF, therapeutic failure of surgery is most likely [9].

Does CBF increase after successful shunting? Kushner *et al.*[17] found that it did not. Graff-Radford *et al.*[18] found that CBF increase does not account for clinical improvement in NPH. Mamo *et al.*[19] think that there is probably no relation between CBF and clinical symptoms. In our study there was a good agreement between CBF SPECT measurement and clinical improvement. This agreement (Kappa = 0.76) was only qualitative, but the quantitative correlation coefficient was 0.51, which is not very useful in clinical practice : only one in two patients will demonstrate quantitative correlation.

We conclude that a large increase in CBF does not warrant a dramatic increase in clinical status, and a small increase in CBF can coexist with good clinical improvement.

Acetazolamide has been used in the treatment of vari diseases such as hypertension, glaucoma, and a diuretic. It has also been used to treat altitude sicknes and hydrocephalus in tuberculous meningitis in child Intracerebral penetration of ACZ is slow (about 1 h) its plasma half life is 5 h[21]. At brain level, ACZ has actions:

- It is a vasodilator via CBF autoregulation

- It reduces CSF production by choroid plexus.

The results of this study suggest that CBF improveme correlate with regression of clinical symptoms as a res of acetazolamide administration. The observed eff might result from the two above mentioned mechanis of action.

Conclusion

In 20 patients with normal pressure hydrocephalus, 14, improved clinically when treated with acetazolamide, a 13/14 also had an increase in regional cerebral blood fl on HMPAO SPECT. Assessment of CBF in norr pressure hydrocephalus treated with acetazolamide off an objective additional test to monitor improvement. can be useful when clinical response is difficult to asse or to help decide whether to stop treatment in n responding patients.

References

1   Anderson, M. Normal pressure hydrocephalus. *B.M.J.* 19 293, 837

2   Ekstedt, J. Drug therapy in adult hydrocephalus. *Excer Medica Intern.* Congress Series NB 1973, 296-390, 127

3   Wikkelsö, C., Andersson, H., Blomstrand, C. *et al.* Norr pressure hydrocephalus : predictive value of cerebrospinal fluid tap-test. *Acta Neurol. Scand.* 198 73, 566

4   Larsson, A., Wikkelsö, C., Bilting, M. and Stephensen, Clinical parameters in 74 consecutive patients shunt operat for normal pressure hydrocephalus. *Acta Neurol. Scand.* 199 84, 475

5   Wikkelsö, C., Andersson, H., Blomstrand. C. *et al.* Clinic computed tomography of the brain in the diagnosis of a. prognosis in normal pressure hydrocephalus. *Neuroradiolo,* 1989, 31, 160

6   Aimard, G., Vighetto, A., Gabet, J.Y. *et al.* Acetazolamide: u alternative à la dérivation dans l'hydrocéphalie à pressi normale ? Résultats préliminaires. *Rev. Neurol.* (Paris). 199 146 (6-7), 437

7   Bonte, F.J., Devous, M.D. and Reisch, J.S. The effect Acetazolamide on regional cerebral blood flow in norm human subjects as measured by single photon emissic computed tomography. *Invest. Radiol.* 1988, 23, 564

Hakim, S. and Adams, R.D. The special clinical problem of symptomatic hydrocephalus with normal cerebrospinal fluid pressure. Observation on cerebrospinal fluid hydrodynamic. *J. Neurol. Sci.* 1965 2, 307

Graff-Radford, N.R., Godersky, J.C. and Jones, M.P. Variables predicting surgical outcome in symptomatic hydrocephalus in the elderly. *Neurology* 1989, 39, 1601

Tamaki, N., Kusunoki, T., Wakabayashi, T. and Matsumoto, S. Cerebral hemodynamics in normal pressure hydrocephalus. *J. Neurosurg.* 1984, 61, 510

Moretti, J.L., Defer, G., Delmon, L. *et al.* Acétazolamide: effet sur la perfusion cérébrale appréciée par la tomoscintigraphie à l'isopropyliodoamphétamine 123I (IAMP-123I). *J. Biophys. Biomec.* 1987, 11, 69

Moretti, J.L., Sergent, A., Louarn, F. *et al.* Cortical perfusion assessment with 123I-isopropyl amphetamine (123I-IAMP) in normal pressure hydrocephalus (NPH). *Eur. J. Nuc. Med.* 1988, 14, 73

Kamiya, K., Yamashita, N., Nagai, H. and Mizawa, I.P. Investigation of normal pressure hydrocephalus by 123I-IMP SPECT. *Neurol. Med. Chir.* 1991, 31, 503

Ishikawa, M., Kikuchi, H., Taki, W. *et al.* Regional cerebral blood flow and oxygen metabolism in normal pressure hydrocephalus after subarachnoid hemorrhage. *Neurol. Med. Chir.* 1989, 29, 382

15 Meyer, J.S., Kitagawa, Y. and Tanahashi, N. Pathogenesis of normal pressure hydrocephalus preliminary observations. *Surg. Neurol.* 1985, 23, 121

16 Larsson, A., Bergh, A.C., Bilting, M. *et al.* Regional cerebral blood flow in normal pressure hydrocephalus. *Eur. J. Nucl. Med.* 1994, 21, 118

17 Kushner, M., Younkin, D., Weinberger, J. *et al.* Cerebral hemodynamics in the diagnosis of normal pressure. *Neurology* 1984, 34, 96

18 Graff-Radford, N.R., Rezai, K., Godersky, J.C. *et al.* Regional cerebral blood flow in normal pressure hydrocephalus. *J. Neurol. Neurosurg. Psychiatry* 1987, 50, 1589

19 Mamo, H.L., Meric, P.C., Ponsin, J.C. *et al.* Cerebral blood flow in normal pressure hydrocephalus. *Stroke* 1987, 18, 1074

20 Lassen, N.A., Friberg, L., Kastrup, J. *et al.* Effects of Acetazolamide on cerebral blood flow and brain tissue oxygenation. *Postgraduate Medical Journal* 1987, 63, 185

21 Maren, T.H. and Robinson, B. The pharmacology of Acetazolamide as related to cerebrospinal fluid and the treatment of hydrocephalus. *Bull. John Hopkins Hospital* 1960, 106, 1

SPECT in Neurology and Psychiatry, edited by P.P. De Deyn, R.A. Dierckx, A. Alavi and B.A. Pickut
© 1997 John Libbey & Company Ltd, pp. 45–48

Benzodiazepine Receptor Distribution in Alzheimer's Disease with ^{123}I-iomazenil by SPECT

Chapter

7

A. Varrone, A. Soricelli, A. Postiglione,
M. Salvatore and N.A. Lassen[*]

Introduction

The loss of cortical synapses in AD involves all types of synapses, including those where γ-amino-butyric-acid (GABA) acts as transmitter substance[1,2]. The synapses presenting the $GABA_A$ receptors are also the site of action of benzodiazepines. Therefore, since $GABA_A$ receptors are present on all cortical neurons[3], radioactively labelled benzodiazepine compounds such as ^{11}C-flumazenil (FMZ) or ^{123}I-iomazenil (IMZ) could be used for quantitating the concentration of $GABA_A$ synapses[4-6].

^{123}I-IMZ used with single photon emission computerised tomography (SPECT) could evaluate $GABA_A$ synapse distribution in the cortex with the advantage that its specific uptake in the brain is >85-90% of the total volume of distribution in the cortex[7]. This implies that the distribution volume (Vd) of ^{123}I-IMZ, i.e. the ratio between brain and plasma concentration at equilibrium, is proportional to the benzodiazepine receptor density, and thus to the number of $GABA_A$ synapses.

The measurement of benzodiazepine receptor density with ^{123}I-IMZ in normal man has already been performed[7,8]. These studies showed that protein binding of ^{123}I-IMZ in plasma and the affinity of ^{123}I-IMZ to the benzodiazepine receptor have little inter-individual variability. In our study, we made the assumption that these factors were not modified in cases of AD, so that the Vd for ^{123}I-IMZ reflects the actual synaptic density in this pathological condition.

The aim of the study was to examine the cortical distribution of ^{123}I-IMZ in AD patients and to investigate whether the Vd for ^{123}I-IMZ was abnormal when compared with that of healthy control subjects.

Methods

Subjects

Six patients (4 M, 2 F, mean age 62.8 ± 6 years, range 59-75 years), with a clinical diagnosis of probable AD according to the NINCDS-ADRDA criteria, were studied[9]. Five normal controls (3 M, 2 F, mean age 61,2 ± 8 years, range 56-69 years) with no clinical evidence of dementia or other neurological diseases were also studied.

University of Naples Federico II, Centro per la Medicina Nucleare del CNR, National Research Council, Via S. Pansini 5, 80131 Napoli, Italy
[*]Department of Nuclear Medicine and Physiology, Bispebjerg Hospital, DK-2400 Copenhagen NV Denmark

Imaging protocol

Six to eight mCi (220-300 MBq) of ^{123}I-IMZ, R016-0154 (Mallinckrodt Medical BV, Petten Holland), were i.v. injected. Prior to the injection, the patients had at least 10 min at rest with their eyes open. Two 30 min SPECT scans were acquired 20 and 180 min after the tracer injection using a brain dedicated high resolution device (Ceraspect, Digital Scintigraphics Inc., MA, USA).

The studies were acquired with a window fixed at 159 keV + 20% and the images were reconstructed using a Butterworth filter (cutoff 1 cm, power factor 10), corrected for attenuation (coefficient = 0.150 cm^{-1}) within an ellipse drawn around the skull and reorientated along the cantho-meatal line. Ten images of 128x128 pixels each, approximately 1 cm thick, were finally displayed.

Arterial samples and cross calibration factor

Approximately 20 min prior the tracer injection a catheter was inserted in the radial artery and two arterial blood samples were collected 20 and 25 min after the intravenous injection of the tracer. The lipophilic fraction containing the tracer was obtained by adding one ml of blood to 2 ml of octanol and mixing. One ml of the extracted fraction was then measured in a well counter to obtain the activity of the tracer in the blood sample. To determine the calibration factor between the SPECT system and the well counter, phantom studies were performed with a 20 cm diameter phantom containing water and 1-2 mCi of ^{123}I using the same acquisition and reconstruction protocols as for the patient studies. Therefore, the average counts per cm^2 were obtained in several slices, and aliquots of the water withdrawn by the phantom were measured in the well counter.

Parametric images of Vd

The images of Vd were obtained following the table look up method[1] and using a two compartmental approach: the data obtained from the two acquired scans, the count rate in the blood sample and the cross calibration factor were used to obtain the parametric images. The Vd images were expressed in millilitres of plasma per millilitres (ml/ml) of brain tissue. Possible misalignment between the two SPECT studies were corrected using a semiautomatic algorithm moving the scan matrix.

As an input curve, we used the average 3-exponential IMZ plasma curve previousely calculated by Abi-Dargham et al.[7] . The curve was then scaled to

Table 1 Values (expressed in ml/ml) from the Vd parametric SPECT images in 5 normal subjects and in 6 patients with moderate severe AD

Values from [123]Iomazenil SPECT Vd images (ml/ml)

		Frontal		Temporal		Parietal		Occipital
		Left	Right	Left	Right	Left	Right	
Controls								
	mean	70.3	75.5	65.7	71.9	70.2	72.5	82.6
	s.d.	11.9	14.3	9.1	17.5	13.4	17.0	18.5
AD patients								
	mean	58.0	56.3	52.7	49.8	50.4	45.7	76.9
	s.d.	15.2	15.6	6.0	2.5	9.0	9.2	15.9
	p<	ns	ns	0.019	0.013	0.017	0.009	ns

the individual patient in the following way: the curve points corresponding to the time of arterial sampling were calculated and the mean ratio of observed to calculated counting rate was used as a scaling factor.

Data analysis

All patients underwent an MRI scan within three weeks from the SPECT scans. The MRI tomograms were used as reference for positioning a standard set of regions of interest (ROI) over the cortical areas on the Vd images. The statistical analysis of the data was performed using Student's t-test.

Results

The mean values obtained from the Vd images indicating the density of benzodiazepine receptors in each region of the cortex both for the normal subjects and the patient population are reported in Table 1.

In normal subjects, the mean Vd values for each cortical region were distributed equally in all cortical regions, with the highest value reported in the occipital area.

In AD patients, the mean Vd values were lower than in the control group in the region analysed, but not in the frontal and occipital areas. Vd in the latter was well preserved, with absolute values similar to those in the normal subjects. A significant reduction (p<0.02) in benzodiazepine receptor was found at the level of the parietal and temporal regions bilaterally, as shown in Figure 1.

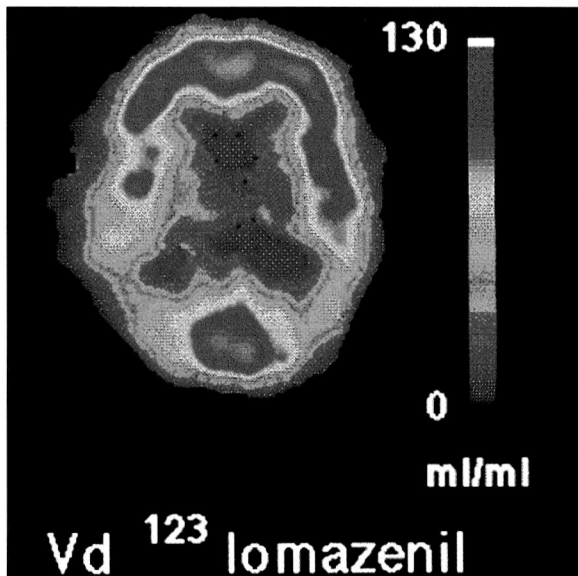

Figure 1 Vd image of [123]Iomazenil in a patient with moderate severe Alzheimer's disease. The image is scaled to the maximum of 120 ml/ml of receptor density. The transaxial slice at the level of the basal ganglia shows a marked involvement of the temporo-parietal regions, bilaterally

have demonstrated a reduction in the cortical synaptic density in AD, and clinicopathological surveys have shown a correlation between synaptic loss and the severity of dementia[18].

In this study we used the table look up method and a protocol of two SPECT scans to obtain parametric images of ^{123}I-IMZ representing the cortical distribution of benzodiazepine receptors. In the group of AD patients, the density of benzodiazepine receptors was significantly reduced in the temporo-parietal cortex compared with the values of the control group. These results indicate a loss of cortical synapses in these associative areas, and are in agreement with the findings obtained from the metabolic and perfusion studies with[18] FDG-PET and ^{99m}Tc-HMPAO SPECT[19,20].

Conclusions

The ^{123}I-IMZ technique can be a valuable procedure for the *in vivo* assessment of synaptic loss in AD. Since this abnormality has been shown to be the factor most clearly related to the severity of the disease, ^{123}I-IMZ can be a reliable agent for the study of the functional state in dementia.

In all studies, basal ganglia and thalami were poorly visualised on the Vd images due to the low benzo-diazepine receptor densities in these regions.

Discussion

Alzheimer's disease is a neurodegenerative disorder characterised by progressive deterioration of memory and cognitive function and is responsible for about 50% of the cases of dementia in the western world[10].

With the extracellular deposition of amyloid and neuritic plaques, the presence of vascular amyloidosis and the intracellular accumulation of neurofibrillary tangles[11-13], the principal histopathological feature associated with the disease is the loss of neuronal cells and their dendritic arborisation with extensive synapse loss[14]. These degenerative changes are most pronounced in the temporo-parietal cortex, in the posterior cingulate gyrus, in the hippocampus and in the amygdala, with involvement of all cortical layers[15].

Many studies reported in recent years were directed at the quantitation of synapses in AD. Electron microscopic[16] and immunohistochemical studies[17]

References

1   Nordberg, A. Neuroreceptor changes in Alzheimer's disease. *Cerebrovasc. Brain Metab. Rev.* 1992, 4, 303

2   Greenmyre, J.T. and Maragos, F. Neurotransmitter receptors in Alzheimer's disease. *Cerebrovasc. Brain Metab. Rev.* 1993, 5, 61

3   Oslen, R.W. The GABA postsynaptic membrane receptor ionophore complex. *Molec. Cell Biochem.* 1981, 39, 261

4   Hunkeler, W., Mohler, H. and Pieri, L. Selective antagonist of benzodiazepines. *Nature* 1981, 290, 514

5   Shintoh, H., Yamasaki, T., Inoue, O. *et al.* Visualization of specific binding sites of benzodiazepine in human brain. *J. Nucl. Med.* 1986, 27, 1593

6   Beer, H.F., Blauentein, P.A., Hasler, P.H. *et al.* In vivo and in vitro evaluation of iodine [123]-RO16-0154: a new imaging agent for SPECT investigations of benzodiazepine receptor. *J. Nucl. Med.* 1990, 31, 1007

7   Abi-Dargham, A., Laurelle, M., Seibyl, J. *et al.* SPECT measurement of benzodiazepine receptors in human brain with iodine-123-iomazenil: kinetic and equilibrium paradigms. *J. Nucl. Med.* 1994, 35, 228

8   Videboek, C., Friberg, L., Holm, S. *et al.* Benzodiazepine receptor equilibrium constants for flumazenil and medazolam determined in humans with single photon emission computer tomography trace ^{123}I-iomazenil. *Europ. J. Pharmacol.* 1993, 249, 43

9 Makhann, G., Drachman, D., Folstein, M. *et al.* Clinical diagnosis of Alzheimer's disease report of the NINCDS-ADRDA work group. *Neurology* 1984, 34, 939

10 Report of the Secretary's Task Force on Alzheimer's Disease, US Department of Health and Human Services, September 1984

11 Terry, R.D., Peck, A., De Teresa, R. *et al.* Some morphometric aspects of the brain in senile dementia of the Alzheimer type. *Ann. Neurol.* 1981, 10, 184

12 Selkoe, D.J. Ageing, amyloid, and Alzheimer's disease. *N. Engl. J. Med.* 1989, 320, 1484

13 Yamaguchi, F., Hirai, S., Morimatso, M. *et al.* A variety of cerebral amyloid deposits in the brains of the Alzheimer-type dementia demonstrated by beta protein immunostaining. *Acta Neuropathol.* 1988, 76, 541

14 De Kosky, S.T. and Bass, N.H. Biochemistry of senile dementia in 'Handbook of Neurochemistry', (Ed. A. Laitha), Plenum Press, New York, USA, 1985, p. 617

15 Brun, A. and Englund, E. Regional pattern of degeneration in Alzheimer's disease: neuronal loss and histopathological grading. *Histopathology* 1981, 5, 549

16 Davies, C.A., Mann, D.M., Sumpter, P.Q. and Yates, P.O. A quantitative morphomteric analysis of the neuronal and synaptic content of the frontal and temporal cortex in patients with Alzheimer's disease. *J. Neurol. Sci.* 1987, 78, 151

17 Schell, S.W., De Kosky, S.T. and Price, D.A. Quantitative assessment of cortical synaptic density in Alzheimer's disease. *Neurobiol. Aging* 1990, 11, 29

18 Terry, R.D., Masliah, E., Salmon, D.P. *et al.* Physical basis of cognitive alterations in Alzheimer's disease: synapse loss is the major correlate of cognitive impairment. *Ann. Neurol.* 1991, 30, 572

19 Rapoport, S.I. Positron emission tomography in Alzheimer's disease in relation to pathogenesis: a critical review. *Cerebrovasc. Brain Metab. Rev.* 1991, 3, 297

20 Waldemar, G. Functional brain imaging with SPECT in normal aging and dementia. *Cerebrovasc. Brain Metab. Rev.* 1995, 7, 89

SPECT in Neurology and Psychiatry, edited by P.P. De Deyn, R.A. Dierckx, A. Alavi and B.A. Pickut
© 1997 John Libbey & Company Ltd, pp. 49–53

rCBF and hCRH-Stimulated ACTH in Alzheimer's Disease

Chapter

8

J.A. Arias, M.L. Cuadrado[*], M.S. Barquero[*], P. Gil[*],
I. Pablos[*] and J.A. Cabranes[*]

Introduction

Neuroendocrine disturbances in Alzheimer's disease (AD) have been reported in many studies and hyperactivity of the hypothalamic-pituitary-adrenal (HPA) axis is one of the most common findings. Indeed, hypercortisolemia and non-suppression in the dexamethasone suppression test occur in a significant percentage of patients suffering from AD[1,2]. Explanations of possible connections between HPA changes and the primary neurodegenerative process are lacking. A lesion in the hippocampal formation, located in the medial aspect of the temporal lobe, might be involved, as it inhibits HPA function in normal conditions[3].

SPECT allows the exploration of blood flow in selected areas of the brain, as a reflection of their function *in vivo*. On the other hand, it is possible to study HPA function by the determination of baseline and stimulated adrenocorticotropin (ACTH) levels after a single administration of human corticotropin-releasing-hormone (hCRH). This test may not only evaluate the hypophyseal condition, but also suprahypophyseal changes acting on the ACTH response[4]. The aim of this study was to examine the potential relationship between HPA functioning, assessed by the CRH stimulation test, and regional cerebral blood flow (rCBF) in inferior parietal and mesial temporal lobes in AD. There is agreement that both cerebral regions show characteristic morphological and functional changes in AD and that these are the regions affected earliest in the disease[5-11]. If there were any cortical influences over HPA activity, this would be expected to be linked with these areas.

Patients and methods

We examined 37 patients (mean age ± s.d., 72.7 ± 9.6 years) suffering from probable AD according to the criteria of the National Institute of Neurological and Communicative Disorders and Stroke and the Alzheimer's Disease and Related Disorders Association (NINCDS-ADRDA)[12]. All subjects met the DSM-III-R criteria for primary degenerative dementia. All participants were medically healthy and none were receiving any therapy known to affect the HPA axis. Dementia severity was assessed by a modified version[13] of the mini mental state examination (MMSE)[14], with the score ranging from 0 to 35. They scored less than 18 on the Hamilton Rating Scale for depression. Consent was given by patients or relatives.

Department of Nuclear Medicine,
Fundacion Jimenez Diaz, Avda
Reyes Catolicos 2,
28040 Madrid, Spain
* Hospital Universitario San
Carlos, Prof. Martin Lagos s/n,
28040 Madrid, Spain

A SPECT scan was obtained 15 min after an intravenous injection of 555-750 MBq of ^{99m}Tc-(hexamethyl propyleneamine oxime) (HMPAO; Ceretec®, Amersham). Patients were instructed to close their eyes and to remain in a physically and psychologically relaxed state for 10 min. Acquisition was performed by a single-head SPECT system (Orbiter® ZLC-75, Siemens) equipped with a high-resolution low energy collimator. Sixty four 20-second frames were obtained over 360° each with a resolution of 64 × 64 pixels. Tomographic images were reconstructed using a Shepp-Logan-Hanning filter, rendering slices two pixels wide (12 mm). No attenuation correction was made. On the appropiate transaxial and coronal slices, we defined two pairs of regions of interest (ROIs): a parietal pair, 4 × 6 pixels wide, and a mesial temporal pair, 3 × 6 pixels wide. These ROIs were selected to include associative cortex in parietal lobes and hippocampal formation in temporal lobes, respectively, in accordance with standard anatomical landmarks in brain atlases. A rectangular ROI in the cerebellum was chosen as a reference. We defined the percentage of uptake in parietal or temporal ROIs as 100 × mean count per pixel in lesion/mean count per pixel in cerebellum. This index was taken as a semiquantitative value of rCBF.

Two days after the SPECT study, a hCRH-stimulated ACTH test was carried out. Blood samples were drawn basally (at 9:00 a.m.) and 30, 45, 60, and 120 min after an intravenous injection of 100 µg hCRH (Corticobiss®, Pharma Bissendorf Peptide GmbH). ACTH was measured by a specific two-site immunoradiometric assay (Nichols Institute Diagnostics). The intra- and interassay coefficients of variation were 3.0% and 7.5%, respectively. The assay sensitivity was 1 pg/ml. ACTH plasma levels were expressed as pg/ml and designated ACTH0, ACTH30, ACTH45, ACTH60 and ACTH120, depending on the time of extraction.

Statistical analysis established the lowest grade polynomial regression that gave a significant ($p<0.05$) value of r. If this value was significant, regression was re-studied by imposing more restricted criteria.

Results

Table 1 summarises the demographic and clinical characteristics, as well as the rCBF and ACTH measurements. Age or duration of the disease was not significantly correlated with any other variable

Table 1 Summary of demographic, clinical, rCBF and ACTH measures

	Mean (s.d.)
n	37
Age (yr)	72.6 (9.7)
Female (%)	72.0
Duration (yr)	3.3 (2.2)
MMSE	18.8 (7.4)
rCBF (%):	
Parietal (both sides)	77.3 (8.0)
Right parietal	77.7 (8.9)
Left parietal	76.0 (8.9)
Temporal (both sides)	64.3 (5.9)
Right temporal	66.3 (6.7)
Left temporal	62.3 (5.5)
ACTH (pg/ml):	
0 min	20.9 (14.5)
30 min	55.7 (44.1)
45 min	57.4 (48.5)
60 min	48.2 (41.6)
120 min	23.4 (16.8)

Table 2 Second grade polynomial correlation coefficients between MMSE and rCBF with ACTH

	ACTH0	ACTH30	ACTH45	ACTH60	ACTH120
Parietal	0.19	0.44[a]	0.61[c]	0.58[b]	0.51[b]
Temporal	0.26	0.22	0.14	0.20	0.29
MMSE	0.08	0.51[b]	0.57[b]	0.56[b]	0.49[b]

n=37; [a], $p<0.05$; [b], $p<0.01$; [c], $p<0.001$

Table 3 Second grade polynomial correlation coefficients between ACTH and parietal rCBF on each side

	ACTH30	ACTH45	ACTH60	ACTH120
Right parietal	0.21	0.45[a]	0.40[a]	0.28
Left parietal	0.60[b]	0.68[c]	0.68[c]	0.66[c]

n=37; [a], $p<0.05$; [b], $p<0.001$; [c], $p<0.0001$

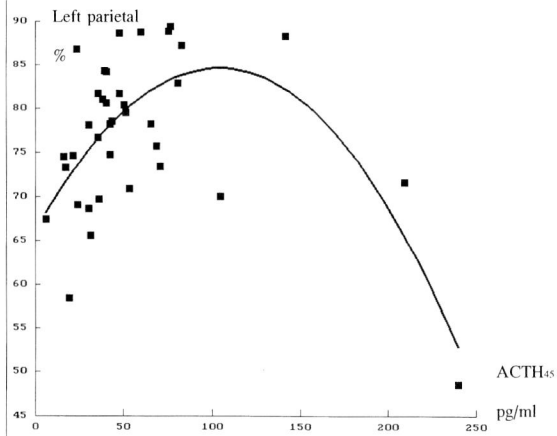

Figure 1 Relationship between ACTH45 and left parietal-to-cerebellar rCBF ratio (n=37). Polynomial regression equation was: $y = 0.0017 x^2 + 0.36 x + 66.1$ ($r = 0.68$, $p = 0.00002$)

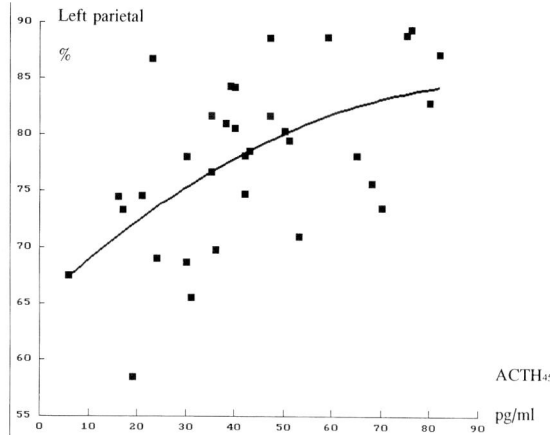

Figure 2 Relationship between ACTH45 and left parietal-to-cerebellar rCBF ratio (n=33). Second grade polynomial regression equation was: $y = -0.0021 x^2 + 0.40 x + 65.0$ ($r = 0.57$, $p = 0.003$). Linear regression equation (not shown in the figure) was: $y = 0.21 x + 68.7$ ($r = 0.56$, $p = 0.0008$)

(data not shown). The MMSE score correlated linearly with parietal rCBF ($r = 0.58$, $p < 0.001$) but not with temporal rCBF ($r = 0.14$, $p =$ n.s.). There was no significant linear correlation (first grade polynomial) between rCBF or MMSE and any of the ACTH concentrations. However, second grade polynomial ($y = ax^2 + bx + c$) correlations between parietal rCBF or MMSE (y-axis) and non-baseline levels of ACTH (x-axis) were all significant (Table 2). Considering each side (Table 3), left parietal rCBF was more involved than right parietal rCBF in the regression. In each graph (Figure 1, ACTH45 as an example), there were a few remote points. Removing four of those points from analysis, rendering n = 33, significant values of r were obtained for a second grade regression again (Table 4 and Figure 2), but in this case a linear regression was also significant.

Table 4 Linear and second grade polynomial correlation coefficients between ACTH and left parietal rCBF

	ACTH30	ACTH45	ACTH60	ACTH120
Left parietal (linear)	0.33	0.56[a]	0.51[b]	0.50[b]
Left parietal (2nd grade)	0.34	0.57[b]	0.51[b]	0.50[c]

n=33; [a], p<0.001; [b], p<0.01; [c], p<0.05

Discussion

There was a relationship between MMSE score, ACTH response and parietal rCBF in our AD patients. This was more evident for left parietal lobe than for right parietal lobe, possibly reflecting asymmetrical damage in AD brains. Association between parietal rCBF and cognitive performance has already been described by many authors.

We found an inverse U-shaped correlation between non-baseline ACTH (x-axis) and parietal rCBF or MMSE (y-axis) when we considered our patients as a whole. In fact, there was a positive correlation between these variables in most patients, the more affected parietal rCBF or MMSE score corresponding to a lower ACTH response. However, some patients with advanced AD exhibited a very high ACTH response, which accounted for the U-shaped curve. In any case, the most striking feature of our results was the link between activity of the HPA axis and parietal rCBF.

It is not easy to establish a causal relationship between these changes. Temporal areas have known neuroanatomical connections with diencephalic nuclei governing the HPA axis and exert an inhibitory influence over them[3]. Therefore, a correlation between temporal rCBF and HPA function could be expected. However, we did not find any traces of temporal/hippocampal involvement in ACTH response. Instead, ACTH values were correlated with parietal rCBF. It has been suggested that reduced parietal blood flow in AD patients might reflect pathological changes in the projection neurones in the parahippocampal gyrus[7]. Nevertheless, such an indirect connection between HPA axis and parietal lobe would not explain our findings, since temporal rCBF did not show correlation with ACTH response.

De Leon et al.[15] found that the amount of cortisol in the recovery phase of the drop in cortisol after glucose administration was related to the degree of hippocampal atrophy measured by computed tomography in AD patients. The hippocampal formation is a small region[16] (5 cm³) and SPECT has a limited resolution for its delimitation. However, mesial temporal lobe CBF can be an acceptable marker of hippocampal function, since lesions in the medial temporal cortex are relatively homogeneous and adjacent structures send predominantly excitatory fibres to hippocampal formation[17]. Perhaps cortisol inhibition with glucose reflects hypothalamic function more directly, whereas ACTH stimulation with CRH gives us an insight into pituitary reserve. It has been hypothesised that disturbances of CRH and acetylcholine, another ACTH modulator, in AD brains might result in a reduced tonic stimulation of corticotropin-producing pituitary cells, which would lead to disminished ACTH stores and impaired maximal secretion[18]. So, the ACTH reserve could reflect the state of higher systems regulating HPA axis. The apparent disparity between de Leon's findings and ours might result from the fact that morphological changes do not parallel functional changes.

From a functional point of view, almost all the damage of the hippocampal formation occurs early in the course of AD. Progression of the disease can be better traced with neuropsychological and functional neuroimaging assessment of other brain areas[19].

Many neurochemical disturbances have been found in AD[20]. It is possible that several factors controlling HPA axis are damaged in AD[21]. If the deficiency of different factors with opposing effects were not equal, the pituitary response could be extremely variable and, therefore, there would be at least two subgroups of patients. This hypothesis is consistent with our findings: as the U-shaped curve shows, patients with advanced AD showed either low ACTH response or high ACTH response. Actually, this non-linear response may account for some of the conflicting results that have been reported in HPA tests of subjects suffering from AD. However, further studies are needed to verify these findings. In fact, as we have stated above, most of our patients showed a linear response between variables.

Clinical studies have shown attentional defects in AD[22,23]. Interestingly, the administration of ACTH and fragments like ACTH4-10 have been followed by an improvement of attentional deficits in patients

diagnosed with AD[24,25]. ACTH does not have a direct effect on memory but allows the individual to keep selective attention[26]. On the other hand, bilateral posterior parietal lesions are associated with impairment in directed and selective attention with hypoarousal states and with unawareness or a failure to act on certain aspects of the environment[27,28]. We suggest that, whatever the cause is, neurodegenerative and endocrine disturbances could coexist and both contribute to the attentional derangement in AD.

Acknowledgements

This work was supported in part by two grants from the Comunidad Autonoma de Madrid: C252/90 (obtained by Prof. J.L. Carreras) and C242/91.

References

1 Davis, K.L., Davis, B.M., Greenwald, B.S. et al. Cortisol and Alzheimer's disease.I: basal studies. Am. J. Psychiatry 1986, 143, 300

2 Greenwald, B.S., Mathe, A.A., Mohs, R.C. et al. Cortisol and Alzheimer's disease.II: dexamethasone suppression, dementia severity, and affective symptoms. Am. J. Psychiatry 1986, 143, 442

3 Jacobson, L. and Sapolsky, R. The role of the hippocampus in feedback regulation of the hypothalamic-pituitary-adrenocortical axis. Endocr. Rev. 1991, 12, 118

4 Schreiber, W., Krieg, J.-C., Bossert, S. et al. Methodological aspects of hCRF-stimulated ACTH and cortisol secretion in healthy subjects. Psychoneuroendocrinology 1988, 13, 487

5 Davis, P.C., Mirra, S.S. and Alazraki, N. The brain of older persons with and without dementia: findings on MR, PET, and SPECT images. A.J.R. 1994, 162, 1267

6 Jernigan, T.L., Salmon, D.P., Butters, N. and Hesselink, J.R. Cerebral structure on MRI, II: specific changes in Alzheimer's and Huntington's diseases. Biol. Psychiatry 1991, 29, 68

7 Jobst, K.A., Smith, A.D., Barker, C.S. et al. Association of atrophy of the medial temporal lobe with reduced blood flow in the posterior parietotemporal cortex in patients with a clinical and pathological diagnosis of Alzheimer's disease. J. Neurol. Neurosurg. Psychiatry 1992, 55, 190

8 Lehericy, S., Baulac, M., Chiras, J. et al. Amygdalohippocampal MR volume measurements in the early stages of Alzheimer's disease. A.J.N.R. 1994, 15, 927

9 Ohnishi, T., Hoshi, H., Nagamachi, S. High resolution SPECT to assess hippocampal perfusion in neuropsychiatric diseases. J. Nucl. Med. 1995, 36, 1163

10 Pearson, G.D., Harris, G.J., Powers, R.E. et al. Quantitative changes in mesial volume, regional cerebral blood flow, and cognition in Alzheimer's disease. Arch. Gen. Psychiatry 1992, 49, 402

11 Stern, Y., Alexander, G.E., Prohovnik, I. and Mayeux, R. Inverse relationship between education and parietotemporal perfusion deficit in Alzheimer's disease. *Ann. Neurol.* 1992, 32, 371

12 McKhann, G., Drachman, D., Folstein, M. *et al.* Clinical diagnosis of Alzheimer's disease: report of the NINCDS-ADRDA Work Group, Department of Health and Human Services Task Force on Alzheimer's disease. *Neurology* 1984, 34, 939

13 Lobo, A. and Ezquerra, J. El mini-examen cognoscitivo: un test sencillo, practico, para detectar alteraciones intelectivas en pacientes medicos. *Actas Luso Esp. Neurol. Psiquiatr.* 1979, 3, 149

14 Folstein, M.F., Folstein, S.E. and McHugh, P.R. 'Mini-mental state': a practical method for grading the mental state of patients for the clinician. *J. Psychiatr. Res.* 1975, 12, 189

15 de Leon, M., McRae, T., Tsai, J.R. *et al.* Abnormal cortisol response in Alzheimer's disease linked to hippocampal atrophy. *Lancet* 1988, 2, 391

16 Watson, C., Andermann, F., Gloor, P. *et al.* Anatomic basis of amygdaloid and hippocampal volume measurement by magnetic resonance imaging. *Neurology* 1992, 42, 1743

17 Braak, H. and Braak, E. The human entorhinal cortex: normal morphology and lamina-specific pathology in various diseases. *Neurosci. Res.* 1992, 15, 6

18 Dodt, C., Dittman, J., Hruby, J. *et al.* Different regulation of adrenocorticotropin and cortisol secretion in young, mentally healthy elderly and patients with senile dementia of Alzheimer's type. *J. Clin. Endocrinol. Metab.* 1991, 72, 272

19 de Toledo-Morrell, L. and Morrell F. Alzheimer's disease: new developments for non-invasive detection of early cases. *Curr. Opin. Neurol. Neurosurg.* 1993, 6, 113

20 Fowler, C.J., O'Neill, C., Winblad, B. and Cowburn, R.F. Neurotransmitter, receptor and signal transduction disturbances in Alzheimer's disease. *Acta Neurol. Scand. Suppl.* 1992, 139, 59

21 Miller, A.H., Sastry, G., Speranza, A.J. *et al.* Lack of association between cortisol hypersecretion and non-suppression on the DST in patients with Alzheimer's disease. *Am. J. Psychiatry* 1994, 151, 267

22 Daffner, K.R., Scinto, L.F.M., Weintraub, S. *et al.* Diminished curiosity in patients with probable Alzheimer's disease as measured by exploratory eye movements. *Neurology* 1992, 42, 320

23 Freed, D.M., Corkin, S., Growdon, J.H. and Nissen, M.J. Selective attention in Alzheimer's disease: characterizing cognitive subgroups of patients. *Neuropsychologia* 1989, 27, 325

24 Heuser, I., Heuser-Link, M., Gotthardt, U. *et al.* Behavioural effects of a synthetic corticotropin 4-9 analog in patients with depression and patients with Alzheimer's disease. *J. Clin. Psychopharmacol.* 1993, 13, 171

25 Nappi, G., Facchinetti, F., Martignoni, E. *et al.* N-terminal ACTH fragments increase the CSF beta-EP content in Alzheimer type dementia. *Acta Neurol. Scand.* 1988, 78, 146

26 Ur, E. Psychological aspects of hypothalamo-pituitary-adrenal activity. *Balliere's Clin. Endocrinol. Metab.* 1991, 5, 79

27 Mennemeier, M., Wertman, E. and Heilman, K.M. Neglect of near peripersonal space. Evidence for multidirectional attentional systems in humans. *Brain* 1992, 115, 37

28 Weinberg, W.A. and Harper, C.R. Vigilance and its disorders. *Neurol. Clin.* 1993, 11, 59

Neuropsychology

SPECT in Neurology and Psychiatry, edited by P.P. De Deyn, R.A. Dierckx, A. Alavi and B.A. Pickut
© 1997 John Libbey & Company Ltd, pp. 57-66

Use of HMPAO to Investigate Memory Function in Patients with Amnesia

Chapter

9

D. Montaldi, A. Mayes[**], A. Barnes[*], L. Wilson[***],
D. Hadley[*], J. Patterson[*] and D. Wyper[*]

Introduction

Organic amnesia is a syndrome in which preservation of intelligence and immediate memory are typically accompanied by varying degrees of anterograde and retrograde amnesia. Anterograde amnesia is a deficit in recalling and recognising post-traumatically encountered facts and events whereas retrograde amnesia is a similar recall and recognition deficit for pre-traumatically encountered facts and events, which should have initially been put normally into memory. This syndrome is caused by lesions to any of three main brain areas that are strongly interconnected: the medial temporal lobes, the midline diencephalon, and the basal forebrain[1]. Organic amnesia is of considerable interest because it seems probable that exposing both the precise location of the lesions that cause it and the precise nature of the functional deficits that underlie it will throw light on how the human brain mediates episodic and semantic memory.

Despite extensive research, it still remains controversial, however, as to: (a) what the precise location of the critical lesions underlying amnesia actually is - for example, within the temporal lobe, although the hippocampus is believed to contribute to amnesia recent evidence[1] suggests that lesions of the parahippocampal and perirhinal cortices also have dramatic effects, and damage to other structures in this region may also affect memory; (b) whether several distinct functional deficits underlie the syndrome although evidence seems to be gradually accumulating that it is indeed heterogeneous; and (c) what the exact nature of the deficit or deficits actually is. In general, amnesic symptoms may be caused by encoding, storage, or retrieval deficits, and these may either apply to all aspects of the fact and event information that patients are impaired at recalling and recognising, or it may only apply to specific aspects of this information. If amnesia is heterogeneous, then more than one deficit of this kind will be implicated, but differently located lesions should be responsible for the distinct deficits.

If the functional deficits and the critical lesions underlying amnesia can be identified, some structures involved in mediating the critical processes may still not be isolated. It may, however, be possible to isolate such structures, if they exist, by using positron emission tomography (PET), single photon emission computed tomography (SPECT), or functional magnetic resonance imaging (fMRI) to measure changes that are associated with level of neuronal activity in patients and normal subjects. There are two main ways in which these procedures can be used. The first and simpler way is to record activity during a resting state in patients with lesions of known location and matched control subjects in order to determine whether the patients show evidence of abnormal

Department of Psychology,
University of Paisley, Paisley,
Scotland, UK
*Institute of Neurological
Sciences, Southern General
Hospital NHS Trust, Glasgow,
Scotland, UK **Department of
Clinical Neurology, University of
Sheffield, Royal Hallamshire
Hospital, Glossop Road, Sheffield,
UK
***Department of Psychology,
University of Stirling, Stirling,
Scotland, UK

metabolic activity in neuronal regions that are structurally intact. For example, Levasseur[2] used PET to examine patients with fairly selective midline thalamic lesions and varying degrees of amnesia following paramedian artery infarcts, and found reduced levels of oxygen metabolism in the cerebral cortex. A similar study[3] of Korsakoff patients, who have midline diencephalic lesions, also found that these patients displayed a widespread reduction in neocortical metabolic activity. If one assumes that these studies indicate that the cortex is likely to be involved in the memory system that mediates episodic and semantic memory, then one plausible interpretation of their results is that certain midline diencephalic regions somehow modulate activity in widespread neocortical areas so that they are better able to lay down long-term episodic and semantic memories. This interpretation is attractive, but its empirical base requires further buttressing because Perani[4] failed to find a similar widespread reduction in neocortical activity in a mixed group of amnesics that included patients with midline diencephalic lesions.

The second way in which the procedures can be used to explore amnesia is through the use of memory challenge techniques in which the pattern of activation produced by the attempted triggering of specific memory processes can be identified and compared in normal people and amnesics. These techniques try to isolate the activation associated with a specific memory process by determining the differences between the blood flow changes produced by a memory task that should involve the relevant memory process and the blood flow changes produced by an otherwise similar task that does not. It is only possible to examine memory processes that are active around the time of acquisition or retrieval because passive long-term retention probably does not involve any detectable patterns of activation or deactivation. If normal subjects show specific and different patterns of activation around the times of encoding and retrieval, then it becomes relevant to ask whether amnesics show similar patterns of activation or whether their activation patterns are abnormal in a way that may or may not depend on the location of the lesion that underlies their memory deficit. The available evidence[5] suggests that amnesics encode information normally so that, if they were found to have abnormal activation patterns associated with memory acquisition processes, this would probably reflect a deficit in the processes responsible for consolidation of information into long-term storage. The activational abnormality should mean that these processes are not occurring to a normal extent and comparison with normal subjects will also reveal within which brain structures they should be occurring. A similar abnormal activation pattern

associated with retrieval would not reveal at what stage memory processing is impaired in amnesic patients unless their memory levels were matched to those of their control subjects. This is because poor amnesic retrieval could reflect an encoding deficit, some kind of storage deficit, or a specific retrieval problem. If amnesic memory levels are matched to those of their control subjects, then any abnormal activation pattern should reflect a disorder that is specific to the way that they retrieve fact and event information.

Although there have been no published comparisons of amnesics with normal subjects using memory challenge tasks, there have been several challenge studies performed at the encoding and retrieval stages of memory with normal subjects. These indicate the presence of different patterns of activation associated with acquisition and retrieval processes and provide a sound basis for comparisons with amnesic patients. In normal subjects, both acquisition and retrieval processes have been associated with posterior and anterior activations. With acquisition, several studies[6-8] using PET have found left frontal cortex activation, but patterns of activation in more posterior regions have varied across studies. It is possible that the left frontal activation reflects the operation of elaborative semantic kinds of encoding process, but this possibility awaits rigorous testing. Although Grady[8] found that encoding was associated with medial temporal cortex (including the hippocampus) activation in young subjects, this has not been found in all studies and the precise conditions that elicit activation in this region need to be determined. One possibility is that hippocampal activation is particularly associated with the short term consolidation of complex associations between items that are represented in different cortical domains, but this possibility needs to be tested formally. Interestingly, Grady[8] noted that old people (who have worse memory than young people) failed to show significant activation in either frontal or medial temporal sites, which suggests that they may have been impaired at encoding and so engaged in less consolidation processing as well.

Studies that have examined retrieval processes using PET have consistently found predominantly right frontal cortex activation and more posterior activation in the region of the cuneus, precuneus and related structures[6,9,10]. It is plausible to argue on general grounds that the right frontal cortex activation represents the operation of some kind of elaborative retrieval process whereas the more posterior activation reflects one or more aspects of successful retrieval such as the operation of visual imagery as has been suggested by Shallice[6]. In support of the role of the right frontal cortex in elaborative aspects of retrieval,

Kapur et al.[9] have shown that the activation found in this region during a recognition task in which only 15% of items were targets was the same as that produced when 85% of the items were targets whereas the cuneus and precuneus showed more activation when 85% of test items were recognition targets. It is not clear whether these results generalise to the presentation of no targets at all[11], but they provide preliminary support for the view that right frontal activation reflects some aspect of memory search whereas more posterior activations reflect one or more aspect of successful retrieval.

In this chapter, we describe a study which examined whether the memory challenge procedures developed with PET can also be used effectively with SPECT in a study using both amnesic and normal subjects. We developed a cued recall retrieval task similar to that employed by Shallice et al.[6] with PET. SPECT scans were analysed using a region of interest (ROI) method following co-registration of the baseline SPECT with MRI and the activation SPECT with the baseline scan. The effect of the co-registration error was evaluated to determine its significance on the end result.

Our study had three main aims. First, we wished to determine in what ways the patterns of activation found in two groups of normal subjects, who differed in their level of cued recall performance, would diverge from each other. Our assumption was that the group with recall near to ceiling levels should show less retrieval search activation (probably in the right frontal cortex) because for them the task was very easy and probably largely automatic. This group should, however, show more activation of the kind associated with successful retrieval (probably in a more posterior site such as the precuneus). Second, we wished to see whether a group of amnesics, whose level of cued recall was matched to that of the control group with weaker cued recall, would show a different pattern of activation from these controls that would either be indicative of a retrieval deficit or possibly of the use of a compensatory retrieval strategy. Finding such differences anteriorly might indicate the presence of a deficit (or possibly a compensatory strategy) in a search or verification process whereas a more posterior activation difference might reflect an abnormality in the activation produced by successful retrieval. As a subsidiary aim, we wished to demonstrate that these differences were specific to the comparison of the amnesics with the control group that was matched to them on cued recall. The better performing cued recall group would not show the same effects. Third, we wished to examine whether abnormal patterns of activation shown by the amnesics would be a function of the location of their underlying lesions.

Methods and procedures

Subjects

Two control groups were used for this study: i) a group of normal subjects who were thoroughly taught the word list used for the recall task and therefore performed near to ceiling levels (the high performance [HP] group); ii) a group of normal subjects who had limited time to assimilate the word list and performed with a recall success rate matched to the amnesics of around 50% (the matched performance [MP] group). All control subjects displayed normal levels of intelligence (Wechsler adult intelligence scale - revised [WAIS-R], National adult reading test [NART]) and memory performance (Warrington recognition test) (Table 1). Six amnesics were used for the study, they varied both in aetiology and lesion location. One amnesic, L.A., had thalamic damage due to bilateral thalamic infarcts. I.S. was an amnesic patient in whom pressure from the presence of a large colloid cyst, suggested medial thalamic and fornix damage. Another amnesic patient, R.M. had a lesion to the left fornix due to the excision of a colloid cyst while another, D.R. suffered damage to the mammillary bodies as a result of a Wernicke-Korsakoff episode. The remaining two amnesics were post-encephalitic patients, displaying parietal damage in one case, J.O. and severe damage to the left medial temporal lobe in the other, R.B. In all cases, 1.5 Tesla MRI scans were carried out to establish the exact site of the lesion. Neuropsychological assessment of the amnesics included measurements of present intelligence (WAIS-R), premorbid intelligence (NART-R), memory function (WMS-R and Warrington recognition test) and naming (Boston naming test).

Cognitive activation tasks

In order to isolate the episodic component of memory function, two separate tasks were developed that were different to but based on, a design by Shallice et al.[6]. The first, the baseline task required subjects to generate words which were semantically associated with high frequency noun stimuli presented to them at a rate of approximately one every 5 s. The demands of the baseline task therefore involved retrieval of semantic information. The second, the memory challenge task required subjects to recall the second word of a previously studied word pair in response to the presentation of the first word. The word pairs were weak semantic associates and consisted of words of high frequency and high concreteness, (e.g. stream - fish, cat - fur, hand - ring). The presentation rate was matched to that of the baseline task. The demands of the memory challenge task therefore involved retrieval of both semantic and episodic information. This design

Table 1 Details of controls and amnesic patients including site of lesion for each amnesic patient and performance scores for intelligence test (WAIS-R), premorbid intelligence (NART-R), memory function (WMS-R and Warrington recognition test) and naming (Boston naming test) for both the control groups and the amnesic group. The 'high' group is trained to produce a near optimal challenge response whereas the 'match' group is performance-matched with the amnesic group for the challenge task

| | Controls | | Amnesic patients | | | | | |
	High	Match	AL	RB	RM	JO	DR	IS
Sex	3M/3F	3M/1F	M	M	M	F	M	F
Age	39-60	42-61	61	59	42	47	56	60
Lesion site			Thal	Tem	Fnx	Par	Mam	Thal
	Mean	Mean						
WAIS:FIQ	106	103	86	114	88	84	93	88
WMS:GEN. MQ			62	79	82	63	89	77
WMS:VERB. MQ			62	68	76	65	63	74
Recognition: words	48	48	33	35	43	32	29	28
Recognition: faces	46	47	29	37	42	32	28	41
Activation tasks								
Baseline%	100	100	100	89	93	77	100	83
Challenge%	93	54	5	56	57	50	18	53

ensured that while both tasks were similar in the cognitive demands they made with respect to verbal output and semantic processing, the challenge task required additional explicit episodic memory processing.

Memory training procedure

Specific memory training procedures were designed to allow both for the manipulation of search effort and retrieval success within the control subjects and for the matching of control subject performance to that of the amnesics. Control subjects were selected for one of two alternative training procedures:

1. High performance procedure: with this procedure, control subjects received repeated presentations of word pairs ensuring 90-100% performance on recall. This procedure was carried out with control group 1 (HP, N=6) and aimed to produce a condition of low search effort and high retrieval success.

2. Matched performance procedure: with this procedure, control subjects received limited presentations of word pairs to ensure a recall performance matched to that of amnesics. This procedure was carried out with control group 2 (PM, N=4) and aimed to produce a condition of high search effort and low retrieval success.

In order to maximise the recall performance of the amnesic subjects during the memory challenge task, extensive training of the word pairs was carried out. The number of presentations ranged from 15 to 27. Where possible, a 50-60% successful retrieval rate was obtained (see Table 1).

Data acquisition

SPECT scans were performed using the SME 810 (Strichman Medical Equipment) Multidetector scanner. This is a section scanner with an in plane resolution of 8 mm and longitudinal resolution of 12 mm. The scan orientation was approximately parallel to the orbito-meatal (OM) line, although this setting was not crucial as the SME software allows 3-D re-orientation of the image data set.

A mean dose of 250 MBq ^{99m}Tc-HMPAO for the control subjects and 500MBq for the amnesic patients was injected intravenously. The acquisition time was increased for the control subjects to compensate for the lower dose administered. Imaging commenced approximately 10 min after injection, and a scan of the whole head was taken. Two sets of scans, baseline and memory challenge, were obtained for all control subjects and the 6 amnesic patients with no less than 24 h between each scan.

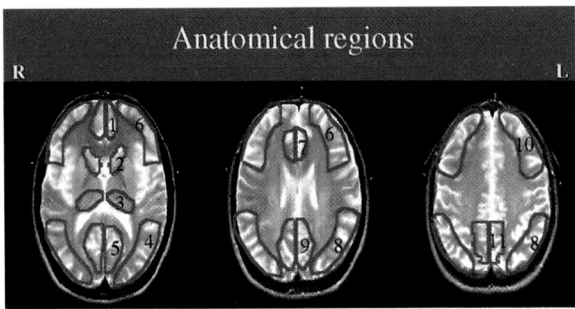

Figure 1 The regions studied superimposed on a normal MR scan. 1. [VF] ventromedial frontal; 2. [Cd] head of caudate; 3. [Th] thalamus; 4. [Occ] occipital; 5. [Calc] calcarine; 6 [LFr] lateral frontal; 7. [Cg] cingulate; 8. [Par] parietal; 9. [Cun] cuneus; 10. [LFr(S)] lateral frontal (superior); 11. [PC] precuneus

Data analysis

The first SPECT scan of each subject was co-registered with that subject's MRI. The second SPECT scan was then co-registered with the first scan. This was done using version 2.9 of the co-registration facility in the SME Neuro 900 software package. The paired image data sets were then used for further analysis. Three sets of ROIs were used to derive quantitative data (Figure 1). For each subject a template of ROIs, based on slices showing the basal ganglia, corpus callosum and centrum semi-ovale, was adjusted according to the appropriate slice of the MR scan. The activity was measured by transferring the templates from the MR scans on to the pair of co-registered SPECT scans.

^{99m}Tc-HMPAO SPECT images cannot produce absolute measurements of cerebral blood flow and a normalising region must be used to compare scans. In this study, data for each ROI were normalised by dividing the average counts per mm^2 of each ROI by the average number of counts per mm^2 in the 6 hemisphere ROIs on all 3 templates. This is more robust than normalising to any single region such as the cerebellum or calcarine cortex[12].

Regional changes in HMPAO uptake were calculated by subtracting the baseline (semantic memory task) activity values from the memory challenge (semantic + episodic memory task) activity values for each ROI to give a difference value (Δa) between the two scans. T-tests were performed to compare the difference values between the groups and Z-scores of these data:

$$z = (\Delta a_A - \Delta \ddot{a}_C) / \sigma \Delta a_C$$

were used to express comparisons of the difference values of the individuals in the amnesic group (Δa_A) with the mean difference values of the performance matched control group ($\Delta \ddot{a}_C$).

Image co-registration

Various methods exist for the co-registration of images within and across modalities. Both prospective techniques using patient immobilisation devices, fiducial markers and stereotactic frames and retrospective techniques such as point landmarks[13], matching spatial moments of 3D volumes[14], correlation of voxel density distributions[15] and matching anatomical surfaces[16-18] have been used. Also, methods to standardise images to compare between subjects rather than within subjects have been developed using anatomical atlases[19,20] or plastic transformations[21]. For this study, a retrospective technique rather than those that require special patient positioning or the use of fiducial markers is preferred as there are problems such as skin movement associated with the attachment of external markers, especially if there is a considerable period between each scan. The commercial co-registration software evaluated here is a purely retrospective technique developed by Hill et al.[17], based on the simplex method.

Extensive investigations regarding the accuracy and precision of co-registration techniques have been published[13,16,18,20-23]. Pelizzari et al.[16] suggest that co-registration of images should be accurate to 1-2 mm but this value will ultimately be limited by the resolution of the imaging technique used. Hill et al.[17] state that precision of their algorithm was measured as 1 mm and 0.5 degrees but Links[24] describes findings that suggest that a change in 1-2 mm in the axial position with respect to the small deep structures can cause more than a 10-20% change in observed counts from these regions. It was therefore necessary for the purposes of this project to establish what effect, if any, the precision of this algorithm might have on the results generated by the study and compare these measurements with the precision of manually co-registered data. Previous techniques to assess the accuracy and precision of automated methods of co-registration have concentrated on positional errors resulting from mis-registration. In this study, it was more appropriate to investigate directly the effect of positional errors on the parameters used in this study i.e. the resulting change in the number of counts in a ROI, and the effect of this on a typical Z-score value.

The method used to investigate the changes produced by mis-registration consisted of producing a sum over all ROIs of differences of Z-scores weighted by the ROI area. The value is an index of precision i.e. small values indicate good precision. Repeated co-

Table 2 Values calculated using the sum of Z-score differences weighted by ROI area as an index of precision. The last entry in the column for auto alignment of SPECT/SPECT and MRI/SPECT images illustrates the difficulty the automated co-registration algorithm had when trying to co-register two images that were mis-aligned to one another by 10 degrees in the sagittal plane

Direction of rotation w.r.t. reference image	SPECT / SPECT		MRI / SPECT	
	auto	manual	auto	manual
10 degree in axial plane	0.03	0.40	0.009	0.239
10 degree in coronal plane	0.04	0.40	0.007	0.430
10 degree in sagittal plane	0.58	0.35	0.010	0.376

registrations, both automated and manual, were carried out after deliberately mis-aligning previously co-registered SPECT/MRI data sets of the same subject and SPECT/SPECT data sets of the same subject scanned on different days. The previous co-registration was undertaken on full brain data sets by first using a manual adjustment to obtain a close approximation and then using the automated co-registration algorithm. The 'real' correspondence cannot be determined but this is of no consequence as this assessment was concerned with variations in correspondence introduced by limitations in the data sets. From the results in Table 2, it can be seen that the automated co-registration is far more precise than the manual co-registration except in the case of initial misalignment in the sagittal plane of ≥10 degrees. In this case the automated co-registration was no better than the manual method. The same problem is evident in the SPECT/MRI co-registration only to a lesser degree. Again the automated method is better than the manual method.

In view of the fact that this algorithm has been described as being sensitive to head boundaries' alignment rather than the internal structures for SPECT brain imaging[17], the effect of co-registering different image volumes, a situation common in MRI and SPECT acquisition, was investigated. Average values for the index of precision calculated for the repeated co-registration of non-equivalent image volumes were 1.31 and 0.75 for the automated and manual co-alignment, respectively, and average values for repeated co-registration of equivalent but reduced image volumes were 1.06 and 0.56 for automated and manual alignment, respectively. In this case the manual co-registration was more consistent than the automated method.

The results listed in Table 2 might be explained by the trapping of the optimisation parameter in a local maximum, which is a common source of error in this type of procedure[17]. The algorithm should work well when starting from a reasonable starting point[16,17]. It may be deduced, therefore, that a misalignment in the sagittal plane of 10 degrees is not a reasonable starting point. For the second set of values used to assess the co-registration of non-equivalent image volumes it can be seen that the manual co-alignment is more precise since an interactive observer can take into account both internal structure and surface boundaries while co-registering. The automated method on the other hand has little to go on once the image volume has been reduced by half. However, once both the image volumes have been reduced by half, precision is improved for the automated method presumably because the two image sets have roughly equivalent surfaces. It is recommended, therefore, that for the purposes of co-registration, whole and matching image volumes should be acquired whenever possible for each subject being investigated.

From these and other assessments of the errors due to limitations in co-registering SPECT with SPECT and SPECT with MRI, we concluded that the SME automated co-registration is superior to manual 'expert' co-registration as long as: 1) the initial sagittal alignment of the two data sets is within 10 degrees and 2) 'whole brain' data sets are available. The typical errors present in this co-registration software produced changes in Z-scores an order of magnitude less than the $Z > 4.0$ criteria used to draw the major conclusions in this study. Most of the images acquired were full data sets and manual adjustment was used only in those cases where a reduced data was obtained.

All co-registrations tested here were intra-subject matching rather than inter-subject matching. The latter involves not only rigid transformations but also some kind of non-linear rescaling to a standardised brain[13,19,21]. In this study individuals were matched to their own MRI, providing a unique atlas for each subject.

Results

In order to investigate the issues addressed in the introduction, the analysis focused on three separate approaches. Firstly, a comparison of the activation patterns between the two control groups, using one-tailed t-tests as this comparison was hypothesis driven. Secondly, a comparison of the amnesic and matched control group using two-tailed t-tests, as this comparison was more exploratory. Finally, an investigation of the individual differences in activation pattern between the amnesics was carried out using Z-scores relative to PM, as a comparative measure of activation.

1. Comparison of activation in the HP and PM groups, (Figures 2 and 3)

(i) Independent t-tests (one-tailed) demonstrated that during the memory challenge task, the HP group displayed significantly greater activation in the left (p=0.01) and right (p=0.05) parietal regions when compared with the PM group. The results also show an increased activation in the HP group in the right precuneus (p=0.01).

(ii) Conversely, the analysis showed a significant increase in activation in the right lateral frontal region in the PM group compared with the HP group (p=0.004).

2. Comparison of activation in amnesic group and PM group, (Figure 4)

(i) Independent t-tests (two-tailed) demonstrated that amnesics show significantly greater left lateral frontal activation (p−0.02) than do the controls. Increased activation in the right calcarine (p=0.02) was also found.

3. Individual differences in activation within the amnesic group, (Figures 5 - 7)

(i) L.A.(5) and R.M.(6) both display the general findings of the amnesic group, but clearly differ with respect to activation of the right ventromedial frontal and parietal regions.

(ii) D.R. (7) by contrast displays clearly increased activation in the right ventromedial frontal region and left cingulate. This individual's results reflect those of the amnesic group with respect to the lateral and high lateral frontal regions but not with respect to the calcarine and precuneus regions.

Discussion

Using HMPAO SPECT imaging, this study investigated the activation patterns found to accompany episodic retrieval in normal controls and amnesics. One principal aim was to replicate the findings of previous PET studies with respect to normal patterns of brain activation. The results of this study achieve this by displaying activation in the right frontal and bilateral parietal as well as in the right precuneus during episodic retrieval, as have previous studies[6,9,10]. Apart from contributing towards the debate concerning the neuroanatomical localisation of the processes involved in memory, these findings suggest that SPECT like PET, is capable of detecting specific neuroactivation associated with isolated cognitive processes.

In order to examine the effect of level of cued recall performance on patterns of activation, retrieval success and search effort were manipulated in the two control groups. Our broad hypothesis held that the group with increased search effort would display right frontal activation, while the group with increased retrieval success would display more posterior patterns of activation. While this hypothesis was upheld by these results we have made no assumptions as to the nature of the search process mediated by the right frontal region. We can conclude that, due to the semantic characteristics of the baseline task and the subtraction technique adopted, the resultant activation most probably reflects the search strategies associated with the retrieval of information relating to a specific event. Previously, in studies in which search effort and retrieval success had not been dissociated, a right frontal activation in episodic retrieval might have been attributed to retrieval success. However, the manipulation carried out in the present study illustrates that when retrieval success is reduced (as in PM) right frontal activation actually increases. Therefore, these findings strongly suggest that right frontal activity, rather than reflecting retrieval success, reflects search effort while posterior activations such as in the precuneus and parietal regions reflect retrieval success.

The most prominent and interesting finding concerning the activation patterns found in the amnesic group was the activation found in the left lateral frontal region and the absence of any activation (and possibly even a trend towards deactivation) in the right lateral frontal region. As mentioned earlier, evidence of the involvement of the left frontal region in encoding semantic information exists[9,10]. Such encoding must inevitably also involve the retrieval of semantic information so our preferred hypothesis for explaining this finding is that the amnesics are not using a normal search strategy. It is possible that as the amnesic group may have no

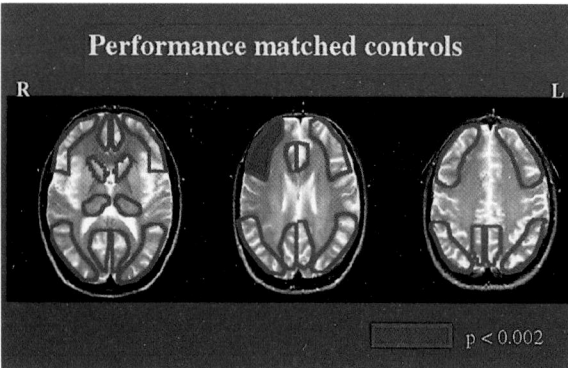

Figure 2 Regional activation of the control group matched to the amnesics for performance compared with the high performance control group

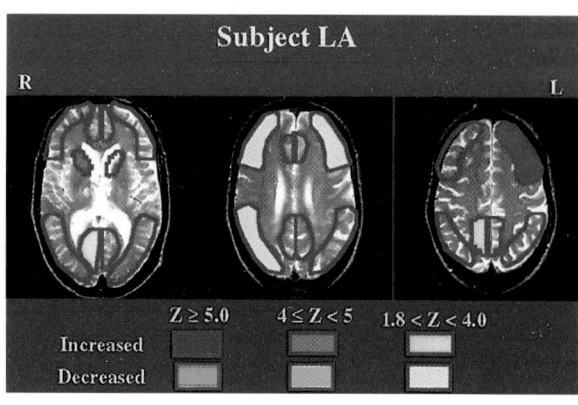

Figure 5 Regional activation for subject LA, who had bilateral thalamic infarcts, compared with the performance matched control group

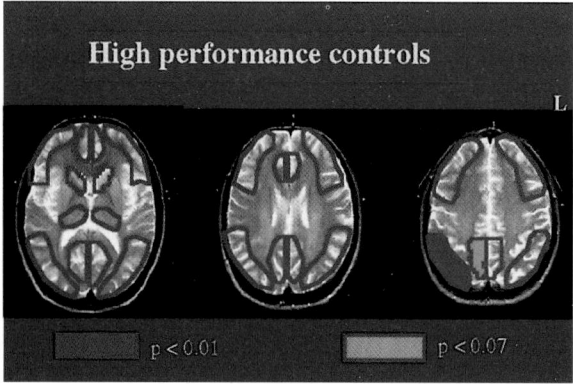

Figure 3 Regional activation of the high performance control group compared with the control group matched to the amnesics for performance

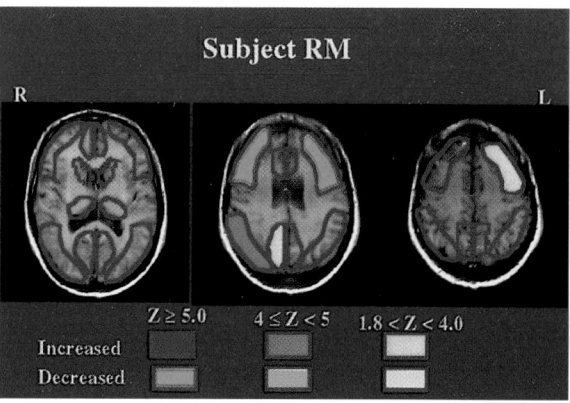

Figure 6 Regional activation for subject RM, who had a lesion to the left fornix, compared with the performance matched control group

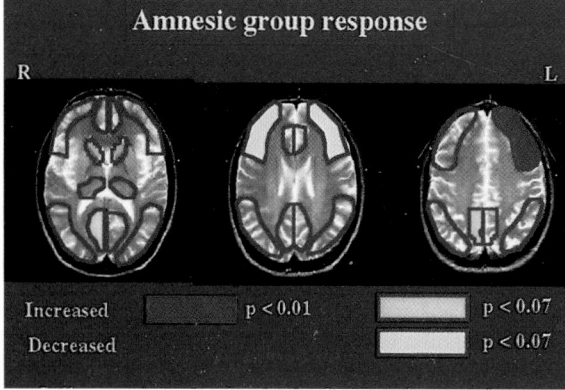

Figure 4 Differences in regional activation between the amnesic group and the performance matched control group

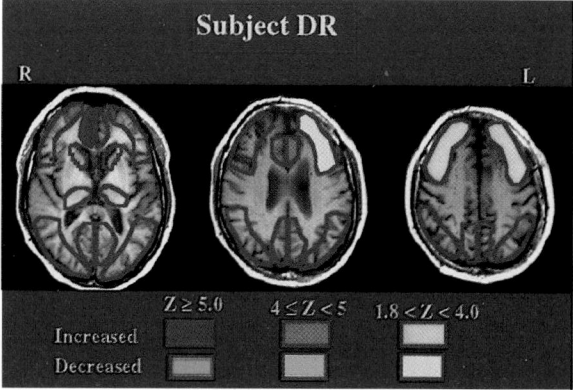

Figure 7 Regional activation for subject DR, who had damage to the mammillary bodies, compared with the performance matched control group

episodes to search for, they turn to a more semantically based search which particularly activates the left frontal cortex. Moreover, they may be retrieving target words implicitly rather than explicitly and therefore to an extent, treating the task as a semantic association task rather than an episodic retrieval task. Their ability to produce a degree of successful retrieval does not, however, reflect the association strength of the word pairs (since this is relatively low) but the implicit priming effect of the memory training procedure. Further to the issue of frontal abnormalities in this amnesic group, it is quite possible that the diencephalic and limbic disconnections evident in many of these patients may themselves be responsible for or contribute towards, the abnormal neuronal activity in the frontal regions. Therefore these frontal abnormalities in activation during episodic retrieval may have two separate but ultimately related, causes; one process-driven in terms of cognitive search strategy and the other, neuronal-driven in terms of the underlying neuroanatomical lesions.

The other region found to be significantly activated in the amnesic group was that of the right calcarine region. Being a posterior region it is tempting to suggest this activation reflects successful retrieval, however there is little, if any empirical or theoretical support for this position. This region most likely contains the striate cortex and therefore there is little reason to believe that it plays a direct part in memory function. Close scrutiny of the calcarine data in all groups showed that the comparison group PM from which the Z-scores were derived, had a particularly small standard deviation for this region. It is therefore possible that the resultant significance in the right calcarine region may be due to methodology (e.g. group size), rather than a reflection of underlying cognitive processes.

The analysis of individual differences in activation pattern in the amnesic group was based on a comparison of Z-scores and revealed two particularly interesting findings. First, differences in the activation of the ventromedial frontal region were found, and, second, differences in the activation of the precuneus were also found. With respect to the ventromedial frontal activation difference across the patients, it is worth pointing out that this region is supposed to receive hippocampal and amygdala projections and has been related[25] to amnesia. In other words, according to Mishkin[25], lesions of this region should produce amnesia in humans. Whether this is true remains to be shown, but it is certainly a region that receives projections from structures such as the hippocampus, damage to which does cause amnesia. It seems likely that the patients who show abnormal activity in this

region all have damage to the hippocampal circuit as well (possibly) as other structures implicated in amnesia. This damage may disrupt the workings of the ventromedial frontal cortex and this may in turn have effects on memory. However, it is clear that sometimes the structural damage causes an increase in activity of the ventromedial frontal cortex and sometimes a decrease. Further parameters need to be specified in order to determine the direction of the effect and it also needs to be determined whether both increased and decreased levels of activation are associated with similar decreases in efficiency. Until this is done, one cannot say whether or not the different patterns of activation in this region reflect functional differences in the amnesic syndrome shown by different patients.

The precuneus activation differences between the patients may indicate a difference in the strategies used by them. If Shallice et al.[6] are correct in postulating that precuneus activation reflects the use of visual imagery accompanying successful retrieval, then more activation may mean that patients are using such imagery to aid verbal recall to a greater extent than normal people, whereas reduced activation should mean that they are using imagery to an abnormally small degree. Of course, the activation is of the right precuneus so this may indicate that the lateralisation of the imagery processing is abnormal.

Future work might compare amnesics who either have fairly selective damage to the hippocampal circuit or to another system in order to determine whether they show distinct patterns of abnormal brain activity both during retrieval and encoding of episodic information. Our study shows that SPECT can usefully be employed in memory challenge studies not only to throw light on episodic memory processes in normal people, but also in amnesics.

References

1   Mayes, A.R. in Human Organic Memory Disorders, Cambridge University Press, Cambridge, UK, 1988

2   Levasseur, M., Baron, J.C., Sette, G. et al. Brain energy metabolism in bilateral median infarcts. Brain 1992, 115, 795

3   Paller, K.A., Acharya, A., Richardson, B.C. et al. Neurophysiological substrates of human memory impairments: altered regional cerebral glucose utilization in alcoholic Korsakoff's syndrome and Alzheimer's disease, as measured by positron emission tomography. Society for Neuroscience Abstracts 1993, 19, 1078

4   Perani, D., Bressi, S., Cappa, S.F. et al. Evidence of multiple memory systems in the human brain. Brain 1993, 116, 903

5   Mayes, A.R., Downes, J.J., Shoqeirat, M. et al. Encoding ability is preserved in amnesics: evidence from a direct test of encoding. Neuropsychologia 1993, 31, 745

6   Shallice, T., Fletcher, P., Frith, C.D. *et al.* Brain regions associated with acquisition and retrieval of verbal episodic memory. *Nature* 1994, 368, 633

7   Kapur, S., Craik, F.I.M., Tulving, E. *et al.* Neuroanatomical correlates of encoding in episodic memory: levels of processing effect. *Proc. Nat. Acad. Sci. USA* 1994, 91, 2008

8   Grady, C.L., McIntosh, A.R., Horwitz *et al.* Age-related reductions in human recognition memory due to impaired coding. *Science* 1995, 269, 218

9   Kapur, S., Craik, F.I.M., Jones, C. *et al.* Functional role of the prefrontal cortex in memory retrieval: A PET study. *NeuroReport* 1995, 6, 1880

10 Tulving, E., Kapur, S., Markowitsch, H.J. *et al.* Neuroanatomical correlates of retrieval in episodic memory: auditory sentence recognition. *Proc. Nat. Acad. Sci.* USA 1994, 91, 2012

11 Fletcher, P.C., Frith, C.D. and Rugg, M.D. The functional neuroanatomy of episodic memory. *Trends in Neuroscience* 1997, 20(5), 213

12 Ebmeier, K.P., Hunter, R., Curran, S.M. *et al.* Effects of a single dose of the acetylcholinesterase inhibitor velnacrine on recognition memory and regional cerebral blood flow in Alzheimer's disease. *Psychopharmacology* 1992, 108, 103

13 Evans, A.C., Collins, D.L., Neelin, P. *et al.* Three-dimensional correlative imaging: applications in human brain mapping in 'Functional neuroimaging, technical foundations', (Eds. R.W. Thatcher, M. Hallett, T. Zeffiro, E. Royjohn and M. Heurta), Academic Press, USA, 1994, p.145

14 Faber, T.L. and E.M. Stokely. Orientation of three-dimensional structures in medical images. *IEEE Trans. Pattern Anal. Machine Intell.* 1988, 10(5), 626

15 Woods, R.P., Mazziotta, J.C. and Cherry, S.R. Optizing activation methods: tomographic mapping of functional cerebral activity in 'Functional neuroimaging, technical foundations', (Eds. R.W. Thatcher, M. Hallett, T. Zeffiro, E. Royjohn and M. Heurta), Academic Press, USA, 1994, p.47

16 Pelizzari, C.A., Levin, D.N., Chen, C. *et al.* Registration of PET and SPECT with MRI by anatomical surface matching in 'Functional neuroimaging, technical foundations', (Eds. R.W. Thatcher, M. Hallett, T. Zeffiro, E. Royjohn and M. Heurta), Academic Press, USA, 1994, p. 233

17 Hill, T.C., Martin, P.J. and Stoddart, H.A. Comparison of manual and automated co-registration of SPECT brain images without the use of external fiducial markers. *Proc. 40th Ann. Meeting Soc. Nuc. Med.* 1993, 34(5), 193P

18 Andersson, J.L.R. A rapid and accurate method to realign PET scans utilizing image edge information *J. Nucl. Med.* 1995, 36(4), 657

19 Fox, P.T., Mikiten, S., Davis, G. and Lancaster, J.L. Brainmap: a database of human functional brain mapping in 'Functional, neuroimaging, technical foundations', (Eds. R.W. Thatcher, M. Hallett, T. Zeffiro, E. Royjohn and M. Heurta), Academic Press, USA, 1994, p. 95

20 Thurfjell, L., Bohm, C., Greitz, T. *et al.* Accuracy and precision in image standardization in intra- and intersubject comparisons in 'Functional neuroimaging, technical foundations', (Eds. R.W. Thatcher, M. Hallett, T. Zeffiro, E. Royjohn and M. Heurta), Academic Press, USA, 1994, p.121

21 Friston, K.J., Frith, C.D., Liddle, P.F. *et al.* Plastci transformation of PET images *J. Comp. Ass. Tomography* 1991, 15(4), 634

22 Magurie, G.Q., Noz, M.E., Rusinek *et al.* Graphics applied to medical image registration. IEEE *Comp. Graph. Appl.* 20-27 March 1991

23 Zubal, I.G., Zhang, L., Tagare, H. and Duncan, J.S. Three-dimensional registration of SPECT and MRI brain images. *Proc. 40th Ann. Meeting Soc. Nuc. Med.* 1993, 34(5), 187P

24 Links, J.M. The influence of positioning in accuracy and precision in emission tomography. *J. Nucl. Med.* 1991, 32(6), 1252

25 Mishkin, M. A memory system in the monkey. *Phil. Trans. Roy. Soc. Lon. B* 1982, 298, 85

SPECT in Neurology and Psychiatry, edited by P.P. De Deyn, R.A. Dierckx, A. Alavi and B.A. Pickut
© 1997 John Libbey & Company Ltd, pp. 67–71

Activation Studies using SPECT

Chapter
10

H.-J. Biersack, E. Klemm, K. Reichmann, C. Menzel and
F. Grünwald

Introduction

HMPAO SPECT has been used in Europe since 1986. Significant improvement of diagnosis using HMPAO SPECT has been achieved in neurology and psychiatry. In neurology the diagnosis of the ictal focus by ictal and interictal brain SPECT has been made possible. As Alzheimer's disease may present with typical bilateral perfusion deficits, a differential diagnosis of other types of dementia became possible. In psychiatry, perfusion deficits were reported in depression, schizophrenia, mood disorders, and obsessive-compulsive disorders[1-4]. Although these findings were not typical for each disease, hypoperfusions of different brain areas such as the temporal and frontal lobes may be an indication of a particular symptom.

To further evaluate the use of brain SPECT, intervention procedures such as acoustic, visual and motoric activation as well as speech and test activation may be used. The results of these procedures are described below.

Acoustic, memory, visual and motor activation

The effect of white noise auditory stimulation on rCBF has been reported previously[5,6]. Fifteen patients with sudden deafness had been treated successfully with dextrane infusion. Auditory stimulation was achieved by simultaneous binaural presentation of white noise (20 dB above threshold). In the non-stimulated condition, typical symmetric IMP uptake images were obtained. With white noise, increased tracer uptake was noted in the temporal regions of both hemispheres. In the majority of cases, auditory stimulation to the right ear resulted in increased activity on the contralateral side. In another study[7], the effects of sentence understanding were investigated. Ten normal male volunteers with normal hearing had 2 IMP SPECT studies, one with ears plugged (basal) and one approximately 2 weeks later. The studies showed increased tracer uptake in association with a speech understanding activation task in the left superior parietal region, with less pronounced effects in the left temporo-parietal region.

Acoustic stimulation was also described in patients with schizophrenia having auditory hallucinations[3]. Studies performed during the hallucinogenic stimulus showed right or left sided temporal lobe hyperperfusion.

Dal Bianco *et al.*[8] published the first report on activation studies using SPECT with isopropyl amphetamine (IMP). He investigated the rCBF changes in memorising verbal and non-verbal acoustic stimuli. One group listened to

Department of Nuclear Medicine,
University of Bonn, Sigmund
Freud Strasse 25, 53127 Bonn,
Germany

nonsense syllables and the other group listened to 300 concrete nouns. The tasks were begun 5 min before injection of IMP, and continued for the whole accumulation procedure (30 min). A resting study was performed separately. The authors reported differences between resting and activation studies. Task performance resulted in marked bilateral activation of the anterior frontal lobes and the left temporal lobe. In response to the nonsense syllable task, there was marked increase of activity in the left anterior basal ganglia, whereas the concrete noun task produced activation of the right temporal lobe as great or greater than that of the left hemisphere.

The effect of rCBF on different types of memory tasks in normal subjects was reported by Goldenberg et al.[9]. Subjects were offered meaningless words, concrete nouns with imagery instructions, abstract nouns, and concrete nouns without imagery instructions. The tracer used was IMP. Imagery instructions produced an asymmetrically large leftward shift of activity. Concrete nouns without the imagery instruction resulted in an asymmetric right hemisphere shift. Moreover, the results of Goldenberg et al.[9] showed that the hippocampus and both inferior temporal regions presented with hyperperfusion after all memory tasks. Lang et al.[10] performed studies with memory tasks consisting of meaningless words, abstract nouns, concrete nouns with no explicit imagery and concrete nouns with explicit imagery. Response to concrete nouns produced significant changes of count rates in the inferior and occipital regions. The regional count rate correlation between midfrontal and superior frontal gyry was stronger for meaningful words than for meaningless words. This may reflect coactivation of the prefrontal cortex

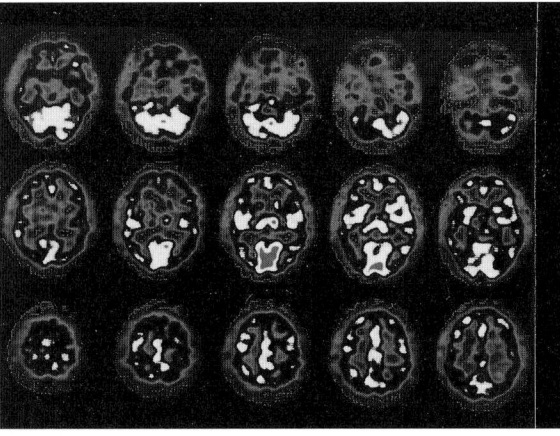

Figure 1 Hyperperfusion of the visual cortex in a patient looking at a complex scene

induced by the meaningfullness of the stimuli. All memory tasks produced the greatest increase in rCBF in the left midfrontal lobe area. In all the studies mentioned an active role of the left hemisphere for processing recognition memory could be shown.

Motor activation may be achieved by asking the patient to make certain movements, especially with his/her finger. This leads to circumscribed increased perfusion in the respective cortical areas. Visual stimulation by asking the patient to look at a complex scene or flickering light, causes hyperactivation of the visual cortex (Figure 1). These studies were used clinically in patients with certain diseases of the visual pathways. A baseline study may be needed to quantitatively evaluate the activation differences. For this purpose, usually a split dose technique (one third of the dose for the baseline study, two thirds of the dose for the activation study) is applied. The patient is then investigated in the same position. A subtraction image (activation minus baseline study) allows delineation of activated brain areas.

Language activation

Despite the importance of activating syntactic knowledge in related words, functional imaging studies on language have focussed mainly on the processing of isolated words rather than sentences.

Tikofsky et al.[11-13] investigated the response of aphasics and normal volunteers to activation with a non-recognition memory task, the Boston naming test (BNT). The BNT requires subjects to give the names of 60 line drawings presented one at a time in a specified order. The studies included IMP SPECT and were performed in chronic aphasics and normal right-handed volunteers. Visual inspection of the images did not show consistent differences between either condition. However, it was speculated that quantitative methods may be useful to detect differences. Using this procedure it was found that, in the left hemisphere, aphasics had a significantly lower cerebral IMP-uptake in the perisylvian region than normals. For the right hemisphere, no difference could be found. Above that, a retrospective study showed significant differences between recovering and deteriorating aphasics.

Former brain lesion studies suggest a different processing of semantic and syntactic structures. In an ethical committee approved study, nine right-handed male volunteers (age 23 to 46 years) were investigated by high resolution SPECT using ^{99m}Tc-ECD as a tracer[14]. The stimulus was to listen either to content words (semantic condition) or to short phrases containing no lexical, but only grammatical information (syntactic condition). Following the resting acquisition after intravenous injection of ECD, stimulation was performed with either the semantic or the syntactic stimulus set binaurally over a period of 5.5 min. The second dose was slowly injected during this period, thus representing the cerebral perfusion pattern during stimulation. The SPECT results were evaluated both semiquantitatively and visually. Quantitative data were expressed as percentage increase (14% or more defined by hyperperfusion) or decrease of counts per voxel normalised to whole brain activity in the stimulation study related to the baseline set. Thus, each subject served as its own control.

Different activation patterns were observed when comparing the two conditions. Hyperperfusion (Figure 2) under syntactical stimulation (n = 4) was seen in the following areas: all 4 superior temporal gyrus (1 left, 3 right), 2 inferior frontal gyrus (1 left, 1 right) and 3 insula (2 left, 1 right). Moreover, 2 subjects had hyperperfusion within the gyrus postcentralis (1 left, 1 right). During semantic stimulation (n = 5), 4 subjects had hyperperfusion (Figure 3) of the medius frontal gyrus (2 left, 2 right), 2 of the superior frontal gyrus, the precentral gyrus and the medius temporal gyrus (each 1 left, 1 both sides), 3 of the right postcentral gyrus, 3 of the insula (1 left, 2 both sides), and 3 of the cuneus (1 right, 2 both sides).

The results of the syntactic stimulation correlate well with experiments demonstrating disabled syntactic processing following lesions of Broca's area and the insula and suggesting the insula to be relevant in the syntactic process. The semantic stimulation reflects involvement of both hemispheres, more prominent on the right side. The hyperperfused regions are not primarily language areas. These findings are consistent with other studies using PET or SPECT, which report activation outside these areas and conclude that semantic processes may be distributed over a network of brain regions. Further studies have to be made to evaluate the differences due to handedness or gender. It may be speculated whether these studies may prove useful in the rehabilitation of aphasia.

Wisconsin card sorting test

The Wisconsin card sorting test[15] was applied in human volunteers as well as in depressed and schizophrenic patients. This test was used to evaluate the stimulation of prefrontal cortical areas with regard to the supposed pathophysiology of the two diseases. Studies in human volunteers (n = 16) showed that right or left sided activation may occur (Figure 4). The same test was applied in a group of depressed (n = 26) and schizophrenic (n = 7) patients. In depressed patients,

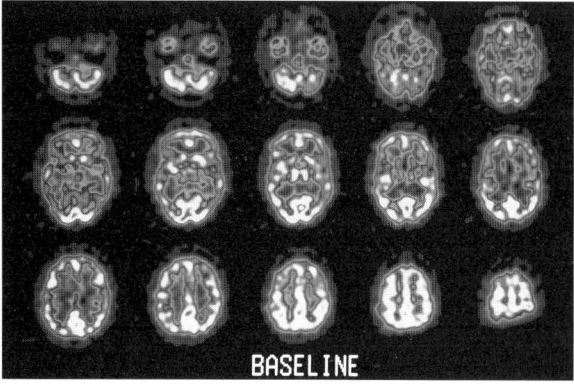

Figure 2a Syntactical stimulation: activation of the right fronto-temporal region (baseline)

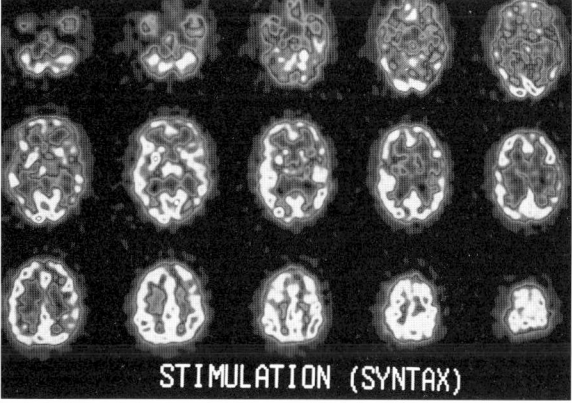

Figure 2b Syntactical stimulation: activation of the right fronto-temporal region (stimulation)

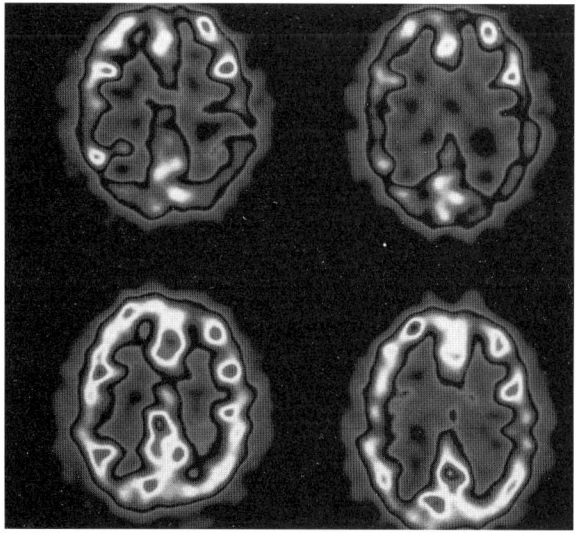

Figure 3 Semantical activation: bilateral activation of the frontal cortex; top, baseline; bottom, stimulation

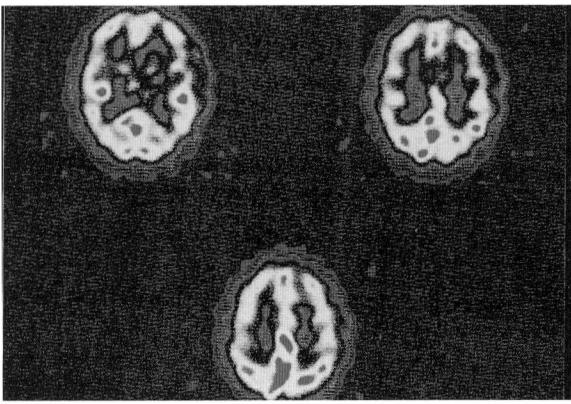

Figure 4a Wisconsin card sorting test in a normal subject: stimulation of the right prefrontal cortex (baseline)

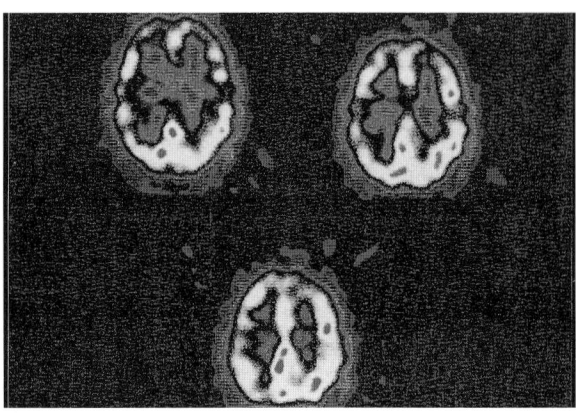

Figure 5a Wisconsin card sorting test in depression: no activation of the (prefrontal) cortex (baseline)

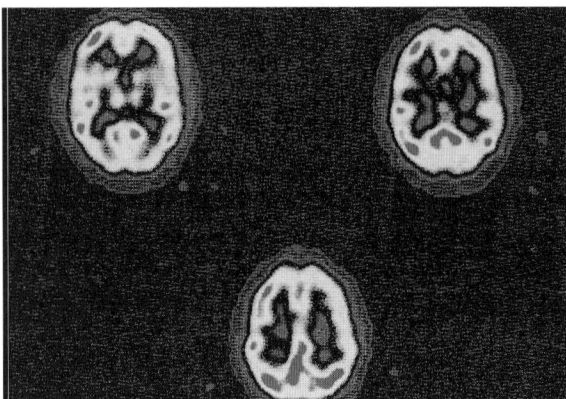

Figure 4b Wisconsin card sorting test in a normal subject: stimulation of the right prefrontal cortex (stimulation)

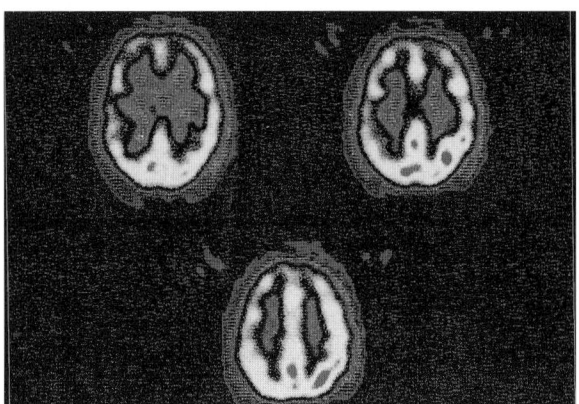

Figure 5b Wisconsin card sorting test in depression: no activation of the (prefrontal) cortex (stimulation)

the Wisconsin card sorting test did not show activation of prefrontal areas in 15 out of 26 patients (Figure 5). In schizophrenics, the same was true for 2 out of 7 patients. However, further studies will be needed to evaluate the results of this test in treated and untreated patients. One of the clinical benefits might be to subgroup patients with psychiatric disorders.

Sleep

Five patients with sleep apnoea and 4 patients with narcolepsy underwent brain SPECT using HMPAO while awake and during sleep[16]. The most prominent finding was a hypoperfusion of the left temporal lobe during sleep (Figure 6), whereas the right temporal lobe did not show significant differences. These data suggest that during sleep, the right temporal lobe remains activated.

Conclusions

These studies give rise to the assumption that activation studies may improve sensitivity of HMPAO or ECD brain SPECT. One of the advantages of high resolution SPECT is that O-15 PET has a good time resolution, but bad spatial resolution. The short accumulation period for HMPAO and ECD allows one to freeze a mental state lasting not longer than 30 - 50 s. A test may be performed during a time period of 5 - 10 min, while the tracer is infused over the same period or injected 1 - 4 min prior to finishing the activation. Moreover, the tracer may be applied outside of the Nuclear Medicine Department, for example under MEG or EEG monitoring (sleep), without affecting the patient. The patient is then transported to Nuclear Medicine to undergo the SPECT study as there is only insignificant tracer washout for a time period of several hours. Thus invasive procedures using arterial

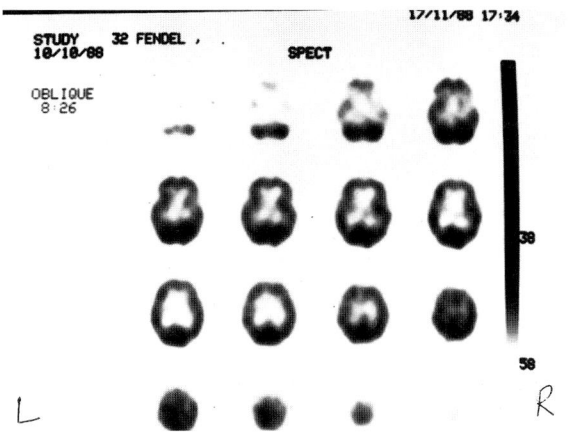

Figure 6a Brain SPECT while awake

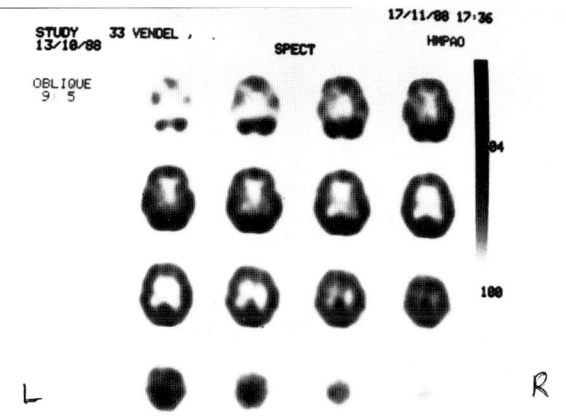

Figure 6b Hypoperfusion of the left temporal lobe during sleep

catheterisation (WADA test, intracarotidal balloon occlusion) may be combined with SPECT. Under clinical conditions, improved aphasia rehabilitation, drug or surgical therapy may be evaluated.

References

1   Andreasen, N.C., Razai, K. and Alliger, R. Hypofrontality in neuroleptic-naive patients and in patients with chronic schizophrenia. *Arch. Gen. Psychiatry* 1992, 49, 943

2   Baxter, L.R., Schwartz, J.M., Phelps, M.E. *et al.* Reduction of prefrontal cortex metabolism common to three types of depression. *Arch. Gen. Psychiatry* 1989, 46, 243

3   Buchsbaum, M.S. Positron emission tomography studies of abnormal glucose metabolism in schizophrenic illness. *Clin. Neurosc.* 1995, 3, 122

4   Rubin, R.T., Villanueva-Meyer, J., Anante, J. *et al.* Regional ^{133}Xe cerebral blood flow and cerebral ^{99m}Tc-HMPAO uptake in unmedicated patients with obsessive-compulsive disorder and matched normal control subjects. *Arch. Gen. Psychiatry* 1992, 49, 695

5   Schadel, A. SPECT studies of the brain with stimulation of the auditory cortex. *Scand. Audiol.* 1988, 30, 177

6   Schadel, A. and Fischer, M. Measurement of regional cerebral blood flow and accentuation of the primary auditory cortex with single photon emission computed tomography. *Arch. Otorhinolarynol.* 1989, 246, 205

7   Craig, C.H., Tikofsky, R.S., Hellman, R.S. *et al.* Single photon emission computed tomography (SPECT): A technique to measure auditory-related changes in regional cerebral blood flow (rCBF). Presented at Issues in Advanced Hearing Aid Research, Los Angeles, USA, 1990

8   Dal Bianco, P., Goldenberg, G., Podreka, I. *et al.* rCBF changes caused by memorizing of verbal and nonverbal acoustic stimuli: a IMP-SPECT study. *J. Neurol.* 1985, 232, 109

9   Goldenberg, G., Podreka, I., Steiner, M. *et al.* Patterns of regional cerebral blood flow related to memorizing of high and low imagery words – an emission computer tomography study. *Neuropsychologia* 1987, 25, 473

10 Lang, W., Lang, M., Goldenberg, G. *et al.* EEG and rCBF evidence for left frontocortical activation when memorizing verbal material in 'Current Trends in Event-Related Potential Research', (Eds. R. Johnson Jr., J.W. Rohrbaugh, R. Parasuraman) (EEG Suppl 40), Elsevier, New York, USA, 1987, p.328

11 Tikofsky, R.S., Hellman, R.S., Collier, B.D. *et al.* Influence of a naming task on SPECT ^{123}I-iodoamphetamine (SPECT/IMP) brain imaging: chronic aphasics vs normals. *J. Nucl. Med.* 197, 28, 559

12 Tikofsky, R.S. Brain SPECT studies: Potential role of cognitive challenge in language and learning disorders. *Adv. Funct. Neuroimaging* 1988, 1, 12

13 Tikofsky, R.S., Hellman, R.S. Brain single photon emission computed tomography: Newer activation and intervention studies. *Sem. Nucl. Med.* 1991, 21, 40

14 Klemm, E., Friederici, A., Pávics, L. and Biersack, H.-J. A study of syntactic and semantic aspects of language processing using ^{99m}Tc-ECD and high resolution SPECT. *J. Nucl. Med.* 1996, 37, 280P

15 Weinberger, D.R., Bergman, K.F. and Zee, R.F. Physiologic dysfunction of dorsolateral prefrontal cortex in schizophrenia. I. Regional cerebral blood flow evidence. *Arch. Gen. Psychiatry.* 1986, 43, 114

16 Biersack, H.-J., Clarenbach, P., Grünwald, F. *et al.* Hirn-SPECT mit ^{99m}Tc-HMPAO im Schlaf. *Nucl. Med.* 1989, 28, 40

SPECT in Neurology and Psychiatry, edited by P.P. De Deyn, R.A. Dierckx, A. Alavi and B.A. Pickut
© 1997 John Libbey & Company Ltd, pp. 73–80

Effects of Cocaine Abuse on Brain Perfusion: Assessment with ^{133}Xe rCBF and ^{99m}Tc-HMPAO and Correlation with Neuropsychological Testing

Chapter
11

I. Mena[*] and T.L. Strickland

Introduction

'Crack' cocaine is one of the most commonly abused psychoactive substances in the United States[1]. Recent studies suggest that there are 5 million regular cocaine users and at least 33 million who are reported to have used the drug[2,3]. Serious medical complications are known to be associated with acute cocaine use even in first-time users. Among the complications are acute myocardial infarction, cardiac arrhythmias, intestinal ischaemia, brain haemorrhage, ischaemic stroke and cerebral vasculitis[4].

Cocaine and other abused substances also produce a wide range of cognitive, behavioural and perfusion changes[5,6]. Neuropsychological studies that have evaluated chronic cocaine abusers suggest significant impairment in learning and memory ability, visuospatial skills, calculations, and abstraction ability. The mechanisms underlying cocaine-induced ischaemic stroke are not well understood. However, several investigators have noted abnormalities of CBF in patients with acute cocaine intoxication through the use of single photon emission computerised tomography (SPECT). Generally these patients demonstrated multi-focal areas of cortical hypoperfusion and scalloping of periventricular regions, indicating that SPECT is sensitive to perfusion abnormalities associated with cocaine use[7,8].

The combined use of ^{133}Xe washout to quantify cerebral blood flow (CBF) and ^{99m}Tc-HMPAO SPECT to obtain a high resolution image of CBF may help delineate the pathophysiological mechanism associated with cocaine induced neurological disease[9]. We report on the incidence of acute cerebrovascular changes in patients with acute cocaine intoxication and assess possible reversibility of perfusion abnormalities observed in patients who have been off the drug for extended time periods.

Most studies have evaluated the sequelae of acute cocaine intoxication on CBF, however, recent investigations[10] suggest that both CBF and cognitive abnormalities may persist following extended periods of drug abstinence, particularly in chronic, long-term users. Moreover, there is evidence that there may be minimal recovery of some cognitive abilities following abstinence, especially recovery of short-term verbal memory deficits. Thus improved understanding of the CBF changes associated with chronic cocaine abuse may help to elucidate long-term neuropsychological sequelae.

[*]Department of Nuclear Medicine, Clinica las Condes, Santiago, Chile
Biobehavioral Research Center, Dept. of Psychiatry, Charles R. Drew University of Medicine and Science and UCLA School of Medicine, Los Angeles, CA 90059, USA

Methods

Three groups of subjects were studied. Group one was composed of 23 patients with acute cocaine intoxication seen within 48 h after consultation in the psychiatric emergency room[9]. For the second group, we randomly selected and evaluated 8 (6 men and 2 women) inpatient long-term cocaine abusers with specific neuropsychological measures, a magnetic resonance image (MRI) and SPECT[10]. All subjects had previously abused freebase cocaine. The mean age of the patients was 32 years ± 2 (mean ± s.d.), and the mean length of drug use was 2.4 years, with an average daily ingestion during the addiction period of 1.8 g of cocaine. The patients were participants in a nine-month, non-hospital based residential treatment unit with strictly enforced visiting privileges. All patients met DSM-III-R criteria for cocaine dependence at the time of admission to the treatment program, underwent detoxification, and each received group and other psychosocial treatment interventions.

This group was studied in order to evaluate the reversibility potential of lesions seen in patients with acute cocaine intoxication. Group three consisted of 10 healthy drug-free normal volunteers[10]. The age range of the cocaine subjects was 32 ± 2 years and normals 31 ± 5 years (mean ± s.d.). At the time of their evaluation, this group of chronic patients did not present any specific neurological or psychiatric complaints. Similarly, none of the patients had a history of serious medical, neurological, or psychiatric disorders, and none were on medication at the time of evaluation. Also, all patients had been 'drug-free' for a minimum of six months and tested seronegative for HIV. Random weekly urine screens were obtained to assure abstinence status.

Neuropsychological evaluation

A subsample of patients (group two) were assessed by a clinical neuropsychologist who administered the following neuropsychological tests: 1) logical and visual reproduction subsets of the Wexler memory scale revised to assess immediate and delayed verbal and figural memory; 2) the Stroop colour interference task (Commali-Kaplan version), a task which requires concentration skills, mental control and response flexibility and is sensitive to frontal system functioning; 3) Trailmaking test, Part B, a complex task requiring both divided and sustained attention to shifting letter and number sequences; 4) Rey tangled lines, a visual tracking and visuomotor processing task; 5) Rey auditory verbal learning test (RAVLT), a measure of learning ability and short-term memory 10 and the controlled oral word association test, a measure of verbal fluency.

All data were scored manually, coded and entered into the computer for further analysis. Each patient's performance was compared with published norms corresponding to their respective age and educational attainment to determine abnormalities.

Neurological examination

All subjects received a comprehensive neurological evaluation by a board certified neurologist.

Magnetic resonance imaging studies in 7 of 8 subjects (T1 and T2 weighted MRI) were obtained with a Picker 1.5 Tesla magnet; axial scans were aligned parallel to the canthomeatal line from skull base to vertex in 10 mm sections.

SPECT: brain functional imaging

All patients were studied with both ^{133}Xe and ^{99m}Tc-HMPAO while awake and in the supine position. Details of the neuro-SPECT procedures can be found in a previous publication[9].

^{133}Xe rCBF

Absolute regional cerebral blood flow (rCBF) was calculated topographically based on the inert gas diffusion principle[11]. The results were expressed in ml/100g/min. rCBF was measured after the inhalation of 30 mCi (1100 MBq) of ^{133}Xe gas, using a brain-dedicated imaging device with high sensitivity collimation (Headtome II, Shimadzu, Kyoto, Japan)[12]. Three transaxial brain slices were obtained simultaneously at 2, 6 and 10 cm parallel to the orbitomeatal (OM) line. The acquisition has three phases: 1) background, 2) inhalation of ^{133}Xe, and 3) a four min washout phase. The total acquisition time was 6 min. A pixel by pixel single exponential model was used to analyse the SPECT data[13]. The resulting images represent rCBF and were displayed using a colour scale coded to ml/100g/min.

All regions of interest (ROIs) were manually placed over the cortex in each slice and all ROIs have the same size, with a diameter of 1.9 cm. The outer edge of the ROI is set in the interface of 45ml/100g/min and the inner edge was defined by the size of the ROI. In slice 1, the regions of interest are the following for each hemisphere: anterior and posterior orbitofrontal, and anterior and posterior temporal. In slice 2, anterior and posterior frontal, anterior and posterior temporal, and anterior and posterior parietal.

Regional CBF analysis was performed by comparing the rCBF results with the results of a group of 10 healthy normal subjects age-matched to the study sample group.

^{99m}Tc-HMPAO

After completing the ^{133}Xe rCBF measurement, each patient received 20 mCi (740 MBq) of ^{99m}Tc-hexamethylpropyleneamine oxime (HMPAO, CeretecTm, Amersham) injected intravenously[9]. Imaging of HMPAO was performed one hour after injection. The antecubital vein of the patient had been cannulated 10 min prior to injection and all patients and controls were maintained in a low ambient light and noise environment during the intravenous injection and brain uptake of phase two min after injection. Normal controls were injected under the same condition.

Regional values for HMPAO were expressed by first, normalisation of all pixel values to the maximal counts in the brain, and second, expressed as average pixel uptake for each region of interest. Normalisation to total brain average pixel count was not performed because this value includes also the areas of abnormal perfusion, and we consider it therefore a weaker standard. All values that fell below the lower 95% confidence interval of the normal subjects were considered abnormal.

In slice 2, the regions of interest were the following for each hemisphere: anterior and posterior frontal, and anterior and posterior temporal. In slice 3, two frontal, two temporal and two occipital ROIs were studied, while in slice 4, three frontal and three parietal ROIs were considered. Slice 5 is the same as slice 4.

Three dimensional display of cortical HMPAO uptake, normalised to maximal activity in the brain was volume normalised and compared with a normal age matched database. The colour scale for display denotes deviations from the mean ± standard deviations of the normal distribution of HMPAO uptake (Figure 1).

Results

Small randomly distributed perfusion defects were observed for both the acute and chronic cocaine users in ^{133}Xe and ^{99m}Tc-HMPAO SPECT studies. The mean CBF for chronic cocaine addicts was 49 ± 8 ml/100g/min and for those with acute cocaine intoxication, 48 ± 3 ml/100g/min. The mean CBF for the normal group was 54 ± 6 ml/100g/min. The difference between normals and cocaine users was significant (p< 0.05), Table 1.

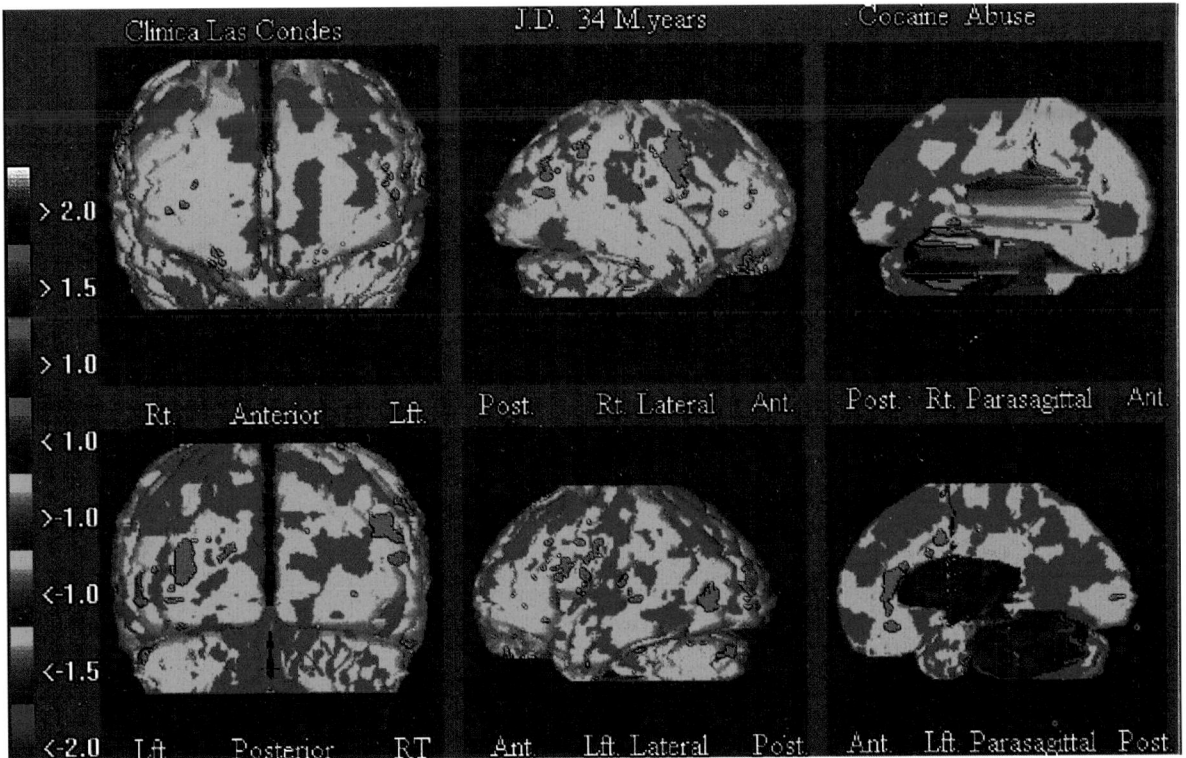

Figure 1 Three dimensional display of cortical ^{99m}Tc-HMPAO uptake normalised to maximal activity in brain, volume normalised and compared with young adult normal database. The colour scale is expressed in standard deviations from the normal mean. Areas in dark blue denote focal, randomly distributed hypoperfusion with a statistical significance of 95% (≤ 2 standard deviations). This abnormality is more marked in the frontal lobes. Areas in green and red are normal

Table 1 Summary of regional analysis of ^{133}Xe cerebral blood flow

Patient number/age (years)/sex	Cortical (M+ SD)	Inferior Frontal	Superior Frontal	Temporal	Parietal
		ml / 100g / min			
1 / 29 / M	47 ± 7[a]	48	50[a]	40[a]	48
2 / 32 / M	45 ± 7[a]	50	49	42[a]	40*
3 / 30 / M	55 ± 5	58	56	51	54
4 / 33 / M	44 ± 6	46[a]	45[a]	39[a]	45[a]
5 / 27 / M	50 ± 7	38[a]	48[a]	51	46[a]
6 / 30 / F	50 ± 8	56	53	45[a]	45[a]
7 / 33 / F	46 ± 7[a]	52	50	44[a]	48
8 / 34 / M	51 ± 6	51	55	51	46[a]
	55 ± 3	55 ± 3	57 ± 3	51 ± 1	51 ± 2

Normal subjects (n = 10; age 31 ± 5 years)

[a], $p < 0.05$. Reprinted from Strickland *et al.*[10], with the permission of the publisher

Locus and severity of hypoperfusion was also assessed. Significant clusters of abnormalities were noted in the anterior left temporal, right temporal, bilateral frontal, with the right showing greater impairment than the left in right parietal areas. For chronic users, the following abnormal results were obtained: left frontal 5 of 8 abnormal studies, uptake 72% ± 11; left occipital lobe 6 of 8 abnormal studies, uptake 87% ± 4; right parietal lobe 7 of 8 abnormal studies, uptake 71% ± 5. The uptake for acute subjects in these areas were 74%, 70% and 70%, respectively. Good correlations between Tc-HMPAO and xenon images were found (Table 2).

Three dimensional display of cortical HMPAO uptake shows dark blue pixels with perfusion below 2 s.d. of the mean of the normals and demonstrates a random distribution of multifocal areas of hypoperfusion that has been described previously as a scalloping pattern of perfusion[9,10]. There is predominance of frontal lobe perfusion impairment (Figure 1, Table 2).

The neuropsychological assessment results reveal impairment in a number of cognitive domains for all patients evaluated. Most notable were deficits in frontal lobe performance. Additionally, the deficits of neuropsychological test performance were generally in agreement with regions of hypoperfusion. Collectively these findings indicate that chronic heavy 'crack' abusers experience significant problems in attention, both divided and sustained, and concentration tasks, learning, visual and verbal memory and word generation ability, Table 3.

Table 2 Summary of clinical, SPECT, and neuropsychological findings

Patient number/ age (years)/ sex	Cocaine use	Other drug use	SPECT findings: hypoperfusion	Neuropsychological findings: deficits
1/29/M	Heavy: >2g/d 6 years	Alcohol occasionally	Severe R temporal	Attention, concentration, new learning, visual and verbal memory, word production, visuomotor integration
2/32/M	Moderate: >1g/d for 3 years	None admitted	Moderate bifrontal bitemporal	Attention, concentration, new learning
3/30/M for 4 years	Heavy: >3g/d occasionally memory, word production,	Alcohol frontotemporal	Extensive new learning, visual	Attention, concentration, visuomotor integration
4/33/M	Heavy: >3g/d for 4 years	Alcohol occasionally	Moderate, R frontal and parietal	Attention, concentration, new learning, word production
5/27/M for 6 years	Heavy: >6g/d marijuana production, visuomotor	Alcohol and and parietal	Severe, bifrontal new learning, word	Attention, concentration, integration
6/30/F	Moderate: >1g/d for 3 years	Marijuana	Moderate, bitemporal, extensive bilateral frontotemporal	Attention, concentration, new learning, word production, visuomotor integration
7/33/F	Moderate: >1g/d for 3 years	None admitted	Some frontal, R>L temporal, R temporal	Attention, concentration, verbal and visual memory, new learning, word production, visuomotor integration
8/34/M	Moderate: >1g/d for 2 years	Alcohol	Moderate, bidorsal frontal, bilateral temporal	Attention, concentration, verbal memory, new learning, word production, visuomotor integration

M = male; F = female; L = left; R = right
Reprinted from Strickland et al.[10], with the permission of the publisher

Table 3 Summary of neuropsychological test results (percentile scores)

Neuropsychological Tests Administered	Patient number / age (years) / sex / education (years)							
	1/29/M/11	2/32/M/11	3/30/M/12	4/33/M/12	5/27/M/12	6/30/F/10	7/33/F/16	8/34/M/11
Verbal Memory (Immediate)	20th	WNL	WNL	35th	WNL	WNL	16th	13th
Verbal Memory (Delayed)	19th	WNL	WNL	WNL	WNL	WNL	24th	14th
Visual Memory (Immediate)	17th	WNL	31st	WNL	—[a]	24th	WNL	WNL
Visual Memory (Delayed)	13th	WNL	44th	WNL	—[a]	25th	9th	WNL
Stroop Interference	25th	1st	1st	3rd	1st	1st	1st	1st
Trail Making Test B	22nd	WNL	WNL	4th	13th	1st	20th	13th
Rey Tangled Lines	1st	WNL	WNL	WNL	35th	1st	1st	1st
RAVLT Total Trial 1-5	1st	39th	29th	32nd	1st	1st	1st	29th
RAVLT Retention	1st	23rd	23rd	23rd	1st	WNL	1st	WNL
Verbal Fluency (FAS)	7th	WNL	WNL	1st	1st	36th	10th	1st

Neuropsychological performance of 8 drug abusers (predominantly cocaine) after a minimum of 6 months' abstinence. Only measures at the 50th percentile or above are identified as within normal limits (WNL). M = male; F = female; RAVLT = Rey Auditory Verbal Learning Test; a, no data

Reprinted from Strickland et al.[10], with the permission of the publisher

The MRI studies were unremarkable in all of the subjects and none demonstrated evidence for stroke or focal brain atrophy. One subject had large ventricles and diffuse brain atrophy, and two subjects had small white matter lesions.

Discussion

Acute cocaine intoxication caused both generalised and focally diminished cerebral blood flow. The most striking abnormalities seen were multifocal small cortical and sometimes deep areas of hypoperfusion. A characteristic and unusual scalloping-pattern of periventricular perfusion was noted[9]. We have previously seen this perfusion pattern in patients with cerebral vasculitis, with AIDS dementia syndrome and exposure to other neurotoxic chemicals i.e. solvents, pesticides and glues. We suspect that this periventricular subcortical hypoperfusion (scalloping) is the manifestation of cerebral vasoconstriction and is a characteristic of cerebral perfusion effects of a vasoconstrictive agent such as cocaine. The scalloping may be due to the constriction of small and medium sized arteries although for reasons that are still undetermined, the deep white matter appears to show selective involvement with cocaine. The second hypothesis is that focal areas of hypoperfusion are secondary to clusters of cells damaged during the acute intense prolonged vasoconstriction induced by cocaine. A primary hypofunction will induce a focal secondary hypoperfusion[9].

Also in the acute cases, large wedge-shaped cortical perfusion defects were frequently seen. These deficits appear to be caused by vasoconstriction of larger arteries or confluence of multiple constricted smaller arteries. This pattern was found in 3 of 4 stroke patients and 2 with TIAs. These large SPECT deficits correlated to focal clinical symptomatology.

Frontal lobe hypoperfusion was found in 70% of the acute patients, which were irritable and disinhibited, both characteristics of patients with frontal lobe dysfunction[9].

A previous study of CBF in cocaine abusers was performed by Volkow[5], who used positron emission computerised tomography to assess cerebral perfusion with oxygen labelled water. Patients from that study were recruited from a drug rehabilitation centre and were by definition without major medical or neurological illness. Our patients differed in this respect as all our acute patients had neurological symptoms. In work-up study, diffuse patchy areas of hypoperfusion were observed and marked hypoperfusion was seen in the prefrontal cortex. Repeat scans performed at 10 days revealed persistent deficits[5]. This has motivated the study of our second group of patients, namely the study on heavy cocaine abusers that were off cocaine for periods of 6 months. The study was conducted in order to ascertain if acute changes induced by cocaine would be reversible. Although abstinent from drug use for at least 6 months, all patients in the chronic group manifested significant cerebral blood flow disturbances and persistent neurocognitive dysfunction. Our findings are consistent with other studies of cocaine, cerebral blood flow and cognition; however, the design of the current study which included a period of verified abstinence from the drug used by the patient, as well as the use of SPECT and neuropsychological assessment to evaluate the long-term sequelae of cocaine use, allow for fewer competing explanations for the outcomes observed.

Although a number of studies using CT or MRI have reported cerebral dysfunction in cocaine abusers, patients with more subtle neuropathology are more difficult to identify with CT or MRI. Holman et al.[8] have demonstrated that SPECT is more sensitive to cerebral abnormalities than CT. In our study, SPECT demonstrated brain perfusion abnormalities which were strongly associated with a neuropsychological deficit observed, although the MRI findings showed only mild atrophy consistent with previous MRI studies of chronic cocaine abusers[14].

In our study, we found significant neuropsychological impairment in our free-base abusing population, particularly on tasks requiring sustained attention and concentration, mental flexibility and speed of mental processing, all tasks related to frontal lobe functioning. Although these findings are preliminary, they suggest adverse and persistent cognitive dysfunction secondary to long-term cocaine use, even after a period of significant abstinence[10].

In summary, our findings reveal: 1) that in acute cocaine exposure, a high percentage of individuals exhibit cerebral focal and diffuse hypoperfusion, the focal abnormalities are of random presentation and present with a scalloping pattern; and 2) even after a clinically significant period of 6 months of drug abstinence, cocaine abusing patients exhibited multifocal regions of diminished cerebral blood flow which is likely to be irreversible. Also, persistent global neuropsychological deficits in attention, concentration, mental control, mental flexibility and learning ability, as well as verbal and visual memory were observed. As the cocaine epidemic expands and the number of users increase, society will potentially be faced with a large number of persons who will pose a new challenge for the health care, rehabilitation, education, employment and judicial system in the United States[10].

References

1 U.S. Department of Health and Human Services news release, 31 August, 1990

2 Adams, E.H. Abuse/availability trends of cocaine in the United States in ' Drug Surveillance Reports', NIDA Division of Epidemiology and Statistical Reports, Rockville, MD, USA, 1982, 2

3 Fishburn, P.M. National Survey on drug abuse: main findings, National Institute of Drug Abuse, 1980 (DHSS publication no. ADM 80-976)

4 Mody, C.K., Miller, B.L., McIntyre, H.B. and Goldberg, M.A. Neurological complications of cocaine abuse. *Neurology* 1991, 38, 1189

5 Volkow, N.D., Fowler, J.S. and Wolf, A.P. Changes in brain glucose metabolism in cocaine dependence and withdrawal. *Am. J. Psychiatry* 1991, 148, 621

6 Manschreck, T.C., Laughery, J.A., Weisstein, C.C. *et al.* Characteristics of freebase cocaine psychosis. *Yale Journal of Biological Medicine* 1989, 61, 115

7 Miller, B.L., Cummings, J.L., Villanueva-Meyer, J. *et al.* Frontal lobe degeneration: clinical, neuropsychological, and SPECT characteristics. *Neurology* 1991, 41, 1374

8 Holman, B.L., Moretti, J.-L. and Hill, T.C. SPECT perfusion imaging in cerebrovascular disease in 'Noninvasive imaging of cerebrovascular disease', Liss, New York, USA, 1989, p. 147

9 Mena, I., Giombetti, R.J., Miller, B.L. *et al.* Cerebral blood flow changes with acute cocaine intoxication: clinical correlations with SPECT, CT and MRI. NIDA *Res. Monograph* 1994, 138, 161

10 Strickland, T.L., Mena, I., Villanueva-Meyer, J. *et al.* Cerebral perfusion and neuropsychological consequences of chronic cocaine use. *J. Neuropsychiatry Clin. Neurosciences* 1993, 5, 419

11 Kety, S.S. Theory and applications of the exchange of inert gas at the lungs and tissues. *Pharmacology Review* 1951, 3, 1

12 Higashi, Y., Yamaoga, N., Ohi, J. *et al.* Development of the Shimadzu single photon emission tomograph for the head, SET-031. *Shimadzu Review* 1985, 42, 59

13 Kanno, I. and Lassen, N.A. Two methods for calculating regional cerebral blood flow from emission computed tomography of inert gas concentrations. *J. Comp. Ass. Tomog.* 1979, 3, 71

14 Pascual-Leone, A., Dhuna, A. and Anderson, D.C. Cerebral atrophy in habitual cocaine abusers: a planimetric CT study. *Neurology* 1991, 41, 34

SPECT in Neurology and Psychiatry, edited by P.P. De Deyn, R.A. Dierckx, A. Alavi and B.A. Pickut
© 1997 John Libbey & Company Ltd, pp. 81-85

Cognitive Stimulations using ^{99m}Tc-HMPAO SPECT: Methodological and Clinical Issues

Chapter
12

O. Migneco, J. Darcourt, Ph. Robert, M. Benoit, F. Thauby,
M. Gray, J. Benoliel and F. Bussiere

Introduction

Emission brain imaging has been widely used in baseline conditions to study various brain diseases. However, emission tomography can also be applied to metabolic or perfusion changes appearing within the brain. Positron emission tomography (PET) is mostly used for brain activation imaging. Techniques such as functional magnetic resonance (FMR) with its high spatial resolution, and magnetoencephalography with its important temporal resolution have been used most recently. Single photon emission computed tomography (SPECT) has also been proposed for stimulation studies, first with ^{133}Xe[1-4], and later with non-diffusable technetium labelled tracers (mainly HMPAO[5]).

Until now, activation studies have been used for research on normal brain mapping or on neuropsychiatric physiopathology. In this paper, we would like to stress the clinical applications of this technique to improve early diagnostic performances. For this clinical aspect, because of its availability, SPECT with a technetium labelled agent such as HMPAO is the tool of choice. At present, at least in Europe, PET and FMR are restricted to a few institutions and are not used for routine clinical work. The clinical rationale is that HMPAO SPECT diagnostic sensitivity is low in the early stage of various chronic neurological diseases. For example, early diagnosis of Alzheimer's disease is a major issue with the advent of the new treatments and remains unreliable with conventional SPECT[6]. Concerning schizophrenia, the findings are controversial and the hypofrontality seems to appear only during frontal lobe stimulation [1]. Therefore, we believe that activation studies, which will 'stress' the brain, could reveal pathological disturbances hidden in the resting state as cardiac stress studies unmask ischaemia that is not detectable in rest studies. Few papers have addressed this issue yet. Among 13 papers reporting on HMPAO SPECT activation studies[7-19], eight deal with brain mapping problems (two with cognitive stimulation), four with physiopathology, exclusively of schizophrenia, and only one with early diagnosis, in this case of Alzheimer's disease [16].

Technical considerations for HMPAO activation SPECT

Due to its biochemical behaviour, HMPAO has many advantages for cognitive stimulation studies. It has a short arterial input allowing activation tasks as short as 3 min and paradigms compatible with patient studies. The HMPAO brain uptake is stable and is not affected by redistribution. Therefore, the activation paradigms can be performed away from the camera room, in a more

University of Nice-Sophia
Antipolis, France

'physiological' environment. Furthermore, this tracer is widely available and, because of its technetium labelling, allows high resolution tomographic images. One of the drawbacks is the difficulty in repeating the studies. Hence only two scans are performed: the activation and the baseline acquisitions. These two studies have to be compared precisely in order to identify and localise the cortical activation. This is problematic and several approaches are possible. First of all, 2 injection protocols can be used: the split dose technique, and the 2 day protocol. In the split dose technique, the baseline study is performed with usually one third of the full dose of HMPAO. After the acquisition has been completed, the stimulation study is performed without moving the patient out of the gantry and injecting the 'remaining' two thirds of the dose. In the 2 day protocol, each study is made on separate days with a full dose each time. The advantages and disadvantages of each technique are reciprocal. With the split dose technique, the patient receives only one full dose of HMPAO, both studies are completed on the same day, and the patient stays in the same position for the 2 acquisitions avoiding the necessity to record two sets of data. On the other hand, the activation paradigm is performed inside the gantry, in a less physiological environment, the statistical count of the first study is low and there is an overlap of both studies. With the 2 day protocol, the patient is exposed to a higher level of radiation, registration of both sets of is needed since both the studies are performed on 2 separate days and the neuro-psychological state can vary. However, the stability of the HMPAO distribution between two studies has been demonstrated[20]. Furthermore, the stimulation paradigm is performed out of the gantry, each study has high statistics, and there is no overlap between both studies. We used 2 day protocols.

Methods of data analysis

We used the Talairach principle[21,22] in order to register the baseline and activation studies and to localise the cortical activation sites.

Talairach principle

The hypothesis is that the individual variability of brain anatomy can be taken into account by proportional transformations independently applied to 6 subvolumes of each hemisphere. These subvolumes are based on three intra-cerebral baselines that have relatively constant relationships with the telencephalic structures. These lines are: (a) a horizontal line joining the upper part of the anterior commissure (CA) to the lower part of the posterior commissure (CP) and extending to the frontal and occipital lobes; and (b) two perpendicular vertical lines, one behind the CA, the VCA, and one in front of the CP, the VCP. These two lines extend to the vertex and to the base of the temporal lobe. Furthermore, a proportional grid system is built on these three baselines and allows the localisation of the brain structures, by their stereotactic coordinates, in Talairach's atlas.

Application to a two dimensional region of interest analysis

Our first approach was a region of interest (ROI) analysis technique[23]. We decided to delineate the ROIs on two 'reconstructed lateral views' (RLV) generated from the tomographic data. These two RLVs, one for each hemisphere, were created with the cortical pixels of the reconstructed transverse slices. The purpose of these RLVs was to decrease the amount of data available for analysis and to match the Talairach atlas layout[21]. The ROIs were drawn automatically using the atlas data on the activation and baseline RLVs (Figure 1). A major problem of this approach was that the CA and CP are not identifiable in brain SPECT. We used neuroanatomical data provided by the literature[22] to calculate the commissural lines from external canthomeatal landmarks. After normalisation for the difference in activity between the two studies using the total counts in the brain, the activation index was calculated for each ROI as follows:

(ROI counts stimulation - ROI counts baseline)/ROI counts baseline

The ROI approach is suitable to test *a priori* hypotheses. Indeed, the choice of ROI definition (Brodman areas, lobe boundaries) depends on the expected topography of the activation sites. Therefore, a pixel by pixel analysis, also referred to as a function of interest approach[3,24], is preferable since it does not need any assumption on the results. For this reason, we moved to a two dimensional pixel by pixel analysis.

Application to a two dimensional pixel by pixel analysis

This approach was applied again on the RLV. For each patient, the base and activation RLV were orientated according to the CACP line, scaled to the total brain activity, normalised for size according to the stereotactic atlas model and analysed on a pixel by pixel basis using the previous activation index formula. The resulting image represents the individual activation map of the subject and is expressed in percentage (with a colour coding from -20% to +20%). Since these individual activation maps are normalised to the brain atlas model, they can be averaged again on a pixel by pixel basis for a group of patients. Therefore, the mean activation map of the group is obtained (Figure 2). The following evolution was the extension of these concepts to a three dimensional approach.

Application to a three dimensional voxel by voxel analysis

Our last processing technique addressed several limitations of the previous two dimensional approaches. One was the superposition of the inner and outer cortices in the two dimensional layout which was solved by a three dimensional handling of the data. The second difficulty was the estimation of the CACP lines from external landmarks, which was replaced by a definition of new lines directly visible on the SPECT data. These lines were: a fronto-occipital line replacing the CACP; a vertical line at the anterior limit of the temporal lobe instead of the VCA; and a vertical plane through the brainstem instead of the VCP. The Talairach principle was applied to this new reference system and validated on 14 normal T1 MRI brain scans showing a satisfactory registration (the error on the commissure localisation was less than 4.3 mm). The last drawback of the previous approaches was the display of the activation maps, which contain a majority of pixels equal to zero, making the identification of brain structures difficult. This was solved by digitising the Talairach atlas so that each activation volume could be displayed on top of this standardised brain shape allowing a better localisation of the activated voxels (Figure 3). This software was developed on Sophy-NXT with the Sopha company (SMV, Buc, France).

Three examples of diagnostic cognitive SPECT activations

Using these different techniques, we studied different groups of patients.

In a first work, we studied seven patients with probable Alzheimer's disease (AD) and five controls. The activation study consisted of a visuospatial task: the patients were asked to search for errors between two drawings. During the baseline study, they were looking at a blank sheet. The resulting activation pattern in the controls involved the primary and associative visual cortex (Brodmann area 19 +13.7% p<0.01) as well as the cerebellum (+11.1% p<0.05) predominantly in the right hemisphere, while AD patients did not exhibit this pattern (Figure 2). These results confirmed the ability of HMPAO SPECT to study brain cognitive activation and support the hypothesis of a limited cognitive reserve capacity (plasticity) in AD[25,26.]

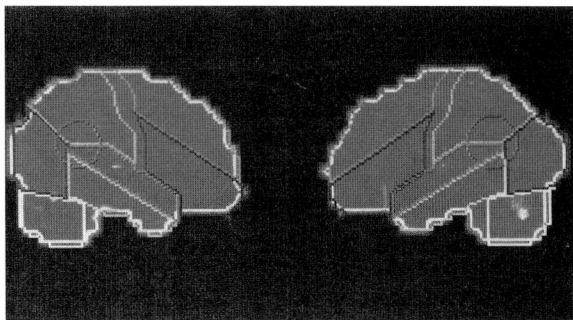

Figure 1 Two dimensional region of interest analysis. The ROIs are automatically delineated on the reconstructed lateral views of each hemisphere using the Talairach atlas

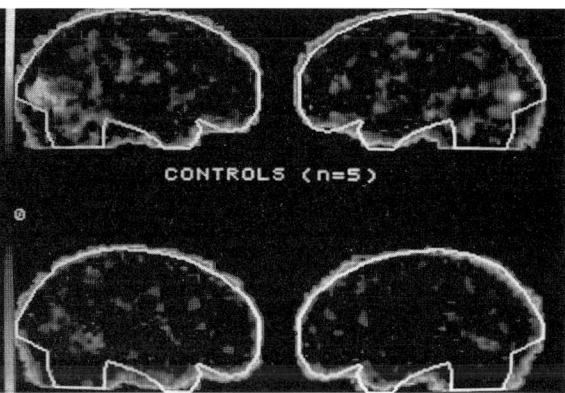

Figure 2 Two dimensional pixel by pixel analysis. Above, the averaged activation map of the control group showing activation of the primary and associative visual cortex as well as the cerebellum predominantly on the right hemisphere during a visuospatial task. Below, Alzheimer patients do not exhibit this pattern

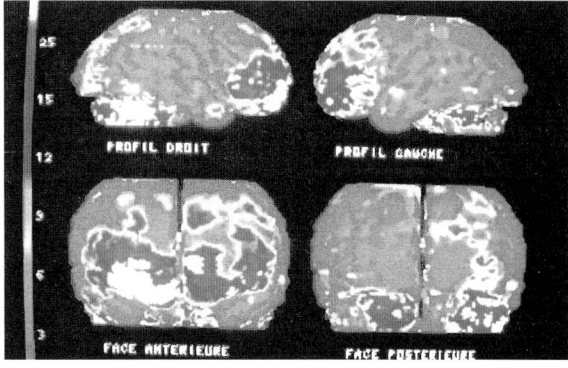

Figure 3 Three dimensional voxel by voxel analysis. Display of the activation map on top of the digitised atlas showing a frontal activation in a normal subject during a verbal fluency task. The colour scale represents the rCBF increase in per cent

The following study gathered 15 non-demented patients with memory complaints[27]. Using the Signoret Memory Battery Scale[28], these patients were separated into two groups: 11 patients had objective memory disorders (OMD), 4 patients had only subjective memory disorders (NOMD). The activation paradigm consisted of a visual memorisation task, namely the Rey's memory efficiency profile (MEP)[29]. This test uses a set of drawings that the patient has to recall. There is a learning step followed by an immediate and delayed recall. The injection of HMPAO for the activation study was made during the learning step. In this case also, during the baseline study, the patients were looking at a blank sheet. The mean activation effect was significantly higher in the right cerebellum (4.8% $p<0.01$) in the NOMD group when compared with the OMD group. Furthermore, there was a significant correlation between the MEP score for immediate recall and the right temporal lobe activation (Spearman correlation coefficient=0.56 $p<0.05$). These results showed that differences in activation can be measured in non-demented patients with mild memory disorders. Follow up of these patients will say whether this test could be used to predict the development of Alzheimer's disease.

Recently, we have studied frontal activation using a categorical verbal fluency test[30]. Preliminary results show a high frontal activation in controls (Figure 3) unlike frontal lobe dementia patients. Comparable results have been obtained by others using PET[31] or ^{133}Xe[32]. Therefore, using the verbal fluency test seems appropriate for studying the frontal lobe.

Conclusion

With appropriate tools, cognitive activation studies with HMPAO are technically feasible in a routine clinical environment. We believe that with proper paradigms, HMPAO SPECT activation can help to improve early diagnosis. It is clear that this is a very important issue especially in Alzheimer's disease since new drugs will only be effective in the early stages of the disease. At present, the appropriate validated brain stress is still to be found, and, unlike coronary artery disease, several tests adapted to each disease will be necessary.

References

1 Weinberger, D.R., Berman, K.F. *et al.* Physiologic dysfunction of dorsolateral prefrontal cortex in schizophrenia. Regional cerebral blood flow evidence. *Arch. Gen. Psychiatry* 1986, 43(2), 114

2 Decety, J., Sjoholm, H. *et al.* The cerebellum participates in mental activity: tomographic measurements of regional cerebral blood flow. *Brain Res.* 1990, 535(2), 313

3 Andreasen N.C., Rezai K. *et al.* Hypofrontality in neuroleptic-naive patients and in patients with chronic schizophrenia. Assessment with xenon 133 single photon emission computed tomography and the Tower of London. *Arch. Gen. Psychiatry* 1992, 49(12), 943

4 Gur, R.E., Jaggi, J.L. *et al.* Cerebral blood flow in schizophrenia: effects of memory processing on regional activation. *Biol. Psychiatry* 1994, 35(1), 3

5 Costa, D.C. and Morgan, G.F. Radiopharmaceuticals for conventional blood-brain barrier and brain perfusion studies in 'New Trends in Nuclear Neurology and Psychiatry, John Libbey & Co. Ltd, London, UK, 1993, p.65

6 Robert, Ph., Migneco, O. *et al.* Regional cerebral blood flow in elderly subjects with and without Alzheimer's disease; study using a HMPAO 99mTc SPECT with an automatized technique. *Dementia* 1992, 3, 15

7 Lang, W., Lang, M. *et al.* DC-potential shifts and regional cerebral blood flow reveal frontal cortex involvement in human visuomotor learning. *Exp. Brain Res.* 1988, 71(2), 353

8 Woods, S.W., Hegeman, I.M. *et al.* Visual stimulation increases technetium-99m-HMPAO distribution in human visual cortex. *J. Nucl. Med.* 1991, 32(2), 210

9 Shedlack, K.J., Hunter, R. *et al.* The pattern of cerebral activity underlying verbal fluency shown by split-dose single photon emission tomography in normal volunteers. *Psychol. Med.* 1991, 21(3), 687

10 Rubin, P., Holm, S. *et al.* Altered modulation of prefrontal and subcortical brain activity in newly diagnosed schizophrenia and schizophreniform disorder. A regional cerebral blood flow study. *Arch. Gen. Psychiatry* 1991, 48(1),987

11 Pantano, P., Di Piero, V. *et al.* Motor stimulation response by technetium-99m hexamethylpropylene amine oxime split-dose method and single photon emission tomography. *Eur. J. Nucl. Med.* 1992, 19(11), 939

12 Ebmeier, K.P., Murray, C.L. *et al.* Unilateral voluntary hand movement and regional cerebral uptake of technetium-99m-exametazine in human control subjects. *J. Nucl. Med.* 1992, 33(9), 1623

13 Le Scao, Y., Jezequel, J. *et al.* Reliability of low-frequency auditory stimulation studies associated with technetium-99m-hexamethylpropylene amine oxime single-photon emission computed tomography. *Eur. J. Nucl. Med.* 1993, 20(5), 387

14 Ryding, E., Ryding, E.L. *et al.* Motor imagery activates the cerebellum regionally. A SPECT rCBF study with 99mTc-HMPAO. *Brain Res. Cogn. Brain Res.* 1993, 1(2), 94

15 Kawasaki, Y., Maeda, Y. *et al.* SPECT analysis of regional cerebral blood flow changes in patients with schizophrenia during the Wisconsin Card Sorting Test. *Schizophr. Res.* 1993, 10(2), 109

16 Riddle, W., O'Carrol, R.E. *et al.* A single photon emission computerised tomography study of regional brain function underlying verbal memory in patients with Alzheimer-type dementia. *Br. J. Psychiatry* 1993, 163, 166

17 Crosson, B., Williamson, D.J. *et al.* A technique to localize activation in the human brain with technetium-99m-HMPAO SPECT: a validation study using visual stimulation. *J. Nucl. Med.* 1994, 35(5), 755

18 Catafau, A.M., Parellada, E. *et al.* Prefrontal and temporal blood flow in schizophrenia: resting and activation technetium-99m-HMPAO SPECT patterns in young neuroleptic-naive patients with acute disease. *J. Nucl. Med.* 1994, 35(6), 935

19 Busatto, G.F., Costa, D.C. *et al.* Regional cerebral blood flow (rCBF) in schizophrenia during verbal memory activation: a 99mTc-HMPAO single photon emission tomography (SPET) study. *Psychol. Med.* 1994, 24(2), 463

20 Deutch, G., Mountz J.M. *et al.* Regional stability of CBF measured by Tc99m-HMPAO SPECT. *J. Nucl. Med.* 1994, 35, 107

21 Talairach, J. and Szikla, G. Atlas d'anatomie stéréotaxique du télencéphale. Masson, Paris, 1967

22 Szikla, G., Bouvier, G. *et al.* Angiography of the human brain cortex. Springer-Verlag, Heidelberg, 1977

23 Talairach, J. and Tournoux, P. Co-planar stereotaxic atlas of the human brain. Georg Thieme Verlag, Stuttgart, 1988

24 Evans, A., Marret, S. *et al.* MRI PET correlative analysis using a volume of interest (VOI) atlas. *J. Cereb. Blood Flow Metab.* 1991, 11, A69

25 Miller, J.D., De Leon, M.J. *et al.* Abnormal temporal lobe response in Alzheimer's disease during cognitive processing as measured by 11C-2-deoxy-D-Glucose and PET. *J. Cereb. Blood Flow Metab.* 1987, 7, 248

26 Kessler, J., Herholz, K. *et al.* Impaired metabolic activation in Alzheimer's disease: a PET study during continuous recognition. *Neuropsychologia* 1991, 29, 229

27 Robert, Ph., Migneco, O. *et al.* A single photon emission computed tomography study of cerebral regional perfusion changes induced by visual memorisation in subjects with mild memory impairment. *Psychiatry Research:* in press

28 Signoret, J.L. Batterie d'efficience amnésique: BEM144, Elsevier, Paris, France, 1991

29 Rey, A. Les troubles de la mémoire et leur examen psychométrique, Bessart, Paris, France, 1966

30 Benton, X.X. Multilingual aphasia examination, University of Iowa Press, 1976

31 Parks, R., Loewenstein, D. *et al.* Cerebral metabolic effects of a verbal fluency test: a PET scan study. *J. Clin. Exp. Neuropsych.* 1988, 10(5), 565

32 Warkentin, S., Passant, U. *et al.* Functional activation of the frontal lobes. *Dementia* 1993, 4, 188

Psychiatry

In Vivo Neuroreceptor Imaging – Methodology and Applications in Neuropsychiatry

Chapter

13

A.R. Lingford-Hughes and L.S. Pilowsky

Introduction

The key step in mediating the actions of neurotransmitters and psychotropic drugs is the interaction between the agent and a receptor. A drug is defined in terms of activity at a particular receptor. For most agents, with the notable exception of steroids, a receptor is a macromolecular protein complex embedded in the plasma membrane, which mediates its signal across the membrane and into the cell. The concept of receptive substances that mediate drug effects was first proposed by Langley and Ehrlich at the turn of the century[1,2]. Drug-receptor interactions have subsequently been characterised and classified. Their biochemical structure and, more recently, molecular genetics are beginning to be elucidated. The characterisation of such drug-receptor interactions is critical in defining a drug's properties and is the starting point for developing more selective, improved pharmacotherapies for neuropsychiatric disorders.

In the classical pharmacological approach, distinct receptor classes were classified through defining the functional activity of agents at the receptor. For example, the particular effects of acetylcholine at the nicotinic and muscarinic receptors (Dale) and separation of the α and β subtypes of the adrenergic receptors (Alquist) was based on their differing activity profiles with different agents[3,4]. An agonist is an agent that invokes a response through receptor occupancy. A partial agonist elicits a similar though less than maximal response. An antagonist occupies the receptor but fails to elicit any response. The blockade may be functional, irreversible, competitive, non-competitive or mixed. Inverse agonists induce a response opposite to that of agonists.

In vitro receptor measurement

The earliest receptor subtypes were distinguished by measuring the functional consequences of agonists and antagonists[3,4]. In the 1970s, the development of radioligand binding techniques allowed detailed pharmacological characterisation of a receptor. Moreover, receptors could be visualised for the first time *in situ*, using autoradiographic techniques[5]. Details of the theory underlying *in vitro* binding characterisation are given elsewhere[6,7], but a brief overview is given here, since knowledge of the principles of the *in vitro* measurement of receptors is fundamental to the understanding of PET and SPECT. Radioligand binding studies involve labelling a compound which interacts with a receptor. In addition to this 'specific' binding in any given tissue, the radioligand will also be present as free ligand, trapped in compartments and bound to non-receptor tissue proteins. These latter three elements constitute non-specific binding. Specific binding, by definition, is a finite measurable quantity,

Institute of Psychiatry,
De -Crespigny Park,
Denmark Hill,
London, SE5 8AF
UK

while non-specific binding is infinite. Thus, in the test tube or on the tissue slice for autoradiography, duplicate incubations are performed with and without a competing ligand. In the absence of the competing ligand, the radioligand will bind to both specific and non-specific binding sites, so that total binding capacity is measured. In the presence of the competing ligand, since all the specific binding sites are occupied by the unlabelled ligand, the non-specific component is measured. Subtraction of non-specific binding from total binding yields the specific binding capacity. A curvilinear relationship is seen between (LR) and (L), with plateau representing the saturable i.e. specific binding of receptors. The concentration of ligand (L) required to occupy half the specific binding sites is a measure of the affinity (K_D) of the ligand for the receptor.

These radioligand binding techniques have been used over the past two decades in human post mortem tissue to characterise the receptors in many neuropsychiatric disorders, and to test and extend hypotheses of aetiology and dysfunction. Their critical role, but also some of the problems inherent in using post mortem tissue, is well illustrated in the field of schizophrenia. The dopamine hypothesis of schizophrenia proposed increased dopaminergic activity in the mesolimbic regions. This was supported by demonstrating an increased density of dopamine (D_2) binding sites[8], but further studies revealed that increased D_2 levels could result from antipsychotic drug treatment[9].

It is important to emphasise that radioligand binding assays pharmacologically describe the receptor binding site but do not necessarily reflect the response generated or the function *in vivo*. The receptor's natural environment of pre- or post-synaptic membrane is altered and neuromodulatory effects from other neurotransmitter systems may be lost. To gain insight into the complexities of receptor function *in vivo*, therefore, animal models have been used. The effects of psychotropic drugs on a variety of animal behavioural paradigms has been a fruitful area of research, but extrapolation to human neuropsychiatric disorders is critically limited with, for example, no satisfactory animal models of depression or schizophrenia. Before the advent of *in vivo* imaging, receptor activity in man could only be inferred for instance from endocrinological profiles which are likely to involve multiple interactions between different receptor systems. SPECT and nuclear medicine techniques have major potential for bridging the gaps between *in vitro* techniques and animal behavioural pharmacology, and for directly investigating the neuropharmacology of neuropsychiatric disorders and their treatment *in vivo*.

In vivo receptor measurement

Traditional receptor theory has been regarded by some as relatively inapplicable to *in vivo* characterisation[6]. The law of mass action of receptor occupancy states that unbound ligand reversibly binds to its receptor at a rate dependent on the concentration of both ligand and receptor. The rate of the dissociation was proportional to the concentration of bound ligand and receptor. At equilibrium, rates of association and dissociation were equal. Clark's model of receptor occupancy also made several other assumptions — among them that the interaction between ligand and receptor was completely reversible, and that all receptors had uniform affinity and were independent of each other — many of which do not hold when delineating receptor characteristics in the brain *in vivo*. The reasons are briefly outlined in Table 1 and have been fully described elsewhere[6], and can, to some extent, be minimised by optimisation of the radioligand's pharmacology and biochemistry.

Radioligand characteristics for use in PET and SPECT

Generally, PET and SPECT ligands are synthesised and their pharmacological profile validated *in vivo* in a number of ways. Isomers of the ligand are given to test stereospecificity of ligand binding[10]. Autoradiographic *ex vivo* and *in vitro* techniques have been used to demonstrate a high correlation between the distribution of receptors by these methods and PET or SPECT[11]. Alternatively, receptor sites can be fully occupied with an unlabelled (cold) ligand known to bind specifically to the receptor of interest, before giving the radioligand e.g. lorazepam given before ^{11}C-flunitrazepam, to characterise the GABA-benzodiazepine receptor

Table 1 Characteristics of PET and SPECT radioligands which challenge the assumption of classical receptor theory[6]

1	Tracer concentrations resulting in less than full occupancy of all available receptors
2	Ligand binding to multiple receptor sites
3	Differential times to reach equilibrium in regions of interest with low and high numbers of receptors
4	Blood brain barrier permeability to ligand
5	Active metabolites of the radioligand interfering with tracer binding
6	Different ratio of white to grey matter in regions of interest
7	Presence of endogenous neurotransmitter/ligands

complex[12]. Alternatively, cold competing ligand, specific to the receptors of interest, can be given after the radioligand, displacing only the radioligand bound to the receptor of interest. This is known as a 'chaser study' and is illustrated by a specific D_2 antagonist, haloperidol, displacing the D_2 radioligand ^{123}I-IBZM from the striatum, which results in increased washout of the radioligand[13]. Thus, *in vivo* in the striatum, ^{123}I-IBZM binds to the D_2 receptor.

Table 2 describes the characteristics of an ideal ligand[6,14].

Radioligands in PET and SPECT

There are now many radioligands available for use with PET and SPECT, the pharmacological profiles of which at the receptors of interest have been well validated. Many more are under development, and some of those available are listed in Table 3.

Since the discovery of multiple dopaminergic receptors — D_1-like (D_1 and D_5) and D_2-like (D_2, D_3, D_4) — their characterisation in terms of molecular genetics and pharmacology continues[16]. Different radioligands give different results in terms of the characterisation of dopaminergic receptors in neuropsychiatric disorders, which may be explained by their distinct pharmacological profiles at the receptor subtypes. ^{11}C-raclopride, for example, previously defined as binding to D_2 receptors, is now known to bind to both D_2 and D_3. Newer ligands that can discriminate between these two subtypes are therefore required if the contribution of particular dopamine receptor subtypes to neuropsychiatric pathology is to be fully understood.

Table 2 Characteristics of an ideal PET and SPECT radioligand

1	Freely diffusible across the blood brain barrier
2	High specificity and selectivity
3	For non-specific ligands, a wide anatomic resolution
4	Low solubility or polar metabolites that do not cross the blood brain barrier
5	Rapid clearance from the blood
6	Rapid association rate
7	High and rapid clearance from non-specific sites
8	Ability to be labelled to high specific activity at about 1% saturation

Techniques for measuring in vivo receptor parameters

Although, as described, the absolute quantification of receptor parameters *in vivo* is problematic, there are several kinetic and equilibrium models that can be applied to generate indices of receptor density (Bmax) and affinity (K_D)[6,17,18]. Early mathematical modelling of radioligand uptake and clearance rates during a scanning experiment to calculate a variety of binding parameters, including K_D and Bmax, influx constants, volume of distribution and specific rate constants, was performed with PET[17,18]. Until recently, such quantification in SPECT was generally limited to empirical approaches such as ratios of activity between regions. Technical issues such as poorer resolution, attenuation and scatter and partial volume effects precluded more sophisticated modelling. Recent advances, such as the use of reference phantoms with which to generate attenuation correction factors, go some way towards overcoming these limitations, and SPECT studies are now generating binding indices comparable to those with PET studies. With ^{123}I-iomazenil SPECT, for example, the *in vivo* receptor density (Bmax) and affinity (K_D) of the GABA-benzodiazepine receptor have been measured and are in good agreement with those obtained by *in vitro* methods[19,20].

The objective of *in vivo* studies performed when validating the pharmacological profile of a radioligand at its receptor is absolute quantification. These studies are generally made in primates, since for technical or ethical considerations, comparable investigations often cannot be performed in man. Although undertaking studies in patients may put further limitations on the feasibility of scanning procedures, absolute over relative quantification may confer no additional information. For instance, changes in the affinity of a ligand for a receptor have not been found in neuropsychiatric disorders investigated by *in vitro* techniques. Rather, any changes in radioligand binding are a consequence of altered receptor density. Thus estimations of receptor density without affinity are generally sufficient for the purpose of testing hypotheses and delineating receptors of interest in neuropsychiatric disorders.

As with *in vitro* binding studies, there are two possible approaches – equilibrium or kinetic models – for the quantification of receptors in PET and SPECT. Both methods use the concept of brain compartments in which the radioligand can be distributed. After injection, the radioligand enters intra- (plasma) and extra-vascular spaces. Within the latter compartment, the radioligand may be free, non-specifically bound (e.g. to proteins) or specifically bound, and this is referred to as the three-compartment model. Specific

Table 3 A selection of ligands commonly used in receptor characterisation in SPECT and PET

Receptor system	SPECT	PET
Dopamine		
D_1	^{123}I-SCH 239482	^{11}C-SCH 23390
		^{11}C-SCH 39166
D_2	2-^{123}I-iodospiperone	N-methyl-^{11}C methyl-spiperone (NMS)
		N-^{18}F-fluoroethyl-spiperone
	^{123}I-iodolisuride	^{76}Br-bromolisuride
	^{123}I-IBZM	^{11}C raclopride
	^{123}I-epidepride	
Uptake site	^{123}I-β-CIT	^{11}C-cocaine
		^{11}C-nomifensine
		^{18}F-GBR
Serotonin		
5-HT$_2$		N-methyl-^{11}C methyl-spiperone (NMS)
	2-^{123}I-iodoketanserin	^{11}C-ketanserin
		^{18}F-setoperone
		^{18}F-altanserin
Uptake site	^{123}I-β-CIT	^{11}C-β-CIT
Monoaminergic nerve terminal		^{11}C- tetrabenzine
Acetylcholine muscarinic		
M_1, M_2, M_3	4-^{123}I-IQNB	^{11}C-scopolamine
	4-^{123}I-iododexetimide	4-^{18}F-fluorodexetimide
ACH-esterase		^{11}C-physostigimine
Opioid		
mu		^{11}C- carfentanil
mu, kappa, delta		^{11}C- diprenorphine
GABA$_A$		
Benzodiazepine	^{123}I-iomazenil	^{11}C-flumazenil

binding sites are saturable and ligands may bind reversibly or irreversibly, rapidly or slowly. Displacement with a 'cold' competitor should result in a rapid decrease in radioligand activity. It is assumed that non-specific binding in tissue is reversible, and on-off binding rates are rapid. The 'cold' competitor should have no effect on the rate of activity washout from such sites. Radioligand distribution between these compartments is time-dependent and rate constants are calculated. The time required for the radioligand to bind to all the receptors within a region is proportional to the number of receptors and, thus, the time taken to reach peak activity is longer in receptor-rich than receptor-poor regions. A full description of all the mathematical models currently used is not given here. The principles underlying equilibrium and kinetic analysis are briefly described. Some of the issues and debates pertaining to aspects of receptor quantification are discussed.

Equilibrium models

This method can only apply to reversibly bound radioligands which attain equilibrium with their receptor within the scanning procedure. Relatively few assumptions are required about the transfer between compartments. Dynamic studies of the uptake and washout of the radioligand display a curvilinear relationship, with a plateau when these two processes are assumed to be in equilibrium. Binding parameters (K_D and Bmax) can be either estimated at the peak (^{11}C-raclopride[21]) or in the plateau region (C-Ro 15 1788[22]). These are 'pseudo-equilibrium' approaches, since the concentration of the radioligand and receptor occupancy will be changing[22]. True equilibrium can be achieved by constant rather than bolus injection paradigms[20,23,24].

Crucial to the quantification of receptor number in equilibrium methods is defining and correcting for the non-specific binding component. It has been calculated for some ligands, e.g. ^{123}I-iomazenil, that this can be ignored[25], but for others, e.g. ^{11}C-flumazenil, the non-specific binding component is significant[26]. A commonly used method is to measure the activity in a region known to be devoid of receptors, in which radioligand uptake represents non-specific (free or bound to intra- and extravascular proteins) binding. Thus in PET and SPECT studies measuring D_2 receptors, radioligand activity either in the cerebellum[21] or frontal cortex[27] has been used to calculate the non-specific binding component.

Traditionally, a semiquantitative index of binding is calculated as the difference or ratio between the region of interest (ROI) and a reference region devoid of receptors[27]. Portrayed graphically, values over the plateau portion of the resulting binding curve represent the saturable component of radioligand binding i.e. the 'specific' binding capacity. Inappropriate areas chosen to represent non-specific binding can have marked effects on calculating the specific binding in the ROI. For ^{11}C-flumazenil PET, overestimation of non-specific activity by using the brain stem results in the calculation of specific binding levels up to 40% lower[24]. The reasons for this include difficulty in accurately defining the brain stem anatomically, and the fact that the brain stem is not devoid of receptors[28]. For ^{123}I-iomazenil SPECT, there are similar problems in identifying a suitable region in which to measure the non-specific binding component. White matter/ventricular regions have been used, but in addition to problems in defining such regions, differences in blood flow to white and grey matter are a concern since the non-specific binding component is known to be affected by blood flow.

An alternative approach has more recently been used to account for regional differences in blood flow which would influence the estimation of total binding capacity. Partial volume effects are also accounted for. Ratios are calculated between the uptake of radioligand at two different time points: an early time period reflecting primarily blood flow and a later time period at equilibrium, reflecting both specific and non-specific binding[29]. Although radioligand activity in the early scanning period will include elements of binding, such scans have been shown to estimate blood flow when the activity profile of ^{123}I-iomazenil is compared with the cerebral perfusion tracer, ^{99}Tc-HMPAO[30].

An important concept in *in vivo* receptor analysis is the volume of distribution. This is defined as the volume of distribution (V_D) of the tracer in the brain and is represented at equilibrium as the concentration of brain (Cb) and plasma (Cp) i.e. $V_D = Cb/Cp$. At equilibrium, the total volume of distribution is the sum of the specific and non-specific volume of distribution[23]. The specific volume of distribution is equal to the level of receptors when experiments are performed at tracer doses and when the equilibrium distribution volume is expressed relative to the free radioligand in plasma. In many studies it is used as an outcome measure[23,24,25] since it also represents B_{max}/K_D.

Multiple studies are needed to obtain the affinity of the ligand for the receptor, K_D. At least two studies are required at different levels of receptor occupancy[23]. This can be achieved with high and low specific ligand activity produced by injecting the radioligand alone (high) or with an unlabelled competitor (low). Scatchard analysis is then used to calculate Bmax and

K_D. As described, this may confer no further useful clinical or research information.

Kinetic analysis

Radioligands with very high affinity bind too avidly to permit quantification in terms of Bmax and K_D invalidating equilibrium analysis[23]. Kinetic models generate quantitative information about the receptor from estimation of rate constants between compartments. The number of compartments actually used in the model depends on the ligand used. Comparisons have been performed in a previous study[25]. The K_1 and K_2 rate constants describe the transfer of radioligand across the blood-brain barrier into and out of the compartment and represent free and non-specifically bound. K_1 is the rate of clearance from plasma to brain and K_2 the reverse. K_3 and K_4 represent the rate constants for association and dissociation from receptors, respectively. K_3 is proportional to the total number of receptors.

In the first kinetic method of receptor quantification, Mintun[31] applied the term 'binding potential' (BP). This was represented by Bmax / K_D and hence reflected both receptor density and the ligand's affinity for the receptor. This analysis took into account the particular kinetics of ^{11}C-NMS at the dopamine receptor and that in tracer amounts, the radioligand cannot occupy all the receptors to generate a true Bmax.

Equilibrium versus kinetic analysis

Comparisons between these two approaches have been performed for ^{11}C-raclopride and ^{123}I-iomazenil. Farde et al.[21] found similar Bmax and K_D values were obtained with different kinetic analyses, and with those produced by equilibrium analysis for ^{11}C-raclopride. Laruelle et al.[19,20] found both Bmax and K_D values calculated by either method in-dependently compared well with in vitro parameters. In addition, there was good agreement between kinetic and equilibrium methods in calculating Bmax.

For ^{123}I-iomazenil, however, the rate of dissociation from the receptor is slow, resulting in large errors in calculating K_4, although the K_3/K_4 ratio was stable. Thus the accuracy and choice of analysis should be validated for each radioligand. For most research and clinical applications, semiquantitative approaches produce adequate binding indices with which to allow hypothesis testing in neuropsychiatric disorders — but it is clearly important to validate these approaches against absolute measures.

Applications of PET and SPECT in neuroreceptor imaging

Receptor characterisation in neuropsychiatric disorders

The ability to measure, in vivo, receptor pharmacology is placing PET and SPECT at the forefront of research defining the psychopharmacology of neuropsychiatric disorders. Research applications include delineating specific receptor populations in neuropsychiatric disorders and exploring correlations between these and clinical indices e.g. symptom response and neuropsychological tests.

Drug challenge and occupancy studies in neuropsychiatric disorders

The effects of psychotropic drugs on neurotransmitter systems can be directly investigated in vivo. With PET and SPECT, the in vivo evaluation of drug treatment and consequently drug development is now available. These strategies depend vitally on the existence of appropriate ligands. There are several ways in which PET and SPECT can assess drug effects at a receptor system. For patients on medication, if the drug is occupying the receptor, then a radioligand with affinity for that particular receptor will be unable to bind. Hence, uptake will be low. The lower the radioligand's uptake, the more receptors are occupied by the drug. Although this is somewhat simplistic and assumes that the drug and radioligand have equivalent affinity for the receptor, it suffices for routine analysis. Using radioligands with affinity for different receptors, a drug's activity can be assessed at multiple receptors.

The relative potency of drugs at a receptor site can be evaluated and compared. Using ^{123}I-iomazenil SPECT, lorazepam at a sedating dose occupied less than 4% of the benzodiazepine receptors available[32]. Similarly, clonazepam has been shown to produce physiological effects (sleep , ataxia, prolongation of P300) at low levels of occupancy as measured by [11]C Ro15-1788-binding[33]. This confirms reports of large receptor reserves for the benzodiazepine receptor[34]. The ability of five different benzodiazepines to displace ^{123}I-iomazenil was compared in vivo[35]. Their in vivo potency in displacing the radioligand correlated reasonably well with their in vitro receptor affinities. The discrepancies (clonazepam and alprazolam) might have been due to different bioavailabilities. This highlights the advantage of in vivo methods for calculating drug potency which take pharmacokinetic issues, such as drug metabolism and lipophilicity in vivo, into account.

PET and SPECT can also be used to assess the response of an endogenous neurotransmitter to drug administration. For instance, amphetamine's ability to release dopamine has been exploited to see whether or not endogenous neurotransmitters can compete with the binding of ^{123}I-IBZM[36], ^{11}C-raclopride[37], or ^{123}I IBF[38] to D_2 receptors. Amphetamine enhanced the washout of the radioligand, thus radioligand D_2 receptor binding was reduced due to the release of dopamine from the presynaptic terminal. Validation that the increase in washout was due to dopamine release came from showing that this effect was abolished by pre-treatment with reserpine which depletes dopamine stores[36]. Other agents that increase the amount of synaptic dopamine such as GBR 12909, a dopamine reuptake inhibitor, and tetrabenazine, which release biogenic amines, also competed for ^{11}C-raclopride binding[37].

The functional interconnectivity between neurotransmitter systems can be investigated using *in vivo* receptor imaging. Striatal ^{11}C-raclopride binding was increased after enhancement of GABAergic function through administration of gamma-vinyl GABA and lorazepam[39]. Thus GABA appears to inhibit dopamine release. In contrast, reduced ^{18}F-NMS and ^{11}C-raclopride binding was seen after challenges by benzotropine and scopolamine[37,40]. This was interpreted as supporting evidence that central cholinergic blockade increases synaptic dopamine levels. To test this further, amphetamine was given to release any dopamine stores. Reduced availability of D_2 receptors for ^{18}F NMS binding was seen, suggesting that benzotropine effects on ^{18}F-NMS binding were related to endogenous dopamine release[41].

Thus, the sensitivity of D_2 radioligands to altered synaptic dopamine levels, permits study of the impact of other neurotransmitter pathways on dopaminergic function. Determination of the neurochemistry underlying side-effects can also be determined. The calcium channel blockers, flunarizine and cinnarizine, which are used to treat a variety of cerebrovascular disorders, induce parkinsonian side effects. ^{123}I-IBZM SPECT revealed that in patients receiving this medication, striatal D_2 receptor-binding availability was reduced by 14-63%[42]. The degree of reduction correlated with the severity of the parkinsonian symptoms. Thus D_2 blockade by these drugs probably underlies their parkinsonian side-effect profile. Farde *et al.*[43] and Nordstrom *et al.*[44] have also demonstrated this effect with typical antipsychotic drugs. Benzodiazepines are known to produce retrograde amnesia and cholinergic systems are involved in memory. A benzodiazepine, triazolam, and ^{11}C NMPB (muscarinic cholinergic receptor ligand) PET were

used to investigate whether or not the amnesic effect involved changes in the cholinergic system[45]. Acutely, triazolam reduced ^{11}C NMPB binding, which could indicate an indirect mechanism for memory impairment by these drugs. Applications of these methods in specific neuropsychiatric diseases are discussed under the relevant sections.

In vivo receptor imaging in neuropsychiatric disorders

The following is a review of PET and SPECT studies elucidating the psychopharmacology of neuro-psychiatric disorders. Both the delineation of abnormalities in receptors and the contribution of *in vivo* imaging to drug evaluation and development is discussed.

Epilepsy

Current models of epilepsy propose that there is an imbalance between excitation and inhibition in the brain. GABA is the principle and ubiquitous inhibitory neurotransmitter in the brain. Clinically, many anti-convulsants enhance GABAergic neurotransmission. Animal and post mortem studies have demonstrated reduced levels of GABA-benzodiazepine receptor in epileptic foci, and have been reproduced by PET and SPECT studies[46,47].

Savic[48], using ^{11}C-flumazenil PET, reported a significant reduction in benzodiazepine receptors in epileptic foci compared to the contralateral homotopic reference region. Seizure frequency has been found to correlate with the reduction in the level of benzo-diazepine receptors. Van Huffelen *et al.*[49] reported over 80% agreement in asymmetry between a ^{123}I-iomazenil SPECT scan and EEG findings. In people with temporal lobe epilepsy, hypometabolism, as measured with ^{18}F-fluorodeoxyglucose, occurs in areas outside epileptic foci, although decreased GABA-benzodiazepine receptor numbers are restricted to the foci[50]. Using ^{123}I-iomazenil SPECT, a reduction in GABA-benzodiazepine receptor levels is reported in epileptogenic areas with no alteration in blood flow[51]. Thus, blood flow or cerebral metabolism appears to be a state marker for peri-ictal activity, while GABA-ben-zodiazepine receptor level may be a stable trait marker.

In addition to giving us information about the possible role of the GABAergic system in the aetiology of epilepsy, *in vivo* imaging has an important, clinically useful application. Neurosurgical treatment is sometimes proposed for severe, intractable cases of epilepsy. Localisation of the focus or foci has previously used PET or SPECT assessment of blood flow or cerebral metabolism. There is now a strong case for quantifying GABA-benzodiazepine receptor levels, since PET and SPECT studies of this receptor appear to be more specific and more accurate in determining epileptic foci than previous methods. *In vivo* receptor imaging has been recommended for clinical use[51,52].

Importantly for such a role, concomitant use of a benzodiazepine, clobazepam, or phenytoin therapy has not been shown to interfere with assessing GABA-benzodiazepine receptor levels in general and partial epilepsy[53,54]. In absence seizures, however, the use of sodium valproate resulted in a reduction of receptor levels[55].

Absence seizures appear to have a different pathophysiological basis to other types of epilepsy, in that use of GABAergic enhancing drugs increases seizure activity. In childhood and juvenile absence epilepsy, no abnormalities of the GABA-benzo-diazepine receptor have been found using ^{11}C-flumazenil PET[55]. Alternative hypotheses include a role for endogenous opioids in such seizure activity. ^{11}C-diprenorphine PET studies showed that endo-genous opioids were released during serial absence seizures in the association area of the brain[56]. In contrast, no changes in ^{11}C-diprenorphine activity were reported in juvenile and childhood absence epilepsy when they were seizure-free[57].

The opiate system has also been investigated in other types of epilepsy. Increased ^{11}C-carfentamil (mu subtype) uptake has been reported in epileptic foci in the temporal neocortex and decreased uptake in the ipsilateral amygdala[58]. In contrast, no differences were seen in the uptake of ^{11}C-diprenorphine (mu, kappa, delta subtypes)[59].

^{123}I-IBZM SPECT has been used to investigate the role of the D_2 receptor in epileptic psychoses. In those epileptic patients with psychosis, decreased striatal ^{123}I-IBZM binding was seen compared with non-psychotic patients[60]. In this study, patients were being treated with a variety of anticonvulsant drugs although none were on vigabatrin, an anticonvulsant associated with the development of psychosis, which had been shown in a previous study to reduce ^{123}I-IBZM binding[61]. These studies support a role for dopaminergic mechanisms in the development of psychosis associated with epilepsy.

In conclusion, SPECT and PET receptor imaging has allowed testing of the hypotheses concerning the aetiology and neuropathology of a number of different epilepsies. An important clinical role in identifying the epileptic focus/foci is emerging.

Dementia

Deficits in many neurotransmitter systems have been found in dementia. Reduced function within the cholinergic system has been the principal focus of research both aetiologically and in terms of drug development. There have been many PET and SPECT studies assessing blood flow and cerebral metabolism in dementias, with such investigations beginning to be used clinically in aiding the diagnosis of different dementia types[62]. Few studies have looked at neuroreceptor changes *in vivo*, however.

Using ^{123}I-QNB, a marker of muscarinic type cholinergic receptors, a single patient study reported a slight decrease in ^{123}I-QNB binding[63]. However dramatic decreases in blood flow may have altered distribution of the ligand contributing to this decrease. Another study of severely demented individuals found decreased levels of ^{123}I-QNB uptake in the superior frontal and parietal regions in two subjects, but in the rest of the sample[6] any decrease could be accounted for by reduced cerebral perfusion[64]. Weinberger *et al.*[65] also reported focal cortical deficits in ^{123}I-QNB levels in the frontal and post temporal cortex in some subjects with Alzheimer's disease and anteriorly in two patients with Pick's disease.

Other receptor systems studied with PET include $5HT_2$ receptors with ^{18}F-setoperone and the GABA-benzodiazepine receptor with ^{11}C-flumazenil. A significant reduction in $5HT_2$ receptors was found in several cortical regions of patients with Alzheimer's disease[66], but no significant changes were found in the GABA-benzodiazepine receptor[67].The dopaminergic system has been investigated in different types of dementia using ^{123}I-IBZM SPECT. A comparison between dementia of the frontal lobe type (DFT) and Alzheimer's dementia reported relative frontal hypoperfusion (^{99}Tc-HMPAO) in both types, but a greater reduction in ^{123}I-IBZM binding in the former[68]. This suggests more pronounced loss of frontocortical dopaminergic systems in DFT than in Alzheimer's. A study comparing striatal D_2 receptors using ^{123}I-IBZM SPECT in patients with Alzheimer's and Lewy Body dementia, reported significantly lower receptor levels in the latter. Levels in those with Alzheimer's disease were comparable to those in healthy controls[69].

Use of neuroreceptor imaging in dementia is in its infancy and can be complicated by alterations in blood flow and perfusion, as has been described. Increasingly, different types of dementia e.g. Alzheimer's, vascular, and Lewy Body, are recognised, and neuroreceptor imaging could help in differentiating them and further elucidating their neuropathologies and aetiologies. Pharmacodynamic studies looking at changes in the cholinergic system after treatment with drugs which enhance cholinergic activity would be of great interest.

Addictions

Pharmacologically, different drugs of abuse act through a variety of neurotransmitter systems e.g. heroin – opiate, amphetamine – monoamine. However, drug addiction is also a result of the fact that the drugs are powerful reinforcers. A midbrain-forebrain-extrapyramidal circuit involving dopamine, opiate and GABA projections has been proposed as the neuroanatomical and psychopharmacological correlate of the concept of reward[70]. *In vivo* imaging can be used to look at both the specific receptor system for individual drugs and this reward loop.

Alcohol

The GABA-benzodiazepine receptor has become an intense focus of research since alcohol shares many pharmacological actions with both barbiturates and benzodiazepines, the receptor binding sites of which lie within this complex. Post mortem studies in alcoholics looking at the GABA-benzodiazepine receptor have been inconclusive[71,72], but functional changes in the GABA-benzodiazepine receptor have been inferred from studies of glucose metabolism and PET and non-alcohol dependent people with and without a family history of alcohol dependency[73,74].

A PET study demonstrated that, acutely, alcohol did not affect binding of ^{11}C-flumazenil[75]. A later study in 5 recently detoxified alcoholics reported wide variability in the number of benzodiazepine receptors, with no change in affinity in the frontal, temporal, occipital and cerebellar cortices[76]. Two patients with higher receptor levels had lower daily alcohol consumption, consumed wine rather than spirits, had a longer drinking episode before detoxification, and suffered more pronounced withdrawal symptoms. This suggests that, with reservations given the small number of subjects, GABAergic abnormalities may be present and could relate to the clinical course of alcohol dependency.

Involvement of the dopaminergic system in alcohol dependence has been investigated in other research spheres. In particular, the D_2 receptor has been the focus of genetic studies. One PET study with ^{11}C-raclopride found decreased striatal D_2 receptor density and affinity in alcoholics who had been abstinent for at least a week. Whether this was primary or secondary to alcohol abuse remained unanswered, but it was suggested that the finding supported a role for D_2

dopaminergic D_2 function in dependence[77]. An alternative approach has been to assess striatal dopamine reuptake sites using β-CIT SPECT in alcoholics abstinent for at least 2 months[78]. Altered striatal dopamine reuptake sites were found, but the direction depended on whether they were violent or non-violent. Lower levels of the reuptake site were reported in non-violent alcoholics, with slightly higher levels in violent alcoholics compared with control subjects. This intriguing finding has yet to be extended to look at violence in other addictive behaviours.

Cocaine

Cocaine inhibits both catecholamine and serotonin reuptake into the presynaptic neuron, but its inhibition of dopamine reuptake appears crucial to the behavioural effects of cocaine[79]. The distribution of the kinetics of cocaine have been examined by ^{11}C-cocaine PET[80]. The tracer showed maximal accumulation in the brain 4-8 min post-injection, with a heterogenous distribution, primarily to the basal ganglia. Pretreatment with a dopamine transporter inhibitor, nomifensine, decreased ^{11}C-cocaine uptake. The same effect was not seen with inhibitors of serotonergic or noradrenergic uptake, supporting evidence that dopamine is fundamental in mediating the effects of cocaine. The timing of cocaine's euphorogenic effects corresponded to binding and release of cocaine from the transporter[81]. A recent study has critically shown that metabolites of ^{11}C-cocaine do not contribute to the PET image obtained[82]. This is significant, since some metabolites bind preferentially to serotonergic uptake sites. Studies of the dopaminergic system after detoxification in chronic cocaine abusers revealed a decrease in ^{18}F-DOPA[83], suggesting reduced dopamine uptake and synthesis. Decreased D_2 receptor levels have also been shown with ^{18}F-NMS, which were maintained for 4 months and were associated with a specific decrease in frontal cortex metabolism[84,85].

The phenomenon of alcohol-enhancing behavioural and toxic effects of cocaine has been investigated. No change in the distribution and pharmacokinetics of ^{11}C-cocaine was found, suggesting that, acutely, this enhancement is not caused by cocaine residing longer in the brain[86].

Amphetamine

Amphetamine acts by releasing stores of noradrenaline and dopamine and to a lesser extent inhibits their reuptake. Use of amphetamine and its derivatives are associated with inducing psychosis. This response has been the basis of many animal models of psychosis, including schizophrenia. ^{11}C-NMS PET has been used to investigate the role of the striatal D_2 receptor and frontal cortical $5HT_2$ receptor in mediating amphetamine-induced psychosis. In people who had experienced methamphetamine-related psychosis, no changes were seen in striatal D_2 receptors, but there was an increase, albeit statistically insignificant, in frontal cortical $5HT_2$ receptors. However the ratio of D_2 to $5HT_2$ receptors was decreased, suggesting altered relative activity may underlie the induction of psychosis[87].

Opiate

Despite two ligands that bind to opiate receptors, ^{11}C-carfentamil and ^{11}C-diprenorphine, no studies have yet been performed in opiate addicts.

Hepatic encephalopathy

Increased GABAergic neurotransmission is involved in hepatic encephalopathy, probably due to the generation of endogenous benzodiazepines[88]. These would be expected to interfere with the exogenous radioligand used to assess receptor number, and result in diminished uptake. However, both PET and SPECT studies, which excluded patients with alcohol-induced cirrhosis, have failed to show this[89,90] – possibly due to the concentration of any endogenous ligands being too low to be detected by *in vivo* imaging. Interestingly, Cluckie *et al.*[90] showed that the uptake of ^{123}I-iomazenil was related to albumin levels, with those with low levels (<35 mg/dl) having higher brain uptake. This reinforces the importance of calculating the free ligand available in interpreting the uptake of radioligands.

Movement disorders

Parkinson's disease and parkinsonism

Parkinson's disease (PD) is associated with degeneration and decreased dopamine in the nigrostriatal pathway. Disruption of this pathway has been shown using ^{18}F-DOPA, with a reduced uptake of 40% in the putamen and of 80% in the caudate[91,92].

The pattern and extent of ^{18}F-DOPA in the striatum can be used to differentiate between Parkinson's disease and 2 other diagnoses which can be difficult to separate clinically, namely multiple system atrophy (MSA) and Steele Richardson Olszewski (SRO), or supranuclear palsy. Accurate diagnosis has obvious importance for prognosis and treatment. Compared with PD, in supranuclear palsy, where nigrostriatal projections are uniformly affected, a similar reduction of ^{18}F-DOPA uptake is seen in the anterior and posterior putamen, but a greater reduction is seen in the caudate[91]. A later study showed that ^{18}F-DOPA reliably discriminated normal from parkinsonian patients and PD from SRO, but that it was not so reliable in distinguishing between PD and MSA[93].

Other markers of the pre-synaptic neuron include ^{11}C-nomifensine and [123]I β-CIT. In PD, ^{11}C-nomifensine uptake is decreased to 40% of that of normal subjects, with relative preservation of activity in the caudate nucleus[92]. Moreover, correlation was shown between asymmetries in movement, ^{18}F-DOPA and ^{11}C-nomifensine activities[92]. In patients with PD, the levels of striatal activity of [123]I β-CIT were reduced, reflecting a 65% loss of presynaptic sites[94]. Consistent with neuropathological studies, a greater loss was seen in the caudate compared with the putamen. Moreover, losses were greater in the striatum contralateral to the side of the body which initially showed symptoms. It is suggested that [123]I β-CIT SPECT imaging has good enough sensitivity for the detection of small changes in dopaminergic activity in the striatum for clinical use in the early diagnosis of PD[95].

With respect to postsynaptic receptors, one study showed no differences in striatal D_1 receptor levels in PD patients with untreated hemiparkinsonism[96]. However, the D_2 receptor is thought to be the receptor to primarily mediate dopaminergic effects on movement. In untreated PD, ^{11}C-NMS revealed no change in striatal D_2 receptor levels[97]. Two studies using ^{11}C-raclopride have shown increased D_2 receptors in the striatum, but also much variation, with some individuals showing no increase[98,99]. In patients with asymmetric PD, D_2 receptors in the putamen contralateral to the motor disability were 10-15% higher than those in the ipsilateral putamen[100,101]. Sawle *et al.*[102] reported that putamen ^{11}C-raclopride uptake was inversely correlated with ^{18}F-DOPA uptake, suggesting upregulation of D_2 receptors in response to decreased pre-synaptic input.

In treated PD, PET and SPECT studies report a decrease in striatal D_2 receptors, whichever radioligand is used[97,98,103,104]. This may be due to the receptor being occupied by the dopamimetic therapy, or because treatment results in a down-regulation of the receptor. Either mechanism may be operating, however oral lisuride, but not L-DOPA therapy, has been shown to reduce ^{11}C-raclopride uptake in the putamen and caudate[105]. The decrease was reversible on lisuride withdrawal, so it appears that the effect was due to competition D_2 receptor sites rather than absolute changes in receptor number. Knowledge of D_2 receptor status may not only help with differential diagnosis but may also predict responsiveness to dopamimetic drugs and help elucidate whether symptoms are due to progression of dopaminergic neuronal loss or a change in D_2 receptor function. Dyskinesia, for example, results from enhanced activity at the D_2 receptor, rather than further neuronal loss.

Clinically, an apomorphine challenge is used to predict the responsiveness of the dopaminergic system in parkinsonism to dopamimetic drugs. A large SPECT study has shown patients who did not respond to apomorphine had lower levels of striatal ^{123}I-IBZM activity than those who did[106]. ^{123}I-IBZM activity predicted responsivity to apomorphine or dopamimetics in about 90% of patients. Patients with clinical diagnoses of progressive nuclear palsy or MSA had reduced ^{123}I-IBZM uptake, which is in accordance with the classic clinical teaching that dopamimetic drugs are ineffective in the treatment of these disorders.

In vivo receptor imaging has a role in the evaluation and development of new therapeutic interventions in PD. Monoamine oxidase B (MAO-B) inhibitors are used in the early treatment of PD. Fowler *et al.* (1993) used the MAO-B tracer ^{11}C L-deprenyl to determine the degree and reversibility of human brain MAO-B inhibition[107]. A MAO-B inhibitor such as RO 19 6237 at a dose of 0.55 mg/kg every 12 h produced a 95% inhibition of brain MAO-B activity, which resolved 36 h after drug discontinuation. Routtinen *et al.*[108] found that peripheral COMT inhibition by drugs such as nitecapone and entacopne increase the bioavailability of ^{18}F-DOPA to the brain. Use of foetal mesencephalic transplants to treat PD has been increasingly realised. Neuroreceptor imaging is well placed to assess the safety and efficacy of the procedure. In some patients, increased ^{18}F-DOPA uptake at sites of implantation parallelled clinical improvement[109,110]. Issues and criticisms surrounding use of ^{18}F-DOPA in this procedure have been recently reviewed[111].

Aside from the many research applications of *in vivo* neuroreceptor imaging, there are potential clinical applications in parkinsonism. These have recently been discussed and include early diagnosis, predicting response to drug treatment or transplant, and distinguishing between different diagnoses which are clinically similar, such as PD and MSA[95,111,112].

Gilles de la Tourette's syndrome

Gilles de la Tourette's syndrome (GTS) is characterised by vocal and motor tics whose neurochemical basis is unknown. The dopaminergic system is likely to be involved, since dopamine antagonists such as haloperidol

decrease tic severity. No change in D_2 receptor levels was seen between controls and unmedicated GTS subjects using ^{123}I-IBZM[113]. Those on haloperidol showed lower levels of ^{123}I-IBZM activity, reflecting drug occupancy of D_2 receptors. Absence of D_2 receptor changes has been confirmed in a more recent study using ^{11}C-raclopride PET[114]. In addition, no changes were seen in ^{18}F-DOPA uptake. Thus, no presynaptic or postsynaptic dopaminergic dysfunction has been shown.

Huntington's disease

Huntington's disease involves degeneration of the basal ganglia. PET and SPECT studies have shown marked reductions bilaterally of D_2 binding[104] and loss of GABAergic binding sites[115]. Such scanning protocols may be useful in diagnosis since loss of D_2 receptors occurred before physical symptoms.

Depression

There are few *in vivo* receptor imaging studies compared with those on blood flow and cerebral perfusion. However, with ligands becoming available for discriminating dopamine and serotonin transporters and receptor subtypes, many hypotheses can now be tested *in vivo*.

Presynaptic function in patients with unipolar depression and mixed drug histories has been studied by measuring uptake of dopamine and serotonin precursors, ^{11}C-L-DOPA and ^{11}C-5-hydroxy-tryptophan(HTP)[116]. Kinetic analysis revealed decreased uptake of both precursors across the blood-brain barrier. Increased use of ^{11}C-5-HTP but not DOPA was seen in the inferomedial prefrontal cortex, more so on the left than the right. Of note in healthy volunteers, tryptophan depletion did not enhance 5-HTP uptake. Decreased D_1 receptor binding in the frontal cortex has been reported using SCH 23390 PET in the dopaminergic system[117]. No changes were seen in D_2 receptor levels in the striatum in people with bipolar disorder using ^{11}C-NMS PET[118]. The dopaminergic system has also been studied in sleep deprivation, which has been used for many years to treat depression. Comparing healthy controls with depressed patients who responded and those that did not, a ^{123}I-IBZM SPECT study showed that responders had reduced levels of ^{123}I-IBZM binding[119]. This suggests that, in those patients who responded to sleep deprivation, dopamine release was enhanced.

The newer generation of antidepressants are the so-called 'serotonin specific reuptake inhibitors' (SSRI). One SPECT study using 2-^{123}I-ketanserin to label 5HT receptors reported higher uptake in the parietal cortex and a greater right-to-left asymmetry in the infero-frontal region of depressed patients[120]. The same group using ^{123}I-IBZM found increased D_2 labelling in the striatum/cerebellar ratio in unipolar depressives[121].

The potential of SPECT/PET neuroreceptor imaging is illustrated by an *in vivo* receptor autoradiographic study. The occupancy of the reuptake site by three SSRIs, fluoxetine, sertraline, and paroxetine, has been studied in mice with ^{125}I-RTI 55[122]. The rate and the duration of occupancy correlated with their pharmacological profiles.

Schizophrenia

PET and SPECT neuroreceptor imaging in schizophrenia has been an extremely fruitful area of research. Not only has the classical dopaminergic hypothesis been tested *in vivo*, but the activity of antipsychotic drugs at different receptors, and the relationship of efficacy and side-effects to receptor occupancy has been explored. Radioligands most commonly used label the D_2 receptor. As has already been described, the discovery of multiple subtypes means that these D_2 ligands may have different profiles at the D_2-like receptors, D_3 and D_4. This might account for the different distributions between the radioligands used. PET and SPECT have an important role in drug development in schizophrenia. This section will be separated into receptor studies of the pathology of schizophrenia and those aimed at drug evaluation and development.

Receptor studies

The classical hypothesis of schizophrenia postulates overactivity within the dopaminergic system. The fact that the potency of antipsychotic drugs correlated with their affinity for the D_2 receptor provided strong support for this theory[123]. The earliest study in schizophrenic patients using [77]Br-bromospiperone reported an 11% increase in the striatum to cerebellar ratio of D_2 receptors[124]. Although antipsychotic-free at the time of the scan, many had previously been treated with antipsychotic medication. This is an important confounder, since *in vitro* such treatment has been shown to result in upregulation of D_2 receptors[9]. In a series of studies of never-medicated schizophrenics using ^{11}C-NMS PET, a two- to three-fold increase in striatal D_2 receptor binding was reported[118,125,126]. However, using ^{11}C-raclopride and saturation rather than kinetic analysis to determine D_2 receptor levels, Farde *et al.*[127] reported no significant differences between drug-naive schizophrenics and healthy controls. This lack of upregulation was also described

by studies using [76]Br bromospiperone[128] and [76]Br bromolisuride[129]. These conflicting results generated much debate and highlight the differences that different methods of quantification and patient populations can bring about.

However, more subtle changes were seen in these studies. A lack of age-related decline in D_2 receptors[128,129] and a greater asymmetry of D_2 receptors with higher levels in the left than right putamen, but not the caudate, were observed[127]. More recently, a ^{123}I-IBZM SPECT study in a group of never-medicated[17] schizophrenic patients who had been antipsychotic-free for over five years[3], similarly found no overall increases in striatal D_2 receptor density, a male-specific left-lateralised asymmetry, and a lack of age-related decline in striatal D_2 receptors[27].

Schizophrenia is a heterogenous disorder with multiple symptoms. Conflicting results may be a reflection of this. Not only are age, sex, laterality and medication status important confounders, but symptom profiles should also be taken into account[27,126]. For instance, in a group of schizophrenics with predominantly negative features, striatal D_2 receptors negatively correlated with blunted affect and alogia[130].

In vivo neuroimaging has provided some support that there is dopaminergic overactivity in schizophrenia. However this evidence comes from using ligands to label the D_2 receptor predominantly in the striatum. The classical hypothesis in fact proposed overactivity within the mesolimbic pathway, not the nigrostriatal pathway. The same D_2 ligands do not visualise extra-striatal receptors well, but the synthesis of ^{123}I-epidepride, a newly developed D_2 ligand, means that extra-striatal D_2 receptors can now be imaged[131], and studies are currently underway using this ligand to quantify extra-striatal D_2 receptors in schizophrenia and their relationship to symptoms.

Other hypotheses about the neurochemical aetiology of schizophrenia have been postulated in the light of inconclusive evidence for the classical dopaminergic hypothesis. Comprehensive pharmacological charac-terisation of clinically efficacious antipsychotic drugs has focussed attention on other neurotransmitter systems, in particular the serotonergic system. One alternative hypothesis proposes that there is a deficit in GABAergic function[132]. In a study of schizophrenics, both medicated and unmedicated, using ^{123}I-iomazenil, activity was reduced in the left medial temporal lobe, which was related to the severity of hallucinations and delusions[133]. This adds to the considerable weight of evidence proposing that abnormalities in the left temporal lobe are fundamental to the psychopathology of schizophrenia.

Drug evaluation and development

Clinically, the potency of antipsychotic drugs was thought to be related to their D_2 affinity. Farde *et al.*[21] using ^{11}C-raclopride PET first showed that treated schizophrenia patients had 84-90% occupancy of the D_2 receptor in their putamen and later went on to report 65-85% occupancy by several different classes of typical antipsychotics. The degree of D_2 occupancy has been correlated with clinical improvement and plasma haloperidol levels[44,134]. After a single dose of haloperidol, a typical antipsychotic, in healthy men, D_2 receptor occupancy was high (>70%) at 3 h and remained so for 27 h[135]. Clinically, an antipsychotic effect from such treatment is not apparent for days to weeks. These results indicate that insufficient D_2 blockade cannot account for the latency. Interestingly though, a side-effect of the medication, akathisia, only occurred at times of maximal occupancy of both D_2 and D_1 receptors[136]. This is important information for the development of new antipsychotic drugs with fewer side-effects.

About 30% of patients do not fully respond to antipsychotic medication[137]. Comparing non-responders and responders in 3 different PET and SPECT studies using a variety of D_2 ligands has shown that the poor response is not due to low D_2 occupancy by antipsychotics[27,138,139,140]. Interestingly, an ^{123}I-IBZM SPECT study revealed that D_2 receptor blockade by antipsychotics was greater in those that responded to treatment than those that did not[141]. Thus, SPECT may be used to provide prognostic information. There is a group of antipsychotic drugs known as 'atypical' due to their low propensity to induce extrapyramidal side-effects[142]. One such atypical, clozapine, has been shown to be clinically efficacious with low D_2 receptor blockade[140,143]. This characteristic may be due to a number of different mechanisms, e.g. concomitant D_1, anticholinergic or serotonergic activity[142]. Investigating its activity at other receptors, clozapine resulted in up to 50% blockade of D_1 receptors[43]. In comparison, haloperidol, a typical antipsychotic drug with high occupancy of D_2 receptors, had zero occupancy of D_1 receptors. Clozapine also has very high occupancy of the $5HT_2$ receptor with ^{11}C NMS PET[144]. This combination of activity at multiple receptor sites may account for clozapine's distinctive treatment profile.

The extrapyramidal side-effects (EPS) of antipsychotic medication are common and can be as devastating as schizophrenia itself. Drug compliance can be severely compromised because of them. EPS are related to the degree of D_2 occupancy in the basal ganglia, with a threshold of 70-80%[44]. Patients with lower levels of occupancy still responded clinically in terms of their

psychosis, but escaped such side-effects. With clozapine, D_2 occupancy was low at 38-63%[143]. These studies have been important in showing that increasing doses of antipsychotic medication may result in debilitating side-effects and not confer any additional antipsychotic effect.

Dysfunction within the serotonergic system in schizophrenia is attracting much attention, since activity at $5HT_2$ receptors may account for the low incidence of EPS. Neuroreceptor PET and SPECT imaging is playing an important role in elucidating the pharmacological profile of new drugs.

Risperidone, another atypical antipsychotic, has a high affinity for both D_2 and $5HT_2$ receptors *in vitro*. Using ^{11}C-raclopride PET to measure striatal D_2 and ^{11}C-NMS PET for neocortical $5HT_2$ receptors, 1 mg of risperidone in healthy volunteers resulted in 50% and 60% occupancy respectively[145]. In schizophrenics receiving clinical doses of risperidone of 4-14 mg, an ^{123}I-IBZM study showed a high level of D_2 occupancy[146], comparable to that in patients on 'typical' antipsychotic medication, but higher than that in patients on clozapine. Remoxipride, another atypical anti-psychotic, showed similarly high occupancy of the striatal D_2 receptor. If, as proposed earlier by Farde *et al.*[21], D_2 occupancy does relate to EPS, then this does not hold true for these atypical drugs[21]. A recent study has used PET to look at receptor occupancy in healthy controls who are poor metabolisers of risperidone metabolites[147], and found that D_2 and $5HT_2$ receptor occupancy was greater and lengthier after 1 mg of risperidone than in normal metabolisers, suggesting that the metabolites are active and may contribute to this drug's clinical profile.

[11]C raclopride PET has been used to establish a minimum dose with which a novel antipsychotic drug, CP-88,059-01, can occupy 65-85% — a degree of occupancy chosen on the basis of Farde's studies (see above). A single dose between 20 and 40 mg produced the required level of occupancy[148], emphasising the power of *in vivo* imaging in enabling the definition of drug dosage regimens *in vivo*.

Conclusions

In vivo receptor measurement by PET and SPECT is a powerful tool in elucidating the aetiology and neurochemistry of neuropsychiatric disorders. In addition, the pharmacological profile, including the side-effects, of psychotropic drugs can be defined. Thus, finally, it is possible to relate neurochemistry to behaviour in living human subjects.

References

1   Langley, J.N. On the physiology of salivary secretion II. On the mutual antagonism of atropin and pilocarpin having special reference to their relations in the submaxillary gland of the cat. *J. Physiol.* 1878, 1, 339

2   Erlich, P. On immunity with special reference to cell life. Croonian Lecture. *Proc. Royal Soc. London* 1900, 66, 424

3   Dale, H.H. On the action of ergotoxine : with special reference to the existence of sympathetic vasodilators. *J. Physiol.* 1914, 65, 219

4   Alquist, R. A study of adrenoreceptors. *Am. J. Physiol.* 1948, 153, 586

5   Young, W.S. and Kuhar, M.J. A new method for receptor autoradiography : 3H opioid receptor in rat brain. *Br. Res.* 1979, 179, 255

6   Kerwin, R.W. and Pilowsky, L. Traditional receptor theory and its application to neuroreceptor measurements in functional imaging. *Eur. J. Nucl. Med.* 1995, 22, 699

7   Taylor, P. and Insel, P.A. Molecular basis of pharmacological selectivity in 'Principles of drug action', (Eds. Pratt and Taylor), 1990, p.1

8   Owen, F., Cross, A.J., Crow, T.J. *et al.* Increased dopamine receptor sensitivity in schizophrenia. *Lancet* 1978, ii, 799

9   Mackay, A.V., Iversen, L.L. and Rossor, M. Increased brain dopamine and dopamine receptors in schizophrenia. *Arch. Gen. Psychiatr.* 1982, 39, 991

10 Kung, H.F., Pan, S., Kung, M-P. *et al.* In vitro and in vivo evaluation of ^{123}I-IBZM: a potential CNS D2 dopamine receptor imaging agent. *J. Nucl. Med.* 1989, 30, 88

11 Sybirska, E., Al-Tikriti, M., Zoghi, S.S. *et al.* SPECT imaging of the benzodiazepine receptor: Autoradiographic comparison of receptor density and radioligand distribution. *Synapse* 1992, 12, 119

12 Comar, D., Maziere, M., Godot, J.M. *et al.* Visualisation of ^{11}C-flunitrazepam displacement in the brain of a live baboon. *Nature* 1979, 280, 329

13 Seibyl, J. P., Woods, S.W., Zoghbi, S.S. *et al.* Dynamic SPECT imaging of dopamine D2 receptors in human subjects with iodine ^{123}I-IBZM. *J. Nucl. Med.* 1992, 33, 1964

14 Stocklin, G. Tracers for metabolic imaging of brain and heart. *Eur. J. Nuclear Med.* 1992, 19, 527

15 Verhoeff, N.P.L.G. Ligands for neuroreceptor imaging by SPECT and PET in Nuclear Medicine in Clinical Diagnosis and Treatment', (Eds. I.P.C. Murray and P.J. Ell), 1994, p. 483

16 Seeman, P. and van Tol, H.H.M. Dopamine receptor pharmacology. *TiPS* 1994, 15, 264

17 Dolan, R., Bench, C. and Friston, K. Positron emission tomography in psychopharmacology. *International Review of Psychiatry* 1990, 2, 427

18 Sedvall, G., Farde, L., Persson, A. and Wiesel, F-A. Imaging of neurotransmitter receptors in the living human brain. *Arch. Gen. Psychiatr.* 1986, 43, 995

19 Laruelle, M., Baldwin, R.M., Rattner, Z. *et al.* SPECT quantification of [^{123}I] iomazenil binding to benzodiazepine receptors in nonhuman primates: I Kinetic modelling of single bolus experiments. *J. Cereb. Blood Flow Metab.* 1994, 14, 439

20 Laruelle, M., Abi-Dargham, A., Al-Tikriti, M.S. *et al.* SPECT quantification of [^{123}I] iomazenil binding to benzodiazepine receptors in nonhuman primates: II Equilibrium analysis of constant infusion experiments and correlation with in vitro parameters. *J. Cereb. Blood Flow Metab.* 1994, 14, 453

21 Farde, L., Eriksson, L., Blomqvist, G. and Halldin, C. Kinetic analysis of central [^{11}C] raclopride binding to D2 dopamine receptors studied by PET - A comparison to the equilibrium analysis. *J. Cereb. Blood Flow Metab.* 1989, 9, 696

22 Pappata, S., Samson, Y., Chavoix, C. *et al.* Regional specific binding of [^{11}C]RO 15 1788 to central type benzodiazepine receptors in human brain : Quantitative evaluation by PET. *J. Cereb. Blood Flow Metab.* 1988, 8, 304

23 Lassen, N.A. Neuroreceptor quantitation in vivo by the steady state principle using constant infusion or bolus injection of radioactive tracers. *J. Cereb. Blood Flow Metab.* 1992, 12, 709

24 Lassen, N.A., Bartenstein, P.A., Lammertsma, A.A. *et al.* Benzodiazepine receptor quantification in vivo in humans using [^{11}C] flumazenil and PET : Application of steady state principle. *J. Cereb. Blood Flow Metab.* 1995, 15, 152

25 Abi-Dargham, A., Gandelman, M., Zoghbi, S.S. *et al..* Reproducibility of SPECT measurement of benzodiazepine receptors in human brain with iodine-123-iomazenil *J. Nucl. Med.* 1995, 36, 167

26 Litton, J-E., Hall, H. and Pauli, S. Saturation analysis in PET - Analysis of errors due to imperfect reference regions. *J. Cereb. Blood Flow Metab.* 1994, 14, 358

27 Pilowsky, L.S., Costa, D.C., Ell, P.J. *et al.* D2 receptor binding in the basal ganglia of antipsychotic free schizophrenic patients - a ^{123}I IBZM single photon emission tomography (SPECT) study. *Br. J. Psychiatr.* 1993, 11

28 Mans, A.M., Kukulka, K.M., McAvoy, K.J. and Rokosz, N.C. Regional distribution and kinetics of three sites on the GABA$_A$ receptor: lack of effect of portacaval shunting. *J. Cereb. Blood Flow Metab.* 1992, 12, 334

29 Busatto, G.F., Pilowsky, L.S., Costa, D.C. *et al. In vivo* imaging of GABAA receptors using sequential whole-volume iodine-123-iomazenil single-photon emission tomography. *Eur. J. Nucl. Med.* 1995, 22, 1

30 Ebmeier, K.P., Lawrie, S.M., O'Caroll, R.E. *et al.* Benzodiazepine binding to the GABAA receptor in schizophrenia - A study using single photon emission tomography (SPET or SPECT) with 123I-iomazenil. *J. Psychopharmacol.* 1995, 12, 177

31 Mintun, M.A., Raichle, M.E., Kilbourn, M.R. *et al.* A quantitative model for the in vivo assessment of drug binding sites with positron emission tomography. *Ann. Neurol.* 1984, 15

32 Sybirska, E., Seibyl, J.P., Bremner, J.D. *et al.* ^{123}I-iomazenil SPECT imaging demonstrates significant benzodiazepine receptor reserve in human and nonhuman primate brain. *Neuropharmacology* 1993, 32, 671

33 Shinotoh, H., Iyo, M., Yamada, T. *et al.* Detection of benzodiazepine receptor occupancy in the human brain by positron emission tomography. *Psychopharmacology* 1989, 99, 202

34 Haefely, W. and Polc, P. Physiology of GABA enhancement by benzodiazepines and barbiturates in 'Benzodiazepine/GABA receptors and Cl-channel. Structural and Functional properties', (Eds. R.W. Ohlsen and J.G. Venter), 1986, p. 97

35 Innis, R.B., Al-Tikriti, M.S., Zoghbi, S.S. *et al.* SPECT imaging of the benzodiazepine receptor : Feasibility of in vivo potency measurements from stepwise displacement curves. *J. Nucl. Med.* 1991, 32, 1754

36 Innis, R.B., Malison, R.T., Al-Tikriti, M. *et al.* Amphetamine-stimulated dopamine release competes in vivo for ^{123}I]IBZM binding to the D2 receptor in nonhuman primates. 1992

37 Dewey, S.L., Smith, G.S., Logan, J. *et al.* Striatal binding of the PET ligand ^{11}C-raclopride is altered by drugs that modify synaptic dopamine levels. *Synapse* 1993, 13, 350

38 Laruelle, M., Al-Tikriti, M., van Dyck, C.H. *et al.* D-amphetamine displacement of ^{123}I IBF equilibrium binding in primates : a new paradigm to investigate amphetamine induced dopamine release. *Schizophren. Res.* 1993, 9, 191

39 Dewey, S.L., Smith, G.S., Logan, J. *et al.* GABAergic inhibition of endogenous dopamine release measured in vivo with ^{11}C-raclopride and positron emission tomography. *J. Neurosci.* 1992, 12, 3773

40 Dewey, S.L., Smith, G.S., Logan, J. *et al.* Effects of central cholinergic blockade on striatal dopamine release measured with positron emission tomography in normal human subjects. *Proc. Natl. Acad. Sci.* 1993, 90, 11816

41 Dewey, S.L., Logan, J., Wolf, A.P. *et al.* Amphetamine induced decreases in ^{18}F-N-methylspiroperidol binding in the baboon brain using positron emission tomography (PET). *Synapse* 1991, 7, 324

42 Brucke, T., Wober, C., Podrecka, I. *et al.* D2 receptor blockade by flunarizine and cinnarizine explains extrapyramidal side effects. A SPECT study. *J. Cereb. Blood Flow Metab.* 1995, 15, 513

43 Farde, L., Nordstrom, A-L., Wiesel, F-A. *et al.* Positron emission tomographic analysis of central D1 and D2 dopamine receptor occupancy in patients treated with classical neuroleptics and clozapine. *Arch. Gen. Psychiatr.* 1992, 49, 538

44 Nordstrom, A-L., Farde, L., Wiesel, F-A. *et al.* Central D2 dopamine receptor occupancy in relation to antipsychotic drug effects : A double blind PET study of schizophrenic patients. *Biol. Psychiatr.* 1993, 33, 227

45 Suhara, T., Inoue, O., Kobayashi, K. *et al.* An acute effect of triazolam on muscarinic cholinergic receptor binding in the human brain measured by positron emission tomography. *Psychopharmacology* 1994, 113, 311

46 Roy, A.E., Bakay, E. and Harris, A.B. Neurotransmitter, receptor and biochemical changes in monkey cortical epileptic foci. *Brain Res.* 1980, 206, 387

47 Savic, I., Persson, A., Roland, P *et al.* In vivo demonstration of reduced benzodiazepine receptor binding in human epileptic foci. *Lancet* 1988, ii, 863

48 Savic, I. and Thorell, J.O. PET shows different pattern of benzodiazepine receptor changes in intractable compared with moderate partial epilepsy. *J. Cereb. Blood Flow Metab.* 1993, 13(suppl 1), S278

49 van Huffelen, A.C., van Isselt, J.W., van Veelen, C.N. *et al.* Identification of the side of epileptic focus with ^{123}I-iomazenil. *Acta. Neurochir.* 1990, Suppl Wien, 50, 95

50 Henry, T.R., Frey, K.A., Scakellares, J.C. *et al.* In vivo cerebral metabolism and central benzodiazepine-receptor binding in temporal lobe epilepsy. *Neurology* 1993, 43, 1998

51 Schubiger, A., Hasler, P.H., Beer, H. *et al.* Evaluation of a multicenter study with iomazenil - a benzodiazepine receptor ligand. *Nucl. Med. Commun.* 1991, 12, 569

52 Savic, I., Ingvar, M. and Stone-Elander, S. Comparison of [11C] flumazenil and [18F]FDG as PET markers of epileptic foci. *J. Neurol. Neurosurg. Psychiatr.* 1993, 56, 615

53 Duncan, S., Gillen, G.J. and Brodie, M.J. Lack of effect of concomitant clobazam on interictal ^{123}I-iomazenil SPECT. *Epilepsy Res.* 1993, 15, 61

54 Savic, I., Pauli, S., Thorell, J-O. and Blomqvist, G. In vivo demonstration of altered benzodiazepine receptor density in patients with generalised epilepsy. *J. Neurol. Neurosurg. Psychiatr.* 1994, 57, 797

55 Prevett, M.C., Lammertsma, A.A., Brooks, D.J. *et al.* Benzodiazepine-GABA$_A$ receptors in idiopathic generalized epilepsy measures with [11C] flumazenil and positron emission tomography. *Epilepsia* 1993, 36(2), 113

56 Bartenstein, P.A., Duncan, J.S., Prevett, M.C. *et al.* Investigation of the opioid system in absence seizures with positron emission tomography. *J. Neurol. Neurosurg. Psychiatr.* 1993, 56, 1295

57 Prevett, M.C., Cunningham, V.J., Brooks D.J. *et al.* Opiate receptors in idiopathic generalised epilepsy measured with [11C] diprenorphine and positron emission tomography. *Epilepsy Res.* 1994, 19, 71

58 Frost, J.J., Mayberg, H.S., Fisher, R.S. *et al.* Mu-opiate receptors measured by positron emission tomography are increased in temporal lobe epilepsy. *Ann. Neurol.* 1988, 23, 231

59 Mayberg, H.S., Sadzot, B., Maltzer, C.C. *et al.* Quantification of mu and non-mu opiate receptors in temporal lobe epilepsy using positron emission tomography. *Ann. Neurol.* 1991, 30, 3

60 Ring, H.A., Trimble, M.R., Costa, D.C. *et al.* Striatal dopamine receptor binding in epileptic psychoses. *Biol. Psychiatr.* 1994, 35, 367

61 Ring, H.A., Trimble, M.R., Costa, D.C. *et al.* Effects of vigabatrin on striatal dopamine receptors: evidence in humans for interactions of GABA and dopamine systems. *J. Neurol. Neurosurg. Psychiatr.* 1992, 55, 758

62 Kerwin, R.W. Functional neuroimaging in Alzheimer's disease: how far should we go? *Eur. J. Nuclear Med.*, 21, 1041

63 Holman, B.L., Gibson, R.E., Hill, T.C. *et al.* Muscarinic acetylcholine receptors in Alzheimer's disease. *J. Am. Med. Assoc.* 1985, 254, 3063

64 Wyper, D.J., Brown, D., Patterson, J. *et al.* Density of acetylcholine receptors in Alzheimer's disease measured in relation to regional blood flow. *J. Cereb. Blood Flow Metab.* 1993, 13(Suppl 1), S1

65 Weinberger, D.R., Mann, U., Gibson, R.E. *et al.* Cerebral muscarinic receptors in primary degenerative dementia as evaluated by SPECT with iodine-123-labeled QNB. *Adv. Neurol.* 1990, 51, 147

66 Blin, J., Baron, J.C., Dubois, B. *et al.* Loss of brain 5-HT2 receptors in Alzheimer's disease. *Brain* 1993, 116, 497

67 Meyer, M., Koeppe, R.A., Frey, K.A. *et al.* Positron emission tomography measures of benzodiazepine binding in Alzheimer's disease. *Arch. Neurol.* 1995, 52, 314

68 Frisoni, G.B., Pizzolato, G., Bianchetti, A. *et al.* Single photon emission computed tomography with [^{99m}Tc]-HMPAO and [^{123}I]-IBZM in Alzheimer's disease and dementia of frontal type : preliminary results. *Acta. Neurol. Scand.* 1994, 89, 199

69 Costa, D.C., Walker, Z. and Katona, C.L.E. Lewy body dementia - dopamine D2 neuroreceptor availability studied with single photon emission tomography. *Eur. J. Nucl. Med.* 1995, 8, 893

70 Koob, G. Drugs of abuse: anatomy, pharmacology and function of reward pathways. *TIPS* 1992, 13, 177

71 Tran, V.T., Snyder, S.H., Major, L.F. and Hawley, R.J. GABA receptors are increased in brains of alcoholics. *Ann. Neurol.* 1980, 9, 289

72 Freund, G. and Ballinger, W.E. Decrease of benzodiazepine receptors in frontal cortex of alcoholics. *Alcohol* 1988, 5, 275

73 Volkow, N.D., Wang, G-J., Hitzemann, R. *et al.* Recovery of brain glucose metabolism in detoxified alcoholics. *Am. J. Psychiatr.* 1994, 151, 178

74 Volkow, N.D., Wang, G-J., Begleiter, H. *et al.* Regional brain metabolic response to lorazepam in subjects at risk for alcoholism. *Alcohol Clin. Exp. Red.* 1995, 19, 510

75 Pauli, S., Liljequist, S., Farde, L. *et al.* PET analysis of alcohol interaction with the brain disposition of [^{11}C] flumazenil. *Psychopharmacology* 1992, 107, 180

76 Litton, J-E., Neiman, J., Pauli, S. *et al.* PET analysis of [^{11}C] flumazenil binding to benzodiazepine receptors in chronic alcohol dependent men and healthy controls. *Psychiatr. Res. Neuroimaging* 1993, 50, 1

77 Hietala, J., West, C., Syvalahti, E. *et al.* Striatal D2 dopamine receptor binding characteristics in vivo in patients with alcohol dependence. *Psychopharmacology* 1994, 116, 285

78 Tiihonen, J., Kuikka, J., Bergstrom, K. *et al.* Altered striatal dopamine re-uptake site densities in habitually violent and non-violent alcoholics. *Nature Medicine* 1995, 1, 654

79 Woolverton, W.L. and Johnson, K.M. Neurobiology of cocaine abuse. *TIPS* 1992, 13, 193

80 Volkow, N.D., Fowler, J.S. and Wolf, A.P. Use of positron emission tomography to study cocaine in the human brain in 'Emerging technologies and new directions in drug abuse research', (Eds. R.S. Rapaka, A. Makriyannis, M.J. Kuhar) National Institute on Drug Abuse, Rockville, MD, Research Monographs: 112, 1991, p.168

81 Cook, C.E., Jeffcoat, R. and Perez-Reyes. M. 'Pharmacokinetic studies of cocaine and phencyclidine in man in Pharmacokinetics and Pharmacodynamics of Psychoactive Drugs', (Eds. J. Barnett and C. Chiang), Foster City, CA, Biomedical Pub., 1985, p. 49

82 Gatley, S.J., Yu, D-W., Fowler, J.S. *et al.* Studies with differentially labelled [^{11}C] cocaine, [^{11}C] nococaine, [^{11}C] benzoylecgonine and [^{11}C]- and 4'[^{18}F] fluorococaine to probe the extent to which [^{11}C] cocaine metabolites contribute to PET images of the baboon brain. *J. Neurochem.* 1994, 62, 1154

83 Baxter, L.R., Schwartz, J.M. and Phelp, M. Localisation of neurochemical effects of cocaine and other stimulants in the human brain. *J. Clin. Psychiatr.* 1988, 49, 23

84 Volkow, N.D., Fowler, J.S., Wolf, A.P. *et al.* Effects of chronic cocaine abuse on postsynaptic dopamine receptors. *Am. J. Psychiatr.* 1990, 147, 719

85 Volkow, N.D., Fowler, J.S., Wang, G-J. *et al.* Decreased dopamine D2 receptor availability is associated with reduced frontal metabolism in cocaine abusers. *Synapse* 1993, 14, 169

86 Fowler, J.S., Volkow, N.D., Logan, J. *et al.* Alcohol intoxication does not change [^{11}C] cocaine phamacokinetics in human brain and heart. *Synapse* 1992, 12, 228

87 Iyo, M., Nishio, M., Fukuda, H. *et al.* Dopamine D2 and serotonergic S2 receptors in susceptibility to metamphetamine psychosis detected by positron emission tomography. *Psychiatry Research: Neuroimaging* 1993, 50, 217

88 Basile, A.S., James, E.A. and Skolnick, P. The pathogenesis and treatment of hepatic encephalopathy: evidence for the involvement of benzodiazepine receptor ligands. *Pharm. Rev.* 1991, 43, 27

89 Samson, Y., Bernan, J., Pappata, S. *et al.* Cerebral uptake of benzodiazepines measured by positron emission tomography in hepatic encephalopathy. *N. Eng. J. Med.* 1987, 316, 414

90 Cluckie, A., Kapcinski, F., Fleminger, S. *et al.* I -123 iomazenil uptake in cirrhosis. *Acta. Psychiat.* 1995, Belgica, 95, suppl 1995, 83

91 Brooks, D.J., Ibanez, V., Sawle, G.V. *et al.* Differing patterns of striatal ^{18}F DOPA uptake in Parkinson's disease, multiple system atrophy and progressive supranuclear palsy. *Ann. Neurol.* 1990, 28, 547

92 Leenders, K.L., Salmon, E.P., Tyrell, P. *et al.* The nigrostriatal dopaminergic system assessed in vivo by positron emission tomography in healthy volunteer subjects and patients with Parkinson's disease. *Arch. Neurol.* 1990, 47, 1290

93 Burns, D.J., Sawle, G.V. and Brooks, D.J. Differential diagnosis of Parkinson's disease, multiple system atrophy, and Steele-Richardson-Olszewski syndrome: discriminant analysis of striatal ^{18}F-dopa PET data. *J. Neurol. Neurosurg. Psychiatr.* 1994, 57, 278

94 Innis, R.B., Seibyl, J.P., Scanley, B.E. *et al.* Single photon emission tomographic imaging demonstrates loss of striatal dopamine transporters in Parkinson's disease. *Proc. Natl. Acad. Sci.* 1993, 90, 11965

95 Innis, R.B. Single-photon emission tomography imaging of dopamine terminal innervation: a potential clinical tool in Parkinson's disease. *Eur. J. Nucl. Med.* 1994, 21, 1

96 Rinne, J.O., Laihinen, A., Nagren, K. *et al.* PET demonstrates different behaviour of striatal dopamine D1 and D2 receptors in early Parkinson's disease. *J. Neurosci. Res.* 1990, 27, 494

97 Leenders, K.L., Herold, S., Palmer, A.J. *et al.* Cerebral dopamine system measured in vivo using PET. *J. Cereb. Blood Flow Metab.* 1985, 5(suppl), S157

98 Brooks, D.J., Ibanez, V., Sawle, G.V. *et al.* Striatal D2 receptor status in Parkinson's disease, striatonigral degeneration, and progressive supranuclear palsy, measured with ^{11}C-raclopride and PET. *Ann. Neurol.* 1992, 31, 184

99 Leenders, K.L., Antonini, A., Schwarz, J. *et al.* Dopamine D2 receptors measured in vivo in patients with Parkinson's disease in 'Tenth international symposium on Parkinson's disease', (Ed. H. Narabayashi), Tokyo, 1991, p. 121

100 Sawle, G.V., Brooks, D.J., Ibanez, V. and Frackowiack, R.S.J. Striatal D2 receptor density is inversely proportional to dopa uptake in untreated Parkinson's disease. *J. Neurol. Neurosurg. Psychiatr.* 1990, 53, 177

101 Rinne, U.K., Laihinen, A., Rinne, J.O. *et al.* Positron emission tomography demonstrates dopamine D2 receptor supersensitivity in the striatum of patients with early Parkinson's disease. *Mov. Disord.* 1990, 5, 55

102 Sawle, G.V., Playford, E.D.l., Brooks, D.J. *et al.* Asymmetrical pre-synaptic and post-synaptic changes in the striatal dopamine projection in dopa naive parkinsonism. *Brain* 1993, 116, 853

103 Weinhard, K., Coenen, H.H., Pawlik, G. *et al.* PET studies of dopamine receptor distribution using [^{18}F]fluoro-ethyl-spiperone: findings in disorders related to the dopaminergic system. *J. Neural Transm.* 1990, Gen. Sect. 81, 195

104 Brucke, T., Podrecka, I., Angelberger, P. *et al.* Dopamine D2 receptor imaging with SPECT:studies in different neuro-psychiatric disorders. *J. Cereb. Blood Flow Metab.* 1991, 11, 220

105 Antonini, A., Schwarz, J., Oertel, W.H. *et al.* [^{11}C] raclopride and positron emission tomography in previously untreated patients with Parkinson's disease. *Neurology* 1994, 44, 1325

106 Schwarz, J., Tatsch, K., Arnold, G. *et al.* ^{123}I-Iodo-benzamide-SPECT in 83 patients with de novo parkinsonism. *Neurology* 1993, 43(suppl 6), S17

107 Fowler, J.S., Volkow, N.D., Logan, J. *et al.* Slow recovery of human brain MAOB after L-deprenyl (Selegine) withdrawal. *Synapse* 1994, 18, 86

108 Routtinnen, H., Rinne, J.O., Laihinen, A. *et al.* The effect of COMT inhibition with entacapone on ^{18}F-6-fluorodopa PET in Parkinson's disease. *J. Cereb. Blood Flow Metab.* 1993, 13, S359

109 Lindvall, O., Rehncrona, S., Brundin, P. *et al.* Human fetal dopamine neurons grafted into the striatum in two patients with severe Parkinson's disease. *Arch. Neurol.* 1989, 46, 615

110 Lindvall, O., Brundin, P., Widner, H. *et al.* Grafts of fetal dopamine neurons survive and improve motor function in Parkinson's disease. *Science* 1990, 247, 574

111 Martin, W.W.R. and Perlmutter, J.S. Assessment of fetal tissue transplantation in Parkinson's disease : does PET play a role? *Neurology* 1994, 44, 1777

112 Brooks, D.J. PET studies on early and differential diagnosis of Parkinson's disease. *Neurology* 1993, 43(suppl 6), S6

113 George, M.S., Robertson, M.M., Costa, D.C. *et al.* Dopamine receptor availability in Tourette's syndrome. *Psychiatr. Res. : Neuroimaging* 1994, 55, 193

114 Turjanski, N., Sawle, G.V., Playford, E.D. *et al.* PET studies of the pre and post-synaptic dopaminergic system in Tourette's syndrome. *J. Neurol. Neurosurg. Psychiatr.* 1994, 57, 688

115 Holthoff, V.A., Koeppe, R.A., Frey, K.A. *et al.* Positron emission tomography measures of benzodiazepine receptors in Huntington's disease. *Ann. Neurol.* 1993, 34, 76

116 Agren, H. and Reibring, L. PET studies of presynaptic monoamine metabolism in depressed patients and healthy volunteers. *Pharmacopsychiatry* 1994, 27, 2

117 Suhara, T., Nakayama, K., Inoue, O. *et al.* D1 dopamine receptor binding in mood disorders measured by positron emission tomography. *Psychopharmacol.* 1992, 106, 14

118 Wong, D.F., Wahner, H.N., Pearlson, G. *et al.* Dopamine receptor binding of C-11-3-N-methylspiperone in the caudate in schizophrenia and bipolar disorder: a preliminary report. *Psychopharmacol Bull.* 1989, 21, 595

119 Ebert, D., Fiestel, H., Kaschka, W. *et al.* Single photon emission computerized tomography assessment of cerebral dopamine D2 receptor blockade in depression before and after sleep deprivation - preliminary results. *Biol. Psychiatr.* 1994, 35, 880

120 D'Haenen, H.A., Bossuyt, A., Mertens, J. *et al.* SPECT imaging of serotonin 2 receptors in depression. *Psychiatr. Res. : Neuroimaging* 1992, 45, 227

121 D'Haenen, H.A. and Bossuyt, A. Dopamine D2 receptors in depression measured with single photon emission computed tomography. *Biol. Psychiatr.* 1994, 35, 128

122 Scheffel, U., Kim, S., Cline, E.J. and Kuhar, M.J. Occupancy of the serotonin transporter by fluoxetine, paroxetine and sertraline: in vivo studies with [125]RTI-55. *Synapse* 1994, 16, 263

123 Peroutka, S.J. and Snyder, S.H. Relationship of neuroleptic drug effects at brain dopamine, serotonin, alpha adrenergic and histamine receptors to clinical potency. *Am. J. Psych.* 1990, 137, 1518

124 Crawley, J.C., Crow, T.J., Johnstone, E.C. *et al.* Uptake of [77]Br-spiperone in the striata of schizophrenic patients and controls. *Nucl. Med. Commun.* 1986, 7, 599

125 Wong, D.F., Wagner, H.N., Tune, L.E. *et al.* Positron emission tomography reveals elevated D2 dopamine receptors in drug-naive schizophrenics. *Science* 1986, 234, 1558

126 Tune, L.E., Wong, D.F., Pearlson, G. *et al.* Dopamine D2 receptor density estimated in schizophrenia : A positron emission tomography study with ^{11}C-N-Methylspiperone. *Psychiatr. Res.* 1993, 49, 219

127 Farde, L., Wiesel, F-A., Stone-Elander, S. *et al.* D2 dopamine receptors in neuroleptic naive schizophrenic patients. *Arch. Gen. Psychiatr.* 1990, 47, 213

128 Martinot, J.L., Peron Magnan, P., Huret, J.D. *et al.* Striatal D2 dopaminergic receptors assessed with positron emission tomography and [76]Br-bromospiperone in untreated schizophrenic patients. *Am. J. Psychiatr.* 1990, 147, 44

129 Martinot, J.L., Paillere-Martinot, M.L., Loch, C. *et al.* The estimated density of D2 striatal receptors in schizophrenia - a study withpositron emission tomography and [76]Br bromolisuride. *Br. J. Psychiatr.* 1991, 158, 346

130 Martinot, J.L., Paillere-Martinot, M.L., Loch, C. *et al.* Central D2 receptors and negative symptoms of schizophrenia. *Br. J. Psychiatr.* 1994, 164, 27

131 Kessler, R.M., Mason, N.S., Votaw, J. R. *et al.* Visualisation of extrastriatal D2 receptors in the human brain. *Eur. J. Pharm.* 1992, 223, 105

132 Stevens, J., Wilson, K. and Foote, W. GABA blockade, dopamine and schizophrenia. *Psychopharmacology* 1974, 39, 105

133 Busatto, G.F., Pilowsky, L.S., Costa, D.C. *et al.* Correlation between reduced *in vivo* benzodiazepine receptor binding and severity of psychotic symptoms in schizophrenics. *Am. J. Psychiatry* 1997, 154, 56

134 Smith, M., Wolf, A.P., Brodie, J.D. *et al.* Serial [^{18}F]N-methylspiperidol PET studies to measure changes in antipsychotic drug D2 receptor occupancy in schizoprenic patients. *Biol. Psychiatr.* 1988, 23, 653

135 Nordstrom, A-L., Farde, L. and Halldin, C. Time course of D2-dopamine receptor occupancy examined by PET after single oral doses of haloperidol. *Psychopharmacology* 1992, 106, 433

136 Farde, L. Selective D1 and D2-dopamine receptor blockade both induces akathisia in humans-a PET study with [^{11}C]SCH 23390 and [^{11}C] raclopride. *Psychopharmacology* 1992, 107, 23

137 Kolakowska, T., Williams, A.O., Ardern, M. *et al.* Schizophrenia with good and poor outcome. I: Early clinical features, response to neuroleptics and signs of organic dysfunction. *Br. J. Psychiatr.* 1985, 146, 229

138 Coppens, H.J., Sloof, C.J., Paans, A.M.J. *et al.* High central D2-dopamine receptor occupancy as assessed with positron emission tomography in medicated but therapeutic resistant schizophrenic patients. *Biol. Psychiatr.* 1991, 29, 629

139 Wolkin, A., Barouche, F., Wolf, A.P. *et al.* Dopamine blockade and clinical response : evidence for two biological subgroups of schizophrenia. *Am. J. Psychiatr.* 1989, 146, 905

140 Pilowsky, L.S., Costa, D.C., Ell, P.J. *et al.* Clozapine, single photon emission tomography and the dopamine D2 receptor blockade hypothesis of schizophrenia. *Lancet* 1992, 340, 199

141 Volk, S., Maul, F-D., Hor, G. *et al.* Dopamine D2 receptor occupancy measured by single photon emission computed tomography with ^{123}I-iodobenzamide in chronic schizophrenia. *Psychiatr. Res. : Imaging* 1994, 55, 111

142 Kerwin R.W. The new atypical antipsychotics. *Br. J. Psychiatr.* 1994, 164, 141

143 Farde, L. and Nordstrom, A-L. PET analysis indicates atypical central dopamine receptor occupancy in clozapine-treated patients. *Br. J. Psychiatr.* 1992, 160(suppl 17), 30

144 Nordstrom, A.L., Farde, L. and Halldin, C. High 5HT2 receptor occupancy in clozapine treated patients demonstrated by PET. *Psychopharmacology*, 110, 365

145 Nyberg, S., Farde, L., Eriksson, L. *et al.* 5-HT2 and D2 dopamine receptor occupancy in the living brain. A PET study with risperidone. *Psychopharmacology* 1993, 110, 265

146 Busatto, G.F., Pilowsky, L.S., Costa, D.C. *et al.* Dopamine D2 receptor blockade in vivo with the novel antipsychotics risperidone and remoxiprode - an ^{123}I-IBZM single photon emission tomography (SPECT) study. *Psychopharmacology* 1995, 117, 55

147 Nyberg, S., Dahl, M-J. and Halldin, C. A PET study of D2 and 5HT-2 receptor occupancy induced by risperidone in poor metabolisers of debrisoquin and risperidone. *Psychopharmacology* 1995, 119, 345

148 Bench, C.J., Lammertsma, A.A., Dolan, R.J. *et al.* Dose dependent occupancy of central dopamine D2 receptors by the novel neuroleptic CP-88,059-01 : a study using positron emission tomography. *Psychopharmacology* 1995, 112, 308

SPECT in Neurology and Psychiatry, edited by P.P. De Deyn, R.A. Dierckx, A. Alavi and B.A. Pickut
© 1997 John Libbey & Company Ltd, pp. 107–115

SPECT Imaging In Primary Mood Disorders

Chapter
14

H.A.H. D'haenen

Introduction

Biological psychiatric research in mood disorders, as in other psychopathological disturbances, has long rested on indicators somewhat removed from the brain (e.g. metabolites of neurotransmitters in cerebrospinal fluid, plasma and/or urine; studies in blood platelets; psychoendocrinological investigation, etc.), which was only directly accessible post mortem. Functional imaging techniques, however, have allowed the direct *in vivo* determination of brain processes, and, thus, the study of the physiopathological substrate of psychopathology.

Single photon emission computerised tomography (SPECT) allows the determination of blood flow and neurochemical processes. Blood flow is of interest since it is closely coupled to the functional activity of brain structures[1]. Changes in neuronal activity can be inferred from changes in regional cerebral blood flow (rCBF). Blood flow studies in the major subtypes of mood disorders are reviewed in this chapter, as are studies addressing the issues of effect of treatment and the correlation of blood flow anomalies with psychopathological variables.

Neuroactivation procedures, which are potentially very interesting but have scarcely been used in mood disorders evaluated with SPECT, will be briefly discussed. The development of radioligands permitting the determination of neuroreceptors *in vivo* are of evident value, for studying the pathophysiological substrate of psychopathological disorders as well as for psychopharmacology, but this will be dealt with elsewhere in the book. Only a few receptor studies have been performed in mood disorders, and these will be reviewed briefly.

Studies of blood flow at rest

Unipolar depression

Most studies have investigated whole brain and/or regional blood flow in this subtype of depression, comparing it with blood flow in normal control subjects. The main findings and confounding variables are displayed in Table 1. Some studies are not included in Table 1 since only the abstract could be considered[2,3]. A reduced flow was demonstrated in all cerebral regions as was a left < right asymmetry in one study[2]. Kawakatsu and Komatani[3] showed a reduced rCBF bilaterally in the frontal and parietal regions, more pronounced on the left.

Department of Psychiatry,
Academic Hospital, Free
University of Brussels (V.U.B.),
Brussels, Belgium

Table 1 Blood flow findings in unipolar depressives compared with normal controls

Reference	Number of patients/controls	Tracer	Patient characteristics	Medication status	Main findings
11	10/6	[133]Xe	RDC[a] endogenous DSM-III[b] melancholia	Not documented	no difference in global flow ↑ flow in left hemisphere
16	10/10	[133]Xe	Newcastle endogenous DSM-III melancholia	On	↑ global flow
6	22/6	^{123}I-IMP	DSM-III major depression	Medication not controlled for	↓ global flow, esp. frontal lobes, ↓ flow in basal ganglia
8	38/8	[133]Xe	RDC major affective disorder (n=34) bipolar affective psychosis (n=4)	20 off medication (since ?) 18 on medication	No difference in global flow. ↑ right frontal flow, higher right ant/post gradient
10	38/16	[133]Xe	RDC MDD[c]	Washout ≥ 10 days	No difference with controls see also text
17	18/12	^{99m}Tc-HMPAO	DSM-III-R[d] MDD> 60 yrs	Not documented	↓ global flow
12	19/14	[133]Xe Therapy resistent	DSM-III unipolar depression DSM-III bipolar depression (n=4)	On	↓ activity in left superior frontal and left parietal cortex
23	10/8	^{99m}Tc-HMPAO	DSM-III-R MDD, melancholic subtype	Washout≥ 14 days	↓ flow in left lower parts of anterolateral prefrontal cortex
41	19/12	^{123}I-IMP subtype (n=8)	DSM-III-R MDD, melancholic (n=14) On (n=5)	Drug free ≥ 10 days temporal lobes	Right > left activity in
7	40/20	^{99m}Tc-HMPAO	20 Newcastle endogenous	15 on medication	↓ flow in temporal, inferior frontal and parietal regions basal ganglia and thalamus
42	14/10	^{99m}Tc-HMPAO	DSM-III-R melancholia Psychotic features (n=3)	Off, since ?	↓ flow in temporal cortex, ↓ left/right ratio prefrontal cortex
9	20/30	^{99m}Tc-HMPAO	DSM-III-R major depression with or without melancholia with or without psychotic features, > 60 years, Newcastle endogenous 14/20	11 on medication	↓ flow in right thalamus and caudate

Table 1 (cont.)

Reference	Number of patients/controls	Tracer	Patient characteristics	Medication status	Main findings
4	47/138	^{133}Xe	RDC definite MDD	13 nonendogenous, 23 endogenous, 11 psychotic, washout $\geq$5 days	see text
5	31/12	^{99m}Tc-HMPAO	DSM-III major depression with (n=13) and without melancholia (n=18)	Washout $\geq$ 14 days	No differences see also text
18	39/20	^{133}Xe, ^{99m}Tc-HMPAO	DSM-III-R MDE[e] > 1 month, > 50 years	Washout $\geq$ 7 days	$\downarrow$ global flow, esp. in males, $\downarrow$ flow in orbital frontal, infero temporal parietal cortex, $\downarrow$ flow in right high frontal, supero temporal and parietal cortex
19	13/11	^{99m}Tc-HMPAO	DSM-III-R MDD	On	$\downarrow$ flow in frontal, anterior temporal cortex, anterior cingulate gyrus, caudate
22	10/9	^{99m}Tc-HMPAO	DSM-III-R MDD, >65 years	On (n=6)	$\downarrow$ flow in parietal, left temporal and left occipital cortex
43	14/38	^{99m}Tc-HMPAO	DSM-III-R MDD	On	Multiple defects, most prevalent in the frontal and temporal lobes, No difference in midcerebral uptake index

[a] Research Diagnostic Criteria; [b], Diagnostic and Statistical Manual of Mental Disorders - third edition; [c], Major Depressive Disorder; [d], Diagnostic and Statistical Manual of Mental Disorders - third edition - revised; [e], Major Depressive Episode

Interestingly, Devous et al.[4] demonstrated, using a multiple regression analysis approach, that different regions exhibited different age-effects on rCBF in different depressive subtypes. These findings must be replicated, of course, but they do pose an interesting methodological challenge. Maes et al.[5] also reported a finding which merits particular attention: while they did not find blood flow differences between depressives and controls, they demonstrated hypoperfusion in the motor frontal and parietal cortex of patients who had been taking benzodiazepines during the study. The effect of psychotropic drugs on blood flow has been addressed in 4 other studies, even though it was not the aim of the investigation: no significant effect of antidepressant drugs on frontal rCBF was demonstrated in one[6], another associated antidepressant drugs with a minor reduction in anterior tracer uptake[7]. Reischies et al.[8] showed that patients taking antidepressants had a lower CBF than unmedicated patients, but did not demonstrate an effect on rCBF. Curran et al.[9] demonstrated a non-significant average effect of treatment with either antidepressants or benzodiazepines, but a manifest interaction with regions of interest (ROI).

Bipolar disorder, depressive episode

Just a few studies have addressed this issue, and most include only a small number of subjects. Reischies et al.[8] included a small minority of bipolar depressed patients, but published no separate data on these subjects. Delvenne et al.[10] (n=8) demonstrated a left < right asymmetry of predominantly cortical flow in a slice that included the basal ganglia, the frontal and occipital poles, compared with unipolar patients as well as with normal controls. There was a trend (p=0.074) for Newcastle scale-defined endogenous depressives (n=11) to show the same lateralisation. There was a significant difference with non-endogenous depressives (n=26; p=0.026).

O'Connell et al.[6] studied 2 bipolar depressives who tended to have a decreased flow compared with controls (n=6), in their right parietal, right temporal and bilateral occipital cortical areas; flow was higher in all cortical areas when compared with major depressives.

Rush et al.[11] studied 6 bipolar I and II depressed subjects and demonstrated no difference with controls. Another study[3] compared 6 bipolar depressed subjects with 20 normal controls, and found no difference in either rCBF or global flow. In Morinobu et al.'s study[12], 4 bipolar depressed subjects were compared with 15 unipolars and 14 volunteers and no differences in mean bilateral hemispheric flow were demonstrated; mean right hemispheric flows were significantly higher

in bipolars than unipolars. Regional left temporal flow was also significantly higher in bipolars than unipolars, but there were no regional differences between bipolars and controls.

Bipolar disorder, manic or mixed episode

In manic (or mixed) patients, a higher flow has been demonstrated globally[11], or in the caudate[6]. Migliorelli et al.[13] studied 5 patients with a manic episode and 7 controls and demonstrated a lower blood flow in the basal portion of the right temporal lobe, a lower perfusion in the right versus left temporal basal cortex and in the right temporal basal versus dorsal cortex. O'Connell et al.[14] studied 11 manic subjects, 21 acute schizophrenic patients and 15 controls. Most patients had abnormal scans, while those of controls were all normal. Hypofrontality, increased flow in temporal lobes, increases and decreases in basal ganglia flow were demonstrated, but did not differentiate between manic and schizophrenic subjects.

Dysthymia

Two studies have addressed this issue[5,15]. One[15], compared 21 dysthymic patients with 21 major depressives and demonstrated a higher flow in the dysthymic subjects in all regions studied, particularly the frontal region. All subjects underwent a psychotropic washout period of at least 5 days, except for chloralhydrate. In the other study, by Maes et al.[5], 12 patients with either dysthymia or an adjustment disorder with depressed mood (n=12) were compared with controls (n=12), after a psychotropic washout of at least 14 days, and no difference was demonstrated.

Correlation of blood flow with psychopathological variables

Fourteen studies which have addressed this issue are reviewed. The most investigated variables have been the severity of depression, mostly measured with the Hamilton Rating Scale for Depression (HRSD), and endogenicity, determined with the Newcastle scale. Most studies have not shown a significant correlation between blood flow and the severity of depression[5,12,15-19]. Interestingly, one small study[16] (n=10) demonstrated that although there was no correlation between the Hamilton Rating Scale for Depression score and cerebral blood flow, there was a significant correlation with the Bech core depression subscale[20]; this correlation disappeared, however, after treatment with ECT. In another study[21], a negative correlation between HRSD scores and blood flow in the anterofrontal and left prefrontal regions was demonstrated, while there was a positive correlation between HRSD scores and occipital flow.

Only 3 studies have looked at correlations with endogenicity: one[22] could not demonstrate any significant correlation, while another[7] demonstrated a significant correlation between Newcastle scale score and a relatively greater tracer uptake in the cingulate and frontal cortex. Moreover, after controlling for the effects of age, medication and Newcastle scale score, a negative correlation was demonstrated between HRSD scores and blood flow in the lower right frontal and right putamen regions. It should be stressed that the significance level was set at p<0.05 while multiple correlations were computed. In yet another study[17], a significant negative correlation was found, after controlling for age and gender, between Newcastle scale score and right and left occipital regions, more significantly on the right side.

Other psychopathological variables investigated have included: psychomotor retardation (one study[15] demonstrating no correlation, and another[19] finding a negative correlation between psychomotor slowing and blood flow in infero frontal, anterior temporal, anterior cingulate and prefrontal cortex); the somatic items of the Montgomery-Asberg Depression Rating Scale[22] (MADRS) (correlated significantly with frontal flow); the anxiety items of the MADRS[22] (significant correlation with the frontal and right occipital flow); hostile suspiciousness—a subscale of the Brief Psychiatric Rating Scale (BPRS) (a positive correlation with right frontal flow)[22]; and psychotic distortion—another BPRS subscale (showing a positive correlation with both right frontal and left occipital flow)[22]. It must be stressed that multiple correlations were computed in 10 subjects, and that the significance level was set at p<0.01. Different correlations were found, some of which were more significant, using a neuroactivation procedure (a Verbal Fluency Task)[22]. These included: a positive correlation between the BPRS global score and left temporal flow and between the withdrawn/depression subscale and left basal ganglia perfusion; a negative correlation between cognitive dysfunction and right occipital, left temporal and left basal ganglia flow; a positive correlation between the suspiciousness sub-scale and right temporal, left parietal, left temporal and left basal ganglia blood flow; and, finally, a positive correlation between the psychotic distortion sub-scale and the right frontal, right basal ganglia, left frontal, left parietal, left occipital and left basal ganglia flow.

One study[19] found no correlation between regional cerebral blood flow and anxiety, apathy or global cognitive function.

Effect of treatment

Table 2 displays relevant information about the different studies. This issue has been addressed in 8 studies. Increases, decreases and no differences in blood flow after treatment have been demonstrated; an increase was demonstrated in most[11,23-26]. Two[11,24] demonstrated an increase in global blood flow, while the 3 others demonstrated a localised increase in blood flow: a small increase in the hypoperfused upper parts of the anterolateral prefrontal cortex[23] and an increase in the left temporal and right parietal regions[25] in responders to a night of sleep deprivation; a bilateral augmentation in the anterior cingulate and putamen and in the right posterior cingulate and thalamus after a successful antidepressant therapy[26].

Rosenberg et al.[16] found normalisation of an abnormally high mean hemispherical flow, with a preferential fall in the frontal lobes, after ECT. Scott et al.[27] found a fall in tracer uptake in the inferior anterior cingulate cortex, especially on the left, after a single ECT. Reischies et al.[8] could not demonstrate any difference in global flow after psychotropic antidepressant treatment, but did find a decrease in left central flow. In two studies[23,28], a relative regional hyperperfusion was shown in responders to sleep deprivation (SD) before SD: in the right and left fronto orbital cortex, with lower parts of the cingulate gyrus, right hippocampus, para-hippocampus, and amygdala, and right and left infratemporal neocortical lobes[23]; this was later confirmed by the same group in another 20 subjects, of whom 11 were responders: a relative hyperperfusion in the right anterior cingulate cortex, in the right and left fronto orbital cortex, in the basal cingulate gyrus and in the hippocampus[28]. In the 1991 study[23], it was demonstrated that, after SD, the relative hyperperfused regions no longer differed from normal controls. In one study[2] (not included in Table 2 since only the abstract was addressed), a globally reduced flow returned to normal when patients were euthymic.

Neuroactivation procedures

Activation studies in mood disorders have been reviewed recently[29], but none of them used SPECT. The basic idea is that the brain is never really at rest, and hence that so-called resting imaging studies' show great variability. The latter might be reduced if the brain is brought in in a more specific activated state. It is also assumed that subtle changes could be enhanced when 'stress' is put on the regions involved. Three types of 'stresses' or probes have been used: sensorimotor, pharmacological and neurobehavioural. The methodological issues have been addressed extensively (e.g. George et al.[30], Ebmeier et al.[31], and Gur et al.[32]).

Table 2 Effect of treatment

Reference	Number of subjects	Medication status at baseline	Medication status after treatment	Response definition	Treatment modality
11	8	On	On, except when ECT	HRSD[b] score ≤ 6	ECT or medication
16	10	On, n=8	On (?)	not documented	medication
8	20	W.O.[a] ≥ 14 days	W.O. ≥ 16 days	Reduction of ≥50% in HRSD[b] score	antidepressants
23	10	On, 2 drug free	idem	Significant difference in HRSD score	ECT
24	9	W.O. ≥ 72 hours	not documented	Reduction of >50% of HRSD score and HRSD <10	ECT (n=5), Nortriptyline (n=4)
44	20	On	On	Reduction of >30% in HRSD score	Sleep deprivation
26	28	≥12 drug free	15 drug free	Well >6 months (retrospective self-report and review case note)	Antidepressants
27	15	On, n=12	idem	Not relevant	Single ECT

[a]Washout; [b], Hamilton rating scale for depression score

George[29] describes 3 kinds of approaches: a functional-geographical approach (depressed patients are imaged while performing tasks that are subserved through brain regions identified as abnormal in depression), a deficit-probing approach (subjects are imaged while performing tasks on which they were shown to be deficient), and a third approach in which subjects are imaged while they are experiencing emotions related to clinical depression.

SPECT activation studies in mood-disordered subjects are still rather scanty: Ebert *et al.*[33] used a somatosensory stimulation paradigm in 6 depressed patients with schizophrenia and 6 depressed patients with major depression. They demonstrated an enhancement of hypofrontality in major depressed subjects in the right inferior frontal lobe and in the right frontal lobe globally, while this occurred in the left dorsolateral prefrontal cortex in schizophrenia. Moreover, in the right inferior parietal lobe an increase in activity was shown in major depressed patients and a decrease in schizophrenic patients. Another study using a verbal fluency test[22] was discussed earlier in the section on correlations with psychopathological variables.

Table 3 Overview of areas involved in regional hypoperfusion

Without further specification	More specifically
Frontal region (2)	left superior frontal cortex, left inferior anterolateral prefrontal cortex, inferior frontal region, orbital frontal cortex, right high frontal cortex
Temporal region (3)	inferior temporal, superior temporal, anterior temporal, left temporal
Parietal region (2)	left parietal cortex
Basal ganglia	caudate, right caudate
Thalamus	right thalamus
Anterior cingulate gyrus	
Left occipital cortex	

Our group[34] has used a depressive mood-induction procedure in normal volunteers. This was a modified Velten procedure which consisted of tape-recorded self-referring depressive statements. A decreased rCBF was demonstrated in the right thalamus. Moreover, after mood induction out of the realm of attention, an increased hippocampal blood flow was shown.

Neuroreceptor studies

Only a few studies have looked at neuroreceptors in mood disorders: 1 on $5HT_2$ receptors[35] and 2 on D_2 receptors[36,37]. A higher uptake of the $5HT_2$ ligand 2-^{123}I-ketanserin was demonstrated bilaterally in the parietal cortex, as was a right > left asymmetry in the infero frontal cortex of depressed patients (n=19) compared with normal volunteers (n=10). This could indicate changes in $5HT_2$ receptors in depression[35]. 2-^{123}I-ketanserin is, however, not an ideal ligand for $5HT_2$ receptors — it suffers, for example, from the same lack of specificity for H_1-histaminergic and α_1-adrenergic receptors as the parent ligand[38] — and these findings are in need of replication using more specific ligands. A potentially interesting new ^{125}I tracer has recently been developed[39].

Using ^{123}I-IBZM as a ligand for D_2 receptors[40], a statistically significant higher basal ganglia/cerebellum uptake ratio was demonstrated in depressed patients (n=21) versus controls (n=11), indicating an increase of D_2 receptor-binding in depression[36].

It must be stressed, however, that results were necessarily expressed as a ratio (binding in the basal ganglia to binding in the cerebellum), so that differences could also reflect differences in non-specific binding in the cerebellum.

In one other study, using the same ligand, the effect of total sleep deprivation on D_2 receptors was studied[37]. These authors did not find significant differences in D_2 receptors between depressives (n=10) and controls (n=5). In this study the relative tracer distribution was calculated as the ratio of counts per voxel in the basal ganglia to counts per voxel in 32 brain ROIs. After total sleep deprivation, it was shown that the relative basal ganglia activity index only decreased significantly on the right in responders. Both studies encourage renewed interest in the involvement of dopamine in depression[21].

Conclusions

Overall, the results of SPECT studies in primary mood disorders are rather discrepant. One of the more consistent findings is a relative regional hypoperfusion in unipolar depression, more particularly in the frontal and temporal regions. The regions involved are displayed in Table 3. Since most studies that have investigated the effect of treatment found an increase in blood flow, it would seem that this hypoperfusion is state-dependent. Anomalies in unipolar major depressed subjects seem different from those in bipolar disorder patients and in dysthymics, although the number of subjects with the latter disorders that have been investigated is still rather small. Studies investigating the correlation of blood flow with severity of depression have mostly been negative, while correlation with endogenicity has been controversial.

Neuroactivation procedures have hardly been used with SPECT, but seem promising tools and will surely be more extensively used in the near future. The development of new receptor ligands also offers interesting new perspectives. Discrepancies are undoubtedly partly due to methodological issues. There is an urgent need to standardise these in order to make interinvestigator comparison of results more reliable. Apart from SPECT methodological aspects, which are dealt with elsewhere, it seems necessary to take into account age, subtype of depression, patient characteristics, medication status, and gender. More longitudinal studies in the same subjects, at different stages of their illness, would be worthwhile.

References

1 Raichle, M.E., Grubb, R.L. Jr., Gado, M.H. *et al.* Correlation between regional cerebral blood flow and oxidative metabolism. *Arch. Neurol.* 1976, 33, 523

2 Kanaya, T. and Yonekawa, M. Regional cerebral blood flow in depression. *Jpn. J. Psychiatr. Neurol.* 1990, 44, 571

3 Kawakatsu, S. and Komatani, A. Xe-133 inhalation single photon emission computerized tomography in manic depressive illness. *Nippon Rinsho.* 1994, 52, 1180

4 Devous, M.D. Sr., Gullion, C.M., Grannemann, B.D. *et al.* Regional cerebral blood flow alterations in unipolar depression. *Psychiatr. Res.* 1993, 50, 233

5 Maes, M., Dierckx, R., Meltzer, H.Y. *et al.* Regional cerebral blood flow in unipolar depression measured with ^{99m}Tc-HMPAO single photon emission computed tomography : negative findings. *Psychiatr. Res. Neuroimaging* 1993, 50, 77

6 O'Connell, R.A., van Heertum, R.L., Billick, S.B. *et al.* Single photon emission computed tomography (SPECT) with [123I] IMP in the differential diagnosis of psychiatric disorders. *J. Neuropsychiatr.* 1989, 1, 145

7 Austin, M-P., Dougall, N., Ross, M. *et al.* Single photon emission tomography with ^{99m}Tc-exametazime in major depression and the pattern of brain activity underlying the psychotic/neurotic continuum. *J. Affect. Dis.* 26, 31

8 Reischies, F.M., Hedde, J.-P. and Drochner, R. Clinical correlates of cerebral blood flow in depression. *Psychiatr Res.* 1989, 29, 323

9 Curran, S.M., Murray, C.M., van Beck, M. *et al.* A single photon emission computerised tomography study of regional brain function in elderly patients with major depression and with Alzheimer-type dementia. *Br. J. Psychiatr.* 1993, 163, 155

10 Delvenne, V., Delecluse, F., Hubain, Ph.P. *et al.* Regional cerebral blood flow in patients with affective disorders. *Br. J. Psychiatr.*1990, 157, 359

11 Rush, A.J., Schlesser, M.A., Stokely, E. *et al.* Cerebral blood flow in depression and mania. *Psychopharmcol. Bull.* 1982, 18, 6

12 Morinobu, S., Sagawa, K., Kawakatsu S. *et al.* Regional cerebral blood flow in refractory depression. *Adv. Neuropsychiatr. Psychopharmcol.* 1991, 2, 65

13 Migliorelli, R., Starkstein, S.E., Teson, A. *et al.* SPECT findings in patients with primary mania. *J. Neuropsychiatr. Clin. Neurosci.* 1993, 5, 379

14 O'Connell, R.A., van Heertum, R.L., Luck, D. *et al.* Single-photon emission computed tomography of the brain in acute mania and schizophrenia. *J. Neuroimaging* 1995, 5, 101

15 Thomas, P., Vaiva, G., Samaille, E. *et al.* Cerebral blood flow in major depression and dysthymia. *J. Affect. Dis.* 1993, 29, 235

16 Rosenberg, R., Vorstrup, S., Andersen, A. and Bolwig, T.G. Effect of ECT on cerebral blood flow in melancholia assessed with SPECT. *Convulsive Ther.* 1988, 4, 62

17 Upadhyaya, A.K., Abou-Saleh, M.T., Wilson, K. *et al.* A study of depression in old age using single-photon emission computerised tomography. *Br. J. Psychiatr.* 1990, 9, 76

18 Lesser, I.M., Mena, I., Boone, K.B. *et al.* Reduction of cerebral blood flow in older depressed patients. *Arch. Gen. Psychiatr.* 1994, 51, 677

19 Mayberg, H.S., Lewis, P.J., Regnold, W. and Wagner H.N. Jr. Paralimbic hypoperfusion in unipolar depression. *J. Nucl. Med.* 1994, 35, 929

20 Bech, P., Bolwig, T.G., Dein, E. *et al.* Quantitative rating of depressive states. *Acta. Psychiatr. Scand.* 1975, 51, 161

21 Willner, P. Dopamine mechanisms in depression and mania in 'Psychopharmacology: the Fourth Generation of Progress', (Eds. F.E. Bloom and D.J. Kupfer), Raven Press, New York, USA, 1995, p.921

22 Philpot, M.P., Banerjee, S., Needham-Bennett, H. *et al.* ^{99m}Tc-HMPAO single photon emission tomography in late life depression : a pilot study of regional cerebral blood flow at rest and during a verbal fluency task. *J. Affect. Dis.* 1993, 28, 233

23 Ebert, D., Feistel, H. and Barocka, A. Effects of sleep deprivation on the limbic system and the frontal lobes in affective disorders: a study with ^{99m}Tc-HMPAO SPECT. *Psychiatr. Res. Neuroimaging* 1991, 40, 247

24 Kumar, A., Mozley, D., Dunham, C. *et al.* Semiquantitative I-123 IMP spect studies in late onset depression before and after treatment. *Int. J. Ger. Psychiatr.* 1991, 6, 775

25 Velten, E. A laboratory task for induction of mood states. *Behav. Res. Ther.* 1968, 6, 473

26 Goodwin, G.M., Austin, M.-P., Dougall, N. *et al.* State changes in brain activity shown by the uptake of ^{99m}Tc-exametazime with single photon emission tomography in major depression before and after treatment. *J. Affect. Dis.* 1993, 29, 243

27 Scott, A.I.F., Dougall, N., Ross, M. *et al.* Short-term effects of electroconvulsive treatment on the uptake of ^{99m}Tc-exametazine into brain in major depression shown with single photon emission tomography. *J. Affect. Dis.* 1994, 30, 27

28 Ebert, D., Feistel, H., Barocka, A. and Kaschka, W. Increased limbic blood flow and total sleep deprivation in major depression. *Psychiatr. Res. Neuroimaging* 1994, 55, 101

29 George, M.S., Ketter, T.A. and Post, R.M. Activation studies in mood disorders. *Psychiatr. Annal* 1994, 24, 648

30 George, M.S., Ring, H.A., Costa, D.C. *et al.* Description and principles of neuroactivation in Neuroactiviation and neuroimaging with SPECT', Springer-Verlag, London, 1991, p141

31 Ebmeier, K.P., Dougall, N.J., Austin M.-P. *et al.* The split-dose technique for the study of psychological and pharmacological activation with the cerebral blood flow marker exametazime and single photon emission computed tomography (SPECT): reproducibility and rater reliability. *Int. J. Methods Psychiatr. Res.* 1991 1, 27

32 Gur, R.C., Erwin, R.J. and Gur, R.E. Neurobehavioral probes for physiologic neuroimaging studies. *Arch. Gen. Psychiatr.* 1992, 49, 409

33 Ebert, D., Feistel, H., Barocka, A. *et al.* A test-retest study of cerebral blood flow during somatosensory stimulation in depressed patients with schizophrenia and major depression. *Eur. Arch. Psychiatr. Clin. Neurosci.* 1993, 242, 250

34 De Raedt, R., D'haenen, H. Everaert, H. *et al.* Cerebral blood flow related to induction of a depressed mood within and out the realm of attention. *Psychiatr. Res. Neuroimaging* 1997, 74, 159

35 D'haenen, H., Bossuyt, A., Mertens, J. *et al.* SPECT imaging of serotonin$_2$ receptors in depression. *Psychiatr. Res. Neuroimaging* 1992, 45, 227

36 D'haenen, H.A. and Bossuyt A. Dopamine D$_2$ receptors in depression measured with single photon emission computed tomography. *Biol. Psychiatr.* 35, 128

37 Ebert, D., Feistel, H., Kaschka, W. *et al.* Single photon emission computerized tomography assessment of cerebral dopamine D$_2$ receptor blockade in depression before and after sleep deprivation - preliminary results. *Biol. Psychiat.* 1994, 35, 880

38 Leysen, J.E., Niemegeers, C.J.E., Van Nueten, J.M. and Laduron, P.M. [3H] ketanserin (R 41 468), a selective 3H-ligand for serotonin2 receptor binding sites. Binding properties, brain distribution, and functional role. *Mol. Pharmacol.* 1982, 21, 301

39 Mertens, J., Terriere, D., Sipido, V. *et al.* Radiosynthesis of a new radioiodinated ligand for serotonin-5HT2-receptors, a promising tracer for g-emission tomography. *J. Lab. Comp. Radiopharmaceut.* 1994, 34, 795

40 Kung, H.F., Alavi, A, Chang, W. *et al.* In vivo SPECT imaging of CNS D-2 dopamine receptors; initial studies with iodine-123-IBZM in humans. *J. Nucl. Med.* 1990, 31, 573

41 Amsterdam, J.D. and Mozley, P.D. Temporal lobe asymmetry with iodoamfetamine (IMP) SPECT imaging in patients with major depression. *J. Affect. Dis.* 1992, 24, 43

42 Yazici, K.M., Kapucu, O., Erbas, B. *et al.* Assessment of changes in regional cerebral blood flow in patients with major depression using the ^{99m}Tc-HMPAO single photon emission tomography method. *Eur. J. Nucl. Med.* 1992, 19, 1038

43 Schwartz, R.B., Komaroff, A.L., Garada, B.M. *et al.* SPECT imaging of the brain: comparison of findings in patients with chronic fatigue syndrome, AIDS dementia complex, and major unipolar depression. *A.J.R.* 1994, 162, 943

44 Volk, S., Kaendler, S.H., Weber, R. *et al.* Evaluation of the effects of total sleep deprivation on cerebral blood flow using single photon emission computerized tomography. *Acta. Psychiatr. Scand.* 1992, 86, 478

SPECT in Neurology and Psychiatry, edited by P.P. De Deyn, R.A. Dierckx, A. Alavi and B.A. Pickut
© 1997 John Libbey & Company Ltd, pp. 117–123

Reduced Frontal Cerebral Blood Flow in Drug-Free Obsessive-Compulsive Disorder (OCD): Preliminary Data of a SPECT Study

Chapter
15

F. Chierichetti, G.L. Bianchin[*], A. Vallerini[*], B. Saitta,
D. Rubello and G. Ferlin

Clinical background

According to DSM-IV[1], obsessive-compulsive disorder (OCD) is characterised by the presence of either obsessions or compulsions. Obsessions are identified by: 1) recurrent and persistent thoughts, impulses or images that are experienced, at some time during the disturbance, as intrusive and inappropriate and that cause marked anxiety or distress; 2) thoughts, impulses or images that are not simply excessive worries about real life problems; 3) the subject attempting to ignore or suppress such thoughts, impulses or images, or to neutralise them with some other thoughts or action; 4) the subject recognising that the obsessional thoughts, impulses or images are a product of his or her own mind.

Compulsions are identified by: 1) repetitive behaviours (e.g. hand-washing, ordering, checking) or mental acts (e.g. praying, counting, repeating words silently) that the person feels driven to perform in response to an obsession, or according to rules that must be applied rigidly; 2) these behaviours or mental acts, although aimed at preventing or reducing distress or preventing some dreaded event or situation, are either connected in a realistic way with what they are designed to neutralise or prevent or are clearly excessive. Besides patients who present the complete obsession-compulsive symptomatology, there are cases of simple obsession, without compulsion, and cases described in 1974 by Rachmann[2] as 'primary obsessive slowness'.

Although the neurological basis of OCD had been suspected in the past century[3], recent and growing experience in clinical psychiatry, pharmacology and brain imaging indicates possible impairment of specific brain areas and of the involved neuronal pathways. It has been reported that more than 90% of OCD patients have 'soft signs' of neurological disorder[4] concomitantly with OCD and true neurological diseases including: lethargic encephalitis (e.g. Schilder[5] and Laplane[6]); Parkinson's disease and parkinsonian syndromes (e.g. Trimble[7]); Huntington's chorea (e.g. Cummings and Cunningham[8]) and Sydenham's chorea (e.g. Swedo[9]); diabetes insipidus (e.g. Barton[10]); brain injury (e.g. Hillbom[11]); epilepsy (e.g. Behar and Fedio[12]); and Gilles de la Tourette's syndrome (e.g. Pauls[13]).

Other observations support the organic hypothesis in OCD:

a) Rapoport[14] found a close similarity between the obsessive-compulsive symptoms in children affected by OCD and the rituals of adult OCD, suggesting that OCD is poorly linked to affective and relational development.

b) The frequency of OCD in mental deficiency conditions, as in Down's syndrome (personal experience), is also in contrast with the psychogenic

Nuclear Medicine-PET Center,
General Hospital, Castelfranco
Veneto, Italy,
*Department of Psychiatry,
General Hospital, Montebelluna,
Italy

interpretation of OCD, which implies unconscious mechanisms in its genesis, suggesting that OCD is poorly linked to intellectual development.

c) The high prevalence of OCD in other psychiatric diseases such as depression (31.7%)[15], schizophrenia (3%)[16], phobic disorders (69%)[17] and anorexia nervosa (37%)[18], indicates that the functional involvement is different. Many biochemical studies observe that OCD may involve impairment of the serotonin neurotransmitter system - the so-called 'serotonin hypothesis' of OCD[19]. In confirmation of these data, an important body of evidence in pharmacological research has proved the therapeutic effect of drugs that are inhibitors of serotonin re-uptake, such as clorimipramine[20], fluoxetine[21], fluvoxamine[22] and sertraline[23].

Brain imaging studies

The introduction of brain imaging techniques (CT, MRI, PET and SPECT) has allowed the *in vivo* study of the pathophysiology of OCD. While anatomical imaging has not yet provided any clear structural findings, PET and SPECT are now revealing many functional impairments that may relate neural function to the specific mental processes of OCD. The differences in the various reports, especially in the early ones, were probably due to poor patient selection. Moreover, some critics, in recent studies, have focused on: a) possible associated depression, which is quite common; b) previous therapeutic treatment, which is a crucial problem when studying psychiatric diseases; c) various scan technologies.

Anatomical imaging

In OCD, CT and MRI have shown not only the involvement of ventricles, basal ganglia and frontal cortex, but also normal patterns. Behar *et al.*[24] reported a higher than expected frequency of relative brain ventricular enlargement in 16 adolescents with OCD at early onset (who had had one or more episodes of major depression, too). In contrast, Insel *et al.*[25] found no differences in the ventricular-brain ratio in a small group of adults with OCD compared with control subjects. Luxemberg *et al.*[26], using quantitative X-ray CT, in 10 males affected by severe primary OCD, showed a significantly smaller volume of the caudate nucleus bilaterally. The same data were recently reported by Robinson *et al.*[27], who also noted no correlation with the severity or duration of the disease. But Kellner *et al.*[28] and Aylward *et al.*[29] found no differences in caudate volumes between OCD patients and controls; Scarone *et al.*[30] reported increased caudate volume in OCD patients, but only on the right side. Lastly, Stein *et al.*[31] found ventricular enlargement but not with any caudate nucleus involvement.

With regard to frontal lobes, an MRI study of Garber *et al.*[32] revealed prolonged T_1 relaxation time in the white matter of the right frontal lobe, arguing cerebral asymmetry (left larger than right). This finding was correlated with the severity of the disease.

Functional imaging

[18]FDG PET

FDG PET has indicated hypermetabolism in many brain areas. The first report (Baxter *et al.*[33]) in 14 adult OCD patients (9 of them also meeting DSM-III criteria for major depression) showed significantly increased metabolism in the left orbital gyrus and, bilaterally, in the caudate nuclei, hypothesising a functional imbalance between caudate nucleus and orbito frontal cortex. Later the same authors[34] studied 10 non-depressed OCD patients, and achieved similar results. Increased metabolism of the left and right orbito frontal cortex was also shown by Nordhal *et al.*[35] and Sawle *et al.*[36]. The latter authors also found no differences in the cingulate cortex between OCD patients and controls, in contrast to Swedo *et al.*[37] and Perani *et al.*[38] who found increased activity in this region and also reported a decrease in cingulate cortex values after serotoninergic treatment. Some other studies that have related OCD and the effects of drugs are: a) Swedo *et al.*[39]: 'in comparison with baseline cerebral glucose metabolism, normalised right and left orbito frontal metabolic rates were significantly decreased after therapy with fluoxetine'; b)Benkelfat *et al.*[40]: 'after clorimipramine, significant decrease in left nucleus caudate activity and in right orbito frontal region'; c) Baxter *et al.*[41] observed decreased metabolism in the head of the right caudate nucleus after fluoxetine.

Opposing results were presented by Martinot *et al.*[42] who, in 16 non-depressed OCD patients, showed a global grey matter hypometabolism and significantly lower FDG uptake in the orbito frontal, lateral and medial frontal, temporal and parieto occipital regions. Interestingly, they did not find any differences between treated and drug-free subjects.

^{15}O-CO_2 PET

Using this technique, Rauch *et al.*[43] studied 8 OCD patients in resting and provoked (symptomatic) states. By subtracting the images, they found a statistically significant increase in cerebral blood flow during the symptomatic state in the right caudate nucleus, left anterior cingulate cortex and bilateral orbito frontal cortex.

Perfusion SPECT

Many authors have reported increased cerebral blood flow in some brain areas using ^{99m}Tc-HMPAO.

In 10 OCD patients, Machlin et al.[44] found 'a significantly higher ratio of medial frontal to whole cortex... no differences in orbito frontal'. The same result, with an interesting outcome, was further reported by Hohen-Saric et al.[45], of the same group, who showed that the ratio of medial frontal to whole-brain blood flow decreased during fluoxetine treatment. Hollander et al.[46] reported an increase in whole cortical blood flow (measured by ^{133}Xe) in 10 OCD patients after administration of the serotonin agonist m-chlorophenylpiperazine (m-CPP). The orbito frontal cortex, dorso parietal and left postero frontal regions were found to be hyperperfused by Rubin et al.[47] who studied 10 OCD males. Interestingly, the same study showed decreased blood flow in the head of the caudate nucleus bilaterally.

However, not only increases have been found. Lucey et al.[48] presented a study of 30 OCD drug-free patients compared with a group of 30 controls. In OCD they found significant hypoperfusion not only in the frontal, temporal and parietal cortex but also in the right caudate nucleus and thalamus, which correlated with the severity of the disease. Decreased blood flow in the temporal cortex was also found by Zohar et al.[49] during exposure to the specific contaminant; its imaginal flooding produced the opposite result.

Materials and methods

For our study on OCD, we enrolled 6 right-handed subjects (mean age 37 ± 12 years, range 23-52), including 4 females and 2 males, who met the DSM-III-R criteria for OCD based on the Structured Clinical Interview for DSM-III-R. Mean duration of disease was 12 ± 4 years and subjects were non-smokers with no previous history of brain injury, epilepsy, drug and/or alcohol abuse. In 2 cases, the onset of OCD was in childhood — it was in early adulthood in the other 4. Patients were submitted to MRI, which showed enlarged ventricles in the 2 childhood onset cases, but was normal in the other 4.

The Yale Brown Obsessive-Compulsive Scale was used to quantify the severity of obsessive and compulsive symptoms: obsession score (items 1 through 5) was 12.1 ± 2.2, while compulsion score (items 6 through 10) was 10.6 ± 2.7. Overall score was

22.7 ± 2.5. Before SPECT, we also excluded anxiety and depression using the Hamilton Rating Scale for anxiety and the 24-item Hamilton Rating Scale for depression.

At the time of the SPECT scan, 3 patients were therapy-free after a 1-week complete drug washout, and the other 3 were drug-naive. The controls were 6 sex- and age-matched, right-handed normal subjects with no previous history of neurological or psychiatric disease. Perfusion SPECT was performed using ^{99m}Tc-HMPAO, injecting 900 MBq of tracer in the resting condition (eyes closed and ears unplugged). Patients were fasting and the scan began within 30 min. A single-head rotating camera (GE 400 AC Starcam) with a resolution of 15 mm (FWHM) on the transaxial slices was used. Patients' heads were positioned along the OM line by a laser device and SPECT data were collected on 360° rotation, recording 64 views of 35 s each, on a 128 x 128 matrix. Reconstruction of transaxial, coronal and sagittal slices was made, after uniformity correction by a filtered back-projection algorithm using a Ramp filter, pre-filter Butterworth (cut-off 0.5 cycles/cm power 10). Images were reconstructed both without and with attenuation correction (coefficients from 0.01-0.12 cm^{-1}). The thickness of the reconstructed slices was 1.2 cm.

We also performed SPECT of a bidimensional brain phantom (2 slices at the level of basal ganglia) filled with 370 MBq of ^{99m}Tc-HMPAO. The same technique (acquisition and reconstruction of raw data) of OCD and controls was used. Reconstructed transaxial slices of the phantom, with the different coefficients of attenuation correction, were visually compared with the equivalent slices of patients and controls. The SPECT studies of OCD and normal subjects were examined visually, by two trained independent observers who considered all slices.

Semi-quantitative analysis was then performed on the transaxial slices of OCD patients and controls, and regions of interest (ROIs), on each hemisphere were positioned using a home-made software program. A stereotactic atlas (Talairach Tournoux, 1988) and each subject's MRI were used as references. Four slices in the OM plane were considered for ROI placement. Cortical and subcortical ROIs (20 per study) with which to define the activity (expressed as mean counting per pixel in the ROI) of cortical lobes, basal ganglia and thalamus, were placed on each slice. The ratio to cerebellum activity, as an internal standard, was then computed for each ROI. The frontal cortex was divided into orbito frontal, medium frontal and upper frontal; the temporal cortex was divided into low temporal and upper temporal. Parietal and occipital ROIs were considered as a whole. Student's t-test for unpaired data was used for statistical analysis.

Results

Visual interpretation of SPECT

Considering the images of the various reconstruction techniques, we divided them into non-attenuated, attenuated by coefficients from 0.01-0.06 cm^{-1}, attenuated by coefficients from 0.06-0.12 cm^{-1}.

1) Non-attenuated images

In normal subjects, perfusion was homogeneous in the various cortical regions. Basal ganglia and thalamus had low uptake (about 10% less on the colour scale) compared with the cortex. The same images were evident for brain phantom slices. In all OCD patients we found mild hypoperfusion in the frontal cortex (10-20% less on the colour scale), more evident in the orbito frontal and prefrontal regions (the latter particularly in the sagittal slices). In the 2 cases of childhood onset, there was patchy distribution of the tracer. Similar findings as in the controls were observed for basal ganglia and thalamus uptake.

2) Attenuation correction from 0.01-0.06 cm^{-1}

Visual examination confirmed the results of the non-attenuated images.

3) Attenuation correction from 0.06-0.12 cm^{-1}

Basal ganglia and thalamus showed the greatest activity in both normal subjects (Figure 1) and brain phantom. The uptake of these regions increased concomitantly with the values of the attenuation correction coefficients. In OCD patients we found the same, but hypoperfusion of the frontal cortex was more evident and extensive in the more attenuated slices (Figure 2).

Semi-quantitative analysis

We considered the same subdivisions according to the different coefficients of attenuation:

1) Non-attenuated images

Low uptake indexes in whole brain were found in OCD patients compared with controls, with statistically significant values (p<0.005) for orbito frontal, upper frontal, and low temporal and the occipital cortex, thalamus and basal ganglia (Figure 3).

2) Attenuation correction from 0.01-0.06 cm^{-1}

Semi-quantitative analysis confirmed previous data.

3) Attenuation correction from 0.06 up 0.12 cm^{-1}

With respect to the results in points 1 and 2, the statistical difference between controls and OCD increased in the orbito frontal and upper frontal cortex regions and in the basal ganglia (p < 0.01) (Figure 4).

Discussion

In our preliminary experience of OCD, admittedly in only six cases, we found decreased perfusion in many

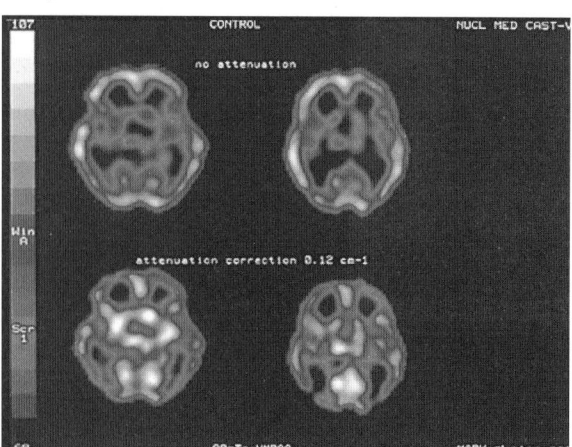

Figure 1 Transaxial slices, in the OM plane, of a control subject, reconstructed both without (upper slices) and with attenuation correction

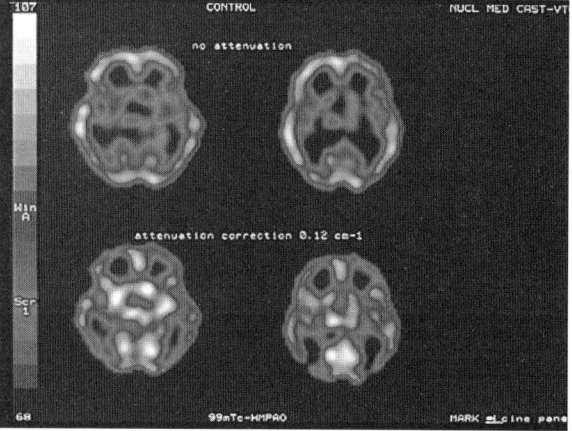

Figure 2 Transaxial slices, in the OM plane, of an OCD patient, reconstructed both without (upper slices) and with attenuation correction

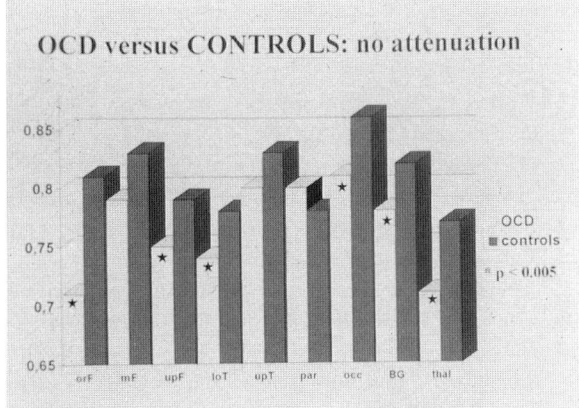

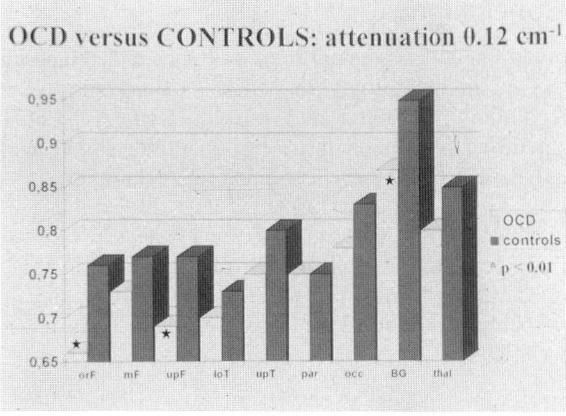

Figure 3 Brain regions (expressed as ratio of the mean values of all ROIs positioned on those regions towards cerebellum) in the non-attenuated transaxial slices of OCD and controls (orF = orbito frontal; mF = medium frontal; upF = upper frontal; loT = low temporal; upT = upper temporal; par = parietal; occ = occipital; BG = basal ganglia; thal = thalamus)

Figure 4 Brain regions (expressed as ratio of the mean values of all ROIs positioned on those regions towards cerebellum) in the attenuated transaxial slices (coefficient value: 0.12 cm^{-1}) of OCD and controls (orF = orbito frontal; mF = medium frontal; upF = upper frontal; loT = low temporal; upT = upper temporal; par = parietal; occ = occipital; BG = basal ganglia; thal = thalamus)

brain regions, evident even by semi-quantitative analysis. These data were confirmed by various reconstruction techniques of SPECT images, although 'heavier' attenuation correction enlarged the gap between the basal ganglia and frontal cortex of OCD and normal subjects. We found no significant right-to-left differences and, when considering drug-naive and drug-free patients, no substantial discrepancies. The same result was obtained when males and females were compared.

One particular finding was patchy distribution of the tracer in the whole cortex of subjects with childhood onset. At this point, it seems useful to mention some pathophysiological considerations. Various imaging studies have shown the involvement principally of the orbito frontal region, the cingulate cortex and the head of caudate nucleus and, as Insel[50] reported in a recent review: 'several authors have suggested that these regions form a circuit that is "hyperactive" in OCD' (Modell[51], Rapoport[52], Baxter[53]). This pathophysiological model is based on the results of those reports showing hyperactivity, generally hypermetabolism, in these brain areas (Baxter [33, 34, 41], Nordhal[35], Swedo[37], Swale[36]). Moreover, many authors report that anti-obsessive treatment produces a reduction in metabolism in the regions with increased activity (Swedo[39], Benkelfat[40]). Our data agree with the involvement of these regions - with the exception of the cingulate cortex, which SPECT can evaluate poorly

- but they do show decreased activity in drug-free and drug-naive conditions.

Possible explanations of our results are as follows. First, our group of patients had had OCD for long periods of time; long-lasting disease may lead to adaptive changes in the neuronal pathways involved. A similar opinion was expressed by Martinot[42], whose patients had long-lasting disease (18±13 yrs), while opposite results were reported by Baxter in a group of subjects who had had the illness for at least 1 year. Second, according to the Yale Brown Obsessive Scale (YBOS) score, our subjects had a severe clinical picture which may be related to a permanent status of internal exposure to the stimulus or, better, of internal flooding, as stated by Zohar[49] (increased blood low during imaginal flooding and decreased flow during real exposure to the specific contaminant object). Third, the difference between our and other authors' experience may reflect different patient selection. For example, our subjects had higher obsession than compulsive scores.

Although the idea of a specific hyperactive neuronal circuit in OCD is very exciting, our data seem to prove that OCD reflects different, discrete and variable functional states involving several brain areas. This hypothesis is probably more in line with the various conflicting results of the literature, and with the complexities of both brain function and human behaviour.

Conclusions

Perfusion SPECT has proved useful in understanding the pathophysiology of OCD. Considering the technology involved and our experience, SPECT should be performed in a semi-quantitative way and compared with other neuroimaging techniques. It is necessary to carry out further *in vivo* studies that will combine anatomical and functional data. So far, our finding of the patchy distribution of the tracer in cases of childhood onset of OCD is interesting and is probably related to the enlarged ventricles highlighted by MRI.

References

1   American Psychiatric Association: Diagnostic and Statistical Manual of Mental Disorders, 4th Edn. American Psychiatric Association, Washington, DC, USA, 1994

2   Rachman, S.J. Primary obsessional slowness. *Beh. Res. Ther.* 1974, 12, 9

3   Tuke, D. Imperative ideas. *Brain* 1894, 17, 179

4   Hollander, E., Schiffman, E., Cohen, B. *et al.* Signs of central nervous system dysfunction in obsessive-compulsive disorder. *Arch. Gen. Psychiatr.* 1990, 47, 27

5   Schilder, P. The organic background of obsessions and compulsions. *Am. J. Psychiatr.* 1938, 94, 1397

6   Laplane, D., Baulac, M., Widlocher, D. and Dubois, B. Psychic akinesia with bilateral lesion of basal ganglia. *J. Neurol. Neurosurg. Psychiatr.* 1984, 47, 377

7   Trimble, M.R. in 'Neuropsychiatry', Wiley, New York, USA, 1981, p.209

8   Cummings, J.L. and Cunningham, F. Obsessive-compulsive disorder in Huntington's disease. *Biol. Psychiatr.* 1992, 31, 263

9   Swedo, S.E., Rapoport, J.L., Cheslow, D.L. *et al.* High prevalence of obsessive-compulsive symptoms in patients with Sydenham's chorea. *Am. J. Psychiatr.* 1989, 146, 246

10   Barton, R. Diabetes insipidus and obsessional neurosis. *Lancet* 1965, 1, 133

11   Hillbom, E. After-effects of brain injuries. *Acta. Psychiatr. Neurol. Scand.* 1960, 35(suppl 142), 125

12   Behar, D.M. and Fedio, P. Quantitative analysis of interictal behavior in temporal lobe epilepsy. *Arch. Neurol.* 1977, 34, 454

13   Pauls, D.L., Towbin, K.E., Lechman, J.F. *et al.* Gilles de la Tourette's Syndrome and obsessive-compulsive disorder: evidence supporting an etiological relationship. *Arch. Gen. Psychiatr.* 1986, 43, 1180

14   Rapoport, J. The boy who couldn't stop washing. The experience and treatment of obsessive-compulsive disorder. New York, USA, New American Library, 1989

15   Robins, L.N., Helzer, J.E. and Weissman, M.M. Lifetime prevalence of specific psychiatric disorders in three sites. *Arch. Gen. Psychiatr.* 1984, 41, 949

16   Black, A. The natural history of obsessional neurosis in 'Obsessional States', (Ed. H.R. Beech), Methuen, London, 1974, p.19

17   Kringlen, E. Obsessional neurotics. A long term follow-up. *Br. J. Psychiatr.* 1965, 111, 709

18   Thiel, A., Broocks, A., Ohlmeyer, M. *et al.* Obsessive-compulsive disorder among patients with anorexia nervosa and bulimia nervosa. *Am. J. Psychiatr.* 1995, 152, 72

19   Murphy, D.L., Zohar, J., Benkelfat C. *et al.* Obsessive-compulsive disorder as a 5-HT subsystem-related behavioural disorder. *Br. J. Psychiatr.* 1989, 155(suppl 8), 15

20   The Clomipramine Collaborative Study Group. Clomipramine in the treatment of patients with obsessive-compulsive disorder. *Arch. Gen. Psychiatr.* 1991, 48, 730

21   Pigott, T.A., Pato, M.T., Bernstein, S.E. *et al.* Controlled comparisons of clomipramine and fluoxetine in the treatment of obsessive-compulsive disorder: behavioural and biological results. *Arch. Gen. Psychiatr.* 1990, 47, 926

22   Goodman, W.K., Price, L.H., Delgado, P.L. *et al.* Specificity of serotonin reuptake inhibitors in the treatment of obsessive-compulsive disorder: comparison of fluvoxamine and desipramine. *Arch. Gen. Psychiatr.* 1990, 47, 577

23   Chouinard, G.F., Goodman, W.K., Greist, J.H. *et al.* Results of a double-blind placebo controlled trial of a new serotonin uptake inhibitor, sertraline, in the treatment of obsessive-compulsive disorder. *Psychopharmacol. Bull.* 1990, 26, 279

24   Behar, D., Rapoport, J.L., Berg, C.J. *et al.* Computerized tomography and neuropsychological test measures in adolescents with obsessive-compulsive disorder. *Am. J. Psychiatr.* 1984, 141, 363

25   Insel, T.R., Donnelly, E.F., Lalakea, M.L. *et al.* Neurological and neuropsychological studies of patients with obsessive-compulsive disorder. *Biol. Psychiatr.* 1983, 18, 741

26   Luxenberg, J.S., Swedo, S.E., Flament, M.F. *et al.* Neuroanatomical abnormalities in obsessive-compulsive disorder detected with quantitative X-ray computed tomography. *Am. J. Psychiatr.* 1988, 145, 1089

27   Robinson, D., Houwei, W., Munne, R.A. *et al.* Reduced caudate nucleus volume in obsessive-compulsive disorder. *Arch. Gen. Psychiatr.* 1995, 52, 393

28   Kellner, C.H., Jolley, R.R., Holgate, R.C. *et al.* Brain MRI in obsessive-compulsive disorder. *Psychiatr. Res.* 1991, 36, 45

29   Aylward, E.H., Schwartz, J., Machlin, S. and Pearlson, G. Bicaudate ratio as a measure of caudate volume on MR images. *Am. J. Neuroradiol.* 1991, 12, 1217

30   Scarone, S., Colombo, C., Livian, S. *et al.* Increased right caudate nucleus size in obsessive-compulsive disorder: detection with magnetic resonance imaging. *Psychiatr. Res. Neuroimaging* 1992, 45, 115

31   Stein, D.J., Hollander, E., Chan, S. *et al.* Computed tomography and neurological soft signs in obsessive-compulsive disorder. *Psychiatr. Res. Neuroimaging* 1993, 50, 143

32 Garber, H.J., Ananth, J.V., Chiu, L.C. *et al.* Nuclear magnetic resonance study of obsessive-compulsive disorder. *Am. J. Psychiatr.* 1989, 146, 1001

33 Baxter, L.R., Phelps, M.E., Mazziotta, J.C. *et al.* Local cerebral glucose metabolism rates in obsessive-compulsive disorder - a comparison with rates in unipolar depression and in normal controls. *Arch. Gen. Psychiatr.* 1987, 44, 211

34 Baxter, L.R.Jr., Schwartz, J.M., Mazziotta, J.C. *et al.* Cerebral glucose metabolism rates in nondepressed patients with obsessive-compulsive disorder. *Am. J. Psychiatr.* 1988, 145, 1560

35 Nordhal, T.E., Benkelfalt, C., Semple, W. *et al.* Cerebral glucose metabolic rates in obsessive-compulsive disorder. *Neuropsychopharmacology* 1989, 2, 23-28.

36 Sawle, G.V., Hymas, N.F., Lees, A.J. and Frackowiak, R.S.J. Obsessional slowness: functional studies with positron emission tomography. *Brain* 1991, 114, 2191

37 Swedo, S.E., Schapiro, M.B., Gady, C.L. *et al.* Cerebral glucose metabolism in childhood onset obsessive-compulsive disorder. *Arch. Gen. Psychiatr.* 1989, 46, 518

38 Perani, D., Colombo, C., Bressi, S. *et al.* (^{18}F)FDG PET study in obsessive-compulsive disorder. A clinical/metabolic correlation study after treatment. *Br. J. Psychiatr.* 1995, 166, 244

39 Swedo, S.E., Pietrini, P., Leonard, H.L. *et al.* Cerebral glucose metabolism in childhood onset obsessive-compulsive disorder: revisualization during pharmacotherapy. *Arch. Gen. Psychiatr.* 1992, 49, 690

40 Benkelfat, C., Nordhal, T.E., Semple, W.E. *et al.* Local cerebral glucose metabolic rates in obsessive-compulsive disorder patients treated with clomipramine. *Arch. Gen. Psychiatr.* 1990, 47, 840

41 Baxter, L.R.Jr., Schwartz, J.M., Bergman, K.S. *et al.* Caudate glucose metabolic rate changes with both drug and behavior therapy for obsessive-compulsive disorder. *Arch. Gen. Psychiatr.* 1992, 49, 681

42 Martinot, J.L., Allilaire, J.F., Mazoyer, B.M. *et al.* Obsessive-compulsive disorder: a clinical, neuropsychological and positron emission tomography study. *Acta. Psychiatr. Scand.* 1990, 82, 233

43 Rauch, S.L., Jenike, M.A., Alpert, N.M. *et al.* Regional cerebral blood flow measured during symptom provocation in obsessive-compulsive disorder using oxygen 15-labelled carbon dioxide and positron emission tomography. *Arch. Gen. Psychiatr.* 1994, 51, 62

44 Machlin, S.R., Harris, G.J., Pearlson, G.D. *et al.* Elevated medial-frontal cerebral blood flow in obsessive-compulsive patients: a SPECT study. *Am. J. Psychiatr.* 1991, 148, 1240

45 Hohen-Saric, R., Pearlson, G.D., Harris, G.J. *et al.* Effects of fluoxetine on regional cerebral blood flow in obsessive-compulsive patients. *Am. J. Psychiatr.* 1991, 148, 1243

46 Hollander, E., DeCaria, C.M., Saoud, J.B. *et al.* M-CPP-activated regional cerebral blood flow in obsessive-compulsive disorder. *Biol. Psychiatr.* 1991, 29, 170A

47 Rubin, R.T., Villanueva-Meyer, J., Ananth, J. *et al.* Regional xenon 133 cerebral blood flow and cerebral technetium ^{99m}Tc HMPAO uptake in unmedicated patients with obsessive-compulsive disorder and age-matched normal control subjects. *Arch. Gen. Psychiatr.* 1992, 49, 695

48 Lucey, J.V., Costa, D.C., Busatto, G.F. *et al.* Regional cerebral blood flow in obsessive-compulsive disorder measured by ^{99m}Tc-HMPAO uptake and single photon emission tomography. *J. Nucl. Med.* 1995, 36(5), 20

49 Zohar, J., Insel, T.R., Berkman, K.F. *et al.* Anxiety and cerebral blood flow during behavioural challenge. Dissociation of central from peripheral and subjective measures. *Arch. Gen. Psychiatr.* 1989, 46, 505

50 Insel, T.R. Toward a neuroanatomy of obsessive-compulsive disorder. *Arch. Gen. Psychiatr.* 1992, 49, 739

51 Modell, J.G., Mountz, J.M., Curtis, G.C. and Greden, J.F. Neurophysiologic dysfunction in basal ganglia/limbic striatal and thalamocortical circuits as a pathogenetic mechanism of obsessive-compulsive disorder. *J. Neuropsychiatr. Clin. Neurosci.* 1989, 1, 27

52 Rapoport, J. Recent advances in obsessive-compulsive disorder. *Neuropsychopharmacology* 1991, 5, 1

53 Baxter, L.R., Schwartz, J.M., Guze, B.H. *et al.* Neuroimaging in obsessive-compulsive disorder: seeking the mediating neuroanatomy in 'Obsessive-Compulsive Disorder: Theory and Management', (Eds. M.A. Jenike, L. Baer, W.E. Minichiello), Mosby Year Book, St Louis, USA, 1990, p.167

SPECT in Neurology and Psychiatry, edited by P.P. De Deyn, R.A. Dierckx, A. Alavi and B.A. Pickut

Experimental Neuroactivation with SPECT in Schizophrenic Patients

Chapter
16

J. Pinkert, I. Gerdsen, R. Fötzsch, W.G. Franke, W. Felber, U. Neumann and L. Oehme

Introduction

A defect in neural transmission and information processing is supposed to be one of the basic pathological disturbances in schizophrenia. Visual, acoustic and olfactory perception, as well as motor control, is affected. Since the early works of Diefendorf and Dodge[1], and later Holzmann[2], the ocular motor system, which can be considered as a model of motor control, became the subject of neuroscientific research to study the neural process underlying schizophrenia. These studies observed disorders of smooth pursuit and saccadic eye movements - which are suspected to indicate an impairment of higher cortical control - in 60-80% of schizophrenic and 30% of other psychiatric patients. This phenomenon has also been regarded as a possible genetic trait marker for schizophrenic vulnerability.

The ocular motor system involves a neuronal network of cortical and subcortical structures. Cortical areas incorporating the frontal (FEF) and supplementary eye fields (SEF), the dorsolateral prefrontal cortex (DLPFC), the posterior parietal cortex (PPC), the medial superior and middle temporal areas and the striate cortex (SC), are all part of this network. Neurons in the FEF, SEF, DLPFC and basal ganglia seem to discharge during saccadic eye movements[3,4]. Neuronal ocular motor pathways with their cortical projections are illustrated in Figures 1 and 2.

Little is known about the pathomorphological substrates responsible for these impairments. To understand more about the functional anatomy of a possible ocular motor system disturbance, Nakashima *et al.*[5] (PET) and Crawford *et al.*[6] (SPECT) have used a reflexive, volitional, memory-guided and antisaccadic paradigm in recent studies in an attempt to identify regions of reduced rCBF in schizophrenic subjects. Their objective was to determine the contribution of prefrontal or other areas to saccadic abnormality and to compare results with reports from lesion studies.

In contrast to these authors, we used the following SPECT study to monitor saccadic intrusions during smooth pursuit eye movements, in order to analyse cortical saccadic control in schizophrenics and patients with affective disorders. Regional blood flow was used as an index of neuronal activity and rCBF values were compared for activation and resting conditions - images were calculated by subtraction of the activation from the resting patterns.

Departments of Nuclear Medicine, Psychiatry, Neurology and Radiology, Dresden University of Technology, Fetscherstrasse 74, Dresden D-01307, Germany

Methods

Thirty patients (21 schizophrenic and 9 depressive subjects) aged 20-60 years were recruited from our psychiatric department. All patients were diagnosed according to DSM-III-R criteria. Psychopathological symptoms were assessed on the Brief Psychiatric Rating Scale (BPRS)[7]. Handedness was defined according to Oldfield. The medication, mainly neuroleptic and antidepressive drugs, remained unchanged between the SPECT examinations. Patients with a history of any neurological disorder or drug abuse were not included. Neuro-ophthalmological and electronystagmographic (EOG) examinations were carried out in all patients with the Nicolet Nystar EOG system (Baloh et al. [8], Depondt[9]).

Following activation with a horizontally oscillating red light point (0.4 Hz) on a light bar over 3 min (Nicolet Nystar Plus Task Design) in a dimmed, quiet room, 750 MBq ^{99m}Tc-ECD were given intravenously via a long venous catheter so that the moment of injection was not noticed by the patient. Stimulation was continued for another 2 min after injection. The second investigation was performed within the next 2 weeks under resting conditions, and again in a dimmed and quiet room — the patient was left in a relaxed position for about 15 min before tracer injection.

SPECT studies were accomplished both at rest and following activation 1 h after injection using a dual-

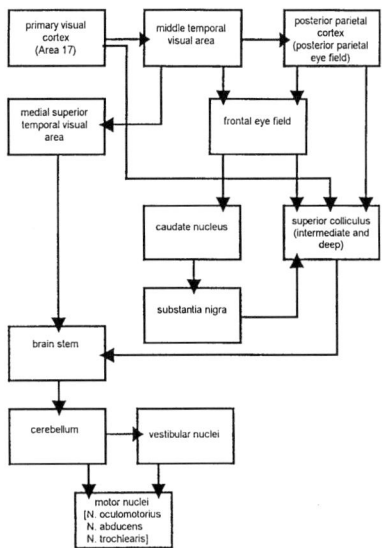

Figure 1 Diagram of ocularmotor neuronal pathways acccording to Goldberg, M.E. *et al.* The ocular motor system in 'Principles of neural science', (Eds. E.R. Kandel *et al.*), Prentice-Hall Int. Inc., 1991, p.660

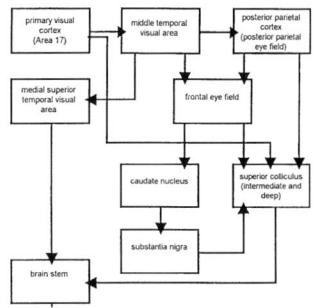

Figure 2 Cortical areas active in ocular movements according to Goldberg, *et al.* (see legend for Figure 1)

head camera equipped with low-energy, high-resolution collimators, with 40 s per frame, and 64 frames on a 64x64 matrix. The resolution of our camera was approximately 10 mm FWHM. After reconstruction with a Butterworth filter an attenuation correction using the CHANG algorithm was performed. A re-orientation in the orbito-meatal line and an image re-registration between the activation and the resting study were made. Neuroactivation images were calculated by subtracting resting from activation patterns. Finally, a 5x5 spatial filter was applied. In order to obtain 25% more counts for the activation image, we multiplied with a variable factor. A slight activity in brain structures obtained by applying this technique is convenient as a landmark for hot spots caused by activation. The activation pattern of all calculated neuroactivation images was visually analysed, also taking into account the SPECT slices from both studies. The increase in the regional count rate in the FEF was determined using the ROI technique at 7.4% ±2 .6 under stimulation.

Results

After subtraction of both images, increased blood flow, indicating neuroactivation, was seen as a hot-spot area in the striatal cortex (SC), frontal eye field (FEF), posterior parietal cortex (PPC) and cerebellum. To a smaller extent and obviously not in all patients, higher rCBF values due to neuroactivation were also observed in the basal ganglia and thalamus. No activation was seen in the dorsolateral prefrontal cortex (DLPFC). This activation pattern is in agreement with the known functional anatomy active during the generation of saccades, visual attentional processing for saccades and visual motion processing. EOG measurements showed reduced mean gain values for schizophrenic and depressive patients (0.74). Reduced enhancement of rCBF values (p<0.05), in several subjects presenting an

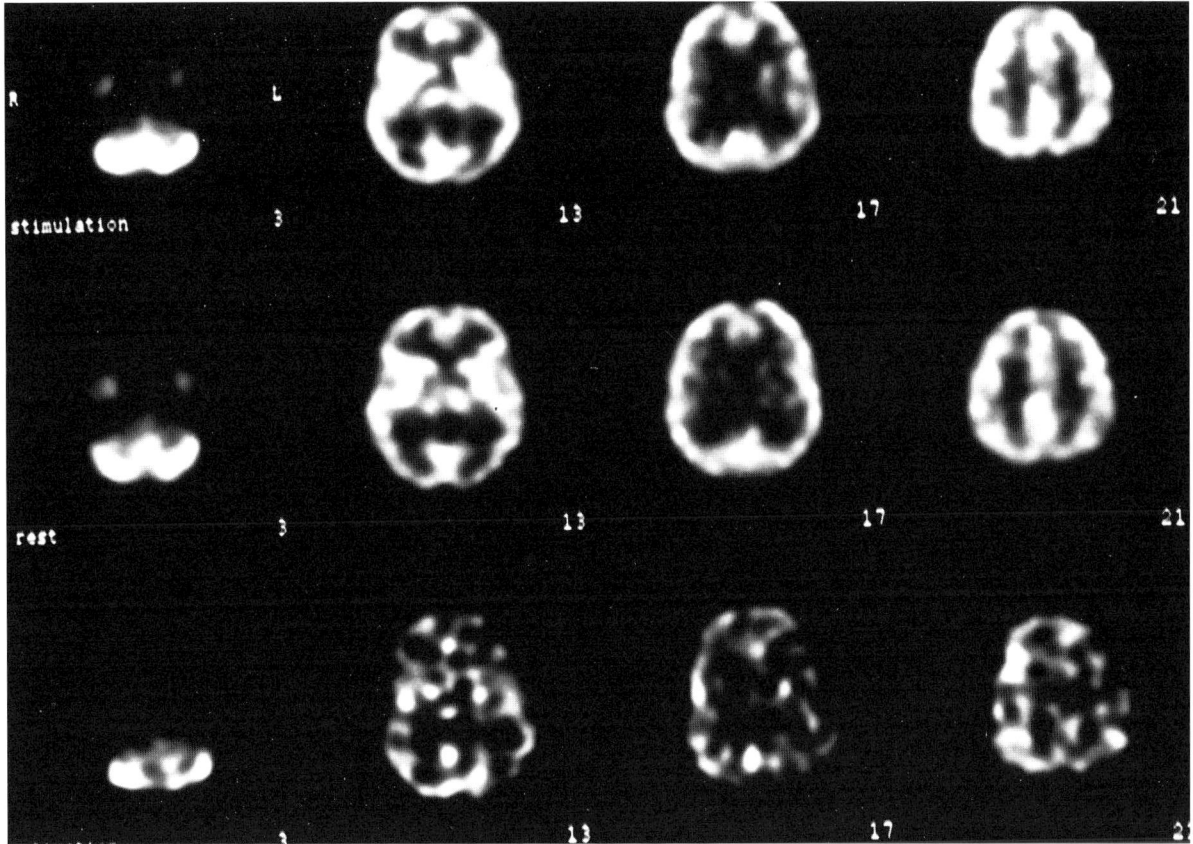

Figure 3 SPECT slices and substraction images of a 37 year old male patient suffering from schizophrenia

increased number of saccadic intrusions, was observed for the frontal eye field (FEF). The SPECT slices and neuroactivation images of a 37-year-old male patient suffering from schizophrenia are shown in Figure 3. Smooth pursuit in this patient was only slightly impaired by saccadic intrusions.

Discussion

Several neuroimaging studies have provided a large amount of data on impaired cerebral activity during eye movements in schizophrenia and speculations have been made about different ocular motor centres and their function in controlling saccades. For cortical control of saccadic eye movements, the important role of the frontal eye field (FEF) has already been well established by both electrical stimulation (Ferrier et al.[10]) and single-unit studies (Goldberg and Bruce,[11]). When comparing the rCBF findings with PET of schizophrenic subjects compared with normal controls, Nakashima et al.[5] also showed a reduced activation in the left dorsolateral prefrontal cortex (DLPFC) during voluntary saccadic tasks and no increase in rCBF values for the frontal eye field (FEF). In contrast, Crawford et al.[6], using an antisaccade paradigm, failed to show any differential rCBF changes with SPECT in the FEF and failed to activate the DLPFC. However, the latter study did have some methodological limitations. It lacked a baseline condition and compared all patients in an activated state only.

So far no SPECT and PET studies including schizophrenic and depressive patients have focussed on the relationship between ocular motor activation and the rate of inappropriate saccades by using a smooth pursuit eye-tracking stimulus as we have done. In both schizophrenic and depressive patients, we identified subgroups with high rates of saccadic intrusions using EOG measurements. Analysis showed that there was an inverse correlation between frontal eye field (FEF) activation and intrusion rate (p<0.05). Our results therefore support the hypothesis that the frontal eye field (FEF) is involved in the control of saccades. In line with the results of Weinberger et al.[12] during prefrontal challenge tasks, no activation was detected in the DLPFC for any patient. He termed this phenomenon, which he observed only in schizophrenic subjects, a 'functional hypofrontality'. Lack of DLPFC activation is in good agreement with concepts of frontal lobe pathology for both schizophrenia and affective disorders (Franzen et al.[13], Berman et al.[14], Dolan et al.[15]).

In addition, our data show that, by using a simple smooth pursuit eye-tracking stimulus, cortical and subcortical structures of the ocular motor system can be activated and detected with single photon emission tomography (SPECT) - despite certain limitations of SPECT methodology (Pinkert et al.[16], Orrison[17]). Image resolution can be considerably improved using a triple-head camera equipped with fan-beam collimators (FWHM 6-7 mm). This allows functional studies with reasonable results, even when PET and MRI facilities are not available or not easily accessible. SPECT studies are less costly and the SPECT environment is well tolerated, even by anxious or psychotic patients.

However, technical improvements in the analysis of our data have to be made. A program for automatic re-registration will be applied to the re-registration of resting and activation procedures, which might reduce artefacts due to insufficant re-registration. A fusion with MRI data and the projection in the standard stereotactic space, as defined by Tailarach and Tournoux[18], will allow the more precise identification of activated structures. In this context, rCBF values will be compared with statistical parametric mapping (SPM95) which is now also available for SPECT activation studies[19].

References

1 Diefendorf, A.R. and Dodge, R. An experimental study of the ocular reaction of the insane from photographic records. *Brain* 1908, 31, 451 2

2. Holzman, P.S., Proctor, L.R. and Hughes, D.W. Eye tracking patterns in schizophrenia. *Science* 1973, 181, 179

3 Buttner-Ennever, J. A. (Ed.) Reviews of Oculomotor Research, Vol 2: Neuroanatomy of the Oculomotor System. Elsevier, Amsterdam, The Netherlands, 1988

4 Leigh, R.J. and Zee, D.S. The neurology of eye movements, 2nd edn., F.A. Davis Company, Philadelphia, USA, 1992

5 Nakashima, Y., Momose, T., Sano, I. et al. Cortical control of saccade in normal and schizophrenic subjects: a PET study using a task-evoked rCBF paradigm. *Schizophr. Res.* 1994, 12, 259

6 Crawford, T.J., Puri, B.K., Nijran, K.S. *et al.* Abnormal saccadic distractibility in patients with schizophrenia: a ^{99m}Tc-HMPAO SPECT study. *Psychol. Med.* 1995, in press

7 Overall, J.E. and Gorham, D.R. The Brief Psychiatric Rating Scale. *Psychol. Rep.* 1962, 10, 799

8 Baloh, R.W., Yee, R.D., Honrubia, V. and Jacobson, K. A comparison of the dynamics of horizontal and vertical smooth pursuit in normal human subjects. *Aviat. Space Environ. Med.* 1986, 1

9 Depondt, M. and Damman, W. Normative data in horizontal ocular motor testing obtained on Nystar Plus system and transmitted to Nicolet by ENT Department, A.Z. St.Jan, B-8000 Brugge, Belgium. Nycolet Nystar Manual, Brugge, Belgium, 1990

10 Ferrier, D. The localisation of function in the brain. *Proc. R. Soc.* 1974, 22, 229

11 Goldberg, M.E. and Bruce, C.J. The role of the arcuate frontal eye fields in the generation of saccadic eye movements. *Prog. Brain Res.* 1986, 64, 143

12 Weinberger, D.R., Bergman, K.F. and Zec, R.F. Physiologic dysfunction of dorso-lateral prefrontal cortex in schizophrenia: I. Regional cerebral blood flow evidence. *Arch. Gen. Psychiatr.* 1986, 43, 114

13 Franzen, G. and Ingvar, D.H. Absence of activation in frontal structures during psychological testing of chronic schizophrenics. *J. Neurol. Neurosurg. Psychiatr.* 1975, 38, 1027

14 Berman, K.F., Zec, R.F. and Weinberger, D.R. Physiologic dysfunction of dorso-lateral prefrontal cortex in schizophrenia: II. role of neuroleptic treatment, attention, and mental effort. *Arch. Gen. Psychiatr.* 1986, 43, 126

15 Dolan, R.L., Bench, C.J., Liddle, F.F. *et al.* Dorsolateral prefrontal cortex dysfunction in the major psychoses; symptom or disease specificity? *J. Neurol. Neurosurg. Psychiatr.* 1993, 56, 1290

16 Pinkert, J., Gerdsen, I., Foetzsch, R. *et al.* Visualization of neuroactivation with SPECT after ocular motor stimulation in schizophrenics with smooth pursuit eye movement disorders. *Eur. J. Nucl. Med.* 1995, 22, 792

17 Orrison, W.W., Lewine, J.D., Sanders, J.A. and Hartshorne, M.F. in 'Functional Brain Imaging', Mosby, St Louis, USA, 1995

18 Tailarach, J. and Tournoux, P. Co-planar stereotaxic atlas of the human brain. Thieme, Stuttgart, Germany, 1988

19 Friston, K.J., Frith, C.D., Liddle, P.F. and Frackowiak, R.S.J. Comparing functional images: The assessment of significant change. *J. Cereb. Blood Flow Metab.* 1991, 1, 690

SPECT in Neurology and Psychiatry, edited by P.P. De Deyn, R.A. Dierckx, A. Alavi and B.A. Pickut
© 1997 John Libbey & Company Ltd, pp. 129–132

D$_2$ Dopamine Receptor Occupancy during Treatment with Neuroleptics in Schizophrenic Patients

Chapter
17

J. Scherer, K. Tatsch*, M. Albus,
M. Konjarczyk, K. Scherer, P. Thielking and
J. Schwarz*

Introduction

Dopamine D$_2$ receptors can be studied *in vivo* using Single Photon Emission Computed Tomography (SPECT) and Positron Emission Tomography (PET) techniques, applying the tracers ^{123}I-IBZM and ^{11}C-raclopride. These substances are substituted benzamides and selectively bind as antagonists to dopamine D$_2$ receptors in the basal ganglia. The striatum contains the highest density of dopamine D$_2$ receptors in the brain[1]. D$_2$ receptors are considered to be located mainly on postsynaptic membranes and as autoreceptors on presynaptic mesencephalo-striatal dopaminergic projections[2]. The disadvantages of SPECT in terms of spatial resolution, scatter and attenuation correction lead to a less accurate quantification of tracer uptake compared with PET. In spite of these limitations, SPECT using ^{123}I-IBZM has been reported to be a specific and safe technique with which to visualise dopamine D$_2$ receptor densities in the human CNS[3,4].

Evaluation of D$_2$ dopamine receptor occupancy is of particular interest in schizophrenia research, since the dopamine hypothesis of schizophrenia suggests that a high degree of D$_2$ dopamine receptor occupancy is usually necessary to obtain an antipsychotic response to neuroleptics[5]. However, since the evaluation of the relatively modest effects of clozapine and other atypical neuroleptics with good antipsychotic efficacy on D$_2$ dopamine receptors and their more pronounced effects on D$_1$ and D$_4$ dopamine receptors[6,7] compared with the typical neuroleptics, it is suggested that the amount of dopamine D$_2$ receptor occupancy of typical and atypical neuroleptics is not exclusively related to their antipsychotic properties[8]. Moreover, PET findings of a higher D$_2$ dopamine receptor occupancy in patients with EPMS suggest that the level of D$_2$ dopamine receptor occupancy is also related to the occurrence of EPMS[6].

The present study aimed to investigate whether or not there is a different dose-response relationship between D$_2$ receptor occupancy and total daily dosage for haloperidol and clozapine, using ^{123}I-iodobenzamide Single Photon Emission Computed Tomography (IBZM SPECT). A second aim was to investigate whether or not D$_2$ receptor occupancy is related to the occurrence of EPMS. We also looked at whether or not it is possible to define a threshold of D$_2$ dopamine receptor occupancy in the striatum, above which drug-induced EPMS can be expected.

State Mental Hospital Haar,
Vockestrasse 72, D 85529 Haar,
Germany
*Klinikum Grosshadern, Ludwig-
Maximilians-University, Munich,
Germany

Methods

Patients

We investigated a total of 27 patients (mean age 39.5 years, range 22-59) who met the diagnostic criteria for schizophrenia according to DSM-III-R and were able to give informed consent: 18 patients were treated with the typical neuroleptic haloperidol in a mean daily dose of 5-21 mg (corresponding to a daily dose of 0.07-0.35 mg/kg body weight); 9 patients were treated with the atypical neuroleptic clozapine in a mean daily dose of 125-400 mg (corresponding to a daily dose of 1.51-6.15 mg/kg body weight). All patients were treated for at least 4 weeks and had a stable daily dosage during the last 2 weeks before the study. One patient treated with clozapine and 4 patients treated with haloperidol additionally received tricyclic antidepressants, while 10 patients treated with haloperidol additionally received biperiden hydrochloride. Besides these drugs, no concomitant medication was administered.

EPMS were recorded according to the rating scale for EPMS also used by Farde et al.[6]. In patients with EPMS, at least one item indicating rigidity on the rating scale for EPMS was rated at 2 or more. Ten controls who had no psychiatric or relevant medical history were matched with patients for gender and age (within 4 years, age range 20-61 years).

Procedure

^{123}I-IBZM SPECT was performed two hours after i.v. injection of 185 MBq IBZM (3-iodo-6-methoxybenzamide, Cygne BV). A rotating dual-head gamma camera (Siemens Rota II, high-resolution collimator) connected to a computer system (Siemens Max Delta, Micro Vax 3400) was used for data acquisition and processing. Data were collected for 60 projections (360° rotation) in a 64x64 matrix with an acquisition time of 50 s per projection. During the acquisition period, the head was firmly fixed in a head rest to prevent any kind of motion. Data processing is described in detail elsewhere[10]. Briefly, transverse images were reconstructed by filtered backprojection (Butterworth filter, cut-off frequency: 0.5 Nyquist) with subsequent computation of coronal slices (slice thickness 6.0 mm). The transverse slices were reorientated according to the orbitomeatal line. Selected transverse slices encompassing the maximum tracer uptake over the striatum were corrected for attenuation. The size of all regions of interest (ROIs) was at least twice FWHM (14 mm) as described elsewhere[10]. Specific tracer uptake was calculated using the ratio: striatal ROI activity/frontal ROI activity, which is usually calculated in SPECT studies.

The values of the left and right striatum of each subject were pooled. The investigator who calculated the striatal/frontal cortex ratio (SFCR) was unaware of patients' diagnoses or drug regimens.

Statistical analysis

To evaluate the relationship between daily dose of neuroleptic and SFCR, a non-linear exponential regression analysis (least square method) with the model (d=daily dosage (mg); w=body weight) was carried out.

$$SFCR = 1 + A \times \exp(B \times d/w)$$

To compare 2 means, a Mann-Whitney Rank Sum Test was applied. All reported p values are based on 2-tailed tests. Differences between groups are expressed as means and 95% CI or range. A 2-tailed p-value <0.05 was taken to indicate significance.

Results

Patients on haloperidol and clozapine were similar in demographic characteristics, disease duration and functional impairment as measured by means of the global assessment scale (GAS). None of the 9 patients treated with clozapine had EPMS. Of the 18 patients treated with haloperidol, 10 had EPMS, and 8 had none. The haloperidol dosage/kg body weight was significantly higher in patients with EPMS (x = 0.17, s.d. = 0.07) than in patients without EPMS (x = 0.11, s.d. = 0.05; ANOVA: dF 1,17; F = 4.9, p<0.05). The SFCR was significantly lower in patients treated with haloperidol with EPMS (x = 1.15, s.d. = 0.05) than in those without EPMS (x = 1.23, s.d. = 0.05; ANOVA: dF 1,17; F = 7.71, p>0.01). Patients treated with haloperidol had a significantly lower SFCR (x = 1.19, s.d. = 0.06) than patients treated with clozapine (x = 1.46, s.d. = 0.05) and controls (x = 1.52, s.d. = 0.06, ANOVA: dF 2,36; F = 141.2, p<0.000).

When the patients investigated were subdivided according to the presence or absence of EPMS, all patients with EPMS were below a threshold of the SFCR of 1.2. All but one patient without EPMS were above this threshold (Chi-square = 23.10, p<0.000). The SFCR of tracer binding in haloperidol-treated patients was significantly lower (x = 1.19, s.d. = 0.06) than that in patients treated with clozapine (x = 1.46, s.d. = 0.05) and controls (x = 1.52, s.d. = 0.06, ANOVA: dF 2,36; F = 141.2, p< 0.000). There is an exponential dose-response relationship between striatal

D$_2$ receptor blockade (as measured by the reduction of the SFCR of tracer binding) and total daily dosage of haloperidol and clozapine, the function of which can be expressed by (SFCR-1) = 0.506 x e$^{-6.86 \text{ mg/kg body weight}}$ for patients treated with haloperidol and by (SFCR-1) = 0.526 x e$^{-0.0458 \text{ mg/kg body weight}}$ for patients treated with clozapine.

Discussion

Our data suggest an exponential dose-response relationship between striatal D$_2$ receptor blockade and total daily dosage of both haloperidol and clozapine. Thus, for haloperidol, we could not just confirm the results of Brücke et al.[4] qualitatively, but achieved a quantitative precision. The established exponential dose-response relationship reflects that changes in receptor occupancy seem to be directly proportional to the level of D$_2$ receptor blockade, i.e. the higher the given receptor occupancy, the higher the increase in dosage necessary to increase D$_2$ receptor occupancy by a constant rate. The exponential dose-response relationship found for clozapine contrasts with the results of Brücke et al.[4], suggesting no relationship between D$_2$ receptor occupancy and total daily clozapine dose. This discrepancy can be attributed to the considerable wider variance in the patients investigated by these authors compared with our sample. Brücke et al.[4] did not report on the length of time patients were on a stable dosage, but our sample's medication remained unchanged for at least 2 weeks before the study. Taking the wider interindividual variance in the clozapine group into account, one can speculate that the more variable bioavailability of clozapine requires a longer stable dosage regimen to come up to equilibrium than haloperidol.

The remarkable planar gradient of the clozapine binding curve reflects the lower D$_2$ receptor occupancy induced by this compound, also demonstrating that even with maaximum doses of clozapine, D$_2$ receptor occupancy remains less than it does with haloperidol. The assumption of a lower D$_2$ dopamine receptor occupancy during clozapine treatment compared with haloperidol treatment is supported by the higher SFCR in patients treated with clozapine than in those treated with haloperidol, and concords with the results of PET studies [6,11,12]. The validity of the dose response curves for both drugs is proven by the assumed SFCR doses of 0 mg/kg body weight being close to the SFCRs found in controls. This finding is in line with data published so far, suggesting no differences in the densities of D$_2$ receptors between schizophrenics and controls[12].

All patients treated with haloperidol had a significantly lower SFCR than controls. In concordance with other authors[4,6], we found a lower D$_2$ dopamine receptor occupancy during clozapine treatment compared with haloperidol treatment. This is supported by the finding that the significantly higher SFCR in the group treated with clozapine is close to that of normal controls. To our knowledge, this is the first direct demonstration by SPECT of the finding already demonstrated by PET[6], that EPMS are quantitatively related to striatal dopamine D$_2$ receptor occupancy. Most importantly, our data suggest the existence of a 'neuroleptic threshold', below which drug-induced EPMS can be expected - namely an SFCR of 1.2. In concordance with PET studies[6], we found that the patients with EPMS had higher D$_2$ dopamine receptor occupancies and therefore a significantly lower SFCR than the patients with no EPMS. Since patients with EPMS had a higher haloperidol dosage compared with patients without EPMS, this finding points at a dose-relationship between the occurrence of EPMS and the level of D$_2$ receptor occupancy.

The absolute counts measured in the frontal cortex did not differ between patient groups, indicating that our results were not influenced by differences in plasma tracer level or brain perfusion, but data on plasma tracer levels were not investigated.

In the sample investigated, only one patient without EPMS was below the threshold. Evaluation of the medical records showed that this patient had received extremely high dosages of haloperidol without ever developing EPMS in the past. Thus, this patient can be regarded as exceptional in terms of the response to neuroleptics. Our data support the hypothesis that the very low incidence of EPMS in patients treated with clozapine is, at least in part, due to the lesser D$_2$ dopamine receptor occupancy[6,7]. The concordant findings on the relationship between the level of D$_2$ receptor occupancy and the occurrence of EPMS between PET and SPECT strongly suggest that IBZM SPECT, a safe procedure which is readily available in nuclear medicine departments, is also a reliable means of demonstrating the in vivo occupancy of dopamine D$_2$ receptors by antipsychotic drugs.

References

1   Dawson, T.M., Gehlert, D.R. and Wamsley, J.K. Quantitative autoradiographic demonstration of high and low affinity agonist binding of D$_2$ dopamine receptors. *Clin. Res.* 1985, 33, 69a

2   Rinne, U.K., Laihinen, A., Rinne, J.O. et al. Positron emission tomography demonstrates dopamine D$_2$ receptor super-sensitivity in the striatum of patients with early

Parkinson's disease. *Mov. Dis.* 1990, 5, 55

3   Kung, H.F., Alavi, A., Chang, W. *et al.* In vivo SPECT imaging of dopamine D₂ receptors: initial studies with ¹²³I-IBZM in humans. *J. Nucl. Med.* 1990, 31, 573

4   Brucke, T., Roth, J., Podreka, l. *et al.* Striatal dopamine D₂-receptor blockade by typical and atypical neuroleptics. *Lancet* (letter) 1992, 339, 497

5   Peroutka, S.J. and Snyder, S.H. Relationship of neuroleptic drug effects at brain dopamine, serotonin, adrenergic and histamine receptors to clinical potency. *Am. J. Psychiatr.* 1980, 137, 1518

6   Farde, l., Nordström, A.L., Wiesel, F.A. *et al.* Positron emission tomographic analysis of central D1 and D₂ dopamine receptor occupancy in patients treated with classical neuroleptics and clozapine. *Arch. Gen. Psychiatr.* 1992, 49, 538

7   Seeman, P. Dopamine receptor sequences. Therapeutic levels of neuroleptics occupy D₂ receptors, clozapine occupies D4. *Neuropsychopharmacology* 1992, 2, 261

8   Pilowsky, L.S., Costa, D.C., Ell, P.J. *et al.* Clozapine, single photon emission tomography, and the D₂ dopamine receptor blockade hypothesis of schizophrenia. *Lancet* 1993, 340, 199

9   Simpson, G.M. and Angus, J.W.S. A rating scale for extra-pyramidal side effects. *Acta. Psychiatr. Scand.* 1970, 45(suppl), 11

10 Tatsch, K., Schwarz, J., Oertel, W.H. and Kirsch, C.M. SPECT imaging of dopamine D₂ receptors with ¹²³I-IBZM: initial experience in controls and patients with Parkinson's syndrome and Wilson's disease. *Nucl. Med. Comm.* 1991, 12, 699

11 Farde, l., Wiesel, F.A., Nordström A.L. and Sedvall, G. D₁- and D₂-dopamine receptor occupancy during treatment with conventional and atypical neuroleptics. *Psychopharmacology* 1989, 99, s28

12 Sedvall, G. The current status of PET scanning with respect to schizophrenia. *Neuropsychopharmacology* 1992, 7(1), 41

SPECT in Neurology and Psychiatry, edited by P.P. De Deyn, R.A. Dierckx, A. Alavi and B.A. Pickut
© 1997 John Libbey & Company Ltd, pp. 133–137

^{99m}Tc-HMPAO Brain SPECT and Psychopathology in Drug-Naive Schizophrenic Patients during the Active Phase and after Treatment

Chapter 18

O. Sabri, R. Erkwoh, M. Schreckenberger, C. Dickmann,
G. Schulz, H.J. Kaiser, U. Buell and H. Saß

Introduction

Recent SPECT/PET studies in schizophrenic patients have shown inconsistent findings of regional cerebral blood flow (rCBF) and glucose consumption (rMRGlu). Hypofrontality was described predominantly in medicated patients with chronic disease[1-7], while hyperfrontality was found mainly in unmedicated patients with acute disease[8-12]. Some groups measured increased metabolism in the basal ganglia[3,6], while others described reduced metabolism in the basal ganglia[13]. Temporal rCBF abnormalities have also been reported in schizophrenia[12]. One crucial handicap in assessing the relationship between schizophrenic symptoms and altered rCBF may be the lack of large groups of patients examined. Studies on rCBF in acute and never-treated schizophrenic patients are still especially rare in the literature.

The goal of this study was to evaluate the relationship between altered rCBF values and negative and positive symptoms in neuroleptic-naive schizophrenic patients and to determine the influence of neuroleptic treatment on brain perfusion and negative or positive symptoms. Since not only frontal or temporal rCBF abnormalities were found, several regions of interest (ROIs) were quantified, including frontal, parietal, temporal, occipital, cingulate, basal ganglia and thalamic areas.

Patients and methods

A total of 23 patients (7 women, mean age 36 years; 16 men, mean age 30 years) never treated with neuroleptics and with first-episode schizophrenic psychosis were recruited. The first examinations were made neuroleptic-naive during the acute, psychotic state. The second examination was performed after neuroleptic treatment and clinical improvement in 21 of the 23 patients. Examinations included measurement of rCBF with ^{99m}Tc-HMPAO SPECT and psychiatric evaluation by PANSS, the positive and negative syndrome scale of schizophrenia.

SPECT was performed 15 min after injection of 740 MBq ^{99m}Tc-HMPAO. In restless patients, up to 20 mg diazepam was given intraveneously 10 min after injection of ^{99m}Tc-HMPAO. The acquisition parameters were 2 x 180° rotations

Departments of Nuclear Medicine
and Psychiatry, Aachen University
of Technology, Aachen, Germany

99mTc-HMPAO-SPECT

schizophrenia

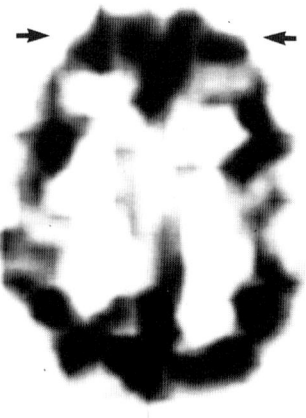

drug naive

99mTc-HMPAO-SPECT

schizophrenia

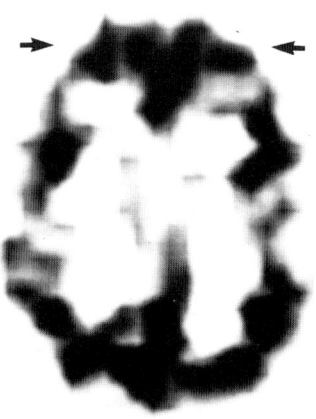

on drug

Figure 1 17-year-old male patient with first-episode schizophrenic psychosis. Left, [99mTc]-HMPAO SPECT in acute, neuroleptic-naive state. High subscores for positive symptoms such as formal thought disorders (Pos2) and grandiosity (Pos5) and low scores for all negative symptoms were observed. Left, bifrontal hyperperfusion (arrows), which normalises after neuroleptic treatment and clinical improvement (right)

in 3° angular steps, and 30 s per view. We used a 128 x 128 matrix, Butterworth filter with n=3.0 and a cut-off frequency of 0.48 for reconstruction (filtered back projection). Attenuation correction was applied by Chang's method. A semiquantitative rCBF evaluation was derived from normalisation to cerebellum. ROIs (98) were defined in 13 canthomeatal slices of 6.25 mm thickness (frontal, temporal, parietal, occipital, cingulate gyri, basal ganglia and thalami). A comparison to 20 control patients was performed and differences of more than 2 s.d. versus these ratios were taken as abnormal, since all ROI values were normally distributed.

All patients underwent recent CT to exclude moderate to severe atrophy, shown to reduce rCBF values severely[14]. PANSS was evaluated by a formalised, semistructured 40 min interview[15]. It scores 33 items, from 1 (normal) to 7 (extremely abnormal). The subscores divide 7 positive symptoms (Pos 1-7), 7 negative symptoms (Neg 1-7), 16 general psychopathological symptoms, and 3 aggression symptoms. The points obtained are then expressed as a percentage of the maximal possible: 0-33% means normal to mildly abnormal, 34-67% is moderately abnormal, and 68-100% indicates severely abnormal

findings. Spearman correlation coefficients and the Wilcoxon test were used for statistical evaluation.

Results

Hyperperfusion was revealed in several cortical ROIs in 8 drug-naive patients. Subsequent to neuroleptic treatment and clinical improvement there was a complete normalisation in 5 of them and partial normalisation in 3. Hypoperfusion revealed in several cortical ROIs in 3 drug-naive patients. After treatment, 2 of them showed complete and 1 partial normalisation. Subsequent to neuroleptic medication, a significant reduction in positive symptoms occurred (PANSS Sum Score of positive symptoms 1-7: from 43 to 9, p<0.0005), but no significant changes in negative symptoms (PANSS Sum Score of negative symptoms 1-7: from 17 to 19, n.s.)(Figures 1-4).

In neuroleptic-naive schizophrenic patients, positive symptoms such as formal thought disorders (Pos 2) and grandiosity (Pos 5) were highly significantly and positively correlated to bifrontal and temporal (r= +0.6, p<0.01) rCBF, while delusional ideas (Pos 1), hallucinatory behaviour (Pos 3) and suspiciousness

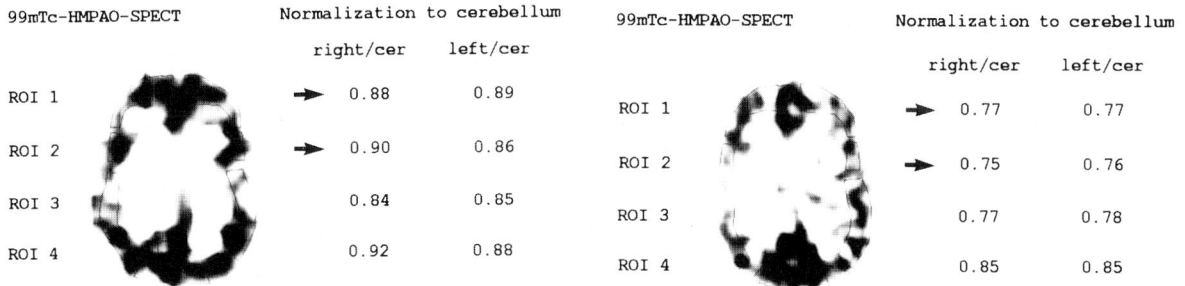

Figure 2 Left, semiquantitative evaluation of rCBF shows increased bifrontal rCBF ratios (0.88, 0.89, 0.90 and 0.86, arrows) in the acute, neuroleptic-naive state. Right, after neuroleptic treatment and clinical improvement, reduction to normal bifrontal rCBF ratios (0.77, 0.77, 0.75 and 0.76, arrows) is observed

(Pos 6) were highly significantly and negatively correlated to bifrontal, left temporal and left parietal rCBF (r= -0.6, p<0.01). Negative symptoms such as stereo-typed ideas (Neg 7) were highly significantly and negatively correlated to bifrontal, bitemporal and left parietal rCBF before treatment (r= -0.6, p<0.01). After neuroleptic treatment and clinical improvement, no significant correlations between residual positive symptoms and rCBF were found. In contrast, all negative symptoms (Neg 1-7) were strongly and highly significantly negatively correlated to rCBF in various ROIs (r= -0.7, p<0.001).

Discussion

The most frequent SPECT/PET pattern reported in schizophrenia is hypofrontality. Some authors have described that any observed rCBF pattern in schizophrenic patients may depend on the medication status of the patients examined[16]. Even in un-medicated schizophrenic patients, totally different rCBF patterns are described. Some groups found hyperfrontality in unmedicated patients with acute disease[12,16]. Catafau et al.[12] found prefrontally in-creased blood flow in neuroleptic-naive schizophrenics and ascribed these findings to positive symptoms. These authors concluded that there is no evidence of hypofrontality in young schizophrenic patients with acute disease who have never been exposed to neuro-leptics[12]. Other researchers measured hypofrontality in neuroleptic-naive patients[17]. It was speculated[12] that there may be a pattern of hyperfrontality at rest and hypofrontality during a prefrontal-linked task. Most frequently it has been supposed that the lack of large numbers of patients examined and the use of a variety of techniques is the reason for these findings[16]. This study clearly demonstrates that hyperfrontality as well as hypofrontality in neuroleptic-naive schizophrenic

patients can be measured and that this does not depend on different techniques, but only on the amount and proportion of different positive symptoms. According to the DSM-III-R criteria, only 1 of the 7 positive symptoms worth more than 5 points in PANSS is needed to diagnose schizophrenia. Thus, without differentiating acute schizophrenics according to the 7 positive symptoms in PANSS, one may classify them in one group, but this does not take into account that formal thought disorders (Pos 2) and grandiosity (Pos 5) are correlating positively to rCBF (therefore leading to hyperfrontality). However delusional ideas (Pos 1), hallucinatory behaviour (Pos 3) and suspiciousness (Pos 6) correlate negatively to rCBF (and therefore contribute to hypofrontality). This is the reason why, considering all neuroleptic-naive schizophrenic patients, hypoperfused, hyperperfused, as well as normal perfused rCBF patterns were found. In other words, the different positive symptoms show opposite rCBF changes, cancelling out deviations. In acute schizophrenics only stereotyped ideas (Neg 7) as a negative symptoms, correlate negatively to rCBF (thus contributing to hypofrontality).

Some studies reported so-called schizophrenic hypotemporality[6]. Since morphological abnormalities in the temporal lobe (mainly on the left side) of schizo-phrenic patients are well known, a link between such abnormalities and left temporal hypoperfusion is assumed[12]. Most recently, our group could demonstrate that, with a method of SPECT/PET resolution in the range of 7-15 mm FWHM, only moderate to severe atrophy significantly reduces the rCBF values measured compared with patients without or with only slight atrophy[14]. Therefore, in the present study, all patients underwent recent CT to exclude moderate to severe atrophy. Nevertheless, we found hypo- as well as hyperperfusion of the temporal lobes in neuroleptic-naive patients, mainly on the left side, depending on the

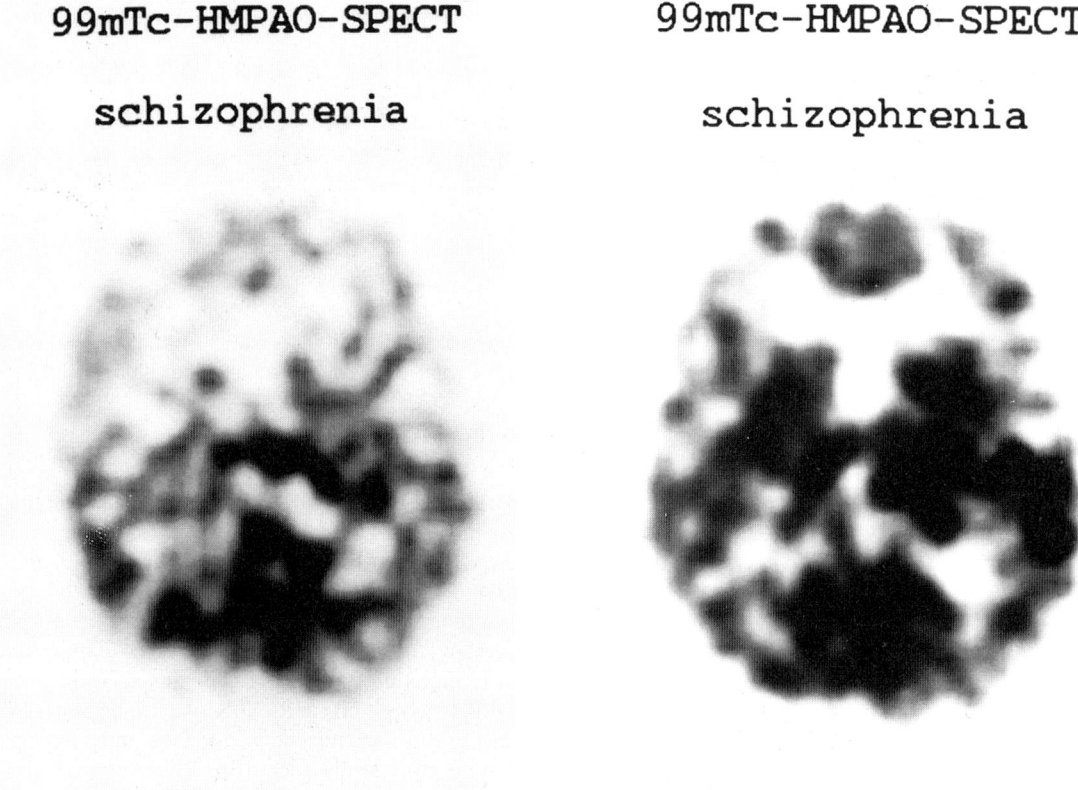

99mTc-HMPAO-SPECT

schizophrenia

drug naive

99mTc-HMPAO-SPECT

schizophrenia

on drug

Figure 3 Female patient (24 yrs) with first-episode schizophrenic psychosis. Left, SPECT in acute, neuroleptic-naive state. High subscores for positive symptoms like delusional ideas (Pos1) and suspiciousness (Pos6) and high subscores for negative symptoms like difficulties in abstract thinking (Neg5) and stereotyped ideas (Neg 7). General cerebral hypoperfusion with exception of the thalami is shown. Right, perfusion normalises after neuroleptic treatment and clinical improvement

99mTc-HMPAO-SPECT — Normalization to cerebellum

	right/cer	left/cer
ROI 1	0.59	0.63
ROI 2	0.68	0.57
ROI 3	0.69	0.69
ROI 4	0.71	0.76
ROI 5	0.68	0.72
ROI 6 →	0.79	0.83

99mTc-HMPAO-SPECT — Normalization to cerebellum

	right/cer	left/cer
ROI 1	0.70	0.71
ROI 2	0.70	0.68
ROI 3	0.75	0.80
ROI 4	0.78	0.81
ROI 5	0.84	0.85
ROI 6 →	0.83	0.85

Figure 4 Semiquantitative evaluation of rCBF shows reduced rCBF ratios except for thalami (left, arrow). Right, after treatment, increase to normal rCBF values

magnitude and proportion of each positive symptom. As for frontal perfusion, some of the positive symptoms correlate positively and some negatively to temporal rCBF. We feel that these rCBF changes are not due to morphological alterations, but correlate to psychopathological alteration. Furthermore, our study demonstrates that, in neuroleptic-naive schizophrenic patients, positive (Pos 6) and negative (Neg 7) symptoms correlated negatively to left parietal rCBF. Most recent studies did not pay much attention to this region, focussing instead primarily on frontal and temporal areas.

Most groups[1-7] have described hypofrontality in medicated schizophrenics. In this study, after neuroleptic medication and clinical improvement (and reduction of positive symptoms), all negative symptoms (1-7) showed a negative correlation to rCBF, which is in good agreement with findings in the literature.

Conclusions

Perfusion changes in several cerebral regions in neuroleptic-naive schizophrenic patients showed highly significant positive or negative correlations to single psychopathological symptoms. This indicates the necessity of subdividing patient groups according to symptomatology before interstudy comparisons. After neuroleptic treatment and clinical improvement in our group, positive symptoms decreased and residual negative symptoms correlated negatively to rCBF in different locations. These findings may explain inconsistent recent results in rCBF patterns in drug-naive schizophrenics.

References

1 Ingvar, D.H. and Franzén, G. Abnormalities of cerebral blood flow distribution in patients with chronic schizophrenia. *Acta. Psychiatr. Scand.* 1974, 50, 425

2 Buchsbaum, M.S., Ingvar, D.H. and Kessler, R. Cerebral glucography with positron tomography. Use in normal subjects and in patients with schizophrenia. *Arch. Gen. Psychiatr.* 1982, 39, 251

3 Brodie, J.D., Christman, D.R. and Corona, J.F. Patterns of metabolic activity in the treatment of schizophrenia. *Ann. Neurol.* 1984, 15, 166

4 Farkas, T., Wolf, A.P., Jaeger, J. *et al.* Regional brain glucose metabolism in chronic schizophrenia. A positron emission transaxial tomographic study. *Arch. Gen. Psychiatr.* 1984, 41, 293

5 DeLisi, L.E., Buchsbaum, M.S. and Holcomb, H.H. Clinical correlates of decreased anteroposterior metabolic gradients in positron emission tomography (PET) of schizophrenic patients. *Am. J. Psychiatr.* 1985, 142, 78

6 Wolkin, A., Jaeger, J. and Brodie, J.D. Persistence of cerebral metabolic abnormalities in chronic schizophrenia as determined by positron emission tomography. *Am. J. Psychiatr.* 1985, 142, 564

7 Lewis, S.W., Ford, R.A., Syed, G.M. *et al.* A controlled study of ^{99m}Tc-HMPAO single-photon emission imaging in chronic schizophrenia. *Psychol. Med.* 1992, 22, 27

8 Volkow, N.D., Brodie, J.D., Wolf, A.P. *et al.* Brain metabolism in patients with schizophrenia before and after acute neuroleptic administration. *J. Neurol. Neurosurg. Psychiatr.* 1986, 49, 1199

9 Wiesel, F.A., Wik, G., Sjögren, I. *et al.* Regional brain glucose metabolism in drug free schizophrenic patients and clinical correlates. *Acta. Psychiatr. Scand.* 1987, 76, 628

10 Szechtman, H., Nahmias, C. and Garnett, E.S. Effect of neuroleptics on altered cerebral glucose metabolism in schizophrenia. *Arch. Gen. Psychiatr.* 1988, 45, 523

11 Cleghorn, J.M., Garnett, E.S. and Nahmias, C. Increased frontal and reduced parietal glucose metabolism in acute untreated schizophrenia. *Psychiatr. Res.* 1989, 28, 119

12 Catafau, A.M., Parellada, E. and Loména, F.J. Prefrontal and temporal blood flow in schizophrenia. *J. Nucl. Med.* 1994, 35, 935

13 Sheppard, G., Manchanda, R. and Gruzelier, J. 15-O positron emission tomographic scanning in predominantly never-treated acute schizophrenic patients. *Lancet* 1983, 2, 1448

14 Sabri, O., Hellwig, D., Kaiser, H.J. *et al.* Effects of Morphological Changes on Perfusion and Metabolism in Cerebral Microangiopathy. *Nucl. Med.* 1995, 34, 50

15 Kay, S.R., Fiszbein, A. and Opler, L.A. The positive and negative syndrome scale (PANSS) for schizophrenia. *Schizophr. Bull.* 1987, 13(2), 261

16 Ebmeier, K.P., Blackwood, D.H.R., Murray, C. *et al.* Single-Photon Computed Tomography with ^{99m}Tc-Exametazime in Unmedicated Schizophrenic Patients. *Biol. Psychiatr.* 1993, 33, 487

17 Andreasen, N.C., Rezai, K. and Alliger, R. Hypofrontality in neuroleptic-naive patients and in patients with chronic schizophrenia. *Arch. Gen. Psychiatry.* 1992, 49, 943

SPECT in Neurology and Psychiatry, edited by P.P. De Deyn, R.A. Dierckx, A. Alavi and B.A. Pickut
© 1997 John Libbey & Company Ltd, pp. 139–146

Cerebral Blood Flow Measured by ^{99m}Tc-HMPAO SPECT in Mood Disorder

Chapter
19

T. Iidaka, T. Nakajima, Y. Suzuki, A. Okazaki, T. Maehara, H. Shiraishi[*] and H. Matsuda[**]

Introduction

CBF in mood disorder has been studied using SPECT and tracers such as ^{99m}Tc-hexamethyl-propylene amine oxime (HMPAO) and ^{123}I-iodoamphetamine (IMP). Semiquantification of radioactivity has been applied to measure CBF in ROIs. The most common method for semiquantification is to use the radioactivity of a non-affected region as a reference. Whole hemispheric, whole slice, cerebellar and occipital cortex radioactivities have been chosen as reference regions in studies at various centres. This inconsistency could be one of several reasons for the discrepancies in the results of these studies.

Until recently, quantification of CBF using SPECT had many methodological limitations. Arterial blood sampling was required when IMP was used as a tracer, and input of the tracer to the brain could not be measured because HMPAO was partially metabolised in the blood vessels. Recently, a non-invasive, simple method for quantitative evaluation of brain perfusion using intravenous radionuclide angiography with ^{99m}Tc-HMPAO was reported[1-3]. Graphical analysis was employed to measure the influx constant of the tracer from the blood to the brain. This value (brain perfusion index) showed a highly significant correlation with CBF obtained from ^{133}Xe SPECT. Lassen's correction was applied to calculate the rCBF from the brain perfusion index (BPI).

In the current study, patients with mood disorder and control subjects with neurosis underwent non-invasive measurement of their CBF. Mean hemispheric CBF and rCBF values were measured, and correlations between these values and the depression scale score (HRSD and SDS) were studied.

Methods

A total of 28 patients with mood disorder and 13 control subjects with neurosis were included. The patients with mood disorder were diagnosed using the DSM-III-R[4]: 9 had bipolar disorder and 19 major depression (M/F: 16/12, mean age ±s.d.: 55.4 ±10.3, range 27-72 years). Controls included 13 neurotic patients with depressive symptoms (M/F: 7/6, mean age ±s.d.: 51.6 ±17.9, range 25-77 years - 6 patients had hypochondriasis, 6 adjustment disorder with depressed mood, and 1 hysterical neurosis). No subjects had organic brain lesions except for 1 with bipolar disorder who had a small venous malformation of the brain. No patients had apparent cognitive impairment. None of the patients with mood disorder had been given electroconvulsive therapy within 6 months of the study. All patients were taking medication (antidepressants, hypnotics, or other psychotropic drugs).

Departments of Psychiatry and Radiology, Kanto Teishin Hospital, 5-9-22, Higashi-Gotanda, Shinagawa-ku, Tokyo, 141, Japan

[*]Department of Psychiatry, Institute of Clinical Medicine, University of Tsukuba, Tsukuba, Japan

[**]Division of Radiology, National Centre Hospital for Mental, Nervous and Muscular Disorders, NCNP, Tokyo, Japan

We evaluated the depressive symptoms using the HRSD (21 items)[5] and the SDS[6], within 2 days of CBF examination. HRSD scores for mood disorder ranged from 2 to 33, compared with 3 to 28 in the controls. SDS scores for mood disorder and controls ranged from 24 to 66 and from 26 to 63, respectively.

Eight patients with mood disorder underwent the examination twice during their clinical course. These patients comprised 4 with bipolar disorder and 4 with major depression (M/F: 4/4, mean age: 56.8 ±10.1, range 41-72 years). Six patients underwent the examination in a depressed state and in remission and 2 did so in depressed and hypomanic states. Informed consent was obtained from all subjects before examination.

CBF measurement

Measurement of CBF was performed using a GE Starcam 3000 (single-head rotating gamma camera) with the patients at rest with their eyes closed. A bolus injection of HMPAO (740 MBq) was given into the right antecubital vein and radionuclide angiography was performed simultaneously for 100 s (1 frame/s). After data acquisition, the mCBF of each hemisphere was computed using graphical analysis on the SPECT console (Figure 1)[1-3]. This method is a simple and non-invasive one for the quantitative evaluation of brain perfusion using intravenous radionuclide angiography with HMPAO. ROIs were drawn on the aortic arch and bilateral brain hemispheres. The activity at the aortic arch was monitored instead of arterial blood sampling. The time activity curves of these ROIs were used for analysis. The graphical approach by plotting the activity curves from each group of data gives the unidirectional influx rate as the slope of a straight line. The influx constants were standardised to provide BPI, which represents the mCBF. As reported previously, the BPI value for each hemisphere showed a highly significant correlation with the mean hemispheric cerebral blood flow measured by the early picture method of ^{133}Xe inhalation[1,2]. We converted the BPI into the CBF value (ml/100 g/min) using the regression equation (y = 2.75x + 17.7) between the two values.

Five minutes after the injection of HMPAO, brain SPECT was performed using a single-head rotating gamma camera. The hemispheric mean SPECT counts were substituted into Lassen's correction algorithm for linearisation correction, using the left hemisphere as a reference region. Twelve irregular ROIs were drawn in two axial SPECT images to calculate rCBF (Figure 2). The regions drawn in the lower image were the lower frontal cortex, temporal cortex, basal ganglia, thalamus on right and left sides, and the lower medial frontal

cortex. The regions in the upper image were the bilateral upper frontal and upper medial frontal cortex. The analyses were performed using software provided by Amersham Japan.

Statistical analysis

The Wilcoxon test (non-parametric, two-tailed) and Spearman's rank order correlation were used for statistical analysis. The Kruskal-Wallis test (non-parametric) was used to compare the three groups. We analysed the data by multiple regression analysis and analysis of covariance (ANACOVA) using a Statistical Analysis System package. The level of statistical significance was set at p<0.05. Numerical values were expressed as mean ±s.d. The value of CBF was represented as ml/100 g/min.

Results

Comparison of mCBF between mood disorder and control

In patients with mood disorder, hemispheric mCBF ranged from 29.1 to 49.6, compared with 37.8 to 53.4 in controls. The patients with mood disorder had significantly lower mCBF bilaterally (Figure 3, right: 38.6 ±5.1 versus 43.9 ±4.9, p<0.01, left: 39.2 ±5.3 versus 44.3 ±4.0, p<0.01) than the controls. There was no significant difference in mean age, HRSD score (mood disorder versus control; 16 ±9.3 versus 11.8 ±7.5, n.s.) or SDS score (47.6 ±11.4 versus 43.0 ±9.2, n.s.) between the two groups. The difference in mCBF between the patients with mood disorder and the controls was still significant (p<0.01) after removing the effects of age, HRSD and SDS score, by ANACOVA (using these variables as covariates).

Correlation between mCBF and depressive symptoms

In all subjects, mCBF in both hemispheres was significantly and negatively correlated with age (right: r= -0.51, p<0.001, left: r= -0.55, p<0.001). HRSD score was significantly correlated with right hemispheric mCBF (r= -0.31, p<0.05), but not with left hemispheric mCBF (r= -0.28, n.s.). The correlation between SDS score and mCBF did not reach statistical significance. In patients with mood disorder, mCBF in both hemispheres was significantly and negatively correlated with age (right: r= -0.44, p<0.01, left: r= -0.48, p<0.01). HRSD score was significantly correlated with right hemispheric mCBF (r= -0.37, p<0.05) but not with left hemispheric mCBF (r= -0.36, n.s.).

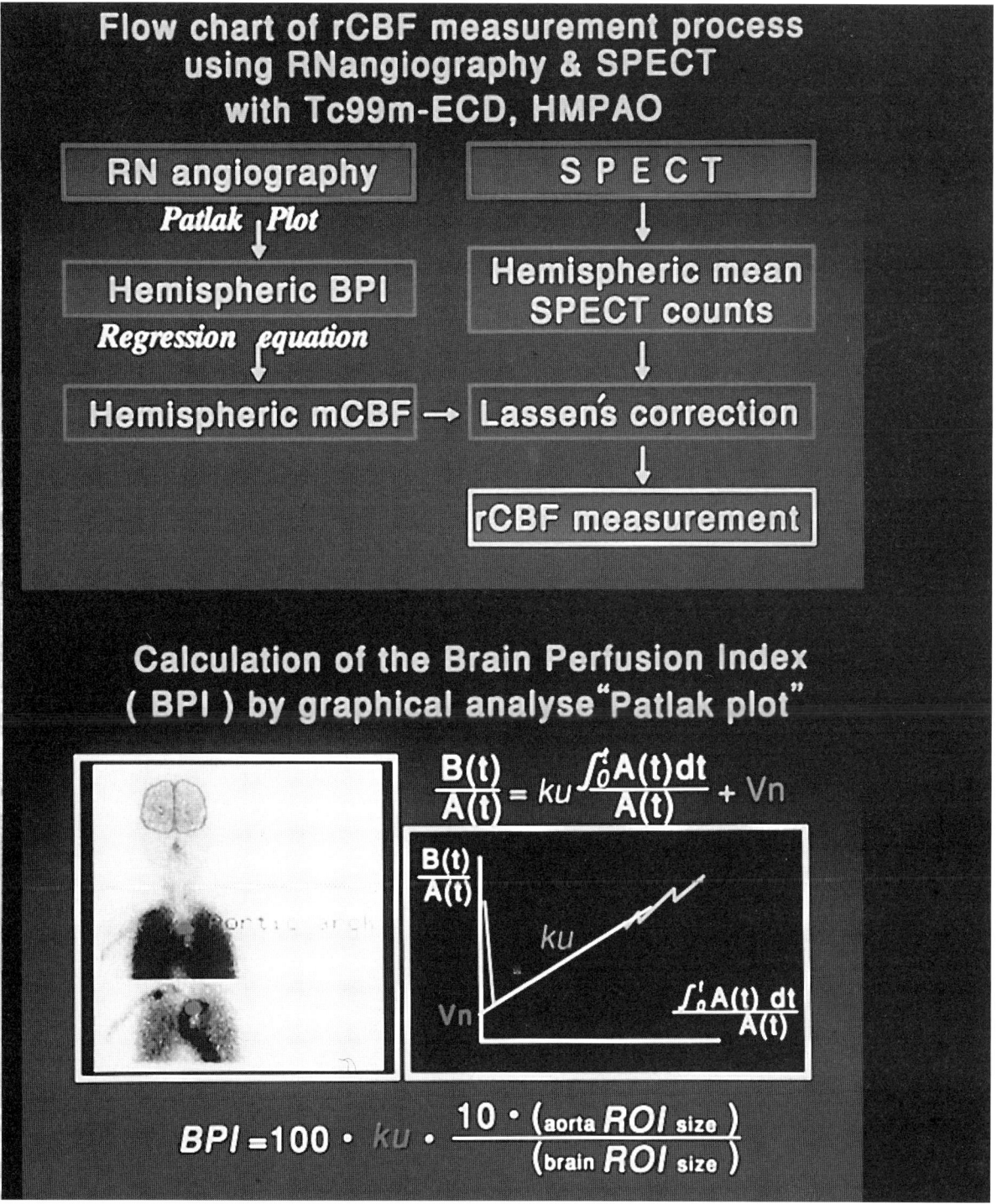

Figure 1 Flow chart of CBF measurement (above). Hemispheric mCBF is computed using regression equation between the brain perfusion index and cerebral blood flow measured by ^{133}Xe SPECT. Hemispheric mean and regional SPECT counts are substituted into Lassen's correction algorithm to obtain rCBF. Calculation of the brain perfusion index by graphical analysis (below). The time-activity curves of bilateral hemispheres (B(t)) and aortic arch (A(t)) are monitored on radionuclide angiography. The graphical approach by plotting the activity curves gives the influx rate (ku) as the slope of a straight line. The influx rate is standardised using the ratio between the size of ROIs to provide brain perfusion index

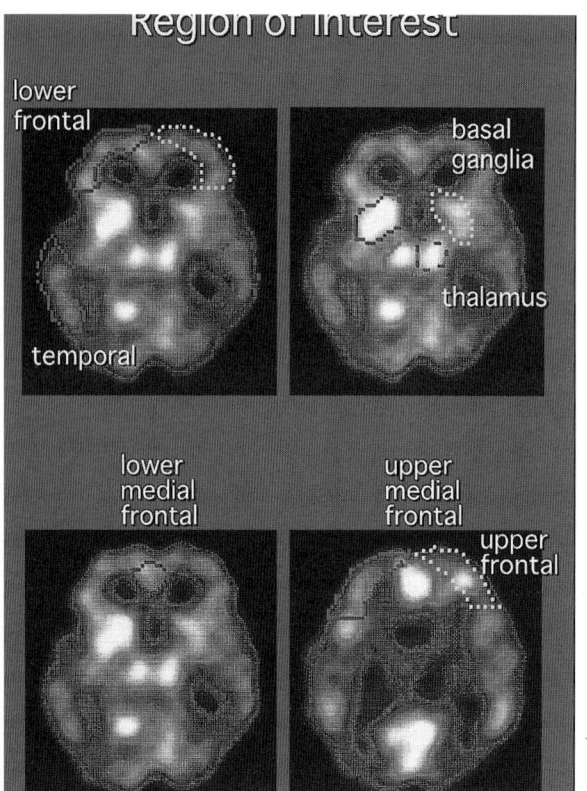

Figure 2 ROIs drawn in two axial SPECT images

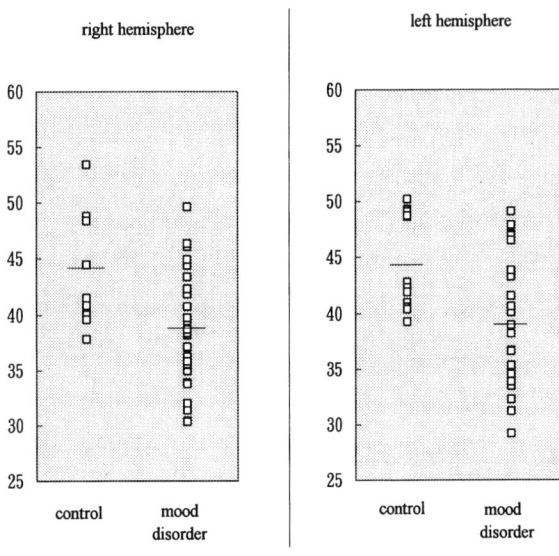

Figure 3 Comparison of bilateral hemispheric mCBF between patients with mood disorder and controls. Horizontal lines represent the mean value. Units are ml/100/ g/min. The patients with mood disorder had significantly (p<0.01) lower mCBF bilaterally

SDS score had no significant correlation with mCBF. In controls, significant negative correlations were found between mCBF and age (right: r= -0.69, p<0.01, left: r= -0.79, p<0.01). No correlation was seen between mCBF and HRSD or SDS in controls.

Multiple regression analysis was performed to remove the effects of age on the correlation between mCBF and HRSD (Table 1). mCBF was used as a dependent variable, and age and HRSD and SDS scores were used as independent variables. In mood disorder, mCBF in both hemispheres had a significantly (p<0.05) negative correlation with HRSD after removing the effect of age. There was no correlation between mCBF and SDS score bilaterally. In controls, there was no correlation between mCBF and HRSD or SDS score.

Changes in mCBF after treatment

We compared mCBF before and after patients' recovery from a depressed state. In 8 patients who underwent CBF examination twice during their course, there was a significant (p<0.01) increase in mCBF bilaterally (Figure 4). In the right and left hemispheres, mCBF increased from 38.1 ±4.9 to 41.6 ±4.6 and from

38.1 ±5 to 42.7 ±4.1, respectively. The mean was 3.5 ±3.6 (range 0.4-10.5) on the right and 4.6 ±3.4 (range 0.2-10.6) on the left. We then tested the intra-observer reliability of the graphical analysis. In 54 hemispheres of 27 subjects, mCBF was measured twice by the same observer (T.I.), and the difference in mCBF between the 2 measurements ranged from 0 to 3.7 (mean: 1.0 ±0.8).

Table 1 Results of multiple regression analysis in patients with mood disorder. Numerical data represent correlation coefficients between CBF and age or depression score. After removal of the age effect, significant correlations between CBF and HRSD score are seen in the bilateral hemispheres and 4 frontal cortices. SDS score had a positive correlation with rCBF in the lower medial frontal cortex

		Age	HRSD score	SDS score
mCBF	right hemisphere	-0.2[a]	-0.35[a]	0.22
	left hemisphere	-0.21[a]	-0.39[a]	0.27
rCBF	right lower frontal	-0.12	-0.68[a]	0.32
	left lower frontal	-0.23	-0.68[a]	0.35
	lower medial frontal	-0.23	-0.91[a]	0.64[a]
	left upper frontal	-0.21	-0.59[a]	0.29

[a], p<0.05

Table 2 Comparison of rCBF in 12 ROIs between the patients with mood disorder and controls (ANACOVA). Units of the numerical data are ml/100 g/min. The patients with mood disorder had significantly lower rCBF in all ROIs

	Mood disorder	Control	p
Right lower frontal	42.1±7.8	50.6±6.6	<0.01
Left lower frontal	43.6±8.1	52.6±7.8	<0.01
Right basal ganglia	61.3±11.2	71.3±9.9	<0.05
Left basal ganglia	57.5±12	68.6±12.9	<0.05
Right thalamus	55.7±13.1	69±14.6	<0.01
Left thalamus	54.3±12.3	65.2±13.3	<0.05
Right temporal	46.1±7.2	55±7.7	<0.01
Left temporal	46.3±8.4	54±7.6	<0.05
Lower medial frontal	52.2±11.2	67.5±13.8	<0.001
Right upper frontal	43.2±7.8	53.1±6.4	<0.0001
Left upper frontal	45.1±8	55.7±7	<0.0001
Upper medial frontal	53.6±10.7	65.9±11.7	<0.01

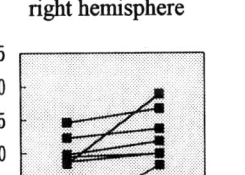
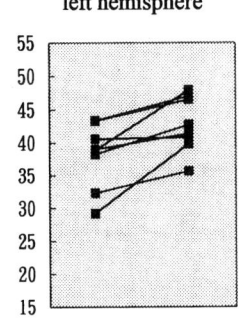

Figure 4 Changes in mCBF before (left) and after (right) treatment in 8 patients with mood disorder. Significant (p<0.01) increases are seen in the bilateral hemispheres. Units are ml/100 g/min

Comparison of rCBF between mood disorder and control

Patients with mood disorder had significantly lower rCBF in all 12 ROIs. The significance still remained after removal of the age effect using ANACOVA (Table 2). We compared rCBF among 13 depressed patients with mood disorder (HRSD score: 15-33), 15 patients with remission of mood disorder (HRSD score: 2-14) and controls. Significant differences in rCBF between controls and depressed patients were found in all 12 ROIs. Between remitted patients and controls, significant (p<0.05) differences were seen in the right temporal and right upper frontal cortices. Between depressed and remitted patients, significant (p<0.05) differences were seen in the bilateral lower frontal cortices.

Correlations between rCBF and depressive symptoms

In all subjects, significant negative correlations between rCBF and age were seen in all 12 ROIs. HRSD score was significantly and negatively correlated with rCBF in both the bilateral lower frontal (right: r= -0.38, p<0.05, left: r= -0.45, p<0.01) and upper frontal (right: r= -0.36, p<0.05, left: r= -0.42, p<0.01) cortices. In patients with mood disorder, significant negative correlations between age and rCBF were seen in the left lower frontal (r= -0.37, p<0.05), right temporal (r= -0.5, p<0.01) and upper medial frontal (r= -0.38, p<0.05) cortices, left basal ganglia (r= -0.53, p<0.01) and bilateral thalamus (right: r= -0.45, p<0.05, left: r= -0.57, p<0.01). HRSD score was significantly and negatively correlated with rCBF in the bilateral lower

frontal (right: r= -0.46, p<0.05, left: r= -0.48, p<0.01) and upper frontal (right: r= -0.37, p<0.05, left: r= -0.41, p<0.05) cortices and right thalamus (r= -0.39, p<0.05) in patients with mood disorder. In controls, no significant correlation was found between HRSD score and rCBF.

We performed multiple regression analysis to remove the effect of age from the correlation between HRSD score and rCBF. In all subjects, significant negative correlations between HRSD score and rCBF were found in the bilateral lower frontal, lower medial frontal, bilateral upper frontal, and upper medial frontal cortices, left basal ganglia and bilateral thalamus. In patients with mood disorder, significant negative correlations between HRSD score and rCBF were found in the bilateral lower frontal, lower medial frontal and left upper frontal cortices (Table 1). In controls, HRSD score was significantly and negatively correlated with rCBF in the left thalamus.

Positive correlations were seen between rCBF in the lower medial frontal cortex and SDS score in all subjects and in patients with mood disorder (Table 1). In controls, SDS score had a positive correlation with rCBF in the bilateral thalamus.

Changes in rCBF after treatment

In the patients with mood disorder who underwent SPECT twice during their clinical course, rCBF in all ROIs except for the lower and upper medial frontal cortices showed significant (p<0.05) increases after treatment. The mean width of the increase ranged from 5 (in the right temporal cortex) to 13.1 (in the left basal ganglia).

Discussion

Mood disorder and cerebral blood flow

Quantitative CBF in patients with mood disorder has been measured by the ^{133}Xe inhalation method. In an early study using this method, patients with depression (medication-free for 2 weeks) and controls were examined[7]. The depressives showed highly reduced values for grey-matter blood flow in both hemispheres compared with controls. The severity of symptoms rated with HRSD was significantly and negatively correlated with CBF. In another study, no significant differences in CBF were found between medicated unipolar depressives and controls in a resting state[8]. However, male patients had a lower CBF than female patients. Although whole hemispheric CBF in the resting state did not differ between subgroups of depressed patients defined by biological markers (REM latency and dexamethasone suppression test) and clinical characteristics (unipolar and bipolar, endogenous and non-endogenous), cortical blood flow was significantly lower in the left hemisphere in bipolar patients than in controls[9]. The depressed group showed a marked reduction in global cortical blood flow, and this reduction was prominent in frontal and temporoparietal areas[10]. In a recent study using Xe, 39 depressed patients over the age of 50 were studied with controls.The depressed patients exhibited a global reduction in CBF compared with the controls, and the orbital frontal and inferior temporal areas were affected bilaterally[11].

Semiquantitative CBF in major depression measured by HMPAO showed reduction of anterior cortical function, and this reduction was related to symptom severity[12]. Significant bilateral increases in CBF were found in the basal ganglia and cingulate region after recovery[13]. Left-sided hypoactivity of the brain has been found using IMP SPECT in patients with mood disorders[14]. The decreases in perfusion were seen in the paralimbic region, specifically the inferior frontal and cingulate cortex. The degree of psychomotor slowing was negatively correlated with frontal and cingulate perfusion[15].

Cerebral metabolic rate measured by PET was significantly lower in patients with bipolar depression and mixed state patients. The whole brain metabolic rates for patients with bipolar depression increased by 4-36% as the patients went from a depressed or mixed state to a euthymic or manic state[16]. Another study of glucose metabolism by PET showed significant left-right prefrontal asymmetry in patients before, but not after, successful treatment. Significant hypofrontality and whole-cortex hypometabolism were also found in

the patients, and these findings persisted in the treated state [17]. In a recent study with PET analysed on a pixel-by-pixel basis, regional CBF was found to decrease in the left anterior cingulate region and the left dorsolateral prefrontal cortex[18]. Three factors of depressive symptoms analysed by factor analysis were correlated with rCBF in the different regions. The factor for anxiety had a positive correlation with rCBF in the posterior cingulate and inferior parietal lobule bilaterally. The factor for retardation and depressed mood had negative correlations with rCBF in the left dorsolateral prefrontal cortex and left angular gyrus. The factor for cognitive performance had a positive correlation with left medial prefrontal cortex[19]. Neuropsychological dysfunction in the patients was closely related to rCBF in the medial prefrontal cortex and frontal polar cortex[20].

Ageing and cerebral blood flow

The influences of ageing on CBF have been the subject of controversy[21]. CBF measured by the ^{133}Xe inhalation method showed a significant negative correlation with advancing age. This age-related decline was greater in the territory of the middle cerebral artery than in other arteries. There were no significant differences in CBF between the right and left hemispheres[22]. In a recent study of CBF measured by SPECT and HMPAO in normal ageing, whole-brain CBF was negatively correlated with age. Regional CBF also declined with age in half of the 20 regions, and these regions included the precentral, frontal, cingulate, temporal and parietal cortex and basal ganglia. Such negative correlations were not seen in the cerebellum or occipital or orbital cortex[2].

In a PET study, mean hemispheric cerebral and grey-matter glucose use was studied in resting healthy subjects. Neither value was correlated significantly with age, nor were any right-left differences. The author indicated that the previously reported decline with age might be due to the inclusion of subjects with cerebrovascular disease[23]. Another report showed no significant relationship between global cerebral blood flow and age.

However, after removal of the variation in global flow, there were many regions that showed a significant negative correlation with age. These included the cingulate, parahippocampal, superior temporal and medial frontal gyri[24]. Cerebral metabolic rate for oxygen and CBF decreased with age at a rate of about 0.5% per year. This result suggested diminished neuronal firing or a decrease in synaptic density with age[25]. Another report showed an age-related decrease in the cerebral metabolic rate of oxygen (0.6% per year) in all 4 lobes bilaterally. In contrast, changes in CBF were less significant because of a larger variance of data[26].

Results of this study

In this study, mean and regional CBF were measured using HMPAO and graphical analysis in patients with mood disorder and in neurotic controls. Although there were no differences in mean HRSD and SDS score between the groups, mCBF was significantly lower bilaterally in mood disorder than in controls. After removal of the effects of age and HRSD and SDS scores by ANACOVA, the difference was still significant. Moreover, rCBF in 12 ROIs drawn in two axial images was significantly lower in mood disorder than in controls. These results indicate that mood disorder has a biological trait of decreased mean and regional CBF as compared with control subjects with neurosis who also show depressive symptoms.

It is known that healthy elderly subjects have more depressive symptoms than younger subjects and that mCBF is highly and significantly correlated with age. Therefore it is necessary to remove the effects of age in the correlation between mCBF and HRSD. We performed multiple regression analysis for this purpose. Although HRSD score and age were significantly correlated with mCBF in both hemispheres, SDS had no correlation with mCBF. These results were seen in all subjects and in patients with mood disorder. In controls, however, only age was correlated significantly with mCBF. This indicates that mCBF decreases with both advancing age and the severity of depressive symptoms. It is noteworthy that mCBF was significantly correlated with HRSD score but not with SDS score. Generally, depressive symptoms are evaluated objectively with HRSD[5] and subjectively with SDS[6]. In clinical testing, the subjective evaluation of symptoms occasionally differs from the objective evaluation[27]. Our results suggest that mCBF measured by this method reflects the objective evaluation of symptoms.

After removal of the age effect, rCBF in the bilateral lower frontal, lower medial frontal and left upper frontal cortices showed significant negative correlations with HRSD score. These negative correlations seen in the frontal region indicate that frontal hypoactivity is closely related to depressive symptoms. These results are consistent with other investigations reported previously. Another finding was a positive correlation between SDS score and rCBF in the lower medial frontal cortex. Activation of the medial frontal region has been observed during tasks that require attention[28]. This region includes part of the

cingulate cortex, and anterior cingulate hyperperfusion has been seen in patients with atypical pain[29]. These results indicate that the central attention system including the cingulate gyrus is activated in patients with mood disorder and chronic pain.

In 8 patients with mood disorder, we measured mCBF before and after treatment. Bilateral hemispheric mCBF increased significantly as the patients recovered from their depressed state to a remitted or hypomanic state. These increases were equivalent to 10% of the mCBF. rCBF in 10 out of 12 ROIs measured in this study showed significant increases after the treatment.

Conclusion

In conclusion, patients with mood disorder have a lower mean and regional CBF than controls, and CBF measured by this non-invasive method contributes to the objective evaluation of depressive symptoms. Although HRSD and SDS have been used for the clinical evaluation of patients' symptoms, the reliability of raters is occasionally questionable and there is a degree of inter-rater variability[27]. Some physiological examinations such as sleep REM latency[30] and the dexamethasone suppression test[31] have been used for diagnostic purposes. However, their correlations with the severity of symptoms are not sufficient for clinical use. mCBF measured using HMPAO and graphical analysis had good inter- and intra-observer reliability when the same protocol is used[1]. A good intra-observer reliability was also confirmed in this study. The difference between the 2 measurements was equivalent to 2% of the mCBF. This non-invasive method is thus useful for the clinical evaluation of mood disorder.

Acknowledgements

We thank Humihide Akita, Yuichi Nakanishi and the nuclear medicine technicians in Kanto Teishin Hospital for their support.

References

1   Matsuda, H., Tsuji, S., Shuke, N. *et al.* A quantitative approach to technetium-99m hexamethylpropylene amine oxime. *Eur. J. Nucl. Med.* 1992, 19, 195

2   Matsuda, H., Tsuji, S., Shuke, N. *et al.* Noninvasive measurements of regional cerebral blood flow using technetium-99m hexamethylprophylene amine oxime. *Eur. J. Nucl. Med.* 1993, 20, 391

3   Patlak, C.S., Blasberg, R.G. and Fenstermacher, J.D. Graphical evaluation of blood-to-brain transfer constants from multiple-time uptake data. *J. Cereb. Blood Flow Metab.* 1983, 3, 1

4   American Psychiatric Association. Diagnostic and Statistical Manual of Mental Disorders (3rd edn, revised). APA, Washington, USA, 1987

5   Hamilton, M. A rating scale for depression. *J. Neurol. Neurosurg. Psychiatr.* 1960, 23, 56

6   Zung, W.W.K. A self-rating depression scale. *Arch. Gen. Psychiatr.* 1965, 12, 63

7   Mathew, R.J., Meyer, J.S., Semchuk, K.M. *et al.* Cerebral blood flow in depression. *Lancet* 1980, 1308

8   Gur, R.E., Skolnick, B.E., Gur, R.C. *et al.* Brain function in psychiatric disorders. *Arch. Gen. Psychiatr.* 1984, 41, 695

9   Delvenne, V., Delecluse, F., Hubain, P.P. *et al.* Regional cerebral blood flow in patients with affective disorders. *Br. J. Psychiatr.* 1990, 157, 359

10   Sackeim, H.A., Prohovnik, I., Moeller, J.R. *et al.* Regional cerebral blood flow in mood disorders. *Arch. Gen. Psychiatr.* 1990, 47, 60

11   Lesser, I.M., Mena, I, Boone, K.B. *et al.* Reduction of cerebral blood flow in older depressed patients. *Arch. Gen. Psychiatr.* 1994, 51, 677

12   Austin, M-P., Dougall, N., Ross, M. *et al.* Single photon emission tomography activity underlying the psychotic / neurotic continuum. *J. Affect. Disord.* 1992, 26, 31

13   Goodwin, G.M., Austin, M.P., Dougall, N. *et al.* State changes in brain activity shown by the uptake of [99mTc]-exametazime with single photon emission tomography in major depression before and after treatment. *J. Affect. Disord.* 1993, 29, 243

14   Iidaka, T., Nakajima, T. and Kawamoto, K. Correlations between cerebral blood flow and depression scale in mood disorder. A study using [123I]-IMP SPECT. *Eur. J. Nucl. Med.* 1994, 21, S110

15   Mayberg, H.S., Lewis, P.J., Regenold, W. and Wagner, H.N. Jr. Paralimbic hypoperfusion in unipolar depression. *J. Nucl. Med.* 1994, 35, 929

16   Baxter, L.R., Phelps, M.E., Mazziotta, J.C., Schwartz, J.M. *et al.* Cerebral metabolic rates for glucose in mood disorders. *Arch. Gen. Psychiatr.* 1985, 42, 441

17   Martinot, J.L., Hardy, P., Feline, A. *et al.* Left prefrontal glucose hypometabolism in the depressed state: A confirmation. *Am. J. Psychiatr.* 1990, 147, 1313

18   Bench, C.J., Friston, K.J., Brown, R.G. *et al.* The anatomy of melancholia-focal abnormalities of cerebral blood flow in major depression. *Psychol. Med.* 1992, 22, 607

19   Bench, C.J., Friston, K.J., Brown, R.G. *et al.* Regional cerebral blood flow in depression measured by positron emission tomography: the relationship with clinical dimensions. *Psychol. Med.* 1993, 23, 579

20   Dolan, R.J., Bench, C.J., Brown, *et al.* Neuropsychological dysfunction in depression: the relationship to regional cerebral blood flow. *Psychol. Med.* 1994, 24, 849

21   Roland, P.E. in 'Brain Activation', Wiley, New York, USA, 1993, p.472

22   Matsuda, H., Maeda, T., Yamada, M. *et al.* Age-matched normal values and topographic maps for regional cerebral blood flow measurements by Xe-133 inhalation. *Stroke* 1984, 15, 336

23   Duara, R., Margolin, R.A., Robertson-Tchabo, E.A. *et al.* Cerebral glucose utilization, as measured with positron emission tomography in 21 resting healthy men between the ages of 21 and 83 years. *Brain* 1983, 106, 761

24   Martin, A.J., Friston, K.J., Colebatch, J.G. and Frackowiak, R.S.J. Decreases in regional cerebral blood flow with normal aging. *J. Cereb. Blood Flow Metab.* 1991, 11, 684

25   Leenders, K.L., Perani, D., Lammertsma, A.A. *et al.* Cerebral blood flow, blood volume and oxygen utilization. *Brain* 1990, 113, 27

26   Marchal, G., Rioux, P., Petit-Taboue, M.C. *et al.* Regional cerebral oxygen consumption, blood flow, and blood volume in healthy human aging. *Arch. Neurol.* 1992, 49, 1013

27   Bech, P. Symptoms and assessment of depression in Handbook of affective disorders, 2nd edn', (Ed. E.S. Paykel), Churchill Livingstone, Edinburgh, Scotland, 1992, p.3

28   Larrue, V., Celsis, P., Bes, A. and Marc-Vergnes, J.P. The functional anatomy of attention in humans: cerebral blood flow changes induced by reading, naming, and the stroop effect. *J. Cereb. Blood Flow Metab.* 1994, 14, 958

29   Delbyshire, S.W.G., Jones, A.K.P., Devani, P. *et al.* Cerebral responses to pain in patients with atypical facial pain measured by positron emission tomography. *J. Neurol. Neurosurg. Psychiatr.* 1984, 57, 1166

30   Buysse, D.J., Kupfer, D.J. Diagnostic and research applications of electroencephalographic sleep studies in depression. *J. Nerv. Ment. Dis.* 1990, 178, 405

31   Miller, K.B., Nelson, J.C. Does the dexamethasone suppression test relate to subtypes, factors, symptoms, or severity? *Arch. Gen. Psychiatr.* 1987, 44, 769

Movement Disorders

SPECT in Neurology and Psychiatry, edited by P.P. De Deyn, R.A. Dierckx, A. Alavi and B.A. Pickut
© 1997 John Libbey & Company Ltd, pp. 149–165

Neuroreceptor Ligand Imaging by SPECT in Parkinsonian Syndromes

Chapter
20

N.P.L.G. Verhoeff*, J. Booij*, R.B. Innis and E.A. van Royen*

Introduction

Parkinsonian syndrome consists of tremor, rigidity, hypokinesia, and postural abnormalities. The major cause of this syndrome is idiopathic Parkinson's disease (IPD), accounting for approximately 60-85% of all cases[1,2]. A clinical hallmark of IPD is its responsiveness to dopaminergic medication[3]. Lewy bodies are observed post mortem in the substantia nigra pars compacta[4,5]. The prevalence of IPD is 84-164 per 100,000 for Caucasians, whereas the annual incidence is 8.7-20 per 100,000[2]. Both increase with age. These figures show that IPD is and will be one of the major neurological causes of morbidity, especially with an increasing mean age of the population.

However, other causes of the parkinsonian syndrome exist that fail to respond to dopaminergic medication. Mutiple system atrophy (MSA) and progressive supranuclear palsy (PSP) may account for up to 15% of all patients with parkinsonian symptoms[1,6,7]. Depending on its main manifestations, MSA includes syndromes such as striatonigral degeneration (SND) with predominantly extrapyramidal symptoms, Shy-Dräger syndrome with mainly autonomic symptomatology, and olivopontocerebellar atrophy (OPCA) with predominantly cerebellar dysfunction[7,8]. The pathology is characterised by argyrophilic inclusions in neurons and glial cells[8,9]. In PSP, which is neuropathologically distinct from MSA, the clinical characteristic is paralysis of vertical gaze[6].

The state of the art of neuroreceptor imaging in nuclear medicine, in neurology and in psychiatry has been discussed previously[10-15]. This article deals with the ligands presently available for imaging patients with the parkinsonian syndrome *in vivo* by single photon emission computed tomography (SPECT) or by positron emission tomography (PET). The emphasis will be on SPECT ligands, as for most nuclear medicine clinics there are several advantages for using this technique[16].

Dopamine D$_2$ receptors

Differential diagnosis between MSA and PSP on the one hand and IPD on the other is considered to be important in view of the differences in prognosis and therapy[6,7,17], although a clinical distinction between IPD and MSA or PSP is sometimes hard to achieve[1,18,19]. X-ray transmission CT, MRI and MR spectroscopy, however, may to some extent contribute to such differential diagnosis. Atrophy of the putamen[20], cerebellar atrophy[21], atrophy of the brainstem[22] and reduction in N-acetyl aspartate and in choline-containing

*Department of Nuclear Medicine, Academic Medical Centre, Amsterdam Zuidoost, The Netherlands
Department of Psychiatry, Yale University School of Medicine, New Haven, and Veterans Affairs Medical Center, West Haven, USA

compounds in the lentiform nucleus[23] have been reported in some cases of MSA. The apomorphine test has been used to predict dopaminergic responsiveness in parkinsonian syndromes[24]. However, inconsistencies have been observed[25].

In this respect, functional imaging of striatal dopamine D_2 receptors *in vivo* may be promising. Little or no response to L-DOPA treatment has previously been coupled to a decreased striatal D_2 receptor density post mortem[26,27]. Indeed, a severe reduction in striatal D_2 receptor binding potential was demonstrated *in vivo* using ^{11}C-raclopride or [76]Br-bromospiperone and PET in IPD patients with a fluctuating response to L-DOPA and in patients with MSA or PSP[28,29]. However, PET is not a suitable technique for larger clinical studies in view of its costs and limited availability. SPECT is less expensive and more available than PET.

Recently, several SPECT studies have confirmed the findings with PET. Using SPECT and ^{123}I-iodolisuride or ^{123}I-iodobenzamide (^{123}I-IBZM), a reduced striatal D_2 receptor binding potential was observed in PSP and MSA patients[30,31], whereas patients with IPD revealed normal values[32,33]. The reduced striatal D_2 receptor binding potential in MSA and PSP probably reflects degeneration of striatal medium spiny neurons, although dopaminergic afferents from the cerebral cortex and from the substantia nigra to the striatum may also contribute. These contributions may, however, be negligible as in rats the striatal D_2 receptor density decreased markedly upon kainic acid lesions of intrinsic neurons in the striatum, but not upon lesions involving the corticostriatal pathway[34]. In IPD only a loss >90% of dopaminergic innervation may result in D_2 receptor upregulation in the putamen[35]. The apparent lack of striatal D_2 receptor upregulation in patients with IPD on ^{123}I-IBZM SPECT may therefore be explained partially by a lower loss of dopaminergic innervation in the patients studied[33]. However, another ^{123}I-IBZM SPECT study in recently diagnosed IPD patients with pronounced unilateral symptoms revealed increased uptake of the tracer in the striatum contralateral to the parkinsonian symptoms[36,37]. In the study of Knable *et al.*[36] the maximal slope of the integral for specific binding, occurring at the time when peak specific binding occurs, was used, resulting in a better estimation of the D_2 receptor binding potential. Using this approach, lateralised differences in the D_2 binding potential were actually correlated with differences in the modified abnormal involuntary movements scale score and in the four subscales (tremor, bradykinesia, rigidity and dystonia).

In two recent studies using ^{123}I-IBZM SPECT and in one study using ^{11}C-methylspiperone PET, the striatal D_2 receptor binding potential actually decreased with longer disease duration[33,38,39]. This may be either an effect of the disease *per se* resulting in transsynaptic degeneration of striatal neurons[38] or of the prolonged use of the dopaminergic medication resulting in down-regulation of D_2 receptors[33,37]. However, the latter is less likely as 3-4 months therapy with L-DOPA or lisuride did not change striatal D_2 receptor density as measured with ^{11}C-raclopride PET[40]. Whether longer duration or dopaminergic therapy (e.g. for several years) leads to D_2 receptor down regulation still needs to be studied longitudinally.

It has been claimed that ^{123}I-IBZM SPECT can actually predict responsiveness to dopaminergic therapy. In a prospective study using ^{123}I-IBZM SPECT in *de novo* parkinsonian patients, similar results were obtained regarding the relation between striatal D_2 receptor binding potential and clinical response to dopaminergic medication[41]. Based on prospective data in 77 untreated patients with the parkinsonian syndrome, a sensitivity of 98% and a specificity of 74% have been calculated in differentiating IPD from MSA and PSP[42].

Dopamine D_2 receptor SPECT or PET can be used in future to create homogeneous patient groups for clinical trials exploring both medical and surgical experimental therapies. In parkinsonian patients, possible additional damage in the connections forming the striato-thalamo-cortical circuit might occur[5,43,44]. This is the clinical basis for therapies with NMDA antagonists such as MK-801, AMPA/kainate antagonists such as NBQX, metabotropic antagonists $\alpha 2$ adrenergic agonists such as clonidine, and muscarinic antagonists such as dexetimide, either alone or in combination with or without apomorphine or other dopamine (D_1) agonists[44,45-49]. These largely experimental therapies could be evaluated in those patients having a striatal D_2 receptor deficiency as demonstrated with e.g. ^{123}I-IBZM SPECT. Moreover, in view of the increasing number of embryonic or foetal mesencephalic brain cell transplantations performed[50-56], and its ethical implications[57-59], imaging of striatal D_2 receptors *in vivo* may be useful in selecting the appropriate patients to undergo such a procedure. It is questionable whether patients displaying a low dopamine D_2 receptor binding potential in the striatum are suitable candidates for transplantation[55,60].

Using unilateral intracaratoid injections of the dopaminergic neurotoxin 1-methyl-4-phenyl-1,2,3,6-tetrahydropyridine (MPTP) in monkeys, a significant increase in striatal dopamine D_2 receptors has been observed at the site of the lesion both post mortem using ^{3}H-sulpiride[61] and *in vivo* using ^{11}C-raclopride and PET[62]. Autoradiography *ex vivo* using ^{123}I-IBZM showed a 10% to 50% increase in D_2 receptor density in the caudate nucleus on the side with the lesion[63].

With ^{123}I-IBZM SPECT an increase in striatal activity of up to 30% was observed *in vivo* at the lesioned side compared with the contralateral side[64]. This may not only be due to D_2 receptor upregulation on the side of the lesion, but also to displacement of ^{123}I-IBZM be enhanced endogenous dopamine release at the contralateral side[65]. At present, experiments are being performed to induce dopamine release by D-amphetamine to assess the relative contribution of the latter component. The MPTP monkey model enables one to follow the time course of possible D_2 receptor upregulation after a presynaptic dopaminergic deficit within a much shorter time-frame than would be the case in clinical studies concerning patients with IPD, in whom the disease progresses more slowly. Moreover, in addition to imaging dopamine uptake sites or L-DOPA conversion, normalisation of the previously upregulated striatal D_2 receptor binding potential after e.g. neurografting of new dopamine-producing cells may be indicative of restoration of the dopaminergic input.

SPECT studies with ^{123}I-IBZM in unilaterally MPTP-lesioned monkeys showed displacement by dopaminergic agonists but did not reveal a linear relationship between striatal D_2 receptor occupancy by dopaminergic agonists and the extent of resulting behavioural corrections[64]. In contrast, a 15% decrease in D_2 receptor binding potential was observed in 8 healthy volunteers when ^{123}I-IBZM was administered via a bolus plus constant infusion and 0.3 mg/kg amphetamine was injected i.v. at 240 min p.i.[66]. The euphoria, alertness and restlessness induced by the D-amphetamine were correlated with the decrease in D_2 binding potential measured with SPECT, most likely induced by release of endogeneous dopamine. The asymmetries measured in the IPD patients by Knable *et al.*[36] were most likely due to a lateralised deficiency of endogenous dopamine and changes in striatal D_2 receptor status.

For detection of more subtle changes in striatal D_2 receptor density without potentially interfering influences of endogenous dopamine release, D_2 receptor ligands providing better signal-to-noise ratios and a more favourable bandwidth of the signal will be needed, e.g. the substituted benzamides ^{123}I-epidepride[67,68] or ^{123}I-NCQ 298[69]. Recently, ^{123}I-IBF SPECT has been performed in patients with IPD, MSA and PSP with results comparable to previous ^{123}I-IBZM studies[70]. However, imaging only took place up to 190 min p.i., at which time a transient equilibrium state of the ligand was not (yet) reached. Imaging for longer periods after the injection of ^{123}I-IBF may be necessary for a more accurate estimation of the striatal D_2 receptor binding potential.

Dopamine D_1 receptors

In patients suffering from IPD, there may be a reduction of dopamine D_1 receptor density in the substantia nigra and putamen. The substantia nigra contains high concentrations of the D_1 receptor but relatively few D_2 receptors, and in the caudate nucleus the density of D_1 receptors is about equal to the density of D_2 receptors[69,71]. Also, most of the dopaminergic agonists used to treat IPD are acting on both D_1 and D_2 receptors. Recently, it has been discussed[29] that the lack of effect of dopaminergic agonists in patients with IPD and other forms of parkinsonism may not only be explained by the slight decrease in D_2 receptor density in the striatum observed. An additional loss of D_1 receptors in the striatum may provide another explanation. Indeed, in a recent PET study, marked losses of both D_1 and D_2 receptors were observed in patients with SND, not responding to dopaminergic therapy[72]. Therefore, studying D_1 receptors in the brain *in vivo* with PET or SPECT, may reveal important information in addition to studying D_2 receptors, both for schizophrenia and parkinsonism, and probably also for other disorders.

In the unilateral MPTP model, striatal D_1 and D_2 receptors respond differently to the decreased dopaminergic input. Therefore, these receptors may also respond in a different way to long-term therapy with dopaminergic agonists in patients with IPD[61]. This has not been studied yet prospectively *in vivo* in IPD patients (as for D_2 receptors). In a patient with PSP, a preservation of striatal D_1 receptors was observed post mortem despite a severe depletion of D_2 receptors[27]. Therefore, in case of a striatal D_2 deficiency observed *in vivo* in patients with MSA or PSP, or in IPD patients with a decreased of fluctuating response to L-DOPA, imaging of D_1 receptors may be indicated in addition, as selective dopamine D_1 agonists might have a therapeutic effect.

^{123}I-SCH 23982, although highly recommended for SPECT studies[73], is not a suitable ligand for D_1 receptor SEPCT in humans[74]. However, Chumpradit *et al.*[75-77] enabled diminished deiodination *in vivo* by moving the iodine from the phenolic group to a non-activated 1-phenyl ring, thereby creating FISCH (iodine at the 4'-position) and TISCH (iodine at the 3'-position). The affinity of FISCH for the D_1 receptor *in vitro* was in the range of that reported for SCH 23390. Studies *in vivo* in monkeys additionally showed a fast uptake for this compound, but also a rapid washout from the brain, leading to low signal/noise ratios[78]. The D_1 receptor affinity of the active ^{125}I-R(+)TISCH isomer was even more favourable and upon application *in vivo* showed a good uptake and a D_1 receptor selective regional distribution in rat[77], non-human

primate[76] and human brain[79]. A 4-iodo-phenyl nitrogen-substituted benzopyran derivative, reported to have a high affinity, selectivity and intrinsic-agonistic activity towards the D_1 receptor[80], might also be of future interest as a D_1 receptor ligand for SPECT, especially as the iodinated substance has maintained agonistic properties. Due to a lower rate of metabolism, ^{11}C-SCH 39166 may be a more interesting D_1 receptor ligand for PET than ^{11}C-SCH 23390[81].

Research *in vitro* concerning D_1 receptor density in humans resulted in conflicting conclusions regarding ageing: either a decrease[82] or no change[83] has been reported. Recently, it has been demonstrated in healthy male volunteers (20-72 years) with ^{11}C-SCH23390 PET that the binding potential of the D_1 receptors in the striatum and frontal cortex decreased by 35% and 39%, respectively, with age[84]. Thus, probably the D_1 receptor density decreases with age. Therefore, age should be taken into account when studying D_1 receptors *in vivo* in patients with the parkinsonian syndrome.

Dopamine transporters

Recently, the presynaptically located transporters for dopamine have been cloned[85-87]. Post mortem studies reported decreased dopamine transporter densities in putamen and caudate nucleus in patients with IPD[88-91]. In addition, post mortem studies have suggested that the striatal dopamine concentration has to be reduced by 80% before mild parkinsonian symptoms start to develop, whereas with a dopamine loss of 90% a severe parkinsonian syndrome occurs[92]. Based on animal models of IPD, it is also believed that, at a very early phase of the disease, the dopaminergic neurons still available are hyperfunctioning so that basal levels of extracellular dopamine are being maintained[93,94].

The development of new pharmacological treatments to retard the progression of IPD[95-97] has increased the need for a reliable outcome measure to assess progressive loss of the dopaminergic system, to monitor the efficacy of treatment and to diagnose the disease during the preclinical phase so that treatments could be implemented before irreversible loss of dopaminergic neurons occurs[98]. The preclinical phase in IPD may be as long as 20 to 40 years. In addition, epidemiologic investigations regarding the cause(s) of IPD would be greatly facilitated by earlier disease detection[99]. For example, screening could take place in subjects suspected to be at risk for developing IPD based on neuropsychological characteristics such as a reduced shifting aptitude as to behaviour that is triggered or guided by self-generated information[100]. Neuro-imaging techniques such as PET and SPECT of

dopamine transporters will provide such objective outcome measures.

Transplantation of embryonic or foetal mesencephalic tissue into patients with the parkinsonian syndrome requires positive striatal D_2 receptor imaging for patient selection as mentioned previously. Clinical improvement has been linked to survival and outgrowth of the dopaminergic cells of the transplant, and these can probably be predicted by ^{18}F-DOPA PET[51,53,54]. Sequential PET scans have shown progressive increases in ^{18}F-DOPA uptake at the site of implantation in two patients with IPD up to 13 months after unilateral putaminal implantation of foetal dopaminergic cells[53,101], and in two patients with MPTP-induced parkinsonism up to 24 months after bilateral implantation in the caudate and putamen of embryonic dopaminergic cells, parallelling clinical improvement[56].

However, to some extent the results with ^{18}F-DOPA PET after embryonic or foetal tissue transplantation are controversial. In one IPD patient showing clinical improvement shortly after transplantation, no increase in ^{18}F-DOPA uptake in the putamen was seen at 9 months after transplantation[51], whereas striatal ^{18}F-DOPA uptake continued to increase markedly in two patients even when they seemed to have reached their maximal recovery[54,56]. Therefore, clinical improvement may precede the improvement of ^{18}F-DOPA uptake visualised with PET and growth of uptake capacity may continue for a very long period. Regarding ^{18}F-DOPA uptake in the unoperated striatal structures after unilateral putaminal implantation, Sawle *et al.*[101] reported a progressive decrease whereas Freed *et al.*[51] and Spencer *et al.*[55] described an increase. These outcomes need further evaluation. Further insights may be given by PET and SPECT studies of dopamine transporters.

PET ligands

Several ligands are available for PET studies of dopamine transporters[102], e.g. ^{11}C-cocaine[103], ^{18}F-GBR 13119[104,105], ^{11}C-nomifensine[62], [11]C- or, possibly, ^{18}F-CFT (11C- or ^{18}F-WIN 35,428)[106-108], and possibly in the future, ^{18}F-fluoromethyl-BTCP[109]. ^{11}C-Nomifensine has been shown to be useful in the study of patients with IPD[110] and MSA[21,111].

The derivative α-dihydrotetrabenazine (TBZOH) inhibits monoamine uptake in all monoaminergic vesicles[112], and may therefore be useful for imaging of presynaptic monoaminergic nerve endings *in vivo*. However, TBZOH has also been reported to block presynaptic and postsynaptic dopamine receptors[113]. Other markers proposed for monoaminergic nerve terminal imaging *in vivo* are ^{11}C-tetrabenazine, which is a potent inhibitor of the vesicular monoamine transporter with higher selectivity for dopaminergic than for serotonergic vesicles[114], reserpine[115] and ^{18}F-α-fluoromethyl-p-tyrosine, a tyrosine hydroxylase-activated decarboxylase suicide inhibitor[116].

SPECT ligands: developments until ^{123}I-CIT

Similar ligands for SPECT would greatly accelerate the possibility for such a preclinical detection because of better accessibility and reduced costs[16]. The potential of SPECT imaging of dopamine transporters as a clinical tool in parkinsonian syndromes (notably IPD) has been reviewed recently[117]. Iodinated derivatives have been proposed for mazindol[118] and cocaine (i.e. [123]I-4'-iodococaine[103] and [125]I-2'-iodococaine[119]. In addition, bupropion and benztropine might be labelled with ^{123}I, although the latter has a relatively high affinity for muscarinic receptors[120]. The new series of substances developed by Gist-Brocades are the only pharmaceuticals with absolute selectivity for the dopamine transporter (i.e. having much less affinity for the serotonin or noradrenaline transporters)[121], but no such ligands have yet been developed for SPECT, though several ^{123}I-labelled derivatives have been reported to be successful *in vitro*[122-124].

SPECT ligands: ^{123}I-CIT

Recently, the ligand [123]I-2ß-carbomethoxy-3ß-(4-iodophenyl)tropane (^{123}I-CIT or ^{123}I-RTI-55) has been developed as a high-affinity SPECT radiotracer of the monoamine transporter with two different affinities unlike mazindol and GBR 12935[127]. The equilibrium binding constants (Kd) of ^{123}I CIT are 0.4 and 18 nm, for the high and low affinity site, respectively, measured *in vitro* in baboon striatum membranes homogenised in a buffer mimicking the composition of cerebrospinal fluid[128]. In squirrel monkeys[107] and in baboons[129] satisfactory results were obtained. ^{123}I-CIT also binds to serotonin transporters with about equivalent affinity as to dopamine transporters; however, in rats the contribution to the signal in the striatum was very limited[130]. In non-human primates similar findings were reported for ^{123}I-CIT SPECT and ^{11}C-CIT PET studies[131-134], as well as for studies using both the active (1R) and inactive (1s) enantiomers of CIT labelled with ^{125}I and [123]I[135]. The vast majority (>90%) of striatal binding is associated with the dopamine transporter, which is consistent with a striatal dopamine/serotonin transporter ratio of >10[117]. Supratherapeutic infusions of L-DOPA with peripheral DOPA-decarboxylase inhibitor did not displace ^{123}I-CIT during the plateau phase of imaging[134]. Peak

whole brain activity was 6%-10% of the injected ^{123}I-CIT activity within the first h p.i. in non-human primates[131] and 14% of the injected activity in healthy volunteers, with about 2% overlying the striatal region[136]. The signal/noise ratios increased from 30 min to 5 h p.i.[132-134]. Metabolites of ^{123}I-CIT probably do not influence the distribution on the SPECT images, as a minor lipophilic metabolite increased to only about 2-4% at 2-7 h p.i.[131,137]. However, this is controversial as higher percentages of lipophilic metabolites have been reported[138]. This deserves further evaluation.

With ^{123}I-CIT SPECT some desirable characteristics of a preclinical marker of later onset of IPD may be met: (1) acceptable clinical-epidemiologic characteristics regarding (a) accessibility and (b) safety of the test (c) reproducibility, (d) precision and accuracy, (e) sensitivity and specificity, and (f) positive and negative predictive values[139]; (2) clinical pathological relevance to the process, implying (a) correlation with onset of sympomatic IPD and with severity of symptoms and (b) correlation with neuronal cell counts or dopamine levels[98]. Taking these criteria into consideration, there are several indications that ^{123}I-CIT SPECT will be a useful marker.

Accessibility. SPECT is a relatively accessible technique in developed countries[16]. Recently, a faster and simplified method for the routine multidose preparations of ^{123}I-CIT has been developed with purification of the labelled compound by solid phase extraction[140].

Safety. Dosimetry in 8 healthy volunteers revealed highest radiation-absorbed doses to the lungs (0.1 mGy/MBq), liver (0.87 mGy/MBq) and lower large intestine (0.053 mGy/MBq)[136]. Thus, the lung is the limiting organ for radiation exposure from ^{123}I-CIT. Based on the radiation dose limit of 50 mSv in a single dose for most organs[141], individuals could receive a single dose of 500 MBq (14 mCi) as an absolute maximum[136].

Reproducibility, precision and accuracy. The most practical clinical measure for the dopamine transporter binding potential is the specific to non-displaceable partition coefficient V_3" (e.g. the ratio of [striatum-occipital] over occipital cortex) during a state of equilibrium, because it requires neither calibration of the camera relative to the injected radioactivity nor any plasma measurements[142]. As 18-24 h after injection of ^{123}I-CIT striatal uptake only increased by 0.5%/h and occipital cortex uptake only decreased by 1.2%/h in 28 healthy volunteers[143], and as after 240 min p.i. the free parent compound in the plasma decreased by only 1%/h in 5 healthy volunteers[142], equilibrium conditions seem to be met during this interval. Simulations using a washout in the occipital cortex of 1%/h showed that V_3" measured between 20 and 24 h after injection was within 6% of the true binding potential[142]. A study consisting of two ^{123}I-CIT SPECT scans separated by 7-14 days in 7 healthy volunteers showed excellent test/retest reproducibility of V_3" with a variablity of 6.8 ± 6.8% and an intraclass correlation coefficient of 0.96[144].

Sensitivity and specificity, and positive and negative predictive values. With kinetic analysis of ^{123}I-CIT SPECT, loss of about 65% striatal dopamine transporters was observed in 5 patients with IPD compared with 5 sex-matched healthy controls with a similar mean age[145]. Greater losses occurred in the putamen than in the caudate, confirming the finding of initial loss of dopaminergic projections in the putamen[146] and there was no overlap between the 2 groups when the striatum/occipital cortex ratios were taken as an estimate for the dopamine transporter binding potential. These results were confirmed by Brücke *et al.*[147].

The V_3", the putamen/caudate ratio and the contralatral/ipsilateral ratio for putamen and caudate were significantly reduced in 28 IPD patients compared with 27 healthy controls[148]. Discriminant function analysis using V_3" for ipsilateral and contralateral caudate and putamen correctly classified 54 of the 55 cases; when age-correction of the data was performed, all cases were correctly identified. Age-corrected V_3" in the putamen contralateral to the side of sign onset provided a particularly good group separation with only 18% unaccounted variance. Similar analyses for the putamen/caudate ratio and the contralateral/ipsilateral ratio for putamen and caudate correctly classified 96% and 80% of the subjects, respectively.

Similar findings were observed with ^{11}C-CIT PET in 9 IPD patients when compared with 3 healthy controls[149]. However, because of the short half-life of ^{11}C, only the first part of a prolonged accumulation process could be visualised. Therefore, CIT may be better suited for SPECT studies than for PET.

It has been suggested that the elevation of the caudate/putamen ratio and marked asymmetry of ^{123}I-CIT activity may be useful in distinguishing IPD from atypical parkinsonian syndromes such as MSA[117,150], as these would usually show a more uniform and symmetrical loss of dopaminergic activity both involving the caudate and putamen, reflected in reduced ^{18}F-DOPA uptake in both nuclei[151-153]. A recent study using ^{123}I-CIT SPECT in MSA patients showed a markedly decreased signal in the striatum (Booij *et al.*, preliminary results). In this study the MSA patients were selected according to their clinical

features (i.e. at least an akinetic-rigid syndrome, with a poor or no response to dopaminomimetics) in combination with a loss of striatal D_2 receptors, as indicated by a reduced signal on ^{123}I-IBZM SPECT[31,33,154,155]. The binding activity of ^{123}I-CIT in both caudate nucleus and putamen decreased significantly when assayed 24 h after injection in comparison to controls (Figure 1). In both IPD and MSA patients a loss of dopamine transporter signal was more dramatic in the putamen than in the caudate nucleus. In a recent PET study, 4 of 10 patients with sporadic OPCA, believed to belong to the spectrum of MSA, had reduced ^{11}C-diprenorphine binding in the putamen individually, whereas only 1 had reduced values in the caudate nucleus[8]. This finding is likely to reflect preferential putaminal involvement by the pathology of MSA. Pathological studies have shown that in MSA the putamen, especially the dorsolateral posterior two thirds, is more severely affected than the caudate nucleus[9,156,157]. Neuronal loss in the substantia nigra in MSA patients has been found to be more severe in the ventrolateral part projecting into the putamen, although the dorsal tier projecting to the caudate is also affected[156]. A more extensive PET study revealed that ^{18}F-DOPA uptake in MSA patients was more heterogeneous, with relative sparing of caudate uptake in some and uniform striatal involvement in others, without clear differences in locomotor disability between patients with mild and those with severe caudate involvement[21]. Thus, there are conflicting reports on whether ^{123}I-CIT SPECT will be able to differentiate between IPD and MSA based on preferential putaminal involvement versus diffuse involvement of both caudate and putamen, respectively.

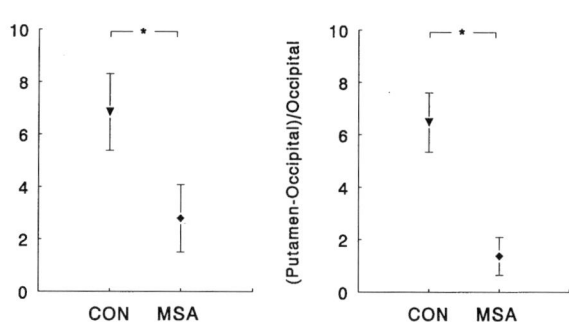

Figure 1 ^{123}I-CIT binding in caudate nucleus and putamen of controls (CON, n=7; mean ± s.d.) and MSA patients (MSA, n=10; mean ± s.d.) 24 h following injection. Data were expressed as relative ratio over occipital cortex value *:p<0.05. For a description of the methods used, see Appendix

Correlation with onset of symptomatic IPD and with severity of symptoms. ^{123}I-CIT SPECT in 5 patients with IPD showed greater losses in the striatum contralateral to the side of the body with intial symptoms[145]. In 8 early IPD patients with exclusively hemi-parkinsonism, ^{123}I-CIT striatal uptake was reduced by about 53% contralateral and by 38% ipsilateral to the clinically symptomatic side, when compared with 8 age and sex matched healthy subjects[150]. The reduction in ^{123}I-CIT uptake was greater in the putamen than in the caudate. These data indicate that ^{123}I-CIT SPECT may be useful in identifying individuals with developing dopaminergic pathology prior to the onset of motor signs.

In 28 L-DOPA-reponsive IPD patients, the degree of abnormal striatal uptake of ^{123}I-CIT, expressed as both ipsilateral and contralateral $V_3"$ in both putamen and caudate, was significantly correlated with the toal Unified Parkinson's Disease Rating Scale (UPDRS) score and with the Hoehn-Yahr stage[148]. Both UPDRS motor subscores and bradykinesia were strongly correlated with the $V_3"$ measures. The uptake in the putamen was relatively more reduced than in the caudate. Also, the asymmetry (based on the side where the parkinsonian signs started) was larger in the putamen than in the caudate.

In a more recent ^{123}I-CIT SPECT study, in small groups of IPD patients discriminated as early (Hoehn and Yahr score 1-2) and late IPD (Hoehn and Yahr score 2.5-4: disease history > 10 years), a stage-dependent decrease of striatal binding was seen [158]. In this study, images were obtained 24 h following intravenous injections of ^{123}I-CIT, and binding of ^{123}I-CIT to the striatum was substantially lower in both early and late IPD as compared with the control group. Moreover, ^{123}I CIT binding to both caudate nucleus and putamen was significantly decreased with IPD stage. Again, the effect was more prominent in the putamen than in the caudate nucleus.

Correlation with neuronal cell counts and dopamine levels. As mentioned above, decreased dopamine transporter densities have been observed in putamen and caudate nucleus in patients with IPD, closely paralelling losses of dopamine[88-91]. Both the decrease of tissue dopamine levels and ^{3}H-CFT binding to the dopamine transporter showed similar medial to lateral gradients in the striatum and more severe losses in the putamen compared with the caudate[90]. ^{123}I-CIT SPECT studies performed in patients with IPD have confirmed the relative selective loss of dopamine transporters in the putamen[145,148,150].

Ageing is associated with a gradual degeneration of dopaminergic neurons and an accompanying loss of

transmitter and transporter. A decrease of about 10%/decade has been described for dopamine transporters in post mortem samples[159,160]. ^{123}I-CIT SPECT in healthy volunteers showed a comparable age-related decline of dopamine transporters of 8%/decade in the striatum[143].

The question remains as to which marker would be more important to establish the status quo *in vivo* of the nigrostriatal pathway: one that assays the surviving neurons, like the markers discussed above, or a dopamine analogue, like ^{18}F-DOPA[101,151,153,161], that might be a better measure for the functional status of the surviving neurons[162]. However, dopamine turnover is increased in animals with nigrostriatal lesions and in post mortem parkinsonian brain. As a result of this enhanced turnover, an increased proportion of radiometabolites may leave the brain of parkinsonian patients, exaggerating the deficits in these patients when measured with ^{18}F-DOPA[117]. The assumption at present is that the number of dopamine transporters per nerve terminal remains constant in IPD, so that a ligand for the dopamine transporter can directly visualise the number of remaining nerve terminals. However, as the loss of dopaminergic neurons reaches a critical threshold, the remaining neurons may compensate by decreasing the amount of dopamine transporters per terminal in order to maintain synaptic dopamine at a certain level[143].

The ^{123}I-CIT SPECT data mentioned above lead to the following conclusions:

1. ^{123}I-CIT striatal outcome measures are reproducible in heallthy controls and in IPD patients.

2. ^{123}I-CIT SPECT in sensitive to age-related loss of dopamine transporters in healthy subjects.

3. Hemi-Parkinson patients demonstrate reduced striatal uptake contralateral and ipsilateral to motor symptoms suggesting ^{123}I-CIT may be sensitive to preclinical changes in dopamine transporters.

4. Disease severity in IPD is correlated with reductions in ^{123}I-CIT striatal uptake.

5. In IPD there is relatively greater reduction in putaminal ^{123}I-CIT uptake than in caudate.

6. Contralateral-ipsilateral asymmetries of striatal ^{123}I-CIT uptake with respect to the side of onset of parkinsonian signs discriminate IPD patients from healthy controls.

7. ^{123}I-CIT SPECT may be able to differentiate between IPD and MSA patients with preferential putaminal involvement on the one hand and MSA

patients with diffuse involvement of both caudate and putamen on the other hand, but may be not be able to differentiate between IPD and MSA *per se*.

8. CIT may be better suited for SPECT studies than for PET.

Finally, ^{123}I-CIT SPECT imaging of dopamine transporters may be useful for: diagnosing early or pre-symptomatic stages of IPD; monitoring progression severity in IPD over time; assessing the efficacy of putative neuroprotective agents; revealing the extent of striatal involvement in IPD and other parkinsonian syndromes; and following growth or rejection of foetal tissue transplanted into IPD patients.

SPECT ligands: beyond ^{123}I-CIT

Several other promising ligands besides ^{123}I-CIT have been developed for dopamine transporter imaging. The isopropyl ester of CIT, 2ß-carboisoproxy-3ß-(4-iodophenyl-tropane (IPCIT or RTI-121), has a 50-100 fold higher selectivity for the dopamine transporter than for the serotonin transporter[163]. However, the non-specific binding of ^{125}I-IPCIT was almost four times that of ^{125}I-CIT in baboon striatum membranes[164] and non-specific uptake in baboon cerebellum *in vivo* was 2 times as large for ^{123}I-IPCIT as for ^{123}I-CIT[135]. The brain uptake of ^{123}I-IPCIT in 2 baboons was about 9% in the first h p.i. and activity levels of areas with moderately dense serotonergic innervation (superior colliculus and thalamus) was equal[164] or only slightly greater than[135] that in the cerebellum. In conclusion, ^{123}I-IPCIT demonstrated *in vivo* a higher dopamine transporter selectivity and a higher level of non-specific uptake than ^{123}I-CIT. For SPECT imaging, ^{123}I-IPCIT is not likely to provide any clear advantage over ^{123}I-CIT.

Several N-Ω-fluoralkyl analogs of CIT have been synthesised[165]. The methyl ester (N-fluoroethyl, methyl ester {CIT-FE} and N-fluoropropyl, methyl ester {CIT-FP}) have a lower affinity for the dopamine transporter than CIT has and thus should allow for faster kinetics, which is prefereable for studies *in vivo*[166]. After labelling with ^{123}I, the methyl esters (CIT-FE and CIT-FP) showed a higher total and specific peak uptake in baboon striatum *in vivo* than the isopropyl esters (N-fluoroethyl, isopropyl ester {IP-CIT-FE} and N-fluoropropyl isopropyl ester {IP-CIT-FP})[167]. ^{123}I-CIT-FE had more rapid striatal kinetics than ^{123}I-CIT-FP, with specific striatal washout rates of 10-14%/peak/h and 4-6%/peak/h, respectively[165,167]. Absorbed radiation dose estimates indicated highest dose rates to urinary bladder wall (0.18 mGy/MBq for ^{123}I-CIT-FE)

and to the intestinal wall (0.24 mGy/MBq for ^{123}I-CIT-FP)[167].

In a study using ^{123}I-CIT-FP in unilateral MPTP-treated non-human primates (Mucaca mulatta, at least 3 year post treatment), the striatal to occipital cortex ratio of radioactivity already reached an average value of 4 at 3 h p.i. In all five MPTP-lesioned monkeys, the striatal uptake on the lesioned side was severely reduced to about 10% of the non-lesioned side (Figure 2 [Booij *et al.*, preliminary results]).

In four healthy volunteers, both ^{123}I-CIT-FE and ^{123}I-CIT-FP demonstrated high brain uptake: on average 7.8% and 6.4% of the injected radioactivity, respectively[166]. Radioactivity concentrated in the striatum over time, reaching a peak within 30 min p.i., with about 14.7%/h washout for ^{123}I-CIT-FE and little or no washout for ^{123}I-CIT-FP. Occipital and midbrain activity showed similar patterns for both tracers, with a peak within 15 min p.i. and rapid washout, followed by stable levels at about 100 min. The average peak striatum/peak midbrain ratio was 7.7 for ^{123}I-CIT-FE and 9.1 for ^{123}I-CIT-FP, thus showing a high selectivity *in vivo* for the dopamine transporter. ^{123}I-CIT-FE would be preferable for kinetic modelling with arterial sampling and would allow comparing SPECT and PET when labelled with ^{18}F, whereas ^{123}I-CIT-FP would be preferable for non-invasive equilibrium analysis[166,168]. It seems likely that both ^{123}I-CIT-FE and ^{123}I-CIT-FP allow imaging *in vivo* in a one-day protocol.

At present a SPECT study is in progress using ^{123}I-CIT-FP dealing with the measurement of loss of striatal dopamine transporters in patients with early (Hoehn and Yahr score 1-2) and late IPD (Hoehn and Yahr score 2.5-4; disease history > 10 years). In the group of 2 controls and 8 patients, assayed at 3 h after the intravenous injection of ^{123}I-CIT-FP, the patients

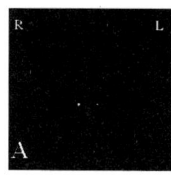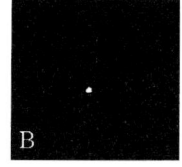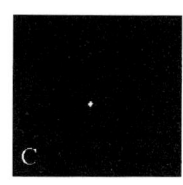

Figure 2 Transverse slices from the monkey brain at the level of the striatum (approximately 1.5 cm above the canthomeatal line) (L = left side and R = right side). In all three images the level of ^{123}I-CIT-FP activity is encoded from low (black) via medium (grey) to high (white) and scaled to the maximum in the slice of the control monkey. A: control monkey; B and C: MPTP-lesioned monkeys, lesion at the left side. For a description of the methods used, please see Appendix

showed reduced signal in both caudate nucleus and putamen (Figure 3 [Booij *et al.*, preliminary results]). From this limited study, it may be concluded that progression of IPD evolves more rapidly in the putamen than in caudate nucleus based on the relatively higher uptake of the latter area in early IPD.

Opiate receptors

[11]C-Diprenorphine PET has claimed to be more consistent in distinguishing striatal degeneration and in distinguishing patient with MSA from those with IPD[169]. Opiate receptors (mainly kappa and delta) are located postsynaptically on striatal neurons[170], and mu receptors are located in striosomes and in striatal matrix[171]. There is controversy over whether they are also found presynaptically on nigrostriatal terminals[170,172,173]. No opioid receptor messenger RNA has been found in nigral neurons[171]. Loss of striatal delta[174], and mu[172] receptors after nigral lesions has been documented but it is known that such lesions can lead to secondary striatal degeneration[175]. A loss of presynaptic opioid receptors could contribute to the positive correlation betwen the reduced putamen ^{18}F-DOPA and ^{11}C-diprenorphine uptake observed recently in patients with sporadic OPCA[8]. However, in 8 patients with IPD the striatal uptake of ^{11}C-diprenorphine was similar to that of healthy controls, which makes a presynaptic localisation of the opioid receptors in IPD less likely[169]. Studies with more specific opioid receptor ligands such as ^{11}C-naltrindole (for delta receptors[176]) and ^{18}F-cyclofoxy (for mu and kappa receptors[177]) could help to determine whether particular opiate receptor subtypes are selectively affected in MSA. Unfortunately, no specific opiate receptors are presently available for SPECT although iodinated derivatives have been developed for sigma opiate receptors (MIPAG and PIPAG[178]).

Muscarinic receptors

Muscarinic (M) receptors can now be studied *in vivo* with SPECT using the specific ligands ^{123}I-quinuclidinyl benzylate[179] or ^{123}I-iododexetimide[180]. This technique may be used to increase the knowledge about which cell types are actually responsible for the reduced D_2 receptor binding potential observed *in vivo* in some patients with the parkinsonian syndrome with a decreased or no response to dopaminergic medication (i.e. with MSA or PSP). Thus, the target cells of the nigrostriatal pathway may by affected differentially and this may vary according to the aetiology of the disease (IPD or MSA/PSP). In case of a degeneration of medium spiny neurons, a reduced M receptor binding potential might be expected[181]. Indeed reduced M cholinergic receptor densities have been observed in caudate specimens from 8 patients with IPD with a fluctuating response to L-DOPA[60]. In case of a degeneration of the cholinergic interneurons, which form a numerical minority in the striatum as compared with the medium spiny neurons[182,183], no change or even an increased expression of M receptors could be expected. Cholinergic neurons were observed to be degenerated in the mesencephalon in autopsy material from 3 patients with PSP[184]. Besides cholinergic interneurons, a cholinergic tract from the parafascicular and centromedian nuclei of the thalamus may innervate the putamen, and its activation may worsen parkinsonian symptomatology[185]. Changes in the function of this tract might also influence the striatal M receptor status.

N-methyl D-aspartate receptors

The non-competitive N-methyl-D-aspartate (NMDA) receptor antagonist ^{125}I-MK-801 has been synthesised and evaluation *in vivo* is still in progress[186]. Should this ligand, labelled with ^{123}I, become available for SPECT studies in humans, then an interesting application may be possible in patients with the parkinsonian syndrome in which glutamatergic function may be disrupted. Due to an increased inhibition of the external globus pallidus, the subthalamic nucleus may become more active[43]. This may, via excitatory amino acids (probably glutamate), stimulate increased activity in the internal globus pallidus, leading in turn to increased inhibition of the thalamus and thalamocortical neurons[187]. Thus, parkinsonian symptoms are associated with the enhanced excitatory amino acid

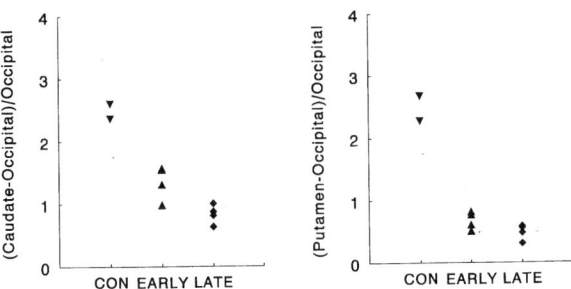

Figure 3 ^{123}I-CIT-FP binding in caudate nucleus and putamen of controls (CON, n=2), early PD (EARLY, n=4) and late PD patients (LATE, n=4) 3 h following injection. Data were expressed as relative ratio over occipital cortex value. For a description of the methods used, please see Appendix

neurotransmisssion in the subthalamo-pallidal pathway[46,47]. Patients with MSA or PSP who fail to show a decreased dopamine D_2 receptor binding potential in the striatum but who have a poor response to dopaminergic medication, might therefore exhibit additional damage in the connections forming the striato-thalamo-cortical circuit[44]. Studies *in vivo* with NMDA antagonists such as ^{123}I-MK-801 may therefore be useful in future in patients with parkinsonian symptoms, especially regarding experimental therapy.

Patients belonging to the dominantly inherited variant of olivopontocerebellar atrophy did not reveal the parkinsonian syndrome, despite marked deficiencies in the dopaminergic system in some of them[188]. However, these patients showed marked reductions in aspartate and glutamate levels throughout the brain, especially in the cerebellar cortex (-40% to -70%). The cerebellar reductions were higher than could be explained by neuronal loss[189]. A similar situation may exist in some patients with the sporadic variant of OPCA as marked deficiencies in striatal uptake of ^{18}F-DOPA have been visualised without marked extrapyramidal symptoms in these patients[8]. Visualising NMDA receptors *in vivo* in these patients may therefore be of interest to study both why these patients have such a high threshold before developing parkinsonian symptoms and how the NMDA receptors respond to chronically reduced levels of stimulating amino acids.

Acknowledgements

The authors thank John P. Seibyl, Departments of Diagnostic Radiology and Psychiatry, and Kenneth L. Marek, Department of Neurology, Yale University School of Medicine, New Haven, as well as colleagues working at the Department of Nuclear Medicine of the Academic Medical Centre, Amsterdam, for their support.

References

1   Hughes, A.J., Daniel, S.E., Kilford, L. and Lees, A.J. Accuracy of clinical diagnosis of idiopathic Parkinson's disease: a clinico-pathological study of 100 cases. *J. Neurol. Neurosurg. Psychiatry* 1992, 55, 1812

2   Speelman, J.D. Parkinson's Disease and Stereotaxic Neurosurgery. *Thesis* University of Amsterdam, 1991, p.11

3   Côté, L, Crutcher, M.D. The Basal Ganglia in 'Principles of Neural Science', (Eds. E.R. Kaudel, J.H. Schwartz, T.H. Jessel) 3rd Edition, New York, Elsevier

4   Perkin, G.D., Hochberg, F.H., Miller, D.C. *et al.* Dementia and Movement Disorders in 'Atlas of Clinical Neurology', Wolfe Publishing, an imprint of Mosby-Year Book Europe Ltd., London, 1993, 6.1

5   Roberts, G.W., Leigh, P.N., Weinberger, D.R. *et al.* Parkinson's Disease in 'Neuropsychiatric Disorders', Wolfe Publishing, an imprint of Mosby-Year book Europe Ltd, London 1993, 9.1

6   Maher, E.R. and Lees, A.J. The clinical features and natural history of the Steele-Richardson-Olszewski syndrome (progressive supranuclear palsy). *Neurology* 1986, 36, 1005

7   Quinn, N. Multiple system atrophy - the nature of the beast. *J. Neurol. Neurosurg. Psychiatry* 1989, special supplement 78

8   Rinne, J.O., Burn, D.J., Mathias, C.J. *et al.* Positron Emission Tomography Studies on the Dopaminergic System and Striatal Opioid Binding in the Olivopontocerebellar Atrophy Variant of Multiple System Atrophy. *Ann.Neurol.* 1995, 37, 568

9   Daniel, S.E. The neuropathology and neurochemistry of multiple system atrophy in 'Autonomic failure: a textbook of clinical disorders of the autonomic nervous system', (Eds. R. Bannister, C.J. Mathias), Oxford University Press, 1992, p.564

10   Costa, D.C., Morgan, G.F., Lassen, N.A. (Eds.) 'New Trends in Nuclear Neurology and Psychiatry', John Libbey & Company Ltd, London, UK, 1993

11   Mazière, B. and Mazière, M. Where have we got to with neuroceptor mapping of the human brain? *Eur. J. Nucl. Med.* 1990, 16, 817

12   Mazière, B. and Mazière, M. Positron emission tomography studies of brain receptors. *Fundam. Clin. Pharmacol.* 1991, 5, 61

13   Mazière, B., Mazière, M., Delforge, J. *et al.* Contribution of positron emission tomography to pharmacokinetic studies in 'New Trends in Pharmacokinetics', (Eds. A. Rescigno, A.K. Thakur), Plenum Press, New York, USA, 1991, 169

14   Verhoeff, N.P.L.G. Pharmacological implications for neuroreceptor imaging. *Eur. J. Nucl. Med.* 1991, 18, 482

15   Verhoeff, N.P.L.G. Ligands for neuroreceptor imaging by single photon emission tomography (SPECT) or positron emission tomography (PET) in 'Nuclear Medicine in Clinical Diagnosis and Treatment', (Eds. I.P.C. Murray, P.J. Ell), Churchill Livingstone, London, UK, 1994, p.483

16   Innis, R.B. and Malison, R.T. Principles of Neuroimaging in ' Comprehensive Textbook of Psychiatry VI, 6th ed.', (Eds. H.I. Kaplan, B.J. Sadock), Williams and Wilkins, Baltimore, USA, 1995, p.89

17   Koller, W.C. Classification of Parkinsonism in 'Handbook of Parkinson's Disease', Marcel Dekker Inc., New York, USA, 1987, p. 51

18   Editorial. Parkinson's disease: one illness of many syndromes? *Lancet* 1992, 339, 1263

19   Marsden, C.D. Parkinson's disease. *Lancet* 1990, 335, 948

20   Pastakia, B., Polinsky, R., Di Chiro, G. *et al.* Multiple system atrophy (Shy-Dräger Syndrome) *M R Imaging Radiol.* 1986, 159, 499

21   Brooks, D.J., Salmon, E.P., Mathias, C.J. *et al.* The relationship between locomotor disability, autonomic dysfunction, and the integrity of the striatal dopaminergic system in patients with multiple system atrophy, pure

autonomic failure, and Parkinson's disease, studies with PET. *Brain* 1990, 113, 1539

22 Staal, A., Meerwaldt, J.D., van Dongen, K.J. *et al.* Non-familial degenerative disease and atrophy of brainstem and cerebellum. Clinical and CT data in 47 patients. *J. Neurol. Sci.* 1990, 95, 259

23 Davie, C.A., Wenning, G.K., Barker, G.J. *et al.* Differentiation of Multiple System Atrophy from Idiopathic Parkinson's Disease Using Proton Magnetic Resonance Spectroscopy. *Ann. Neurol.* 1995, 37, 204

24 Hughes, A.J., Lees, A.J., Stern, G.M. *et al.* Apomorphine test to predict domaminergic responsiveness in Parkinsonian syndromes. *Lancet* 1990, 336, 32

25 Stieger, M.J., Quinn, N.P. and Marsden, C.D. The clinical use of apomorphine in Parkinson's disease. *J. Neurol.* 1992, 239, 389

26 Rinne, U.K. Brain neurotransmitter receptors in Parkinson's disease in 'Movement Disorders', (Eds. C.D. Marsden, S. Fahn), Butterworth & Co. (Publishers) Ltd, London, 1982, p. 59

27 Pascual, J., Berciano, J, Grijalba, B. *et al.* Dopamine D_1 and D_2 Receptors in 'Progressive Supranuclear Palsy: An Autoradiographic Study', *Ann. Neurol.* 1992, 32, 703

28 Baron J.C., Mazière, B., Loc'h, C. *et al.* Loss of Striatal [^{76}Br]Bromospiperone Binding Sites Demonstrated by Positron Tomography in Progressive Supranuclear Palsy. *J. Cereb. Blood Flow Metab.* 1986, 6, 131

29 Brooks, D.J., Sawle, G.V., Playford, E.D. *et al.* Striatal D_2 Receptor Status in Patients with Parkinson's Disease, Striatonigral Degeneration and Progressive Supranuclear Palsy, Measured with ^{11}C-Raclopride and Positron Emission Tomography. *Ann. Neurol.* 1992, 31, 184

30 Chabriat, H., Levasseur, M., Vidailhet, M. *et al.* In-Vivo SPECT Imaging of D_2 Receptor with Iodine-Iodolisuride: Results in Supranuclear Palsy. *J. Nucl. Med.* 1992, 33, 1481

31 van Royen, E.A., Verhoeff, N.P.L.G., Speelman, J.D. *et al.* Multiple System Atrophy and Progressive Supranuclear Palsy. Diminished Striatal D_2 Dopamine Receptor Activity Demonstrated by ^{123}I-IBZM Single Photon Emission Computed Tomography. *Arch. Neurol.* 1993, 50, 513

32 Brücke, T., Podreka, I., Angelberger, P. *et al.* Dopamine D_2 Receptor Imaging with SPECT: Studies in Different Neuropsychiatric Disorders. *J. Cereb. Blood Flow Metab.* 1994, 11, 220

33 Verhoeff, N.P.L.G., Speelman, J.D., Kuiper, M.A. *et al.* Clinical significance of dopamine D_2 receptor imaging with ^{123}I-iodobenzamide SPECT in patients with parkinsonian syndromes in 'SPECT in Neurology and Psychiatry', (Eds. P.P. De Deyn, R.A. Dierckx, A. Alavi and B.A. Pickut), John Libbey & Co. Ltd, London, UK, 1997, p.167

34 Trugman, J.M., Geary, W.A.I.I., Wooten, G.F. *et al.* Localization of D-2 dopamine receptors to intrinsic striatal neurones by quantitative autoradiography. *Nature* 1996, 323, 267

35 Riederer, P., Sofic, E., Konradi, C. *et al.* The Role of Dopamine in the Control of Neurobiological Functions in 'The role of brain dopamine basic and clinical aspects of neuroscience, (Eds. E. Flückiger, E.E. Muller), Springer Verlag, Berlin, Germany, 1989, 3, p.1

36 Knable, M.B., Jones, D.W., Copola, R. *et al.* Lateralized Differences in Iodine-123-IBZM Uptake in Basal Ganglia in Asymmetric Parkinson's Disease. *J. Nucl. Med.* 1995, 36, 1216

37 Laulumaa, .V, Kuikka, J.T., Soininen, H. *et al.* Imaging of D_2 Dopamine Receptors of Patients With Parkinson's Disease Using Single Photon Emission Computed Tomography and Iodobenzamide I 123. *Arch. Neurol.* 1993, 50, 509

38 Nadeau, S.E., Couch, M.W., Devane, L. *et al.* Regional Analysis of D_2 Dopamine Receptors in Parkinson's Disease Using SPECT and Iodine-123-Iodobenzamide. *J. Nucl. Med.* 1995, 36, 384

39 Rutgers, A.W.F., Lakke, J.P.W.F., Paans, A.M.J. *et al.* Tracing of dopamine receptors in hemi-parkinsonism with positron emission tomography (PET). *J. Neurolog. Sci.* 1987, 80, 237

40 Antonini, A., Schwarz, J., Oertel, W.H. *et al.* [^{11}C]raclopride and positron emission tomography in previously untreated patients with Parkinson's disease: influence of L-DOPA and Iisuride therapy on striatal dopmaine D_2-receptors. *Neurology* 1994, 44, 1325

41 Schwarz, J., Tatsch, K., Arnold, G. *et al.* ^{123}I-iodobenzamide SPECT predicts dopaminergic responsiveness in patients with de novo parkinsonism. *Neurology* 1992, 41, 556

42 Tatsch, K., Schwarz, J., Oertel, W.H. *et al.* Dopamine D_2 receptor imaging with I-123 IBZM SPECT to differentiate idiopathic from other parkinson syndromes. *J. Nucl. Med.* 1992, 33, 917

43 Alexander, G.E. and Crutcher, M.D. Functional architecture of basal ganglia circuits: neural substrates for parallel processing. *Trends Neurosci.* 1990, 13, 266

44 Wichmann, T., Vick, J. and DeLong, M.R. Parkinson's Disease and the Basal Ganglia: Lessons from the Laboratory and from Neurosurgery. *The Neuroscientist* 1995, 1, 236

45 Carlsson, M. and Carlsson, A. Interactions between glutamatergic and monoaminergic systems within the basal ganglia - implications for schizophrenia and Parkinson's disease. *Trends Neurosci.* 1990, 13, 272

46 Crossman, A.R. Hypothesis on the Pathophysiological Mechanisms that Underlie Levodopa-or Dopamine Agonist-Induced Dyskinesia in Parkinson's Disease: Implications for Future Strategies in Treatment. *Movement Disorders* 1990, 5, 100

47 Crossman, A.R., Mitchell, I.J., Brotchie, J.M. *et al.* Excitatory Amino Acid Transmission of Subthalamic Nucleus Efferents: Relationship to Hyperkinetic Movement Disorders and to Parkinsonism in 'Excitatory Amino Acids', (Ed. RP Simon), Fidia Research Foundation Symposium Series, Thieme Medical Publishers, Inc., New York, 1992, volume 9, p.199

48 Greenamyre, J.T., Klockgether, T., Turski, L. *et al.* Glutamate Receptor Antagonism as a Novel Therapeutic Approach in Parkinson's Disease in 'Excitatory Amino Acids', (Ed. R.P. Simon), Fidia Research Foundation Symposium Series, Thieme Medical Publishers, Inc., New York, 1992, volume 9, p.195

49 Turski, L., Bressler, K., Rettig, K.J. *et al.* Protection of substantia nigra from MPP+ neurotoxicity by N-methyl-D-aspartate antagonists. *Nature* 1991, 349, 414

50 Fahn, S. Fetal-tissue transplants in Parkinson's disease. *N. Eng. J. Med.* 1992, 327, 1589

51 Freed, C.R., Breeze, R.E., Rosenberg, N.L. *et al.* Survival of implanted fetal dopamine cells and neurologic improvement 12 to 16 months after transplantation for Parkinson's disease. *N. Eng. J. Med.* 1992, 327, 1549

52 Lindvall, O. Prospects of transplantation in human neurodegenerative diseases. *Trends Neurosci.* 1991, 14, 376

53 Lindvall, H., Brundin, P., Widner, H. *et al.* Grafts of foetal dopamine neurons survive and improve motor function in Parkinson's disease. *Science* 1990, 247, 574

54 Lindvall, O., Widner, H., Rehcrona, S. *et al.* Transplantation of foetal dopamine neurons in Parkinson's disease - one year clinical and neurophysiological observations in two patients with putaminal implants. *Ann. Neurol.* 1992, 31, 155

55 Spencer, D.D., Robbins, R.J., Naftolin, F. *et al.* Unilateral transplantation of human fetal mesencephalic tissue into the caudate nucleus of patients with Parkinson's disease. *N. Eng. J. Med.* 1992, 327, 1541

56 Widner, H., Tetrud, J., Rechcrona, S. *et al.* Bilateral fetal mesencephalic grafting in two patients with parkinsonism induced by 1-methyl-4-pheynl-1,2,3,6-tetrahydropyridine (MPTP). *N. Eng. J. Med.* 1992, 327, 1556

57 Gary, D.J., Caplan, A.L., Vawter, D.E. *et al.* Sounding Board. Are there really alternatives to the use of foetal tissue from elective abortions in transplantation research? *N. Eng. J. Med.* 1992, 327, 1592

58 Hoffer, B.J. and Olson, L. Ethical issues in brain-cell transplantation. *Trends Neurosci.* 1991, 14, 384

59 Kassirer, J. and Angell, M. The use of foetal tissue in research on Parkinson's disease. *N. Eng. J. Med.* 1992, 237, 1591

60 Ahlskog, J.E., Richelson, E., Nelson, A. *et al.* Reduced D_2 Dopamine and Muscarinic Cholinergic Receptor Densities in Caudate Specimens from Fluctuating Parkinsonian Patients. *Ann. Neurol.* 1991, 30, 185

61 Graham, W.C., Clarke, C.E., Boyce, S. *et al.* Autoradiographic studies in animal models of hemi-parkinsonism reveal dopamine D_2 but not D_1 receptor supersensitivity. II. Unilateral intra-carotid infusion of MPTP in the monkey (Macaca fasicularis). *Brain Research* 1990, 514, 103

62 Leenders, K.L., Aquilonius, S.M., Bergström, K. *et al.* Unilateral MPTP lesion in a rhesus monkey: effects on the striatal dopaminergic system measured in vivo with PET using various novel tracers. *Brain Research* 1988, 445, 61

63 Chiueh, C.C. Dopamine in the Extrapyramidal Motor Function. A study based upon the MPTP-Induced Primate Model of Parkinsonism in 'Central Determinants of Aged-related Declines in Motor Function', (Ed. J.A. Joseph), Ann. NY. Acad. Sci., New York, USA, 1988, 515, 226

64 Vermeulen, R.J., Drukarch, B., Verhoeff, N.P.L.G. *et al.* No Direct Correlation Between Behaviourally Active Doses of the Dopamine D_2 Agonist LY 17155 and Displacement of [^{123}I]IBZM as Measured with SPECT in MPTP Monkeys. *Synapse* 1994, 17, 115

65 Innis, R.B., Malison, R.T. *et al.* Amphetamine-Stimulated Dopamine Release Competes In Vivo for [^{123}IBZM Binding to the D_2 Receptor in Non-human primates. *Synapse* 1992, 10, 177

66 Laruelle, M., Abi-Dargham, A., van Dyck, C.H. *et al.* SPECT imaging of Striatal Dopamine Release after Amphetamine Challenge. *J. Nucl. Med.* 1995, 36, 1182

67 Kessler, R.M., Ansari, M.S., De Paulis, T. *et al.* High Affinity Dopamine D_2 Receptor Radioligands. 1. Regional Rat Brain Distribution of Iodinated Benzamides. *J. Nucl. Med.* 1991, 32, 1593

68 Votaw, J.R., Ansari, M.S., Mason, N.S. *et al.* Dosimetry of Iodine-123-Epidepride: A Dopamine D_2 Receptor Ligand. *J. Nucl. Med.* 1995, 36, 1316

69 Hall, H., Farde, L. and Sedvall, G. Human dopamine receptor subtypes - in vitro binding analysis using ^{3}H-SCH 23390 and ^{3}H-raclopride. *J. Neurol. Trans.* 1988, 73, 7

70 Buck, A., Westera, G., Sutter, M. *et al.* Iodine-123-IBF SPECT Evaluation of Extrapyramidal Diseases. *J. Nucl. Med.* 1995, 36, 1196

71 Kebabian, J.W., Agui, T., van Oene, J.C. *et al.* The D_1 dopamine receptor: new perspectives. *Trends Pharmacol. Sci.* 1996, 7, 96

72 Shinotoh, H., Inoue, O., Suzuki, K. *et al.* Dopamine D_1 and D_2 receptor imaging in Parkinson's disease and striato-nigral degeneration by PET. *J. Nucl. Med.* 1992, 33, 917

73 Friedman, E. and Neumeyer, J.L. Neurochemicals for the Neuroscientist. RBI Catalog/Handbook. Research Biochemicals Incorporated, Natick, MA, USA, 1992, 60

74 Verhoeff, N.P.L.G., Bekier, A., Beer, H.F. *et al.* ^{123}I-SCH 23982 is not suitable for dopamine D_1 receptor imaging in vivo in the human brain. *Nucl. Med. Commun.* 1193, 14, 137

75 Chumpradit, S., Billings, J., Kung, J. *et al.* An improved CNS D-1 dopamine receptor imaging ligand:[I-123](+-) FISCH. *J. Nucl. Med.* 1989, 30, 803

76 Chumpradit, S., Billings, J., Kung, J. R(+) and S(-)TISCH: new CNS D-1 dopamine receptor ligands. *J. Nucl. Med.* 1990, 31, 899

77 Chumpradit, S., Billings, J. and Kung, J. *et al.* Synthesis and Resolution of (±)-7-Chloro-8-hydroxy-1-(3'-iodophenyl)-3-methyl-2,3,4,5-tetrahydro-1H-3-benzazepine (TISCH): A High Affinity and Selective iodinated Ligand for CNS D₁ Dopamine Receptor. *J. Med. Chem.* 1991, 34, 877

78 Billings, J., Kung, M.P., Chumpradit, S. *et al.* Characterisation of a new CNS D-I dopamine receptor imaging ligand: [I-123](±)FISCH. *J. Nucl. Med.* 1989, 30, 830

79 Kung, H.F., Kung, M.P., Billings, J. *et al.* In vivo study of I-123 TISCH: a new D₁ dopamine receptor imaging agent. *J. Nucl. Med.* 1991, 32, 1069

80 DeNinno, M.P., Schoenleber, R., Perner, R.J. *et al.* Synthesis and Dopaminergic Activity of 3-Substituted 1-(Aminomethyl)-3,4-dihydro-5,6-dihydroxy-1H-2-benzopyrans: Characterization of an Auxiliary Binding Region in the D₁ Receptor. *J. Med. Chem.* 1991, 34, 2561

81 Halldin, C., Farde, L., Barnett, A. *et al.* Synthesis of [C]SCH 39166, a new selective D-I dopamine receptor ligand for PET in Eckelman W.C., Ksenia, D., Kucynski, B. *et al.* Eighth International Symposium of Radiopharmaceutical Chemistry Princeton University, Princeton, New Jersey, USA, 1990, p.357

82 Seeman, P., Bzowej, N.J., Guan, H.C. *et al.* Human brain dopamine receptors in children and ageing adults. *Synapse* 1987, 1, 399

83 Rinne, J.O. Muscarinic and dopaminergic receptors in the ageing human brain. *Brain Res.* 1987, 404, 162

84 Suhara, T., Fukuda, H., Inouse, O. *et al.* Age-related changes in human D₁ dopamine receptors measured by positron emission tomography. *Psychopharmacology* 1991, 103, 41

85 Fuller, R.W. Biogenic Amine Transporters. *Neurotransmissions* 1993, IX(2), 1

86 Uhl, G.R. Neurotransmitter transporters (plus): a promising new gene family. *Trends Neurosci.* 1992, 15, 265

87 Uhl, G.R. and Hartig, P.R. Transporter explosion: update on uptake. *Trends Pharmacol. Sci.* 1992, 13, 421

88 Hirai, M., Kitamura, N., Hashumoto, T. *et al.* [³H]GBR-12935 binding sites in human striatal membrane: binding characteristics and changes in parkinsonians and schizophrenics. *Jpn. J. Pharmacol.* 1988, 47, 237

89 Janowsky, A., Vocci, F., Berger, P. *et al.* [³H]GBR-12935 binding to the dopamine transporter is decreased in the caudate nucleus in Parkinson's disease. *J. Neurochem.* 1987, 49, 617

90 Kaufman, M.J. and Madras, B.K. Severe depletion of cocaine recognition sites associated with the dopamine transporter in Parkinson's diseased striatum. *Synapse* 1991, 9, 43

91 Maloteaux, J.M., Vanisberg, M.A., Laterre, C. *et al.* [³H]GBR-12935 binding to dopamine uptake sites: subcellular localization and reduction in Parkinson's disease and progressive supranuclear palsy. *Eur. J. Pharmacol.* 1988, 156, 133

92 Hornykiewicz, O. Imbalance of brain monoamines and clinical disorders. *Prog. Brain Res.* 1982, 55, 419

93 Robinson, T.E. and Whislaw, I.Q. Normalization of extracellular dopamine in striatum following recovery from a partial unilateral 6-OHDA lesion of the substantia nigra: a microdialysis study in freely moving rats. *Brain Res.* 1988, 450, 209

94 Zigmond, M.J., Abercrombie, E.D. and Stricker, E.M. Partial damage to nigrostriatal bundle: compensatory changes and the action of L-DOPA. *J. Neural. Transm.* 1990, 29, 217

95 Elizan, T.S., Yahr, M.D., Moros, D.A. *et al.* Selegiline Use to Prevent Progression of Parkinson's Disease. Experience in 22 De Novo Patients. *Arch. Neurol.* 1989, 46, 1275

96 Elizan, T.S., Yahr, M.D., Moros, D.A. *et al.* Selegiline as an Adjunct to Conventional Levodopa Therapy in Parkinson's Disease: Experience With This Type B Monoamine Oxidase Inhibitor in 200 Patients. *Arch. Neurol.* 1989, 46, 1280

97 The Parkinson Study Group. Effect of deprenyl on the progression of disability in early Parkinson's disease. *N. Eng. J. Med.* 1989, 321, 1364

98 Ellenberg, J.H. Preclinical detection in studies of the etiology, natural history, and treatment of Parkinson's disease. *Neurology* 1991, 41, 14

99 Langston, J.W. and Koller, W.C. The next frontier in Parkinson's disease: Presymptomatic detection. *Neurology* 1991, 41, 5

100 Cools, A.R. Role of Neostriatal and Mesostriatal or Meslimbic Dopaminergic Fibres in Parkinson's Disease with and without Dementia: Prospects, Concepts and Facts. *Jpn J. Psychopharmacol.* 1990, 10, 15

101 Sawle, G.V., Bloomfield, P.M., Björklund, A. *et al.* Transplantation of Fetal Dopamine Neurons in Parkinson's Disease: PET [¹⁸F]6-L-Fluorodopa Studies in Two Patients with Putaminal Implants. *Ann. Neurol.* 1992, 31, 166

102 Mazière, B., Coenen, H.H., Haldin, C. *et al.* PET Radiologands for Dopamine Receptors and Re-uptake Sites: Chemistry and Biochemistry. *Nucl. Med. Biol.* 1992, 497

103 Fowler, J.S., Volkow, N.D., Wolf, A.P. *et al.* Mapping cocaine binding sites in human and baboon in vivo. *Synapse* 1989, 4, 371

104 Kilbourn, M.R., Carey, J.E., Koeppe, R.A. *et al.* Biodistribution, Dosimetry, Metabolism and monkey PET Studies of [¹⁸F]GBR 13119. Imaging the Dopamine Uptake System In Vivo. *Nucl. Med. Biol.* 1989, 16, 569

105 Kilbourn, M.R., Mulholland, G.K., Sherman, P.S. *et al.* In vivo binding of the dopamine uptake inhibitor (using) [F]-GBR 13119 in MPTP-treated C57BL/6 mice. *Nucl. Med. Biol.* 1991, 18, 803

106 Hantraye, P., Brownell, A.L., Elmalch, D. *et al.* Dopamine fober detection by [¹¹C]-CFT and PET in a primate model of parkinsonism. *NeuroReport* 1992, 3, 265

107 Kaufman, M.J. and Madras, B.K. Distribution of Cocaine Recognition Sites in Monkey Brain: II. Ex Vivo Autoradiography With [³H]CFT and [¹²⁵I]RTI-55. *Synapse* 1992, 12, 99

108 Scheffel, U., Boja, J.W. and Kuhar, M.J. Cocaine receptors: in vivo labelling with ^{3}H-(-)cocaine, ^{3}H-WIN 35,065-2, and ^{3}H-WIN 35, 428. *Synapse* 1989, 4, 390

109 Ponchant, M., Crouzel, C., Kamenka, J.M. *et al.* [^{18}F]-3-fluoromethyl-N[2-benzothienyl)-cyclohexyl]-piperidine, a potent radioligand for the dopamine re-uptake complex. Abstracts IXth Int.Symp.Radiopharm.Chem. Paris. 1992, p. 255

110 Tedroff, J., Aquilonius, S.M., Laihinen, A. *et al.* Striatal kinetics of [^{11}C]-(+)-nomifensine and 6-[^{18}F]fluoro-L-DOPA in Parkinson's disease measured with Positron Emission Tomography. *Acta Neurol. Scand.* 1990, 81, 24

111 Salmon, E.P., Brooks, D.J., Mathias, C.J. *et al.* Studies on the integrity of the dopamine system in Shy-Dräger syndrome and pure autonomic failure using ^{11}C-nomifensine and PET. *Neurology* 1989, 39(1), 204

112 Scherman, D., Desnos, C., Darchen, F. *et al.* Striatal Dopamine Deficiency in Parkinson's Disease: Role of Ageing. *Ann. Neurol.* 1989, 26, 551

113 Jankovic, J. The neurology of tics in 'Movement Disorders', (Eds. C.D. Marsden, S. Fahn), Butterworth & Co. (Publishers) Ltd, London, UK, 1987, p. 383

114 Dasilva, J.N., Kilbourn, M.R., Mangner, T.J. *et al.* Synthesis of [^{11}C]-Tetrabenazine and a [^{11}C]methoxy derivative of a-Dihydrotetrabenazine for PET-imaging of monoaminergic nerve terminals. Abstracts IXth Int.Symp.Radiopharm. Chem. Paris, France, 1992, p.257

115 Murrin, L.C., Enna, S.J., Kuhar, M.J. Autoradiographic localisation of [^{3}H]reserpine binding sites in rat brain. *J. Pharmacol. Exp. Ther.* 1977, 203, 564

116 Dejesus, O.T., Murali, D. *et al.* Sythesis of [F-18-]-labelled a-fluoromethyl-p-tyrosine. A tyrosine hydroxylase-activated decarboxylase suicide inhibitor with potential as imaging agent for dopmine for nerve terminals. Abstracts IXth Int.Symp.Radiopharm.Chem. Paris, France, 1992, p.260

117 Innis, R.B. SPECT Imaging of Dopamine Terminal Innervation: Potential Clinical Tool in Parkinson's disease. *Eur. J. Nucl. Med.* 1994, 21, 1

118 Galinier, E., Garreau, L., Frangin, Y. *et al.* Synthesis of halogenated analogues of 5-94-chlofephenyl)-2,3-dihydro-5-hydroxy-5H-imadaxo(2,1-a)isoindole or mazindol as new dopamine uptake carrier ligands. Abstracts IXth Int.Symp.Radiopharm.Chem.Paris. 1992, p. 217

119 Basmadjian, G.P., Mills, S.L., Kanvinde, M. *et al.* Radioiodinated tropeines: search for a molecular probe for the characterization of the cocaine receptor. *J. Nucl. Med.* 1990, 3, 899

120 Cooper, J.R., Bloom, F.E., Roth, R.H. *et al.* in 'The Biochemical Basis of Neuropharmacology', Oxford University Press, New York, 7th Edition, 1996

121 van der Zee, P., Koger, H.S., Gootjes, J. *et al.* Aryl 1,4-dialk(en)piperazines as selective and very potent inhibitors of dopmaine uptake. *Eur. J. Med. Chem.* 1980, 15, 363

122 Foulon, C., Garreau, L., Chalon, S. *et al.* Synthesis and in vitro binding properties of halogenated analogues of GBR as new dopamine uptake carrier ligands. *Nucl. Med. Biol.* 1992, 19, 597

123 Grigoriadis, D.E., Wilson, A.A. *et al.* Dopamine transport sites labelled by a novel photoaffinity probe: ^{125}I-DEEP. *J. Neurosci.* 1989, 9, 2664

124 Hanson, R., Byon, C., Matsushita, F. *et al.* Radiosynthesis of (I-125) N-iodoallyl nor GBR 12935. Abstracts IXth Int.Symp.Rad.Pharm.Chem. Paris, France, 1992, p. 246

125 Boja, J.W., Patel, A., Carrol, F.I. *et al.* [^{125}I]-RTI-55: A potent ligand for dopamine transporters. *Eur. J. Pharmacol.* 1994, 194, 133

126 Neumeyer, J.L., Wang, S., Millius, R.A. *et al.* [^{123}I]-2ß-Carbomethoxy-3ß-(4-iodophenyl)tropane: High-Affinity SPECT Radiotracer of Monoamine Reuptake Sites in Brain. *J. Med. Chem.* 1991, 34, 3144

127 Carrol, F.L., Lewis, A.H., Boja, J.W. *et al.* Cocaine receptor: Biochemical characterization and structure-activity relationships of cocaine analogues at the dopamine transporter. *J. Med. Chem.* 1992, 35, 969

128 Laruelle, M., Giddings, S.S., Zea-Ponce, Y. *et al.* Methyl 3ß-(4-[^{125}I]Iodophenyl)Tropane-2ß-Carboxylate In Vitro Binding to Dopamine and Serotonin Transporters Under "Physiological" Conditions. *J. Neurochem.* 1994, 62, 978

129 Shaya, E.K., Scheffel, U., Dannals, R.F. *et al.* In Vivo Imaging of Dopamine reuptake Sites in the Primate Brain Using Single Photon Emission Computed Tomography (SPECT) and Iodine-123 Labelled RTI-55. *Synapse* 1992, 10, 169

130 Scheffel, U., Dannals, R.F., Cline, E.J. *et al.* [$^{123/125}$I]RTI-55, an In Vivo Label for the Serotonin Transporter. *Synapse* 1992, 11, 134

131 Baldwin, R.M., Zea-Ponce, Y., Zoghbi, S.S. *et al.* Evaluation of the Monoamine Uptake Site Ligand [^{123}I]Methyl 3ß-(4-Iodophenyl)tropane-2ß-carboxylate([^{123}I]ß-CIT) in Non-human Primates: Pharmacokinetics, Biodistribution, and SPECT Brain imaging Coregistered with MRI. *Nucl. Med. Biol.* 1993, 20, 597

132 Halldin, C., Farde, L., Müller, L. *et al.* Preparation of (^{11}C)ß-CIT, a new ligand for imaging cocaine binding sites by PET. *Eur. J. Nucl. Med.* 1992, 19, 592

133 Laruelle, M., Baldwin, R.M., Zea-Ponce, Y. *et al.* SPECT imagin of monoamine transporter sites with ^{123}I-CIT in non-human primates brain. *J. Nucl. Med.* 1992, 33, 945

134 Laruelle, M., Baldwin, R.M., Madison, R.T. *et al.* SPECT imaging of Dopamine and Serotonin Transporters with [123]ß-CIT: Pharmacological Characterisation of Brain Uptake in Non-human Primates. *Synapse* 1993, 13, 295

135 Scanley, B.E., Baldwin, R.M., Laruelle, M. *et al.* Active and Inactive Enantiomers of 2ß-Carbomethoxy-3ß-(4-iodophenyl)tropane: Comparisons Using Homogenate Binding and Single Photon Emission Computed Tomographic Imaging. *Mol. Pharmacol.* 1994, 45, 136

136 Seibyl, J.P., Wallace, E., Smith, E.O. *et al.* Whole-Body Biodistribution, Radiation, Absorbed Dose and Brain SPECT Imaging with Iodine-123-ß-CIT in Healthy Human Subjects. *J. Nucl. Med.* 1994, 35, 764

137 Scanley, B.E., Al-Tikriti, M.S., Gandelman, M.S. *et al.* Comparison of [^{123}I]ß-CIT and [^{123}I]IPCIT as single-photon emission tomography radiotracers for the dopamine transporter in non-human primates. *Eur. J. Nucl. Med.* 1995, 22, 4

138 Bergström, K.A., Halldin, C., Kuikka, J.T. *et al.* Lipophilic metabolite of [123I]ß-CIT in human plasma may obstruct quantification of the dopamine transporter. *Synapse* 1995, 19, 297

139 Sackett, D.L., Haynes, R.B. and Tugwell, P. in 'Clinical Epidemiology. A basic science for clinical medicine', Little Brown and Company, Toronto, Canada, 1985

140 Zea-Ponce, Y., Baldwin, R.M., Laruelle, M. *et al.* Simplified Multidose Preparation of Iodine-123-ß-CIT: A marker for Dopamine Transporters. *J. Nucl. Med.* 1995, 36, 525

141 United States General Services Administration. Code of Federal Regulations. Chapter 21, Part 361. Prescription drugs for humans generally recognized as safe and effetive and not misbranded: drugs used in research. US Government Printing Office, Washington DC, USA, 1992, p.221

142 Laruelle, M., Wallace, E., Seibyl, J.P. *et al.* Graphical, Kinetic and Equilibrium Analyses of In Vivo [^{123}I]ß-CIT Binding to Dopamine Transporters in Healthy Human Subjects. *J. Cereb. Blood Flow Metab.* 1994, 14, 982

143 van Dyck, C.H., Seibyl, J.P., Malison, R.T. *et al.* Age-Related Decline in Dopamine Transporter Binding in Humane Striatum with [^{123}I]ß-CIT SPECT. *J. Nucl. Med.* 1995, 36, 1175

144 Seibyl, J.P., Laruelle, M., Van Dyck, C.H. *et al.* Reproducibility of [^{123}I]ß-CIT SPECT brain measurement of dopamine transporters in healthy human subjects. *J. Nucl. Med.* 1996, 37, 222

145 Innis, R.B., Seibyl, J.P., Scanley, B.E. *et al.* Single photon emission computed tomographic imaging demonstrates loss of striatal dopamine transporters in parkinson disease. *Proc. Natl. Acad. Sci. USA* 1993, 90, 11965

146 Kish, S.J., Shannak, K. and Hornykiewics, O. Uneven pattern of dopamine loss in the striatum of patients with idiopathic Parkinson's disease. *N. Eng. J. Med.* 1988, 318, 876

147 Brücke, T., Kornhuber, J., Angelberger, P. *et al.* SPECT imaging of dopamine and serotinin transporters with [^{123}I]ß-CIT. Binding kinetics in human brain. *J. Neural Transm. [Gen.Sect.]* 1993, 94, 137

148 Seibyl, J.P., Marek, K.L., Quinlan, D. *et al.* Decreased SPECT [^{123}I]ß-CIT striatal uptake correlates with symptom severity in idiopathic Parkinson's disease. *Ann. Neurol.* 1995, 38, 589

149 Laihinen, A.O., Rinne, J.O., Nagren, K.A. *et al.* PET studies on Brain Monoamine Transporters with Carbon I1-ß-CIT in Parkinson's Disease. *J. Nucl. Med.* 1995, 36, 1263

150 Marek, K.L., Seibyl, J.P., Zoghbi, S.S. *et al.* ^{123}I-beta-CIT SPECT imaging demonstrates bilateral loss of dopamine transporters in hemi-Parkinson's disease. *Neurology* 1995, in press

151 Brooks, D.J. Functional imaging in relation to parkinsonian sydromes. *J. Neurol. Sci.* 1993, 115, 1

152 Brooks, D.J., Ibanez, V., Sawle, G.V. *et al.* Differing patterns of striatal ^{18}F-DOPA uptake in Parkinson's disease, multiple system atrophy and progressive supranuclear palsy. *Ann. Neurol.* 1990, 28, 547

153 Sawle, G.V. Nuclear medicine and the management of patients with Parkinson's movement disorders in 'Nuclear Medicine in Clinical Diagnosis and Treatment', (Eds. IPC Murray, PJEll), Churchill Livingstone, London, UK, 1994, p. 589

154 Churchyard, A., Donnan, G.A., Hughes, A. *et al.* G-DOPA resistance in multiple-system atrophy: loss of postsynaptic D_2 receptors. *Ann. Neurol.* 1993, 34, 219

155 Schulz, J.B., Klockgether, T., Peterson, D. *et al.* Multiple system atrophy: natural history, MRI, morphology and dopamine receptor imaging with ^{123}I-IBZM-SPECT. *J. Neurol. Neurosurg. Psychiatry* 1994, 57, 1047

156 Fearnley, J.M. and Lees. A.J. Striatonigral degeneration: a clinico-pathological study. *Brain* 1990, 113, 1823

157 Spokes, E.G.S., Bannister, R. and Oppenheimer, D.R. Multiple system atrophy with autonomic failure. Clinical, histological and neurochemical observations on four cases. *J. Neurol. Sci.* 1979, 43, 50

158 Vermeulen, R.J., Wolters, E.Ch., Tissingh, G. *et al.* ^{123}I-beta-CIT binding with SPECT in controls, early and late Parkinson's disease. *Nucl. Med. Biol.* 1995, 22, 985

159 De Keyser, J.D., Ebinger, G. and Vauquelin, G. Age-related changes in the human nigrostriatal dopaminergic system. *Ann. Neurol.* 1990, 27, 157

160 Zelnik, N., Angel, I., Paul, S.M. *et al.* Decreased density of human striatal dopamine uptake sites with age. *Eur. J. Pharmacol.* 1986, 126, 175

161 Sawle, G.V., Wroe, S.J., Lees, A.J. *et al.* The Identification of presymptomatic Parkinsonism: Clinical and [^{18}F]DOPA Positron Emission Tomography Studies in an Irish Kindred. *Ann. Neurol.* 1992, 32, 609

162 Kilbourn, M.R., Shades of Grey: Radiopharmaceutical Chemistry in the 1990s and Beyond. *Nucl. Med. Biol.* 1992, 19, 603

163 Boja, J.W., McNeill, R.M., Lewin, A.H. *et al.* Selective dopamine transporter inhibition by cocaine analogs. *Neuroreport* 1992, 3, 984

164 Al-Tikriti, M.S., Zea-Ponce, Y., Baldwin, R.M. *et al.* Characterization of the Dopamine Transporter in Non-human Primate Brain: Homogenate Binding, Whole Body Imaging and Ex Vivo Autoradiography Using [^{125}I] and [^{123}I]IPCIT. *Nucl. Med. Biol.* 1995, 22, 649

165 Neumeyer, J.L., Wang, S., Gao, Y. *et al.* N-omega-Fluoroalkyl Analogs of (1R)-2ß-Carbomethoxy-3ß (4-iodphenyl)tropane (ß-CIT): Radiotracers for Positron Emission Tomography and Single Photon Emission Computed Tomography Imaging of Dopamine Transporters. *J. Med. Chem.* 1994, 37, 1558

166 Abi-Dargham, A., Gandelman, M.S., DeErasquin, G.A. *et al.* Single Photon Emission Computed Tomographic Imaging of Dopamine Transporters In Human Brain With [123]N-omega-Fluoroalkyl-2ß-Carbyomethoxy-3ß-(4-Iodophenyl) Nortropanes. *J. Nucl. Med.* 1996, 37, 1129

167 Baldwin, R.M., Zea-Ponce, Y., Al-Tikriti, M.S. *et al.* Regional Brain Uptake and Pharmacokinetics of [123I]N-omega-Fluoralkyl-2ß-carboxy-3ß-(4-iodophanyl) nortropane Esters in Baboons. *Nucl. Med. Biol.* 1995, 22, 211

168 Kuikka, J.T., Bergström K.A., Ahonen, A. *et al.* Comparison of iodine-123 labelled 2ß-carbomethoxy-3ß-(-4 iodophenyl)tropane and 2ß-carbomethoxy-3ß-(4 iodophenyl)-N-(3-fluoropropyl)nortropane for imaging of the dopamine transporter in the living human brain. *Eur. J. Nucl. Med.* 1995, 22, 356

169 Burn, D.J., Mathias, C.J., Quinn, N. *et al.* Striatal opiate receptor binding in Parkinson's disease and multiple system atrophy: ^{11}C-diprenorphine study. *Neurology* 1992, 43, S454

170 Murrin, L.C., Coyle, J.T. and Kuhar, M.J. Striatal opiate receptors: pre- and postsynaptic localization. *Life Sci.* 1980, 27, 1175

171 Mansour, A., Fox, C.A., Thompson, R.C. *et al.* Mu-Opioid receptor mRNA expression in the rat CNS: comparison to mu-receptor binding. *Brain Res.* 1994, 643, 245

172 Pollard, H., Llorens, C., Schwarz, J.C. *et al.* Localization of opiate receptors and enkephalins in the rat striatum in relationship with the nigrostriatal dopaminergic system: lesion studies. *Brain Res.* 1978, 151, 392

173 Bodnar, R.J., Clark, J.A., Cooper, M.L. *et al.* Loss of striatal mu1 opiate binding by substantia nigra lesions in the rat. *Life Sci.* 1988, 43, 1697

174 Trovero, F., Herve, D., Desban, M. *et al.* Striatal opiate mu-receptors are not located on dopamine nerve endings in the rat. *Neuroscience* 1990, 39, 313

175 Eghbali, M., Santoro, C., Parades, W. *et al.* Visualisation of multiple opioid-receptor types in rat striatum after specific mesencephalic lesions. *Proc. Acad. Sci. USA* 1987, 84, 6582

176 Lever, J.R., Scheffel, U., Kinter, C.M. *et al.* In vivo binding of NI'-9[11C]methyl)naltrindole to delta-opioid receptors in mouse brain. *Eur. J. Pharmacol.* 1992, 216, 459

177 Kawai, R., Channing, M.A., Rice, K.L. *et al.* Opiate receptor subtype discrimination in vivo using cylofoxy and the site-specific alkylation agent beta-FNA. *J. Cereb. Blood Flow Metab.* 1991, 11(2), S872

178 Wilson, A.A., Sheffel, U., Stathis, M. *et al.* Synthesis and biodistribution of two I-125 labelled sigma receptor ligands. *J. Nucl. Med.* 1990, 31, 797

179 Weinberger, D.R., Gibson, R., Coppola, R. *et al.* The Distribution of Cerebral Muscarinic Acetylcholine Receptors In Vivo in Patients With Dementia. *Arch. Neurol.* 1991, 48, 169

180 Müller-Gärtner, H.W., Wilson, A.A., Dannals, R.F. *et al.* Imaging Muscarinic Cholinergic Receptors in Human Brain In Vivo with SPECT. [123I]4-Iododexetimide, and [123I]4-Iodolevetimide. *J. Cereb. Blood Flow Metab.* 1992, 12, 562

181 Smith, A.D. and Bolam, J.P. The neural network of the basal ganglia as revealed by the study of synaptic connections of identified neurones. *Trends Neurosci.* 1990, 13, 259

182 Groenewegen, H.J., Berendse, H.W., Meredith, G.E. *et al.* Functional Anatomy of the Ventral, Limbic System-Innervated Striatum in 'The Mesolimbic Dopamine: from motivation to action', (Eds. P. Willner, Scheel-Krüger), John Wiley & Sons Ltd, London, UK, 1991, p. 19

183 Ruberg, M., Javoy-Agid, F., Hirsch, E. *et al.* Dopaminergic and cholinergic lesions in progressive supranuclear palsy. *Annals of Neurology* 1987, 18, 523

184 Juncos, J.L., Hirsch, E.C., Malessa, S. *et al.* Mesencephalic cholinergic nuclei in progressive supranuclear palsy. *Neurology* 1991, 41, 25

185 Calne, D.B. Parkinsonism - physiology and pharmacology. *Br. Med. J.* 1971, 3, 693

186 Wieland, D.M., Kilbourn, M.R., Yang, D.J. *et al.* NMDA Receptor Channels: Labelling of MK-801 with Iodine-125 and Fluorine-18. *Appl. Radoat. Isot.* 1988, 39, 1219

187 Bergman, H., Wichmann, T. and DeLong, M.R. Reversal of Experimental Parkinsonism by Lesions of the Subthalamic Nucleus. *Science* 1990, 249, 1436

188 Kish, S.J., Robitaille, Y., El-Awar, M. *et al.* Striatal monoamine neutrotransmitters and metabolites in dominantly inherited olivopontocerebellar atrophy. *Neurology* 1992, 42, 1573

189 Kish, S.J., Robitaille, Y, El-Awar, M *et al.* Brain amino acid reductions in one family with chromosome 6p linked dominantly inherited olivopontocerebellar atrophy. *Ann. Neurol.* 1991, 30, 780

190 Gerlach, M., Riederer, P., Youdim, M.B.H. The pharmacology of L-deprenyl. *Eur. J. Pharmacol-Mol. Parmacol. Sect.* 1992, 226, 97

191 Verhoeff, N.P.L.G., Kapucu, O., Sokole-Busemann, E. *et al.* Quantification of dopamine D_2 receptor binding potential in the striatum with ^{123}I-IBZM SPECT: technical and inter-observer variability. *J. Nucl. Med.* 1993, 34, 2076

192 Matsui, T., and Hirano A. in 'An atlas of the human brain for computerized tomography', Gustave Fisher Verlag, Stuttgart, Germany, 1978

193 Farde, L., Von Bahr, C. Distribution of remoxipride to the human brain and central D_2-dopamine receptor binding examined *in vivo* by PET. *Acta Psychiatr. Scand.* 1990, 82, 67

Appendix: Methods of ^{123}I-CIT and ^{123}I-CIT-FP SPECT studies

SPECT Camera. In all SPECT studies a brain-dedicated SPECT system, Strichman Medical Equipment 810X was used. The energy level was set at 135-190 keV. Data acquisition took place in a 128-128 matrix. The images were reconstructed with a variable filter, according to the level of counts per slice. The measured concentration of radioactivity was expressed as Strichman Medical Units (SMUs): 1 SMU = 1 Bq/ml as specificied by Strichman Medical Equipment Inc.

SPECT studies. Prior to all experiments, humans and monkeys received potassium iodide orally in order to prevent thyroid uptake of free radioactive iodine. PD and MSA patients were asked to stop deprenyl (selegeline) one week prior to the experiment, since this compound is metabolised into L-amphetamine, which might compete for the dopamine transporter[190]. L-DOPA therapy was continued, since Laruelle *et al.*[133] showed that acute administration of a large dose of L-DOPA (50 mg/kg iv) had no influence on specific CIT binding.

Twenty-four hours following injection of ^{123}I-CIT, 12 slices or less, starting at and parallel to the canthomeatal line were acquired for 300 s, with an interslice distance of 10 mm. For ^{123}I-CIT-FP the acquisition of data started 3 h following injection. Twelve slices or less starting at and parallel to the canthomeatal line were acquired for 300 s in the human studies, and for 150 s in the monkey studies.

For SPECT scanning, the monkeys were anaesthesised via an intramuscular injection of a mixture of ketamine-HCI (0.1 mg/kg), acepromazine maleate (0.02 mg/kg) and atropine sulphate (0.05 mg/kg). Anaesthesia was maintained with hourly injections of ketamine (0.1 mg/kg i.m.). During scanning, the heads of both monkeys and humans were fixed with bandage.

Calculation of data. Regions of interest (RIOs) for striatum were defined in control monkeys on the basis of the 60% isocontour line, as validated in previous phantom studies with the SME 810 SPECT camera[191]. ROIs of the occipital cortex were manually defined as described previously[64]. All data were decay-corrected to the time of injection of radioactivity.

For human analysis of caudate nucleus and putamen ^{123}I-CIT binding and ^{123}I-CIT-FP binding, the slice with the highest activity was selected and standard regions of interest, according to the stereoatactic atlas of Matsui and Hirano[192] were applied. In all the experiments a quantification protocol was used[193], in order to estimate the specific striatal ^{123}I-CIT or ^{123}I-CIT-FP binding potential.

^{123}I-CIT or ^{123}I-CIT-FP binding potential = (ROI-OCC)/OCC.

SPECT in Neurology and Psychiatry, edited by P.P. De Deyn, R.A. Dierckx, A. Alavi and B.A. Pickut
© 1997 John Libbey & Company Ltd, pp. 167–179

Clinical Significance of Dopamine D$_2$-Receptor Imaging with ^{123}I-Iodobenzamide SPECT in Patients with Parkinsonian Syndromes

Chapter
21

N.P.L.G. Verhoeff, J.D. Speelman[°], M.A. Kuiper[*],
E.A. van Royen[°], Ö. Kapucu[°], G.J. Boer[**], A.G.M. Janssen[†]
and E. Ch. Wolters[*]

Introduction

The parkinsonian syndrome consists of tremor, rigidity, hypokinesia and postural abnormalities. The major cause of this syndrome is idiopathic Parkinson's disease (IPD), which accounts for approximately 60-85% of all cases[1]. A clinical hallmark of IPD is its responsiveness to dopaminergic medication[2].

However, other causes of the parkinsonian syndrome exist that fail to respond to dopaminergic medication. Multiple system atrophy (MSA) and progressive supranuclear palsy (PSP) may account for up to 15% of all patients with parkinsonian signs[3,4]. Depending on its main manifestations, MSA includes syndromes such as striatonigral degeneration with predominantly extrapyramidal signs, Shy-Dräger syndrome with mainly autonomic symptomatology, and olivopontocerebellar atrophy with predominantly cerebellar dysfunction[4]. In PSP, which is neuropathologically distinct from MSA, the clinical characteristic is paralysis of vertical gaze[3].

Differential diagnosis between MSA and PSP on the one hand and IPD on the other is considered important because of the differences in prognosis and therapy[3,4], but a clinical distinction between IPD and MSA or PSP is sometimes hard to achieve[1]. X-ray transmission CT or MRI can to some extent contribute to such differential diagnosis.

Atrophy of the putamen[5], cerebellar atrophy[6], and atrophy of the brainstem[7] have been reported in some cases of MSA. The apomorphine test has been used to predict dopaminergic responsiveness in parkinsonian syndromes[8].

However, inconsistencies have been observed[9], and functional imaging of striatal dopamine D$_2$-receptors *in vivo* may be promising in this respect. Little or no response to L-DOPA treatment has previously been coupled to a decreased striatal D$_2$-receptor density post mortem[10]. Indeed, a severe reduction in striatal D$_2$-receptor binding potential was demonstrated *in vivo* using ^{11}C-raclopride or ^{76}Br-bromospiperone and positron emission tomography (PET) in IPD patients with a fluctuating response to L-DOPA and in patients with MSA or PSP[11]. Unfortunately, PET is not suitable for use in larger clinical studies because of its costs and limited availability. Single photon emission computerised tomography (SPECT) is less expensive and more readily available.

University School of Medicine, New Haven, and Veterans Affairs Medical Center, West Haven, USA
°Departments of Nuclear Medicine and Neurology, Academic Medical Centre, Amsterdam Zuidoost, The Netherlands
*Free University Hospital, Amsterdam
**Netherlands Institute for Brain Research, Amsterdam
†Cygne b.v., Technical University, Eindhoven

Table 1 Individual data from the 42 patients with parkinsonian syndrome. Gender, age, outcome of ^{123}I IBZM SPECT and Columbia Scale, and findings with CT and/or MRI are presented

Patient no.	Group[a]	Sex (M1,F2)	Age (yrs)	Duration (yrs)	IBZM SPECT ST/OC	ST L/R	Columbia Scale Total	Axial	Extremities	CT and/or MRI Study	Findings. NP=No anatomical imaging performed because of lack of clinical indication
1	IPD	1	78	3	1.69	0.96	32	14	18	CT	Normal
2	IPD	1	64	1	1.57	1.04	16	9	7	NP	NP
3	IPD	2	58	3	2.10	0.88	11	4	7	CT	Normal
4	IPD	1	57	2	1.85	1.07	6	5	1	NP	NP
5	IPD	1	70	2	2.07	0.95	25	11	14	NP	NP
6	IPD	1	75	5	1.52	1.00	31	15	16	NP	NP
7	IPD	2	35	3	2.44	0.98	17	8	9	CT+MRI	Normal
8	IPD	1	65	4	1.62	0.98	4	3	1	NP	NP
9	IPD	2	76	3	1.73	1.10	39	23	16	CT	Normal
10	IPD	1	50	5	1.79	1.02	14	8	6	NP	NP
11	IPD+M	1	62	3	1.68	0.95	20	9	11	CT	Normal
12	IPD+M	1	44	7	2.47	0.96	23	9	14	CT	Normal
13	IPD+M	1	53	13	1.45	1.00	40	17	23	NP	NP
14	IPD+M	1	36	3	1.90	0.97	15	9	6	CT	Normal
15	IPD+M	2	50	21	1.60	1.00	36	12	24	NP	NP
16	IPD+M	1	68	9	1.75	0.99	18	14	4	NP	NP
17	IPD+M	1	72	14	1.69	1.15	39	8	31	NP	NP
18	IPD+M	1	67	5	1.92	0.93	38	18	20	CT	Slight global atrophy
19	IPD+M	1	50	10	1.77	1.00	14	6	8	CT	Lacunar infarction left basal ganglia
20	IPD+M	1	34	2	2.03	1.03	17	6	11	CT+MRI	Normal
21	IPD+M	2	45	3	1.80	0.96	26	7	19	NP	NP
22	MSA	2	53	5	1.14	1.05	34	20	14	CT	Hypodense lesion right temporal lobe, tissue loss cerebellar hemispheres
23	MSA	2	69	3	1.46	1.10	69	28	41	CT	Hydrocephalus, subcortical arteriosclerotic encephalopathy, hypodense lesion left parietal lobe
24	MSA	1	72	4	1.33	0.96	30	16	14	CT	Normal
25	MSA	1	53	3	1.45	1.00	24	14	10	MRI	Wide peripontine cisterns, cerebellar atrophy
26	MSA	2	65	4	1.31	1.04	32	19	13	CT	Normal
27	MSA	2	58	6	1.17	1.14	39	15	24	CT	Slight global atrophy
28	MSA	1	49	2	1.51	1.02	24	8	16	CT	Normal

SPECT Section 4: Movement Disorders

Chapter 21 – Clinical Significance of Dopamine D$_2$-Receptor Imaging with ^{123}I-Iodobenzamide SPECT in Patients with Parkinsonian Syndromes

Table 1 (continued)

Patient no.	Group	Sex (M1,F2)	Age (yrs)	Duration (yrs)	IBZM SPECT ST/OC	IBZM SPECT ST L/R	Columbia Scale Total	Columbia Scale Axial	Columbia Scale Extremities	CT and/or MRI Study	Findings. NP=No anatomical imaging performed because of lack of clinical indication
28	MSA	1	49	2	1.51	1.02	24	8	16	CT	Normal
29	MSA	1	48	1	1.69	1.06	20	10	10	CT	Bilaterally hypodense lesions in globus pallidus
30	MSA	2	80	39	1.75	1.05	22	16	6	NP	NP
31	MSA	2	82	2	1.36	1.19	26	15	11	MRI	Dilated ventricles, global atrophy, lesions white matter and basal ganglia on T$_2$- images
32	MSA	1	55	2	1.77	0.97	38	20	18	CT	Atrophy cerebellum and brain stem
33	MSA	1	74	5	1.62	1.00	14	10	4	NP	NP
34	MSA	2	26	7	1.81	0.95	37	19	18	MRI	Accumulation of iron in globus pallidus
35	MSA	1	66	6	1.46	0.93	31	17	14	MRI	Normal
36	MSA	1	48	4	1.66	0.98	22	10	12	CT+MRI	Tiny calcification directly above right caudate nucleus
37	MSA	1	68	6	1.68	0.95	45	31	14	CT	Global supratentorial tissue loss, calcifications in basilar artery
38	MSA	1	55	5	1.34	1.07	48	24	24	NP	NP
39	MSA	1	80	4	1.47	1.11	18	18	0	CT	Normal
40	PSP	1	39	15	1.78	1.06	34	11	23	CT	Slight atrophy brain stem and cerebellum
41	PSP	2	75	5	1.61	1.17	44	28	16	MRI	Dilated ventricles. No abnormalities in striatum or mesencephalon
42	PSP	2	69	6	1.22	0.97	17	7	10	NP	NP

[a]IPD, idiopathic Parkinson's disease; M, dopaminergic medication; MSA, multiple system atrophy

Recently, several SPECT studies have confirmed findings with PET. Using SPECT and ^{123}I iodolisuride or $[^{123}$I](S)-N-[(1-ethyl-2-pyrrolidinyl)]methyl-2-hydroxy-3-iodo-6-methoxybenzamide (^{123}I-IBZM), a reduced striatal D_2-receptor binding potential was observed in PSP and MSA patients[12,13]. It has, moreover, been claimed that ^{123}I-IBZM SPECT can predict responsiveness to dopaminergic therapy in *de novo* parkinsonian patients[14].

The aim of our present study was to determine the relationship between the striatal D_2-receptor binding potential, measured *in vivo* with ^{123}I-IBZM SPECT, and the various clinical signs related to the parkinsonian syndrome, measured with the Columbia University Parkinson Rating Scale[15]. The hypothesis tested was whether or not hypofunctioning striatal D_2-receptors are linked to a reduced ability to switch postures with the help of static proprioceptive stimuli[16].

Table 2 Subject characteristics and ratios obtained with ^{123}I-IBZM SPECT. For age and ratios the following are given: (1) mean ± s.d, (2) range, and p-values of the Mann-Whitney U test comparing each patient subgroup with the following groups: (3) controls, (4) IPD, and (5) IPD+M

		Controls (n = 10)	IPD (n = 10)	IPD+M (n = 11)	MSA (n = 21)
Male/Female		6/4	7/3	9/2	12/9
Age (yrs)	1	54 ± 10	63 ± 13	53 ± 13	61 ± 15
	2	40 - 71	35 - 78	34 - 72	26 - 82
	3		0.082	0.86	0.11
	4			0.091	0.72
	5				0.084
ST/OC ratio	1	1.86±0.1	1.84±0.29	1.82±0.27	1.50±0.21
	2	1.61-2.25	1.52-2.44	1.45-2.47	1.14-1.81
	3		0.45	0.40	0.0002[a]
	4			0.97	0.0035[a]
	5				0.0027[a]
ST L/R ratio	1	0.98±0.04	1.00±0.06	1.00±0.06	1.04±0.07
	2	0.89-1.04	0.88-1.10	0.93-1.15	0.94-1.19
	3		0.79	0.72	0.083
	4			0.65	0.25
	5				0.11

Using the Bonferroni procedure with p<0.05 as level of significance: [a], significant: p<0.0083 for the Mann-Whitney U-test

Subjects, materials and methods

Subjects

Subject groups: (1) IPD: 10 *de novo* patients with a positive apomorphine test, clinically diagnosed as probable IPD[1]; (2) IPD+M: 11 patients with IPD effectively treated with dopaminergic medication; (3) MSA: 18 patients clinically diagnosed as MSA plus 3 patients clinically suffering from PSP[4], all with a negative or doubtful apomorphine test or with either a poor long-term response to dopaminergic medication or none at all; (4) controls: 10 age-matched subjects without parkinsonian signs and without dopaminergic medication. Characteristics are shown in Tables 1 and 2.

Exclusion criteria for patients and controls were: (1) liver, kidney, endocrine, haematologic and/or cardio-vascular diseases; (2) dependence on psychotropic substances, except for caffeine and nicotine; (3) allergy or hypersensitivity to iodine or drugs; (4) lack of contraceptive use among fertile women.

The severity of the various aspects of the parkinsonian syndromes was evaluated semiquantitatively by using the Columbia Scale that relates increasing severity of parkinsonian signs (tremor, rigidity, bradykinesia, and gait-balance dysfunction) to a five-point numeric scale[15]. The Columbia Scale contains 11 items for axial signs and 4 items for non-axial signs over the extremities. Patients on dopaminergic medication were scored in their 'off' periods. Neuro-imaging with ^{123}I-IBZM SPECT was performed at least 12 h after the last dose of dopaminergic medication. The interval between clinical rating with the Columbia Scale and neuroimaging was less than 1 month.

Each subject had given informed consent after approval had been obtained from the Medical Ethical Committee at the Academic Medical Centre.

^{123}I-IBZM SPECT

The methodology of the ^{123}I-IBZM SPECT has already been described[13]. The thyroid was blocked in younger patients and controls using potassium iodide. Dopaminergic medication was stopped at least 12 h before the SPECT. A total activity of 185 MBq of ^{123}I-IBZM (specific activity 222 MBq/nmol) was administered intravenously and the SPECT performed with a high-sensitivity, high-resolution, multi-detector system, the SME 810 (Strichman Medical Equipment Inc., Medfield, MA, USA). A multi-slice study was carried out 120-180 min after injection, with 5-min slices acquired from the cantho-meatal line to the vertex and spaced by 10 mm. Images were

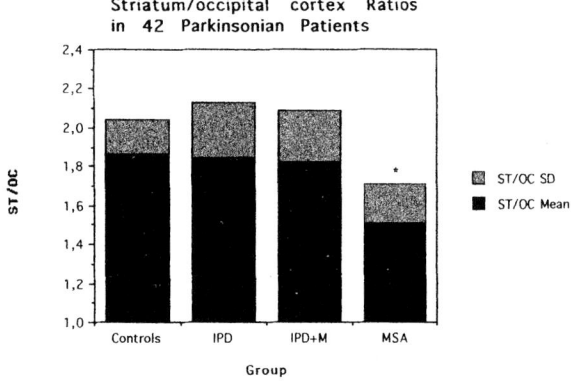

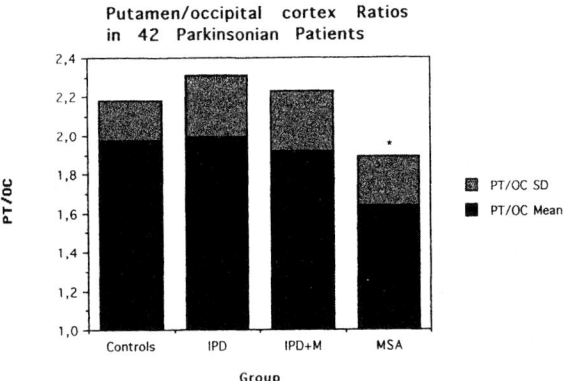

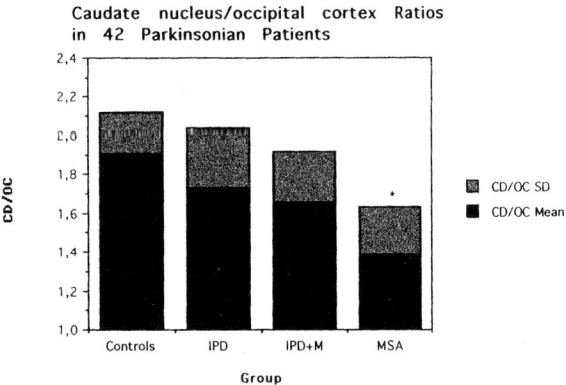

Figure 1 Results of ^{123}I-IBZM SPECT n 10 age-matched control subjects, 10 patients with idiopathic Parkinson's disease (IPD), 11 patients with idiopathic Parkinson's disease on dopaminergic medication (IPD+M), and in a combined group (MSA) of 18 patients with MSA and 3 patients with PSP. Top, striatum/occipital cortex ratio; middle, putamen/occipital cortex ratio; bottom, caudate nucleus/occipital cortex ratio. data are mean ± s.d. *: Significant with p<0.0083 for the Mann-Whitney U-test when compared with the other groups (according to the Bonferroni procedure with p<0.05)

reconstructed in the highest resolution mode with 1 iteration, using a dedicated software programme (Strichman Medical Equipment Inc., version 2.65, 1990). Uniform attenuation equal to that of water was assumed in an ellipse automatically drawn around the brain.

The procedure for semiquantification of D_2-receptor binding potential has been described elsewhere[17]. After reconstruction of the transversal slices, the two slices showing the highest striatal radioactivity were selected. Fixed regions of interest derived from a stereotaxic brain atlas[18] were optimally fitted over the striatum (ST),

Table 3 Results obtained with the Columbia Scale. In the 3 columns on the left, the data are given as mean ± s.d. In the 3 columns on the right, the p-values of the Mann-Whitney U-test are given

Columbia Scale item	IPD	IPD+M	MSA	IPD vs.	IPD vs.	IPD+M vs.
	(n = 10)	(n = 11)	(n = 21)	IPD+M	MSA	MSA
Disease duration	3.1 ± 1.4	8.1 ± 6.0	6.4 ± 8.2	0.031[a]	0.074	0.24
Facial expression	1.7 ± 0.7	1.9 ± 0.7	2.0 ± 0.9	0.48	0.28	0.64
Seborrhoea	1.1 ± 0.9	0.6 ± 0.5	0.8 ± 0.8	0.18	0.37	0.67
Salivation	0.5 ± 0.5	0.9 ± 0.8	1.3 ± 1.0	0.25	0.020[a]	0.24
Speech	1.2 ± 0.8	1.1 ± 0.7	2.0 ± 1.0	0.70	0.031[a]	0.012[a]
Head-tremor	0.0 ± 0.0	0.1 ± 0.3	0.0 ± 0.0	0.32	1.0	0.15
Head-rigidity	0.4 ± 0.5	0.7 ± 1.0	1.1 ± 1.2	0.58	0.15	0.44
Rising	0.6 ± 0.7	0.7 ± 0.8	2.0 ± 1.0	0.73	0.0007[b]	0.0017[b]
Posture	0.7 ± 1.1	0.9 ± 0.7	2.0 ± 1.2	0.33	0.010[a]	0.014[a]
Stability	1.0 ± 1.1	0.7 ± 0.6	1.7 ± 1.3	0.65	0.16	0.036[a]
Gait	1.2 ± 0.8	1.0 ± 0.6	1.8 ± 1.3	0.64	0.16	0.058
Bradykinesia	1.6 ± 0.7	1.6 ± 0.5	2.1 ± 0.9	0.75	0.11	0.12
Total axial	10.0± 6.1	10.5± 4.2	17.0± 6.7	0.62	0.0077[a]	0.0048[a]
Total r extr.	4.2 ± 4.0	7.3 ± 4.9	7.2 ± 4.6	0.13	0.090	0.94
Total l extr.	5.3 ± 3.8	8.5 ± 6.2	7.7 ± 4.6	0.16	0.23	0.43
Total extre-mities	9.5 ± 6.2	15.5± 8.5	14.9± 8.5	0.10	0.12	0.81
Total Columbia Rating Scale	19.5± 11.8	26.0±10.3	31.8±12.9	0.15	0.019[a]	0.25
Total tremor	1.3 ± 1.2	3.1 ± 3.3	1.0 ± 1.9	0.18	0.17	0.034[a]
Total rigidity	3.6 ± 3.0	5.2 ± 3.4	3.9 ± 4.0	0.29	0.97	0.22
Total RAM[c]	2.6 ± 2.4	5.7 ± 3.0	6.8 ± 4.0	0.018	0.0057[a]	0.47
Total dexterity	2.0 ± 1.9	1.5 ± 1.9	3.1 ± 2.3	0.54	0.19	0.061

Using the Bonferroni procedure with p<0.05 as level of significance: [a], trend towards significance: 0.0024< p<0.05 for the Mann-Whitney U-test; [b], significant: p<0.0024 for the Mann-Whitney U-test; rapid alternating movements

putamen (PT) and caudate nucleus (CD). Fixed regions of interest derived from a neuroanatomical atlas[19] were placed over the occipital cortex (OC) in the same slices. The values of the count density in the regions of interest derived from the two slices were then averaged.

Ratios of striatal count density divided by occipital count density (ST/OC) were then calculated in order to estimate D_2-receptor binding potential. Striatal left/right (ST L/R) ratios were also calculated. Similar ratios were calculated for the PT and CD.

Statistical analysis

The semiquantitative estimates for the D_2-receptor binding potential based on the ^{123}I-IBZM SPECT in the

Table 4 Results of the Spearman rank correlation test between ST/OC, PT/OC and CD/OC ratios and corresponding Columbia Scale items in 42 patients with parkinsonian symptoms. The correlation coefficient rho and its p-value are given

Columbia Scale item	ST/OC rho	p	PT/OC rho	p	CD/OC rho	p
Age	-0.37	0.017[a]	-0.32	0.38	-0.25	0.11
Disease duration	-0.09	0.57	-0.14	0.37	-0.19	0.24
Facial expression	-0.23	0.15	-0.17	0.29	-0.12	0.45
Seborrhoea	-0.06	0.68	-0.00	0.98	-0.12	0.42
Salivation	-0.34	0.031[a]	-0.29	0.06	-0.25	0.11
Speech	-0.30	0.057[a]	-0.21	0.16	-0.31	0.046[a]
Head-tremor	+0.09	0.55	+0.04	0.80	+0.18	0.27
Head-rigidity	-0.02	0.89	-0.04	0.82	-0.19	0.23
Rising	-0.47	0.0029[a]	-0.42	0.0071[a]	-0.37	0.019[a]
Posture	-0.40	0.01[a]	-0.35	0.027[a]	-0.33	0.033[a]
Stability	-0.22	0.17	-0.17	0.29	-0.25	0.10
Gait	-0.33	0.033[a]	-0.28	0.08	-0.27	0.087
Bradykinesia	-0.18	0.24	-0.15	0.34	-0.22	0.16
Total axial	-0.41	0.0084[a]	-0.34	0.028[a]	-0.37	0.017[a]
Total extremities	-0.19	0.23	-0.21	0.18	-0.26	0.090
Total Columbia Rating Scale	-0.34	0.031[a]	-0.32	0.038[a]	-0.38	0.014[a]
Total tremor	+0.07	0.64	0.00	1.00	-0.05	0.74
Total rigidity	-0.01	0.96	-0.02	0.92	-0.16	0.032
Total RAM[b]	-0.33	0.036[a]	-0.33	0.04	-0.36	0.022[a]
Total dexterity	-0.17	0.28	-0.13	0.40	-0.04	0.78

Using the Bonferroni procedure with p<0.05 as level of significance: [a], trend towards significance: 0.0025< p<0.05 for the rank correlation; [b], rapid alternating movements

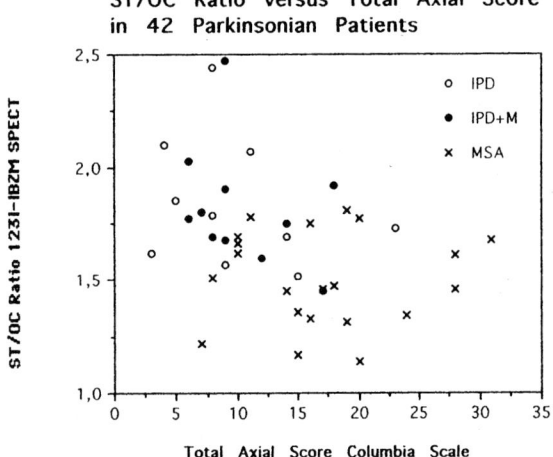

ST/OC Ratio versus Total Axial Score in 42 Parkinsonian Patients

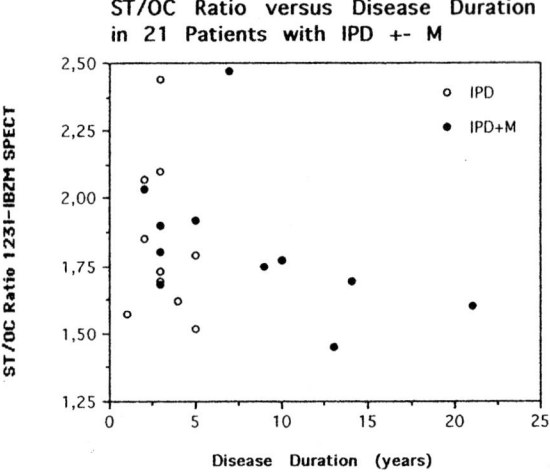

ST/OC Ratio versus Disease Duration in 21 Patients with IPD +- M

Figure 2 Relation of striatum/occipital cortex ratio obtained with ^{123}I-IBZM SPECT with total axial score on the Columbia Scale in 10 patients with idiopathic Parkinson's disease (IPD), 11 patients with idiopathic Parkinson's disease on dopaminergic medication (IPD+M), and in a combined group (MSA) of 18 patients with MSA and 3 patients with PSP

Figure 3 Relation of striatum/occipital cortex ratio obtained with ^{123}I-IBZM SPECT with duration of disease in 10 patients with idiopathic Parkinson's disease (IPD) and in 11 patients with idiopathic Parkinson's disease on dopaminergic medication (IPD+M)

various groups were compared using the Mann-Whitney U-test[20]. This was also applied to compare the clinical variables rated using the Columbia Scale between the patient subgroups.

The SPECT and Columbia Scale data were correlated with Spearman's rank correlation test[20]. The L/R ratios for the ST, PT and CD were correlated similarly with L/R ratios and L-R subtractions derived from the Columbia Scale scores concerning signs in the extremities. This was performed for the whole patient group as well as the various subgroups. All non-parametric tests were performed on a MacIntosh IIci computer using StatView[TM]II (Abacus Concepts, Inc., Berkely, CA, USA).

The Bonferroni procedure was applied to each set of comparisons to obtain a significance level of p<0.05 for each comparison[21]. For each single comparison the outcome was considered significant if its actual p value was lower than that calculated using the Bonferroni correction. A trend towards significance was assumed if the actual p-value was higher than the value calculated using the Bonferroni correction but lower than 0.05.

Results

The results of ^{123}I-IBZM SPECT for the control group and the patient subgroups are given in Tables 1 and 2

and Figure 1. The ST/OC, PT/OC and CD/OC ratios were significantly lower in the MSA group than in the other patient groups and the controls.

The results of the Columbia Scale for the patient subgroups are shown in Table 3. Total Columbia Rating Scale and total axial sign scores tended to be more severe in the MSA group than in the patients with IPD or IPD+M.

The results of the Spearman rank correlation test between the ST/OC, PT/OC and CD/OC ratios obtained with ^{123}I-IBZM SPECT and the Columbia Scale scores for all 42 patients with parkinsonian signs are given in Table 4. A trend towards significance was observed, especially for the correlation between the ST/OC ratio and both total axial signs and total outcome of the Columbia Scale (Figure 2). Except for total rapid alternating movements (RAM), no significant correlations were observed between the ratios obtained with SPECT and signs of the extremities. Similar results were obtained for the PT/OC and CD/OC ratios.

When the patient subgroups were analysed separately, the IPD+M group displayed a trend towards a significant correlation between disease duration and the ST/OC and PT/OC ratios (rho = -0.61; p= 0.052 and rho = -0.62; p= 0.049, respectively). This trend remained when the 21 patients with IPD and IPD+M were combined (rho = -0.45; p= 0.049) (Figure 3).

Furthermore, trends for significant correlations were observed in this combined group for the PT/OC ratios versus gait (rho = -0.50; p= 0.024) and bradykinesia (rho = -0.43; p= 0.053). The subgroups showed no other significant correlations.

No significant correlations were observed when the Spearman rank correlation test was applied to the ST L/R, PT L/R and CD L/R ratios obtained with ^{123}I-IBZM SPECT versus the L/R ratios and L-R subtractions of the Columbia Scale scores of the extremities for all 42 patients or for the various subgroups.

Discussion

Applying ratios is a common procedure in SPECT with ^{123}I-IBZM[14,22] or ^{123}I-iodolisuride[12]. The use of ratios has also been validated for clinical purposes by comparison with parameters for the striatal D$_2$-receptor binding potential derived from compartment models in PET[23]. Both the cerebellum[12] and the frontal cortex[14,22] have been used as denominators in the ratio as estimations of the 'free plus non-specifically bound' ligand concentration in the SPECT estimation of striatal D$_2$-receptor binding potential in parkinsonian patients. We preferred the occipital cortex as a reference region in our present study, since: frontal lobe dysfunction has been reported in IPD patients with depressive disorders[24]; frontal hypoperfusion has been described in PSP[25]; and cerebellar atrophy has been associated with MSA[6].

Our results agreed with those of Brücke et al.[22], in that no changes in dopamine D$_2$-receptor binding potential were observed in the IPD patients compared with controls. Increased D$_2$ receptor densities have been observed in striata obtained post mortem from patients with IPD[26], and the reason for the discrepancy is unclear. The increased densities may be the outcome of the very late stages of IPD alone[27], but this is not in accordance with the current trend in our data that D$_2$-receptor binding potential decreases in patients with long-term disease in the IPD+M group. Our data support Brücke et al.'s[22] and Leenders'[23] observations that uptake in L-DOPA-treated IPD patients is reduced D$_2$, but are in conflict with the findings of Rutgers et al.[28]. It is possible, therefore, that L-DOPA treatment results in dopamine receptor down-regulation[29], but it is difficult to separate this effect from that of the progress of the disease. Antonini et al.[30] recently showed that a short duration of L-DOPA therapy does not result in diminished dopamine D$_2$-receptor tracer uptake. Nadeau et al.[31] obtained significant inverse correlations between D$_2$-receptor binding in the ventral caudate and L-DOPA dosage, as well as between D$_2$-receptor binding in the anterior putamen and disease duration. Thus, L-DOPA may well result in reduced tracer uptake by competitive inhibition in those areas still most capable of producing dopamine, rather than in D$_2$-receptor down-regulation. A longer duration of IPD may result in more trans-synaptic degeneration in the most affected areas with decreased D$_2$-receptor expression, rather than in D$_2$ upregulation[31].

The reduced striatal D$_2$-receptor binding potential in the MSA group confirms the findings reported previously[13]. Schelosky et al.[32] also demonstrated higher ^{123}I-IBZM binding in IPD patients than in MSA or PSP patients, but the overlap between IPD patients and MSA or PSP patients was considerable in their study. Our study shows similar results. Eight of our 18 MSA patients have a striatal ^{123}I-IBZM uptake within 2 s.d. of the normal mean, and one of the IPD+M patients falls below the normal range. Thus, the sensitivity of ^{123}I-IBZM SPECT in discriminating IPD from other parkinsonian syndromes on an individual basis is limited. We studied too few subjects with PSP to be able to discuss MSA and PSP patients separately but, based on the current ^{123}I-IBZM SPECT data, differentiation of PSP from MSA seems unlikely.

Our results are also in agreement with those of Schwarz et al.[14], who, using ^{123}I-IBZM SPECT with a double-headed rotating gamma-camera in de novo parkinsonian patients, reported a positive predictive value for response to oral dopaminergic therapy of 86% and to apomorphine of 72%, and negative predictive values of 86% and 89%, respectively. Schelosky et al.[32] also demonstrated significantly higher binding of ^{123}I-IBZM in apomorphine responders than in non-responders.

However, the lack of responsiveness to L-DOPA in some parkinsonian patients may not result from D$_2$-receptor loss alone[11,27]. Other factors, such as: (1) insufficient metabolism of L-DOPA by remaining intact dopaminergic nerve terminals[33] as well as adjacent nondopaminergic cells[2]; (2) the variable pharma-cokinetics of L-DOPA; (3) disturbed receptor-effector coupling[27]; and (4) damaged efferent connections from the basal ganglia[34]; may also be important. In cases (1) and (2), with still enough D$_2$-receptors in the striatum, dopaminergic agonists rather than dopamine precursors may improve the parkinsonian disability[9]. In case (3) a decreased affinity of the D$_2$-receptor for agonists may play a part[35]. The labelled agonist ^{11}C-apomorphine may prove useful in discovering such defects in future PET studies[36]. In case (4), it is not known exactly which efferent connections are involved. Dopamine D$_2$-receptor imaging in vivo may help to define whether striato-thalamo-cortical circuits are deficient. For instance, D_2-receptors are mainly located on medium spiny neurones, forming the first connection in the indirect striato-thalamo-cortical circuits[37,38]. Striatal D_2-receptors may moreover also be present on D_1-receptor-expressing striatal neurons, as part of the direct striato-thalamo-cortical circuits[39], on cholinergic interneurones[38], on nigrostriatal terminals[27] and on corticostriatal terminals[40].

In trying to define patients who will not respond to dopaminergic therapy, one should strive for maximal specificity, in order not to withhold any potentially beneficial treatment. Based on our study, the likelihood of a negative response is 100% at ST/OC ratios of ^{123}I-IBZM SPECT below 1.45. Schelosky *et al.*[32] also concluded that a reliable prediction can be made only in patients with an abnormally low ^{123}I-IBZM binding. Using such criteria, homogeneous patient groups could be created for clinical trials testing experimental medication[41] or neuro-transplantation[42]. In clinical practice, it might not be unreasonable to do a ^{123}I-IBZM SPECT study on patients with a negative response to both an oral L-DOPA test and an apomorphine test. If one then found that the D_2-receptor binding potential was normal or just below the normal range, then this would encourage a prolonged trial of chronic dopaminergic medication (it is known that false-negatives may occur in *de novo* IPD patients to acute challenges in a small percentage of cases[43]).

In our study the semiquantitative estimates for the striatal D_2-receptor binding potential were mainly correlated with axial signs such as rising from a chair, posture, gait, and speech. Furthermore, a trend towards significant correlation was observed for the total axial Columbia Scale score as well as for the general Columbia Scale score. These correlations are in accordance with a conceptual framework linking hypofunctioning striatal D_2-receptors that mainly affect the indirect striato-thalamo-cortical circuit[37,38], on the one hand with a reduced ability to switch postures, and on the other with an ability to switch motor patterns with the help of static (tonic) proprioceptive stimuli[16]. This concept also postulates that, before reaching this state of advanced striatal pathology, a reduced shifting aptitude exists with respect to behaviour guided by self-generated information, which is followed by changes at the level of motor expression. This hypothesis may be tested prospectively in future, using more sensitive ligands for D_2-receptor imaging *in vivo*[44] — in subjects without overt IPD but who show abnormalities when sensitive neuropsychometric methods are applied, as well as in primates with subclinical damage to the nigrostriatal system by MPTP[45].

We observed a significant correlation between D_2 binding potential and bradykinesia for the 21 patients in the IPD and IPD+M groups. In patients with IPD+M, significant correlations between ^{18}F-DOPA uptake measured with PET have not only been observed for bradykinesia as determined with the modified Columbia Scale, but also for total score, tremor, bradykinesia, rigidity, stability, and gait[46]. Tremor and rigidity, more related to the extremities than to the trunk, showed no correlation with the SPECT findings, either for the whole group or for the patient subgroups, in our study.

In patients with MSA, significant correlations were observed in the putamen (but not in the caudate) between ^{18}F-DOPA influx constants as measured by PET and both Hoehn and Yahr disability scores and duration of locomotor disability[10]. We did not observe any correlation between the ST/OC, PT/OC or CD/OC ratios based on ^{123}I-IBZM uptake and the scores on the Columbia Scale for the group of 21 patients with MSA or PSP.

Taken together, the correlations above seem to indicate that, in patients with the parkinsonian syndrome, postsynaptic dopaminergic dysfunction is mainly linked to axial signs, while presynaptic dopaminergic dysfunction is linked to both axial and non-axial signs, such as tremor. Since self-reports of disability are strongly correlated with deficiencies of purposeful movement (bradykinesia, gait disturbance, abnormal posture), but not at all correlated with tremor, both of which are assessed with the Columbia scale[15], it seems that postsynaptic dopaminergic dysfunction may be particularly related to difficulties in performing daily living activities. In contrast to presynaptic dopaminergic dysfunction, which correlates well with the signs, the postsynaptic change may give rise to an 'all or none' effect: below a certain D_2-receptor density in the ST, severe axial signs will arise and MSA or PSP will be diagnosed. Another possibility is that there is no causal relationship between axial signs and striatal D_2-receptor binding potential. The association of impaired gait or inability to switch postures with low ^{123}I-IBZM uptake may simply reflect a different pathology which also involves other brain stem and frontal connections. Combined imaging of striatal dopamine D_2-receptors, L-DOPA uptake and glucose metabolism (e.g. by using ^{18}F-DOPA and ^{18}F-FDG PET, respectively) may provide a much sharper clustering of patient groups with different parkinsonian syndromes.

No correlation between L/R ratios for ST, PT or CD derived from the ^{123}I-IBZM SPECT and L/R ratios for items from the Columbia Scale was observed. These findings are in agreement with some older D_2-receptor PET studies[28], but not with more recent PET studies showing increments in striatal ^{11}C-raclopride binding potential contralateral to the side of parkinsonian signs[47], especially in the putamen. These increments have also been observed in unilaterally MPTP-lesioned monkeys[48]. The present lack of correlation between the asymmetries mentioned above may either be due to modest sign lateralisation in our patients or to insufficient sensitivity of the applied technique. Recent ^{123}I-IBZM SPECT studies in unilaterally MPTP-treated monkeys in our group revealed an increase in the striatal D_2-receptor binding potential of up to 30% *in vivo* at the lesioned side[49]. This shows that our technique is able to detect striatal D_2-receptor asymmetries due to a decreased dopaminergic input, and this is supported by other ^{123}I-IBZM SPECT studies in recently diagnosed IPD patients that revealed increased uptake of the tracer in the striatum contralateral to the parkinsonian signs[50,51]. As the patients in the studies of Laulumaa *et al.*[50] and Knable *et al.*[51] mainly had unilateral signs, it is likely that modest sign lateralisation in the patients in our study is the main reason for the failure to find a correlation.

Conclusions

A significant correlation has been observed between a low striatal dopamine D_2-receptor binding potential determined using ^{123}I-IBZM SPECT and axial parkinsonian signs rated by the Columbia Scale. These findings are partially in concert with current pathophysiological models. ^{123}I-IBZM SPECT may be used clinically: (a) to monitor whether or not lack of response to dopaminergic medication is due to a deficiency of striatal D_2-receptors; (b) to predict whether or not a patient with parkinsonism is likely to respond to dopaminergic medication; (c) to select those patients unlikely to respond to dopaminergic medication for clinical trials in which experimental therapeutic strategems can be tested; (d) to exclude patients with a severely decreased striatal D_2-receptor binding potential from clinical trials in which D_2 dopaminergic medication is tested and from transplantation with dopaminergic cells.

Acknowledgements

The authors thank Cygne B.V., Technical University Eindhoven, for providing the ^{123}I-IBZM for free, and Mrs G.E.E. van Noppen for her additional comments. This study was supported by grants from the Queen Beatrix Foundation, the Dutch Organization for Scientific Research (NWO), and from the Sandoz Research Foundation.

References

1   Hughes, A.J., Daniel, S.E., Kilford, L., Lees, A.J. Accuracy of clinical diagnosis of idiopathic Parkinson's disease: a clinico-pathological study of 100 cases. *J. Neurol. Neurosurg. Psychiatr.* 1992, 55, 181

2   Côté, L. and Crutcher, M.D. The Basal Ganglia in Principles of Neural Science, 3rd Edn', (Eds. E.R. Kandel, J.H. Schwartz and T.M. Jessell), Elsevier, New York, USA, 1992, p.647

3   Maher, E.R. and Lees, A.J. The clinical features and natural history of the Steele-Richardson-Olszewski syndrome (progressive supranuclear palsy). *Neurology* 1986, 36, 1005

4   Quinn, N. Multiple system atrophy - the nature of the beast. *J. Neurol. Neurosurg. Psychiatr.* 1989, special supplement, 78

5   Pastakia, B., Polinsky, R., Di Chiro, G. *et al.* Multiple system atrophy (Shy-Dräger Syndrome): MR Imaging. *Radiol.* 1986, 159, 499

6   Brooks, D.J., Salmon, E.P., Mathias, C.J. *et al.* The relationship between locomotor disability, autonomic dysfunction, and the integrity of the striatal dopaminergic system in patients with multiple system atrophy, pure autonomic failure, and Parkinson's disease, studied with PET. *Brain* 1990, 113, 1539

7   Staal, A., Meerwaldt, J.D., van Dongen, K.J. *et al.* On-familial degenerative disease and atrophy of brainstem and cerebellum. Clinical and CT data in 47 patients. *J. Neurol. Sci.* 1990, 95, 259

8   Hughes, A.J., Lees, A.J. and Stern, G.M. Apomorphine test to predict dopaminergic responsiveness in parkinsonian syndromes. *Lancet* 1990, 336, 32

9   Steiger, M.J., Quinn, N.P. and Marsden, C.D. The clinical use of apomorphine in Parkinson's disease. *J. Neurol.* 1992, 239, 389

10 Pascual, J., Berciano, J., Grijalba, B. *et al.* Dopamine D1 and D2 receptors in progressive supranuclear palsy: an autoradiographic study. *Ann. Neurol.* 1992, 32, 703

11 Brooks, D.J., Ibanez, V., Sawle, G.V. *et al.* Striatal D2 receptor status in patients with Parkinson's disease, striatonigral degeneration, and progressive supranuclear palsy, measured with ^{11}C-raclopride and positron emission tomography. *Ann. Neurol.* 1992, 31, 184

12 Chabriat, H., Levasseur, M., Vidailhet, M. *et al.* In vivo SPECT imaging of D2 receptor with iodine-iodolisuride: results in supranuclear palsy. *J. Nucl. Med.* 1992, 33, 1481

13 van Royen, E.A., Verhoeff, N.P.L.G., Speelman, J.D. *et al.* Multiple system atrophy and progressive supranuclear palsy. Diminished striatal D2 dopamine receptor activity demonstrated by ^{123}I-IBZM single photon emission computed tomography. *Arch. Neurol.* 1993, 50, 513

14 Schwarz, J., Tatsch, K., Arnold, G. *et al.* ^{123}I-iodobenzamide SPECT predicts dopaminergic responsiveness in patients with de novo parkinsonism. *Neurology* 1992, 42, 556

15 Montgomery, G.K., Reynolds, N.C. Jr. and Warren, R.M. Special article - qualitative assessment of Parkinson's

disease: study of reliability and data reduction with an abbreviated Columbia Scale. *Clin. Neuropharmacol.* 1985, 8, 83

16 Cools, A.R. Role of neostriatal and mesostriatal or mesolimbic dopaminergic fibers in Parkinson's disease with and without dementia: prospects, concepts and facts. *Jpn. J. Psychopharmacol.* 1990, 10, 15

17 Verhoeff, N.P.L.G., Kapucu, O., Sokole-Busemann, E. *et al.* Estimation of dopamine D2 receptor binding potential in the striatum with iodine-123-IBZM SPECT: technical and interobserver variability. *J. Nucl. Med.* 1993, 34, 2076

18 Schaltenbrand, G. and Wahren, W. Atlas for stereotaxy of the human brain. Georg Thieme Publishers, Stuttgart, Germany, 1977

19 Matsui, T. and Hirano, A. An atlas of the human brain for computerised tomography. Gustav Fischer Verlag, Stuttgart, Germany, 1978

20 Armitage, P. and Berry, G. Statistical methods in medical research, 2nd Edn. Blackwell Scientific Publ, Oxford, UK, 1987, p.408

21 Wassertheil-Smoller, S. Biostatistics and epidemiology. A primer for health professionals. Springer-Verlag, New York, USA, 1990, p.49

22 Brücke, T., Podreka, I., Angelberger, P. *et al.* Dopamine D2 receptor imaging with SPECT: studies in different neuropsychiatric disorders. *J. Cereb. Blood Flow. Metab.* 1991, 11, 220

23 Leenders, K.L. Movement disorders. A study with positron emission tomography. Thesis. Amsterdam: Free University, 1986

24 Cummings, J.L. Depression and Parkinson's disease: a review. *Am. J. Psychiatr.* 1992, 149, 443

25 Johnson, K.A., Sperling, R.A., Holman, B.L. *et al.* Cerebral perfusion in progressive supranuclear palsy. *J. Nucl. Med.* 1992, 33, 704

26 Seeman, P., Bzowej, N.H., Guan, H.C. *et al.* Human brain D1 and D2 dopamine receptors in schizophrenia, Alzheimer's, Parkinson's, and Huntington's diseases. *Neuropsychopharmacol.* 1987, 1, 5

27 Riederer, P., Sofic, E., Konradi, C. *et al.* The role of dopamine in the control of neurobiological functions in 'The role of brain dopamine. Basic and clinical aspects of neuroscience, vol 3', (Eds. E. Flückiger, E.E. Müller and M.O. Thorner), Springer Verlag, Berlin, Germany, 1989, p.1

28 Rutgers, A.W.F., Lakke, J.P.W.F., Paans, A.M.J. *et al.* Tracing of dopamine receptors in hemiparkinsonism with positron emission tomography (PET). *J. Neurol. Sci.* 1987, 80, 237

29 Guttman, M. and Seeman, P. L-DOPA reverses the elevated density of D2 dopamine receptors in Parkinson-diseased striatum. *J. Neural Transm.* 1985, 64, 93

30 Antonini, A., Schwarz, J., Oertel, W.H. *et al.* [^{11}C]raclopride and positron emission tomography in previously untreated patients with Parkinson's disease: influence of L-dopa and lisuride therapy on striatal dopamine D2-receptors. *Neurology* 1994, 44, 1325

31 Nadeau, S.E., Couch, M.W., Devane, L. and Shukla, S.S. Regional analysis of D2 dopamine receptors in Parkinson's disease using SPECT and iodine-123-iodobenzamide. *J. Nucl. Med.* 1995, 36, 384

32 Schelosky, L., Hierholzer, J., Wissel, J. *et al.* Correlation of clinical response in apomorphine test with D2-receptor status as demonstrated by ^{123}I IBZM-SPECT. *Mov. Dis.* 1993, 8, 453

33 Leenders, K.L., Salmon, E.P., Tyrrell, P. *et al.* The nigrostriatal dopaminergic system assessed in vivo by positron emission tomography in healthy volunteer subjects and patients with Parkinson's disease. *Arch. Neurol.* 1990, 47, 1290

34 Agid, Y., Javoy-Agid, F., Ruberg, M. *et al.* Biochemistry of neurotransmitters in Parkinson's disease in Movement disorders', (Eds. C.D. Marsden, S. Fahn), Butterworths, London, UK, 1986, p166

35 Aquilonius, S.M. What has PET told us about Parkinson's disease? *Acta. Neurol. Scand.* 1991, 84(Suppl 136), 37

36 Zijlstra, S. Positron emission tomography of cerebral dopamine receptors. Synthesis and evaluation of potential agonists and drug response in schizophrenia. Thesis. University of Groningen, 1993

37 Gerfen, C.R. The neostriatal mosaic: multiple levels of compartmental organization. *Trends Neurosci.* 1992, 15, 133

38 Groenewegen, H.J., Roeling, T.A.P., Voorn, P., and Berendse, H.W. The parallel arrangement of basal ganglia-thalamocortical circuits: a neuronal substrate for the role of dopamine in motor and cognitive functions in Mental dysfunction in Parkinson's disease', (Eds. E.Ch. Wolters and P. Scheltens), Free University, Amsterdam, Holland, 1993, p.3

39 Surmeier, D.J., Reiner, A., Levine, M.S. and Ariano, M.A. Are neostriatal dopamine receptors co-localized? *Trends Neurosci.* 1993, 16, 299

40 Snyder, S.H. The dopamine connection. *Nature* 1990, 347, 121

41 Turski, L., Bressler, K., Rettig, K.J. *et al.* Protection of substantia nigra from MPP+ neurotoxicity by N-methyl-D-aspartate antagonists. *Nature* 1991, 349, 414

42 Sawle, G.V., Bloomfield, P.M., Björklund, A. *et al.* Transplantation of fetal dopamine neurons in Parkinson's disease: PET [^{18}F]6-L-fluorodopa Studies in two patients with putaminal implants. *Ann. Neurol.* 1992, 31, 166

43 Steiger, M.J., Quinn, N.P. and Marsden, C.D. The clinical use of apomorphine in Parkinson's disease. *J. Neurol.* 1992, 239, 389

44 Kessler, R.M., Ansari, M.S., de Paulis, T. *et al.* High affinity dopamine D2 receptor radioligands. 1. Regional rat brain distribution of iodinated benzamides. *J. Nucl. Med.* 1991, 32, 1593

45 Burns, R.S. Subclinical damage to the nigrostriatal dopamine system by MPTP as a model of preclinical Parkinson's disease: a review. *Acta. Neurol. Scand.* 1991, 84(Suppl 136), 29

46 Snow, B.J., Schulzer, M., Martin, W.R.W. *et al.* PET studies of the relationship between dopaminergic deficit and motor performance in Parkinson's disease. *Neurology* 1991, 41 (Suppl 1), 359

47 Sawle, G.V., Brooks, D.J., Ibanez, V. and Frackowiak, R.S.J. Striatal D2 receptor density is inversely proportional to DOPA uptake in untreated hemi-Parkinson's disease: a positron emission tomography study. *J. Neurol. Neurosurg. Psychiatr.* 1990, 53, 177

48 Leenders, K.L., Aquilonius, S.M., Bergström, K. *et al.* Unilateral MPTP lesion in a rhesus monkey: effects on the striatal dopaminergic system measured in vivo with PET using various novel tracers. *Brain Res.* 1988, 445, 61

49 Vermeulen, R.J., Drukarch, B., Verhoeff, N.P.L.G. *et al.* No direct correlation between behaviorally active doses of the dopamine D2 agonist LY 171555 and displacement of [^{123}I]IBZM as measured with SPECT in MPTP monkeys. *Synapse* 1994, 17, 115

50 Laulumaa, V., Kuikka, J.T., Soininen, H. *et al.* Imaging of D2 dopamine receptors of patients with Parkinson's disease using single photon emission computed tomography and iodobenzamide I 123. *Arch. Neurol.* 1993, 50, 509

51 Knable, M.B., Jones, D.W., Copola, R. *et al.* Lateralized differences in iodine-123-IBZM uptake in the basal ganglia in asymmetric Parkinson's disease. *J. Nucl. Med.* 1995, 36, 1216

SPECT in Neurology and Psychiatry, edited by P.P. De Deyn, R.A. Dierckx, A. Alavi and B.A. Pickut

Brain SPECT ^{123}I-IBZM Distribution Analysis in the Differentiation of Patients with Parkinsonian Syndromes

Chapter

22

M.S. Rebel

Introduction

The differential diagnosis of the Parkinson's syndromes is difficult to make on clinical grounds alone at the onset of symptoms[1]. Parkinson's syndromes are currently subclassified according to three major categories[2]:

1. Idiopathic Parkinson's disease (idiopathic parkinsonian syndrome, IPS);
2. Secondary parkinsonism; and
3. Parkinsonism in neural system degenerations (e.g. multiple system atrophy, MSA; progressive supranuclear palsy, PSP; autosomal dominant cerebellar ataxia; Huntington's chorea).

Parkinson's syndromes are the third most common neurological disorders[3] and, as the prognosis and treatment of IPS differs markedly from those of MSA and PSP, a reliable and cost-effective method with which to differentiate patients with Parkinson's syndromes at the onset of symptoms is desirable.

Today, several radiotracers are available for the study of dopamine D_2-receptors *in vivo* in the human brain by SPECT (single photon emission computed tomography) or PET (positron emission tomography). Concerns over the costs of diagnostic procedures are increasing[4], and ^{123}I-IBZM (iodobenzamide) SPECT seems to be a cost-effective, non-invasive diagnostic tool with which to differentiate patients with Parkinson's syndrome. Unfortunately, the analysis of ^{123}I-IBZM SPECT scans is not yet completely reliable. The present approach to SPECT scan analysis compares user-defined regions of interest (ROIs) and is far from satisfactory when applied to ^{123}I-IBZM SPECT scans; the human brain and IBZM kinetics are obviously too complex to be described adequately by 2-dimensional ROIs — at least, no statistically stable results can be achieved with the ROI-approach[5,6].

The aim of this study was to develop a reliable method of analysis for ^{123}I-IBZM distribution in the human brain, to better differentiate patients with Parkinson's syndromes.

Wolfgang Müller-Schauenburg, Tuebingen, Germany

Methods

Patients

Over a period of 20 months, a total of 55 patients (21 female, 34 male) with Parkinson's syndromes were examined at the department of nuclear medicine at the University of Tuebingen, Germany. Patients with the following neurological diagnoses were included in the study:

Idiopathic Parkinson's syndrome (idiopathic Parkinson's disease — IPS, n=30, Hoehn and Yahr I 22/30, Hoehn and Yahr II 8/30)

Multiple System Atrophy (MSA) which was divided into MSA with predominant cerebellar symptoms (MSAc, n=11) and MSA with predominant parkinsonian symptoms (MSAp, n=7)

Progressive Supranuclear Palsy (PSP, n=7).

The mean age of this group of patients was 59.8 years with a SD of 7.8 years. None of them were taking any centrally acting drugs likely to interfere with the ^{123}I-IBZM SPECT scan.

Data acquisition

Sodium pertechnetate was given 2 h before the scan to block thyroid uptake of ^{123}I-IBZM. ^{123}I-labelled IBZM (^{123}I (S)-IBZM, 185 MBq, Cygne BV a specific dopamine D_2-receptor antagonist[7]) was used for visualisation of dopamine D_2-receptor density. Patients were placed in a supine position and the orbito-meatal (OM) line used as a reference with which to position the patient in the gantry.

SPECT data acquisition was started 90 min p.i. using a Picker Dyna Scan twin-headed camera with a general purpose (GP) collimator. Sixty-four views (of 40 s duration) were taken over a 360° rotation of the camera. The time needed to take 2 x 64 views (one full circle of the twin-headed camera) was about 45 min.

Reconstruction of images

Only one of the two data-sets was used (i.e. data of only one camera head) for the reconstruction and analysis of the SPECT data. SPECT image reconstruction was performed on a Picker Odyssey, using standard filtered backprojection (Ramp filter, slope = 1) and transverse reconstruction with a resulting slice thickness of 6.4 mm — resulting pixel-dimensions were 6.4 by 6.4 mm. Transverse slices were 9-point filtered (4-2-1) and corrected for attenuation.

Selection of the brain volume for analysis

To define the brain volume for the analysis of ^{123}I-IBZM distribution, a 10-slice (64 mm) wide region enclosing the basal ganglia was selected. To eliminate noise from outside the brain which might influence analysis, the outline of the brain was selected and the value of all voxels outside the specified volume set to zero (a 0-mask is applied to the set of selected transverse slices). For analysis of the intensity distribution in the selected brain volume, the intensity values of the voxels in the 10 slices were exported as an ASCII file (with 'Region-draw','Region-apply' and 'Pixel-report' of the Odyssey's PIXIE-Picker International X Window Imaging Environment). A distribution curve (histogram) of number of voxels against intensity was generated using the UNIX commands 'sort -n' and 'uniq -c'. Alternatively, (e.g. in a non-UNIX environment) another algorithm (Matlab[The Math Works]) that does not have to sort the data-array first (see appendix) can be used.

The resulting array was (like the one generated by the UNIX sort -n and uniq -c) not continuous — i.e. not every possible intensity-value is represented. The 'missing' values were interpolated to create a continuous range of intensity values — the correction is 'facultative' and distorts the original information, but only to a negligible degree. To reduce noise in the data, the distribution curve was 3-point filtered (1-2-1). To correct for different brain volumes, the area under the curve was normalised.

The distribution curve represents the distribution of ^{123}I-IBZM in the basal ganglia (striatum) and the 'non-specific' distribution of ^{123}I-IBZM and/or its metabolites in the surrounding brain tissue. Regions of high-intensity values on transversal slices correspond to high-intensity values of the distribution curve, while the background in SPECT images corresponds to 'medium' intensities on the distribution curve.

Scaling of intensities

A general problem of attributing a greyscale or colourmap to images is deciding whether to normalise the maximum intensity to 100% (intensity value) as is the standard approach to viewing SPECT data, or to normalise the intensity data (represented by the distribution curve) with respect to the 'background' intensity, which facilitates inter- and intra-individual comparisons. We applied both methods: the former as a quick and simple means of comparing results with other applications that scale images to 100% (e.g. the Picker Odyssey default setting), the latter to enable us to perform inter- and intra-individual comparisons. Figure 1 scales the maximum intensities of MSAc and

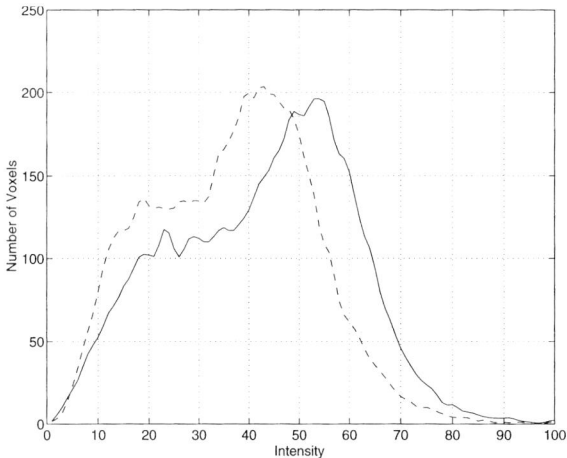

Figure 1 MSAc (solid line) and MSAp (dashed line), maximum intensities scaled to 100%

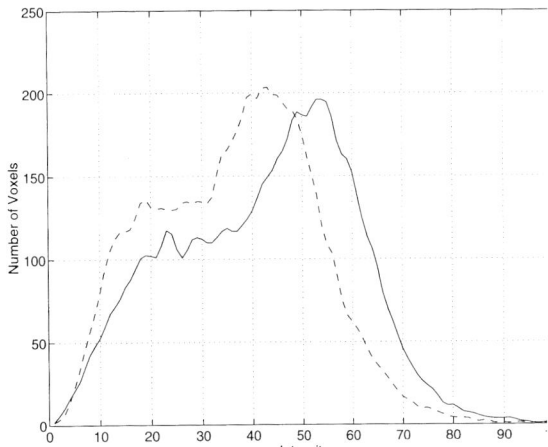

Figure 2 MSAc (solid line) and MSAp (dashed line), distribution curves scaled to background

MSAp to 100%, and the result, due to a higher maximum intensity (respective to MSAc), is a shift of MSAp (the dashed line) to the left (towards the lower intensities). Such distortion of the shape of the distribution curves is avoided when the distribution curves are scaled respective to background intensity, as shown in Figure 2, in which the similarity between MSAc and MSAp is obvious.

Reference curves

To compare the distribution curves of/from individual patients with the reference curves of the different diagnoses, a 'mean' distribution curve was generated from some individual distribution curves for each diagnosis.

Automated allocation to a diagnosis

To reduce observer interaction we implemented an automated allocation of the individual distribution curve to a diagnosis. The comparison of the individual distribution curve with different reference curves can be made with the determination of the degree of similarity by a chi-square test in 80 of 100 data points (from intensity value 10 to 90 per cent if the maximum intensity is scaled to 100% — the first 10% are not useful for a chi-square test because noise can contribute to a substantial part of the data, and the last 10% is similar for all shapes of distribution curve). If the distribution curve is scaled respective to background intensity, the region for the chi-square test must be selected according to the value to which the background value is set. Alternatively, a mathematical model of the form of two exponential functions can be fitted to the distribution curve. An allocation to a

diagnosis can be made by comparing the factors of the model with a reference 'library'.

Results

We found three significantly different shapes of distribution curve for the group of four diagnoses:

- IPS (Figure 3)
- MSAc and MSAp (Figures 4 and 5)
- PSP (Figure 6)

MSAc and MSAp are of similar shape but differ in their absolute intensity (position on the x-axis) (Figure 2). MSAp is in the same position as IPS, but differs markedly in shape.

We found the following 'overlaps' of initial neurological diagnoses and results obtained with the analysis of the distribution of ^{123}I-IBZM and its metabolite(s) in the human brain: IPS 23/30, MSAc 9/11, MSAp 5/7, PSP 6/7.

In a follow-up study of one patient initially diagnosed as IPS, the IBZM SPECT analysis of MSA was confirmed; on the ^{123}I-IBZM SPECT re-scan, a marked reduction of IBZM uptake in the basal ganglia could be seen (result of distribution analysis: MSA).

Elements of the distribution curve

To determine the elements of the distribution curve, ^{123}I-IBZM SPECT images were compared with MRI images with an image overlay tool. The following structures could be assigned to regions of the distribution curve:

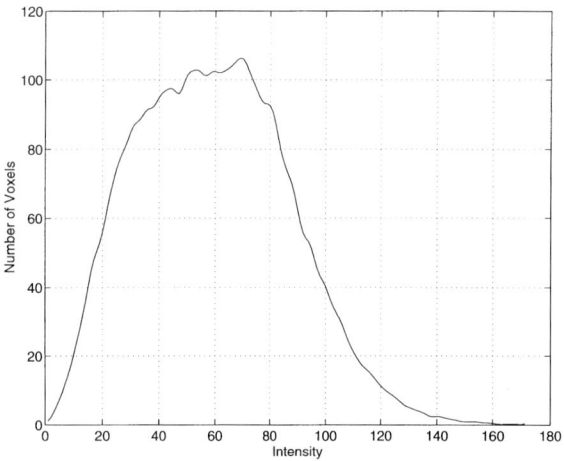

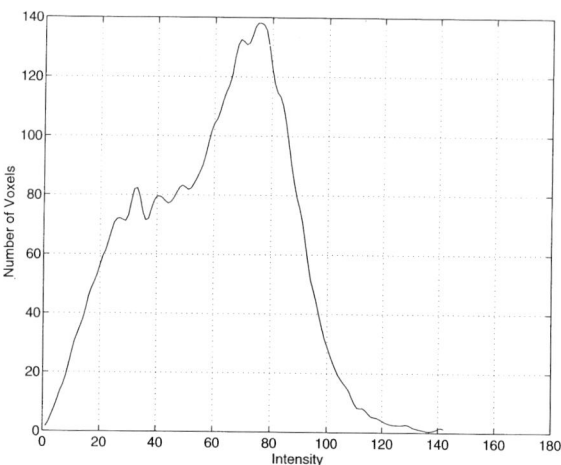

Figure 3 Reference curve IPS, distribution curve scaled to background

Figure 4 Reference curve MSAc, distribution curve scaled to background

1. Region of highest intensities in the distribution curve: basal ganglia (striatum)
2. Region of high intensities: brain grey matter
3. Region of lower to medium intensities: brain white matter.

In the region of lower intensity, noise can comprise a substantial part of the distribution curve.

Discussion

The standard approach to the analysis of IBZM SPECT image data is still a 2-dimensional 'ROI' (region of interest) approach. The region of interest (the striatum) is compared with the mean intensity in a 'background' ROI for which the frontal cortex is mostly used. This approach has a tendency towards unstable intensity values due to the small number of pixels/voxels in the ROIs, and results in unstable overall results. The user interaction required to select slices and to draw ROIs also adds to the statistical uncertainty of the overall results. To overcome the problems associated with small amounts of pixels/voxels, the 2-dimensional ROI was expanded to a 3-dimensional one, enclosing the whole brain volume around the basal ganglia.

Scaling the maximum intensity to 100% (as is usual in a default setting) does not allow for inter- and intra-individual comparisons, because the focus in

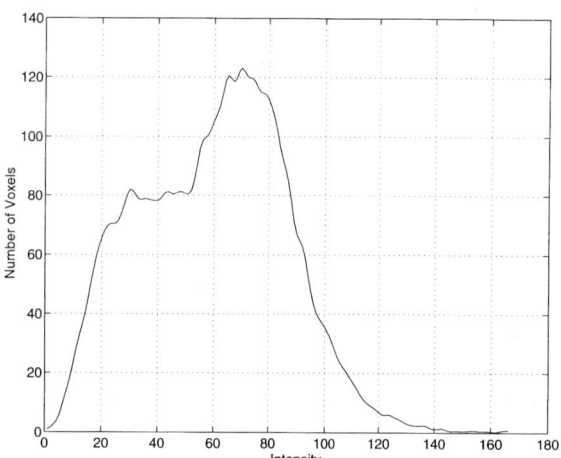

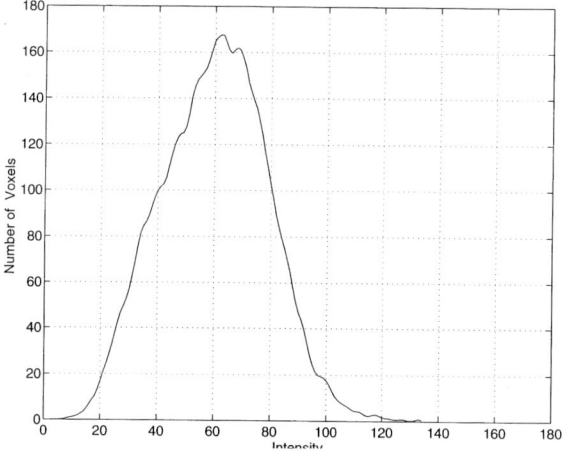

Figure 5 Reference curve MSAp, distribution curve scaled to background

Figure 6 Reference curve PSP, distribution curve scaled to background

^{123}I-IBZM SPECT analysis is on maximum intensities — which change with the progression of the Parkinson's syndromes. To enable inter- and intra-individual comparisons, background intensity should instead be the anchor or reference against which the striatal binding of ^{123}I-IBZM is compared. This background-reference can be determined by fitting an exponential function (Gaussian normal distribution) to the area of the highest intensity frequency of the distribution curve.

The region used as a basis for the discrimination of the different Parkinson's syndromes can not yet be linked to a specific anatomical region in the brain. Dynamic ^{123}I-IBZM SPECT studies will probably be able to answer questions about the shape of the distribution curves. Further studies are needed to fully understand IBZM kinetics, since possible IBZM metabolites can account for the differences in distribution curves in the different Parkinson's syndromes.

Although the effect of ^{123}I-IBZM SPECT distribution curve analysis is not fully understood, it is a very promising approach to the differential diagnosis of Parkinson's syndromes.

Outlook

We tested this method of ^{123}I-IBZM SPECT distribution analysis on IBZM SPECT scans of patients with autosomal dominant cerebellar ataxia (ADCA, n=11) and Huntington's chorea (ChH, n=4). A shape similar to that of PSP patients was found in ADCA patients, and a shape similar to that of IPS patients in ChH patients. As the number of patients is still very small and the ADCA group is heterogeneous, further studies are needed to include these diagnoses in the routine analysis method.

At present we are implementing new algorithms in an attempt to better differentiate the different shapes without having to compare with reference curves. Another project is applying the IBZM distribution analysis to IBZM SPECT scans of patients with hemiparkinsonism in order to detect uptake differences between the right and left basal ganglia.

References

1   Rajput, A.H., Rozdilsky and B., Rayput, A. Accuracy of clinical diagnosis in parkinsonism - a prospective study. *Can. J. Neurol. Sci.* 1991, 18, 275

2   Poewe, W. Clinical features, diagnosis, and imaging of parkinsonian syndromes. *Curr. Opin. Neurol. Neurosurg.* 1993, 6, 333

3   Harding, A.E. Movement disorders in 'Brain's diseases of the nervous system, 10th edn', (Ed. J. Walton), J. Oxford Medical Publishing, Oxford, New York, Tokyo, 1993, p.393

4   Gershon, D. Is there a future for PET? *Nat. Med.* 1995, 1, 494

5   Schelosky, L., Hierholzer, J., Wissel, J. *et al.* Correlation of clinical response in apomorphine test with D2-receptor status as demonstrated by ^{123}I IBZM-SPECT; *Mov. Dis.* 1993, 8, 453

6   Nadeau, S.E., Couch, M.W., Devane, C.L. and Shukla, S.S. Regional analysis of D2 dopamine receptors in Parkinson's disease using SPECT and iodine-123-iodobenzamide. *J. Nucl. Med.* 1995, 36, 384

7   Kung, H.F., Kasliwal, R., Pan, S. *et al.* Dopamine D2 receptor imaging radiopharmaceuticals: synthesis, radiolabeling, and in vitro binding of (R)-(+)- and (S)-(-)-3-iodo-2-hydroxy-6-methoxy-N-[(1-ethyl-2-pyrrolidinyl)-methyl]benzamide. *J. Med. Chem.* 1988, 31, 1039

Appendix

Example for a MATLAB macro as an alternative for the UNIX commands 'sort' and 'count':

Input = data-array of (integer) intensity values; specify borders for non-integers and modify the algorithm;

Output = number of voxels at the intensity of the index

[c_row c_column]=size(input); %dimension of input

maximum_intensity=max(input);

Output=[]; %initialisation of Output

%create an array of the correct length which is filled with zeros

Output(1,:) = zeros(1,maximum_intensity);

help_value = 0;

for n = 1 : c_column

help_value = input(1,n);

if help_value>0

Output(help_value) = Output(help_value)+1;

end

SPECT in Neurology and Psychiatry, edited by P.P. De Deyn, R.A. Dierckx, A. Alavi and B.A. Pickut
© 1997 John Libbey & Company Ltd. pp. 187–194

The Application of [123I]β-CIT and SPECT in the Diagnosis of Movement Disorders

Chapter
23

S. Asenbaum, T. Brücke, W. Pirker,
S. Wenger, I. Podreka and D. Lüder

Introduction

Parkinson's disease (PD) is characterised by a loss of pigmented cells in the substantia nigra and the presence of Lewy bodies[1], whereas in multiple system atrophy (MSA), including striatonigral degeneration, olivopontocerebellar atrophy and the Shy-Drager syndrome, a degeneration without inclusion bodies occurs in the basal ganglia, pontine nuclei, olives, cerebellum and intermediolateral columns of the spinal cord[2]. Nevertheless the existence of parkinsonian symptoms in both diseases makes a differential diagnosis sometimes difficult.

Essential tremor (ET) is usually defined by a postural or kinetic tremor of the hands, head or other parts of the body in the 4- to 9 Hz range[3]. A relationship of this disease to other movement disorders such as PD or dystonia (DT) has been discussed repeatedly[4-10], but neuropathological data did not confirm an association between ET and PD. In contrast to PD, no histological abnormalities have been found in ET[10].

Clinically PD is characterised by resting tremor, rigidity, bradykinesia and postural instability[11]. Additionally, postural tremor similar to that in ET may occur[7]. As patients with ET on the other side often demonstrate a resting tremor component[12] as well, a differentiation of these diseases on clinical parameters may be difficult in some cases.

Postural tremor may also be associated with familial or sporadic dystonia[3,13]. This tremor shows distinct clinical and electromyographic features, but as it can appear without dystonic symptoms[14], differential diagnosis might be difficult. However Dürr *et al.*[5] were able to exclude a genetic entity between ET and DT. Furthermore, dystonic symptoms can occur in several movement disorders together with parkinsonian features[15-19].

Recently a new radiotracer has been developed, labelled with 123I for single photon emission tomography (SPECT): 2β-carbomethoxy-3β(4-iodophenyl) tropane (β-CIT[20], also designated as RTI-55[21]) which is a cocaine derivative, binding selectively to monoamine transporters. In the striatum, specific binding occurs almost exclusively to dopamine (DA) transporters, and binding in the brainstem seems to belong mainly to serotonin (5HT) transporters[22]. In previous studies[23-27], a reduction of striatal β-CIT binding has been demonstrated in patients with PD, reflecting the degeneration of dopaminergic nigrostriatal neurons in this disease.

University of Vienna, Wahringer Gurtel 18-20, A-1090 Wien, Austria

The aim of the present study was to investigate the use of β-CIT and SPECT in the differential diagnosis of movement disorders. The first question was, whether this method offers a new opportunity in differentiating MSA against PD. Secondly the application of β-CIT should be examined in ET, as in early stages of PD and based on clincial data alone a differentiation between these two diseases might be difficult. Furthermore, the question of a predisposition of patients with ET to parkinsonism should be investigated by demonstrating a possible subclinical lesion of dopaminergic nigrostriatal pathways. Additionally, the integrity of the nigrostriatal system should be examined in DT respectively in dystonic tremor, so as to distinguish idiopathic DT from other possible existing movement disorders with dystonic symptoms.

Materials and methods

Patients

Eleven healthy volunteers (2 female, age range 24-72 years, mean age 47), 30 patients with idiopathic PD (12 female, age range 42-82 years, mean age 63), 23 patients with ET (12 female, age range 31-83 years, mean age 60), 4 patients with multiple system atrophy (3 female, age range 49-72 years, mean age 60) and 5 patients with dystonia (3 female, age range 28-52 years, mean age 47) were investigated with β-CIT and SPECT. The volunteers were free of medication and had no neuropsychiatric disorders in their history. The patients were examined neurologically by three experienced physicians (T.B., W.P., S.W.). In the case of PD and MSA respectively, the severity of the disease was classified according to Hoehn and Yahr (H/Y)[11]. None of the patients showed neurological symptoms other than those listed.

PD: 15 of the patients ranged in H/Y stage I, 6 in stage II and 9 in stage III. Nine patients were untreated or stopped therapy 24 h before tracer administration. The remaining 21 patients were allowed to take antiparkinsonian medication with L-DOPA/decarboxylase inhibitor of various doses, in some cases in combination with dopamine agonists or amantadin and anticholinergic drugs except benztropine. Three patients were treated with a low dose neuroleptic medication, and two with a tetracyclic antidepressant. Therapy with l-(-)-deprenyl was withdrawn at least 18 h before β-CIT application.

MSA: The clinical data are listed in Table 1. Four patients were classified in H/Y stage III, 1 pt in H/Y IV. A previous assessment of postsynaptic D_2 receptor density with benzamides had revealed a degeneration of striatal neurons. In one patient, magnetic resonance tomography demonstrated an atrophy of the cerebellum and the midbrain areas. All patients were under antiparkinsonian (see above) as well as antidepressant therapy with 5HT re-uptake blockers.

ET: The clinical data are listed in Table 2. According to the diagnostic criteria of the Tremor Investigation Group[28] 9 patients were classified as definite ET, 4 patients as probable and 10 patients as possible ET. None received tremor therapy. Cerebral computed tomography (cCT) was normal in all cases.

DT: The clinical data are listed in Table 3. One patient was under antidepressant therapy with a 5HT re-uptake blocker together with a tetracyclic antidepressant. No abnormalities were seen in cCT.

The study was approved by the local ethical committee and informed consent was obtained from each person.

Table 1 Clinical data of patients with multiple system atrophy

Number	Age,gender	EPS[a]	Cereb.[b]	Auton.[c]	Pyr.[d]	H/Y	Dur.[e]
1	63,f	+		+	+	III	5
2	57,f	+	+	+		III	2
3	49,m		+	++	+	IV	5
4	72,f	++	+	+	+	III	2

[a], extrapyramidal symptoms; [b], cerebellar symptoms; [c], autonomic failure; [d], pyramidal signs; [e], duration of the disease

Table 2 Clinical data of patients with essential tremor, classified into definite, probable or possible essential tremor

Number	Age,gender	Postural tremor	Kinetic tremor	Resting tremor	Local.[a]	Dur.[b]	Fam.hist[c]	Remarks
Definite								
1	74,m	++	++	+	U,M	10	-	
2	76,f	+	+	+	U,r>l	10	+	
3	72,f	+		+	U	5	-	
4	83,m	++	++	+	U,l>r	70	+	
5	56,m	+			U	45	+	
6	51,f	+	+		U	10	+	
7	63,m	+	+		U,L	40	+	
8	81,m	++	+	+	U	10	-	
9	34,m	+		+	U,l>r	10	-	
Probable								
1	31,m	+	+		U,H	4	+	
2	61,f	+	+	+	U,r>l	3	n.k.	
3	68,m	+		+	U,r>l	3	-	
4	43,f	+		+	U,H	4	n.k.	
Possible								
1	47,f	+		+	U,r>l	2	+	
2	74,f	+	+	++	U	1	n.k.	
3	33,m	++	+		U,r>l	0.25	-	
4	58,f	+	+		U ,r>l	2	-	PD+[d]
5	72,f	++	+	++	U,H	1	n.k.	
6	67,f	+			U,l<r	0.25	-	
7	72,m	+		+	U	0.5	-	
8	76,f	+		+	U	0.3	-	
9	39,f	+		+	U	1	-	
10	48,m	+		+	U	0.4	-	

[a], tremor localisation, A: U/L, upper/lower extremities; l, left; r, right; M, mouth; H, head; [b], duration of the disease; [c], familial history of essential tremor: n.k., not known; [d], positive familial history of Parkinson's disease

SPECT investigation

After blockade of thyroid uptake, subjects received a mean dose of 3.76 mCi (139 MBq) (range 2.57-5.38 mCi) of [123I]β-CIT intravenously as a bolus. All subjects were investigated 20 h after tracer administration. SPECT studies were performed with a triple-headed rotating scintillation camera (Siemens Multispect 3, FWHM 9 mm) equipped with medium-energy collimators and a dedicated computer system. Images lasted for 40 min (40 s per frame), so that 180 frames in a step and shoot mode were collected. The subject's head was positioned in a head holder using a crossed laser beam system for repositioning. Parallel to the cantho-meatal plane 3.5 mm thick cross sections were reconstructed by filtered back projection in 128x128 matrices using a Butterworth filter. Attenuation correction was then performed with a uniform attenuation coefficient of 0.12/cm after manual drawing an ellipse around the head contour.

Regions of interest (ROI) were drawn manually on single slice views by one investigator (A.S.) over the right and left striatum (size: 40-45 pixels each) and the cerebellum respectively (size: 50-55 pixels each), using a brain atlas for help. Striatal ROIs were drawn on the slice with highest activity, cerebellar ROIs on the slice of best visualisation, usually 10 slices below the striatum. Right and left cerebellar values were pooled together, as well as striatal values. Cerebellar values were taken as reference, as previous studies[24] as well as post mortem studies[7,29] had shown very low densities of DA and 5HT transporters in this region. For semiquantification, two different methods of describing brain activity were applied: 1) the ratio target over cerebellum minus 1 (which is specific/non-specific binding) based on average counts/pixel values as a measure of specific binding was calculated ([total non-specific activity/non-specific activity=total/non-specific activity-1], according to Leenders *et al.*[30]); 2) age-matched control values were obtained from regression analysis of the data of the volunteers. The percentage deviation of each patient's ratio from these age matched control values was calculated.

Statistics

The ratios of the striatal ROIs were compared between the groups of ET as well as between the control group and the patient groups using an one-way ANOVA. Additionally, patients with PD in H/Y stage I were compared with ET patients, and patients in H/Y III with the MSA group.

Results

Visual evaluation

In all patients with PD, high activities could be seen in the caudate nucleus, whereas the putamen could hardly be differentiated. Three patients with MSA demonstrated a similar Parkinsonian binding pattern. In one patient (number 3), an overall reduced striatal ß-CIT binding was evident. No abnormalities in the visualisation of the basal ganglia could be detected in ET or DT (see Figures 1 and 2).

Comparison between ET groups

The mean ratios of the three ET groups did not differ significantly (definite ET: r=7.8, probable ET: r=9.9, possible ET: r=9.0; F=2.9, p<0.08), so that for further calculations the values of the ET patients were pooled together.

Table 3 Clinical data of patients with dystonia

Number	Age,gender	Local.[a]	Dur.[b]	Remarks
1	28,m	torticoll	6	fam +[c]
2	52,f	torticoll,bleph	6	
3	49,f	torticoll	5	
4	32,m	U,r	1	
5	39,f	U,r	4	

[a], localization: torticoll, toricollis spasticus; bleph, blepharospasm; U, upper extremities; r, right; [b], duration of the disease; [c], positive familial history of dystonia

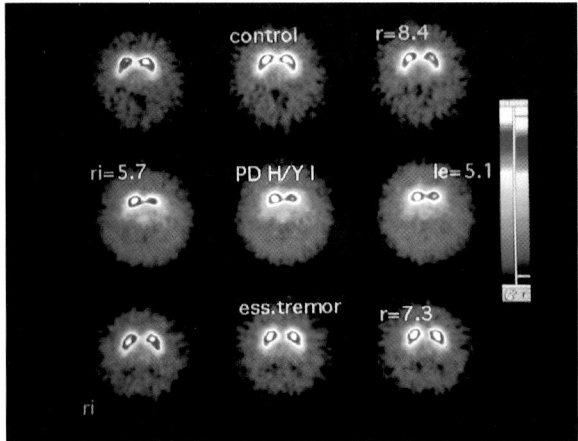

Figure 1 [123I]β-CIT SPECT study of a control person (first row), a patient with Parkinson´s disease (PD) in stage Hoehn and Yahr (H/Y) I (second row) and a patient with essential (ess.) tremor (third row). Studies are scaled on their own maximum. The ratio striatum/cerebellum is listed for each patient, for the patient with PD additionally for the left (le) and right (ri) side

Comparison PD / MSA / ET / DT versus control group

The comparison of the ratio striatum/cerebellum between the investigated groups is shown in Figure 3 (control: r=7.46(+-1.2); PD: r=3.8(+-1.0); ET: r=8.72(+-1.7); MSA: r=2.90(+-0.2); DT: r=9.1(+-3.6)).

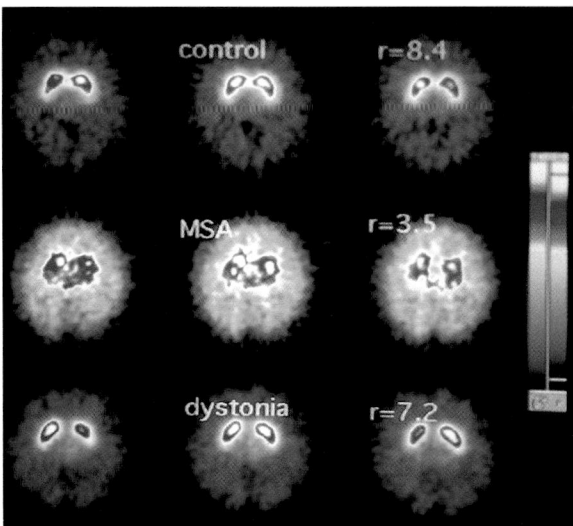

Figure 2 [123I]β-CIT SPECT study of a control person (first row), a patient with multiple system atrophy (MSA) (second row) and a patient with dystonia (third row). Studies are scaled on their own maximum. The ratio striatum/cerebellum is listed for each patient

ANOVA between the groups was significant (F=40.0, p<0.0001). Values of controls or patients with ET or DT did not differ significantly, but were significantly higher than values of patients with PD or MSA (f.e.: control versus PD: F=19.4, p<0.0001; PD versus ET: F=36.1, p<0.0001; control versus ET: F=0.06, n.s.; control versus DT: F=0.02, n.s.; PD versus MSA: F=0.05, n.s.). Additionally, a significant difference was found between PD patients in H/Y I and patients with ET (F=14.8, p<0.04), whereas no difference was obvious between PD patients in H/Y III and patients with MSA (F=0.01, n.s.).

Patients with PD demonstrated a percentage decrease of β-CIT binding in the striatum of 44% in comparison to age corresponding control values. Patients with MSA showed a decrease of 58%.

Discussion

Parkinson´s disease has been investigated repeatedly with PET and various tracers such as ^{18}F-DOPA[30-32] or DA transporter labelling substances[30,32-34]. In these studies, a reduction of DOPA decarboxylase activity could have been delineated. A reduction of DA reuptake sites in the striatum, mainly in the posterior putamen, could be demonstrated, indicating a degeneration of dopaminergic nigrostriatal pathways. Similar results in PD have been obtained recently with SPECT using the cocaine derivative β-CIT[23,24,26,27]. Patients with PD demonstrate a significantly reduced specific β-CIT binding as a measure of dopaminergic nerve terminals in the striatum, mainly in the putamen, which correlates with the severity of the disease[25].

In the present study this method has been applied in patients with MSA, and it was possible to show a significantly reduced striatal β-CIT binding. Specific binding did not differ between PD patients and MSA, respectively, between PD in H/Y III and MSA, although lower ratios and a more pronounced reduction in comparison to age-related norm values were found in the MSA group. Brooks *et al.*[31] also described a more pronounced reduction of striatal ^{18}F-DOPA uptake in MSA than in PD within the same range of locomotor disability classified according to Hoehn and Yahr. In a PET investigation with S-[11C]nomifensine, which binds to DA transporters, a diminished specific binding in the basal ganglia was evident in PD and MSA[32].

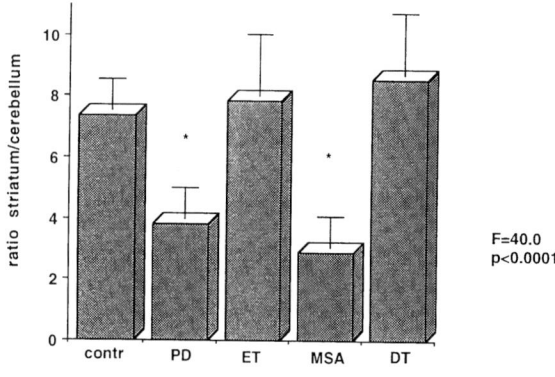

Figure 3 Comparison of the ratio striatum/cerebellum as a measure of specific binding between control persons (contr), patients with Parkinson's disease (PD), essential tremor (ET), multiple system atrophy (MSA) and dystonia (DT). (*) indicates a significant difference with at least p<0.001

In PD, regional distribution of ^{18}F-DOPA or S-[^{11}C]nomifensine shows a distinct pattern with maximal reduction of tracer uptake in the posterior putamen with relative sparing of the caudate[30-33] caused by a pronounced degeneration of the ventrolateral sustantia nigra[35,36]. In contrast to PD the evaluation in MSA demonstrated a more heterogeneous pattern of regional tracer distribution in the striatum[31,32]. This finding has been obtained visually only in 1 out of 4 patients in the present study. The investigated patient with MSA (clinically an olivopontocerebellar degeneration) did not demonstrate a classical PD pattern of striatal β-CIT binding, but a more diffuse reduction of tracer uptake. This would be in accordance with pathological data, where a more global nigral degeneration is described[37], consequently leading to a more widespread disruption of the dopaminergic nigrostriatal system. For confirmation of this result in the remaining 3 patients with MSA, a separate evaluation of β-CIT binding in the caudate and the putamen would be necessary.

Investigations with β-CIT and SPECT did not demonstrate any abnormality in ET. Specific binding, even when compared with age-related norm values, as well as the striatal binding pattern, was similar to the control group. No differences existed between the ET groups classified according to the recommendations of the Tremor Investigation Group[28]. β-CIT and SPECT therefore offer a valuable tool in diagnosing ET even in uncertain cases i.e. with short duration of the disease or in patients with other neurological disorders. Normal dopaminergic function has been described before in patients with familial ET using ^{18}F-DOPA[38].

Furthermore, a clear distinction of striatal β-CIT binding as well as the binding pattern, was evident between PD even in stage H/Y I and ET. No sign of nigrostriatal degeneration was obvious in ET. This makes an early differentiation of PD/ET possible. The results do not give evidence for an association between ET and PD, and are in accordance with experimental animal studies, which suggest the inferior olive rather than the extrapyramidal system as the principal generator of postural tremor[39,40]. No subclinical involvement of the nigrostriatal pathways could be found in the investigated patients with ET. Brooks et al.[38] have described reduced ^{18}F-DOPA uptake in the putamen in one patient with sporadic postural tremor, who developed PD symptoms later on. As the applied method in the present study has already been successful in demonstrating a subclinical affection of the nigrostriatal dopaminergic system contralateral to the clinically unaffected side in hemiparkinsonism[25], it might be argued that the patients in this study did not seem to have a higher predisposition for PD. This finding supports epidemiological studies, where no higher risk for PD was found in patients with ET[4,9], but contradicts clinical experience that cases with a history of essential tremor sometimes actually do develop PD.

Patients with DT, which can be regarded as idiopathic due to the absence of other neurological abnormalities and normal CT scans, showed no pathological changes of dopaminergic nigrostriatal pathways. Striatal β-CIT binding did not differ between DT and the control group.

Besides the idiopathic form of dystonia, various pathogenic mechanisms for symptomatic dystonia have been described, for example alterations of the basal ganglia, the thalamus or the peripheral nervous system. Dystonia can be found additionally in other movement disorders. DT is described in early-onset parkinsonism[15], juvenile-onset parkinsonism with DT[16,17], hemiparkinsonism-hemiatrophy[18], progressive supranuclear palsy (PSP) or MSA[19]. In a case study, Lewy bodies could be found post mortem in the substantia nigra in a patient with Meige syndrome[41]. In all these cases, an investigation with β-CIT and SPECT would be helpful in demonstrating or excluding a dopaminergic lesion underlying the dystonic symptoms. It has already been possible to differentiate successfully another dystonic disease from PD i.e. the DOPA-responsive dystonia from PD, using ^{18}F-DOPA and PET[42].

In conclusion β-CIT and SPECT has proven to be a new and valuable tool in the investigation of movement disorders. Reduced specific binding can be found in PD and MSA, whereas no abnormalities are evident in ET or DT. Even in the early stages of PD, a dopaminergic lesion can be detected mainly in the putamen. Similar findings are obtained in MSA, but here a more diffusely altered binding pattern than in PD could be seen as well. Both, resting and postural tremor may occur in PD and ET, which can make clinical differentiation difficult. The application of β-CIT allows an earlier differential diagnosis between PD and ET. In dystonic syndromes β-CIT can help to distinguish between idiopathic and symptomatic DT forms.

References

1   Duvoisin, R. and Golbe, L.I. Towards a definition of Parkinson´s disease. *Neurology* 1989, 39, 746

2   Daniel, S.E. The neuropathology and neurochemistry of multiple system atrophy in ' Autonomic failure: a textbook of clinical disorders of the autonomic nervous system', (Eds. R. Bannister, C.J. Mathias), Oxford University Press, Oxford, UK, 1992, p. 564

3   Hubble, J., Busenbark, K. and Koller, W.C. Essential tremor. *Clin. Neuropharmacol.* 1989, 12, 453

4   Cleeves, L., Findley, L.J. and Koller, W. Lack of association between essential tremor and Parkinson´s disease. *Ann. Neurol.* 1988, 24, 23

5   Dürr, A., Stevanin, G., Jedynak, C.P. *et al.* Familial essential tremor and idiopathic torsion dystonia are different genetic entities. *Neurology* 1993, 43, 2212

6   Geraghty, J.J., Jankovic, J. and Zetusky, W.J. Association between essential tremor and Parkinson´s disease. *Ann. Neurol.* 1985, 17, 329

7   Koller,W.C., Overfield, B.V. and Barter, R. Tremor in early Parkinson's disease. *Clin. Neuropharmacol.* 1989, 12, 293

8   Koller, W.C., Busenbark, K. and Miner, K. The relationship of essential tremor to other movement disorders: report on 678 patients. *Ann. Neurol.* 1994, 35, 717

9   Pahwa, R. and Koller, W.C. Is there a relationship between Parkinson's disease and essential tremor? *Clin. Neuropharmacol.* 1993, 16, 30

10 Rajput, A.H., Rodilsky, B., Ang., and Rajput, A. Significance of Parkinsonian manifestations in essential tremor. *Can. J. Neurol. Sci.* 1993, 20, 114

11 Hoehn, M.M. and Yahr, M.D. Parkinsonism: onset, progression, and mortality. *Neurology* 1967, 17, 427

12 Salisachs, P. and Findley, L.J. Problems in differential diagnosis of essential tremor in 'Movement Disorders: Tremor', (Eds. L.J. Findley and R. Capildeo), MacMillan Press, London, UK, 1984, p.214

13 Yanagisawa, N., Goto, A. and Narabayashi, H. Familial dystonia musculorum deformans and tremor. *J. Neurol. Sci.* 1972, 16, 125

14 Jedynak, C.P., Bonnet, A.M. and Agid, Y. Tremor and idiopathic dystonia. *Movement Disorders* 1991, 6, 230

15 Dwork, A.J., Balmaceda, C., Fazzini, E.A. *et al.* Dominantly inherited, early-onset parkinsonism: neuropathology of a new form. *Neurology* 1993, 43, 69

16 Gibb, W.R. Neuropathology of the substantia nigra. *Eur. Neurol.* 1991, 31(1), 48

17 Gibb, W.R. New pathological observations in juvenile onset parkinsonism with dystonia. *Neurology* 1991, 41, 820

18 Giladi, N., Burke, R.E., Kostic, V. *et al.* Hemiparkinsonism-hemiatrophy syndrome; clinical and neuroradiological features. *Neurology* 1991, 40, 1731

19 Rivest, J., Quinn, N. and Marsden, C.D. Dystonia in Parkinson's disease, multiple system atrophy, and progressive supranuclear palsy. *Neurology* 1990, 40, 1571

20 Neumayer, J.L., Wang, S., Milius, R.A. *et al.* [^{123}I]2β-carboxymethoxy-3β-(4-iodophenyl)trpane (β-CIT): high affinity SPECT radiotracer of monoamine re-uptake sites in brain. *J. Med. Chem.* 1991, 34,3144

21 Shaya, E.K., Scheffel, U., Dannals, R.F. *et al.* In vivo imaging of dopamine reuptake sites in the primate brain using single photon emission computed tomography (SPECT) and iodine-123 labeled RTI-55. *Synapse* 1992, 10, 169

22 Laruelle, M., Baldwin, R.M., Malinson, R.T. *et al.* SPECT imaging of dopamine and serotonin transporters with [123I]β-CIT: pharmacological characterization of brain uptake in non-human primates. *Synapse* 1993, 13, 295

23 Asenbaum, S., Brücke, T., Pozzera, A. *et al.* Degeneration of striatal dopaminergic neurons in Parkinson´s disease visualized and quantified by [123I]ß-CIT and SPECT. *Eur. J. Nucl. Med.* 1994, 21, 848

24 Brücke, T., Kornhuber, J., Angelberger, P. *et al.* SPECT imaging of dopamine and serotonin transporters with [123I]ß-CIT. Binding kinetics in the human brain. *J. Neural. Transm. [GenSect]* 1993, 94, 137

25 Brücke, T., Asenbaum, S., Pirker, W. *et al.* Quantification of the dopaminergic nerve cell loss in Parkinson´s disease with [123I]β-CIT and SPECT. *J. Cereb. Blood Flow Metab.* 1995, 10(1), 37

26 Innis, R.B., Seibyl, J.P., Scanley, B.E. *et al.* Single photon emission computed tomographic imaging demonstrates loss of striatal dopamine transporters in Parkinson's disease. *Proc. Natl. Acad. Sci. USA* 1993, 90, 11965

27 Kuikka, J.T., Bergstrom, K.A., Vanninen, E. *et al.* Initial experiences with single photon emission tomography using iodine-123-labelled 2β-carbomethoxy-3β-(4-iodophenyl)-tropane in human brain. *Eur. J. Nucl. Med.* 1993, 20, 783

28 Findley, L.J. Classification of tremors. *J. Clin. Neurophysiol.* 1996, 13, 122

29 DeKeyser, J., DeBacker, J.-P., Ebinger, G. and Vauquelin, G. [3H]GBR-12935 binding to dopamine uptake sites in the human brain. *J. Neurochem.* 1989, 53, 1400

30 Leenders, K.L., Salmon, E.P., Tyrrell, P. *et al.* The nigrostriatal dopaminergic system assessed in vivo by positron emission tomography in healthy volunteer subjects and patients with Parkinson's disease. *Arch. Neurol.* 1990, 47, 1290

31 Brooks, D.J., Ibanez, V., Sawle, G.V. *et al.* Differing patterns of striatal ^{18}F-dopa uptake in Parkinson's disease, multiple system atrophy, and progressive supranuclear palsy. *Ann. Neurol.* 1990, 28, 547

32 Brooks, D.J., Salmon, E.P., Mathias, C.J. *et al.* The relationship between locomotor disability, autonomic dysfunction, and the integrity of the striatal dopaminergic system in patients with multiple system atrophy, pure autonomic failure, and Parkinson's disease, studied with PET. *Brain* 1990, 113, 1539

33 Frost, J.J., Rosier, A.J., Reich, S.G. *et al.* Positron emission tomography imaging of the dopamine transporter with 11C-WIN 35,428 reveals marked declines in mild Parkinson's disease. *Ann. Neurol.* 1993, 3, 423

34 Kaufman, M.J. and Madras, B.K. Severe depletion of cocaine recognition sites associated with the dopamine transporter in Parkinson's diseased striatum. *Synapse* 1991, 49, 43

35 German, D.C., Manaye, K., Smith, W.K. *et al.* Midbrain dopaminergic cell loss in Parkinson's disease: computer visualization. *Ann. Neurol.* 1989, 26, 507

36 Goto, S., Hirano, A. and Matsumoto, S. Subdivisional involvement of nigrostriatal loop in idiopathic Parkinson´s disease and striatonigral degeneration. *Ann. Neurol.* 1989, 26, 766

37 Bannister, R. and Oppenheimer, D.R. Degenerative diseases of the nervous system associated with autonomic failure. *Brain* 1972, 95, 457

38 Brooks, D.J., Playford, E.D., Ibanez, V. *et al.* Isolated tremor and disruption of the nigrostriatal dopaminergic system: an ^{18}F-dopa PET study. *Neurology* 1992, 42, 1554

39 Lamarre, Y. and Joffroy, A.J. Experimental tremor in the monkey: activity of thalamic and precentral cortical neurons in the absence of peripheral feedback. *Adv. Neurol.* 1979, 24, 109

40 Poirier, L.J., Sourkes, T.L., Bouvier, G. *et al.* Striatal amines, experimental tremor, and the effect of harmaline in the monkey. *Brain* 1966, 89, 37

41 Mark, M.H., Sage, J.I., Dickson, D.W. *et al.* Meige syndrome in the spectrum of Lewy body disease. *Neurology* 1994, 44, 1432

42 Turjanski, N., Bhatia, K., Burn, D.J. *et al.* Comparison of striatal ^{18}F-dopa uptake in adult-onset dystonia-parkinsonism, Parkinson's disease, and dopa-responsive dystonia. *Neurology* 1993, 43, 1563

SPECT in Neurology and Psychiatry, edited by P.P. De Deyn, R.A. Dierckx, A. Alavi and B.A. Pickut

Quantification of Dopaminergic Nerve Cell Loss in Parkinson's Disease and Ageing with [^{123}I]β-CIT and SPECT

Chapter

24

T. Brücke, S. Asenbaum, W. Pirker, S. Djamshidian,
S. Wenger, Ch. Wöber, Ch. Müller, I. Podreka and
P. Angelberger*

Introduction

Over the past decade, imaging of the presynaptic part of the dopaminergic nigrostriatal system has been a domain of PET. Several PET studies[1-5] using ^{18}F-DOPA as a tracer demonstrated the dopaminergic degeneration in Parkinson's disease (PD) *in vivo* and showed a good correlation with clinical parameters. Only recently has a group of cocaine analogues with very high affinity for dopamine transporters located on dopaminergic terminals been described[6]. These compounds can also be labelled with gamma-emitting isotopes and can thus be used for SPECT. Although PET remains the gold standard for studies of *in vivo* receptor function, SPECT has the advantage of wider applicability and, thus, greater clinical use.

PD is a slowly progressing neurodegenerative disorder with a loss of dopaminergic neurons in the substantia nigra which leads to a loss of dopaminergic nerve endings and to a marked reduction of the dopamine content in the striatum. It is characterised by symptoms such as resting tremor, akinesia, rigidity and postural instability. Typically, symptoms start asymmetrically on one body-side, gradually affect both sides, and usually respond well to L-DOPA. Although these symptoms are very characteristic, the differential diagnosis to other extrapyramidal syndromes can, in many cases, be difficult. A clinico-pathological study recently reported that the clinical diagnosis of PD was only correct in about 80% of cases — even when strict diagnostic criteria had been used[7]. It may be that this figure would be even lower for those patients diagnosed by physicians less familiar with the disorder. It is clinical experience that many patients with vascular encephalopathies and also patients with essential tremor are misdiagnosed as PD and have often received unnecessary antiparkinsonian treatment for years. Thus, there is a real need for an objective diagnostic test for PD.

Because the evaluation of disease progression based on clinical neurological examinations is often difficult due to the effects of antiparkinsonian treatment, there is also a need for an objective measure of dopaminergic nerve cell loss *in vivo* with which to assess the course of disease progression and evaluate possible neuroprotective strategies.

Dopamine transporters are located presynaptically on the dopaminergic nerve endings that are lost in PD — demonstrated *in vitro* in post mortem human brain studies[8,9]. The labelling of these transporter sites *in vivo* can thus be used to measure the integrity of the nigrostriatal dopaminergic system. A loss of dopamine uptake sites in PD has been described *in vivo* with the PET ligand [^{11}C]nomifensine[10,11]. PET studies with one of the cocaine derivatives

University of Vienna and Seibersdorf Research Centre, Austria mentioned above, the [^{11}C]-labelled tropane analogue WIN 35428 (CFT), have also demonstrated reduced binding in patients with PD [12]. 2-β-Carbomethoxy-3-β-(4-iodophenyl)-tropane (β-CIT, RTI 55) is an iodinated analogue of the originally described fluoro-derivative CFT, which has the advantage of further increased affinity for monoamine transporters and low non-specific binding [13,14]. This tracer has been extensively characterised in animal experiments [15-19], and its binding studied in post mortem human brain samples [20,21].

SPECT studies with [^{123}I]-labelled β-CIT in patients with PD have shown that it is possible to visualise and quantify the loss of dopaminergic nerve endings in this disorder and that the results correlate well with clinical measures of disease severity, motor impairment and asymmetry of symptomatology [22-31]. The aim of the present study was to extend the findings in a larger number of patients and to correlate subscores of different symptoms with [^{123}I]β-CIT binding data.

Another aspect of the present work was to study the effects of ageing on the presynaptic part of the dopaminergic system. Ageing is associated with a loss in motor function which probably reflects an age-related decline of the function of the nigrostriatal dopaminergic system [32]. *In vitro*, such changes have been described on the pre- and postsynaptic sides, and these findings have been replicated by *in vivo* imaging studies. Most of the latter have concentrated on the postsynaptic side where a decline of D$_2$ receptor density with age has consistently been described [33,34]. Changes of the presynaptic part of the dopaminergic system with ageing have been studied using ^{18}F-DOPA and PET, but the results have been contradictory [35-37]. One SPECT study using [^{123}I]β-CIT clearly demonstrated a dopamine transporter loss with increasing age, thus confirming previous post mortem results [38], and similar findings have been reported in preliminary form by our own group [29].

Subjects and methods

Patients and controls

The control group consisted of 13 healthy volunteers and patients with peripheral neurological disorders (7 volunteers, 6 patients; 7 male, 6 female; average age 51.1 ±20.4, range 26-75 yrs).

A large group of patients with PD was studied (n=113; 75 male, 38 female; average age 65.2 ±11.5, range 39-85 yrs). All fulfilled Hughes *et al.*'s clinical criteria for the diagnosis of PD [7] and were responsive to L-DOPA. Enough clinical information was available

Table 1 Clinical data of controls and patients

Groups	n	Age (range)	m/f
Controls	13	51.1 ± 20.4 (26-75)	7/6
Parkinson (stage 1 - 5)	113	65.2 ± 11.5 (39-85)	75/38
Essential tremor	21	62.9 ± 10.6 (46 - 85)	9/12

in 80 patients to determine disease severity according to Hoehn and Yahr [39]: 29 patients were in stage I (mean age 62.5 yrs), 8 in stage II (mean age 60.3 yrs), 27 in stage III (mean age 68.2 yrs), 14 in stage IV (mean age 67.9 yrs) and 2 in stage V (mean age 74 yrs). Of these 80, 61 were rated with the Unified Parkinson's Disease Rating Scale (UPDRS) [40] at the time of their SPECT examination. Patients were allowed to take antiparkinsonian medication on the day of tracer administration with the exception of L-deprenyl and benztropine which were stopped at least 18 h before. Patients on antiparkinsonian medication had their clinical ratings performed in the early afternoon.

The influence of increasing age was also examined in a group of patients with essential tremor (n=21; 9 male, 12 female; average age: 62.9 ±10.6, range 46-85 yrs). Detailed clinical criteria are described in another chapter of this book [41].

Table 1 lists the demographic data of both control and patient groups. The study was approved by the local ethics committee and informed consent obtained from each subject.

SPECT study

After blockade of thyroid uptake with 600 mg sodium perchlorate orally 30 min before tracer application, subjects received a mean dose of 140 MBq (3.8mCi) (range 104-222MBq; 2.6-5.4 mCi) of [^{123}I]β-CIT i.v. as a bolus.

SPECT studies were performed using a 3-headed rotating scintillation camera (Siemens Multispect 3, FWHM 9mm) equipped with medium-energy collimators. The subject's head was positioned in the head holder by means of a crossed laser beam system.

Because earlier studies in our group had shown a binding equilibrium at this time-point [25,31], the patients and all controls were studied 20 h after i.v. injection of the tracer. Imaging lasted 40 min. For each scan a total of 180 frames (40 s per frame) was obtained in a step-and-shoot mode. Cross-sections with a thickness of 3.5 mm orientated parallel to the cantho-meatal plane were reconstructed by filtered back projection (Butterworth filter cutoff frequency 0.7, order 7) in 128 x 128 matrices. Attenuation correction was performed with a uniform attenuation coefficient of 0.12/cm, after manually drawing an ellipse around the head contour. Irregular regions of interest (ROIs) were drawn manually on single slice views in areas corresponding to the left and right striatum (size: 40 to 45 pixels each) and the cerebellar hemispheres on either side (55 to 60 pixels each). All ROIs were drawn with the help of a brain atlas by the same examiner. Counts in striatal regions were calculated in several consecutive 3.5 mm-thick axial slices and the highest value for each striatum was taken to avoid tilting errors. The two striatal ROIs were pooled together and average counts per pixel calculated.

Cerebellar ROIs were drawn on the slice of best visualisation, usually 10 slices below the maximal activity in the striatum and in the two adjacent slices. Left and right cerebellar values were pooled and the average values from the 3 slices taken as the reference region. Cerebellar activity was assumed to represent non-specific bound and free radioactivity because it is known that the cerebellum has a very low density of dopamine and 5HT transporters. A ratio was calculated between average count-rates in the striatum and the cerebellum for analysis. This ratio minus 1 represents specific/non-displaceable binding and, during a period of binding equilibrium, it is directly related to the binding potential. Patients' data were compared with age-corrected control values obtained via regression analysis of control group data according to the formula: $y = -0.036x + 9.067$, where y = age-corrected ratio and x = age of patient. The percentage deviation of each patient's ratio from this age-corrected control value was calculated.

Statistics

Binding ratios of controls and patients were compared with a 2-tailed student's t-test for unpaired samples, and contra-and ipsilateral striata in hemiparkinsonian patients with a t-test for paired samples. Clinical rating scores and disease severity scores as well as age were correlated to the [123I]β-CIT binding ratios with regression analysis. A one-way ANOVA was used to evaluate differences between the PD groups with different disease severities and between contra- and ipsilateral striata in patients with hemiparkinsonism and controls.

Values are given as mean ±s.d. (range), and $p<0.05$ was considered statistically significant.

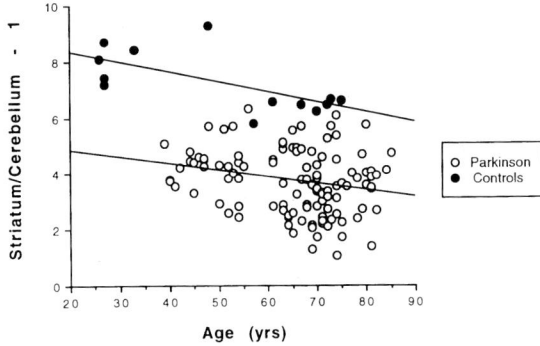

Figure 1 Specific/non-displaceable (Striatum/Cerebellum -1) binding ratio of [123I]β-CIT in the whole striatum (left and right pooled together) in the control group (filled circles, n=13) and in patients with Parkinson's disease (open circles, n=113) plotted against age. A marked reduction of the ratio is seen in the patient group (3.71 ±1.15 versus 7.22 ±1.08; p<0.0001; patients versus controls) with overlap in only a few cases with hemiparkinsonism. A significant age-dependent decline in [123I]β-CIT binding was found in the control goup (4.9% of the mean ratio per decade; R= -0.68; p=0.01) and was also seen less significantly in the PD group (R= -0.2; p=0.036)

Results

Figure 1 gives the results in the total group of PD patients (n=113). There was a highly significant difference between the PD group compared with the controls (n=13) in the specific/non-displaceable binding ratio of the whole striatum (left and right pooled together), and almost no overlap of data (3.71 ±1.15 versus 7.22 ±1.08; p<0.0001; PD versus controls). The percentage reduction compared with age-corrected values was 45%.

A significant age-dependent decline in [123I]β-CIT binding was found in the control goup (4.9% of the mean ratio per decade; R =-0.68; p=0.01) and was also seen, less significantly, in the PD group (R =-0.2; p=0.036).

In hemiparkinsonian patients (n=29), the comparison of specific/non-displaceable binding in the whole striatum contralaterally and ipsilaterally to the affected body side revealed a highly significant difference (4.05 ±0.76 and 4.79±0.096; p=0.0001; contra-and ipsilaterally, respectively). Ratios were also significantly reduced on both sides in comparison to controls (p=0.0001). The percentage reduction compared with age-corrected values was 41% contralaterally and 30% ipsilaterally (Figure 2).

Figure 3 shows the correlation of [123I]β-CIT binding ratios and disease severity according to Hoehn and

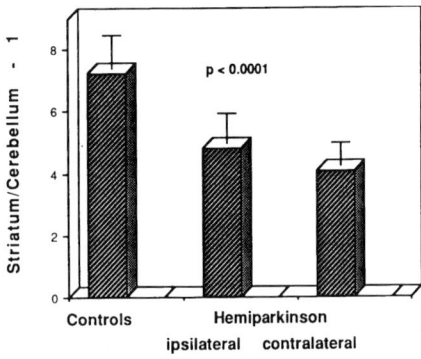

Figure 2 Specific/non-displaceable striatal binding ratio of [^{123}I]β-CIT in controls and patients with hemiparkinsonism (n=29) ipsi-and contralaterally to the affected body side. Reduction on the ipsilateral side 30% and on the contralateral side 41% of age-corrected control values (4.79 ±0.096 ipsi, 4.05 ±0.76 contra; p=0.0001; mean ±s.d.)

Yahr. A highly significant negative correlation was found (R =-0.66; p=0.0001). ANOVA also revealed a highly significant difference between groups (F = 15.9; p=0.0001; group 1 versus 3, 4 and 5, group 2 versus 4 and 5, group 3 versus 4 and 5). Reductions compared with age-corrected values were 35% in stage 1, 46% in stage 2, 48% in stage 3, 62% in stage 4 and 72% in stage 5.

Comparing clinical findings as assessed with the UPDRS rating scale with [^{123}I]β-CIT binding ratios

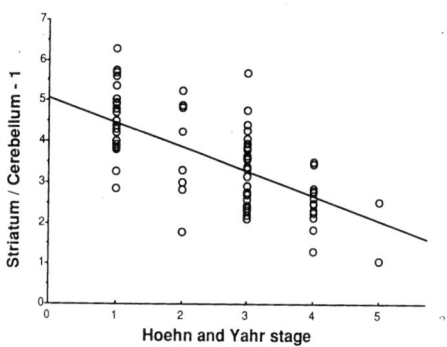

Figure 3 Correlation of specific/non-displaceable striatal binding of [^{123}I]β-CIT and disease severity according to Hoehn and Yahr (n=80). A highly significant negative correlation is found (R= -0.66; p=0.0001). ANOVA also reveals a highly significant difference between groups (F = 15.9; p=0.0001; group 1 versus 3, 4 and 5, group 2 versus 4 and 5, group 3 versus 4 and 5). Reductions to age-corrected values are 35% in stage 1, 46% in stage 2, 48% in stage 3, 62% in stage 4 and 72% in stage 5

revealed highly significant negative correlations with rigidity (R =-0.38; p=0.0027), akinesia (R =-0.38; p=0.0025) and axial symptoms (R =-0.52; p=0.0001), but no correlation with tremor scores (R -0.15; n.s.) (Figure 4). Total UPDRS motor scores and activities of daily living scores were also highly negatively correlated with [^{123}I]β-CIT binding (R =-0.42; p=0.0007 and R -0.55; p=0.0004, respectively) (Figure 5). No gender differences were observed.

A significant age-dependent decline of [^{123}I]β-CIT binding was also found in the group of patients with essential tremor (R =-0.56, p=0.009). The reduction in binding ratio was larger than in the control group (10% of the mean ratio per decade), but the age-range of these patients was somewhat smaller than that of the controls (46-85 compared with 26-75yrs) (Figure 6). However, when controls and essential tremor patients were pooled together, the decline was calculated as 4.6% per decade.

Discussion

β-CIT is a ligand with high affinity for dopamine-and serotonin uptake sites[13,14,42,19]. *In vivo* studies in primates have shown that its binding in the striatum is practically exclusive to dopamine transporters[18].

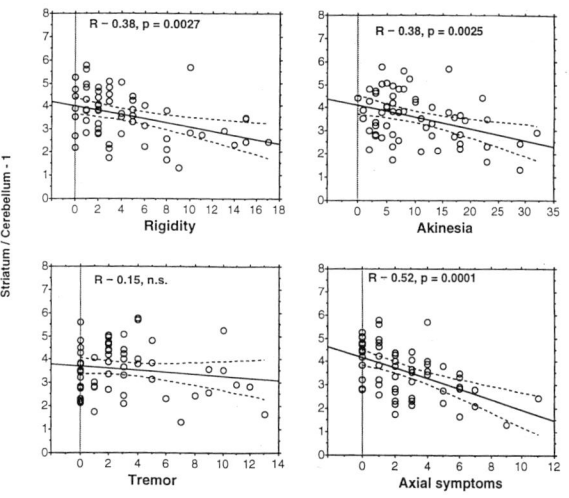

Figure 4 Correlations of specific/non-displaceable striatal binding of [^{123}I]β-CIT and different subscores of the UPDRS rating scale for Parkinson's disease (n=61). Highly significant negative correlations with akinesia, rigidity and axial symptoms but no correlation with tremor scores are found. Dotted lines indicate 95% confidence intervals for the true mean of the binding ratios

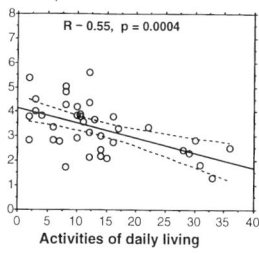

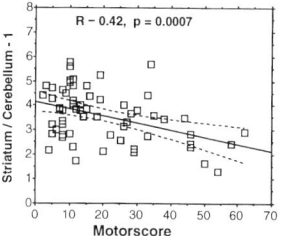

Figure 5 Correlations of specific/non-displaceable striatal binding of [123I]β-CIT and activities of daily living (n=38) and total motorscores (n=61) from the UPDRS rating scale showing highly significant negative correlations. Dotted lines indicate 95% confidence intervals for the true mean of the binding ratios

Studies in our own group demonstrated no reduction of striatal [123I]β-CIT binding in patients treated with the selective serotonin reuptake inhibitor citalopram, thus indicating that the striatal signal after i.v. application of

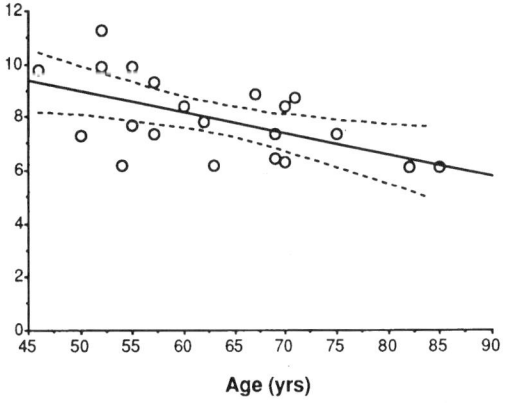

Figure 6 Correlation of specific/non-displaceable striatal binding of [123I]β-CIT and age in 21 patients with essential tremor. A significant age-dependent decline of [123I]β-CIT binding was found (10% of the mean ratio per decade; R= -0.56; p=0.0086). There is no significant difference in binding ratios between these patients and normal controls (7.95 ±1.51 versus 7.22 ±1.08). Dotted lines indicate 95% confidence intervals for the true mean of the binding ratios

this ligand is due to the dopamine uptake sites and is not influenced to a measurable degree by serotonin transporters[43]. Kinetic studies have shown that [123I]β-CIT reaches its maximal specific binding in the striatum around 20 h after injection[23,24]. These slow kinetics have been considered a disadvantage with respect to clinical use and have prompted the search for derivatives with faster brain uptake[44,45]. However, β-CIT does have the advantage of reaching a true binding equilibrium that is stable over several hours and makes it possible to use a simple ratio method for quantification of the results. With most other ligands, such a binding equilibrium — crucial for quantification — can only be achieved with a bolus/infusion application[46]. A comparison of different methods of evaluation of *in vivo* [123I]β-CIT binding with graphical, kinetic and equilibrium analyses has proven the validity of using a simple ratio of specific/non-displaceable binding on day 2 after application during a period of binding equilibrium[47]. Such thorough evaluations have not been performed with other CIT derivatives, but it has been suggested that the loss of dopamine transporters in PD might be overestimated with ligands with faster uptake and faster washout which do not reach a binding equilibrium — FP-CIT, the fluoro-propyl derivative of CIT, for example[44]. Furthermore, a good reproducibility of [123I]β-CIT SPECT measurements in test retest experiments, suggesting that this is a reliable and reproducible method for the *in vivo* measurement of dopamine transporters in the brain, has been demonstrated[48].

In the present study [123I]β-CIT and SPECT were used to examine dopamine transporter density in the striatum as a measure for the loss of dopaminergic nerve endings in PD and ageing. In a large group of PD patients, the overall loss of dopamine transporters in the striatum (both sides pooled together) was found to be reduced by 45% compared with the age-corrected value. Figure 1 shows that there is an excellent separation between controls and PD patients with an overlap in only two cases. Visual and subregional analysis in these two patients with hemiparkinsonism also made a distinction possible.

Several previous SPECT studies with [123I]β-CIT have shown a reduction in striatal binding in patients with PD[22-24], as well as a good correlation with clinical parameters[25-31]. In the present study the severity of the disease and of several symptoms such as akinesia, rigidity, axial symptoms and tremor were compared with the SPECT findings. In line with a study by Seibyl *et al.*[27], excellent correlations were found with all symptoms except tremor, suggesting that the reduction in striatal [123I]β-CIT binding is a good measure for the loss of nigro-striatal dopaminergic neurons which causes akinesia and rigidity, and that tremor is not directly related to this dopaminergic lesion. In fact, post mortem studies in patients with tremor-dominant PD show that dopaminergic neurons in the substantia nigra pars compacta are less affected than in cases with akinetic-rigid subtypes, and that neurons in the retrorubal field (A8) are more severely degenerated in these patients (K. Jellinger, personal communication).

Correlations with clinical parameters such as disease severity, asymmetry of symptoms, and severity of bradykinesia, and *in vivo* indices of dopaminergic function have also been described in ^{18}F-DOPA PET studies in smaller numbers of PD patients[2-5]. In a subregional analysis of [^{123}I]β-CIT binding in caudate and putamen in patients with mild-to-moderate and moderate-to-severe disease, a putaminal loss of 54% and 63% of dopamine terminals, respectively, was calculated[49]. Almost exactly the same findings have been published for the loss of ^{18}F-DOPA influx constants in the putamen in PD patients[3]. These results contrast with post mortem studies of dopamine concentrations in the striatum that have described reductions of 90% or more[50,51]. An explanation for this discrepancy may be that many dopaminergic neurons are still morphologically intact and also have a relatively preserved aromatic amino acid decarboxylase activity — measured with ^{18}F-DOPA, but a marked decrease in tyrosine hydroxylase, the rate-limiting enzyme of dopamine synthesis. Post mortem results that prove that the percentage of surviving dopaminergic neurons in the substantia nigra of PD patients is higher than expected from measurements of dopamine concentration in the striatum are in line with this hypothesis[52-54]. This offers hope for possible neuroprotective treatments in PD, which will have a better chance of success if a larger proportion of dopaminergic neurons is still surviving in patients in whom the disease is already clinically manifest.

However, the validity of [^{123}I]β-CIT SPECT as a measure of dopaminergic nerve cell loss in the substantia nigra may be confounded. It is possible that regulatory changes in the dopamine transporters might accompany changes in the concentration of dopamine in the synaptic cleft[55-57]. It might be conceivable that a compensatory decrease in dopamine transporters accompanies a loss of dopamine in PD. This would lead to overestimation of nerve cell loss in *in vivo* studies of the dopamine transporter. It is also possible, however, that surviving nigrostriatal dopaminergic axons in PD undergo axonal sprouting affecting SPECT results in the opposite way. Different subpopulations of dopaminergic neurons in the midbrain also seem to express synaptic dopamine transporters to different degrees, and it has been hypothesised that neurons with higher levels of expression might be more susceptible to the degenerative process of PD[58]. Neurons with a primarily lower expression rate of dopamine transporters would be more likely to survive, again leading to over-estimation of nerve cell loss in [^{123}I]β-CIT studies. Despite this, the high correlation of clinical symptoms and SPECT results in the present and previous studies[25-31] nevertheless suggests that [^{123}I]β-CIT is a good measure of the degree of dopaminergic nigrostriatal degeneration.

The second part of this study deals with the effect of ageing on dopamine transporters. It is shown that there is a significant age-related decline in the control group and patients with essential tremor. This is in line with previous post mortem studies in the human brain[59-61], SPECT[38,62] and PET results[11,32]. A dopamine transporter loss of about 10% per decade had been calculated from post mortem studies, which is in the range of the SPECT findings of van Dyck *et al.*[38] (8%). We also found a 10% loss per decade in essential tremor patients. Similar findings have been obtained by our group in patients with major depression (Pirker, unpublished results). The results in our normal control group suggest a slower decline of about 5% per decade — the estimated rate of decline of dopaminergic neurons in the substantia nigra from post mortem studies of normal human brain[63]. However, since the number of normal controls in the present study is relatively small, we should not place too much emphasis on these differences in decline rate. The most probable reason for the finding of decreased [^{123}I]β-CIT binding is an age-related loss of dopaminergic terminals (although it is important to remember that regulatory changes in the dopamine uptake sites might also play a role).

Our own observations from a subregional analysis of caudate and putamen in the control group (data not included in the present study) suggest no differences in decline rates of [^{123}I]β-CIT binding in caudate and putamen. In an extension of their previous report, van Dyck *et al.*[62] report similar findings in a large group of normal controls and also describe a correlation with neuropsychological tests of motor performance. A primary and predominant lesion of dopaminergic neurons projecting to the putamen has been described in PD[50]. This suggests different mechanisms of dopaminergic nerve cell loss in ageing and PD, and was also evident from visual analysis of all PD cases in the present study.

In conclusion, our results show that [^{123}I]β-CIT SPECT is a sensitive and reliable method for the *in vivo* assessment of dopaminergic function, enabling quantification of the degree of dopaminergic degeneration in PD and ageing. Findings in PD are highly correlated with clinical symptoms and with measures of disease severity. Therefore [^{123}I]β-CIT SPECT can be used as a diagnostic test and as a measure of the degree of dopaminergic degeneration which will be useful in longitudinal studies of disease progression and in the evaluation of possible neuroprotective strategies.

References

1   Garnett, E.S., Nahmias, C. and Firnau, G. Central dopaminergic pathways in hemiparkinsonism examined by positron emission tomography. *Can. J. Neurol. Sci.* 1984, 11, 174

2   Leenders, K.L., Salmon, E.P., Tyrrell, P. *et al.* The nigrostriatal dopaminergic system assessed *in vivo* by positron emission tomography in healthy volunteer subjects and patients with Parkinson's disease. *Arch. Neurol.* 1990, 47, 1290

3   Brooks, D.J., Ibanez, V., Sawle, G.V. *et al.* Differing patterns of striatal ^{18}F-dopa uptake in Parkinson's disease, multiple system atrophy, and progressive supranuclear palsy. *Ann. Neurol.* 1990, 28, 547

4   Eidelberg, D., Moeller, J.R., Dhawan, V. *et al.* The metabolic anatomy of Parkinson's disease: complementary [^{18}F] fluorodesoxyglucose and [^{18}F] fluorodopa positron emission tomographic studies. *Mov. Dis.* 1990, 5, 203

5   Otsuka, M., Ichiya, Y., Hosokawa, S. *et al.* Striatal blood flow, glucose metabolism and ^{18}F-DOPA uptake: difference in Parkinson's disease and atypical parkinsonism. *J. Neurol. Neurosurg. Psychiatr.* 1991, 54, 898

6   Madras, B.K., Spealman, R.D., Fahey, M.A. *et al.* Cocaine receptors labelled by 2β-carbomethoxy-3β-(4-fluorophenyl)tropane. *Mol. Pharmacol.* 1989, 36, 518

7   Hughes, A.J., Daniel, S.E., Kilford, L. *et al.* Accuracy of clinical diagnosis of idiopathic Parkinson's disease: a clinico-pathological study of 100 cases. *J. Neurol. Neurosurg. Psychiatr.* 1992, 55(3), 181

8   Pimoule, C., Schoemaker, H., Javoy-Agid, F. *et al.* Decrease in [3H]cocaine binding to the dopamine transporter in Parkinson's disease. *Eur. J. Pharmacol.* 1983, 95, 145

9   Janowsy, A., Vocci, F., Berger, P. *et al.* [3H]GBR-12935 binding to the dopamine transporter is decreased in the caudate nucleus in Parkinson's disease. *J. Neurochem.* 1987, 49, 617

10 Aquilonius, S.M., Bergström, K., Eckernäs, S.A. *et al. In vivo* evaluation of striatal dopamine reuptake sites using 11C-nomifensine and positron emission tomography. *Acta. Neurol. Scand.* 1987, 76, 283

11 Tedroff, J., Aquilonius, S.M., Hartvig, P. *et al.* Monoamine reuptake sites in the human brain evaluated *in vivo* by means of 11C-nomifensine and positron emission tomography: the effects of age and Parkinson's disease. *Acta. Neurol. Scand.* 1988, 77, 192

12 Frost, J.J., Rosier, A.J. and Reich, S.G. Positron emission tomography imaging of the dopamine transporter with 11C-WIN 35428 reveals marked declines in mild Parkinson's disease. *Ann. Neurol.* 1993, 34, 423

13 Boja, J.W., Patel, A., Carroll, F.I. *et al.* [125I]RTI-55: a potent ligand for dopamine transporters. *Eur. J. Pharmacol.* 1991, 194, 133

14 Neumeyer, J.L., Wang, S., Milius, R.A. *et al.* [^{123}I]2β-carbomethoxy-3β-(4-iodophenyl)tropane (β-CIT): high-affinity SPECT radiotracer of monoamine re-uptake sites in brain. *J. Med. Chem.* 1991, 34, 3144

15 Innis, R.B., Baldwin, R., Sybirska, E. *et al.* Single photon emission computed tomography imaging of monoamine reuptake sites in primate brain with [^{123}I]CIT. *Eur. J. Pharmacol.* 1991, 299, 369

16 Scheffel, U., Dannals, R.F., Cline, E.J. *et al.* [$^{123/125}$I]RTI-55, an *in vivo* label for the serotonin transporter. *Synapse* 1992, 11, 134

17 Shaya, E.K., Scheffel, U., Dannals, R.F. *et al. In vivo* imaging of dopamine uptake sites in primate brain using single photon emission tomography (SPECT) and iodine-123-labelled RTI-55. *Synapse* 1992, 10, 169

18 Laruelle, M., Baldwin, R.M., Malison, R.T. *et al.* SPECT imaging of dopamine and serotonin transporters with [^{123}I]β-CIT: pharmacological characterization of brain uptake in nonhuman primates. *Synapse* 1993, 13, 295

19 Laruelle, M., Giddings, S., Zea-Ponce, Y. *et al.* Methyl 3β-(4-[125I]iodophenyl) tropane-2β-carboxylate *in vitro* binding to dopamine and serotonin transporters under 'physiological' conditions. *J. Neurochem.* 1994, 62, 978

20 Farde, L., Halldin, C., Müller, L. *et al.* PET study of [11C]β-CIT binding to monoamine transporters in the monkey and human brain. *Synapse* 1994, 16, 93

21 Staley, J.K., Basile, M., Flynn, D.D. and Mash, D.C. Visualizing dopamine and serotonin transporters in the human brain with the potent cocaine analogue [125]RTI-55: *in vitro* binding and autoradiographic characterization. *J. Neurochem.* 1994, 62, 549

22 Kuikka, J.T., Bergström, K.A., Vanninen, E. *et al.* Initial experience with single photon emission tomography using iodine-123-labelled 2β-carbomethoxy-3β-(4 iodo-phenyl)tropane in human brain. *Eur. J. Nucl. Med.* 1993, 20, 783

23 Brücke, T., Kornhuber, J., Angelberger, P. *et al.* SPECT imaging of dopamine and serotonin transporters with [^{123}I]β-CIT. Binding kinetics in the human brain. *J. Neural. Transm. [GenSect]* 1993, 94, 137

24 Innis, R.B., Seibyl, J.P., Scanley, B.E. *et al.* Single photon emission computed tomographic imaging demonstrates loss of striatal dopamine transporters in Parkinson's disease. *Proc. Natl. Acad. Sci. USA.* 1993, 90, 11965

25 Brücke, T., Asenbaum, S., Pozzera, A. *et al.* Dopaminergic nerve cell loss in Parkinson's disease quantified with [^{123}I]β-CIT and SPECT correlates with clinical findings. *Mov. Disord.* 1994, 9(S1), 120

26 Marek, K.L., Seibyl, J.P., Sandridge, B. *et al.* SPECT imaging demonstrates striatal dopamine transporter loss in hemiparkinsonism. *Soc. Neurosci. Abstr.* 1994, 20, 1780

27 Seibyl, J.P., Marek, K.L., Quinlan, D. *et al.* Decreased single photon emission computed tomographic [^{123}I]β-CIT striatal uptake correlates with symptom severity in Parkinson's disease. *Ann. Neurol.* 1995, 38, 589

28 Rinne, J.O., Kuikka, J.T., Bergström, K.A. and Rinne, U.K. Striatal dopamine transporter in different disability stages of Parkinson's disease studied with [^{123}I]β-CIT SPECT. *Parkinsonism and Related Disorders* 1995, 1(1), 47

29 Brücke, T., Asenbaum, S., Pirker, W. *et al.* Quantification of the dopaminergic nerve cell loss in Parkinson's disease with [^{123}I]β-CIT and SPECT. *J. Cereb. Blood Flow Metab.* 1995, 15(Suppl 1), S37

30 Marek, K.L., Seibyl, J.P., Zoghbi, S. *et al.* [^{123}I]β-CIT/SPECT imaging demonstrates bilateral loss of dopamine transporters in hemi-Parkinson's disease. *Neurology* 1996, 46, 231

31 Asenbaum, S., Brücke, T., Pirker, W. *et al.* Imaging of dopamine transporters with [^{123}I]β-CIT and SPECT in Parkinson's disease. *J. Nucl. Med.* 1997, 38, 1

32 Volkow, N.D., Ding, Y-S., Fowler, J.S. *et al.* Dopamine transporters decrease with age. *J. Nucl. Med.* 1996, 37, 554

33 Wong, D.F., Wagner, H.N. Jr., Dannals, R.F. *et al.* Effects of age on dopamine and serotonin receptors measured by positron emission tomography in the living brain. *Science* 1984, 226, 1393

34 Brücke, T., Podreka, I., Angelberger, P. *et al.* Dopamine D_2 receptor imaging with SPECT. Studies in different neuropsychiatric disorders. *J. Cereb. Blood Flow Metab.* 1991, 11, 220

35 Martin, W.R.W., Palmer, M.R., Patlak, C.S. *et al.* Nigrostriatal function in humans studied with positron emission tomography. *Ann. Neurol.* 1989, 26, 535

36 Sawle, G.V., Colebatch, J.G., Shah, A. *et al.* Striatal function in normal ageing -implications for Parkinson's disease. *Ann. Neurol.* 1990, 28, 799

37 Eidelberg, D., Takikawa, S. and Dhawan, V. Striatal ^{18}F-DOPA uptake: absence of an ageing effect. *J. Cereb. Blood Flow Metab.* 1993, 13, 881

38 van Dyck, C.H., Seibyl, J.P., Malison, R.T. *et al.* Age-related decline in striatal transporter binding with iodine-123-β-CIT SPECT. *J. Nucl. Med.* 1995, 36, 1175

39 Hoehn, M.M. and Yahr, M.D. Parkinsonism: onset, progression and mortality. *Neurology* 1967, 6, 253

40 Fahn, S., Elton, R., and members of the Unified Parkinson's Disease Rating Scale development committee. Unified Parkinson's disease rating scale in 'Recent developments in Parkinson's disease', (Eds. S. Fahn, C.D. Marsden, D.B. Calne *et al.*), Macmillan Healthcare Information, New York, USA, 1987, 2, p.153

41 Asenbaum, S., Brücke, T., Pirker, W. *et al.* The application of [^{123}I]β-CIT and SPECT in the diagnosis of movement disorders in 'SPECT in Neurology and Psychiatry', (Eds. P.P. De Deyn, R.A. Dierckx, A. Alavi and B. Pickut), John Libby & Co. Ltd, London, 1997, p.187

42 Boja, J.W., Mitchell, W.M., Patel, A. *et al.* High affinity binding of [125I]RTI-55 to dopamine and serotonin transporters in rat brain. *Synapse* 1992, 12, 27

43 Pirker, W., Asenbaum, S., Kasper, S. *et al.* β-CIT SPECT demonstrates blockade of 5HT-uptake sites by citalopram in the human brain *in vivo. J. Neural. Transm. [Gen Sect]* 1995, 100, 247

44 Seibyl, J., Marek, K., Sheff, K. *et al.* Comparison of [^{123}I]FP-CIT and [^{123}I]β-CIT for SPECT imaging of dopamine transporters in Parkinson's disease. *J. Nucl. Med.* 1996, 37, 133P

45 Malison, R.T., Vessotskie, J., Kung, M.P. *et al.* Striatal dopamine transporter imaging in non-human primates with ^{123}I-IPT SPECT. *J. Nucl. Med.* 1995, 36, 2290

46 Carson, R.E., Channing, M.A., Blasberg, R.G. *et al.* Comparison of bolus and infusion methods for receptor quantification: application to [^{18}F]Cyclofoxy and positron emission tomography. *J. Cereb. Blood Flow Metab.* 1993, 13, 24

47 Laruelle, M., Wallace, E., Seibyl, J.P. *et al.* Graphical, kinetic and equilibrium analyses of *in vivo* [^{123}I]β-CIT binding to dopamine transporters in healthy human subjects. *J. Cereb. Blood Flow Metab.* 1994, 14, 982

48 Seibyl, J.P., Laruelle, M., van Dyck, C.H. *et al.* Reproducibility of iodine-^{123}-β-CIT SPECT brain measurement of dopamine transporters. *J. Nucl. Med.* 1996, 37, 222

49 Brücke, T., Asenbaum, S., Pirker, W. *et al.* Measurement of the dopaminergic degeneration in Parkinson's disease with [^{123}I]β-CIT and SPECT. Correlation with clinical findings and comparison with multiple system atrophy and progressive supranuclear palsy. *J. Neural Transm.* 1997, 50, 9

50 Bernheimer, H., Birkmayer, W., Hornykiewicz, O. *et al.* Brain dopamine and the syndromes of Parkinson and Huntington. *J. Neurol. Sci.* 1973, 20, 415

51 Kish, S.J., Shannar, K. and Hornykiewicz, O. Uneven pattern of dopamine loss in the striatum of patients with idiopathic Parkinson's disease. Pathophysiological and clinical implications. *N. Engl. J. Med.* 1988, 318, 876

52 German, D.C., Manaye, K., Smith, W.K. *et al.* Midbrain dopaminergic cell loss in Parkinson's disease: computer visualization. *Ann. Neurol.* 1989, 26, 507

53 Goto, S., Hirano, A. and Matsumoto, S. Subdivisional involvement of nigrostriatal loop in idiopathic Parkinson's disease and striatonigral degeneration. *Ann. Neurol.* 1989, 26, 766

54 Rinne, J.O., Rummukainen, J., Paljarvi, L. and Rinne, U.K. Dementia in Parkinson's disease is related to neuronal loss in the medial substantia nigra. *Ann. Neurol.* 1989, 26, 47

55 Kilbourn, M.R., Sherman, P.S. and Pisani, T. Repeated reserpine administration reduces *in vivo* [18F]GBR-13119 binding to the dopamine uptake site. *Eur. J. Pharmacol.* 1992, 216, 109

56 Wilson, J.M., Nobrega, J.N., Carroll, M.E. *et al.* Heterogeneous subregional binding patterns of 3H-WIN 35,428 and 3H-GBR 12,935 are differentially regulated by chronic cocaine self-administration. *J. Neurosci.* 1994, 14, 2966

57 Malison, R.T., Wallace, E.A., Best, S. *et al.* SPECT imaging of dopamine transporters in cocaine-dependent and healthy control subjects with [123I]β-CIT. *Soc. Neurosci. Abstr.* 1994, 20(2), 1625

58 Pifl, C. and Uhl, G.R. Dopamine transporter: state of the art in parkinsonism. *Mov. Dis.* 1996, 11(S1), 22

59 Allard, P. and Marcusson, J.O. Age-correlated loss of dopamine uptake sites with [3H]GBR-12935 in human putamen. *Neurobiol. Age.* 1989, 10, 661

60 Zelnik, N., Angel, I., Paul, S.M. and Kleinman, J.E. Decreased density of human striatal dopamine uptake sites with age. *Eur. J. Pharmacol.* 1986, 126, 175

61 de Keyser, J.D., Ebinger, G. and Vauquelin, G. Age-related changes in the human nigrostriatal dopaminergic system. *Ann. Neurol.* 1990, 27, 157

62 van Dyck, C.H., Seibyl, J.P., Laruelle, M. *et al.* Age-related decline in dopamine transporters with I-123-β-CIT SPECT: analysis of gender striatal subregions and neuropsychological correlates. *Soc. Neurosci. Abstr.* 1996, 22(2), 1201

63 Fearnley, J.M. and Lees, A.J. Ageing and Parkinson's disease: substantia nigra regional selectivity. *Brain* 1991, 114, 2283

Epilepsy

SPECT in Neurology and Psychiatry, edited by P.P. De Deyn, R.A. Dierckx, A. Alavi and B.A. Pickut
© 1997 John Libbey & Company Ltd, pp. 207–217

Biochemical and Functional Imaging for Adult Partial Epilepsy: PET or SPECT?

Chapter
25

B. Sadzot, R.M.C. Debets[*] and G. Franck

Introduction

The International Classification of the Epilepsies recognises 2 broad types of epilepsy: generalised, which remains poorly understood, and partial, in which the first clinical and electroencephalographic changes indicate initial activation of a system of neurons limited to part of one cerebral hemisphere. The past decade has witnessed dramatic improvements in neuroimaging techniques. Structural and functional scans now often reveal discrete alterations associated with the epileptic focus and have thus become increasingly indispensable in the non-invasive evaluation of epileptic patients[1]. Their impact is so important that they are now part of the diagnosis of 'mesial epilepsy syndrome', the most frequent form of partial epilepsy and a syndrome accessible to surgical treatment[2]. Magnetic resonance imaging (MRI) provides exquisite anatomical detail, particularly important when studying the hippocampus, an area of the brain often involved in the MTS syndrome[3].

Single photon emission computed tomography (SPECT) and positron emission tomography (PET) are used to assess the functional status of the brain. They do not have the anatomical precision of MRI, but have proved very useful in the work-up of epileptic patients being considered for surgery, because they reveal localised functional alterations related to the epileptic focus.

This chapter will give an overview of the contribution of PET in partial epilepsy but will limit its scope to adult partial epilepsy, since child epilepsy is, in many respects, a quite different subject.

Technical considerations

PET is based upon the detection of radioactive tracers and computerised tomographic reconstruction methods. It permits the non-invasive measurement of the regional biodistribution of a radiotracer in a slice of organ at any time after its administration and the monitoring of its regional kinetics. The measured radioactive concentrations can be translated into colour-coded images and, with an appropriate calibration, it is also possible to quantify the true regional tracer concentration at any given time.

Department of Neurology, CHU Sart Tilman, B. 35, 4000, Liege, Belgium
[*]Centrum voor Epilepsiebestrijding, Heemstede, The Netherlands

PET has several other important advantages. First, it is a highly sensitive method, far more so than MRI: tracer concentrations as low as 0.1-1 nM can be measured, which is important, as neuroreceptors exist in nanomolar concentrations; only small amounts of radioligand can be administered to avoid receptor saturation. Second, it is a non-invasive method of radiation detection which makes it possible to repeat measurements: during the course of a disease, and before and after a treatment, or a behavioural paradigm. The third advantage is related to the nature of the radioactive tracers. They are similar to (or slightly modified versions of) natural, biologically active molecules or pharmaceuticals, and their fate within the organism is known. This knowledge allows the development of mathematical models describing the behaviour of the ligand after its introduction into the organism and, thus, the transformation of radioactive concentrations into biologically meaningful parameters. The measurements made are highly specific to the biological system of interest, so that high signal-to-noise ratios and images with high contrast result. Tracers are labelled with positron-emitting isotopes produced by a nearby cyclotron. The isotopes have the advantage of a short half-life (Table 1), which limits the radiation dose to the subject. Moreover, background activity variation from one study to the next is not an overiding problem and sequential studies are possible.

Although many biochemical and physiological parameters can be studied *in vivo* with PET, in epileptic patients, it has mainly been used to study blood flow, oxygen and glucose consumption, and neuroreceptors (Table 1). PET methods developed to image these parameters usually require a steady state in the patient's condition. They are not designed to study short-time events such as epileptic fits. Measurement of glucose consumption, for example, requires a pre-scan incubation period (or steady state) of 30-45 min after tracer administration. During this time, [18]FDG is trapped and accumulates in cells as a function of hexokinase activity. The [18]FDG scan reflects cerebral glucose metabolism during the uptake, weighted towards the beginning of that period - primarily the first 10 min after injection. Because of this, the method

Table 1 Major radioactive tracers used to study epileptic patients with PET or SPECT

	Tracer	Isotope	Half life	Positron range (mm)	Parameter	Reference
PET	$C^{15}O_2$-$H_2{}^{15}O$	[15]O	123 sec	8.2	Blood flow	38
PET	[15]O	[15]O	123 sec	8.2	Oxygen consumption	37
PET	[18]FDG	[18]F	109.7 min	2.4	Glucose consumption	10
PET	3-^{18}F-acetylcyclofoxy	[18]F	109.7 min	2.4	Mu, delta and kappa opiate R	29
PET	^{11}C-carfentanil	[11]C	20.4 min	4.1	Mu opiate R	41
PET	^{11}C-diprenorphine	[11]C	20.4 min	4.1	Mu, delta and kappa opiate R	42
PET	^{11}C-flumazenil	[11]C	20.4 min	4.1	Benzodiazepine R	47
PET	^{11}C-methionine	[11]C	20.4 min	4.1	Protein synthesis	51
SPECT	^{123}I-IMP	[123]I	13h	-	Blood flow	77
SPECT	^{123}I-iomazenil	[123]I	13h	-	Benzodiazepine R	47
SPECT	^{123}I-iododexetimide	[123]I	13h	-	Cholinergic R	75
SPECT	^{99m}Tc-ECD	[99m]Tc	6h	-	Blood flow	78
SPECT	^{99m}Tc-HMPAO	[99m]Tc	6h	-	Blood flow	59

HMPAO: hexamethyl-propyleneamineoxime; IMP: I-N-isopropyl-iodoamphetamine; ECD:ethyl cysteinate dimer or bicisate; R: receptors.
Positron range: distance between the place where a positron is emitted and the place where it annihilates

Table 2 Comparative merits of neuroimaging techniques used in the non-invasive evaluation of epileptic patients (adapted from references 43 and 80)

	SPECT	PET	MRI
Resolution	10-15 mm	5-10 mm	1-3 mm
Availability	Widespread	Limited	Universal
Quantification	Problematic	Yes	Some
Complexity	Moderate	High	Routine
Risk	Radiation	Radiation	Gadolinium
Interictal	Yes	Yes	Yes
Ictal	Yes-Reasonable	No-Fortuitous	No
Function	Limited	Yes	Soon?
Anatomy	No	No	Yes
Blood flow	Yes	Yes	No
Metabolism	No	Yes	Some
Receptors	Some	Yes	No
Drug distribution	No	Some	Yes
Sensitivity	50-70%	>80%	60-70%

underestimates changes in metabolic rates associated with changes in cerebral function of short duration[4]. PET is designed for studying compliant patients during the interictal state. Few ictal PET studies have been reported and they will not be discussed here.

Another important limitation of PET is its spatial resolution. The first tomographs had an in-plane resolution of 15 mm. This has been reduced to 5-10 mm in most recent machines but, because of the physics of positron decay (positron range, Table 1), it will never be possible to reach the resolution of MRI. One of the consequences of the limited spatial resolution is the so-called partial volume effect, which can be defined as an averaging of the signal between adjacent areas. This effect concerns structures smaller than approximately twice the spatial resolution of the system[5], but the latest tomographs also have better spatial sampling. Up to 30 slices can be acquired simultaneously, which allows the entire brain volume to be scanned at once. Studies can be resliced in the coronal plane, which is particularly useful for imaging the amygdalo-hippocampal complex[6].

Single photon emission tomography (SPECT) is based on different technology and other isotopes. Because of the lower cost of the cameras, it is more widely available. The isotopes have a longer half-life, do not need to be produced by an on-site cyclotron, and are commercially available. Compared with PET, SPECT is characterised by lower performances in terms of both spatial and temporal resolution (Table 2). Spatial resolution is crucial to sensitivity, a point illustrated by the following: with the old single-slice ECAT scanner (in-plane resolution of 16 mm), the yield of positive scans in a large epileptic population was 52%[7]; this increased to 86% with the multislice CTI-831 (in-plane resolution of 5 mm). Improvement in the spatial resolution of the PET camera has resulted in higher sensitivity. With limited spatial resolution and the resulting partial-volume effect, the apparent size of the hypometabolic (hypoperfused) zone is increased, but the degree of hypometabolism (hypoperfusion) is underestimated.

With SPECT, true isotope concentrations in a slice cannot be measured for technical reasons and quantification remains difficult. Fewer tracers are available; they allow measurement of blood flow or, more recently, some neuroreceptors (Table 1). Of the blood flow tracers, ^{99m}Tc-HMPAO is the most widely used. It is a lipophilic amine with a rapid brain uptake: 85% of brain uptake occurs on the first pass after i.v. injection. Uptake is proportional to blood flow at the time of administration, and is complete within 2 min. Once inside the brain, ^{99m}Tc-HMPAO forms a hydrophilic compound which cannot cross back across the blood-brain barrier, and the tracer is essentially trapped in cells - less than 5% is redistributed after 8 h. The nearly constant maintenance of HMPAO brain activity over several hours provides ideal conditions for equilibrium imaging: distant from clinical events and with a pre-scan delay[8,9].

Glucose metabolism

[18]FDG is the standard PET method for patients with partial epilepsy. Because of the methodological and technical considerations mentioned above, the vast majority of all [18]FDG PET studies have been carried out during the interictal state.

Temporal lobe epilepsy (mesial epilepsy syndrome)

It is now well established that in more than 80% of patients with temporal lobe epilepsy, [18]FDG PET shows a regional decrease in brain glucose metabolism[10-21]. The PET may, however, be normal, even in patients with a well defined EEG focus. Conversely, PET may show an area of decreased CMRGlu in patients with a non-localising EEG or IC-EEG[11,12]. The hypometabolism may be regional or lobar and usually has a progressive demarcation from the normal cortex. It may also be more widespread and multilobar, with the lobe of seizure onset usually being the most hypometabolic[18]. The hypometabolic region may include an area of more severe hypometabolism and a sharp demarcation from the adjacent cortex that often corresponds to a structural lesion. Because the site of seizure onset always lies within a demonstrated hypometabolic area, the hypometabolism is always on the side of the brain with the epileptic focus and false lateralisations are exceptional[7,18,22,23].

Glucose metabolism is usually vast, affecting the entire temporal lobe and, sometimes, extratemporal areas as well (homolateral adjacent cortex and thalamus)[18,22,24,25]. In the first PET studies, the mean asymmetry in the lateral cortex (−20%) was larger than that in the mesial part of the temporal lobe (−10%)[12,18,20,26,27] - even though most temporal lobe epilepsies (TLE) arise from the amygdalo-hippocampal complex[18,22,28]. With the newest tomographs and their improved resolution, however, the measured asymmetry in lateral and mesial temporal cortexes is now similar[29-31].

For therapeutic reasons, it is particularly important to sort out TLE patients with a mesial epilepsy syndrome from those with seizures originating in the lateral neocortex or with widespread seizure onset, but the issue has received little attention so far. In a group of patients studied with IC-EEG recordings, we did not find any metabolic difference beween patients with

mesiotemporal seizure onset and those with more widespread ictal onset (mesiotemporal and temporal neocortical)[18]. However, Hajek et al.[17] found that patients with seizure of lateral (neocortical) temporal origin had pronounced hypometabolism in the lateral temporal cortex but quite normal metabolic activity in the mesiobasal temporal lobe, while patients with mesiotemporal sclerosis had hypometabolism in both the mesial and the lateral cortex. Henry et al.[32] observed mesial and lateral temporal hypometabolism not only in mesiotemporal epilepsy, but also in patients with neocortical seizures. Thus far, mesiolateral temporal hypometabolism cannot be considered evidence for limbic versus neocortical epileptic focus.

The relationship between surgical outcome and temporal lobe hypometabolism is also important, but still debated. Part of the problem is that, in the few series addressing this question, surgical results are excellent and 'non-significantly improved' patients are few. At UCLA, the presence or absence of metabolic defect did not appear to predict post-operative outcome[33], and similar conclusions have been reported by others. Chee et al.[19] and Theodore et al.[24] found no difference in outcome between those patients with an abnormal PET and those with a non-localising PET. Patients of Swartz et al.[22] all had a very good outcome, but more than expected had an extratemporal area of hypometabolism in the relatively 'poor' group; the authors suggested that extent of hypometabolism may be a determinant of outcome. For Radtke et al.[31], an abnormal preoperative PET correlated strongly with a positive outcome after temporal lobectomy. The authors found no association between the location of the hypometabolism (mesial versus lateral temporal lobe) and outcome.

Manno et al.[34] followed 43 patients after temporal lobectomy. Those with hypometabolism restricted to the temporal lobe were more likely to be seizure-free at 1 year after temporal lobectomy than those with other PET findings (normal, multilobar, or extratemporal metabolism); those with restricted mesial temporal hypometabolism were as likely to be seizure-free after temporal lobectomy as patients with diffuse (mesial and lateral) temporal lobe hypometabolism; 3 patients with visually assessed extratemporal or multilobar hypometabolism continued to have seizures after temporal lobectomy.

Extratemporal epilepsies

Surprisingly, only a few metabolic studies of non-lesional partial epilepsies of neocortical origin have been confirmed by IC-EEG[7,18,32,35]. The regional patterns of interictal hypometabolism are thus not as well characterised as those of mesial temporal lobe epilepsy. However, it is well established that [18]FDG PET is more often normal than it is in TLE, just as it is with MRI. A lobar hypometabolism has seldom been reported in the presence of a normal MRI, but it is good indication of the lobe of seizure onset. Multilobar hypometabolism (including temporal hypometabolism) has also been observed[7,32,36], yielding less valuable or even misleading information. Engel *et al.*[7] reported 2 patients with predominantly temporal lobe hypometabolism with a seizure frontal onset during IC-EEG. Thus, temporal lobe hypometabolism can be seen in patients with seizures arising from non-temporal structures. In 6 patients with frontal lobe epilepsy confirmed by IC-EEG, we found 3 patients with a hypometabolism limited to the frontal lobe (Figure 1) and 2 patients with a fronto temporal hypometabolism; one patient with bilateral seizure foci had a normal PET study. In such patients - with documented extratemporal epilepsies - PET appears less helpful, but more metabolic data are needed.

Blood flow studies with PET

Few blood flow studies have also been carried out interictally with PET in TLE patients. Those that have shown a reduction in blood flow in the temporal lobe with the epileptic focus[37,38]. [18]FDG PET has, however, largely superceded these studies for this indication. Oxygen-15 emits positrons that are more energetic than those from fluorine-18 (1.72 versus 0.64 MeV) meaning that the positron range is longer for oxygen-15 than for fluorine-18 (8.2 versus 2.39 mm). Images obtained with oxygen-15-labelled molecules are more fuzzy and have a poorer spatial resolution and higher statistical noise than images obtained with fluorine-18-labelled compounds. Regional brain asymmetries in normal controls are larger with $H_2^{15}O$ than with [18]FDG.

Leiderman *et al.*[39] investigated 28 patients with medically intractable partial epilepsy undergoing presurgical evaluation with PET using both [18]FDG and $H_2^{15}O$. Of the 15 patients who had surgery or subdural electrodes, 3 showed falsely lateralising $H_2^{15}O$-PET and 4 were normal. Only one [18]FDG PET was normal, and there was no discordant lateralisation. [18]FDG PET is more sensitive and specific for the lateralisation and localisation of the epileptogenic area than methods using [15]O. CBF measurements with $H_2^{15}O$ should not be used to select patients for temporal lobectomy.

Receptor studies with PET

Highly specific maps (autoradiographies) of the major receptors in the brain (serotonin, dopamine, opiate, etc) have been obtained using PET with high-affinity, selective radioligands. Brain receptor studies may result in a better knowledge of the biochemistry of the epileptic focus; they might also be of clinical interest. Like [18]FDG PET, receptor imaging may help localise dysfunctional areas that have some relationship with the epileptic focus.

Opiate receptors

Animal models[40] suggest that opioid peptides are important in seizure control and termination. Opiate receptors were first studied in patients with CPS using PET and the selective and extremely potent mu opiate-agonist ^{11}C-carfentanil (^{11}C-CFN). ^{11}C-CFN binding was increased in the lateral temporal cortex, at a distance from the presumed epileptic focus, and was decreased in the amygdala, probably reflecting tissue damage[41]. While interpretation of these findings is not straightforward, if one considers that endogenous opiates inhibit epileptiform discharges, increased ^{11}C-CFN binding could be explained either by an increased liberation of endogenous ligand, inducing a compensatory increase in receptor density, or by a decrease in liberation of the endogenous ligand. This is, at least, the first indication that endogenous opioids may play a role in seizure disorders in humans. No significant changes and no specific binding patterns were observed for TLE patients as a group with ^{11}C-diprenorphine[42] or with 3-^{18}F-acetylcyclofoxy[43], even though some individual patients appeared to have higher binding in the temporal lobe ipsilateral to the EEG focus. These are less specific opiate ligands that bind with the same high affinity to mu (delta) and kappa receptors. Opposite changes in mu and kappa receptors might explain the conflicting findings[42], but specific ligands for delta and kappa receptors that may help answer this interesting question are being developed.

Benzodiazepine receptors

Autoradiographies of hippocampi resected from subjects with mesiotemporal lobe epilepsy have revealed regionally specific decreases in 3H-flumazenil binding to the $GABA_A$-BZ receptor complex. This decreased binding seemed to parallel the neuronal cell loss associated with mesial temporal sclerosis and it was therefore tempting to study these receptors *in vivo* with PET in epileptic patients.

The BZ receptor antagonist ^{11}C-flumazenil is an excellent PET ligand with a high affinity and a low non-specific binding[44,45]. A further advantage is that a simple interpretation of its late uptake images is

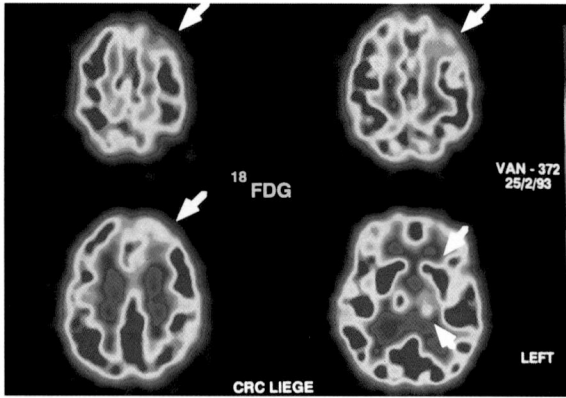

Figure 1 Seizure semeiology suggestive of a frontal lobe epilepsy with frequent, short-lasting spectacular seizures. Surface interictal and ictal EEG showed a left frontal focus. MRI revealed a small area of cortical dysplasia deep in a frontal sulcus, with a thicker layer of grey matter at its base. PET showed an area of glucose hypometabolism in the antero-superior region of the left frontal lobe, corresponding well with MRI and EEG

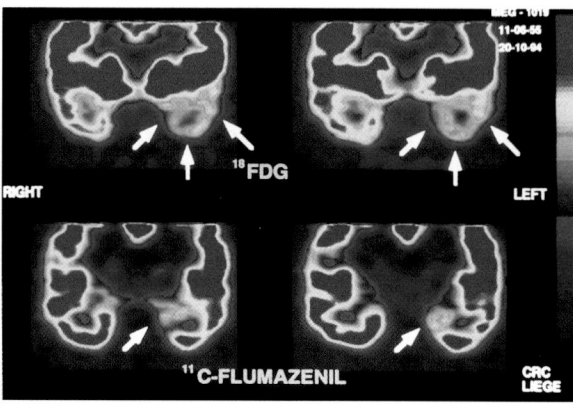

Figure 2 Typical example of a young woman with a long history of complex partial seizures. Surface EEG consistently showed a left temporal EEG focus, ictally and interictally. MRI revealed a slight left hippocampal atrophy. Glucose metabolism is decreased in each part of temporal cortex (mesial, basal and lateral) while ^{11}C-flumazenil binding is decreased only in the left hippocampus. A temporal lobectomy is considered, without preliminary intracranial EEG recordings

sufficient for clinical purposes and that compartmental modelling does not seem mandatory[46]. Savic *et al.* were the first to report the *in vivo* demonstration of reduced BZ receptor density in a limited area corresponding to the (presumed) epileptic focus[47].

Given the short half-life of ^{11}C and the rapid dissociation of the ^{11}C-flumazenil-receptor complex, it is possible to study ^{11}C-flumazenil binding and glucose consumption in the same compliant individual during the same PET session. Such an approach allows a direct comparison of these 2 biochemical parameters. Henry *et al.* and ourselves[25,30] have shown that patients with TLE are characterised, on the epileptogenic side, by a reduction in ^{11}C-flumazenil binding which is limited to the mesial temporal region (-15% on average), with little change in the lateral temporal cortex. Glucose metabolism is reduced to the same magnitude but is more extensive, affecting not only the mesial area but also the lateral temporal cortex and, sometimes, extratemporal areas. The decreased ^{11}C-flumazenil uptake in the hippocampus is particularly well demonstrated on the coronal planes. A representative example of these combined studies is shown in Figure 2. This pattern has been observed in more than 90% of 23 consecutive patients who later underwent a temporal lobectomy; 19 of them were diagnosed with mesial temporal sclerosis[48].

Both ^{11}C-flumazenil and [18]FDG are very sensitive markers of TLE. The area of decreased ^{11}C-flumazenil binding is spatially more limited and could have a closer relationship with the epileptic focus than the area of glucose hypometabolism. Several explanations of this reduced binding are theoretically possible but, currently, the favourite hypothesis is that ^{11}C-flumazenil simply reflects the loss of neurons in the hippocampus expressing this receptor. The accuracy of this hypothesis will be better appreciated when patients with documented extra-hippocampal epilepsy have been investigated. It will then be possible to define the respective advantages and roles of [18]FDG and ^{11}C-flumazenil in the non-invasive exploration of patients with CPS.

Other parameters

Monoamine oxidase B

PET may also be used to detect and highlight the gliosis associated with mesiotemporal sclerosis. ^{11}C-deprenyl and ^{11}C-deuterium-deprenyl have been used *in vivo* with PET to label monoamine oxidase B, an enzyme located on astrocytes[49]. In a recent work[50], the uptake of ^{11}C-deuterium-deprenyl - initially considered a marker of gliosis, was markedly increased throughout the temporal lobe that harboured a mesially situated epileptic focus in 7 patients with a unilateral focus. The extent of this increased binding, larger than the mesiotemporal sclerosis, suggests that it is not purely a glial marker. However, given the high sensitivity of MRI in detecting gliosis, this new PET method might be of limited interest.

Table 3 Respective merits of interictal PET and ictal PET

	Interictal PET	Ictal SPECT
Requirements	Outpatient	Inpatient + videoEEG
Temporal resolution	Poor	Good
Preferential indication	MRI normal	Rapid spread of ictal EEG activity
Complexity	Moderate	High < organisation - logistics >
Cost	High	High < organisation - logistics >
Sensitivity	High	High

These tests are redundant if EEG and MRI + one of these tests are congruent; they are complementary if there is no congruence or if one of them is not localising

^{11}C-methionine

This PET tracer is an amino acid used to evaluate protein synthesis. It accumulates markedly in brain tumours, even in those of low grade, and can be used in patients with partial epilepsy and a brain lesion of questionable nature[51].

The value of SPECT

Because of its lower cost, and the ease of radiopharmaceutical preparation, SPECT is more widely available than PET. There is, therefore, considerable interest in whether or not SPECT is as sensitive and useful as PET in the presurgical protocols of patients with partial epilepsy.

Blood flow

Interictal blood flow SPECT studies with ^{123}I-IMP or ^{99m}Tc-HMPAO in TLE patients have yielded highly variable results. Patients have often been less rigorously screened than in PET studies, and patients with gross anatomical lesions have often been included. Moreover, different SPECT technologies have been used. All three factors may explain why the sensitivity of SPECT reputedly varies between 80%[52-56] and less than 50%[57-60]. Regardless, sensitivity is substantially less than that of PET. Another concern is the frequency of false lateralisations with SPECT[54,55,57,59,61], and of side changes in relative hypoperfusion between repeated scans[52,59,62]. When present, the degree of hypoperfusion is lower than the asymmetry reported with PET. Experienced workers in the field[59] have suggested that interictal SPECT is

unreliable. The lower performance compared with PET is explained by technical factors.

PET and SPECT have seldom been carried out in the same patients, but Stefan et al.[16] evaluated both imaging methods in 10 patients with TLE, 7 of whom had a unilateral EEG focus and a normal CT scan. All 7 patients had an area of hypometabolism on PET, while only 3 showed corresponding SPECT abnormalities; in an additional patient, SPECT lateralisation differed from that obtained with either PET or MRI. In another group of TLE patients with normal MRI, SPECT was abnormal in 20% and PET in 80% but, when MRI was abnormal, sensitivity was similarly high (90 and 100%, respectively)[60]. The spatial resolution of the SPECT camera was lower than that of the PET camera (14 versus 7 mm in plane, respectively). The metabolic abnormalities not detected by SPECT were always mildly intense and restricted to the most anterior part of the lateral temporal cortex. These results again emphasise the importance of technical factors.

As we have seen, SPECT is more suited than PET to ictal studies, defined as studies in which injection of the radiopharmaceutical is done during the seizure, or up to 30 s following termination, and several authors have taken advantage of this potential. Their studies[63-66] have shown various regional blood flow patterns, a function of the timing between isotope injection and EEG activity, and are described in detail in other chapters. Peri-ictal scans must be interpreted with knowledge of the characteristic changes in blood flow (the 'switch') accompanying ictal and postictal activity, and with a strict documentation of the temporal relationship between the time of injection and

EEG activity. They offer reliable localisation in more than 70% of cases[67-69], and false lateralisation seems to occur less frequently than with interictal scans. Peri-ictal scanning is a useful tool, yielding information complementary to that provided by the ictal EEG, which cannot always be interpreted. At present, only one study[70] directly compares interictal [18]FDG PET and ictal HMPAO SPECT in the same TLE patients (n=35) - both methods were found reliable and very sensitive for the lateralisation of temporal lobe seizure foci (Table 3). Ictal SPECT seemed slightly superior to interictal PET, particularly in the few patients not showing MRI abnormalities. There was no evidence that patients need both functional imaging techniques when one test is congruent with EEG and MRI. In easy cases, they are both redundant, but they may have complementary roles when localisation is difficult - ictal SPECT, for example, may be useful in patients not showing MRI abormality, while interictal PET is helpful in patients showing a rapid controlateral spread of seizure activity on EEG recordings.

Receptors

Attempts to label receptors with SPECT have recently been reported. ^{123}I-iomazenil (a ^{123}I-flumazenil derivative) is used in several centres to label benzodiazepine receptors with SPECT. 'Positive findings' have been reported in 75-100% of patients with partial epilepsy[71-73]. The area of reduced binding was large and its anatomical localisation approximate. Furthermore, when directly compared with blood flow studies, benzodiazepine receptor mapping with SPECT did not seem to offer any advantages over HMPAO SPECT in the detection of epileptic foci[72,73].

Muscarinic acetylcholine receptors have been labelled with SPECT and [123]I- iododexetimide[74]. In 4 subjects with normal MRI (including hippocampal volume measurements), ^{123}I-iododexetimide binding in the anterior hippocampus ipsilateral to the electrical focus was reduced by an average of 40% compared with the contralateral hippocampus, and was symmetrical in other temporal regions. Perfusion measured with HMPAO was reduced in hippocampus, amygdala and anterior temporal lobe ipsilateral to the seizure focus, but to a lesser degree[75]. These interesting and promising findings must be extended and confirmed in a larger group of patients.

Conclusions

Epileptologists have greatly benefited from progress in neuroimaging techniques in recent years. In more than half of patients with partial seizures, it is now possible to detect, non-invasively, structural abnormalities that are often highly correlated with the epileptogenic zone. In experienced hands, and with dedicated protocols, MRI and PET now have similar sensitivities, but it must be stressed that EEG remains, and will remain, absolutely indispensible in the confirmation of the epileptic nature of the disorder being considered. It is not yet clear whether PET can provide indispensible information on the management of epileptic patients with abnormal MRI - it may be recommended only for patients with a normal MRI. At present, it is useful as a source of independent information, since it is the accumulation of information from various sources that currently helps epileptologists formulate hypotheses about location. PET also shows the extent of functional disturbances (which might be relevant). In mesiotemporal epilepsy, ^{11}C-flumazenil-PET shows a binding defect limited to the hippocampus, probably reflecting the neuronal loss characterising the epileptic focus. The relative indications for [18]FDG and ^{11}C-flumazenil have yet to be defined.

The reliability of interictal SPECT is still hampered by poor spatial resolution but, with better cameras, it could reach the accuracy of [18]FDG PET. Ictal SPECT is an interesting alternative when PET is not available. These functional modalities have a bright future in epilepsy.

References

1   Engel, J. Jr. Update on the surgical treatment of the epilepsies. *Neurology* 1993, 43, 1612

2   Engel, J. Jr., Henry, T.R. and Risinger, M.W. The role of positron emission tomography in the presurgical evaluation of temporal lobe epilepsy in 'Epilepsy surgery', (Ed. H. Lüders), Raven Press, New York, USA, 1991, p.231

3   Jackson, G.D. New techniques in magnetic resonance in epilepsy. *Epilepsia* 1994, 35, S2

4   Phelps, M.E., Huang, S.C., Hoffman, E.J. *et al.* Tomographic measurements of local cerebral glucose metabolic rate in humans with [F18]-2-fluoro-2-deoxy-D-glucose: validation of method. *Ann. Neurol.* 1979, 6, 371

5   Hoffman, E.J., Huang, S.C. and Phelps, M.E. Quantitation in positron emission computed tomography. 1. Effect of object size. *J. Comput. Assist. Tomogr.* 1979, 3, 299

6   Jackson, G.D., Berkovic, S.F., Tress, B.M. *et al.* Hippocampal sclerosis can be reliably detected by magnetic resonance imaging. *Neurology* 1990, 40, 1869

7   Engel, J. Jr., Henry, T.R., Risinger, M.W. *et al.* Presurgical evaluation for partial epilepsy: relative contribution of chronic depth-electrode recordings versus FDG-PET and scalp-sphenoidal ictal EEG. *Neurology* 1990, 40, 1670

8   Anderson, A.R., Friberg, H., Lassen, N.A. *et al.* Serial studies of cerebral blood flow using ^{99m}Tc-HMPAO: a comparison with 133Xe. *Nucl. Med. Commun.* 1987, 8, 549

9   Neirinckx, R.D., Canning, L.R., Piper, I.M. *et al.* Technetium ^{99m} D,l-HM-PO: a new radiopharmaceutical for SPECT imaging of regional cerebral blood perfusion. *J. Nucl. Med.* 1987, 28, 191

10 Kuhl, D.E., Engel, J. Jr., Phelps, M.E. and Selin, C. Epileptic patterns of local cerebral metabolism and perfusion in humans determined by emission computed tomography of ^{18}FDG and 13NH3. *Ann. Neurol.* 1980, 8, 348

11 Engel, J. Jr., Kuhl, D.E., Phelps, M.E. and Crandall, P.H. Comparative localization of epileptic foci in partial epilepsy by PCT and EEG. *Ann. Neurol.* 1982, 12, 529

12 Abou-Khalil, B.W., Siegel, G.J., Sackellares, J.C. *et al.* Positron emission tomography studies of cerebral glucose metabolism in chronic partial epilepsy. *Ann. Neurol.* 1987, 22, 480

13 Theodore, W.H., Newmark, M.E., Sato, S. *et al.* [^{18}F]fluorodeoxyglucose positron emission tomography in refractory complex partial seizures. *Ann. Neurol.* 1983, 14, 429

14 Theodore, W.H., Fishbein, D., Dubinsky, R. Patterns of cerebral glucose metabolism in patients with partial seizures. *Neurology* 1988, 38, 1201

15 Holmes, M.D., Kelly K. and Theodore, W.H. Complex partial seizures. Correlation of clinical and metabolic features. *Arch. Neurol.* 1988, 45, 1191

16 Stefan, H., Pawlik, G., Böcher-Schwarz, H.G. *et al.* Functional and morphological abnormalities in temporal lobe epilepsy: a comparison of interictal and ictal EEG, CT, MRI, SPECT and PET. *J. Neurol.* 1987, 234, 377

17 Hajek, M., Antonini, A., Leenders, K.L. and Wieser, H.G. Mesiobasal versus lateral temporal lobe epilepsy: metabolic differences in the temporal lobe shown by interictal ^{18}F-FDG positron emission tomography. *Neurology* 1993, 43, 79

18 Sadzot, B., Debets, R.M., Maquet, P. *et al.* Regional brain glucose metabolism in patients with complex partial seizures investigated by intracranial EEG. *Epilepsy Res.* 1992, 12, 121

19 Chee, M.W.L., Morris, H.H III., Antar, M.A. *et al.* Presurgical evaluation of temporal lobe epilepsy using interictal temporal spikes and positron emission tomography. *Arch. Neurol.* 1993, 50, 45

20 Henry, T.R., Mazziotta, J.C., Engel, J. Jr. *et al.* Quantifying interictal metabolic activity in human temporal lobe epilepsy. *J. Cereb. Blood Flow Metab.* 1990, 10, 748

21 Salanova, V., Morris, H.H., Rehm, P. *et al.* Comparison of the intracarotid amobarbital procedure and interictal cerebral 18F-fluorodeoxyglucose positron emission tomography scans in refractory temporal lobe epilepsy. *Epilepsia* 1992, 33, 635

22 Swartz, B.E., Tomiyasu, U., Delgado-Escueta, A.V. *et al.* Neuroimaging in temporal lobe epilepsy: test sensitivity and relationships to pathology and post-surgical outcome. *Epilepsia* 1992, 33, 624

23 Sperling, M.R., Alavi, A., Reivich, M. *et al.* False lateralization of temporal lobe epilepsy with FDG positron emission tomography. *Epilepsia* 1995, 36, 722

24 Theodore, W.H., Katz, D., Kufta, C. *et al.* Pathology of temporal lobe foci: correlation with CT, MRI and PET. *Neurology* 1990, 40, 797

25 Henry, T.R., Mazziotta, J.C., Engel, J. Jr. Interictal metabolic anatomy of mesial temporal lobe epilepsy. *Arch. Neurol.* 1993, 50, 582

26 Sackellares, J.C., Siegel, G.J., Abou-Khalil, B.W. *et al.* Differences between lateral and mesial temporal metabolism interictally in epilepsy of mesial temporal origin. *Neurology* 1990, 40, 1420

27 DeLaPena, R., Perlman, S.B., Levine, R. *et al.* PET scan findings in patients with temporal lobe epilepsy of mesial temporal origin. *J. Nucl. Med.* 1992, 33, 1014

28 Spencer, S.S., Spencer, D.D., Williamson, P.D. *et al.* Combined depth and subdural electrode investigation in uncontrolled epilepsy. *Neurology* 1990, 40, 74

29 Theodore, W.H. MRI, PET, SPECT. Interrelations, technical limits, and unanswered questions. *Epilepsy Res.* 1992, 5, 127

30 Sadzot, B., Debets, R.M., Delfiore, G. *et al.* Decrease of ^{11}C-flumazenil binding is more localized than glucose hypometabolism in patients with TLE studied by PET. *Neurology* 1994, 44(Suppl 2), A351

31 Radtke, R.A., Hanson, M.W., Hoffman, J.M. *et al.* Temporal lobe hypometabolism on PET: predictor of seizure control after temporal lobectomy. *Neurology* 1993, 43, 1088

32 Henry, T.R., Sutherling, W.W., Engel, J. Jr. *et al.* Interictal cerebral metabolism in partial epilepsies of neocortical origin. *Epilepsy Res.* 1991, 10, 174

33 Engel, J.Jr, Babb T.L. and Phelps M.E. Contribution of positron emission tomography to understanding mechanisms of epilepsy in 'Fundamental Mechanisms of Human Brain Function', (Eds J. Engel, Jr, *et al.*), Raven Press, New York, 1987, p.209

34 Manno, E.M., Sperling, M.R., Ding, X. *et al.* Predictors of outcome after anterior temporal lobectomy: positron emission tomography. *Neurology* 1994, 44, 2331

35 Radtke, R.A., Hanson, M.W., Hoffman, J.M. *et al.* Positron emission tomography: comparison of clinical utility in temporal lobe and extratemporal epilepsy. *J. Epilepsy* 1994, 7, 27

36 Swartz, B.E., Halgren, E., Delgado-Escueta, A.V. *et al.* Neuroimaging in patients with seizures of probable frontal lobe origin. *Epilepsia* 1989, 30, 547

37 Bernardi, S., Trimble, M.R., Frackowiak, R.S.J. *et al.* An interictal study of partial epilepsy using positron emission tomography and the oxygen-15 inhalation technique. *J. Neurol. Neurosurg. Psychiatr.* 1983, 46, 473

38 Franck, G., Sadzot, B., Salmon, E. *et al.* Regional blood flow and metabolic rates in human focal epilepsy and status epilepticus in 'Advances in neurology: basic mechanisms of the epilepsies, vol 44', (Eds. A.V. Delgado-Escueta A.A. Ward Jr, D.M. Woodbury and R.J. Porter), Raven Press, New York, USA, 1986, p.935

39 Leiderman, D.B., Balish, M., Sato, S. *et al.* Comparison of PET measurements of cerebral blood flow and glucose metabolism for the localization of human epileptic foci. *Epilepsy Res.* 1992, 13, 153

40 Tortella, F.C. Endogenous opioid peptides and epilepsy: quieting the seizing brain. *Trends Pharmacol. Sci.* 1988, 9, 366

41 Frost, J.J., Mayberg, H.S., Fisher, R.S. *et al.* Mu-opiate receptors measured by positron emission tomography are increased in temporal lobe epilepsy. *Ann. Neurol.* 1986, 23, 231

42 Mayberg, H.S., Sadzot, B., Cidis Meltzer, C.C. *et al.* Quantification of mu and non-mu opiate receptors in temporal lobe epilepsy using positron emission tomography. *Ann. Neurol.* 1991, 30, 3

43 Theodore, W.H., Carson, R.E., Andreasen, P. *et al.* PET imaging of opiate receptor binding in human epilepsy using [^{18}F]cyclofoxy. *Epilepsy Res.* 1992, 13, 129

44 Persson, A., Ehrin, E., Eriksson, L. *et al.* Imaging of [^{11}C]-labelled Ro 15-1788 binding to benzodiazepine receptors in the human brain by positron emission tomography. *J. Psychiat. Res.* 1985, 19, 609

45 Samson, Y., Hantraye, P., Baron, J.C. *et al.* Kinetics and displacement of [^{11}C]Ro 15-1788, a benzodiazepine antagonist, studied in human brain in vivo by positron emission tomography. *Eur. J. Pharmacol.* 1985, 110, 247

46 Savic, I., Ingvar, M., Stone-Elander, S. Comparison of [^{11}C]flumazenil and [^{18}F]FDG as PET markers of epileptic foci. *J. Neurol. Neurosurg. Psychiatry* 1993, 56, 615

47 Savic, I., Persson, A., Roland, P. *et al.* In vivo demonstration of reduced benzodiazepine receptor binding in human epileptic foci. *Lancet* 1988, 2, 863

48 Debets, R.M.C., Sadzot, B., van Isselt, J.W. *et al.* Is ^{11}C-flumazenil PET superior to ^{18}FDG PET and ^{123}I-iomazenil SPECT in presurgical evaluation of temporal epilepsy? *J. Neurol. Neurosurg. Psychiatry* 1997, 62, 141

49 Fowler, J.S., Wolf, A.P., MacGregor, R.R. *et al.* Mechanistic positron emission tomography studies: demonstration of a deuterium isotope effect in the monoamine oxidase-catalyzed binding of ^{11}C-L-deprenyl in living baboon brain. *J. Neurochem.* 1988, 51, 1524

50 Kumlien, E., Bergström, M., Lilja, A. *et al.* Positron emission tomography with [^{11}C]deuterium-deprenyl in temporal lobe epilepsy. *Epilepsia* 1995, 36, 712

51 Derlon, J.M., Bourdet, C., Bustany, P. *et al.* [^{11}C]L-methionine uptake in gliomas. *Neurosurgery* 1989, 25, 720

52 Biersack, H.J., Reichmann, K., Winkler, C. *et al.* ^{99m}Tc-labelled hexamethylpropyleneamine oxime photon emission scans in epilepsy [letter]. *Lancet* 1985, 2(8469-70), 1436

53 Podreka, I., Suess, E., Goldenberg, G. *et al.* Initial experience with technetium-99m HM-PAO brain SPECT. *J. Nucl. Med.* 1987, 28, 1657

54 Ryding, E., Rosén, Elmqvist, D. and Ingvar, D.H. SPECT measurements with ^{99m}Tc-HM-PAO in focal epilepsy. *J. Cereb. Blood Flow Metab.* 1988, 8, S95

55 Cordes, M., Christe, W., Henkes, H., Delavier, U. *et al.* Focal epilepsies: HMPAO SPECT compared with MR, and EEG. *J. Computed Assist. Tomogr.* 1990, 14, 402

56 Andersen, A.R., Waldemar, G., Dam, M. *et al.* SPECT in the presurgical evaluation of patients with temporal lobe epilepsy. A preliminary report. *Acta. Neurochir.* 1990, Supplement 50, 80

57 Duncan, S., Gillen, G., Adams, F.G. *et al.* Interictal HMPAO SPECT: a routine investigation in patients with medically intractable complex partial seizures? *Epilepsy Res.* 1992, 13, 83

58 Jabbari, B., van Nostrand, D., Gunderson, C.H. *et al.* EEG and neuroimaging localization in partial epilepsy. *EEG Cli. Neurophysiol.* 1991, 79, 108

59 Rowe, C.C., Berkovic, S.F., Austin, M.C. *et al.* Visual and quantitative analysis of interictal SPECT with technetium-99m-HMPAO in temporal lobe epilepsy. *J. Nucl. Med.* 1991, 32, 1688

60 Ryvlin, P., Garcia-Larrea, L., Philippon, B. *et al.* High signal intensity on T2-weighted MRI correlates with hypoperfusion in temporal lobe epilepsy. *Epilepsia* 1992, 33, 28

61 Grünwald, F., Durwen, H.F., Bockisch, A. *et al.* Technetium-99m-HMPAO brain SPECT in medically intractable temporal lobe epilepsy: a postoperative evaluation. *J. Nucl. Med.* 1991, 32, 388

62 Homan, R.W., Devous, M.D., LeRoy, R.F. and Bonte, F.J. Interictal focal cerebral blood flow elevations in partial seizures. *Neurology* 1989, 39(Suppl1), 300

63 Stefan, H., Bauer, J., Feistel, H. *et al.* Regional cerebral blood flow during focal seizures of temporal and frontocentral onset. *Ann. Neurol.* 1990, 27, 162

64 Rowe, C.C., Berkovic, S.F., Austin, M. *et al.* Postictal SPECT in epilepsy. *Lancet* 1989, 1(8634), 389

65 Shen, W., Lee, B.I., Park, H.M. *et al.* HIPDM-SPECT brain imaging in the presurgical evaluation of patients with intractable seizures. *J. Nucl. Med.* 1990, 31, 1280

66 Lee, B.I., Markand, O.N., Siddiqui, A.R. *et al.* Single photon emission computed tomography (SPECT) brain imaging using HIPDM: intractable complex partial seizures. *Neurology* 1986, 36, 1471

67 Duncan, R., Patterson, J., Roberts, R. *et al.* Ictal/postictal SPECT in the pre-surgical localisation of complex partial seizures. *J. Neurol. Neurosurg. Psychiatr.* 1993, 56, 141

68 Newton, M.R., Berkovic, S.F., Austin, M.C. *et al.* Ictal postictal and interictal single-photon emission tomography in the lateralization of temporal lobe epilepsy. *Eur. J. Nucl. Med.* 1994, 21, 1067

69 Newton, M.R., Berkovic, S.F., Austin, M.C. *et al.* SPECT in the localisation of extratemporal and temporal seizure foci. *J. Neurol. Neurosurg. Psychiatr.* 1995, 59, 26

70 Ho, S.S., Berkovic, S.F., Berlangieri, S.U. *et al.* Comparison of ictal SPECT and interictal PET in the presurgical evaluation of temporal lobe epilepsy. *Ann. Neurol.* 1995, 37, 738

71 van Huffelen, A.C., van Isselt, J.W., van Veelen, C.W. *et al.* Identification of the side of epileptic focus with ^{123}I-Iomazenil SPECT. A comparison with [18]FDG-PET and ictal EEG findings in patients with medically intractable complex partial seizures. *Acta. Neurochir.* 1990, Supplement 50, 95

72 Cordes, M., Henkes, H., Ferstl, F. *et al.* Evaluation of focal epilepsy: a SPECT scanning comparison of [123]-I-iomazenil versus HM-PAO. *Am. J. Neuroradiol.* 1992, 13, 249

73 Bartenstein, P., Ludolph, A., Schober, O. *et al.* Benzodiazepine receptors and cerebral blood flow in partial epilepsy. *Eur. J. Nucl. Med.* 1991, 18, 111

74 Wilson, A.A., Dannals, R.F., Ravert, H.T. *et al.* Synthesis and biological evaluation of [125I]- and [^{123}I]-4-iododexetimide, a potent muscarinic cholinergic receptor antagonist. *J. Med. Chem.* 1989, 32, 105

75 Müller-Gärtner, H.W., Wilson, A.A., Dannals, R.F. *et al.* Imaging muscarinic cholinergic receptors in human brain in vivo with SPECT, [^{123}I]4-iododexetimide, and [^{123}I]4-iodolevetimide. *J. Cereb. Blood Flow Metab.* 1992, 12, 562

76 Henry, T.R., Engel, J. Jr., Sutherling, W.W. *et al.* Correlation of structural and metabolic imaging with electrographic localization and histopathology in refractory complex partial epilepsy. *Epilepsia* 1987, 28, 601

77 Kawamura, M., Murase, K., Kataoka, M. *et al.* Early and delayed I-[123] IMP SPECT in epileptic patients with partial seizures and normal CT. *Clin. Nucl. Med.* 1991, 6, 839

78 Menzel, C., Grünwald, F., Pavics, L. *et al.* Brain single-photon emission tomography using technetium-99m bicisate (ECD) in a case of complex partial seizure. *Eur. J. Nucl. Med.* 1994, 21, 1244

79 Rowe, C.C., Berkovic, S.F., Austin, M. *et al.* Patterns of postictal blood flow in temporal lobe epilepsy: qualitative and quantitative analysis. *Neurology* 1991, 41, 1096

80 Spencer, S.S. The relative contribution of MRI, SPECT and PET imaging in epilepsy. *Epilepsia* 1994, 35(Suppl 6), S72

SPECT in Neurology and Psychiatry, edited by P.P. De Deyn, R.A. Dierckx, A. Alavi and B.A. Pickut
© 1997 John Libbey & Company Ltd, pp. 219–224

Ictal 99mTc-HMPAO SPECT and 123I-Iododexetimide SPECT in Temporal Lobe Epilepsy

Chapter
26

C. Rowe, K. Boundy, M. Kitchener, L. Barnden, M. Kassiou*,
A. Katsifis* and R. Lambrecht*

Introduction

Australia has a population of 18 million and is served by 8 epilepsy surgery centres, all of which use ictal SPECT imaging routinely in the pre-operative localisation of seizure foci. This valuable technique has gained worldwide acceptance, despite the logistic difficulties of radiopharmaceutical administration during seizure.

The first ictal SPECT report appeared in 1983 - a small number of interictal and ictal studies using 123I-IMP and a single-slice SPECT instrument had been performed at Massachusetts General Hospital[1]. However, the findings were not applied to clinical practice and no further studies were performed. In 1988, a group at the University of Indiana published the results of ictal SPECT with 123I-HIPDM and began to use ictal SPECT clinically in their seizure surgery program[2]. In 1989, the Austin Hospital group from Melbourne published a post-ictal SPECT series with 99mTc-HMPAO[3]. Since then, both groups have published extensively on ictal and postictal SPECT imaging[4-11]. Other centres - including Glasgow[12], Erlangen-Nurnberg[13], and the Melbourne Royal Children's Hospital[14] - have also reported ictal SPECT results from series of 15 or more patients with unilateral Temporal Lobe Epilepsy (TLE). The results of ictal or early postictal SPECT studies in more than 260 patients with unilateral TLE proven by ictal electroencephalography (EEG) or by seizure-free surgical outcome have now been published.

Ictal SPECT correctly identifies the seizure focus in 80-95% of patients with incorrect lateralisation reported in 1-5% of studies. Early postictal injection is less accurate but still identifies seizure focus in 70%; results appear to be better in those patients with hippocampal sclerosis as their underlying pathology. These results are clearly superior to the reported literature on interictal SPECT (Figure 1). The current literature contains reports on interictal SPECT covering over 350 patients with refractory temporal lobe epilepsy. Interictal SPECT showed temporal lobe hypoperfusion on the side of the seizure focus in 60% of these patients[4,8,10,15-23]. Contralateral hypoperfusion leading to incorrect lateralisation was present in 7%, a figure similar to PET results[24-26]. A recent comparison of ictal SPECT with interictal FDG PET showed that ictal SPECT had superior sensitivity[27].

Departments of Nuclear Medicine and Neurology, The Queen Elizabeth Hospital, Adelaide, South Australia 5011
*Australian Nuclear Science and Technology Organization, Sydney, Australia

Definitions and technique

True ictal studies are obtained with injection during the seizure but many authors have also included injection within 30 s of seizure completion. Early postictal studies are obtained by injection within 4 min of seizure completion, even though changes may persist in some patients for 10 min or more. Given the variability of this period, some authors use the term peri-ictal to refer to the ictal and early postictal phases.

The high first-pass extraction of ^{99m}Tc-HMPAO with prolonged retention makes imaging of ictal cerebral blood flow feasible with this widely available agent. ^{123}I-iodoamphetamine and ^{123}I-HIPDM are also suitable radiopharmaceuticals for ictal SPECT imaging and their greater stability removes the need for reconstitution immediately before injection, but these compounds are not readily available. Medical staff, nursing staff, and electroencephalography technicians have all been employed to reconstitute ^{99m}Tc-HMPAO at the bedside and give the ictal injection. The recent introduction of stabilised 'Ceretec' and Ethyl Cysteinate Dimer (ECD, 'Neurolyte') allows even faster injection, because these compounds can be reconstituted at the beginning of the day for later immediate injection.

Patterns of ictal and post-ictal CBF

Almost all patients with unilateral temporal lobe seizures will show hyperperfusion of the involved temporal lobe when given an ictal injection. The area of hyperperfusion is variable and may be seen predominantly in the anterior pole, lateral cortex or medial temporal lobe. Often it is extensive and involves the anterior half of the temporal lobe. Hyperperfusion of the ipsilateral basal ganglia is common and correlates well with dystonic posturing of the contralateral arm during the seizure[6]. Hyperperfusion may also be seen in the ipsilateral thalamus and remote areas of the cortex. Secondarily generalised seizures will show predominantly unilateral temporal lobe hyperperfusion if the focal component of the seizure lasts at least 15 s or if the seizure remains predominantly hemigeneralised. In such circumstances, hyperperfusion is more widespread and may be seen in the temporal lobe, ipsilateral motor cortex, basal ganglia and thalamus, and contralateral cerebellar cortex. Ictal hyperperfusion is seen both with mesial temporal sclerosis and seizures due to structural lesions such as low-grade temporal lobe tumours.

The area of ictal hyperperfusion is usually surrounded by hypoperfusion. The latter becomes the predominant feature in the postictal period and may extend widely to involve the entire ipsilateral hemisphere and sometimes the contralateral temporal lobe. Postictal hyper-perfusion, if present, is usually restricted to the antero-medial temporal lobe and not seen more than 5 min after seizure completion[5,8,10]. The timing of the switch from an ictal to a postictal pattern of perfusion varies from individual to individual, as does the duration of the postictal change.

Postictal changes are more frequently bilateral and this feature plus rapid resolution of CBF changes in some individuals accounts for the reduced sensitivity of post-ictal imaging compared with ictal injection. The earlier the injection, the greater the chance of detecting useful blood flow changes. Injection more than 5 min from seizure completion will substantially reduce sensitivity.

Bilateral temporal lobe ictal hyperperfusion from a unilateral focus is rare, despite the fact that spread of seizure activity to the contralateral temporal lobe is commonly seen with depth electrode recordings.

When does ictal SPECT fail?

The commonest reason for an inconclusive ictal SPECT study is a short seizure, especially one of extratemporal origin. The magnitude and duration of hyperperfusion is related to seizure duration. It resolves quickly after a short seizure and also quickly after an extratemporal seizure. True ictal injection is required under these circumstances and the increasing availability of stabilised 'Ceretec' and ECD will make this logistically easier to achieve.

Early secondary generalisation of a seizure can also lead to difficulty in interpreting an ictal SPECT. In most cases, lateralisation of the focus can still be achieved, since hyperperfusion tends to remain lateralised (see above).

Bilateral temporal lobe hyperperfusion is occasionally observed, mostly in patients with features suggestive of bilateral temporal lobe pathology, such as severe verbal and non-verbal memory impairment, or bilateral hippocampal atrophy on MRI. Such patients usually require depth electrode studies, since scalp ictal EEG is mostly unhelpful.

The clinical role of ictal SPECT

Ictal SPECT studies can be achieved in at least 80% of patients during the video-EEG monitoring phase of the surgical work-up. Clear localisation of the seizure focus with ictal SPECT is usually possible, even when scalp ictal EEG is unhelpful due to muscle artefact or simultaneous bilateral appearance of epileptiform electrical activity. A single ictal SPECT study will usually be sufficient, provided the history and ictal clinical and EEG features do not suggest more than one seizure type or possible bilateral foci. In such circumstances, multiple ictal SPECT studies may be needed. Correlation of ictal SPECT localisation with the seizure focus defined by ictal EEG is superior to interictal SPECT, PET, and MRI[27,28]. However, the relative accuracy of each of these modalities in predicting a seizure-free surgical outcome is not clearly defined. This issue is complicated by the variety of reasons for failed surgery - including inadequate resection of the hippocampus, the presence of bilateral foci, and the presence of an undetected extratemporal focus.

Muscarinic cholinergic neuroreceptor imaging with ^{123}I-iododexetimide (IDEX) SPECT in temporal lobe epilepsy

A variety of neuroreceptors have been imaged with SPECT and PET in patients with partial epilepsy. These techniques have demonstrated focal changes in benzodiazepine[28-30], and opiate receptors at the seizure focus[31,32]. The cholinergic system plays a modulatory role in neuronal excitation and also appears to be disturbed at seizure foci. Animal kindling models of epilepsy have shown a reduction in muscarinic cholinergic receptors (mAChR) at the site of seizure focus[33-35], and muscarinic cholinergic receptors are reduced in concentration in temporal lobectomy specimens[36]. *In vivo* imaging of cholinergic neuroreceptors can be performed with PET[37] or SPECT[38-40]. Iododexetimide (IDEX) has recently been developed for SPECT imaging of mAChR[39]. It was produced from dexetimide, a long-acting anticholinergic pharmaceutical used for many years in the treatment of Parkinson's disease and tardive dyskinesia. It was radioiodinated in 1989 and validated as a mAChR SPECT ligand, by Müller-Gartner *et al.* at Johns Hopkins Hospital, Baltimore[39]. Regional brain uptake reflects the known distribution of mAChR[39,40]. Non-specific binding of IDEX slowly clears from the brain, while specific binding remains[40]. Consequently, IDEX SPECT images best reflect the mACh receptor distribution and density when acquired 6 or more hours post-injection[39,40]. Radiation dosimetry calculations show that it is safe for human studies[40]. A preliminary report of a reduction in uptake of IDEX in the medial temporal lobe in 4 patients with temporal lobe epilepsy was published in 1993 by the Johns Hopkins group[41].

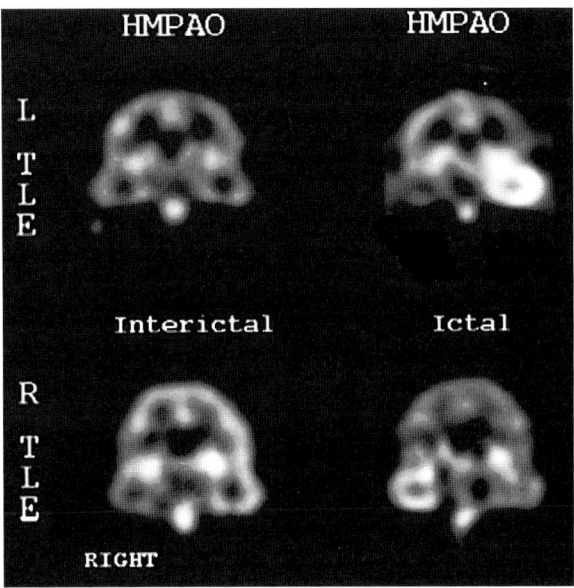

Figure 1 Interictal and ictal ^{99m}Tc-HMPAO SPECT. Coronal slices are shown from interictal (left) and ictal (right) studies from two patients. The top row is from a patient with left TLE. The interictal study showed no perfusion asymmetry but the ictal study revealed left temporal lobe hyperperfusion. Note the relative hypoperfusion of adjacent frontoparietal cortex and the contralateral temporal lobe. The bottom studies are from a patient with right TLE. Interictal hypoperfusion and ictal hypoperfusion are seen. Both patients had histologically proven hippocampal sclerosis

We performed a study to assess mAChR imaging with IDEX SPECT in temporal lobe epilepsy and to examine the relationship of changes in mAChR to seizure focus, and to interictal cerebral blood flow SPECT and MRI findings.

Methods

We studied 18 people with proven intractable unilateral temporal lobe epilepsy with IDEX SPECT. All subjects underwent MRI, interictal EEG, ictal video-surface EEG, neuropsychological evaluation, and interictal and ictal HMPAO SPECT. The location of the seizure focus was determined from these investigations, with greatest weight given to the results of ictal EEG and ictal SPECT.

IDEX was produced by the Biomedicine and Health Program of the Australian Nuclear Science and Technology Organisation in Sydney with 97% radiochemical purity, and a specific activity of >2,000mCi/μmol. IDEX was transported overnight to Adelaide for use the following morning. IDEX SPECT was performed on full medication and interictally (>48h since last seizure). Standard potassium iodide solution (1.5g) was given half an hour before injection of 120-185 MBq of IDEX, with the brain SPECT 6 h later.

SPECT scans were performed with ultra-high resolution fan-beam collimators on a triple-headed gamma camera (TRIAD) with 20% photopeaked window. SPECT acquisition was of 72 angles, into a 128 x 64 matrix (3.56 mm pixel size) for 30 s per view. The projection data was prefiltered in 2 dimensions with a Metz filter. Images were reconstructed to produce coronal slices perpendicular to the temporal lobe. Image analysis was performed by applying a standard template to the coronal slices, using the anterior-posterior brainstem as a guide to the portions of the hippocampus, with 2 slices (3.56 mm/slice) each through the amygdala, and the anterior, mid- and posterior hippocampus. Square ROIs (regions of interest) were placed over the lateral and medial temporal lobes. An asymmetry index (100 times the difference in counts in the two areas/average of the two sides) was calculated for the amygdala, hippocampal region and lateral temporal cortex. Asymmetry indices were also calculated for the HMPAO studies. Studies were also reviewed by 3 blinded clinicians who recorded focal reductions in perfusion or IDEX binding. A consensus rating was reached on each study of normal, possible or definite temporal lobe abnormality.

MRI was performed on a Siemens 1.0 Tesla IMPACT scanner, with routine T_1 and T_2 axial sequences, followed by fine slices (2-3 mm) coronal to the plane of the temporal lobe using T_1 3D MP-RAGE sequence and T_2 fast spin echo. Scans were reported by a radiologist blinded to all other localising data.

Results

Blinded visual inspection of interictal HMPAO SPECT in the unilateral cases showed hypoperfusion at the focus in (9/18) 50% of cases, and indicated the incorrect temporal lobe in 4. The remaining 5 interictal HMPAO studies were inconclusive. Blinded review of the MRI scans showed definite changes of unilateral hippocampal sclerosis in 13 of the 18 cases, while the hippocampi were considered normal or inconclusive in 5.

Blinded visual analysis of IDEX scans identified the correct side of the seizure focus in 14 of the 18 cases, while 3 were inconclusive and one showed the most marked IDEX reduction contralateral to the focus. This patient had bilateral reduction of IDEX binding and

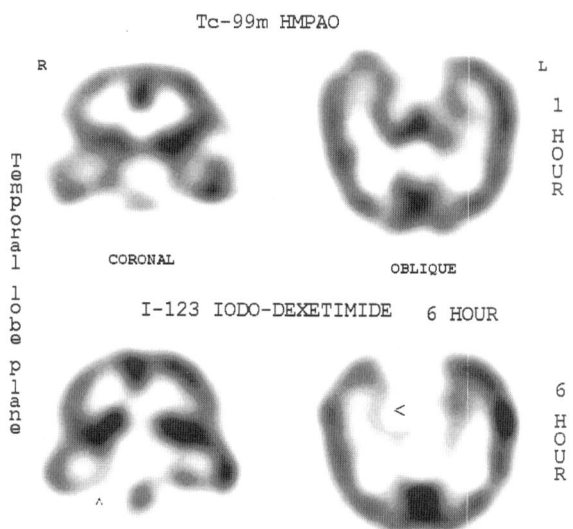

Figure 2 ^{99m}Tc-HMPAO SPECT. The top images show a slight reduction in right anterior temporal lobe interictal perfusion on ^{99m}Tc-HMPAO SPECT. The bottom row are ^{123}I-IDEX SPECT images from the same patient that clearly show a reduction in binding to muscasrinic cholinergic receptors in the right medial temporal region. Hippocampal sclerosis was proven at operation in the right temporal lobe

was excluded from surgery due to severe global memory impairment. IDEX SPECT showed reduced temporal lobe binding in 4 of the 5 normal/inconclusive MRI cases.

The IDEX asymmetry index showed reduced binding in the medial temporal lobe on the side of the focus in all but one case. The reduction of medial temporal IDEX binding averaged 19% ±12.1 and ranged from 1.4 to 40%. The asymmetry index in the region of the amygdala was smaller, 11.3% ±6.4, and the lateral temporal neocortex recorded the smallest reduction, 7.6% ±12.1. In contrast, cerebral blood flow was uniformly reduced throughout the epileptogenic temporal lobe by about 10%. The reduction of IDEX in the medial temporal region was significantly greater than the reduction in blood flow as measured with HMPAO SPECT (p=0.02, Wilcoxon signed ranks test) (Figure 2).

Fourteen of the patients have undergone anterior temporal lobectomy. Histological examination of resected material revealed hippocampal sclerosis in 12. One showed neuronal heterotopia and one was normal. All patients have experienced a >90% reduction in seizure frequency.

Discussion

Our data demonstrate a reduction in muscarinic cholinergic receptors in the medial temporal region containing the seizure focus, with asymmetry of IDEX binding almost twice as great as that of HMPAO binding. The area of reduced IDEX binding was also more localised than the area of reduced CBF. Almost all of our patients had histological or MRI evidence of hippocampal sclerosis, so it is not surprising to find reduced neuroreceptor numbers in this region. It is well established that the reduction in CBF and metabolism seen in TLE exceeds the area of histological abnormality. Several patients showed a focal reduction in medial temporal lobe IDEX binding without clear MRI evidence of hippocampal sclerosis. In these cases evidence of hippocampal sclerosis was found in the resected material.

IDEX can be produced with high specific activity and high synthetic yield (50-70%). Its stability permits use up to a day after production and the high brain uptake (8% of the injected dose) gives high quality images with low injected doses. The prolonged retention permits washout of early blood flow-dependent non-specific binding before imaging, so that arterial sampling and detailed mathematical corrections are not needed to obtain images of specific binding.

The clinical role of IDEX SPECT in seizure localisation is not yet defined but it may have a useful role in patients with normal or equivocal MRI findings. Further studies in such patients are required.

References

1   Magistretti, P.L. and Uren, R.F. Cerebral blood flow patterns in epilepsy in ' Epilepsy: an update on research and therapy', (Ed. G. Nistico), Alan R Liss, New York, USA, 1983, p.241

2   Lee, B.I., Markand, O.N., Wellman, H.N. *et al.* HIPDM-SPECT in patients with medically intractable complex partial seizures: ictal study. *Arch. Neurol.* 1988, 45, 397

3   Rowe, C.C., Berkovic, S.F., Sia, S.T.B. *et al.* Localization of epileptic foci with post-ictal SPECT. *Ann. Neurol.* 1989, 26, 660

4   Markand, O.N., Salanova, V., Worth, R.M. *et al.* Ictal brain imaging in presurgical evaluation of patients with medically intractable complex partial seizures. *Acta. Neurol. Scand.* 1984, suppl 152, 137

5   Newton, M.R., Berkovic, S.F., Austin, M.C. *et al.* Post-ictal switch in blood flow distribution and temporal lobe seizures. *J. Neurol. Neurosurg. Psychiatr.* 1992, 55, 891

6   Newton, M.R., Berkovic, S.F., Austin, M.C. *et al.* Dystonia, clinical lateralization, and regional blood flow changes in temporal lobe seizures. *Neurology* 1992, 42, 371

7   Newton, M.R., Austin, M.C., Chan, J.G. *et al.* Ictal SPECT using Tc-99m HMPAO: methods for rapid preparation and optimal deployment of tracer during spontaneous seizures. *J. Nucl. Med.* 1993, 34, 666

8   Newton, M.R., Berkovic, S.F., Austin, M.C. *et al.* Ictal, post-ictal and interictal SPECT in the lateralization of temporal lobe epilepsy. *Eur. J. Nucl. Med.* 1994, 21, 1067

9   Newton, M.R., Berkovic, S.F., Austin, M.C. *et al.* SPECT in the localization of extratemporal and temporal seizure foci. *J. Neurol. Neurosurg. Psychiatr.* 1995, 59, 26

10 Rowe, C.C., Berkovic, S.F., Austin, M.C. *et al.* Patterns of post-ictal cerebral blood flow in temporal lobe epilepsy: qualitative and quantitative analysis. *Neurology* 1991, 41, 1096

11 Shen, W., Lee, B.I., Park, H.M. *et al.* HIPDM SPECT brain imaging in the presurgical evaluation of patients with intractable seizures. *J. Nucl. Med.* 1990, 31, 1280

12 Duncan, R., Patterson, J., Roberts, R. *et al.* Ictal/post-ictal SPECT in the presurgical localization of complex partial seizures. *J. Neurol. Neurosurg. Psychiatr.* 1993, 56, 141

13 Weis, M., Feistel, H. and Stefan, H. Utility of ictal SPECT: peri-ictal, post-ictal. *Acta. Neurol. Scand.* 1994, (suppl 152), 145

14 Harvey, A.S., Bowe, J.M., Hopkins, I.J. *et al.* Ictal 99mTc-HMPAO SPECT in children with temporal lobe epilepsy. *Epilepsia* 1993, 35(suppl 6), S72

15 Andersen, A.R., Waldemar, G., Dam, M. *et al.* SPECT in the presurgical evaluation of patients with temporal lobe epilepsy - a preliminary report. *Acta. Neurochirurgica.* 1990, 50(Suppl), 80

16 Bauer, J., Stefan, H., Feistel, H. *et al.* Ictal and interictal SPECT measurements using Tc-99m HMPAO in patients suffering from temporal lobe epilepsies. *Nervarzt.* 1991, 62, 745

17 Dietrich, M.E., Bergen, D., Smith, M.C. *et al.* Correlation of abnormalities of interictal n-isopropyl-p-iodoamphetamine single photon emission tomography with focus of seizure onset in complex partial seizure disorders. *Epilepsia* 1991, 32, 187

18 Grunwald, F., Durwen, H.F., Bockisch, A. *et al.* Technetium-99m-HMPAO brain SPECT in medically intractable temporal lobe epilepsy: a postoperative evaluation. *J. Nuc. Med.* 1991, 32, 388

19 Hajek, M., Siegel, A.M., Haldemann R. *et al.* Value of HMPAO SPECT in selective temporal lobe surgery for epilepsy. *J. Epilepsy* 1991, 4, 43

20 Ryding, E., Rosen, I., Elmqvist, D. and Ingvar, D.H. SPECT measurements with Tc-99m HMPAO in focal epilepsy. *J. Cereb. Blood Flow Metab.* 1988, 18(suppl 1), 95

21 Ryvlin, P.R., Philippon, B., Cinotti, L. *et al.* Functional neuroimaging strategy in temporal lobe epilepsy: a comparative study of FDG-PET and Tc-99m HMPAO SPECT. *Ann. Neurol.* 1992, 31, 650

22 Stefan, H., Pawlik, G., Bocher-Schwarz. *et al.* Functional and morphological abnormalities in temporal lobe epilepsy:

a comparison of interictal and ictal EEG, CT, MRI, SPECT, and PET. *J. Neurol.* 1987, 234, 377

23 Stefan, H., Bauer, J., Feistel, H. *et al.* Regional cerebral blood flow during focal seizures of temporal and frontocentral onset. *Ann. Neurol.* 1990, 27, 162

24 Engel, J. The use of PET scanning in epilepsy. *Ann. Neurol.* 1984, 15, 180

25 Mazziotta, J.C. and Phelps, M.E. Positron emission studies of the brain in 'Positron emission tomography and autoradiography; principles and applications for the brain and heart', (Eds. M.E. Phelps, J.C. Mazziotta and H.R. Schelbert), Raven Press, New York, 1986, p.493

26 Theodore, W.H., Fishbein, D. and Dubinsky, R. Patterns of cerebral glucose metabolism in patients with partial seizures. *Neurology* 1988, 38, 1201

27 Ho, S.S., Berkovic, S.F., Berlangieri, S.U. *et al.* Comparison of ictal SPECT and interictal PET in the presurgical evaluation of temporal lobe epilepsy. *Ann. Neurol.* 1995, 37, 738

28 Ferstl, F.J., Cordes, M., Cordes, I. *et al.* 123-I-iomazenil SPECT in patients with focal epilepsies - a comparative study with 99m Tc-HMPAO SPECT, CT and MR in Neuroreceptor mechanisms in brain', (Ed. S. Kito), Plenum Press, New York, USA, 1991, p.405

29 Bartenstein, P., Ludolph, A., Schober, O. *et al.* Benzodiazepine receptors and cerebral blood flow in partial epilepsy. *Eur. J. Nucl. Med.* 1990, 18, 111

30 Savic, I., Persson, A., Roland, P. *et al.* In vivo demonstration of reduced benzodiazepine receptor binding in human epileptic foci. *Lancet* 1988, 2, 863

31 Frost, J.J., Mayberg, H.S., Fisher, R.S. *et al.* Mu-opiate receptors measured by positron emission tomography are increased in temporal lobe epilepsy. *Ann. Neurol.* 1988, 23, 231

32 Mayberg, H.S., Sadzot, B., Meltzer, C.C. *et al.* Quantification of Mu and non-Mu opiate receptors in temporal lobe epilepsy using positron emission tomography. *Ann. Neurol.* 1991, 30, 3

33 Byrne, M.C., Gottlieb, R. and McNamara, J.O. Amygdala kindling induces muscarinic cholinergic receptor decline in a highly specific distribution within the limbic system. *Exp. Neurol.* 1980, 69, 85

34 McNamara, J.O. Muscarinic cholinergic receptors participate in the kindling models of epilepsy. *Brain Res.* 1978, 154, 415

35 Yaari, Y. and Jensen, M.S. Two types of epileptic foci generating brief and sustained paroxysms in the in vitro rat hippocampus in Neurotransmitters in epilepsy (Epilepsy Res, suppl 8)', (Eds. G. Avanzini, J. Engel Jr, R. Fariello and U. Heinemann), Elsevier, 1992, 33, p.263

36 Wyler, A.R., Nadi, N.S. and Porter, R.J. Acetylcholine, GABA, benzodiazepine, and glutamate receptors in the temporal lobe of epileptic patients. *Neurology* 1987, 37(suppl 1), 103 (abstract)

37 Wilson, A.A., Scheffel, U.A., Dannals, R.F. *et al.* In vivo biodistribution of two (^{18}F)-labelled muscarinic cholinergic receptor ligands: 2-(^{18}F)-and 4-(^{18}F)-fluorodexetimide. *Life Sci.* 1991, 48, 1385

38 Eckelman, W.C., Eng, R., Rzeszitarski, W.J. *et al.* Use of 3-quinuclidinyl 4-iodobenzilate as a receptor binding tracer. *J. Nucl. Med.* 1985, 26, 637

39 Müller-Gartner, H.W., Wilson, A.A., Dannals, R.F. *et al.* Imaging muscarinic cholinergic receptors in human brain in vivo with SPECT, I-123-4-iododexetimide. *J. Cereb. Blood Flow Metab.* 1992, 12, 562

40 Boundy, K.L., Barnden, L.R., Rowe, C.C. *et al.* Human dosimetry and normal brain distribution of iodine-123-iododexetimide: a SPECT imaging agent for cholinergic muscarinic neuroreceptors. *J. Nucl. Med.* 1995, 36, 1332

41 Müller-Gartner, H.W., Mayberg, H.S., Fisher, R.S. *et al.* Decreased hippocampal muscarinic cholinergic receptor binding measured by 123-iododexetimide and single photon emission computed tomography in epilepsy. *Ann. Neurol.* 1993, 34, 235

SPECT in Neurology and Psychiatry, edited by P.P. De Deyn, R.A. Dierckx, A. Alavi and B.A. Pickut
© 1997 John Libbey & Company Ltd, pp. 225–231

rCBF Changes in Seizures Originating Outside Mesial Temporal Structures

Chapter
27

R. Duncan

Introduction

Most focal epilepsies in adults originate in the mesial temporal lobe structures, and cause a relatively well described clinical syndrome of complex partial seizures with or without secondary generalised seizure[1]. In the past, the term 'complex partial epilepsy' has been widely used to denote temporal lobe epilepsy, illustrating the extent to which complex partial seizures have been assumed to arise in the mesial temporal lobe. In recent years, with the increasing use of surgical treatment for epilepsy and the consequent widening of interest in localisation of seizure origin, it has become increasingly recognised that a proportion of complex partial seizures originate outside the mesial temporal lobe structures, and the electrical and clinical features of these seizures are becoming better defined[2]. The proportion is, according to most authorities, about 20%, but remains the subject of debate. It is important to obtain reasonably certain pre-surgical localisation for any focal seizure disorder, but there is additional reasoning behind the division of mesial temporal seizures from others. Most centres use relatively standardised presurgical assessments and surgical strategies for mesial temporal epilepsies, but other focal epilepsies require a much more individual approach, and often require greater epileptological expertise, and more invasive presurgical EEG investigation.

This chapter gives an account of the use of SPECT in the detection of interictal, ictal and postictal changes in rCBF in extratemporal epilepsies. The term 'extratemporal', although succinct, has been avoided in the title of this chapter because, strictly speaking, it excludes lateral temporal seizures, which will be dealt with in this chapter.

Interictal rCBF in extratemporal epilepsies

There has been limited study of interictal rCBF in extratemporal epilepsies. Two series, which excluded lesional cases, have shown low sensitivity compared with mesial temporal epilepsies[3,4], and our recent series showed that only 3/30 patients with confirmed extratemporal epilepsies had an abnormal interictal rCBF unassociated with structural abnormality on MRI. Although the data remain scant, therefore, it seems likely that the localising sensitivity of interictal HMPAO SPECT will turn out to be lower in extratemporal than in temporal epilepsies (unsurprisingly, the sensitivity of interictal PET in this situation also seems low[5]).

Institute of Neurological Sciences, Southern General Hospital, Glasgow G51 4TF, Scotland

Ictal rCBF in focal seizures

Extratemporal, particularly frontal, seizures can present practical problems in the use of ictal SPECT; these relate both to the biology of the seizure, and to the characteristics of SPECT rCBF tracers.

The temporal sampling of an image of rCBF is determined by the behaviour of the tracer. Before that is an issue, however, the seizure has to be recognised, and the injection mixed and given. The tracer then has to reach the brain from the vein into which it was injected and be taken up and fixed. Transit time from arm to brain is approximately 15 s, and the uptake period approximately 40 s (for HMPAO)[6]. The rCBF image acquired is approximately averaged over this 40 s period, and will reflect any rCBF changes of sufficient magnitude, extent, or duration that have taken place during the 40 s.

It is often assumed that the time-course of ictal changes in rCBF is the same as that of EEG changes, but this is not always the case - the obvious example being the persistence of mesial temporal hyperperfusion for several minutes after mesial temporal lobe seizures have finished. Our experience, and that of at least one other group[4], suggests that ictal hyperperfusion does persist after shorter seizures, but for a shorter time, which would support observations made by Penfield in the thirties[7]. Our experience suggests that changes in rCBF may sometimes be detected when HMPAO has been injected toward the end of a seizure lasting 20 s, but that the injection has to be given at or near seizure onset with seizures shorter than this. This is only possible if the seizure can be provoked, or if it occurs very frequently and the injection can be pre-mixed, and the syringe connected to the cannula ready to inject. The new rCBF tracer ^{99m}Tc-ECD (Bicisate - Neurolite, Dupont Pharma[8]) is stable for several hours, and may well be useful for seizures that are short but frequent. HMPAO can be rendered stable by mixing with cobalt chloride, but this product is unlicensed. Regardless of all this, it is important to remember that the main cause of tracer injection delay is failure to recognise and notify the seizure. There is little point in saving the 10-15 s it takes to mix the tracer when the person who is to perform the injection can only arrive at the bedside 1 min after seizure recognition.

Successful use of ictal SPECT in short seizures is difficult, and requires attention to all aspects of the organisation and logistics of tracer injection. It also needs to be recognised that the technique may simply not be capable of capturing very short seizures - those lasting 10 s or less - since even when injection is at onset, the tracer may not arrive in the brain in sufficient quantities before the ictal rCBF changes resolve.

Ictal rCBF changes in seizures originating outside mesial temporal lobe structures

There is relatively little material in the literature on rCBF changes in seizures originating outside the mesial temporal structures. Nonetheless, work that has been published shows patterns of perfusion clearly different from those seen during mesial temporal seizures[4,8-14]. This chapter will deal with seizures originating in the frontal lobe, the lateral temporal lobe, the temporo-parieto-occipital junction (TPOJ), the parietal lobe, and the occipital lobe.

Corollary localising data for some ictal SPECT observations may not include what some would regard as definitive (invasive) EEG data, but this is sometimes unavoidable. Not all extratemporal seizures are operable. If the non-invasive data suggests, for example, that seizures originate in the dominant frontal operculum or TPOJ, then it is unlikely that an excision will be considered for functional reasons. In such an event, submitting the patient to the trauma and risk of invasive EEG recording is not usually justifiable, and confirmatory evidence of SPECT localisation will instead have to rely on the clinical semiology of the seizure, interictal and ictal surface EEGs, and MRI. The gold standard localisation, i.e. the successful result of an excision that has not been restricted for functional or technical reasons, may also be unfeasible.

However, whatever its value as a localising investigation, the images of the whole brain that SPECT can provide are capable of showing changes in subcortical structures and other areas not usually sampled by EEG electrodes. When such observations are correlated with well observed seizure semiology and electrophysiology, SPECT certainly has the potential to improve our understanding of the dynamics of seizures and their clinical correlates.

Seizures originating in the lateral temporal lobe

There are currently no data in the literature, and the author's experience is limited to 2 ictal studies in patients with evidence of anterolateral temporal lobe seizures. One showed hyperperfusion of the lateral temporal cortex with ipsilateral mesial hypoperfusion, the other showed hyperperfusion of the whole temporal lobe, but with a clear lateral predominance. In neither case was the localisation confirmed by invasive EEG recording or by the result of a lateral temporal resection, so the observations remain unconfirmed. Posterolateral temporal seizures are probably a subset of TPOJ seizures.

Seizures originating in the area of the temporo-parieto-occipital junction

Seizures originating in the area of the temporo-parieto-occipital junction (TPOJ) are not extensively described, except in the French literature[15]. Because limbic structures are often involved early in the seizure by propagation of the ictal discharge, seizures in this area may be difficult to distinguish clinically and electrically from those of mesial temporal origin. However, it is important to make the distinction, since standard temporal lobe resections are unlikely to affect TPOJ seizures, and the TPOJ itself is not amenable to resection on the dominant side. In our experience, TPOJ seizures are a more common reason for failure of temporal lobectomy than orbital frontal seizures, which are clinically rather more distinct. TPOJ seizures are characterised by seizure discharge involving neighbouring areas of the temporal, parietal and occipital lobes: vertiginous sensations[16], visual hallucinations[17], head and truncal version and gyration[18,19], oculoclonus and blinking[18], result. Later in the seizure, features suggesting mesial temporal propagation, such as oro-alimentary and gestural automatisms[18,20], may also be seen, and massive postictal aphasia can occur. Although both interictal and ictal discharges can be clearly distinguished (being localised more posteriorly) from those arising from medial temporal epileptogenic zones, lateralisation may be made difficult by rapid involvement of the contralateral TPOJ in seizure discharge.

The rCBF changes may consist of an isolated focus of hyperperfusion at the TPOJ, or may involve the ipsilateral temporal lobe (Figure 1). When this is the case, hyperperfusion extends anteriorly into the anterolateral temporal cortex. Perfusion of the mesial structures is variable - in some cases reduced, in some increased, but never to as great a degree as perfusion of the lateral cortex. In the seizures studied so far, we have not seen the typical pattern of mesial temporal seizures - hyperperfusion roughly equal in both the mesial and lateral cortex, but it is important to allow for the attenuation correction applied during image reconstruction. There is variable hyperperfusion of the anterolateral temporal lobe structures, and mesial temporal structures are hyperperfused to a lesser degree, or even hypoperfused. There may also be a small area of hyperperfusion in the contralateral parietal lobe, seemingly correlating with bilateralisation of the seizure discharge.

Frontal lobe seizures

Frontal lobe seizures can present considerable localisation difficulties. The frontal lobe is a large structure in which seizure discharges can spread and bilateralise very rapidly, so that invasive EEG monitoring is often necessary. Although seizures can be very frequent, their brevity poses problems for rCBF SPECT, and many seizures are simply too short to be captured by this method.

Seizures originating in the frontal lobes seem to be associated with a variety of ictal changes[4,9,10,13]. Although it is difficult to make generalisations from the small amount of data published, they all have perfusion abnormalities distinct from those seen in mesial temporal lobe seizures, and apparently consistent with the site of origin of the seizure within the frontal lobe (where this is known).

At its simplest, a single focal area of hyperperfusion is seen (Figure 2), but the rCBF disturbances are, in some cases, much more complex. The frontal hyperperfusion itself may be bilateral or widespread (Figure 3), and associated hyperperfusion of subcortical structures such as the basal ganglia, thalamus and cerebellum seems to be common (Figure 4). One further interesting characteristic of frontal seizures is the pattern of ictal hypoperfusion, which seems to be as variable as the pattern of hyperperfusion. There is often none at all, but hypoperfusion may even involve the hemisphere contralateral to the frontal hyperperfusion (Figure 3). Ipsilateral hypoperfusion may also be seen.

All these data serve to demonstrate that perfusion patterns in frontal lobe seizures are variable and can be complex, and that the associated images require very careful interpretation. In particular, they suggest that it may be dangerous to draw any conclusions from images that seem to show hypoperfusion alone, since the imager may not have detected a small or mildly abnormal area of hyperperfusion in the contralateral frontal lobe.

Parietal lobe seizures

Little has been published, but pure parietal lobe seizures seem to be associated simply with localised hyperperfusion in the parietal lobe (Figure 5)[12]. As Figure 5 shows, the changes can be subtle.

Occipital lobe seizures

There are no series reported in the literature, and the author's experience is limited to a few cases of occipital hyperperfusion, an example of which is shown in Figure 6. As in TPOJ seizures, ipsilateral temporal lobe structures may also be involved.

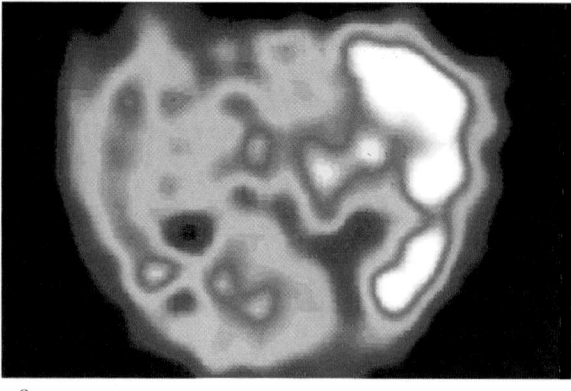

a

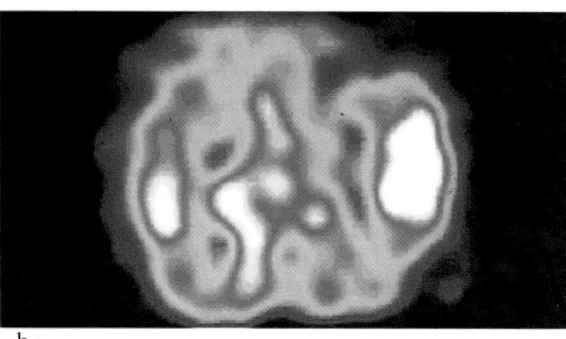

b

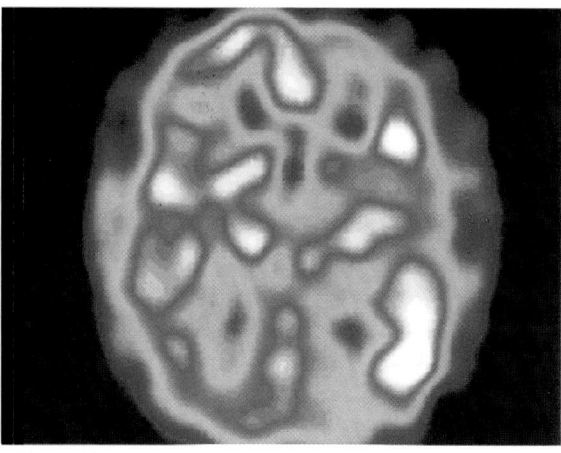

c

Figure 1 a, HMPAO SPECT, injection during seizure originating in the left TPOJ. Axial slice in the plane of the long axis of the temporal lobe showing hyperperfusion of the left temporal lobe, more marked in the lateral cortex and pole. b, Same dataset. Posterior coronal slice showing hyperperfuions of the area of the left TPOJ, with a small contralateral area of hyperperfusion (seen in approximately 50% of cases studied so far). c, Same dataset. Flat axial slice showing hypoperfusion of the left hemisphere. Hyperperfusion of the TPOJ is also shown, with an area of hyperperfusion in the lateral frontal cortex (seen in a minority of cases so far)

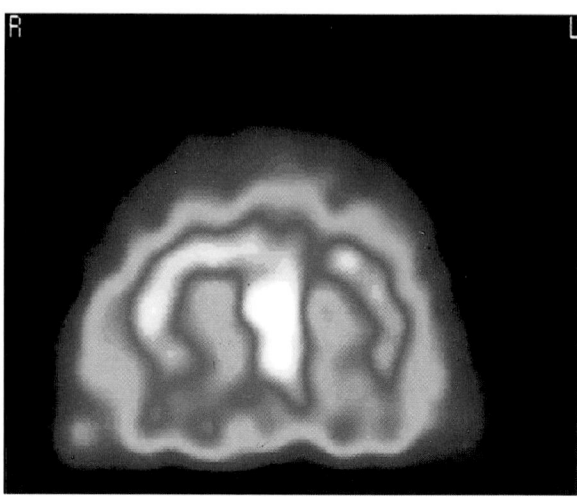

Figure 2 HMPAO SPECT, injection during seizure of left mesial frontal origin. Anterior coronal slice showing hyperperfusion of the mesial frontal cortex, which cannot be lateralised from the SPECT image

Interpretation of periictal rCBF images

Image interpretation presents particular problems in the context of periictal rCBF changes, since these can be complex, and only fully assessed through comparison of periictal and interictal images. When the only

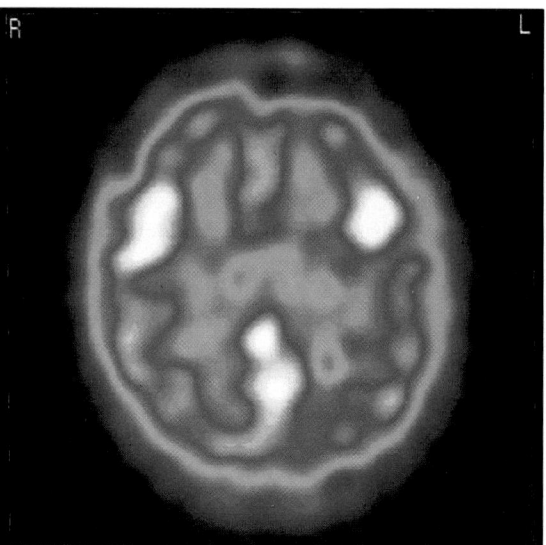

Figure 3 HMPAO SPECT, injection during seizure of left lateral frontal origin. Axial slice showing bilateral hyperperfusion of the lateral frontal cortex and hypoperfusion of the left hemisphere

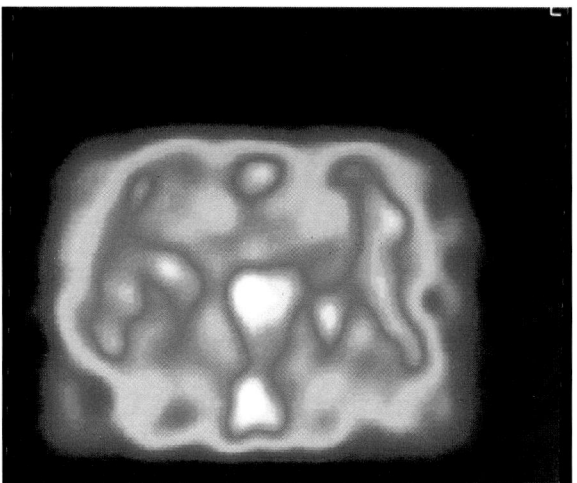

Figure 4 Same dataset as Figure 2. Coronal slice showing bilateral hyperperfusion of the thalamus extending into the brainstem

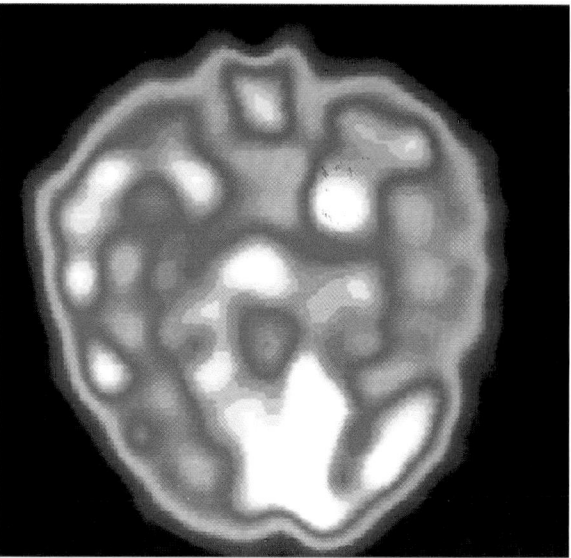

Figure 6 HMPAO SPECT, injection at end of seizure of left occipital origin. Axial slice in the long axis of the temporal lobe showing hyperperfusion of the mesial and lateral occipital cortex on the left. There is also hypoperfusion of the ipsilateral lateral temporal cortex, and a small area of hyperperfusion of the mesial temporal cortex (i.e. the temporal lobe is showing a pattern typical of that seen in the postictal phase of a mesial temporal lobe seizure)

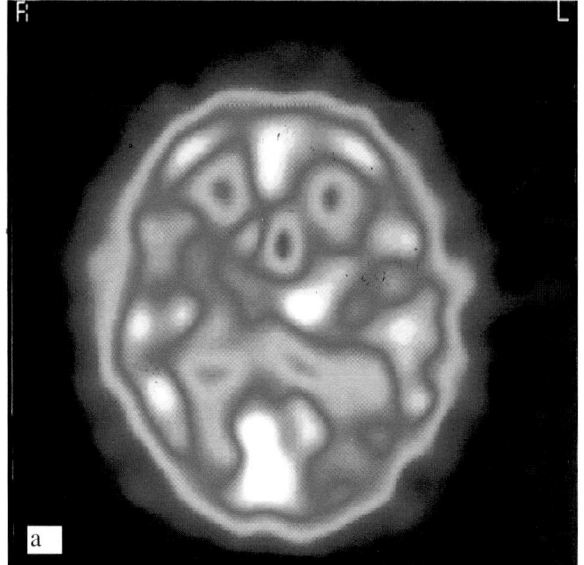

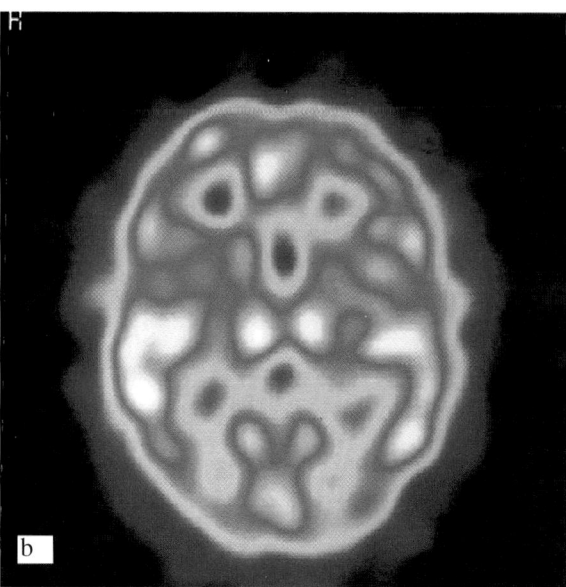

Figure 5 a, Interictal HMPAO SPECT in patient with right parietal seizures. Axial slice showing perfusion pattern within normal limits. b, HMPAO SPECT, injection during seizure in the same patient. Equivalent axial slice to a, showing subtle hyperperfusion of right parietal lobe

change seen is a localised area of hyperperfusion, interpretation is relatively straightforward - perhaps not simply a case of deciding that the seizure originates at the 'bright spot' on the scan. The process of interpretation can be conceptually divided into 2 stages:

1. Identifying the abnormalities seen on interictal and periictal scans and the changes seen with respect to the interictal scan
2. Explaining the changes seen by means of a hypothesis of seizure origin and spread.

The first stage primarily requires imaging (nuclear medicine, clinical physics, neuroradiology) expertise, while the second stage requires the input of someone who has experience in epileptology, and, in particular, understands the pathophysiology of seizure genesis and spread. It is the author's experience that, when changes are complex, more than one possible hypothesis of localisation and spread needs to be considered in order to explain the rCBF changes.

Place of HMPAO SPECT in a programme for the neurosurgery of epilepsy - extratemporal seizures

Already published data suggest that ictal rCBF changes can be used as a major localising criterion in mesial temporal seizures - certainly when the treatment offered is temporal lobectomy rather than more restricted excision. It would, in the author's opinion, be unnecessary to subject a patient to invasive EEG recordings in cases where ictal HMPAO SPECT had already shown hyperperfusion of one temporal lobe, and when injection had clearly been carried out during the patient's habitual seizure. One group[3,4] has already greatly reduced the proportion of their patients undergoing invasive EEG monitoring using this technique, and mesial temporal lobe seizures, which represent most adult epilepsies, are a major indication.

There is not yet enough published data to use rCBF SPECT findings as a major localising criterion in seizures of extratemporal origin, despite promising preliminary data. Moreover, especially in frontal lobe seizures, ictal changes may be complex and require careful interpretation. More also needs to be learnt about the changes associated with seizures originating in different extratemporal structures. However, in centres with experience of surgical treatment it would be reasonable to add ictal SPECT data to all other data (clinical, structural imaging, surface ictal, interictal EEG, etc.) with which the hypothesis of seizure origin and spread is constructed, allowing the design of a strategy of invasive monitoring.

Acknowledgements

The SPECT imager used to acquire images in Glasgow patients was funded by the Wellcome Trust. Some of the data on which this chapter is based, particularly the section on TPOJ seizures, were acquired at the epilepsy unit of Professor P. Chauvel, CHRU Pontchaillou, 35033 Rennes Cedex, France. Acquisitions were carried out with the help of Professor P. Bourguet of the Centre Eugene Marquis at the same site.

References

1 Weiser, H.G., Engel, J., Williamson, P.D. *et al.* Surgically remediable temporal lobe syndromes in Surgical treatment of the epilepsies, 2nd edn.' (Ed. J. Engel), Raven Press, New York, USA, 1993, p.49

2 Williamson, P.D. and Spencer, S.S. Clinical and EEG features of complex partial seizures of extratemporal origin. *Epilepsia* 1986, 27(suppl 2), S46

3 Duncan, R. Epilepsy, cerebral blood flow and cerebral metabolic rate. *Cerebrovasc. Brain Metab. Rev.* 1992, 4, 105

4 Newton, M.R., Berkovic, S.F., Austin, M.C. *et al.* SPECT in the localisation of extratemporal and temporal seizure foci. *J. Neurol. Neurosurg. Psychiatr.* 1995, 59, 26

5 Henry, T.R., Sutherling, W.W., Engel, J. *et al.* Interictal cerebral metabolism in partial epilepsies of neocortical origin. *Epilepsy Res.* 1991, 10, 174

6 Andersen, A.R., Friberg, H., Schmidt, J.F. *et al.* Quantitative measurements of cerebral blood flow using SPECT and Tc99m D,L-HMPAO compared to Xenon-133. *J. Cereb. Blood Flow Metab.* 1988, 8(Suppl 1), S69

7 Gibbs, F.A., Lennox, W.G. and Gibbs, E.L. Cerebral blood flow preceding and accompanying seizures in man. *Arch. Neurol. Psychiat.* 1934, 32, 257

8 Friberg, L., Andersen, A.R., Lassen, N.A. *et al.* Retention of [99mTc] bicisate in the human brain after intracarotid injection. *J. Cereb. Blood Flow Metab.* 1994, 14(Suppl 1), S19

9 Marks, D.A., Katz, A., Hoffer, P. and Spencer, S.S. Localisation of extratemporal epileptic foci during ictal single photon emission computed tomography. *Ann. Neurol.* 1992, 31, 250

10. Harvey, A.S., Hopkins, I.J., Bowe, J.M. *et al.* Frontal lobe epilepsy: clinical seizure characteristics and localisation with ictal [99mTc]-HMPAO SPECT. *Neurology* 1993, 43, 1966

11 Stefan, H., Bauer, J., Feistel, H. *et al.* Regional cerebral blood flow during focal seizures of temporal and frontal central onset. *Ann. Neurol.* 1990, 27, 162

12 Ho, S.S., Berkovic, S.F., Newton, M.R. *et al.* Ictal [99mTc] HMPAO SPECT findings in parietal lobe epilepsy. *Epilepsia* 1993, 34(Suppl 2), 112

13 Duncan, R., Patterson, J., Hadley, D.M. *et al.* Ictal HMPAO SPECT in frontal lobe seizures. *Epilepsia* 1993, 34(Suppl 2), 174

14 Duncan, R., Patterson, J., Roberts, R. *et al.* rCBF during posterior seizures: an HMPAO SPECT study. *J. Neurol. Neurosurg. Psychiatr.* (abstract: in press)

15 Bancaud, J. Sémiologie clinique des crises épileptiques d'origine temporale. *Rev. Neurol.* 1987, 143, 392

16 Sveinbjronsdottir, S. and Duncan, J. Parietal and occipital lobe epilepsy: a review. *Epilepsia* 1993, 34, 493

17 Koelmel, H.W. Complex visual hallucinations in the hemianopic field. *J. Neurol. Neurosurg. Psychiatr.* 1985, 48, 29

18 Haecan, H., Penfield, W., Bertrand, C. and Malmo, R. The syndrome of apractognosia due to lesions of the minor hemisphere. *Arch. Neurol. Psychiatr.* 1956, 75, 400

19 Wyllie, E., Luders, H., Morris, H.H. *et al.* The lateralising significance of versive head and eye movements during epileptic seizures. *Neurology* 1986, 36, 606

20 Ajmone-Marsan, C. and Goldhammer, L. Clinical ictal patterns and electrographic data in cases of partial seizure of fronto-central-parietal origin in 'Epilepsy: its phenomena in man', (Ed. M.A.B. Brazier), Academic Press, New York, USA, 1973, p.235

SPECT in Neurology and Psychiatry, edited by P.P. De Deyn, R.A. Dierckx, A. Alavi and B.A. Pickut
© 1997 John Libbey & Company Ltd, pp. 233–246

HMPAO SPECT and Video -EEG Monitoring in Candidates for Surgical Treatment of Epilepsy

Chapter
28

I. Podreka, C. Baumgartner[†], A. Olbrich[†], A. Relič,
U. Pietrzyk[*], W. Serles[†], K. Novak[†], D. Wimberger[**],
S. Aull[†], G. Lindinger[†], S. Lurger[†], T. Brücke[†], E. Punz and
V. Stellamor

Introduction

Quantitative or semiquantitative measurement of regional cerebral blood flow (rCBF) by single photon emission computerised tomography (SPECT) or positron emission tomography (PET) is an established procedure for the detection of impaired brain function or tissue abnormalities, which are not visualised by conventional magnetic resonance imaging (MRI). Both techniques are used together with routine EEG, video-EEG, MRI and neuropsychological testing, including the WADA test, for lateralisation of the epileptogenic focus and estimation of a possible postoperative disturbance of higher brain functions in candidates for surgical epilepsy treatment.

From many studies published during the past 15 years it is well known that patients suffering from temporal lobe seizures (TLE) exhibit decreased rCBF in the epileptogenic zone interictally (this term is defined as the time where EEG does not show epileptogenic discharges and no clinical sign of an ongoing seizure is observable). During a partial seizure, rCBF is increased in brain areas responsible for seizure onset and seizure propagation. However, in the SPECT literature, interest was mainly focussed towards the visible interictal side differences of tracer uptake or detection of unilateral ictal and postictal rCBF changes[1-3] in patients with temporal lobe eplilepsy. To our knowledge, no attempt has been made so far to apply systematically a semiquantitative method, which would allow a more detailed evaluation of SPECT studies and to correlate seizure semiology to rCBF changes. Furthermore, there are no SPECT or PET reports on rCBF changes in the preictal state.

In this paper, we give an overview of our combined video-EEG and SPECT investigations on a small cohort of patients suffering from refractory TLE or extratemporal (ETE) seizures, who were candidates for surgery. Due to effective patient management, we were able to perform SPECT studies in seizure free periods, during seizures, psychotic episodes and, in one case, preictally.

Neurologie Rudolfstiftung, Wien, Austria
[†]Neurologische Universitätsklinik Wien, Austria
[*]Max Planck Institut für Neurologische Forschung, Köln, Germany
[**]Abteilung für Neuroradiologie der Universitätsklinik für Radiologie, Wien, Austria

Patients and methods

Eighteen patients (9 males, 9 females), 19-63 years of age (mean 29.3 ± 7.4 years) were investigated. Fifteen suffered from TLE and 3 patients had ETE. Patient data seizure aetiology and MRI findings are shown in Table 1. Four patients had idiopathic seizures (patients U.S., H.S., B.M. and D.M.) while in the remaining 14 cases the following factors responsible for seizure development could be identified: perinatal •injury (patients K.P. and C.R.), febrile convulsions (patients B.H., H.G. and H.R.), meningitis or encephalitis (patients L.B., G.I., G.D., M.G.), benign tumour (patients R.H. and E.H.), vaccination (patient R.S.), premature birth (patient B.B.) and postoperative defect (patient Z.M., operation of a benign astrocytoma in childhood). MRI was normal in 5 subjects, hippocampal atrophy was observed in 4 cases, hippocampal sclerosis in 1 patient, atrophy of the temporal lobe or of one hemisphere in 2 patients and 2 patients had a postoperative defect (partial resection of one temporal lobe, operated benign astrocytoma). Heterotopia or dyplasia was observed in 2 cases and in 2 patients a benign tumour in the temporal lobe was detected (hamartoma or cavernoma).

Video-EEG recording (Pegasus-Video-EEG-Monitoring-System, Electric Medical Systems-Korneuburg) lasted for 2-7 days (mean 5 days). Gold disc electrodes were placed according to an extended International 10-20 System with additional electrodes over the frontocentral regions[4]. All channels were referenced to a common vertex electrode (Pz) that allowed off-line reformatting of the data in any desired montage. Data were amplified (x 20.000) and filtered (bandpass 1 to 70 Hz) using Grass 12A5 amplifiers (Grass Instruments, Quincy, MA), digitised at a sampling rate of 256 Hz (12 bits) and stored digitally for off-line data analysis[5]. Anticonvulsive therapy was reduced stepwise and then stopped in order to enable seizure registration, SPECT was performed with a 3-headed rotating scintillation camera (Siemens Multispect3) equipped with HRES collimators. The spatial resolution of the system is 6-7 mm FWHM in the reconstructional plane. Projections were obtained in 2° step and shoot mode (25 sec/angle) and images were reconstructed in 128 x 128 matrices by filtered back projection (Butterworth filter cut of 0.9).

Each patient had an interictal SPECT investigation. In 14 instances the second SPECT study was obtained during a seizure. HMPAO (18-22 mCi, 666-814 MBq) was injected i.v. within 12-56 s after EEG- and clinically proven seizure onset. Four patients suffering from TLE were studied during a psychotic episode and 1 case by occasion, 15 min prior to seizure onset.

In order to ensure comparison of identical anatomical structures, two individual SPECT studies (in patient H.S., three SPECT studies) and MRI images were realigned by using an appropriate interactive technique for three-dimensional image registration[6]. Thereafter 9 adjacent, 10.4 mm thick cross-sections covering the entire brain were chosen for further evaluation. One hundred and seven regions of interest (ROIs, Figure 1) were first drawn on interictal SPECT images and then transferred to correspondent ictal cross-sections. Normalised values of rCBF (regional indices = RIs) were expressed by the ratio between the mean counts/voxel of a specific ROI and the mean counts/ voxel of all ROIs. An RI change of at least 12% between two SPECT studies was regarded to be significant.

Results

Interictal SPECT and interictal EEG

Thirteen patients suffering from TLE (86.7%) had a visually detectable low tracer deposition in the temporal regions and 2 had a normal SPECT finding (see Table 2). In 8 instances, a clear unilateral abnormality in the medial and/or lateral portion of one temporal lobe, i.e. low perfusion, could be recognised, while in 5 cases a low tracer uptake was observed in both temporal regions. The last finding is obviously dependent on experience in interpreting SPECT images. Taking into account that the investigator responsible for SPECT interpretation was blinded for the EEG results, a fairly good comparison between the two methods was achieved. The 8 patients with unilateral temporal hypoperfusion had on the same side 80%-100% of the totally recorded interictal spikes. Three of the 5 patients with assumed bilateral SPECT abnormalities showed clearly bilateral spike activity on EEG (patients K.P., G.D. and M.G.), 1 case mainly unilateral spikes (patient B.H.) and in 1 patient (patient C.D.), no spikes could be detected. In the 2 patients with a normal SPECT finding, no focus lateralisation could be achieved by EEG.

Interictal and ictal SPECT

Interictal and ictal RI-values were compared for the whole TLE-group studied during a seizure (n=12). Figure 2 shows the results. Significantly increased rCBF (paired t-test, two tailed) was found in right medio-temporal and laterotemporal ROIs (slice 2: ITr1, MTr1), in the right cerebellum (CBr2) and both thalamic ROIs (slice 5: THr1, THl1). Significant rCBF decreases were seen only in frontal ROIs (slice 5:

Table 1 Patients and clinical data

Patient	Gender	Age	Duration (years)	Seizure type[a]	Aetiology	MRI
Temporal lobe seizures						
K.P.	m	36	35	CPS without and with sG	hypoxic brain damage	left hippocampal atrophy
B.H.	m	32	22	CPS with questionable sG	fever convulsions	left hippocampal sclerosis
U.S.	m	30	21	CPS without and with sG	unknown	normal
H.S.	f	29	12	CPS	unknown	heterotopia left opercular region
H.G.	m	30	21	CPS without and with sG	fever convulsions	right hippocampal atrophy
L.B.	f	25	21	CPS	meningoencephalitis	atrophy of the right temporal lobe
B.M.	f	30	22	CPS without and with sG	unknown	partial resection of the right temporal lobe
D.M.	f	20	12	CPS without and with sG	unknown	left hemiatrophy
G.I.	f	36	18	CPS without and with sG	meningitis	right hippocampal atrophy
H.R.	m	31	26	CPS without and with sG	fever convulsion	left hippocampal atrophy
G.D.	m	24	16	SPS and CPS	encephalitis	normal
M.G.	f	36	23	CPS without and with sG	meningitis	normal
R.H.	m	50	14	CPS without and with sG	expansive lesion	right hippocampal hamartoma or dysplasia
C.R.	m	28	21	CPS without and with sG	perinatal injury	normal
E.H.	m	63	31	CPS without sG	expansive lesion	cavernoma
Extratemporal seizures						
R.S.	f	19	18	NMS without and with sG	vaccination	normal
Z.M.	f	27	6	CPS of parietal origin	st.p. left parietal astrocytoma	left parietal defect
B.B.	m	19	15	frontal seizures	premature birth	right orbito-frontal heterotopia

[a]SPS, simple partial seizures; CPS, complex partial seizures; sG, secondary generalisation; NMS, negative motor seizures

Table 2 Comparison of visually estimated interictal and ictal SPECT findings with interictal spike activity and ictal EEG

Patient[a]	Gender	Age	Duration	Seizure type	Interictal SPECT		EEG(%)		ictal SPECT[a]		Seizures	ictal EEG
					left	right	left	right	left	right	n	
K.P.[b]	m	36	35	CPS without and with sG	++	+	55	45	++	++	20	20 LT
B.H.[b]	m	32	22	CPS with questionable sG	++	+	96	4	++	++	4	4 SOI
U.S.[b]	m	30	21	CPS without and with sG	0	0	0	0	?	?	2	1 SOI 1 SOI ->RT
H.S.[c]	f	29	12	CPS	0	0	60	40	++	++	6	5 SOI 1 SOI ->RT
H.G.	f	30	21	CPS without and with sG	0	+	2	98	0	++	6	3 SOI ->RT, 3 SOI
L.B.[d]	f	25	21	CPS	0	++	0	100	0	++	9	9 RT
B.M.	f	30	22	CPS without and with sG	0	++	0	100	0	++	5	4 SOI 1 RT
D.M.	f	20	12	CPS without and with sG	0	++	0	100	0	++	15	15 SOI
G.I.	f	36	18	CPS without and with sG	0	++	0	100	0	++	6	5 RT 1 SOI ->RT
H.R.	m	31	26	CPS without and with sG	+	0	100	0	++	0	6	6 SOI ->LT
G.D.	m	24	16	SPS and CPS	+	+	50	50	0	+	6	5 RT 1 LT
M.G.	f	36	23	CPS without and with sG	+	+	55	45	+	0?	7	7 SOI
R.H.	m	50	14	CPS without and with sG	+	0	80	20	++	++	4	1 RT 3 LT
C.D.	m	28	21	CPS without and with sG	+	+	0	0	++	++	4	2 RH 2 bi-occipital >L+R
E.H.	m	63	31	CPS without sG	++	0	100	0	++	0	11	11 LT

SPECT 0, normal; +, moderately abnormal; ++, clearly abnormal. EEG %, percentage side distribution of recorded interictal spikes; n, number of registered seizures; RT, right temporal; LT, left temporal; SOI, seizure onset inconclusive; ->, lateralizing to one side; [a], patients state during SPECT investigation: [b], periictal psychosis; [c], periictal psychosis as well as ictal SPECT; [d], 15 min before seizure onset (preictal); CPS, complex partial seizures; SPS, simple partial seizures; sG, secondary generalisation

REGIONS OF INTEREST

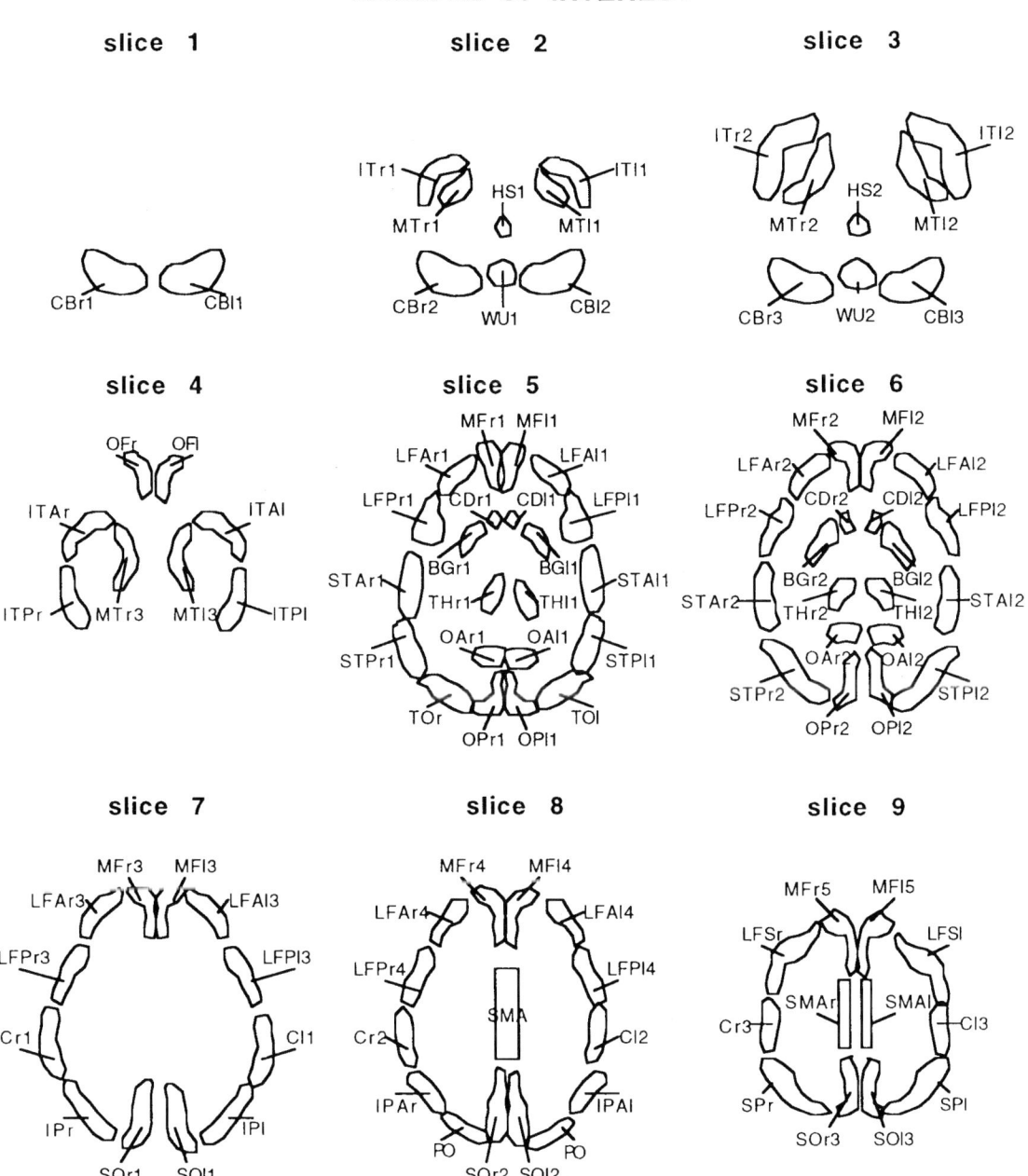

Figure 1 CB1-3=cerebellum, WU1-2=vermis, HS1-2=brain stem, IT1-2=inf.temp, MT1-3=medio -temporal, ITA=inf. temporal ant, ITP=inf. temporal post, MF1-5=medio-frontal, LFA1-4=lat. front. ant, LFP1-4=lat.front.post, STA1-2=sup. temp. post, TO=temporo-occipital, OP1-2=occipital post, OA1-2=occipital ant, CD1-2=nucl. caudatus, BG1-2=Striatum, TH1-2=thalamus, C1-3=central region, IP=inf. parietal, IPA=inf. patietal ant, PO=parieto-occipital, SO1-3=sup. occipital, SP=sup. parietal, SMA=supplementary motor area, r=right, l=left

ICTAL rCBF CHANGES IN PATIENTS WITH TEMPORAL LOBE EPILEPSY

slice 1

slice 2

p=0.0383

p=0.0467

p=0.033

slice 3

slice 4

slice 5

p=0.0002*

p=0.0135

p=0.0316

p=0.0135

slice 6

p=0.0079

p=0.0138

p=0.0277

L

slice 7

p=0.0051

p=0.0447

p=0.0381

slice 8

p=0.0007

p=0.0019

p=0.0308

slice 9

Figure 2 rCBF changes between the interictal and ictal state in TLE patients (paired t-test) *persisting significance after Bonferroni-correction (p<0.05)

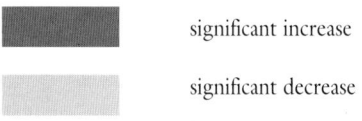

significant increase

significant decrease

MFr1, LFAr1; slice 6: MFr2, MF12, LFPr2; slice 7: MFr3, LFAr3, LFAl3; slice 8: MFr4, MFl4, LFPr4). After correction for multiple comparisons (Bonferroni), only a significant result was obtained in the right medio-frontal ROI (slice 5: MFr1, p <0.05).

Preictal SPECT

As we have emphasised, one patient (patient L.B.) had HMPAO injected 15 min prior to seizure onset. Investigators were waiting for the whole morning in order to obtain an ictal SPECT investigation but the patient did not have a seizure. In the afternoon it was decided to administer the already reconstituted tracer. When the patient was positioned for scanning a partial complex seizure occurred. Figure 3 shows interictal and preictal SPECT images. It is clearly visible that rCBF is elevated in the right medio-temporal and latero-temporal cortex. RI increases are mainly seen in right temporal ROIs and only 1 orbito-frontal ROI was seen on 4 slices from bottom to the top (slice 2: MRrQ 38.5%, ITr1 56.5%; slice 3: MTr2 27.2%, ITr2 35.2%; slice 4: OFr 13%, MTr3 17.5%, ITAr 30.6%, ITPr 13.8%; slice 5: STAr1 14.1%, STPr1 21.2%).

Periictal psychosis and SPECT findings

Four patients were investigated during a psychotic state of various intensity. Two of them (patients K.P. and B.H.) developed paranoid ideas, delusions, and were anxious and restless. Here SPECT revealed a relative increase of HMPAO deposition in both medio-temporal and medio-frontal ROIs. In patient K.P. the following percentage increases between the interictal and psychotic state were found (values within brackets (<12%) are considered not to be significant rCBF changes): slice 2: ROI ITr1/ITl1 +30.6% / 89.4%, ROI MTr1/MTl1 +27.2% / 47.7%; slice 3: ROI ITr2/ITl2 +22.5% / 35.4%, ROI MTr2/MTl2 +(7.0%) / 29.9%; slice 4: ROI OFr/OFl +13.9% / 18.4%, ROI MTR3/MTl3 (7.3%) / 22.6%; slice 5: ROI MFr1/MFl1 12.7% / (10.3%),. ROI LFAr1/LFAl1 (-0.8%) / 37.6%, ROI LFPr1/LFPl1 (5.7%) / 14.5%, ROI STAr1/STAl1 (2.1%) 20.7%.

Comparison of SPECT studies obtained in patient B.H. gave similar relative percentage rCBF changes: slice 2: ROI ITr1/ITl1 +26.1% / 23.3%, ROI MTr1/MTl1 +12.1% / 18.0%; slice 3: ROI ITr2/ITl2 +20.2% / 14.3%, ROI MTr2/MTl2 +13.2% / 12.0%; slice 4: ROI OFr/OFl (9.2%) / 22.0%, ROI ITAr/ITAl -19.2 / 12.0; slice 5: ROI LFAr1/LFAl1 (11.9%) / 21.9%, ROI STAr1/STAl1 (-2.5%) / +20.4: slice 6: ROI MFr2/MFl2 (-1.1%) / +13.9%; slice 7: ROI LFAr.LFAl3 +(1.1%) / 12.6%.

The other 2 patients had a less pronounced psychotic symptomatology, with anxiety and irritability, and were reproachful towards physicians and nurses. rCBF changes obtained in patient H.S. were also localised in the medial and lateral portion of both temporal lobes (slice 2: ROI ITr1/ITl1 +18.7% / 18.5%, ROI MTr1/MTl1 +22.8% / (9.5%); slice 3: ROI MTr2/MTl2 +13.1% / 14.8%; slice 4: ROI MTr3/MT13 17.4% / (8.3%)). However, these rCBF changes were of lower magnitude than those observed in the previous two cases and the RIs calculated from the ictal SPECT in the same patient (Figure 4). Patient U.S. showed the lowest range of relative rCBF changes between the interictal and psychotic state (slice 2: re/li ROI ITr1/ITl1 +12.1% / -18.6%; slice 3: ROI MTr2/MTl2 12.9% / (-4.4%); slice 4: ROI ITAr/ITAl (5.7%) / +16.5%; slice 5: ROI MFr1/MFl1 +18.8% / (2.9%), ROI STPr1/STPl1 +13.0% / (1.9%). ROI CDr1/CDl1 +16.3% / (5.7%); slice 6: ROI MFr2/MFl2 +15% / (5.7%); slice 9: ROI LFSr/FLSl +12.2% / (11.5%)). Figure 5 summarises the findings in these four patients. Relative rCBF increases above 12% were seen in 10.1% of all ROIs, while in only 2.8% of the ROIs relative rCBF decreased more than 12% of the interictal RI value.

Comparison of RIs obtained interictally and during the psychotic state by paired t-test indicated several significant changes in relative rCBF distribution. Significant t-values are given in Table 3. It is evident that a redistribution of rCBF occurred with a relative increase in the temporal lobes (slices 2 and 4) and a relative rCBF decrease directed towards occipital ROIs in higher cross-sections. These comparisons assist us in the formulation of a hypothesis for future investigations and cannot be considered as a definitive result, due to the small number of subjects investigated.

Extratemporal seizures

Three patients were suffering from extratemporal epilepsy. One had frequent seizures (up to 30 seizures/day) of frontal lobe origin (patient B.B.) with sudden flexion of the body, version of head to the left, speech arrest and absence of postictal amnesia. Video-EEG was in this case inconclusive but the ictal SPECT investigation (Figure 6) revealed a clearly increased tracer deposition in the right orbito-frontal region. Implanted subdural grid-electrodes proved seizure onset exactly in this area. After surgery, the patient is seizure free. Histological examination of the removed tissue showed heterotopia in the orbito-frontal white matter.

The second patient (R.S.) had, in addition to tonic - clonic seizures, negative motor seizures, with sudden

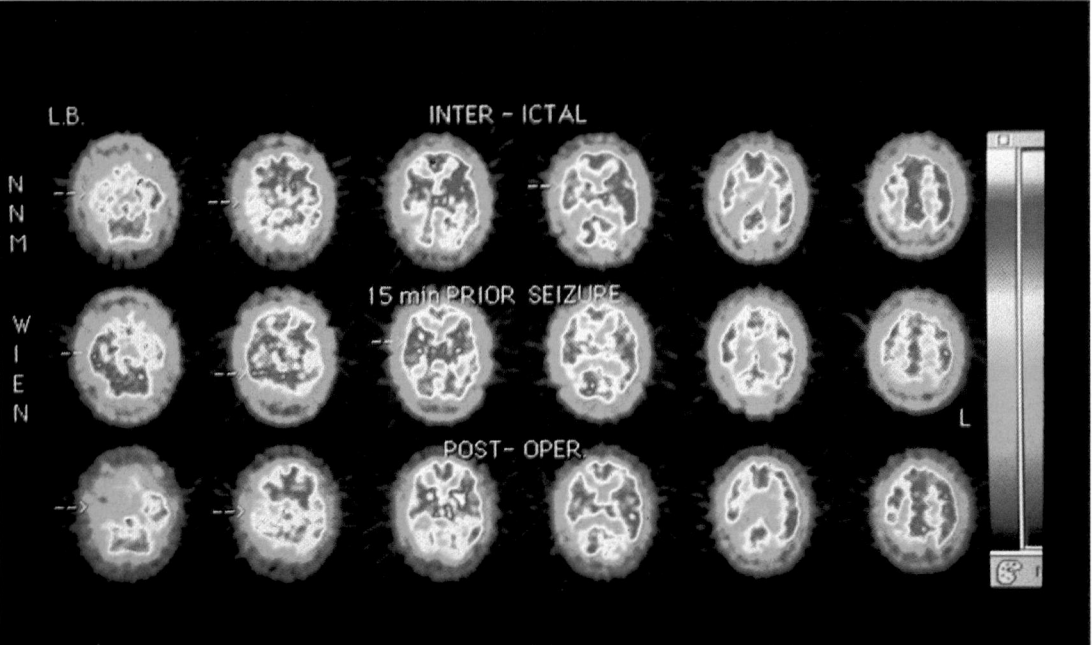

Figure 3 3 HMPAO SPECT studies (interictal, 15 min before seizure onset and postoperative). The increase of tracer deposition is clearly visible in the second row (arrows) when compared with the interictal study, which shows a relative decrease of tracer uptake (arrows first row). After surgery (amygdalohippcampectomy) low HMPAO uptake is visible not only in the medial portion of the temporal lobe but also in the neocortial areas (third row, arrows)

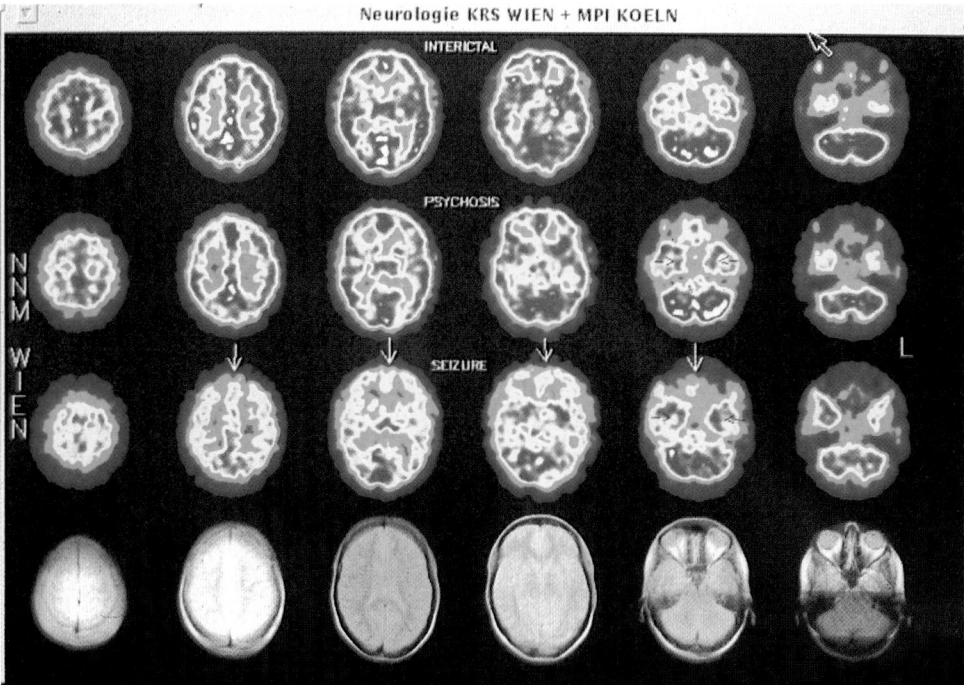

Figure 4 3 HMPAO SPECT studies in a seizure-free state (first row), during a psychotic period (second row) and during a seizure (third row). The interictal study shows no abnormality. During psychosis an increased tracer deposition is visible in both medio-temporal areas (fifth slice from the left, black arrows). The latter is more pronounced during the seizure (fifth slice from the left), while frontal relative rCBF is decreased (second - fifth slice from the left, white arrows). MRI sections of identical thickness as SPECT images are shown in the fourth row

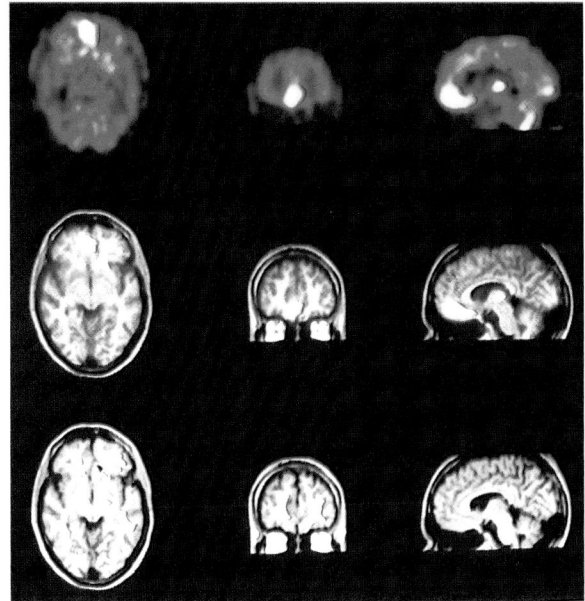

Figure 6 Identical cross sections (transversal, coronal, saggital) of ictal SPECT (first row) and MRI (second row). Coregistration is shown in the second row. The arrow in the transversal MRI-section indicates the region where dysgenesis was found intraoperatively and where the seizure had its origin as shown in SPECT images

repetitive losses of postural tone of the right upper limb and without any impairment of consciousness. SPECT revealed during this condition an increased HMPAO uptake in the left prefrontal cortex and to a lesser extent also in the parietal cortex. Interictal as well as the EEG during epileptic negative myoclonus showed frequent frontal spikes in electrodes FC1 and F1. The case has been reported extensively by Baumgartner et al.[7].

Patient Z.M. had focal seizures, which were occasionally generalised. The epileptogenic focus was assumed to be in the tissue surrounding a postoperative (a benign astrocytoma was removed at 2 years of age) lesion in the left central and parietal region. Interictal SPECT showed low tracer uptake in the known lesion but also in the left medio-temporal tissue. Ictal SPECT indicated a relative increase of rCBF in the parieto-central area as well as in both medial portions of the temporal lobe, more pronounced on the left and in the left anterior basal gaglia. Seizure onset was characterised by a motionless stare, followed by a version of the head to the right and jerks of the left upper limb. If generalisation occurred, tonic - clonic jerks on both sides were observed. EEG indicated a seizure onset in the left centro-parietal region. However, in this case dual pathology could not be excluded and the patient did not undergo surgery.

Table 3 Comparison of regional indices (RIs) between the interictal and psychotic state (paired t-test, two tailed) in 4 subjects

Slice	ROI	RI interictal	RI psychosis	t	p
2	ITr1	0.690 ± 0.044	0.844 ± 0.035	- 6.181	0.0085
2	MTr1	0.798 ± 0.062	0.935 ± 0.043	- 4.514	0.020
3	ITr2	0.833 ± 0.035	0.954 ± 0.025	- 4.185	0.0249
3	MTr2	0.870 ± 0.042	0.970 ± 0.070	- 6.833	0.0064
5	OPr1	1.068 ± 0.077	1.012 ± 0.067	3.302	0.045
6	OPr2	1.076 ± 0.037	0.970 ± 0.032	6.024	0.0092
6	MF12	0.991 ± 0.054	1.076 ± 0.055	- 4.124	0.0259
7	SOr1	1.100 ± 0.036	1.046 ± 0.029	4.764	0.0176
7	SOl1	1.139 ± 0.023	1.097 ± 0.031	3.483	0.04
8	POr	1.062 ± 0.058	0.982 ± 0.053	5.755	0.0104
8	SOr2	1.096 ± 0.049	1.012 ± 0.065	7.099	0.0057
8	Cl2	1.010 ± 0.039	0.977 ±0.037	3.664	0.0351
8	POl	1.037 ± 0.032	0.956 ± 0.027	4.277	0.0235
9	SPr	1.005 ± 0.045	0.945 ± 0.036	3.416	0.042
9	SOr3	1.047 ± 0.021	0.970 ± 0.023	3.649	0.0355
9	SMAr	1.048 ± 0.045	0.965 ± 0.043	19.378	0.0003

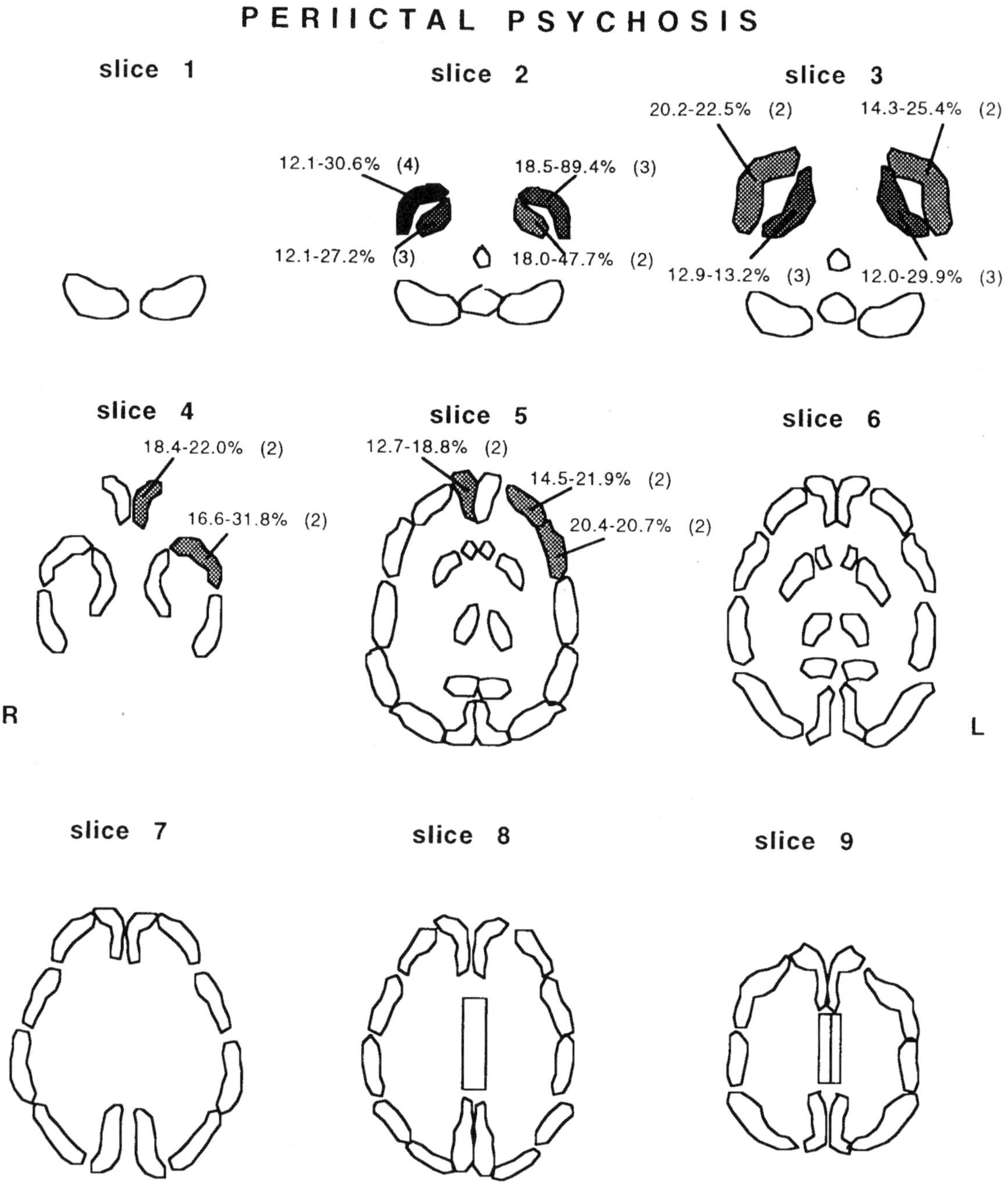

PERIICTAL PSYCHOSIS

slice 1

slice 2

slice 3

20.2-22.5% (2)

14.3-25.4% (2)

12.1-30.6% (4)

18.5-89.4% (3)

12.1-27.2% (3)

18.0-47.7% (2)

12.9-13.2% (3)

12.0-29.9% (3)

slice 4

18.4-22.0% (2)

16.6-31.8% (2)

slice 5

12.7-18.8% (2)

14.5-21.9% (2)

20.4-20.7% (2)

slice 6

R

L

slice 7

slice 8

slice 9

Figure 5 Comparison of relative rCBF between the interictal and psychotic state in 4 patients
Changes are given in %

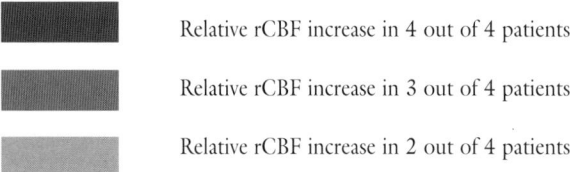

Relative rCBF increase in 4 out of 4 patients

Relative rCBF increase in 3 out of 4 patients

Relative rCBF increase in 2 out of 4 patients

Seizure semiology and ictal SPECT

Since the seizures were recorded on tape, we were able to compare retrospectively seizure symptoms and ictal rCBF patterns visualised by SPECT. At present this has been done in a descriptive manner, without usage of a statistical approach. Table 4 shows our observations. Complete postictal amnesia was associated with increased rCBF in both medio-temporal areas, while in cases with partial amnesia, only one medio-temporal region was involved in the seizure. Dystonic movements of one upper limb correlated with increased rCBF in the contralateral striatum, tonic - clonic jerks on one side with activation of the contralateral central region. In one patient who exhibited a retroflection of the head during a partial complex seizure, a circumscribed increase of relative rCBF located in the midline was observed, suggesting the involvement of the supplementary motor area (SMA). A symmetrical increase of relative rCBF was also seen in the striatum on both sides. As has been mentioned earlier, anterior flection of the body, rotation of the head, short impairment of consciousness, was associated with a contralateral orbito-frontal and ipsilateral cerebellar rCBF increase.

Discussion

Epilepsy is a neurological disease, which manifests itself with a vast range of symptoms such as impaired consciousness, jerks, automatisms, memory impairment, short- and long lasting convulsions, headache, irritability, delusions, hallucinations and vegetative symptoms. Although clinically well studied, little is known about the mechanisms underlying seizure onset and seizure propogation. Seizure classification relies on: the semiology of the epileptic event; the age of the patient; and characteristic EEG patterns. Terms such as periictal psychosis and subclinical seizures are used routinely in our daily clinical work, and are based more or less on clinical observations. Spike activity recorded on EEG is probably related to changes in brain tissue cytoarchitecture, as appearance of mossy fibres and loss of inhibitory terminals, especially in hippocampal formations[8].

The development of imaging techniques such as CT, MRI and ECT during the past 15 years has lead to a marked improvement in the visualisation of structural brain tissue pathology such as hippocampal atrophy or sclerosis, pachygyria, dysgenesis and other brain tissue lesions. Functional brain imaging (PET, SPECT) has revealed metabolic or rCBF abnormalities in apparently normal brain structures in seizure patients. However, the question arises as to whether images obtained with these techniques in a well coordinated clinical setting (in particular SPECT) do contain more information about rCBF patterns related to brain function, seizure propagation and perhaps indirectly, to underlying tissue histopathology, in patients suffering from epilepsy.

The progress in brain imaging was paralleled by new concepts of treatment. New antiepileptic drugs are

Table 4 Observed symptoms during the seizure and ictal rCBF increase

Symptoms	n	Activated brain regions
complete postictal amnesia	7	medio-temporal cortex on both sides
partial postictal amnesia	8	medio-temporal cortex on one side
dystonic movement of upper limb	4	contralateral striatum
unilateral jerks of upper limb	3	contralateral precentral cortex
version of the head	4	contralateral latero-frontal cortex
retroflection of the head	1	SMA, medio-frontal cortex, striatum on both sides
body anteflection	1	orbito-frontal cortex, contralateral cerebellum
psychosis	4	medio-, latero-temporal-, medio-frontal cortex, absent frontal 'deactivation'

permanently developed and the surgical approach in treating seizure patients has become a well established therapy, with the goal to remove a small brain tissue volume containing the so called epileptogenic focus, thus achieving cessation of seizures.

Since SPECT is cyclotron independent, it can be used easily at any time of the day for the study of rCBF changes that may occur in seizure patients. Although the kinetics of the tracers used, such as HMPAO or ECD, are not fully elucidated, the interictal and ictal tracer distribution patterns resemble those known from quantitative procedures such as FDG-PET. However, the major obstacle for the widespread acceptance of SPECT as a reliable clinical tool is the heterogeneity of reported results. This is mainly due to a large variability in spatial resolution of the employed camera systems, imaging modalities and evaluation procedures. In addition, the interpretation of unknown phenomena seen on SPECT images and related to pathological brain function, can be difficult and uncertain.

The percentage of visually estimated abnormal interictal rCBF patterns (86.7%) found in our TLE-patients compares well or is even higher than the numbers reported in the literature. Rowe et al.[1] found 38% abnormal interictal SPECT investigations in 51 TLE-patients. When postictal SPECT was carried out, correct lateralisation was obtained in 69%. In a further study[2], calculation of asymmetry indices yielded a better lateralisation (48%) of the epileptogenic zone than visual estimation (38%), but specificity was higher for the latter one (86% versus 81%). In PET studies, hypometabolic areas in the temporal lobe were found in 60%-80%[9,10].

However, when ictal and postical SPECT findings were considered, positive lateralising findings were obtained in approximately 90%[11,13]. We found in all investigated subjects relative rCBF increases during the seizure, which were in some instances not only restricted in one temporal lobe (neocortex + archicortex), but were also present in the contralateral medial temporal region, containing mainly archicortical structures. In estimating these rCBF changes, the chosen semiquantitative approach was extremely helpful. Such findings have to our knowledge, not yet been reported in the SPECT or PET literature. They emphasise the importance of conducting interictal and ictal SPECT studies in the same subject and the need for semiquantification. The result itself is not so surprising, since post mortem studies of patients suffering from TLE have shown that bilateral asymmetric hippocampal cell loss is present[14,15]. On the other hand, intrahippocampal recordings indicated bilateral independent interictal spikes[16]. On the basis of these results, there is evidence that the ictal rCBF pattern reflects typical tissue changes with cell loss and synaptic reorganisation (mossy fibres) which are not seen by other imaging techniques, and are detectable only in part by quantitative (interictal) imaging as PET, due to the variability of CMRGlu or rCBF values in small tissue volumes. The fairly good correlation between the uni- or bilateral distribution of interictal spike activity and uni- or bilateral ictal rCBF increase in our patient sample speaks in favour of this hypothesis.

It was interesting to observe that in the preictal phase, 15 min prior to the onset of a seizure, relative rCBF is increased by 13% - 57% in the epileptogenic zone (medical and lateral temporal cortex) with absent epileptogenic activity on the EEG recording. Weinand et al.[17] measured temporal cortical rCBF with subdural thermal diffusion flowmetry CBF probes in seizure patients. One of their results indicated an rCBF increase preceeding a seizure by 20 min in the epileptic and by 10 min in the non-epileptic temporal lobe. The pathophysiological basis of this phenomenon is unknown, and further experimental and clinical studies have to be conducted, in order to clarify the time course of rCBF dynamics related to seizure onset and behavioural instability sometimes encountered in epilepsy patients.

The rCBF pattern found in patients who exhibited psychotic symptoms resembled ictal SPECT findings, but differed in two points: the elevation of rCBF did not reach the magnitude of the ictal one (Figure 4) and involved also medio-frontal areas; frontal relative rCBF decrease, as it was seen in ictal SPECT images, was absent. Only a few reports on rCBF dynamics visualised by SPECT in psychotic seizure patients are available, and the results are somewhat contradictory. Kan et al.[18] observed in sequential investigations an rCBF decrease in the left temporal lobe during a psychotic state in one patient. A second subject exhibited decreased rCBF in the right temporal lobe during a depressive phase, which was reversed after release of symptoms. When compared with baseline SPECT studies, increased rCBF in the left limbic system areas was recorded in one patient and symmetrical rCBF in a second patient suffering from TLE and schizophrenia-like psychosis[19]. Gallhofer et al.[20] measured rCBF, $rCMRO_2$, OER in TLE-patients with psychotic episodes (6 patients off and 6 patients on neuroleptic therapy), 5 seizure patients without psychotic symptoms and 5 controls. However, the results obtained were quite heterogeneous and did not allow a clear interpretation. In our small patient sample, 3 out of 4 subjects showed a bilateral relative rCBF increase mainly in the medial portions of the temporal lobe and 2 of them in medio-frontal areas, which also contain parts of the cingulate gyrus. The intensity of the psychotic symptoms paralleled the extent of rCBF changes.

In the small number of subjects investigated who suffered from ETE it was possible to localise the epileptogenic zone according to the SPECT findings. In one patient with frontal lobe seizures (patient B.B.), SPECT was helpful in the decision where to place subdural grid electrodes. Invasive EEG recordings have proven here that the seizure originated exactly in the area exhibiting high rCBF on SPECT images. In the case with negative motor seizures (patient R.S.), SPECT and EEG gave congruent results. The application of both techniques enhanced the reliability of the data concerning the topographical origin of this disturbance. The third patient (patient Z.M.) suffering from partial complex seizures was not operated upon since SPECT indicated possible dual pathology.

In conclusion, a SPECT device with good spatial resolution, a sophisticated SPECT study evaluation and excellent logistical, as well as patient management enabled us to observe four rCBF patterns in TLE patients: increased rCBF in one temporal lobe and in both temporal lobes during a seizure; elevated rCBF in the preictal state (15 min) prior to seizure onset located in the presumed epileptogenic zone; uni- or bitemporal and predominantly medial rCBF increases in periictal psychosis, which extend also to medial frontal regions. In extratemporal seizures, SPECT is helpful in localising the epileptogenic focus and for the study of dual seizure pathology. Due to the improvement in spatial resolution and the unrestricted availability of the tracers employed, SPECT offers at present a unique possiblity to observe routinely brain function related rCBF patterns in seizure patients. In future, when the data from a larger patient cohort are available, our interest will be focussed towards the study of common features between interictal spike activity and ictal rCBF patterns as well as the clinical relevance of such studies for the postsurgical outcome of seizure patients.

References

1   Rowe, C.C., Berkovic, S.F., Austin, M.C. *et al.* Patterns of postictal cerebral blood flow in temporal lobe epilepsy. *Neurology* 1991, 41, 1096

2   Rowe, C.C., Berkovic, S.F., Austin, M.C. *et al.* Visual and quantitative analysis of interictal SPECT with Technetium [99m]-HMPAO in temporal lobe epilepsy. *Nucl. Med.* 1991, 32, 1688

3   Stephan, H., Pawlik, G., Böcher-Schwarz, H.G. *et al.* Functional and morphological abnormalities in temporal lobe epilepsy: a comparison of interictal and ictal EEG, CT, MRI, SPECT and PET. *Neurol.* 1987, 234, 377

4   Sharbrough, F., Chatrian, G.E., Lesser, R.P. *et al.* American Electroencephalographic Society guidelines for standard electrode position nomenclature. *J. Clin. Neurophysiol.* 1991, 8, 200

5   Lindinger, G., Benninger, F., Baumgartner, C. *et al.* Überwachungssystem für die prächirugische Epilepsie-diagnostik, in 'Epilepsie '93 Berlin: Deutsche Sektion der Internationalen Liga gegen Epilepsie,' (eds. H. Stefan, R. Canger, G. Speil), 1994, p.276

6   Pietrzyk, U., Herholz, K., Fink, G. *et al.* An interactive technique for three-dimensional image registration: validation for PET, SPECT, MRI and CT brains studies. *J. Nucl. Med.* 1994, 35, 2011

7   Baumgartner, C., Podreka, I. and Olbrich, A. Epileptic negative myoclonus: an EEG-single photon emission CT study indicating involvement of premotor cortex. *Neurology* 1996, 46, 753

8   Babb, T. and Pretorius, J.K. Patologic substrates of epilepsy in 'The Treatment of Epilepsy. Principles and Practice, (ed. Elaine Wyllie), Lea and Febiger, Philadelphia, USA. 1993, p.55

9   Theodore, W.W., Dorwart, R., Holmes, M. *et al.* Neuroimaging in refractory partial seizures. Comparison of PET, CT and MRI. *Neurology* 1986, 36, 750

10   Engel, J.J., Henry, T.R., Risinger, M.W. *et al.* Presurgical evaluation for partial epilepsy: relative contributions of chronic depth-electrode recordings versus FDG-PET and scalp sphenoidal ictal EEG. *Neurology* 1990, 40, 1670

11   Shen, W., Lee, B.I., Park, H.M. *et al.* HIPDM-SPECT brain imaging in the presurgical evaluation of patients with intractable seizures. *J. Nucl. Med.* 1990, 31, 1280

12   Rowe, C.C., Berkovic, S.F., Sia, S.T. *et al.* Localization of epileptic foci with postictal single photon emission tomography. *Ann. Neurol.* 1989, 26, 660

13   Duncan, R., Patterson, J., Roberts, R. and Hadley, D.M. Ictal/postictal SPECT in the pre-surgical localisation of complex partial seizures. *J. Neurol. Neurosurg. Psychiatry* 1993, 56, 141

14   Margerison, H. and Corsellis, J.A.N. Epilepsy and the temporal lobes. *Brain* 1966, 89, 499

15   Babb, T.L. Research on the anatomy and pathology of epileptic tissue in 'Epilepsy Surgery', (Ed. H. Lüders), Raven Press, New York, USA, 1991, p.719

16   Engel, R. Jr, Crandall, P.H. and Rausch, R. The partial epilepsies in 'The Clinical Neurosciences', (Ed. R.N. Rosenberg), Churchill Livingstone, New York, USA, 1983, p.1349

17   Weinland, M.E., Carter, LP, Patton, D.D. *et al.* Long-term surface cortical cerebral blood flow monitoring in temporal lobe epilepsy. *Neurosurgery* 1994, 35, 657

18 Kan, R., Watanabe, M., Takahashi, R. *et al.* Serial changes of n-isopropyl-p-iodoamphetamine single photon emission computed tomography in two epileptic psychotics. *Jpn J. Psychiatry Neuro.* 1994, 48, 567

19 Jibiki, I., Maeda, T., Kubota, T. and Yamaguchi, N. 123-IMP SPECT brain imaging in epileptic psychosis: A study of two cases of temporal lobe epilepsy with schizophrenia-like syndrome. *Neuropsychobiology* 1993, 28, 207

20 Galhofer, B., Trimble, M.R., Frackowiak, R. *et al.* A study of cerebral blood flow and metabolism in epileptic psychosis using positron emission tomography and oxygen. *J. Neurol. Neurosurg. Psychiatry* 1985, 48, 201

SPECT in Neurology and Psychiatry, edited by P.P. De Deyn, R.A. Dierckx, A. Alavi and B.A. Pickut
© 1997 John Libbey & Company Ltd, pp. 247–253

Non-invasive Cerebral Blood Flow Measurement using ^{99m}Tc-hexamethylpropylene amine oxime (HMPAO) and SPECT in Interictal Temporal Lobe Epilepsy

Chapter
29

H. Matsuda, T. Fukuchi[*], T. Onuma and S. Ishida

Introduction

Changes in cerebral blood flow (CBF) in epilepsy patients are of interest because of their involvement in the pathogenesis of neurological damage during seizures. Interictal single photon emission computed tomography (SPECT) studies are reportedly less significant than either ictal or postictal studies[1-4], but have only been analysed using qualitative or semi-quantitative methods. We had already developed a non-invasive method of regional CBF (rCBF) measurement with ^{99m}Tc-hexamethylpropylene amine oxime (^{99m}Tc-HMPAO) that does not involve blood sampling[5,6]. In this chapter, we describe the application of this non-invasive method to patients with interictal temporal lobe epilepsy.

Materials and methods

We studied 43 patients (20 male, 23 female) with a definite clinical diagnosis of temporal lobe epilepsy. Their ages ranged from 17 to 66 (mean 34.4) years. The duration of their seizure disorder ranged from 4 to 41 (mean 19.3) years, and their age at onset ranged from 2 to 43 (mean 15.2) years. Seizure frequency was classified into three categories: 1-11 per year, 1-4 per month, and >4 per month. Lateralisation of the electroencephalogram (EEG) focus was determined by standard scalp EEGs and simultaneous EEG-video recordings. Patients were treated with 6 major anticonvulsant drugs (phenytoin; 22 cases, phenobarbital; 5 cases, carbamazepine; 35 cases, valproate; 4 cases, clonazepam; 9 cases, and zonisamide; 3 cases) at the time of the SPECT scan. Six cases had received monotherapy with carbamazepine, and the rest had had polytherapy. In the present study, the effects of anticonvulsant drugs on CBF were investigated with special reference to phenytoin.

All patients were examined by magnetic resonance imaging (MRI) using a 1.0T unit (Shimadzu, SMT-100X, Kyoto, Japan) or a 2.0T unit (Philips Medical Systems, GYROSCAN S15A, Best, Netherlands). Detection of MRI abnormalities was based on the presence or absence of unilateral hippocampal

National Center Hospital for Mental, Nervous, and Muscular disorders, NCNP, 4-1-1, Ogawahigashi, Kodaira, Tokyo 187, Japan
[*]Department of Psychiatry, Aichi Medical College, Nagoya, Japan

atrophy with high signal intensity on T_2-weighted images. No subjects had had previous surgery, head injury, encephalitis, progressive neurological disorder, or evidence of a mass lesion or vascular malformation on MRI.

Patients, who had been seizure-free for at least 24 h, underwent non-invasive measurements of rCBF using [99mTc] hexamethylpropylene amine oxime ([99mTc]-HMPAO, [Ceretec] Amersham Corporation, Tokyo, Japan). Two underwent follow-up studies after changes of their anticonvulsant drugs. Thus, a total of 45 measurements was performed. Time activity curves for the aortic arch and brain were analysed to get a brain perfusion index (BPI)[4] using a graphical approach after the bolus injection of 555 MBq of [99mTc]-HMPAO. Mean cerebral blood flow (mCBF) was calculated from BPI using a previously reported linear regression equation[4].

SPECT imaging was carried out using a high-resolution SPECT system with three-head rotating cameras (Siemens Gammasonics Inc, Multispect3, Hoffman Estates, IL, USA). Acquisition of projection data was started from 10 min after injection and lasted for 20 min. Data were accumulated for 24 angles ($5°$ step, total $120°$, with 50 s per angle) for each detector. A Shepp and Logan filter with a 0.85 cycles per cm cut-off frequency was used for image reconstruction in a 128x128 image matrix. Transaxial slices parallel to the long axis of the temporal lobes were reconstructed for evaluation of the temporal lobes. Coronal slices were reconstructed perpendicular to this axis. Attenuation correction was performed using Chang's method. These SPECT images were then converted to rCBF images by application of Lassen's correction algorithm[7]. SPECT data were reported by two different investigators, each blinded to all other data. Detection of SPECT abnormalities was based on visual analysis of side-to-side asymmetry in the temporal regions of at least two contiguous planes. The side with low perfusion was determined as the epileptic focus side on the SPECT scan.

Regions of interest (ROIs) were drawn over 4 homotypic regions of the bilateral temporal lobes in rCBF SPECT images, as shown in Figure 1 - mesial temporal regions included the area of amygdaloid and anterior hippocampus, temporal pole regions, lateral temporal regions, and temporal base regions. An asymmetry flow index (AI) - determined by the equation 200 x |R-L| / (R+L) - was calculated for each pair of bilateral ROIs.

We analysed data by analysis of covariate (ANACOVA), using the Statistical Analysis System. We considered statistical significance at $p<0.05$. The numerical value was expressed as mean ±s.d. The value of cerebral blood flow was represented as ml/100 g/min.

Results

In all subjects mCBF showed significant negative correlation with age ($r= -0.614$, $p<0.0001$) and duration of illness ($r= -0.513$, $p<0.001$), but not with age at onset ($r= -0.253$, $p=0.093$, Table 1). Mean cerebellar blood flow (mCblBF) showed no significant negative correlation with age ($r= -0.234$, $p=0.120$), but was weakly correlated with duration of illness ($r= -0.325$, $p=0.028$, Table 1).

MRI abnormalities were detected in 16 of 43 patients (37%), while SPECT abnormalities were detected in 35 of 45 scans (78%). The images were classified into 4 categories: negative SPECT with negative MRI (type A, 8 scans), positive SPECT with negative MRI (type B, 21 scans), positive SPECT with positive MRI (type C, 14 scans), and negative SPECT with positive MRI (type D, 2 scans). The focus side between SPECT and MRI was concordant in all cases with type C. Accordance of the focus side between EEG and

Table 1 Correlation of brain blood flow with age, duration of seizure disorder, and the age at onset of seizure

	Age (34.8 ± 12.4 years old)	Duration of seizure disorder (19.2 ± 10.2 years)	Age at onset (15.2 ± 9.9 years)
mCBF (43.4 ± 5.9 ml/100g/min)	-0.614[a]	-0.521[a]	-0.252
mCblBF (64.2 ± 12.6 ml/100g/min	-0.234	-0.325[b]	-0.031

[a], 0.01>p; [b], 0.05>p>0.01; mCBF: mean cerebral blood flow, mCblBF: mean cerebellar blood flow

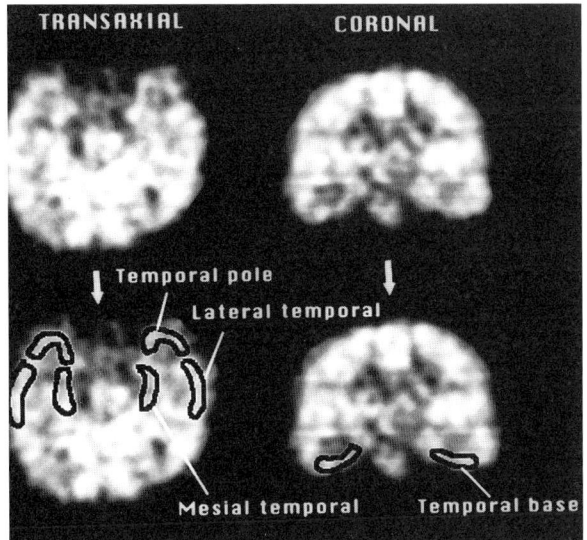

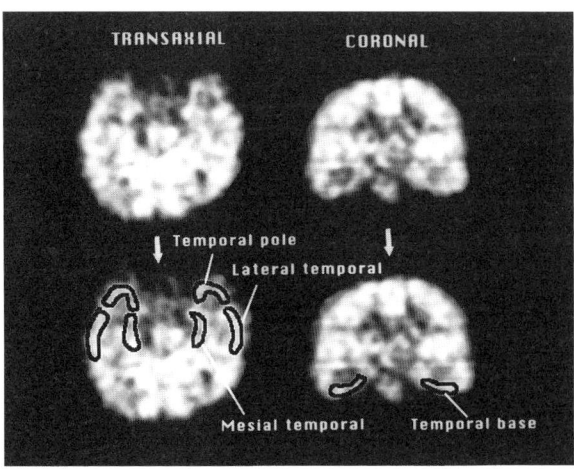

Figure 1 Regions of interest (ROIs) drawn over four homotypic regions of the bilateral temporal lobes in transaxial and coronal images of rCBF SPECT; mesial temporal regions to include the area of amygdaloid and anterior hippocampus, temporal pole regions, lateral temporal regions, and temporal base regions

Figure 2 Representative images in a case with interictal temporal lobe epilepsy showing positive SPECT and negative MRI findings (an image type of B). Hypoperfusion is observed in the mesial temporal, temporal pole, and temporal base regions on the right side (arrows)

SPECT was low in type B (47%), while that between EEG and MRI was extremely high in types C and D (94%, Table 2). Representative MRI and SPECT images of types B, C, and D are shown in Figures 2-4.

From these results, we see that the effects of age need to be taken into consideration. ANACOVA results for: effects of seizure frequency, antiepileptic drugs with special reference to phenytoin, and image types on mCBF, mCblBF, rCBF, and side-to-side AI in temporal regions, are shown in Table 3.

Seizure frequency had no influence on flow values or AI (Table 4).

Patients taking phenytoin had significantly (p<0.05) lower mCBF (mean 8.6%) and lower mCblBF (mean 11.9%) values than those not taking phenytoin after removal of the effects of age (Table 5). A significant reduction of rCBF in those taking phenytoin was also observed in temporal pole and lateral temporal regions contralateral to the focus side (Table 5).

Image types had significant influence on rCBF in the mesial temporal region ipsilateral to the focus side (p<0.05), rCBF in the lateral temporal region ipsilateral to the focus side (p<0.05), AI in the mesial temporal region (p<0.01), AI in the temporal pole region (p<0.05), and AI in the temporal base region (p<0.05) (Table 6). A gradual reduction was observed from type A to type C in temporal rCBF values ipsilateral to the

focus side, while a gradual elevation was shown from type A to type C in temporal AI values.

Discussion

Compared with previous interictal studies of temporal lobe epilepsy, SPECT abnormalities were common in the present study[8-11]. This may be partly due to our application of a high resolution SPECT system dedicated to brain imaging. Although there was a good correlation between visual and semiquantitative analyses using AI in SPECT images, discordance of the epileptic focus side between SPECT and EEG was high

Table 2 Image types and accordance rate of the focus side between EEG and SPECT or MRI

	SPECT (-)	SPECT (+)	Total
MRI (-)	Type A 0% (0/8)	Type B 47% (10/21)	
MRI (+)	Type D 100% (2/2)	Type C 93% (13/14)	94% (15/16)
Total		66% (23/35)	

(scan number with accordance/total scan number)

Table 3 Results of ANACOVA for analysing the effects of seizure frequency, antiepileptic drugs with special reference to phenytoin, and image types on mCBF, mCblBF, rCBF, and side-to-side AI in temporal regions (F-value)

			Age	Seizure Frequency	Phenytoin	Image type
Whole Cerebrum	mCBF		26.14[a]	0	5.11[b]	0.83
Mesial temporal region	rCBF	ipsilateral	2.13	1.79	2.57	4.05[b]
	rCBF	contralateral	2.7	0.26	3.92	1.17
	ASI		0.59	3.07	0.73	5.04[a]
Temporal pole region	rCBF	ipsilateral	4.85[b]	1.00	2.75	1.87
	rCBF	contralateral	8.40[a]	0.52	7.37[a]	0.57
	ASI		3.02	0.80	3.34	3.07[b]
Lateral temporal region	rCBF	ipsilateral	2.78	1.58	1.2	3.00[b]
	rCBF	contralateral	6.76[b]	1.13	7.73[a]	1.64
	ASI		0.12	0.65	3.29	1.75
Temporal base region	rCBF	ipsilateral	4.53[b]	0.40	0.24	2.00
	rCBF	contralateral	3.80	0.06	3.44	1.17
	ASI		0.07	1.66	0.33	2.98[b]
Cerebellum	mCblBF		2.43	0.01	4.70[b]	0.54

[a], $0.01 > p$; [b], $0.05 > p > 0.01$

ipsilateral; ipsilateral to the epileptic focus side: contralateral; contralateral to the epileptic focus side: rCBF; regional cerebral blood flow: AI; asymmetry index

Table 4 Effects of seizure frequency on mCBF, rCBF and AI

			Seizure Frequency		
			1-11 per year N=11	1-4 per month N=16	>4 per month N=18
Whole Cerebrum	mCBF		43.8 ± 1.5	42.8 ± 1.2	43.6 ± 1.2
Mesial temporal region	rCBF	ipsilateral	38.0 ± 1.9	36.9 ± 1.6	39.4 ± 1.6
	rCBF	contralateral	42.8 ± 2.0	42.7 ± 1.7	43.4 ± 1.6
	AI		12.1 ± 3.0	17.6 ± 2.5	11.5 ± 2.4
Temporal pole region	rCBF	ipsilateral	35.6 ± 1.7	33.3 ± 1.4	35.4 ± 1.3
	rCBF	contralateral	37.3 ± 1.9	37.4 ± 1.6	38.9 ± 1.6
	AI		7.4 ± 2.4	10.4 ± 1.9	11.9 ± 1.9
Lateral temporal region	rCBF	ipsilateral	47.7 ± 2.3	43.7 ± 1.9	46.9 ± 1.9
	rCBF	contralateral	49.4 ± 2.8	47.7 ± 2.3	52.0 ± 2.2
	AI		8.1 ± 3.2	12.4 ± 2.6	11.0 ± 2.6
Temporal base region	rCBF	ipsilateral	36.0 ± 2.3	33.3 ± 1.9	35.1 ± 1.8
	rCBF	contralateral	39.1 ± 2.1	39.0 ± 1.7	38.8 ± 1.7
	AI		8.9 ± 4.8	19.3 ± 4.0	13.6 ± 3.9
Cerebellum	mCblBF		63.5 ± 4.1	64.0 ± 3.3	64.9 ± 3.3

mCBF, mCblBF, rCBF; ml/100g/min

Table 5 Effects of ingestion of phenytoin on mCBF, mCblBF, rCBF and AI

			Phenytoin (-) N=22	Phenytoin (+) N=23
Whole cerebrum	mCBF		45.3 ± 1.2	41.5 ± 1.1
Mesial temporal region	rCBF	ipsilateral	39.8 ± 1.5	36.6 ± 1.4
	rCBF	contralateral	45.3 ± 1.6	40.8 ± 1.4
	AI		14.7 ± 2.3	13.1 ± 2.1
Temporal pole region	rCBF	ipsilateral	36.3 ± 1.3	33.2 ± 1.2
	rCBF	contralateral	40.6 ± 1.5	35.4 ± 1.4
	AI		12.3 ± 1.8	8.4 ± 1.7
Lateral temporal region	rCBF	ipsilateral	47.1 ± 1.8	44.8 ± 1.7
	rCBF	contralateral	53.0 ± 1.2	46.8 ± 1.9
	AI		13.5 ± 2.5	8.2 ± 2.3
Temporal base region	rCBF	ipsilateral	35.9 ± 1.8	33.6 ± 1.6
	rCBF	contralateral	41.3 ± 1.6	36.7 ± 1.5
	AI		14.7 ± 3.7	14.2 ± 3.4
Cerebellum	mCblBF		68.4 ± 3.2	60.3 ± 2.9

Table 6 Effects of image types of SPECT and MRI findings on mCBF, mCblBF, rCBF and AI

			Type A SPECT(-)MRI(-) N=8	Type B SPECT(+)MRI(-) N=21	Type C SPECT(+)MRI(+) N=14	Type D SPECT(-)MRI(+) N=2
Whole Cerebrum	mCBF		45.2 ± 1.7	43.0 ± 1.0	43.2 ± 1.3	41.5 ± 3.3
Mesial temporal region	rCBF	ipsilateral	41.4 ± 2.1	39.3 ± 1.3	34.4 ± 1.6	40.9 ± 4.2
	rCBF	contralateral	43.8 ± 2.3	44.2 ± 1.4	41.4 ± 1.7	37.9 ± 4.5
	ASI		6.3 ± 3.4	13.2 ± 2.1	20.0 ± 2.5	7.8 ± 6.6
Temporal pole region	rCBF	ipsilateral	38.5 ± 1.9	34.6 ± 1.1	32.6 ± 1.4	35.3 ± 3.7
	rCBF	contralateral	40.3 ± 2.2	37.8 ± 1.3	37.0 ± 1.6	37.0 ± 4.3
	ASI		5.0 ± 2.7	10.9 ± 1.6	13.2 ± 2.1	4.4 ± 5.3
Lateral temporal region	rCBF	ipsilateral	50.3 ± 2.6	45.6 ± 1.6	42.9 ± 1.9	53.7 ± 5.0
	rCBF	contralateral	49.5 ± 3.0	50.3 ± 1.8	48.7 ± 2.2	53.9 ± 5.8
	ASI		5.6 ± 3.6	11.9 ± 2.2	13.4 ± 2.7	1.6 ± 7.1
Temporal base region	rCBF	ipsilateral	37.7 ± 2.6	36.0 ± 1.6	32.0 ± 1.9	28.6 ± 5.1
	rCBF	contralateral	39.3 ± 2.4	39.7 ± 1.4	38.9 ± 1.8	30.1 ± 4.7
	ASI		4.7 ± 5.5	12.3 ± 3.3	22.8 ± 4.1	18.2 ± 10.7
Cerebellum	mCblBF		62.7 ± 4.7	63.6 ± 3.8	66.7 ± 3.5	60.0 ± 9.0

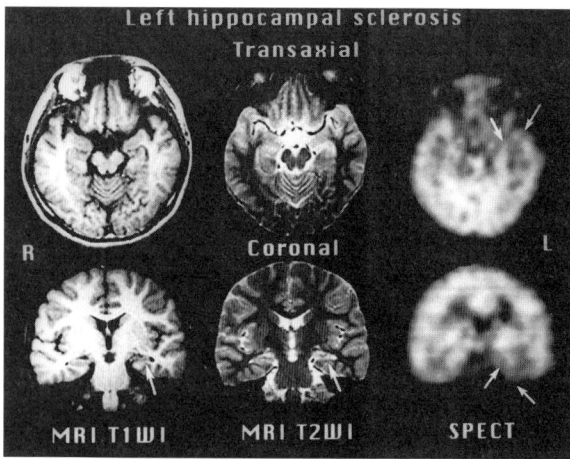

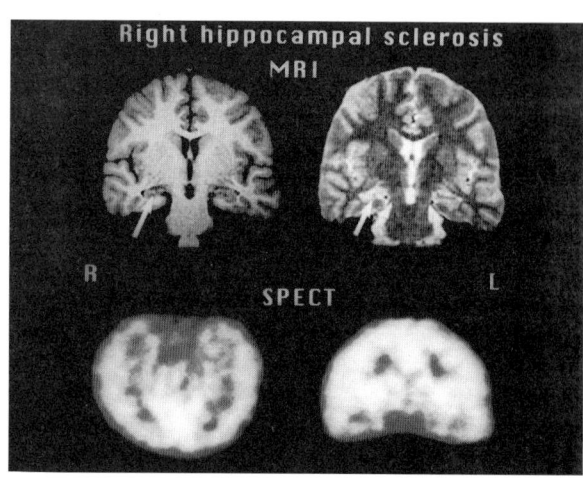

Figure 3 Representative images showing positive SPECT and positive MRI findings (an image type of C). Left temporomesial sclerosis is observed on MRI (arrows). SPECT images demonstrate hypoperfusion in the mesial temporal, temporal pole, and temporal base regions on the same side (arrows)

Figure 4 Representative images showing negative SPECT and positive MRI findings (an image type of D). Right temporomesial sclerosis is observed on MRI (arrows). SPECT images do not show any abnormality

in the image type of B with negative MRI findings. This may partly result from a false lateralisation by routine EEG. Sammaritano *et al.*[12] explained this false finding by suggesting that the discharge originating from the damaged area has a very low voltage and only reaches a voltage sufficient to be detected by scalp EEG when it projects to contralateral normal regions[11]. Ictal or postictal SPECT[1-4] studies may be necessary for more correct definition of the focus side in cases with negative MRI findings. On the contrary, extremely high accordance of the focus side between MRI and EEG was observed in the image types of C and D with positive MRI findings. Although high reliability of MRI abnormalities has been reported in definition of the focus side[13,14], the present study shows that sensitivity is not high in the detection of hippocampal sclerosis. The image type of C showed lower rCBF ipsilateral to the focus side and greater AI values in the temporal region than type A or B. Similar results were reported by Ryvlin *et al.*[15]. Temporomesial lesions detectable by MRI may be more severely damaged and cause more widespread functional depression in the adjacent area than lesions without MRI abnormalities. The reason for negative SPECT findings with positive MRI findings must be further elucidated in a larger number of type D cases.

There have been several reports on the effects of phenytoin on brain metabolism and blood flow in epileptic patients[16-19]. Theodore *et al.*[16,17] reported a 13% lower cerebral and an 18% lower cerebellar metabolic rate for glucose (CMR_{glu}) in patients on

phenytoin. Bernardi *et al.*[19] reported an 18% lower mCBF and an 18% lower hemispheric mean cerebral metabolic rate for oxygen ($CMRO_2$) in 10 epileptic patients - six of whom were taking phenytoin at the time of the scan. They reported extensive abnormalities in $CMRO_2$ and CBF, affecting regions contralateral as well as ipsilateral to the EEG epileptic focus. Our results also showed an 8.6% lower mCBF and an 11.9% lower mCblBF in patients taking phenytoin. Smaller reductions compared with previous results may be attributed to the possibility that some of phenytoin's effect may have been masked by other drugs the patients were taking and that the other drugs may mildly reduce CBF. With reference to normal control values reported by us[6], 12% and 18% reductions in mCBF and mCblBF, respectively, were observed in patients on phenytoin. In the present study, reduction in rCBF was greater on the contralateral side to the focus than the ipsilateral side, and, consequently, the ingestion of phenytoin reduced side-to-side flow asymmetry in the temporal region.

It is not yet clear whether seizures themselves can lead to decreased cerebral or cerebellar metabolism, but seizures do lead to brain damage. Pathological changes in the cerebellum in patients with seizure disorders were noted before phenytoin was introduced[20]. Moreover, the current study showed an inverse correlation between length of seizure history and mCBF or mCblBF. Although similar results between the length of history and CMR_{glu} were reported by Theodore *et al.*[18], seizure frequency did not significantly influence our findings. Previous studies of MR_{glu} in epilepsy have not shown an effect for either interictal EEG spike frequency or seizure frequency on PET results[21], and patients with primarily generalised absence or generalised tonic-clonic seizures have been reported to have normal interictal CMR_{glu}[22-24]. Some investigators have also suggested that phenytoin leads to decreased performance on neuropsychological tests even at blood levels within the therapeutic range and without other signs of toxicity. A double-blind, crossover study found improved cognitive performance in patients with carbamazepine compared with phenytoin[25]. Although the effect of phenytoin is still difficult to distinguish from that of the seizure, our results suggest that phenytoin plays a secondary role in inducing cerebral and cerebellar hypoperfusion.

In conclusion, non-invasive cerebral blood flow measurements using ^{99m}Tc-HMPAO may give useful information on the pathophysiology of the epileptic focus and its adjacent area and also on the effects of antiepileptic drugs on brain function in interictal temporal lobe epilepsy.

References

1 Rowe, C.C., Berkovic, S.F., McKay, W.J. *et al.* Patterns of postictal cerebral blood flow in temporal lobe epilepsy: qualitative and quantitative analysis. *Neurology* 1991, 41, 1096

2 Duncan, R., Patterson, J., Roberts, R. *et al.* Ictal/postictal SPECT in the pre-surgical localisation of complex partial seizures. *J. Neurol. Neurosurg. Psychiatr.* 1993, 56, 141

3 Harvey, A.S., Bowe, J.M., Hopkins, I.J. *et al.* Ictal ^{99m}Tc-HMPAO single photon emission computed tomography in children with temporal lobe epilepsy. *Epilepsia* 1993, 34, 869

4 Newton, R.M., Berkovic, S.F., Austin, M.C. *et al.* Ictal postictal and interictal single-photon emission tomography in the lateralization of temporal lobe epilepsy. *Eur. J. Nucl. Med.* 1994, 21, 1067

5 Matsuda, H., Tsuji, S., Shuke, N. *et al.* A quantitative approach to technetium-99m hexamethylpropylene amine oxime. *Eur. J. Nucl. Med.* 1992, 19, 195

6 Matsuda, H., Tsuji, S., Shuke, N. *et al.* Noninvasive measurements of regional cerebral blood flow using technetium-99m hexamethylpropylene amine oxime. *Eur. J. Nucl. Med.* 1993, 20, 391

7 Lassen, N.A., Andersen, A.R., Freiberg, L. *et al.* The retention of [^{99m}Tc]-D,L-HMPAO in the human brain after intracarotid bolus injection: a kinetic analysis. *J. Cereb. Blood Flow Metab.* 1988, 8(Suppl 1), S44

8 Andersen, A.R., Gram, L., Kjaer, L. *et al.* SPECT in partial epilepsy: identifying side of the focus. *Acta. Neurol. Scand.* 1988, 78(Suppl 117), S90

9 Lee, B.I., Markand, O.N., Wellman, H.N. *et al.* HIPDM-SPECT in patients with medically intractable complex partial seizures. *Arch. Neurol.* 1988, 45, 397

10 Rowe, C.C., Berkovic, S.F. and Austin, M.C. Visual and quantitative analysis of interictal SPECT with technetium-99m-HMPAO in temporal lobe epilepsy. *J. Nucl. Med.* 1991, 32, 1688

11 Duncan, R. Epilepsy, cerebral blood flow, and cerebral metabolic rate. *Cerebrovasc. Brain Metabol. Rev.* 1992, 4, 105

12 Sammaritano, M., de Lotbiniere, A., Andermann, F. *et al.* False lateralization by surface EEG of seizure onset in patients with temporal lobe epilespy and gross focal cerebral lesions. *Ann. Neurol.* 1987, 21, 361

13 Franceschi, M., Triulzi, F., Ferini-Strambi, L. *et al.* Focal cerebral lesions found by magnetic resonance imaging in cryptogenic nonrefractory temporal lobe epilepsy patients. *Epilepsia* 1989, 30, 540

14 Sperling, M.R., Wilson, G., Engel, J. *et al.* Magnetic resonance imaging in intractable partial epilepsy: correlative studies. *Ann. Neurol.* 1986, 20, 57

15 Ryvlin, P., Garcia-Larrea, L., Philippon, B. *et al.* High signal intensity on T2-weighted MRI correlates with hypoperfusion in temporal lobe epilepsy. *Epilepsia* 1992, 33, 28

16 Theodore, W.H., Bairamiand, D., Newmark, M.E. *et al.* Effects of phenytoin on human cerebral glucose metabolism. *J. Cereb. Blood Flow Metabol.* 1986, 6, 315

17 Theodore, W.H., Fishbein, D., Deitz, M. and Baldwin, P. Complex partial seizures: cerebellar metabolism. *Epilepsia* 1987, 28, 319

18 Theodore, W.H., Fishbein, D. and Dubinsky, R. Patterns of cerebral glucose metabolism in patients with partial seizures. *Neurology* 1988, 38, 1201

19 Bernardi, S., Trimble, M.R., Frackowiack, R.S.J. *et al.* An interictal study of partial epilepsy using positron emission tomography and the oxygen-15 inhalation method. *J. Neurol. Neurosurg. Psychiatr.* 1983, 46, 473

20 Margerison, J.H. and Corsellis, J.A.N. Epilepsy and the temporal lobes: a clinical, electroencephalographic, and neuropathologic study of the brain in epilepsy, with particular reference to the temporal lobes. *Brain* 1966, 89, 499

21 Engel, J., Kuhl, D.E., Phelps, M.E. and Mazziota, J.C. Interictal cerebral glucose metabolism and its relation to EEG changes. *Ann. Neurol.* 1982, 12, 510

22 Engel, J., Lubens, P., Kuhl D.E. and Phelps, M.E. Local cerebral metabolic rate for glucose during petit mal absences. *Ann. Neurol.* 1985, 17, 121

23 Theodore, W.H., Brooks, R., Margolin, R. *et al.* Positron emission tomography in generalized seizures. *Neurology* 1985, 35, 684

24 Ochs, R.F., Gloor, P., Tyler, J.F. *et al.* Effect of generalized spike-and-wave discharge on glucose metabolism measured by positron emission tomography. *Ann. Neurol.* 1987, 21, 458

25 Dodrill, C.R. and Troupin, A.S. Psychotropic effects of carbamazepine in epilepsy: a double-blind comparison with phenytoin. *Neurology* 1982, 27, 1023

SPECT in Neurology and Psychiatry, edited by P.P. De Deyn, R.A. Dierckx, A. Alavi and B.A. Pickut

Abnormalities of GABA$_A$ Receptor Density and Blood Flow in the Temporal Lobe of Drug-Naive Patients with Newly Diagnosed Focal Epilepsy: First Results

Chapter
30

T. Kuwert, S.R.G. Stodieck, C. Puskás, B. Diehl, Z. Puskás, B. Vollet, G. Schuierer, E.B. Ringelstein and O. Schober

Introduction

A reduction in GABA$_A$ receptor density (GRD) and regional cerebral blood flow (rCBF) frequently occurs in the temporal cortex of patients with chronic or medically refractory focal epilepsy (for reviews, see Cook and Kilpatrick[1] and Spencer[2]). Limited evidence exists on these variables in drug-naive patients with newly diagnosed focal epilepsies. The aim of this study was to investigate temporal GRD and rCBF in previously untreated patients with newly diagnosed epilepsy.

Methods

Subjects

A total of 20 drug-naive patients with newly diagnosed focal epilepsy were included in the study. There were 15 women and 5 men in the group, mean age 37±14.7 yrs. All patients received a complete diagnostic work-up, including history, clinical examination, lumbar puncture, and electroencephalography (EEG) with various activating procedures. MRI scans performed on a 1.5 T magnetom SP 63 did not show significant abnormalities in the temporal lobe of any patient. A total of 10 patients with clearly psychogenic attacks (6 women, 4 men, aged 36.5±18 yrs) served as controls. MRI and EEG were unremarkable in these subjects.

SPECT data acquisition

All but 4 subjects were studied on 2 separate days in the same month, the remaining 4 were studied at intervals of 2 and 3 months. Single photon emission tomography (SPECT) was performed with the triple-head camera, Multispect 3 (Siemens - Gammasonics, USA), equipped with medium-energy, parallel-hole collimators for the determination of GRD and with low-energy parallel-hole collimators for the determination of rCBF[3]. System resolution was 12 mm and 7 mm full width at half maximum (FWHM) at 10 cm distance, respectively.

Departments of Nuclear Medicine, Neurology, and the Institute of Clinical Radiology, Westfälische Wilhelms-Universität Münster, Germany

Imaging was started 90 min after intravenous injection of 150 MBq ^{123}I-iomazenil (iomazenil), and 15 min after injection of 740 MBq ^{99m}Tc-ethyl cysteinate dimer (ECD). One hundred and twenty views (3x40; 3.75°/step), each registered over 45 s, were recorded into a 128x128 matrix format that corresponded to a pixel dimension of 3.56x3.56 mm on a 360° rotation. Transaxial tomograms were reconstructed without prefiltering, using filtered back-projection with a Butterworth filter of seventh order and a cut-off frequency of 0.4 Nyquist. Attenuation correction was first order, applying Chang's[4] method with a coefficient of 0.11. In-plane resolution of the reconstructed images was 14 mm FWHM for iomazenil SPECT and 8 mm for ECD SPECT, while slice thickness after reslicing was approximately 7 mm.

Data analysis

All images were coronally reformatted for quantitative data analysis; 5 consecutive coronal slices were then selected for further evaluation, the most anterior slice representing the temporal pole. Regional analysis of uptake values was performed without knowledge of

patients' clinical data. Comparing the SPECT images to coronal slices of a neuro-anatomic atlas[5], 3 irregular regions of interest (ROIs) were placed on the lateral, basal, and medial temporal cortex on the right side of each slice. These 3 ROIs were then mirrored to the left side and manually adjusted to the cortical ribbon. This procedure yielded 6 ROIs per coronal slice, amounting to 30 ROIs per patient. The average count rate in each ROI was then related to its contralateral counterpart. As a first approach to data analysis, a significant unilateral reduction was defined as the occurrence of differences >10% in at least 4 adjacent ROIs for iomazenil SPECT and at least 3 adjacent ROIs for ECD SPECT. These cut-off values were chosen with reference to the values obtained in the 10 control subjects. A temporal asymmetry amounting to more than 10% was not detected in more than 3 adjacent ROIs for iomazenil SPECT subjects and in more than 2 adjacent ROIs for ECD SPECT subjects (Figure 1).

Results

In 10 of the 20 patients studied, a pathological reduction in either rCBF or GRD or both was detected (Figure 1). There was no significant correlation beween rCBF and GRD with respect to the number of adjacent regions exhibiting an rCBF or GRD asymmetry of >10% (Spearman's correlation coefficient: r = -0.13, p>0.05).

Discussion

The data presented here are preliminary; this term applies particularly to their statistical analysis which could be improved by using calculated confidence limits rather than an arbitrarily chosen threshold and by taking the multivariate structure of the database into account[6]. Nevertheless, in 10 of the 20 patients studied, we detected 10% asymmetries of rCBF or GRD in more than 2 or 3 (respectively) adjacent ROIs. None of the controls exhibited this abnormality, which indicates that drug-naive patients with newly diagnosed focal epilepsies may also exhibit pathologically reduced rCBF and GRD in their temporal lobes. Until now, only a few authors have investigated rCBF or GRD in such a patient group. Although Venz et al.[7] reported focally reduced GRD and rCBF in several of their 13 patients with untreated epilepsy, their patients were not compared with controls.

The focal reductions of rCBF and GRD detected in our patients involved approximately one-fifth to one-half of the temporal lobe and were thus smaller than those reported for medically refractory patients. Franceschi et al.[8] compared the interictal rCBF of medically

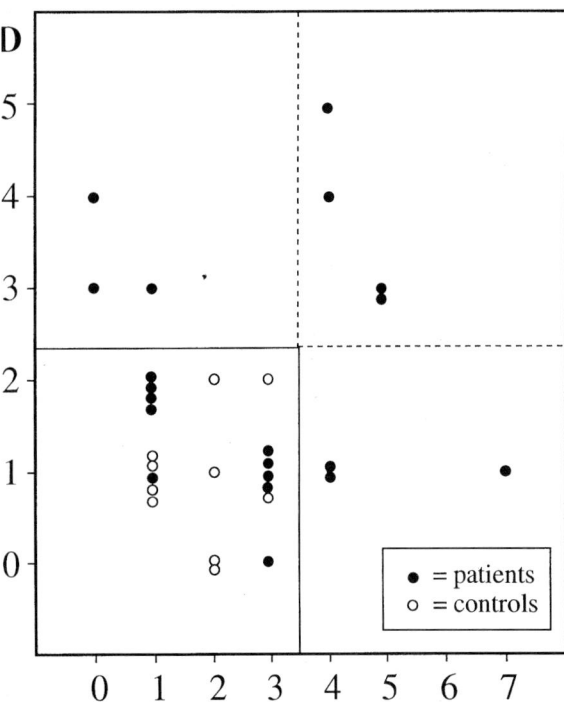

Figure 1 ECD-SPECT versus lomazenil-SPECT: plot of the number of adjacent ROIS exhibiting an asymmetry of more than 10% in twenty drug-naive patients with newly diagnosed focal epilepsies

controlled epileptic patients with that of medically refractory subjects, and found that focally reduced rCBF was more frequent in the latter group. This corresponds to preliminary results obtained using ^{18}F-fluorodeoxy glucose and positron emission tomography[9,10], and suggests that abnormalities of rCBF and GRD may develop or accentuate during the course of the disease. Alternatively, patients with medically refractory epilepsy may experience a more severe reduction in these variables at disease onset than patients in whom seizures are medically controlled. If this is the case, SPECT with iomazenil or ECD may have prognostic significance in focal epilepsy and may help to further differentiate these disorders.

Interestingly, we found no correlation between iomazenil and ECD SPECT with respect to the number of adjacent ROIs exhibiting an asymmetry >10%. This contrasts with results obtained by Bartenstein *et al.*[11] and Cordes *et al.*[12], who reported parallel decreases in these two variables in most patients. Again, differences in the selection of patients may be responsible for the discrepancy - both the latter authors studied medically treated patients with chronic focal epilepsy. In conclusion, drug-naive patients with newly diagnosed focal epilepsies may also experience a reduction in temporal rCBF or GRD. Further studies of these variables in this group of patients will lead to better understanding of the pathogenesis of focal epilepsies. The potential usefulness of iomazenil and ECD SPECT in the assessment of the prognosis of individual patients also merits further consideration.

Acknowledgements

The authors gratefully acknowledge the technical support rendered by Ms Eugenie Rickert, Ms Christine Papenberg, and Ms Martina Telgmann, and Mr Thomas Isokeit's help with the illustration.

References

1 Cook, M.J. and Kilpatrick, C. Imaging in epilepsy. *Curr. Opin. Neurol.* 1994, 7, 123

2 Spencer, S. The relative contributions of MRI, SPECT, and PET imaging in epilepsy. *Epilepsia* 1994, 35, S72

3 Kuikka, J.T., Tenhunen-Eskelinen, M., Jurvelin, J. and Kiliänen, H. Physical performance of the Siemens Multi SPECT 3 gamma camera. *Nucl. Med. Commun.* 1993, 14, 490

4 Chang, L.T. A method for attenuation correction in radionuclide computed tomography. *IEEE. Trans. Nucl. Sci.* 1978, NS-26/2, 2780

5 Talairach, J. and Tournoux, P. Co-planar stereotaxic atlas of the human brain, Thieme Medical Publishers, Stuttgart, Germany, 1988

6 McCrory, S.J. and Ford, I. Multivariate analysis of SPECT images with illustrations in Alzheimer's disease. *Stat. Med.* 1991, 10, 1711

7 Venz, S., Cordes, M., Schmitz, B. *et al.* ^{123}I-iomazenil und ^{99m}Tc-HMPAO in der Diagnostik fokaler Epilepsien: Vergleich von unbehandelten und behandelten Patienten. *Nucl. Med.* 1994, 33, 1

8 Franceschi, M., Messa, C., Ferini-Strambi, L. *et al.* SPECT imaging of cerebral perfusion in patients with non-refractory temporal lobe epilepsy. *Acta. Neurol. Scand.* 1993, 87, 268

9 Hosokawa, S., Kato, M., Goto, I. *et al.* Positron emission tomography in partial epilepsy and its relation to clinical and EEG findings. *Jpn. J. Psychiatr. Neurol.* 1988, 42, 616

10 Henry, T.R., Frey, K.A., Sackellares, J.C. *et al.* Positron emission tomography in 'Surgical treatment of the epilepsies', (Ed. J. Jr. Engel), Raven Press, New York, USA, 1993, p.211

11 Bartenstein, P., Ludolph, A., Schober, O. *et al.* Benzodiazepine receptors and cerebral blood flow in partial epilepsy. *Eur. J. Nucl. Med.* 1991, 18, 111

12 Cordes, M., Henkes, H., Ferstl, F. *et al.* Evaluation of focal epilepsy: a SPECT scanning comparison of [123]-I-iomazenil versus HMPAO. *A. J. N. R.* 1992, 13, 249

SPECT in Neurology and Psychiatry, edited by P.P. De Deyn, R.A. Dierckx, A. Alavi and B.A. Pickut
© 1997 John Libbey & Company Ltd, pp. 259–265

Functional Neuroimaging with CGU-PET and rCBF SPECT: Targeting the Epileptogenic Focus

Chapter

31

C. Menzel, F. Grünwald, A. Hufnagel, L. Pavics,
K. Reichmann, J. Ruhlmann, C.E. Elger and H.J. Biersack

Introduction

Functional neuroimaging with Positron Emission Tomography (PET) and Single Photon Emission Computed Tomography (SPECT) have been used in patients suffering from epilepsy for almost two decades now. Since their initial application in the late 1970s, these methods have been continuously challenged, mostly by technological advances in either tomographs or radiopharmaceuticals. The development of magnetic resonance imaging (MRI) during the 1980s also had great impact on the changing clinical role of functional neuroimaging[1]. In fact, in the imaging field, the process of innovation has outpaced the progress of clinical evaluation, so that more imaging procedures and even more radiotracers are now available than real indications for their application. Different centres have tended to apply different methodologies and have surprisingly shown in numerous studies that there are multiple approaches to the problem of functional neuroimaging in epilepsy. Debate has been very necessary, but there is still a lack of synthesis. While it is clear that functional neuroimaging using PET and SPECT allows tracking of the working brain and its pathophysiology, application in epilepsy remains complex. One major consideration is that the increasing spatial resolution of the newer systems has increased the sensitivity of both PET and SPECT[2,3], but that the evidence to date has not been adequately analysed. This problem will form the mainstay of the following chapter, which will also focus on missing links in the evaluation of some methods. Data will be presented on ictal and interictal imaging of regional cerebral blood flow (rCBF) using ^{99m}Tc-HMPAO[4] and ^{99m}Tc-ECD SPECT[5], interictal cerebral glucose use (CGU) using ^{18}F-DG PET, and aspects of morphology revealed by MRI and of function revealed by the electroencephalogram (EEG).

Methods

SPECT

The DSI Ceraspect annular crystal ring SPECT system is currently used in our centre. The camera consists of a stationary annular crystal/photomultiplier assembly and the only rotating part of the system is a cylindrical collimator, which is divided into three parallel hole sections. The spatial resolution of the system is about 8 mm. The data acquisition time was 30 min, acquiring 120 projections within a 512x64 matrix. Scatter correction and back projection was performed with a Butterworth filter (cut-off 0.9 cm) and attenuation correction with Chang's method, using an attenuation coefficient equal to 0.15 cm E-1.

Departments of Nuclear Medicine and Epileptology, University of Bonn, Sigmund Freud Strasse 25, 53127 Bonn, Germany

Routinely, colour-coded transaxial (canthomeatal), sagittal and coronal slices were recalculated at a slice thickness of 4 pixels (1 pixel = 1.67 mm). Transaxial slices following a temporal angulation were also recalculated at a slice thickness of 1 pixel.

^{99m}Tc-HMPAO and ^{99m}Tc-ECD were reconstituted according to the manufacturer's instructions. In interictal and ictal studies, the applied dose was approximately 740 MBq (20 mCi) per study. Where ^{99m}Tc-HMPAO was used, data acquisition started no earlier than 10 min after injection, and where ^{99m}Tc-ECD scans were used, no earlier than 30 min, but preferably 45 min post-injection (in order to allow sufficient tracer washout from the soft-tissue). We used data acquired using an ADAC Genesys (FWHM 10 mm), an Elscint A 409 (FWHM appr. 16 mm) and a Picker Dyna (FWHM appr. 18 mm) system for retrospective comparison of the sensitivities of low- and high-resolution SPECT. Details of the acquisition parameters and systems are described elsewhere[3].

PET

PET scanning was performed with the Siemens ECAT EXACT 921-47, which provides an estimated spatial resolution of 5 mm under clinical conditions. The system is run as a satellite PET centre model. ^{18}F-deoxyglucose was supplied by the German nuclear research center at Jülich, and the dose applied was 296-370 MBq (8-10 mCi). Data acquisition was started 30 min after i.v. injection of the tracer. Filtered back-projection made with a ramp filter and attenuation correction (Chang's method) was used. Image reconstruction and evaluation followed the same protocol as described above. No quantitative or semi-quantitative data were obtained.

MRI

All patients received an MRI of the brain, mainly with a 1.5 Tesla Philips Gyroscan ACS II. Regardless of the available clinical information, a standard protocol was used in epilepsy. This consisted of sequences including sagittal T1w-spin echo (SE), transaxial and coronal T1w-inversion recovery (IR) or TIR, transaxial double-echo SE (proton density - and T2w-SE) and coronal T2w-TSE. The angulation of transaxial sequences followed the most probable focus site: e.g. in cases of suspected temporal lobe epilepsy an angulation following the long axis of the temporal lobe, and in cases of non-temporal epilepsy an angulation following the canthomeatal line. This protocol was made within 30 min; details of the applied sequences are given elsewhere[6]. According to the results of the protocol,

and individual clinical data, additional sequences were sometimes applied. Gadolinium DTPA-enhanced sequences were used in suspected malignancy, vascular malformation or encephalitis, for example, and T2w-FFE sequences where a history of cerebral trauma had been given. In patients with focal epilepsy and normal results for the above-mentioned sequences, an additional coronal (or sagittal) double-echo sequence at a slice thickness of 3 mm was performed.

Electroencephalography (EEG) and chronical electrocorticography (ECoG)

All patients underwent ictal and interictal surface EEG, mostly with simultaneous video-monitoring. Electrodes were applied according to the international 10/20 system and included sphenoidal electrodes in patients with suspected temporomesial seizure onset. In patients who underwent ECoG, strips and/or grids were implanted over the region of interest (ROI), partly including bitemporal hippocampal depth electrodes. Interpretation of the data followed the criteria previously described by Gloor[7]. Here, EEG/ECoG information obtained was used in its entirety in the possible depiction of focus sites, and for correlation only with imaging results.

Patient populations

All patients had focal epilepsy; 4 groups of patients are detailed here. Due to advancing technology, the passage of time, and time-sparing presurgical evaluation, intrasubject comparison of methods was possible in only a minority of patients (the second group). First, 53 patients suffering from temporal lobe epilepsy were evaluated. These patients received interictal studies using ^{99m}Tc-HMPAO. Second, 12 patients suffering temporal and frontal lobe epilepsy underwent intra-subject comparison of high-resolution (DSI Ceraspect) rCBF SPECT using ^{99m}Tc-ECD and ^{18}F-DG PET (Siemens ECAT EXACT 921-47). Third, 50 patients with temporal lobe epilepsy were evaluated interictally using ^{18}F-DG PET. EEG and MRI were only available for 33 of these patients and, thus, the sensitivity of ^{18}F-DG PET in all patients was calculated according to whether or not the study was informative, as well as in the subgroup of patients in whom correct localisation could be proven by correlation with other techniques. The sensitivity results for this group are compared with those of the group investigated by interictal high-resolution SPECT and ^{99m}Tc-HMPAO or ^{99m}Tc-ECD.

Fourth, data on the interictal and ictal evaluation of 25 patients suffering focal epilepsy of suspected temporal and frontal onset and using ^{99m}Tc-ECD is

Table 1 Clinical data and methodology of the different subgroups of patients

	Group 1	Group 2	Group 3	Group 4
Number of patients	53	12	50	25
Sex (m: f)	28:25	7:5	29:21	14:11
Age (mean yrs)	32	33	33	35
Frontal focus	0	3	0	7
Temporal focus	53	9	50	18
Tracer used	HMPAO	ECD/FDG	FDG	ECD
Tomograph used	different	Ceraspect/ECAT	ECAT	Ceraspect
MRI correlation	yes	yes	partly	yes
EEG correlation	yes	yes	yes	yes
Postsurgical results	yes	partly	no	partly

presented (Table 1). We focused primarily on the differences in sensitivity brought about by using different techniques and tracers. Specificity was calculated for ictal studies only.

Results

If possible, the results of the presurgical work-up are subdivided according to correlation of the SPECT or PET results with those of EEG and MRI.

Results of rCBF SPECT using ^{99m}Tc-HMPAO and SPECT systems of different spatial resolution

Retrospectively, the imaging results of 53 adult patients suffering temporal lobe epilepsy were compared according to the SPECT systems used, the results of MRI and EEG, and the postsurgical decrease in seizure frequency. Two groups are analysed: those using SPECT systems of moderate spatial resolution (Picker Dyna, Elscint A 409), which provide FWHM of 16-18 mm, and those using high-resolution SPECT systems (ADAC Genesys, DSI Ceraspect), which provide FWHM of 8-10 mm in clinical situations. In all, 34 patients were evaluated with low- to moderate-resolution SPECT systems (m:f = 19:17, mean age 33.6 years, range 18-52) and 19 evaluated with present-time high-resolution SPECT systems (m:f = 10:9, mean age 29.3 years, range 18-49) (Table 2).

The overall sensitivity of interictal ^{99m}Tc-HMPAO SPECT increased from 69% with low-resolution SPECT systems to 84% with high-resolution SPECT systems. The interictal studies were considered true-

positive if a hypoperfusion was detected within the temporal lobe that was EEG- or ECoG-proven to carry the focus and if surgery was consequently performed on this side. Additional areas of ipsilateral hypoperfusion involving either the frontal or the parietal lobe were seen in 15 patients. Low-resolution SPECT systems were used in 12 of these studies. If the studies are considered non-localising and thus false-negative, the sensitivity of interictal rCBF SPECT would be 39% for the low-resolution and 63% for the high-resolution SPECT systems. Lateralisation was, however, correct in these patients. A worse post-surgical outcome with respect to seizure frequency would have been an issue in this group, but a correlation could not be established.

Table 2 Results of the presurgical work-up of patients suffering from temporal lobe epilepsy, according to different SPECT systems applied

	Low-resolution	High-resolution
Complete match	16	12
Match of SPECT and EEG MRI normal or inconclusive	9	4
Match of MRI and EEG SPECT normal or inconclusive	4	0
EEG only MRI and SPECT normal or inconclusive	5	3
Total	34	19

Complete match resembles agreement of EEG, MRI and SPECT on focus site

Table 3 Intra-subject comparison of rCBF SPECT and ^{18}F-DG PET with respect to MRI and EEG results

	EEG	MRI	SPECT ictal	SPECT interictal	FDG-PET
# 1	bi F	L F	R F	R F	L F
# 2	R F	R F	n.d.	normal	normal
# 3	R T	normal	n.d.	R T	R T
# 4	R T	R T	R T	normal	normal
# 5	R T	R T	n.d.	R T	R T
# 6	bi T (R > L)	R T	L T-	L T-	normal
# 7	R T	R T	R T	normal	R T
# 8	L T	L T	L T	L T	normal
# 9	bi T (R >>L)	normal	n.d.	R T	L T+
# 10	L F	L F	L F	L F	L F
# 11	R T	normal	R T	R T	R T
# 12	L T	normal	L T	L T	L T
Sensitivity		66 %	87 %	66 %	66 %

L : left, R : right, F : frontal, T : temporal, - : considered false positive, +: considered true-positive, as EEG was bitemporal

However, ECoG was performed more frequently, and showed cortical hypoperfusion that involved areas exceeding the temporal lobe.

Intra-subject comparison of ictal/interictal ^{99m}Tc-ECD SPECT and interictal ^{18}F-DG PET

Both the interictal rCBF SPECT using ^{99m}Tc-ECD and the interictal ^{18}F-DG PET were made in 12 patients. In 8 of them, an additional ictal rCBF SPECT study was performed with the same tracer. On the basis of the complete presurgical investigation, 3 patients suffered frontal lobe epilepsy while 9 had temporal lobe epilepsies.

Within this small group of patients and without post-surgical data for follow up with respect to a decrease in seizure frequency, the typical problems encountered in evaluation of functional imaging methodology can be demonstrated. Using the evaluation in Table 3 no differences in the sensitivity of interictal rCBF SPECT and ^{18}F-DG PET can be demonstrated. Estimating sensitivity without post-surgical data allows calculations of, for example, an ictal SPECT finding sensitivity of 100% (or 8 / 8 cases), if case number 6 is included (this patient actually presented with a rare seizure of left temporal onset at the time of investigation), or a sensitivity of 75% for the interictal

rCBF SPECT, suggesting that this method was better than ^{18}F-DG PET (the sensitivity of which could drop to 58% if the assessment of patient number 9 is considered false-negative). Except for 2 patients with bilateral EEG-abnormalities, cerebral blood flow and cerebral glucose use located pathology in the same cortical region. The interictal rCBF SPECT study was informative in 2 patients, while ^{18}F-DG PET failed to demonstrate pathology (in one case, indicating the opposite). Although both functional imaging procedures were positive in some patients with normal MRI, both failed to show pathology in certain cases with a clearly positive MRI. No conclusion as to a clearly superior functional imaging procedure could be drawn in these patients.

Imaging results of ^{18}F-DG PET in patients suffering temporal lobe epilepsy

In all, 50 patients who underwent interictal ^{18}F-DG PET were evaluated with EEG. The EEG results, however, could only be cross-checked and correlated with MRI in 33 of them. No post-surgical data are currently available for this group. The overall sensitivity of ^{18}F-DG PET in the depiction of disturbed cortical glucose metabolism in the 50 patients was 82%. Those patients who could be evaluated in more detail are presented in Table 4. In 24/33 cases or 73%,

Table 4 Results of ^{18}F-DG PET in 33 patients suffering from temporal lobe epilepsy

	Number of patients
Complete match	N = 20
Match EEG / PET MRI normal	N = 4
Match EEG / MRI PET normal	N = 5
EEG only MRI and PET normal	N = 1
Match PET / MRI EEG unclear (artefacts)	N = 1
Cases unclear (no matches)	N = 2

the ^{18}F-DG PET clearly demonstrated an area of regional hypometabolism according to EEG results. There was evidence of a ganglioglioma in the left temporal lobe of the case in whom artefacts had left the surface EEG unclear, and a corresponding area of hypometabolism on the PET scan. The other two cases deemed unclear showed discrepancies of MRI, PET and EEG results. If the PET scans of the latter 3 patients are to be considered accurate, PET sensitivity could be as high as 85%. We have already mentioned that the sensitivity calculation should ideally involve postsurgical data, but the PET results demonstrated here do seem to be within the expected range (Table 4). Surprisingly, those patients who had a normal ^{18}F-DG PET scan and corresponding EEG and MRI results (n = 5) all showed hippocampal sclerosis and atrophy on their MRIs, which ranged from slight to severe.

Ictal and interictal rCBF SPECT using ^{99m}Tc-ECD

So far investigations have been performed during the ictal and interictal phases of 25 patients with focal epilepsy. Because of the *in vitro* stability of ^{99m}Tc-ECD, injections could be given more rapidly than rCBF injections. Injection latency was 2-20 s after seizure onset, which was determined by either EEG or the appearance of clinical signs typical of the seizure onset. On the basis of the EEG, 7 patients were seen to suffer from frontal lobe epilepsy. MRI showed focal pathology in 4 of them, but was normal in the remaining 3. Eighteen patients had temporal lobe epilepsy and the MRI positively identified a circumscribed temporal pathology in 14 of them, showed widespread pathology involving the entire

temporal and frontal lobes in one of them, and was normal in the remaining 3.

The interictal rCBF SPECT showed temporal hypoperfusion corresponding to the EEG in 83% of (15 of 18) patients with temporal lobe epilepsy (Table 5). In frontal lobe epilepsy, however, only 43% of (3 of 7) true-positive and EEG-related hypoperfusions were found. Ictal investigations detected the involved lobe in 100% of (18 of 18) cases of temporal lobe epilepsy and in 71% (5 of 7) cases of frontal lobe epilepsy. Circumscribed or focal areas of hyperperfusion were seen in 64% of cases of hyperperfusion that affected larger parts of a lobe. In temporal lobe epilepsy these hyperperfused foci were localised temporolaterally in just 4 of 10 cases of ECoG-proven temporomesial onset of the epilepsy. In contrast, patients with focal hyperperfusion in frontal lobe epilepsy also showed a proven generator focus at this site. So far, the phenomenon of a shift of maximum perfusion away from the generator focus has not been seen.

Discussion

Two major approaches to the functional neuroimaging of patients suffering partial epilepsy can be distinguished. There are those that target brain receptors of, for example, the benzodiazepine-type and those that evaluate cortical metabolism and perfusion using either PET or SPECT. Trying to gather and compare the results of experience with these techniques remains difficult - some factors, clinical experience, for example, are immeasureable. This difficulty with audit is enhanced by the complexity of epilepsy and its investigation, but must be overcome if indications for the application of functional neuroimaging are to be worked out. As is shown above, even the measurement of 'sensitivities' in epilepsy remains difficult and subject to bias. More attention should be paid to post-surgical results in this respect. While there are innumerable publications in the field of epilepsy imaging to date, only a handful present data on post-surgical follow-up[3,8].

Table 5 Comparison of sensitivity to an EEG-correlated area of hypometabolism or hypoperfusion in high-resolution rCBF SPECT and rCGU PET during interictal evaluation of partial epilepsies of temporal lobe onset

	rCBF SPECT	rCBF SPECT	rCGU PET
N	19	18	50
Tracer	^{99m}Tc-HMPAO	^{99m}Tc-ECD	^{18}F-DG
Sensitivity	84 %	83 %	82 %

The measurement of specificity depends on the comparison of a baseline interictal study with ictal studies, because it is seemingly difficult to convincingly obtain false-positive results from an interictal study alone. As a consequence, quite apart from superior imaging results, the ictal study remains desirable in the investigation of patients suffering from epilepsy. However, there are known logistical difficulties in performing routine ictal studies, and these must be overcome. One approach might be the introduction of automatic or, at least, semi-automatic devices for ictal deployment of the tracer[9]. A tracer with high *in vitro* stability is needed, and, since the introduction of ^{99m}Tc-ECD, is now available (to be followed commercially in the near future by ^{99m}Tc-HMPAO)[10].

Ictal deployment of a tracer leads to two further considerations. First, the injection of a tracer-bolus needs to be performed under controlled clinical circumstances. This can only be achieved if constant EEG monitoring is available, and was not done in all ictal studies presented here (despite this, the generator focus was detected in many patients). Second, the tracer used needs a high first-pass extraction and no considerable cortical uptake thereafter. Both the established rCBF SPECT tracers match this condition to an acceptable level. Furthermore, tracer washout should not occur with time or, failing this, the contrast of a hyperperfused generator focus should not decrease with time compared with normal cortical uptake. ^{99m}Tc-HMPAO seems to have a favourable retention; serial SPECT shows that, with ^{99m}Tc-ECD, the contrast of a hyperperfusion with the surrounding cortex does not decrease with time[11].

One result of these facts is that ^{18}F-DG PET is less than suitable for ictal imaging in epilepsy. Furthermore, for reasons of tracer metabolism, interictal ^{18}F-DG studies need continuous EEG monitoring for at least the 30 min that follow injection. Because of time resolution, this remains a major problem of CGU PET but is less of a problem for rCBF SPECT. There has been some discussion as to whether or not rCGU and rCBF are correlated in epilepsy and, thus, which tracer model would be better suited for epilepsy imaging, but no convincing data are yet published to show that cerebral metabolism and cerebral blood flow would not be closely correlated in most clinical situations[12,13]. Specifically with respect to the interictal phase of the disease, and in agreement with the intra-subject comparison presented here, no differences could be shown[14]. Some authors argue that there is an uncoupling of rCGU and rCBF during interictal evaluation, while others suggest that this phenomenon would be, if relevant at all, restricted to certain,

especially ictal and early postictal phases[15]. With respect to the inter-subject correlation mentioned here, there seems to be no major difference in sensitivity, so long as high-resolution SPECT systems are used. There were, however, some patients in whom one method was informative, and the other normal or inconclusive, and a possible explanation, since these studies were made without EEG control, is that there is indeed influential subclinical epileptogenic activity. This leads us to the conclusion that EEG monitoring is also desirable during interictal functional neuroimaging. Given the fact that modern systems are already relatively sensitive, this compromise between logistical demand and clinical routine may be allowed.

During evaluation of the data and with respect to the literature, similarities can be found when fully morphological information (MRI) and fully functional information (EEG) are compared with the results of functional neuroimaging in epilepsy. A lesion described by MRI and suspected to be epileptogenic is regularly associated with a regional disturbance of perfusion and metabolism, if certain diseases such as highly malignant tumours or inflammatory processes are not taken into account. This explains why interictal studies, although they are truly functional studies, show a strong relationship with morphology[16]. This also resembles the generally accepted theory that these procedures are more sensitive than MRI because they also show the effects of the lesion itself and its dysfunctional influence on related cortical structures. These findings and this theory imply something already realised by MRI, namely that regional cortical hypoperfusion and hypometabolism are fairly sensitive, but that the epileptogenicity of those lesions still needs to be proven. Interictal functional imaging is currently, therefore, most effective in patients with partial epilepsy and a normal MRI scan. The intrinsic proof that the generator focus resides in the vicinity of a MRI-lesion remains to be shown by ECoG, sometimes by EEG, or by ictal rCBF SPECT only.

Regional disturbances of cortical function (rCGU/rCBF) during interictal investigation are frequently relatively large[17]. Whether or not these areas of hypometabolism or hypoperfusion respectively correlate with the epileptogenic area that extends and possibly surrounds the generator focus remains to be shown. So far, no attempts have been made to correlate lesion size and the regional degree of pathology within functional studies with their impact on, for example, post-surgical seizure control used as an indirect measure of their clinical relevance. One recent study using ^{18}F-DG PET claimed that hypometabolism exceeding the area of surgical resection might be responsible for the minor decrease in seizure frequency afterwards. These aspects need to be evaluated with a quantitative approach for rCBF SPECT. If semi-quantitative techniques are used instead, a well established and age-related cohort of normal controls is needed. These studies have recently been made for ^{18}F-DG PET in a considerable number of patients[18].

An alternative technique with which to obtain this information is the ictal rCBF SPECT study, made under surface EEG control. This method spares the patient a stressful ECoG, as long as certain conditions are met, namely: a focal MRI lesion matched by a focally increased tracer uptake in the ictal rCBF SPECT and a proven switch of perfusion compared with the interictal study. The surface EEG is still needed to support findings. Given its limited spatial resolution, the required information is a fitting unifocal ictal discharge within the target area of the methods outlined above. Interictal studies can contribute additionally, as they present the only way of using imaging to include or exclude further involvement of more distant cortical structures.

The situation changes in patients with a normal MRI scan. Whether or not the diagnostic process outlined can be equally applied to these patients is highly speculative. Presently, the techniques seem more important as guides for invasive ECoG[19]. The primary aim in such a situation is to find the cortical area suspected to carry the focus. Interictal functional imaging is well suited to this. Electrode implantation can be limited to the absolutely necessary strips, grids and depth electrodes, only if the preceeding investigation is specific, i.e. made with ictal rCBF SPECT. In our experience it is mostly only the affected lobe that can be demonstrated by SPECT in such patients - the identification of focal abnormalities remains rare and subject to uncertainty, since the secondary outspread of discharges can not be distinguished from the epileptogenic focus itself.

References

1 Kuzniecky, R.I. and Jackson, G.D. Magnetic resonance in epilepsy, Raven Press, New York, 1994

2 Henry, T.R., Engel, J. and Mazziotta, J.C. Clinical evaluation of interictal fluorine-18-fluorodeoxyglucose PET in partial epilepsy. *J. Nucl. Med.* 1993, 34, 1892

3 Menzel, C., Hufnagel, A., Grünwald, F. *et al.* The relevance of interictal rCBF brain SPECT in temporal lobe epilepsy. *Ann. Nucl. Med.* 1995 (in press)

4 Andersen, A.R. 99m-Tc-D,L-hexamethylene-propylene-amine oxime (99mTc-HMPAO): basic kinetic studies of a tracer of cerebral blood flow. Cerebrovasc. *Brain Metab. Rev.* 1989, 1, 288

5 Walovitch, R.C., Franceschi, M., Picard, M. *et al.*
Metabolism of 99mTc-L,L-ethyl cysteinate dimer in healthy volunteers. *Neuropharmacol.* 1991, 30, 283

6 Menzel, C., Grünwald, F., Pavics, L. *et al.* Brain single-photon emission tomography using Tc-99m bicisate (ECD) in a case of complex partial seizure. *Eur. J. Nucl. Med.* 1994, 21, 1243

7 Gloor, P. in 'Contributions of electroencephalography and electrocorticography to the neurosurgical treatment of epilepsies', Raven Press, New York, USA, 1987, p.553

8 Grünwald, F., Durwen, H.F., Bockisch, A. *et al.* Technetium-99m-HMPAO brain SPECT in medically intractable temporal lobe epilepsy: a postoperative evaluation. *J. Nucl. Med.* 1991, 32, 388

9 Alksne, J.F., Tecoma, E., Iragui-Madoz, V. *et al.* Development of a device to facilitate routine ictal SPECT studies [Abstract]. *Epilepsia* 1993, 34, 139

10 Kuikka, J.T. and Berkovic, S.F. Localization of epileptic foci by single-photon emission tomography with new radiotracers. *Eur. J. Nucl. Med.* 1994, 21, 1173

11 Grünwald, F., Menzel, C., Pavics, L. *et al.* Ictal and interictal brain SPECT imaging in epilepsy using technetium-99m-ECD. *J. Nucl. Med.* 1994, 35, 1896

12 Kuhl, D.E., Engel, J., Phelps, M.E. and Selin, C. Epileptic patterns of local cerebral metabolism and perfusion in humans determinated by emission computed tomography of 18-FDG and 13-NH3. *Ann. Neurol.* 1980, 8, 348

13 Lebrun-Gradie, P., Baron, J.C., Soussaline, F. *et al.* Coupling between regional blood flow and oxygen utilisation in the normal human brain. *Arch. Neurol.* 1983, 40, 230

14 Leiderman, D.B., Balish, M., Sato, S. *et al.* Comparison of PET measurements of cerebral blood flow and glucose metabolism for the localization of human epileptogenic foci. *Epilepsy Res.* 1992, 13, 650

15 Ackermann, R.F., Lear, J.L., Meredith, W. and Engel, J. Uncoupling of hippocampal metabolism and blood flow during amygdala-kindled seizures in rats. *Soc. Neurosci.* 1982, 8, 90

16 Menzel, C., Grünwald, F., Hufnagel, A. *et al.* Vergleich der HMPAO-Hirn-SPECT mit kernspintomographischen Befunden bei 126 Patienten mit Epilepsie [Abstract]. *Nukl. Med.* 1994, 33, A9

17 Ryvlin, P., Cinotti, L., Froment, J.C. *et al.* Metabolic patterns associated with non-specific magnetic resonance imaging abnormalities in temporal lobe epilepsy. *Brain* 1991, 114, 2363

18 Loessner, A., Alavi, A., Lewandrowski, D. *et al.* Regional cerebral function determined by FDG-PET in healthy volunteers: normal patterns and changes with age. *J. Nucl. Med.* 1995, 36, 1141

19 Henry, T.R., Sutherling, W.W., Engel, J. *et al.* Interictal cerebral metabolism in partial epilepsies of neocortical origin. *Epilepsy Res.* 1991, 10, 174

SPECT in Neurology and Psychiatry, edited by P.P. De Deyn, R.A. Dierckx, A. Alavi and B.A. Pickut
© 1997 John Libbey & Company Ltd, pp. 267-271

Cryptogenetic Temporal Lobe Epilepsies: Combined Use of EEG, MRI and HMPAO SPECT for Focus Detection

D. Giobbe and G.C. Castellano[*]

# Chapter 32

Introduction

According to Keranen *et al.*[1], partial complex seizures account for 23% of all epileptic seizures. In many of these cases, an aetiological factor and an anatomical lesion are evident (secondary epilepsy). Nevertheless, not infrequently, both these features are lacking. These last forms, in conformity with the 1989 revised classification of the International League Against Epilepsy (ILAE[2]), are included among the cryptogenetic epilepsies, that is epilepsies presumed to be symptomatic but without aetiological evidence. In these cases, localised EEG abnormalities at the start of the epileptic seizure are usually considered the most indicative for diagnosis and identification of the focus. However, EEG recordings from the scalp may be unreliable and provide erroneous localisation. For these reasons additional investigations seem advisable. Among them the imaging techniques appear to be the most suitable. In large studies, MRI proved much more sensitive that CT and was particularly appropriate for detecting the subtle anatomical lesions which frequently underlie the epileptic focus[3-9]. PET examinations have shown increased cerebral blood flow in the ictal phase as well as discrete foci of hypometabolism in the interictal phase[10,11]. Nevertheless PET, due to the high costs and complexity, is confined to a limited number of centres. SPECT, however, is widely available. This investigation has been used for over a decade to image regional cerebral blood flow (rCBF) in epilepsy, and generally demonstrates hyperperfusion at the focus ictally and hypoperfusion interictally[12,13]. Interictal studies are easy to perform and are more suitable for patients who are not candidates for surgery. Thus combined use of this methodology with MRI and EEG seemed a proper approach for the identification of the focus and a more accurate diagnosis in patients affected by non-refractory crytogenetic temporal lobe epilepsies (TLE).

Methods

Patients

Our study comprises 52 consecutive subjects affected by cryptogenetic TLE, 30 males and 22 females, mean age 34 years (range 14-75 years), who were referred to the Neurology Department of the Ospedale Maria Vittoria of Turin from 1 January 1990 to 30 March 1995. Their mean epilepsy duration was 7 years (range 3 days-28 years) and the mean age of onset 27 years (range 6-74 years). The 24 patients were affected by psychomotor complex partial seizures (automatisms), 15 by absences, 1 by psychosensorial complex partial seizures (vertigo), 4 by affective complex partial seizures; and 6 by complex partial

Neurology Department O. Maria Vittoria, Turin, Italy
*Serv. Med. Nucleare, Turin University, Italy

seizures of several types. The partial seizures were sometimes followed by secondary generalisation in 15 patients. The frequency of seizures was higher than 1 per day in 1 patient, between 1 per day and 1 per month in 25, lower than 1 per month in 26. At the moment of our first visit, 37 patients were in monotherapy (carbamazepine 28, phenobarbital 6, clonazepam 3), 6 were in polytherapy and 9 were not treated at all. Only subjects with normal neurological examinations and normal CT brain scans were included in the study. All the patients were subjected to neuropsychological evaluation, EEG, HMPAO-SPECT. In 32 cases, MRI was performed additionally.

Neuropsychological evaluation

This was carried out employing the mini mental state examination (MMSE). Scores lower than 24 were considered pathological.

EEG

This was performed by means of a Neurograph 14 OTE Biomedica device with 14 channels. Electrodes were positioned according to the 10/20 system. The recordings were carried out both at rest and during the usual activating procedures (hyperventilation and photic stimulation). Only scalp and interictal recordings were performed.

Functional imaging

SPECT studies of regional cerebral blood flow (rCBF) were carried out using at least 925 MBq ^{99m}Tc-HMPAO i.v., starting 15 min after injection. Patients were positioned supine with an immobilised head and with the orbito-meatal line perpendicular to the collimator. Acquisitions were performed by means of a single head rotating gamma camera (GE 400T), equipped with a low energy (LE) ultra high resolution (UHR) collimator, on line with a dedicated computer (GE STAR II). Sixty-four views (each over 25 s) were acquired on 360° into 64x64 pixel matrix, setting a 140 Kev 20% window, recording at least 2000 Kcounts.

Raw data were filtered with a Butterworth filter (cut-off frequency = 0.5 cycles/cm, slope = 15), the two pixel -1.2 cm thick transaxial slices were reconstructed by filtered back - projection algorithm using a Ramp filter. Images were corrected for attenuation (coefficient = 0.12 cm^{-1}).

Transaxial images were evaluated both qualitatively and semiquantitatively. Semiquantitative analysis was performed on the significant sections by putting ten, two by two symmetric, equal (8x8 pixels) square

regions of interest (ROIs) on cerebral cortex and two, equal to the preceeding ones, on cerebellar lobes. Percentage activity ratios were then calculated between: a) symmetric ROIs counts (normal range from 90 to 110); b) each cortical ROI counts and mid cerebellar ROI counts (cortico cerebellar ratio C/C). Asymmetries greater than 10% were considered significant. The statistical significance was evaluated by student's test for unpaired groups. The execution time after the last seizure was less than 1 week in 13 patients, between 1 week and 1 month in 19, higher than 1 month in 20. The interval between EEG and SPECT was less than 24 h in all the subjects.

Magnetic resonance imaging (MRI)

An Esatom MR 5000 0.5 Tesla unit was employed. Axial sections of 8 mm in intermediate echo and T_2W1 (SE, TR 2100, TE 50,100, 2 mm gap) and 5 mm coronal sections in T_1 (FFE, TR 400, TE 17, angle 90, no gap), intermediate echo and T_2 (SE, TR 2100, TE 50,100 1 mm gap) were carried out. The coronal sections were orientated at a slightly oblique angle in order to be perpendicular to the major axis of the temporal lobe for a better anatomical definition of the hippocampal formations.

Results

The MMSE proved normal in all the patients (scores > 24). The EEG showed temporal abnormalities in 34 subjects (65%): focal spikes in 11 patients, focal sharp waves in 10 and focal slow activity in 20. HMPAO SPECT with qualititave analysis (QA) detected low uptake areas in 39 subjects (75%), and a high uptake area in the patient with more than 1 seizure per day (2%). HMPAO SPECT with semiquantitative analysis (SQA) with calculation of the activity ratio between homologous cortical areas proved abnormal only in 20 individuals (38%).

With both these types of analysis HMPAO SPECT was more often positive in the patients with more frequent seizures and with the longer duration of disease (Table 1). Also a short interval between the last seizure and the time of execution of the SPECT correlated positively with the sensitivity of the examination (Table 1). On the contrary, no influence of the type of therapy or of secondary generalisation was observed. Moreover, no relationship was demonstrated between asymmetry values and clinical symptomatology.

HMPAO SPECT with SQA and calculation of the ratio between cortical and cerebellar activities (C/C ratio) showed significantly lower values in foci in comparison with homologous areas of normal controls

Table 1 Relationship between SPECT positivity and clinical features

Seizure frequency	>1 month 25/26	< 1 month 16/26
Epilepsy duration	< 5 years 19/32	> 5 years 19/20
Secondary generalisation	yes 10/15	no 30/37
Execution time after last seizure	<1 week 12/13	>1 week 29/39

Table 2 Statistical evaluation of differences in C/C ratio between foci and normal homologous areas. Student's t test for unpaired groups was employed

	N	Mean	1 s.d.
Controls	15	82.4	±2.7
Foci of the pts.	52	74.7[a]	±5.6

[a], p< 0.0001

(74.6 ± 5.7 versus 82.4 ± 2.7 p<0.0001) (Table 2). No relationship was detected between C/C values in foci and severity of the clinical symptomatology.

MRI showed abnormalities in 14 patients out of 32 (44.%). An MTS was observed in 6 subjects, grey matter heterotopias in 3, an MCA aneurysm in 1, punctate white matter T_2 hyperintensities in 2, and larger white matter T_2 hyperintensities in 2. EEG and QA SPECT were in agreement in 35 out of 52 cases (67%), EEG and SQA SPECT in 20 out of 52 (38%), QA SPECT and MRI in 18 out of 32 (56%), SQA SPECT and MRI in 26 out of 32 (81%) (Table 3).

Discussion

The pathological substrate in patients operated on for intractable TLE consists of vascular malformations, slow growing tumours and hamartomas in 20-30% of cases and by mesial temporal sclerosis in 70-80%[4,6,14]. All these lesions may be too small to be identified using a CT investigation. MRI has shown, in previous studies, a greater sensitivity[4-6,8] than CT, as it proved positive in almost all the arterovenous malformations, slow growing tumours and hamartomas, as well as in 70% of MTS[4,9,15]. Other possible findings include grey matter heterotopias, more frequently localised near the cortical mantle and the ventricles, small cysts of the transverse and hippocampal fissures, gliosis areas, aspecific leucoencephalopathies.

Table 3 Concordance between SPECT, EEG and MRI

Concordance EEG - QA SPECT	36/52	69%
Concordance EEG - SQA SPECT	20/52	38%
Concordance MRI - QA SPECT	17/32	53%
Concordance MRI - SQA SPECT	26/32	81%

Among our patients, all with negative CT, MRI showed 6 MTS, 3 grey matter heterotopias, 1 MCA aneurysm, 2 punctate white matter hyperintensities and 2 larger white matter intensities. If we do not consider punctate hyperintensities, which were observed in people older than 50 years and are probably an aspecific finding, MRI proved positive in 37.5% of cases, which would otherwise not be recognised.

The increase of cerebral blood flow in the focus during partial seizures was observed repeatedly by means of intraoperative measurements and PET and SPECT studies[10,16]. Our case of increased uptake in the patient with frequent seizures, besides confirming these previous data, is of interest as the examination was performed interictally. An electric seizure without clinical correlates may be hypothesised.

PET studies have shown that during interictal periods there is a hypometabolism in the affected temporal lobe[10,11,17]. The first SPECT studies, performed with different tracers, such as IMP, HIPDM and HMPAO, have shown hypoperfusion areas corresponding to the EEG foci in most patients[11,12,18-20]. However, the number of patients was small. In addition, subsequent reports with less promising results have appeared[21-24].

The analysis of our data shows far different sensitivities between QA and SQA SPECT (77 versus 38%). The sensitivity of the former is similar to the overall sensitivity of the technique, as reported by several studies[12,24-28]; the sensitivity of the latter is similar to that reported by Rowe et al. for interictal studies. This low sensitivity may be related to the fact that we considered significant an activity difference between homologous cortical areas if it was higher than 10%. This is probably an important factor if we consider that a decrease of this threshold to 9%, as suggested by other authors[12] would have increased the sensitivity to 56%. However, in our opinion, a higher threshold is better in order to obtain a better specificity. For the same reason SQA SPECT data are more reliable than QA.

In conclusion, among our patients, MRI demonstrated an anatomical abnormality responsible for the clinical symptomatology in more than one third of cases. Due to this observation and to literature data[4-6,8,14], which underline its capability to detect tumours otherwise not identifiable, we consider MRI the method of choice for the examination of patients with cryptogenetic TLE.

SPECT with semiquantitative analysis, while less sensitive, showed a much better agreement with MRI (81 versus 56%) than SPECT with qualitative analysis. This is relevant, as MRI demonstrated a high rate of correct seizure localisation and a low rate of incorrect lateralisation in a previous surgical study[29]. It may be concluded that, due to specificity limits, qualitative analysis should always be performed in association with semiquantitative analysis. This last methodology, while of limited value in preoperative evaluation because of its low sensitivity, seems useful in patients with non-refractory epilepsy, as in more than one third of patients it provides additional, reliable information for the detection of the focus. Further improvements may be obtained employing multihead and dedicated brain SPECT systems.

References

1 Keranen, T., Sillanpaa, M. and Riekkinen, P.J. Distribution of seizure types in an epileptic population. *Epilepsia* 1988, 29, 1

2 Commission on Classification and Terminology of the International League Against Epilepsy proposed for revised classification of epilepsies and epileptic syndromes. *Epilepsia* 1989, 30(4), 389

3 Bronen, R.A., Cheung, G. *et al.* Mesial temporal sclerosis: comparison of MR, CT, angiography, EEG and pathology. *A. J. N. R.* 1989, 10, 897

4 Brooks, B.S., King, D.W. *et al.* MR imaging in patients with intractable complex partial epileptic seizures. *A. J. N. R.* 1990, 11, 93

5 Jabbari, B. and Gunderson, C.H. Magnetic resonance imaging in partial complex epilepsy. *Arch. Neurol.* 1986, 43, 869

6 Kuzniecky, R., De La Sayette., *et al.* Magnetic resonance imaging in temporal lobe epilepsy: pathological correlations. *Ann. Neurol.* 1987, 22, 341

7 Omson, M.J., Kispert, D.B. *et al.* Cryptic structural lesions in refractory partial epilepsy: MR imaging and CT studies. *Radiology* 1986, 160, 215

8 Schorner, W., Meenke, H.J. and Felix, R. Temporal lobe epilepsy: comparison of CT and MR imaging. *AJNR* 1987, 8, 773

9 Sperling, M.R., Sutherling, W.W. and Nuwer, M.R. New techniques for evaluating patients for epilepsy surgery, in 'Surgical treatment of the epilepsies', (Ed. J. Engel, Jr.), Raven Press, New York, USA, 1987, p.235

10 Engel, J. Jr., Brown, W.J., Kuhl, D.E. *et al.* Pathological findings underlying focal temporal lobe hypometabolism in partial epilepsy. *Ann. Neurol.* 1982, 12, 518

11 Henry, T.R., Mazziotta. J.C. and Engel, J. Jr. Interictal metabolic anatomy of mesial temporal lobe epilepsy. *Arch. Neurol.* 1993, 50(6), 582

12 Anderson, A.R. and Lassen, N.A. Single-photon emission computed tomography in temporal lope epilepsy, in 'Comprehensive epileptology', (Eds. M. Dam and L. Gram, Raven Press, New York, USA, 1991, p.375

13 Zubal, I.G., Spencer, S.S., Iman, K. *et al.* Difference images calculated from ictal and interictal ^{99m}Tc HMPAO SPECT scans of epilepsy. *J. Nucl. Med.* 1995, 36(4), 684

14 Bracchi, M., Saviardo, M. and Casazza, M. Diagnostic protocol of epilepsy. *Riv. di Neuroradiologia* 1990, 3(2), 77

15 Heinz, E.R, Heinz, TR *et al.* Efficacy of MR versus CT in epilepsy. *Arch. Neurol.* 1989, 43, 869

16 Ingvar, D.H. Regional cerebral blood flow in focal cortical epilepsy. *Stroke* 1993, 4, 359

17 Mazziotta, J.C., and Engel, J. The use and impact of positron computer tomography scanning in epilepsy. *Epilepsia* 1984, 25(2), 86

18 Jibiki, I., Kubota, T., Fujimoto, K. *et al.* Regional relationships between focal hypofixation images in 123I-IMP single photon emission computed tomography and epileptic EEFG foci in interictal periods in patients with partial epilepsy. *Eur. Neurol.* 1991, 31(6), 360

19 Lee, B.I., Markand, O.N., Wellman, H.N. *et al.* HIPDM SPECT brain imaging in partial onset secondarily generalized tonic-clonic seizures. *Epilepsia* 1987, 28, 305

20 Magistretti, P.L. and Uren, R.F. CBF patterns in epilepsy in 'Epilepsy: an update on research and therapy', (Ed. G. Nistico), Alan R. Liss, New York, USA, p.241

21 Franceschi, M., Messa. C., Ferini-Strambi, L. *et al.* SPET imaging of cerebral perfusion in patients with non-refractory temporal lobe epilepsy. *Act. Neurol. Scand.* 1993, 87(4), 267

22 Rowe, C.C., Berkovic, S.F., Austin, M.C. *et al.* Visual and quantitative analysis of interictal SPECT with technetium-^{99m}-HMPAO in temporal lobe epilepsy. *J. Nucl. Med.* 1991, 32(9), 1688

23 Ryvlin, P., Philippon, B., Cinotti, L. *et al.* Functional neuroimaging strategy in temporal lobe epilepsy: a comparative study of 18FDG-PET and ^{99m}Tc-HMPAO-SPECT. *Ann. Neurol.* 1992, 31(6), 650

24 Stefan, H., Kuhnen, C., Biersack, H.J. *et al.* Initial experience with 99mTc SPECT in patients with focal epilepsy. *Epilepsy Res.* 1987, 1, 134

25 Biersack, H.J., Linke, D., Brassel, F. *et al.* ^{99m}Tc HMPAO brain SPECT and the WADA test. *J. Nucl. Med.* 1987, 28, 592

26 Buell, U., Stimer, H. and Ferbert, D. Cerebral blood flow/volume SPECT with ^{99m}Tc labelled HMPAO and red blood cells in cerebrovascular disease or epilepsy. *J. Nucl. Med.* 1987, 28, 600

27 Podreka, I., Suess, E., Goldenberg, G. *et al.* Initial experience with ^{99m}Tc HM-PAO brain SPECT. *J. Neurol. Med.* 1987, 28, 1857

28 Wellmann, H.N., Lee, B., Mock, B. *et al.* HIPDM imaging in the localization of complex partial seizure foci. *J. Nucl. Med.* 1987, 28, 600

29 Jack, C.R,. Jr, Mullan, B,P., Sharbrough, F.W. *et al.* Intractable non lesional epilepsy of temporal lobe origin: lateralization by interictal SPECT versus MRI. *Neurology* 1994, 44(5), 829

Paediatrics

SPECT in Neurology and Psychiatry, edited by P.P. De Deyn, R.A. Dierckx, A. Alavi and B.A. Pickut

^{99m}Tc-HMPAO SPECT in Paediatric Neurology

Chapter
33

R. Denays

Introduction

There are only a limited number of papers published on the applications of ^{99m}Tc-HMPAO brain SPECT in the field of paediatric neurology. This is probably at least partly due to the technical, ethical and interpretive problems specific to this age group. The first half of this chapter discusses the problems, the second the current status of HMPAO SPECT in the clinical strategy.

Specific problems

Radiation exposure

The tracer currently used in most departments for evaluation of regional cerebral blood flow is ^{99m}Tc-HMPAO. In children, the dose of the tracer is adapted as a function of body size but is, per kilo body weight, higher than in adults. In neonates, the recommended administered dose is 100 MBq, which is, per kilo body weight, 3 times greater than that of adults[1]. In order to avoid unnecessary radiation exposure, the clinical indications should therefore be carefully evaluated (although the radiation dose will be acceptable, because the tracer is technetium).

Drug sedation

Wrapping the child in a comfortable vacuum cushion is, in our experience, usually sufficient to avoid any movement that could produce artefacts of reconstruction. However, drug sedation is mandatory in some uncooperative children, generally those between 8 months and 4 years of age. Ideally, drug sedation should be administered after tracer injection to avoid any possible influence on cerebral blood flow distribution.

Criteria of normality

What is a normal HMPAO SPECT study in a child? The answer to this question depends on age. Theoretically, therefore, there is a need to explore normal children of different ages. This is, of course, ethically unacceptable, and one way round the problem is to use patients who, retrospectively, might reasonably be considered as normals[2,3].

Department of Neurology, New Paul Brien Hospital, Rue du Foyer Schaerbeekois 36, 1030 Bruxelles, Belgium

Cerebral maturation

The general evolution of scintigraphic patterns due to brain maturation as a function of age has been studied in a qualitative manner by Rubinstein *et al.*[2]. Six typical SPECT patterns with more or less thalamic and/or cortical activity were individualised. In prematures, there is a marked predominance of thalamic activity over cortical areas, and the development of cortical activity follows a strict sequence. First, there is an increase in sensorimotor activity around 40 weeks of gestational age, second there is an increase in occipital activity around 44 weeks, and finally there is an increase in frontal activity beginning at 2 months. The adult-like pattern is reached at 1 year. In clinical practice, neglecting these changing patterns, particularly in children younger than 1 year, can lead to gross misinterpretation of images. An example was given in our previous work in which bilateral severe thalamic lesions in a neonate led to distribution of the tracer in intact cortical areas and thus gave rise to an adult-like pattern[4].

The cerebral maturation process was evaluated semi-quantitatively by activity indexes between the cortical areas and a reference area (the thalamus or the cerebellum in the neonate and the cerebellum or the occipital area in the older child)[3]. Significant changes in some of these indexes were observed in the neonatal period and in the first months of life. For example, compared with values observed in neonates with a gestational age of 33-36 weeks, a significant increase was found for parietal cortex/cerebellar index, parietal cortex/thalamus index, occipital cortex/cerebellar index and occipital cortex/thalamus index at the gestational age of 39-40 weeks. In older children some subtle modifications, not seen by simple visual inspection, were shown by these indexes - a progressive increase in prefrontal activity compared with the occipital area until 11-15 years of age, for example.

Right-left distribution

In children, as in adults, the distribution of the tracer in the 2 hemispheres is more or less, but not entirely, symmetrical. So what is the maximal right-left difference that can be considered normal? In reality it varies from 5 to 15%, and is dependent on the width or region of interest (ROI), the type of equipment, and the techniques of reconstruction. Each centre must therefore establish its own normal criteria.

Spatial resolution and partial volume effect

The relatively poor spatial resolution generally observed with a single-head gamma camera in adults is even more pronounced in children because of the small volume of the child's head. Poor resolution is particularly evident in the neonate, and precise localisation in this age group should not be expected. Also in neonates, important asymmetry can be produced by partial volume effects in cases of mild ventricular dilatation[4].

Clinical applications

The high-risk neonate

Despite constant progress in neonatal intensive care, hypoxic events remain an important cause of neurological morbidity. The topography of the lesions differs as a function of gestational age. In preterms, lesions are usually located in the white matter adjacent to the external angles of the lateral ventricles (periventricular leucomalacia) and/or in the germinal matrix (subependymal haemorrhage) with or without intraventricular or parenchymal bleedings. Such lesions are usually well defined by ultrasound. In full-term neonates, hypoxic lesions are usually located in the watershed areas of the major cerebral arteries, that is, the parasagittal and parieto occipital areas, and in the basal ganglia. Ultrasound and CT scans are usually non-contributive, but SPECT was found to be more sensitive in lesion detection in preliminary studies[4,5]. In a prospective study of 88 high-risk neonates (45 term newborns and 43 preterms), we found that asymmetrical distribution of HMPAO had no predictive value for further neurological outcome[6]. On the contrary, the antero-posterior distribution of the tracer had a clear predictive value (sensitivity: 70%, specificity: 100%, precision: 96.5%). However, this does not mean that SPECT should be performed in all high-risk neonates. In fact, conventional investigations (neurological examination, electroencephalogram (EEG), and ultrasound scan) had a very good negative or positive predictive value when concordant. It was only when these 3 examinations were discordant (in approximately one-third of cases) that SPECT provided additional predictive information. Examples of SPECT in neonates are shown in Figure 1.

Cerebral palsy

The outcome of cerebral palsied children is extremely variable and dependent on the severity of the motor handicap and the presence of associated disabilities such as mental retardation or speech impairment. Early and adequate treatment (e.g. physiotherapy or orthophonic support) may contribute to the final prognosis. Despite the continuing development of

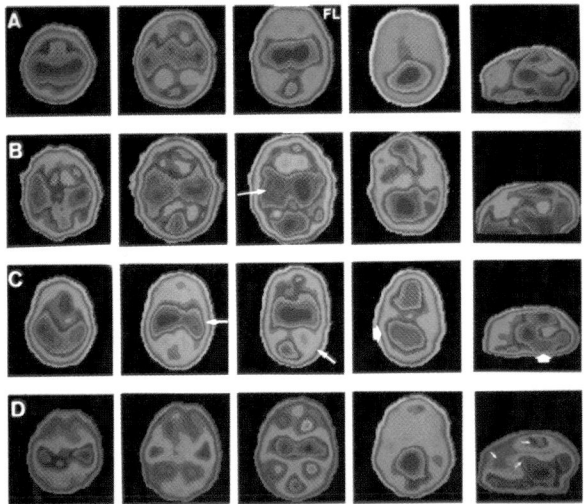

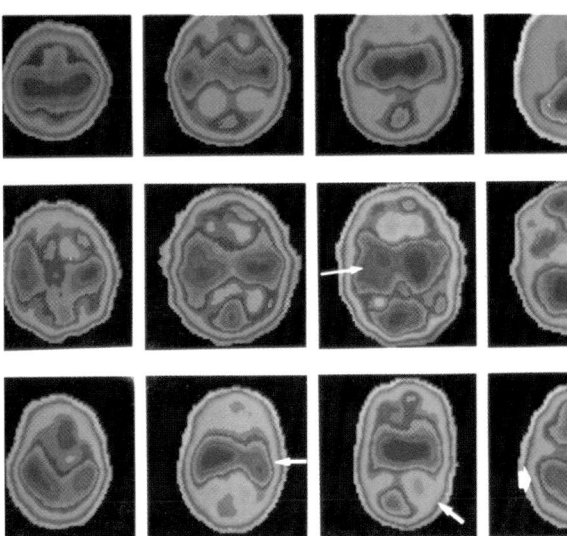

Figure 1 Transaxial and mediosagittal views obtained in 4 high risk neonates. a, Normal neonatal SPECT study. Note high uptake in thalamus, cerebellum and sensorimotor cortex; b, right thalamic hypoactivity; c, left sensorimotor hypoactivity and bilateral cerebellar hypoperfusion; d, marked bilateral decrease of activity in sensorimotor, frontal and thalamic areas. Normal cerebellar perfusion

Figure 3 Child with severe mental retardation. SPECT demonstrates bilateral prefrontal hypoactivity

cerebral investigation techniques, it is often impossible to get an early and complete evaluation of existing disabilities. In cases of congenital hemiplegia, the unilateral hypoperfusion seen on SPECT is often similar to CT scan findings (often a porencephalic cyst in the area of the middle cerebral artery), although it may be observed in the absence of any structural anomaly[7]. The absence of crossed cerebellar diaschisis, even in hemiplegic child patients with large congenital porencephalic cysts, is intriguing (Figure 2). It could be related either to the absence of functional deafferentation of the contralateral cerebellum because of incomplete myelinisation of the corticoponto-cerebellar tracts, or functional recovery of the cerebellum due to inherent plasticity. In spastic diplegia or quadriplegia, SPECT usually shows regional bilateral anomalies in the motor, parietal and

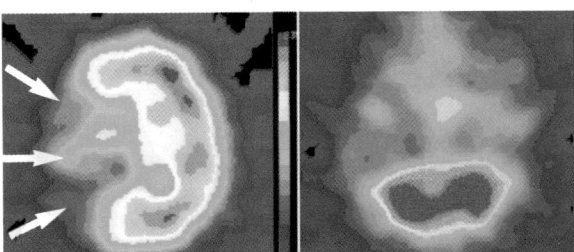

Figure 2 Child with congenital left hemiplegia. Note the large right sylvian SPECT hypoperfusion and the absence of crossed cerebellar diaschisis

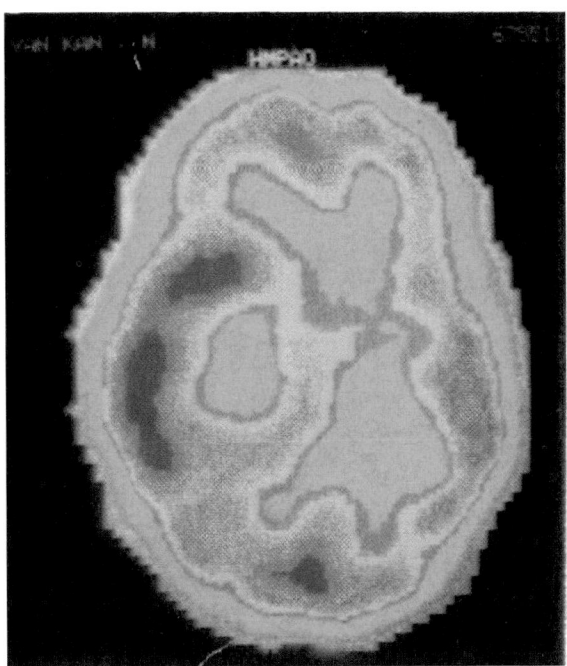

Figure 4 Ictal SPECT study showing right temporal hyperperfusion in a child with complex partial seizures and right epileptogenic focus

prefrontal areas (Figure 3), while a CT scan only shows diffuse cerebral atrophy[7]. However, it is not yet confirmed that these additional anomalies are relevant, nor that they correspond to specific neurological handicaps.

Congenital dysphasia and other congenital or acquired neuropsychological disturbances

Congenital dysphasia is a developmental language disorder that remains unexplained by deafness, phonation disorder, mental retardation, neurological lesion, or psychiatric disease. The aetiology of this disorder has long been debated. It was previously considered to have a psychological origin, but current opinion is that it is usually the result of organic cerebral lesions, the nature of which remains unknown in the absence of demonstrable structural abnormality. In a study of 14 children with congenital dysphasia[8], we found left frontal or left posterior temporo-parietal SPECT hypoperfusion in 11, which suggests that congenital dysphasia, like acquired aphasia, could be due to specific impairment of those cerebral areas devoted to language functions. A right frontal anomaly was also observed in some patients, which could be related to other deficits – particularly attention disturbances – that were present. Similar findings (anomalies in the language areas and the right frontal cortex) have recently been reported by Valenzuela et al.[9]. Findings of physiopathological interest have also een found in other congenital or acquired neuropsychological disturbances. O'Tuama et al.[10] found a temporal anomaly in their 5 patients with Landau-Kleffner syndrome. According to them, their results suggest the temporal anomaly is independently responsible for language disorder and seizures. In autism, a dysfunction of the temporal lobe, usually the left lobe, might also play a part[11], and in attention deficit disorder, a fronto temporal anomaly can often be demonstrated, usually on the right side[12]. In Down's syndrome, as in Alzheimer's, the temporo parietal and the parieto occipital areas are preferentially involved[13]. Finally, in Rett syndrome, Uvebrandt et al.[14] found hypoperfusion of the frontal lobes and the upper brainstem.

Epilepsy

There have been many studies in epileptic disorders in which interictal SPECT anomalies have been revealed by CT scan or MRI[15-19]. CBF anomalies have even been observed by Dierckx et al.[20] in simple febrile convulsions, which questions the real significance and usefulness of interictal SPECT in epilepsy. In contrast, despite considerable practical limitations, ictal SPECT studies represent one of the most interesting clinical

applications of SPECT in children. Cross et al.[21] found focal ictal hyperperfusion, corresponding to focal interictal hypoperfusion, in 12 of 14 children with intractable epilepsy (Figure 4).

Acute neurological illness

Early changes have been described with SPECT even before structural lesions appear on CT or MRI, particularly in cases of acute cerebrovascular disease or focal encephalitis[22-25]. However, these anomalies are often non-specific, and the hyperfixation or the hypofixation no better distinguished[26]. In cases of fever, however, demonstration of a hyperfixation increases suspicion of herpes encephalitis[27].

Monitoring therapy

One of the most promising uses of SPECT could be its contribution to the monitoring of therapy. Vera et al.[28] studied children receiving cytarabine for acute leukemia, and found that a SPECT anomaly was often the only objective imaging feature of the neurotoxicity of cytarabine.

In a technique using extracorporal membrane oxygenation in neonates, Park et al.[29] had to ligate the right common carotid artery. They found SPECT very useful in evaluating the effect of this ligation on cerebral perfusion. SPECT is also, undoubtedly, very useful in the confirmation of brain death, as it gives early confirmation of the absence of any significant brain perfusion[30].

Conclusions

It is clear that further improvement is required before SPECT use can become widespread and better in children. This improvement might include: improved resolution of images and decreased time of acquisition with the use of 2- or 3-head gamma cameras; an improved signal to noise ratio and decreased radiation dose with the use of new tracers such as ECD; improved standardisation of technique in order to obtain more reliable normal criteria.

From a clinical point of view, it is clear that SPECT currently has only a very limited number of clear indications in children: brain death, ictal studies of refractory epilepsy, and high-risk neonates with discordant conventional test results. Although promising and interesting preliminary results have been found in various other situations: cerebral palsy, neuropsychological disturbance, acute deficit, and therapy monitoring, true clinical usefulness still has to be demonstrated.

References

1 Piepsz, A., Hahn, K., Roca, I. *et al.* A radiopharmaceuticals schedule for imaging in paediatrics. *Eur. J. Nucl. Med.* 1990, 17, 127

2 Rubinstein, M., Denays, R., Ham, H.R. *et al.* Functional imaging of brain maturation in humans using iodine-123 iodoamphetamine and SPECT. *J. Nucl. Med.* 1989, 12, 1982

3 Denays, R., Ham, H., Tondeur, M. *et al.* Detection of bilateral and symmetrical anomalies in technetium-99m-HMPAO brain SPECT studies. *J. Nucl. Med.* 1992, 33, 485

4 Denays, R., Vanpachterbeke, T., Tondeur, M. *et al.* Brain single photon emission computed tomography in neonates. *J. Nucl. Med.* 1989, 30, 1337

5 Uvebrant, P., Bjure, J., Hedstrom, A. and Ekholm S. Brain single photon emission computed tomography (SPECT) in neuropediatrics. *Neuropediatrics* 1991, 22, 3

6 Denays, R., Vanpachterbeke, T., Toppet, V. *et al.* Prediction of cerebral palsy in high-risk neonates: a Tc-99m HMPAO SPECT study. *J. Nucl. Med.* 1993, 34, 1223

7 Denays, R., Tondeur, M., Toppet, V. *et al.* Cerebral palsy: initial experience with Tc-99m HMPAO SPECT of the brain. *Radiology* 1990, 175, 111

8 Denays, R., Tondeur, M., Foulon, M. *et al.* Regional brain blood flow in congenital dysphasia: studies with technetium-99m HMPAO SPECT. *J. Nucl. Med.* 1989, 30, 1825

9 Valenzuela, H., Roca, I., Aguade, S. *et al.* Brain SPECT in specific language disorders in '2nd European symposium on pediatric nuclear medicine', (Ed. I. Roca), Barcelona, Spain, 1995, p.63

10 O'Tuama, L.A., Urion, D.K., Janicek, M.J. *et al.* Regional cerebral perfusion in Landau-Kleffner syndrome and related childhood aphasias. *J. Nucl. Med.* 1992, 33, 1758

11 Gillberg, I.C., Bjure, J., Uvebrant, P. *et al.* SPECT (single photon emission computed tomography) in 31 children and adolescents with autism and autistic-like conditions. *Eur. Child Adolesc. Psych.* 1993, 2, 50

12 Dom, L., Dierckx, R., Callens, N. *et al.* Regional cerebral blood flow in children with attention-deficit disorder: a Tc-99m HMPAO SPECT study in 14 children. Buenos Aires: 6th Congress of the International Child Association, 1992

13 Kao, C.H., Wang, P.Y., Wang, S.J. *et al.* Regional cerebral blood flow of Alzheimer's disease-like pattern in young patients with Down's syndrome detected by 99Tc m-HMPAO brain SPECT. *Nucl. Med. Comm.* 1993, 14, 47

14 Yoshikawa, H., Fueki, N., Suzuki, H. *et al.* Cerebral blood flow and oxygen metabolism in the Rett syndrome. *Brain Dev.* 1992, 14(suppl), 69

15 Denays, R., Rubinstein, M. and Ham, H. Single photon emission computed tomography in seizure disorders. *Arch. Dis. Child.* 1988, 63, 1184

16 Gelfand, M.J. and Stowens, D.W. I-123 iofetamine single photon emission tomography in school-age children with difficult-to-control seizures. *Clin. Nucl. Med.* 1989, 14, 675

17 Iivanainen, M., Launes, J., Pihko, H. *et al.* Single-photon emission computed tomography of brain perfusion: analysis of 60 paediatric cases. *Dev. Med. Child Neurol.* 1990, 32, 63

18 Abdel-dayem, H.M., Nawaz, M.K., Hassoon, M.M. *et al.* Cerebral perfusion abnormalities in therapy-resistant epilepsy in mentally retarded pediatric patients. Comparison between EEG, X-ray CT, and Tc-99m HMPAO. *Clin. Nucl. Med.* 1991, 16, 557

19 Adams, C., Hwang, P.A., Gilday, D.L. *et al.* Comparison of SPECT, EEG, CT, MRI, and pathology in partial epilepsy. *Pediatr. Neurol.* 1992, 8, 97

20 Dierckx, R.A., Melis, K., Dom, L. *et al.* Technetium-99m hexamethylpropylene amine oxime single photon emission tomography in febrile convulsions. *Eur. J. Nucl. Med.* 1992, 19, 278

21 Cross, J.H., Gordon, I., Todd-Pokropek, A. *et al.* Ictal and interictal regional cerebral blood flow in focal epilepsy of childhood. *Eur. J. Nucl. Med.* 1994, 21(suppl), 71

22 Nara, T., Nozaki, H. and Nishimoto, H. Brain perfusion in acute encephalitis: relation to prognosis studied using SPECT. *Pediatr. Neurol.* 1990, 6, 422

23 Fujii, Y., Kuriyama, M., Konoshi, Y. and Sudo M. MRI and SPECT in influenzal encephalitis. *Pediatr. Neurol.* 1992, 8, 133

24 Shirasaka, Y., Ito, M., Okuno, T. *et al.* Sequential 123-I-IMP-SPECT in acute infantile hemiplegia. *Pediatr. Neurol.* 1989, 5, 306

25 Shahar, E., Gilday, D., Hwang, P.A. *et al.* Pediatric cerebrovascular disease. Alterations of cerebral blood flow detected by Tc 99m- HMPAO SPECT. *Arch. Neurol.* 1990, 47, 578

26 Meyer M.A. Focal high uptake of HMPAO in brain perfusion studies: a clue in the diagnosis of encephalitis *J. Nucl. Med.* 1990, 31, 1094

27 Launes, J., Nikkinen, P., Lindroth, L. *et al.* Diagnosis of acute herpes simplex encephalitis by brain perfusion single photon emission computed tomography. *Lancet* 1988, 2, 1188

28 Vera, P., Bonnin, F., Stievenart, J.L. *et al.* Neurologic toxicity of cytarabine high-dose (ara-C HD): 99m Tc-HMPAO SPECT scan abnormalities in children. 2nd European Symposium on Paediatric Nuclear Medicine, (Ed. I. Roca), Barcelona, Spain, 1995, p.69

29 Park, C.H., Spitzer, A.R., Desai, H.J. *et al.* Brain SPECT in neonates following extracorporal membrane oxygenation: evaluation of technique and preliminary results. *J. Nucl. Med.* 1992, 33, 1943

30 Galaske, R.G., Schober, O. and Heyer, R. 99mTc-HMPAO and 123 I-amphetamine cerebral scintigraphy: a new, non invasive method in determination of brain death in children. *Eur. J. Nucl. Med.* 1988, 14, 446

SPECT in Neurology and Psychiatry, edited by P.P. De Deyn, R.A. Dierckx, A. Alavi and B.A. Pickut
© 1997 John Libbey & Company Ltd, pp. 281–286

Brain Perfusion Imaging with ^{99m}Tc-ECD in Normal Children: Quantitative Analysis and Database Mapping

Chapter
34

C. Schiepers, A. Verbruggen, J. Hegge,
P. Casaer and M. De Roo

Introduction

Brain perfusion imaging with ^{99m}Tc-labelled radiopharmaceuticals has become a routine procedure in most clinics for the diagnosis and follow-up of various neurological disorders such as dementia, stroke, vascular disease and epilepsy. Most experience so far has been obtained with ^{99m}Tc-HMPAO. Walovitch et al.[1,2] introduced the complex of ^{99m}Tc with L,L-ethyl-cysteinate-dimer (^{99m}Tc-ECD) as an alternative brain perfusion agent. The superior characteristics of the ^{99m}Tc label for tomographic imaging when compared with the ^{123}I label of older brain perfusion radiopharmaceuticals (HIPDM, IMP) have been well documented[3,4].

The perfusion patterns of ^{99m}Tc-ECD in normal adult volunteers have been reported in multicentre trials by Holman et al.[5] and Vallabhajosula et al.[6]. The dosimetric data and biokinetic behaviour of the radiopharmaceuticals are well known. The main advantages of ^{99m}Tc-ECD over ^{99m}Tc-HMPAO concern the somewhat higher brain uptake, a higher contrast between white and grey matter, and the greatly increased clearance from the body by the kidneys. The radiation dose to the brain is slightly higher for ^{99m}Tc-ECD than ^{99m}Tc-HMPAO because of this higher brain uptake. The radiation dose to other organs, with the exception of the bladder wall, is lower, but an adequate fluid intake and frequent voiding may significantly decrease the bladder dose.

The normal brain distribution pattern of ^{99m}Tc-ECD in children is not well known. Brain maturation and changes in cerebral flow with age have been studied by Chiron et al.[7] using ^{133}Xe, and by Rubinstein et al.[8] using IMP. Chugani et al.[9] investigated brain glucose metabolism using ^{18}F-FDG, and elegantly demonstrated the influence of age. In general, there is an increased perfusion and metabolism of subcortical over cortical areas in the young. Denays et al. studied neonates likely to develop cerebral palsy using ^{99m}Tc-HMPAO and ^{123}I-IMP[10], and also studied brain maturation in very young infants using ^{99m}Tc-HMPAO[11]. They found the highest perfusion in sensori-motor zones, the visual cortex and the striatum.

We were interested in the 'normal' pattern of ^{99m}Tc-ECD in children. For obvious ethical reasons normal, healthy children and/or their parents could not be asked to participate. Therefore, we retrospectively reviewed all tomographic studies and clinical charts and selected those children that were finally diagnosed as normal, i.e. disease-free. The children were referred to nuclear medicine for brain perfusion imaging in the workup for febrile convulsions. If epilepsy could be ruled out, their brain perfusion would resemble the pattern of normal volunteers as closely as possible.

Nuclear Medicine and Neuro-paediatric departments, University Hospital Gasthuisberg, Leuven, Belgium

Methods

Radiopharmaceutical

L,L-Ethylcysteinate dimer (L,L-ECD) dihydrochloride was synthesised according to a published procedure[12]. ^{99m}Tc-L,L-ECD was prepared by reconstitution of home-made lyophilised labelling kits containing 1.0 mg ECD.2HCl and 0.07 mg $SnCl_2.2H_2O$, with 1.85 GBq ^{99m}Tc in the form of sodium pertechnetate in a volume of 3 ml saline, adjusted to pH 7.4 with phosphate buffer. The preparation was analysed for radiochemical purity (RCP) using previously published procedures[13].

Patient preparation

The lights in the scanner room were dimmed and the children allowed about 15 min to get accustomed to this. ^{99m}Tc-ECD with a RCP >95% was administered intravenously in a dose of 10-25 MBq/kg. Acquisition was started 10 min later. Young children were usually sedated with a cocktail of Largactil and Luminal i.m. (both in a dose of 1 mg/kg) plus a pentobarbital suppo (dose 30 mg/kg), which caused an extra delay of 15-30 min.

Acquisition

Images were acquired with a dedicated brain scanner (SME 810, Strichman Medical Systems, MA, USA). This is a single-slice machine with 12 detectors that scan the head. This scanner has a high sensitivity and a resolution of 6 mm FWHM for ^{99m}Tc and our collimator set. Slices were acquired sequentially, and a stack of 2D transaxial slices obtained. Acquisition time was 240-300 s per slice, with a relative distance of 10-12 mm. Images were reconstructed using a deconvolution technique with 2 iterations. Attenuation correction was applied using a best-fitting elliptical contour and constant attenuation coefficient of 0.16 cm^{-1}. Patients' heads were positioned parallel to the inferior orbito-meatal line, and about 8-10 slices were acquired.

All studies were reprocessed using commercial software (Neuro-900, Strichman Medical Systems, MA, USA) that became available in 1992. The transaxial slices were interpolated to a 3D volume set of images in a 128x128x128 cube, which amounts to a voxel size of 1.6 mm. In order to obtain a 'standardised' brain presentation, a new set of reorientated slices was created. All data were resampled into 12 mm-thick slices and reorientated along the approximate AC-PC line. Friston et al.[14] have shown good correlation between the plane drawn

through the thalami and both caudate nuclei on ^{18}F-FDG PET images and MR-images (a deviation of <1°). Under normal circumstances, the basal ganglia can be easily determined and rotated to such an extent that coronal cuts have the caudate nuclei in a horizontal plane and sagittal slices have the thalamus and caudate in one plane.

Analysis

On the set of standardised brain cuts, regions were drawn manually for further analysis. Pairs of regions were drawn as shown in Table 1. The count density of these regions was analysed for regional asymmetries. A normalisation was performed to compare regional uptake between patients. A program was developed that performs the quantitative analysis and deals with display and database handling of results.

Quantitative analysis

A set of macros was written in a commercial spreadsheet (Microsoft EXCEL) for the evaluation of left-right differences, perfusion indices and database mapping. An outline of this program (QUANTO) is given in Figure 1. In short, the statistics of the regions drawn over the various areas are pasted to a worksheet. This worksheet functions as data input for the program. The first step is a conversion of the data from the Neuro-900 to EXCEL format. Second, the data are organised in an intermediary file, in which calculations such as slice-averaging, left-right comparison, normalisation of counts etc, can be performed.

The program computes perfusion indices for grey matter, deep grey, and cerebellar structures. Uptake values are also calculated by volume averaging of the contributions of all cortical areas, and database mapping is supplied. Databases can be set up for different parameters: radiopharmaceutical, age, sex, normalisation area (cerebellum, cortex), and type of region statistic (maximum, average, median counts).

Under normal circumstances, the program supplies three different outputs for the referring physician (Figure 2):

1. numeric display of uptake, and area-weighted mean of the various regions
2. graphic display of regional uptake and right-to-left ratios
3. database map.

Various databases have been established for ^{99m}Tc-ECD, according to the age groups outlined below. Figure 3 gives a schematic representation of the

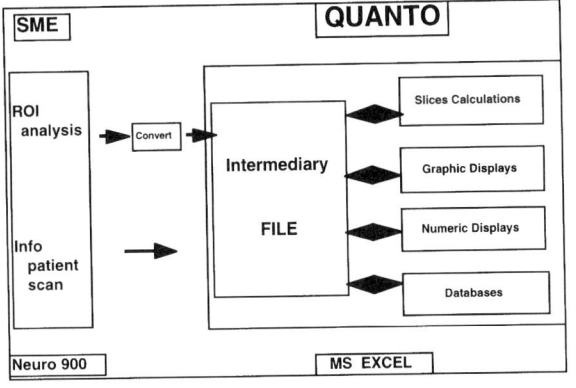

Figure 1 Schematic representation of the QUANTO program. Region statistics, relevant patient and acquisition information are transferred from the NEURO-900 program into the intermediary file. Macros inside the program are available for manipulations of individual slices, regions, and variables. Graphical and numerical displays, as well as database maps, are generated

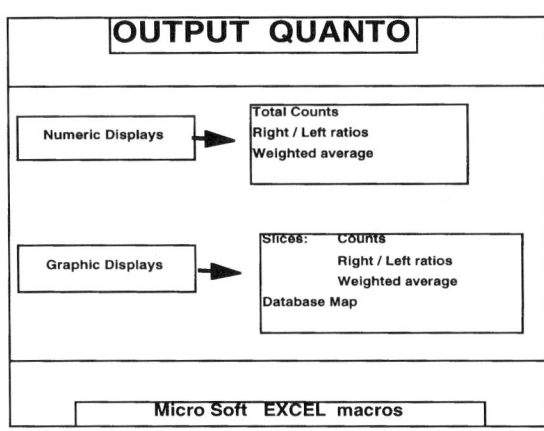

Figure 2 Schematic representation of the QUANTO output. Data from the intermediary file are reprocessed and displayed in the desired format. Macros computed left/right ratios, area-weighted count densities, perform normalisations and map the results onto the database values of the specific age group

variables needed to create a particular database. In a separate module, the criterion for normal can be set (e.g. ±2 s.d.). The currently available age groups for ^{99m}Tc-ECD are also given.

Population

Between August 1988 and August 1992, 88 children referred for brain perfusion imaging were included in the study. They all had a normal perfusion pattern, as read independently by 2 experienced physicians in nuclear medicine (CS, MDR), and the perfusion study was finally classified as normal if the child fulfilled the following criteria:

1. EEG normal at time of admission
2. brain CT normal at time of admission
3. no psychomotor retardation
4. clinical follow-up negative for 1 year after admission.

Table 1 Eleven pairs of regions of interest (ROI) drawn over the cortex, deep grey structures and cerebellum

Zone	ROI	Abbreviation	Code
Hemisphere	both white and grey matter	Hemi	HE
Cortex	fronto medial	FrM	FM
	fronto-lateral	FrL	FL
	sensory-motor	RoI	Ro
	parietal/lateral-occipital	Pa-Oc	OL
	medial-occipital	OcM	OM
	temporal	Temp	TM
Basal ganglia	caudate nucleus	NuC	NC
	lentiform nucleus	NuL	NL
Thalamus		Thal	TH
Cerebellum	grey matter	Cer	OE

Table 2 Databases of normal children, i.e. negative patients, for brain perfusion imaging with ^{99m}Tc-ECD

Group	N	Age in years		
		Range	Mean	s.d.
1 Toddlers	5	1.3 - 2.3	1.9	0.5
2 Children	6	4.8 - 8.7	6.7	1.7
3 Teenagers	5	10.5 - 15.4	13.0	2.2

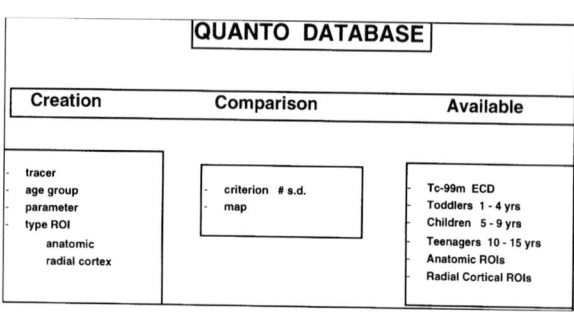

Figure 3 Schematic representation of the setup of database generation and mapping. On the left, pertinent variables such as tracer, age group, and ROI drawing are entered, as well as the relevant parameters for database definition, such as normalisation area, and counts-variable (average, median, maximum). During normal operation, the comparison criterion has to be (pre)defined along with the age group of the actual study. The program automatically detects the parameters and variables that were processed, i.e. normalisation to the cortex, area-weighted mean of all ROIs in the study, average cps/pix etc., and thus automatically generates all maps possible. Currently available databases are shown on the right

Sixteen 'negative' patients fulfilled the above conditions: 13 boys and 3 girls. All infants studied were abnormal and could not be entered in the database. Data were reprocessed and arbitrarily assigned to 3 age clusters: 1-4, 5-9 and 10-15 years. Mean age and standard deviation in each age group are given in Table 2.

Statistics

Results are expressed as the average number of counts per pixel in each region. Left-to-right ratios were computed to evaluate regional changes. A perfusion index was determined by normalising the count density to a specific ROI, i.e. cerebellum or cortex. Paired two-tailed t-tests were applied to evaluate the significance of differences between these parameters ($p < 0.05$).

Results

Detailed inspection revealed that there were no statistically significant differences between corresponding regions in the right and left hemisphere. This finding was true for every child and, therefore, ipsi- and contralateral ROI results were averaged. In Figures 4 and 5 the results are given for the 3 age clusters after normalisation to the cerebellum and cortex, respectively. In both figures, the highest uptake ratio is found for the medial occipital cortex and striatum. The influence of age is clearly different for the 2 normalisation methods. Normalisation to the cerebellum reveals the highest uptake in the visual cortex and basal ganglia of toddlers (group 1, 1-4 years), and the differences between age groups 1 and 3 are significant. After normalisation to the cortex, the above effect disappears. In age group 1 in Figure 5, the lowest uptake ratios are found, surprisingly, for the visual cortex and the cerebellum. Age group 2 has the highest uptake in the striatum relative to the cortex. Note the clear increase of cerebellar uptake with age.

In Figure 6, the graphic output of QUANTO with respect to regional uptake, i.e. the area weighted average count density, is given. The data of left and right ROIs are dealt with separately in these displays. On the left and right hand side of the display the measured count density is given for each individual ROI. In the middle, the right/left ratio is given with 0.05 interval lines highlighted. We usually accept ratios between 0.9 and 1.1 as being within the normal range. This type of display can be generated for every plane of the study, as well as each processed set of planes, or for the area-weighted average uptake of the entire brain as in Figure 6.

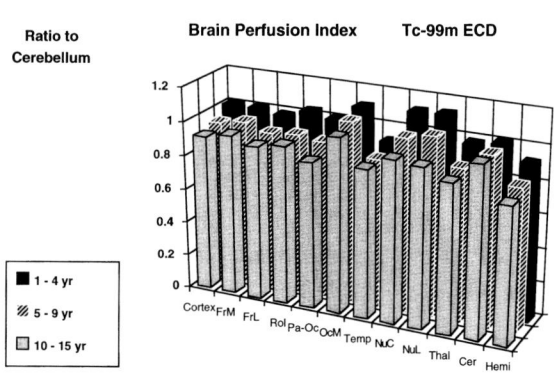

Figure 4 Perfusion index of the three different age groups. Average uptake values have been normalised to the cerebellum. Note the clear decrease in the striatum (caudate and lentiform nuclei) as age increases. The medial occipital ROI has the highest uptake, in part related to open eyes during the ^{99m}Tc-ECD injection. For abbreviations see Table 1

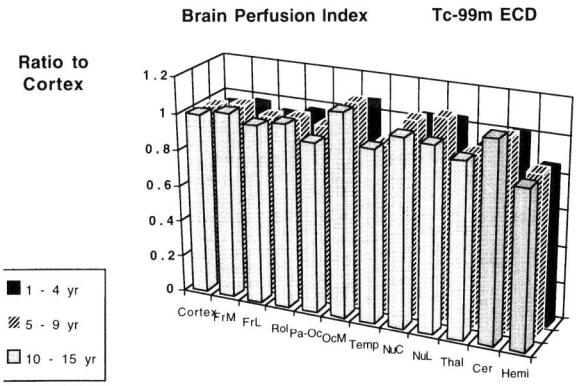

Figure 5 Perfusion index of the three different age groups. Average uptake values have been normalised to the cortex, i.e. weighted average of all grey matter. See Table 1 for abbreviations of regions

Finally, a perfusion index is calculated, i.e. the count density normalised to a specific ROI. The perfusion indices of the above selected normal children were entered in the database for ^{99m}Tc-ECD. Thus, the perfusion patterns of new paediatric patients can be mapped onto the age-specific database. Here, too, various options are available: normalisation to the cerebellum, ipsi- or contralateral hemisphere, or the entire cortex. The type of count density may be indicated as well, i.e. average, maximum or median counts within the ROI. Just as for the R/L comparison, data are presented for both hemispheres independently. In Figure 7, the perfusion indices of a normal teenager

are mapped onto the database. As upper and lower limits, ±1.5 s.d. around the mean are given. The medial occipital cortex has the highest index, corresponding to the highest uptake. Relative hyperfrontality is seen, expressed by the slightly higher uptake values in the frontal cortex compared with the parietal and temporal zones.

Discussion

This survey assessed the normal paediatric perfusion pattern through retrospective analysis of brain imaging studies acquired with ^{99m}Tc-ECD. Basically, these are 'negative' patients who are considered to represent the normal brain pattern of toddlers, children and teenagers. More than 200 perfusion studies were reviewed, and none of the children experienced adverse reactions. As mentioned in the introduction, dosimetry estimates in the literature clearly favour ^{99m}Tc-ECD over ^{99m}Tc-HMPAO. The slightly higher bladder dose may be reduced by urging children to drink and void frequently. In addition, the low *in vitro* stability of ^{99m}Tc-HMPAO is a major disadvantage, especially if rapid injections are required as is the case in ictal epilepsy imaging. Therefore, we think that ^{99m}Tc-ECD is the radiopharmaceutical of choice for the neuro-paediatric population.

We did not observe uptake differences of more than 12% in individual children between left- and right-sided ROIs. Therefore, we kept our historical 10% variation as the limit of normal. Since we are interested in comparing the perfusion patterns of children, we do not want to depend on differences in the dose administered, the time and delay of acquisition (in case

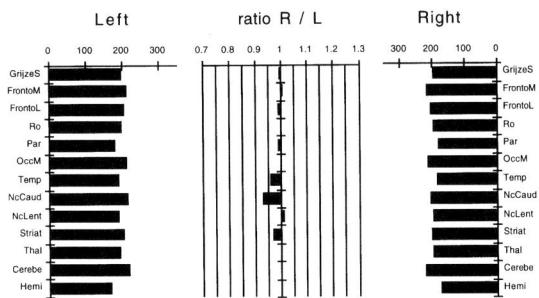

Figure 6 Output of the quantification program. The measured count density (cps/pix) for the regions (see Table 1 for abbreviations) in the left and right hemisphere is given in the outside panels. The right/left ratio is displayed in the middle with lines indicating 0.5 steps. In this way, the quantitative pattern may be 'grasped' in one glance, and significant asymmetries are immediately obvious

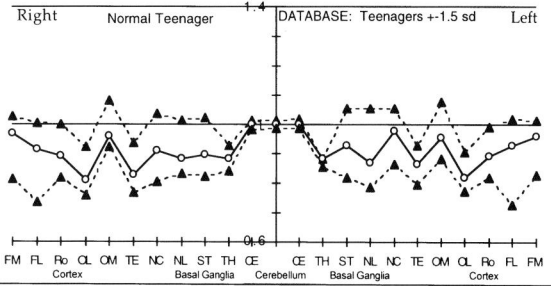

Figure 7 Map of the perfusion index in the indicated regions (full line) onto the database (see Table 1 for ROI codes). Upper and lower limit (dotted lines through triangles) are 1.5 s.d. above and below the mean of that ROI. Note that the visual cortex has the highest index, and the difference between basal ganglia and cortex has disappeared, contrary to the pattern in young children (see Figures 4 and 5)

of sedation), etc. A normalisation step is therefore necessary. The uptake ratio, or perfusion index, is usually calculated with respect to the cerebellum, but we have observed that this does not seem optimal in young children. Apparently, the maturation of perfusion of the cerebellum is different to that of the cortex in the young. Perfusion indices were also quite comparable in individual children. The s.d. for the regions varied between 0.01 and 0.09; i.e. <10%.

Some controversy has been reported over tracer fixation in the brain and washout differences. The initial loss of ^{99m}Tc-ECD would exceed that of ^{99m}Tc-HMPAO and would adversely effect image quality. Walovitch et al.[2] have shown that this loss in brain uptake amounts to <25% over 4 h, with 11.7% during the first half-hour, in normal volunteers. However, the uptake mechanisms of ^{99m}Tc-ECD are definitely different to those of ^{99m}Tc-HMPAO and, in general, appear slower - as has been indicated by ictal perfusion studies[15]. Biersack et al.[15] have shown that ^{99m}Tc-ECD is an effective marker for perfusion imaging in epilepsy and can be used both for ictal and interictal studies[15].

Although we did not encounter problems related to the early start of the acquisition, present knowledge of the biokinetics of ^{99m}Tc-ECD suggests that a 10 min delay is too short and an interval of at least 30 min is recommended.

Conclusions

^{99m}Tc-ECD is a safe brain imaging agent for paediatric applications. The radiation dose is acceptable and compares favourably with that of other available agents. The perfusion pattern is different in toddlers and teenagers, obviating the need for quantification to assess 'normal'. A quantitative program, QUANTO, has been developed, which permits user-friendly interaction and produces easily interpretable displays of regional perfusion asymmetries, and database comparison with specific age-clusters.

References

1 Walovitch, R.C., Hill, T.C., Garrity, S.T. et al. Characterization of technetium-99m-L,L-ECD for brain perfusion imaging. Part 1. Pharmacology of technetium-99m

ECD in nonhuman primates. J. Nucl. Med. 1989, 30, 1892

2 Walovitch, R.C., Franceschi, M., Picard, M. et al. Metabolism of ^{99m}Tc-L,L-ethyl-cysteinate dimer in healthy volunteers. Neuropharmacology 1991, 30, 283

3 Lassen, N.A. Imaging brain infarcts by single-photon emission tomography with new tracers. Eur. J. Nucl. Med. 1994, 21, 189

4 Verbruggen, A.M. Radiopharmaceuticals: state of the art. Eur. J. Nucl. Med. 1990, 17, 346

5 Holman, B.L., Hellman, R.S., Goldsmith, S.J. et al. Biodistribution, dosimetry, and clinical evaluation of technetium-99m ethyl cysteinate dimer in normal subjects and in patients with chronic cerebral infarction. J. Nucl. Med. 1989, 30, 1018

6 Vallabhajosula, S., Zimmerman, R.E., Picard, et al. Technetium-99m ECD: a new brain imaging agent: in vivo kinetics and biodistribution studies in normal human subjects. J. Nucl. Med. 1989, 30, 599

7 Chiron, C., Raynaud, C., Maziere, B. et al. Changes in regional cerebral blood flow during brain maturation in children and adolescents. J. Nucl. Med. 1992, 33, 696

8 Rubinstein, M., Denays, R., Ham, H.R. et al. Functional imaging of brain maturation in humans using iodine-123 iodoamphetamine and SPECT. J. Nucl. Med. 1989, 30, 1982

9 Chugani, H.T., Phelps, M.E. and Maziotta, J.C. Positron emission tomography study of human brain function development. Ann. Neurol. 1987, 22, 487

10 Denays, R., Pachterbeke, T., Tondeur, M. et al. Brain single photon emission computed tomography in neonates. J. Nucl. Med. 1989, 30, 1337

11 Denays, R., Tondeur, M., Foulon, M. et al. Regional brain blood flow in congenital dysphasia: studies with technetium-99m HMPAO SPECT. J. Nucl. Med. 1989, 30, 1825

12 Blondeau, P., Berse, C. and Gravel, D. Dimerization of an inter-mediate during the sodium in liquid ammonia reduction of L-thiazolidine-4-carboxilic acid. Can. J. Chem. 1967, 45, 49

13 van Nerom, C., Bormans, G., Crombez, D. et al. Radiochemical analysis of ^{99m}Tc-ECD by TLC and HPLC in 'Technetium and rhenium in chemistry and nuclear medicine 3', (Eds. M. Nicolini, G. Bandoli, U. Mazzi), Cortina Int, Verona, Italy, 1990, p.525

14 Friston, K.J., Passingham, R.E., Nutt, J.G. et al. Localization in PET images: direct fitting of the intercommissural (AC-PC) line. J. Cereb. Blood Flow Metab. 1989, 9, 690

15 Grunwald, F., Menzel, C., Pavics, L. et al. Ictal and interictal brain SPECT imaging in epilepsy using technetium-99m-ECD. J. Nucl. Med. 1994, 35, 189

SPECT in Neurology and Psychiatry, edited by P.P. De Deyn, R.A. Dierckx, A. Alavi and B.A. Pickut

Comparison of Cerebral Perfusion and Quantitative EEG in Children with Supratentorial Brain Lesions

Chapter
35

L. Sztriha, A.R. Al Suhaili[*], M. Towsey, V. Prais[*], D. Alpsan, A. Bener and Y.M. Berjawi[*]

Introduction

The investigation of regional cerebral blood flow by SPECT has proved a useful tool in the assessment of various brain disorders[1]. Although most SPECT investigations have been performed on adults, the number of publications on the use of SPECT in children is increasing[2].

The value of interictal, ictal and immediate postictal SPECT in temporal lobe epilepsy in adults has been widely assessed[1,3,4], and ictal SPECT has also proved useful in the localisation of extratemporal epileptic foci[5]. In the presurgical evaluation of children with partial epilepsy of various aetiologies (tumour, cyst, cortical dysplasia, mesial temporal sclerosis, Sturge-Weber syndrome, hemangioma), SPECT was considered a valuable additional diagnostic procedure, although surgical decisions were mostly influenced by EEG findings and neuroradiological abnormalities[6]. Several SPECT studies have been performed on adult patients with stroke[1], traumatic brain injury[1,7,8], and psychiatric disorders[1]. SPECT can also give additional information in some metabolic diseases, such as MELAS syndrome (mitochondrial encephalomyopathy with lactic acidosis and stroke)[9].

Quantitative EEG techniques and topographic mapping of scalp electrical activity have proved valuable for the objective evaluation of background electrical activity[10]. Frequency analysis has been widely used in patients with cerebrovascular disease, epilepsy, mass lesions and psychiatric disorders[10].

Since there is a close relationship between oxygen metabolism and rhythmic electrical activity recorded by EEG[11], a correlation between blood flow and quantified EEG features is to be expected. This relationship has been clearly demonstrated in adult patients with stroke[12,13], and partial epilepsy[14].

The aim of this study was to compare the results of brain SPECT and quantified EEG in a small group of children with heterogeneous supratentorial lesions. The data gained by spectral analysis of the EEG records appear more suitable for comparison with the results of a functional brain imaging technique than the data of a scoring system based on visual EEG interpretation. In this preliminary study we wished to confirm that the relationship between blood perfusion and EEG spectral content found in adults also exists in children. We were not trying to assess the sensitivity nor specificity of either technique alone in the localisation of supratentorial lesions.

Faculty of Medicine and Health Sciences, United Arab Emirates University, P>O>Box 17666, Al Ain, United Arab Emirates
*Department of Nuclear Medicine, Tawam Hospital, United Arab Emirates

Methods

Eight patients (2 female and 6 male, aged 8-11 years) with supratentorial focal brain lesions were studied by ^{99m}Tc-HMPAO SPECT and EEG (conventional and frequency analysis). All patients were examined by X-ray CT. The interval between investigations was never longer than 6 months. Table 1 shows the patients' data. Patients 1-7 were treated with carbamazepine, 20 mg/kg.

The control group for SPECT contained 9 children (7 female, 2 male, aged 8-12 years). Entirely normal children cannot be studied with SPECT for ethical reasons, therefore the controls were selected from a group of patients with transient neurological symptoms who were found to be completely normal during follow up. This control group was used to help identify abnormal regions in the SPECT images of our 8 patients. A different group of 20 normal children (12 female and 8 male, aged 8-13 years) served as controls for EEG quantification.

All patients had CT of the head with 10 mm transaxial slices from the base of the skull to the vertex without and with the administration of intravenous contrast material.

^{99m}Tc-HMPAO (20 MBq/kg, maximum 550 MBq, Ceretec, Amersham) was given intravenously when the patients were quiet. SPECT scans were performed within 2 h of the HMPAO injection, using a single-head rotating gamma camera (GE 400 AC) and a low-energy, high-resolution parallel hole collimator. Acquisition was obtained in a 64x64 matrix over 360°. Transaxial, coronal and sagittal slices were reconstructed by filtered back projection (Butterworth filter) after uniformity and attenuation correction (Chang's method). Visual and semiquantitative analyses were performed.

A commercially available software, Cortiqual, produced by Lamourex et al.[15], was used for objective semiquantitative analysis of the SPECT data. This mapping technique, which depicts the distribution of the tracer in the cortical layer of the brain, is essentially similar to the technique used by geographers to describe the surface of the earth. Since both the brain and the earth have two hemispheres, equatorial and hemispherical maps of the brain can be generated using a system similar to that used in geography. The mid-sagittal plane of the brain is defined. The centre of the brain, which is required for the construction of maps, is located on this mid-sagittal plane, approximately half-way from the front to the rear on an axis which is perpendicular to the mid-sagittal slice and runs through the right and left mid-temporal areas. A cortical layer of constant thickness (24 mm in our study) is defined by

the computer, and equatorial and hemispherical maps of isotope uptake are produced.

On the equatorial maps, the frontal area is at the top of the map, the occipital area is in the mid-portion, and the cerebellum at the bottom. The hemispherical maps look like side views of the brain from left and right (Figure 1). Regions of interest (ROIs), corresponding to specific brain regions, are delineated by the computer and a template shows the different cerebral areas as follows: 1 anterior frontal; 2 mid frontal; 3 posterior frontal; 4 parietal; 5 temporo parietal; 6 temporo occipital; 7 perisylvian; 8 temporal; 9 cerebellar. Uptake values in each region are expressed in terms of mean counts and different ratios can be calculated using these values.

In this work, cortical/cerebellar ratios were calculated as mean counts in each cortical segment divided by the mean count in the cerebellum, while asymmetry indices were calculated as segmental uptake differences divided by the average of both segments -

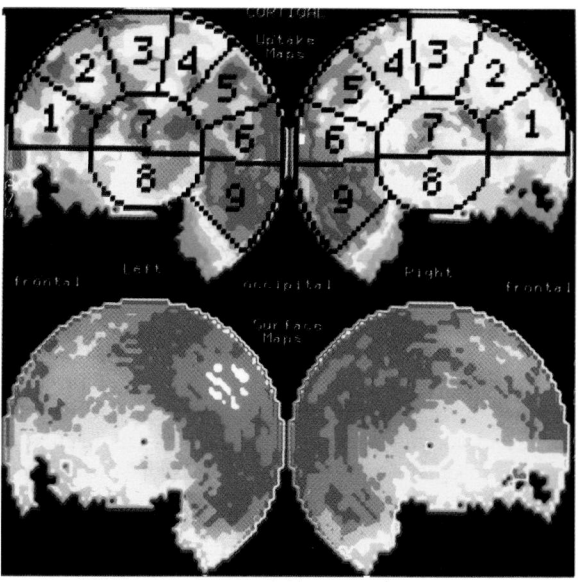

Figure 1 SPECT, uptake and surface maps of Patient 2 with traumatic brain injury as constructed by Cortiqual. Regions on the uptake maps and corresponding EEG electrodes are as follows: 1. anterior frontal - Fp1, Fp2; 2. mid frontal - F3, F4; 3. posterior frontal - C3, C4; 4. parietal - P3, P4; 5. temporo parietal - (no corresponding electrode); 6. temporo occipital - O1, O2; 7. perisylvian - (no corresponding electrode); 8. temporal - T3, T4; 9. cerebellar (no corresponding electrode). These maps are lateral views of the hemispheres. Low perfusion in the right hemisphere is clearly seen

Table 1 Patients' data

No	Age/Sex	Age at onset	Clinical diagnosis	CT	SPECT[a] Supratentorial region of hypoperfusion	EEG (Visual interpretation)
1	8y F	4m	Hemiconvulsion-hemiplegia-epilepsy syndrome (Left hemiplegia)	Dilated R lateral ventricle	R fronto parieto occipital	Diffuse slowing, more prominent on R side, epileptiform discharges over R temporo centro parietal areas
2	10y M	8y	Traumatic brain injury L hemiplegia Epilepsy	Post-traumatic brain atrophy with dilatation of both lateral ventricles	R fronto parieto occipital	Diffuse slowing, more prominent on R side, epileptiform discharges over R fronto centro temporal areas
3	11y M	not known	Tumour cerebri Epilepsy	L parietal tumour	L parieto occipital	Diffuse slowing, more prominent on L side, epileptiform discharges over L fronto parieto temporal areas
4	10y M	Pre-natal	L temporal cyst Epilepsy	L temporal cyst	L temporal	Diffuse slowing, epileptiform discharges over L occipital area
5	9y M	1y	Meningitis Hemiconvulsion-left hemiplegia-epilepsy-syndrome	Moderately dilated lateral ventricles	Normal	Diffuse slowing, epileptiform discharges over L frontal area
6	11y F	Peri-natal (?)	R hemiplegia Epilepsy	Small porencephalic cysts in the L internal capsule and lentiform nucleus	L thalamus, basal ganglia	Epileptiform discharges over L centro temporal area
7	8y M	1y	Congenital heart disease Stroke Epilepsy	Small porencephalic cysts in the L internal capsule and lentiform nucleus	L frontal, thalamus, basal ganglia	Epileptic discharges over L temporal area
8	12y M	12y	MELAS syndrome L occipital stroke	L occipital hypodensity	L occipital	Diffuse slowing

[a] L = left, R = right   Regions, where the cortical/cerebellar ratio and asymmetry index are outside mean ± 2 s.d. of control values

i.e. (R-L)/(0.5x(R+L)). The mean and standard deviation of the cortical/cerebellar ratios and asymmetry indices for the control group were calculated. Patient values outside 2 s.d. of the control group were regarded as abnormal.

The EEG was recorded in the awake, supine state, and patients were stimulated verbally, as required, to prevent drowsiness. Silver/silver chloride electrodes were placed according to the international 10/20 system. A linked ear reference and forehead ground were employed. Electrode impedances were less than 5 k Ohm. Recording and analysis were performed with a Bio-Logic System. Amplified signals were bandpass filtered from 0.3 to 30Hz, digitised at 256 samples/s with 8-bit resolution. Acquisition periods were 20 min. Data were stored on optical disks for later analysis. The same records were visually interpreted on a SVGA computer screen.

Thirty artefact-free 2 s epochs (a total of 60 s) were selected for FFT spectral analysis in 4 frequency bands (delta: 1.50-3.50 Hz, theta: 4.00-7.50 Hz, alpha: 8.00-12.5 Hz and beta: 13-24 Hz). These epochs did not contain epileptiform discharges.

The following EEG power indices were calculated epoch by epoch at each electrode site and averaged over all epochs; absolute power, alpha/delta ratio, alpha/theta ratio, relative power (ratio between one specific band and the sum of all bands at the same electrode site), power normalised for the total scalp (ratio between the power in one specific frequency band and total power summed over all electrodes) and asymmetry indexes, (R-L)/(0.5x(R+L)), of absolute power in homologous electrodes.

This gives a total of 429 EEG indices for each patient. It is necessary to transform some of these indices before carrying out further statistical analysis because they are unlikely to be normally distributed. Absolute power and the A/D, A/T ratios were transformed using ln(X). Relative powers were transformed using ln(X/(1-X)). It was not necessary to transform the asymmetry ratios because they were already normally distributed.

All 429 indices for the 20 children in the control group were tested for normal distribution of the transformed indices using a chi-squared goodness of fit test. At the 95% confidence level, only 12 of the 429 indices were not normally distributed and 9 of these were indices of beta- power. By chance alone, one would expect 21 of these indices to be non-normally distributed at this level of confidence. Z-scores[16] for all 429 indices of each patient were calculated using the means and standard deviations of the controls. Z-scores exceeding ±3.0 were used to identify regions of abnormality.

SPECT indices from each area of the computer-produced template were compared with EEG indices derived from corresponding electrodes. (Figure 1; anterior frontal: Fp1, Fp2; mid frontal: F3, F4; posterior frontal: C3, C4; parietal: P3, P4; temporal: T3, T4 and temporo occipital: O1, O2). The correlation coefficients between SPECT and EEG indices were calculated using a commercial graphing software.

Results

Individual patient results are summarised in Tables 1 and 2.

Patient 1

This patient with hemiconvulsion-hemiplegia-epilepsy syndrome had left hemiplegia. Moderate dilation of the right lateral ventricle was seen on CT, while visual interpretation of the EEG showed diffuse slowing, more prominent over the right hemisphere, and epileptiform discharges in the right temporo centro parietal areas. SPECT revealed right fronto parieto occipital hypoperfusion. Spectral analysis of the EEG confirmed the increase in absolute delta-theta power over the entire scalp and the significant asymmetry over the frontal areas with more abundant theta power over the right side. An increase in absolute alpha power over the right frontal area and an increase in absolute beta power over the entire right hemisphere were observed, while a decrease in relative alpha power was seen over the right temporo parieto occipital areas.

Patient 2

This patient who suffered traumatic brain injury was epileptic. The CT detected moderate diffuse brain atrophy. EEG by visual interpretation showed diffuse slowing, more prominent over the entire right hemisphere, and epileptiform discharges in the right fronto centro temporal areas. A marked hypoperfusion was found by SPECT in the entire right hemisphere (Figures 1 and 2). Quantitative EEG analysis confirmed the diffuse increase in delta-theta absolute and relative powers (Table 2 and Figure 3), while the asymmetry in the slow waves proved significant only over the fronto central areas. An increase in absolute alpha power was seen in the right frontal area, while a decrease in relative alpha-beta power was observed over the entire scalp.

Patient 3

This patient with tumour in the left parietal area and partial epilepsy showed diffuse slowing on the EEG,

Table 2 Abnormalities in quantitative EEG features

	Absolute power[a]				Relative power[a]				Asymmetry index[a] (absolute power) (R-L)/0.5(R+L)			
	Delta	Theta	Alpha	Beta	Delta	Theta	Alpha	Beta	Delta	Theta	Alpha	Beta
1	↑total	↑total	↑F_4,F_8	↑Fp_2,C_4,P_4,O_2,F_8,T_6	↑O_2,O_1	–	↓P_4,O_2,T_4	–	–	↑Fp_2,F_4	↑Fp_2,F_4	↑O_2
2	↑total	↑total	↑Fp_2,F_4	–	↑P_4,O_2,T_6,P_3,O_1	↑C_4,P_4,C_3,T_3,T_5	↓total	↓total	↑Fp_2,F_4,F_8	↑Fp_2,F_4,C_4,F_8	↑Fp_2,F_4,F_8	–
3	↑total	↑total	–	–	↑$C_4,P_4,O_2,F_8,T_4,T_6,C_3,P_3,O_1,F_7,T_3,T_5$	–	↓total	↓$Fp1,F_3,C_3,P_3,O_1,F_7,T_3,T_5$	↓F_4,P_4,O_1,T_6	–	↑C_4,P_4	↑$Fp_2,F_4,C_4,P_4,O_2,F_8,T_6$
4	↑C_4,P_4,C_3,P_3,T_5	↑$F_4,C_4,P_4,O_2,F_8,T_4,T_6,C_3,P_3,O_1,T_5$	–	–	–	↑$Fp_2,F_4,C_4,P_4,O_2,F_8,T_4,T_6,Fp_1,C_3,P_3,O_1,F_7,T_5$	↓P_3,O_1	–	–	–	–	–
5	↑$C_4,P_4,O_2,T_6,F_3,C_3,P_3,O_1,T_5$	↑$F_4,C_4,P_4,F_8,C_3,P_3,O_1,T_5$	–	–	↑O_2,O_1	↑C_4,P_4,T_4,C_3,T_3	↓$P_4,O_2,T_6,C_3,P_3,O_1,T_5$	↓, P_4,O_2,P_3,O_1,T_5	–	–	–	–
6	↓F_4,F_8	–	–	↑Fp_2,Fp_1,F_7	–	–	–	↑$Fp_2,F_4,F_8,Fp_1,F_3,F_7$	–	–	–	–
7	↑T_4,T_6	–	–	–	–	–	–	–	–	–	–	–
8	↑$F_4,C_4,P_4,T_4,F_3,C_3,P_3$	–	↓O_2,T_6,Fp_1,P_3,O_1,F_7	–	↑$F_4,C_4,P_4,O_2,F_8,T_4,T_6,C_3,P_3,O_1,F_7,T_5$	–	↓ total	–	–	–	–	–

[a] Absolute power, relative power and asymmetry index values in these regions are outside ±3s.d. of control values

more prominent on the left side, and epileptiform discharges in the left fronto parieto temporal areas. Marked hypoperfusion was found by SPECT at the tumour site. Quantitative EEG analysis showed an increase in absolute delta-theta power over the entire scalp and an increase in relative delta power over both hemispheres. The asymmetry index was negative due to increased left parieto temporo occipital delta power. A significant decrease in relative beta activity over the affected left hemisphere was observed. This reduced beta activity over the left side gave rise to a higher positive asymmetry index. SPECT circumscribed the tumour rather well, while the EEG abnormalities were diffuse and had a lateralising value only.

Patient 4

This patient, with a left temporal cyst and epilepsy, showed bilateral diffuse slowing on the conventional EEG record. Quantification found this slowing to be due to a bilateral increase in absolute delta and theta powers, and relative theta powers. Relative alpha power was decreased over the left parieto occipital area, but the asymmetry indices were not significantly abnormal.

Patient 5

This patient developed hemiconvulsion, left hemiplegia and epilepsy following meningitis. CT showed dilated lateral ventricles presumably due to leukomalacia. Diffuse slowing with left frontal

epileptiform discharges were observed on the routine EEG. SPECT was normal. Bilateral increases in absolute delta and theta powers and decreases in relative alpha and beta powers were the most striking EEG abnormalities.

Patients 6 and 7

These patients with right hemiplegia had small porencephalic cysts in the left internal capsule and lentiform nucleus and showed normal EEG background activity, with left centro temporal and temporal discharges respectively, on visual analysis. A decrease in absolute delta and an increase in frontal beta power were observed in Patient 6, while an increase in temporal absolute delta power was seen in Patient 7. Asymmetry indices were not significantly abnormal in these 2 patients. SPECT showed hypoperfusion in the left thalamus and basal ganglia in both cases and left frontal hypoperfusion in Patient 7.

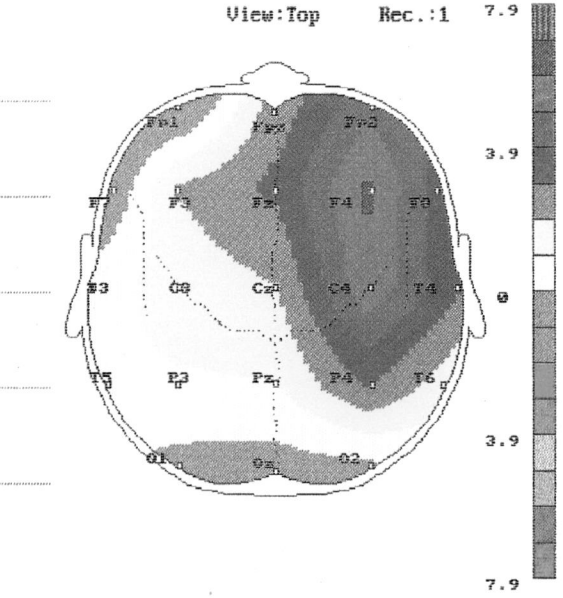

Figure 3 EEG topographic map of Patient 2. Figure illustrates the distribution of theta power normalised to the entire scalp (as defined in methods section). There was a bilateral increase in the absolute and relative theta power in this patient which was more prominent over the right hemisphere, as revealed by the asymmetry index. This asymmetry can be more clearly visualised by mapping normalised power values. The numbers on the scale indicate z-scores (see text). Right is on the viewer's right

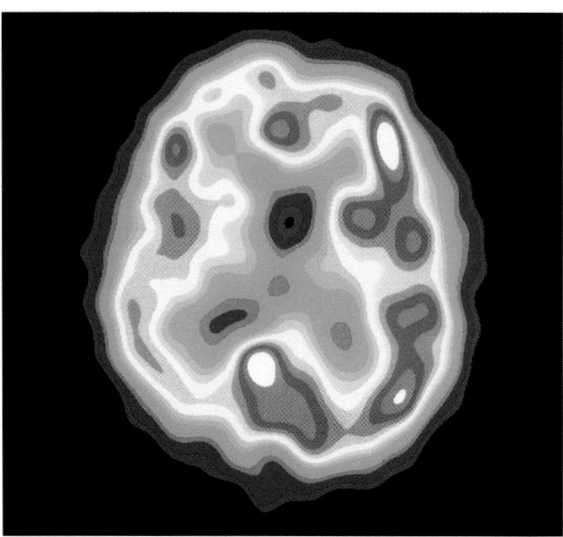

Figure 2 SPECT, transaxial slice of Patient 2. Hypoperfusion can be seen in the right hemisphere. Right is on the viewer's left

Patient 8

This patient had MELAS syndrome and a left occipital stroke with bilateral diffuse slowing on conventional EEG. SPECT revealed left occipital hypoperfusion. EEG quantification showed an increase in absolute and relative delta powers associated with reduced alpha power without asymmetry.

When the indices from all electrode sites over all patients were combined, a significant negative correlation was found between the SPECT cortical/cerebellar ratios and z-scores of EEG power in all 4 frequency bands. A positive correlation was found between SPECT cortical/cerebellar ratios and z-scores of alpha/theta ratios (Table 3). There was a negative correlation between SPECT asymmetry indices and z-scores of EEG delta asymmetry indices (Figure 4).

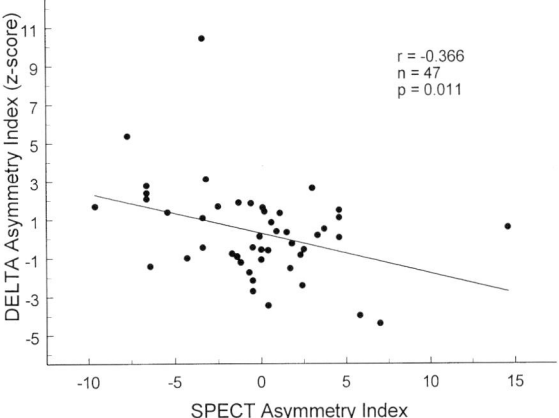

Figure 4 Scattergram of correlation between SPECT asymmetry indices and z-scores of EEG asymmetry indices in the delta band

Discussion

The results of our study in children broadly confirm the results of previous studies in adults[11-14]. A negative correlation between perfusion and absolute delta and theta powers, a negative correlation between perfusion and relative theta power, and a positive correlation between perfusion and the alpha/theta ratio all indicate that a decrease in blood flow of varying aetiology is associated with an increase in the slow wave content of the EEG. However, the EEG slowing was rather

Table 3 Correlation coefficients for z-score of EEG indices on SPECT indices (cortical/cerebellar ratio)

EEG Index	r	p(Ho)	
Delta Abs. Power	- 0.381	0.0004	
Theta Abs. Power	- 0.442	<0.0001	
Alpha Abs. Power	- 0.437	<0.0001	
Beta Abs. Power	- 0.292	0.008	
Alpha/Delta Ratio	+ 0.201	0.071	n.s.
Alpha/Theta Ratio	+ 0.241	0.030	
Delta Rel. Power	- 0.130	0.244	n.s.
Theta Rel. Power	- 0.224	0.043	
Alpha Rel. Power	+ 0.185	0.097	n.s.
Beta Rel. Power	+ 0.303	0.006	
Delta Norm. Power	- 0.213	0.055	n.s.
Theta Norm. Power	- 0.267	0.015	
Alpha Norm. Power	+ 0.060	0.592	n.s.
Beta Norm. Power	+ 0.255	0.021	

n=82, Abs.: absolute, Rel.: relative, Norm.: normalised

widespread in most of our patients, and extended to the contralateral hemisphere so that the asymmetry indices - using 3 s.d. as the threshold for abnormality - had lateralising value only in Patients 1-3.

Several methodological issues are raised in this comparative study. The first is the remote effects that focal brain lesions can have on other parts of the brain, making it difficult to use measures of abnormality to localise a structural lesion. Because of high neural interconnectivity, such effects are well known in EEG[17]. It is probably for this reason that abnormal asymmetry values were observed in only 3 of our patients, despite the fact that all of them had severe unilateral lesions. A related problem can arise with SPECT: abnormalities in blood flow distant from the focal lesion (known as diaschisis) can confound the interpretation of cortical/cerebellar ratios[18]. This phenomenon was observed in Patient 7, in whom cortical hypoperfusion was associated with small, deep subcortical lesions. Although the effect of diaschisis on the EEG has not yet been studied, there was no background EEG abnormality in Patient 7 corresponding to the diaschisis. Cerebellar diaschisis was not observed in this study, thus justifying the use of the cerebellum as a SPECT reference.

A second methodological issue is the matching of EEG electrode sites to SPECT ROIs. SPECT produces real tomograms after reconstruction of the slices, while EEG records electrical activity from the surface of the scalp alone. Our SPECT computer software permitted us to calculate uptake values for relatively large segments of the cortex through its entire depth, and we attempted to match these cortical segments to EEG electrode sites. Such matching cannot be exact and involves some arbitrary decisions that reduce the correlations that might exist between the two modalities.

A third limitation of this preliminary study is the small size of the patient group and the heterogenous locations of their severe supratentorial lesions. This is the reason we believed it necessary to present the results patient by patient.

SPECT results

Seven patients (Patients 1-7) in our group had complex partial seizures of extratemporal origin. Brain pathology was identified by CT and SPECT showed hypoperfusion either corresponding to the lesion (Patients 3 and 4) or more widespread than the area detected by CT. (Patients 1, 2, 6 and 7). SPECT studies on patients with a remote history of traumatic brain injury have revealed such abnormalities in cerebral perfusion that were not obvious on the basis of MRI or CT images[7,8]. These abnormalities can be responsible for the clinical symptoms. The unilateral low perfusion in Patient 2 is more prominent than expected on the basis of CT images and reflects marked functional deterioration. Low perfusion in brain tumours[19], in small deep infarcts[18] and in MELAS syndrome[9] has previously been reported. Interictal SPECT studies on patients with extratemporal epileptic foci revealed a widespread ipsilateral hemispheric decrease in regional cerebral blood flow[5]. We conclude that low perfusion ipsilateral to the extratemporal epileptic foci in Patients 1 and 2 may be attributed to both the epileptic activity (as interictal hypoperfusion) and the structural lesions found by CT.

EEG results

Salinsky et al.[20] tested the sensitivity and specificity of quantified EEG frequency analysis versus conventional EEG interpretation in patients with CT- or MRI-verified focal brain lesions. They found the two methods complimentary when background activity was normal or mildly abnormal. Nuwer[21] found that EEG frequency analysis was useful in lateralising the epileptic focus in several patients with complex partial seizures. In our cases, this attempt was successful only in Patients 1-3. Visual interpretation correctly identified the background EEG abnormalities in all patients, while quantification confirmed these abnormalities and provided us with objective data for comparison with SPECT data.

An unexpected feature of our results is the slight but nevertheless significant increase in absolute alpha and beta powers with decreasing perfusion (Table 3). An increase in the activity of all frequency bands on spike-free epochs within and adjacent to an active epileptic focus has been demonstrated by Hughes et al.[22]. Although this increase was most often seen in the delta and beta-2 (16-30 Hz) frequency ranges, an increase was also observed in the theta, alpha and beta-1 (12-16 Hz) frequencies in several cases. Since 7 of our patients had an active epileptic focus, the increase in alpha and beta powers in relation to decreased perfusion could be attributed to epileptic activity.

Comparison of SPECT and EEG

Several attempts have been made to find correlations between regional cerebral blood flow and quantitative EEG[12-14] in adults. The relationship between cerebral blood flow and quantitative EEG parameters in brain infarction has already been extensively studied. Tolonen and Sulg[13] found a high negative correlation between ^{133}Xe regional cerebral blood flow and delta activity on EEG in patients with infarcts in the territory of the middle cerebral artery. Their results were basically confirmed by Nagata[12], who made comparisons between cerebral blood flow, oxygen metabolic rate and EEG power spectral indices in patients with chronic cerebral infarction. PET data of perfusion and oxygen consumption showed a negative correlation with delta and theta activity and a positive correlation with alpha activity. Z-transformation of the EEG data was performed, and the correlation between PET data and z-scores was also high. Although brain lesions can exert remote effects on brain function, Nagata[12] found that, in general, EEG parameters corresponded to cortical blood flow and metabolism beneath the scalp electrode. Differences between cortical and small subcortical infarcts are not discussed in this study. In the two cases with old, small and deep infarcts (Patients 6 and 7), EEG background activity was normal according to visual interpretation, the abnormalities revealed by quantification were ambiguous in some regions, but SPECT clearly showed localised hypoperfusion.

In partial epilepsy, Jibiki et al.[14] described a negative correlation between absolute values of blood flow and relative theta power and a positive correlation between blood flow and relative alpha power interictally. Our results are in accord with these data.

In conclusion, our results indicate that there are correlations between regional cerebral blood flow and quantitatively analysed EEG background activity in children with various supratentorial lesions. The statistical analysis indicates that decreased blood flow is coupled with an increased amount of slow wave activity on EEG. These results complement previous findings in adults with stroke and partial epilepsy.

Acknowledgements

The authors wish to thank Zs. Sánta and D. Sabatini for technical assistance and Ms P. Roberts for preparing the manuscript. This study was supported by grants from FMHS, United Arab Emirates University (16/95 and CP/96/01) and the Hungarian Research Fund (OTKA, T5091).

References

1   Holman, B.L. and Devous, M.D. Sr. Functional brain SPECT: the emergence of a powerful clinical method. *J. Nucl. Med.* 1992, 33, 1888

2   Uvebrant, P., Bjure, J., Hedstrom, A. and Ekholm, S. Brain single photon emission computed tomography (SPECT) in neuropediatrics. *Neuropediatrics* 1991, 22, 3

3   Rowe, C.C., Berkovic, S.F., Austin, M.C. *et al.* Postictal SPECT in epilepsy. *Lancet* 1989, 1, 389

4   Rowe, C.C., Berkovic, S.F., Austin, M.C. *et al.* Visual and quantitative analysis of interictal SPECT with Technetium-99m-HMPAO in temporal lobe epilepsy. *J. Nucl. Med.* 1991, 32, 1688

5   Marks, D.A., Katz, A., Hoffer, P. and Spencer, S.S. Localization of extratemporal epileptic foci during ictal single photon emission computed tomography. *Ann. Neurol.* 1992, 31, 250

6   Adams, C., Hwang, P.A., Gilday, D.L. *et al.* Comparison of SPECT, EEG, CT, MRI, and pathology in partial epilepsy. *Pediatr. Neurol.* 1992, 8, 97

7   Gray, B.G., Masanori, I., Chung, D-G. *et al.* Technetium-99m-HMPAO SPECT in the evaluation of patients with a remote history of traumatic brain injury: a comparison with X-ray computed tomography. *J. Nucl. Med.* 1992, 33, 52

8   Ichise, M. Chung, D-G. Wang, P. et al. Technetium-99m-HMPAO SPECT, CT and MRI in the evaluation of patients with chronic traumatic brain injury: a correlation with neuropsychological performance. *J. Nucl. Med.* 1994, 35, 217

9   Satoh, M., Ishikawa, N., Yoshizawa, T. *et al.* N-isopropyl-p-[123I]iodoamphetamine SPECT in MELAS syndrome: comparison with CT and MR imaging. *J. Comput. Assist. Tomogr.* 1991, 15, 77

10 Nuwer, M.R. Quantitative EEG: II. Frequency analysis and topographic mapping in clinical settings. *J. Clin. Neurophysiol.* 1988, 5, 45

11 Obrist, W.D., Soledoff, L., Lassen, N.A. *et al.* Relation of EEG to cerebral blood flow and metabolism in old age. *Electroenceph. Clin. Neurophysiol.* 1963, 15, 610

12 Nagata, K. Topographic EEG mapping in cerebrovascular disease. *Brain Topography* 1989, 2, 119

13 Tolonen, U. and Sulg, I.A. Comparison of quantitative EEG parameters from four different analysis techniques in evaluation of relationships between EEG and CBF in brain infarction. *Electroenceph. Clin. Neurophysiol.* 1981, 51, 177

14 Jibiki, I., Kurokawa, K., Fukushima, T. *et al.* Correlations between quantitative EEG and regional cerebral blood flow (SPECT) in patients with partial epilepsy. *Neuropsychobiology* 1994, 30, 46

15 Lamourex, G., Dupont, R.M., Ashburn, W.L. and Halpern, S.E. 'CORT-EX': a program for quantitative analysis of brain SPECT data. *J. Nucl. Med.* 1990, 31, 1862

16 Duffy, F.H., Bartels, P.H. and Burchfiel, J.L. Significance probability mapping: an aid in the topographic analysis of brain electrical activity. *Electroenceph. Clin. Neurophysiol.* 1981, 51, 455

17 Sharbrough, F.W. Nonspecific abnormal EEG patterns in 'Electroencephalography. Basic principles, clinical applications, and related fields. 3rd edn.', (Eds. E. Niedermeyer and F.L. da Silva), Williams and Wilkins, Baltimore, USA ,1993, p.197

18 Bowler, J.V., Costa, D.C., Jones, B.E. *et al.* High resolution SPECT, small deep infarcts and diaschisis. *J. Roy. Soc. Med.* 1992, 85, 142

19 Langen, K-J., Herzog, H., Kuwert, T. *et al.* Tomographic studies of rCBF with [99mTc]-HM-PAO SPECT in patients with brain tumors: comparison with C15O2 continuous inhalation technique and PET. *J. Cereb. Blood Flow Metab.* 1988, 8, S90

20 Salinsky, M.C., Oken, B.S., Kramer, R.E. and Morehead, L. A comparison of quantitative EEG frequency analysis and conventional EEG in patients with focal brain lesions. *Electroenceph. Clin. Neurophysiol.* 1992, 83, 358

21 Nuwer, M.R. Frequency analysis and topographic mapping of EEG and evoked potentials in epilepsy. *Electroenceph. Clin. Neurophysiol.* 1988, 69, 118

22 Hughes, J.R., Taber, J.E. and Fino, J.J. The effect of spikes and spike-free epochs on topographic brain maps. *Clin. Electroencephalogr.* 1991, 22, 150

Cerebrovascular Disorders

SPECT in Neurology and Psychiatry, edited by P.P. De Deyn, R.A. Dierckx, A. Alavi and B.A. Pickut
© 1997 John Libbey & Company Ltd, pp. 299–305

Cerebral Blood Flow by SPECT in Ischaemic Stroke

Chapter
36

B. Sperling and N.A. Lassen

Introduction

Given the high incidence and severe disability of ischaemic stroke, it is not surprising that tomographic measurement of CBF is increasingly used with the aim of improving diagnosis, selecting treatment or evaluating prognosis[1]. This paper will describe CBF methods based on SPECT and give an outline of results obtained in typical cases with emphasis on infarct reperfusion due to thrombolysis, whether spontaneously occurring or therapeutically induced.

HMPAO

Several radioactive tracers can be used for measuring CBF by SPECT. A key role must be assigned to HMPAO, hexamethylenepropylamine oxime labelled with ^{99m}Tc, as this tracer is widely used and is well suited for SPECT imaging. We shall assume that the general properties of HMPAO are well known to the reader, and focus on aspects of special importance for its use in ischaemic stroke.

The retention of HMPAO is due to its conversion to a hydrophilic form that cannot diffuse freely across the cell membranes. The conversion is catalysed by glutathione and probably occurs mainly inside the mitochondria. An infarct develops into an area of necrosis of all cells with loss of all mitochondria within the first couple of days. Hence one might expect failure of HMPAO ('hypofixation') retention in infarcted tissue. In a recent study using ^{133}Xe SPECT to measure CBF, we found evidence of this phenomenon up to about 10 days after stroke onset. The degree of hypofixation was, however, quite moderate (Figure 1), amounting to about 10% both in infarcts with persistent ischaemia and in infarcts with reperfusion hyperaemia (luxury perfusion).

After 10 days and for some weeks thereafter the opposite phenomenon is observed[2]. Now the infarct area shows up as an area with somewhat increased HMPAO retention ('hyperfixation') relative to CBF as recorded by ^{133}Xe (Figure 2). We are puzzled by this phenomenon and are currently exploring its mechanism. Perhaps accumulation of the hydrophilic form of HMPAO entering across the lesioned blood-brain barrier of the late subacute phase plays a role. The magnitude of HMPAO hyperfixation is on average about 20%, but shows considerable variation. It affects infarct areas with reperfusion as documented using ^{133}Xe. In other words, a 'hot spot' on the HMPAO image corresponding to a CT or MR infarct is evidence of thrombolysis, although the degree of 'luxury perfusion is exaggerated by HMPAO after day 10, approximately.

Department of Clinical Physiology and Nuclear Medicine, Bispebjerg Hospital, Copenhagen, Denmark

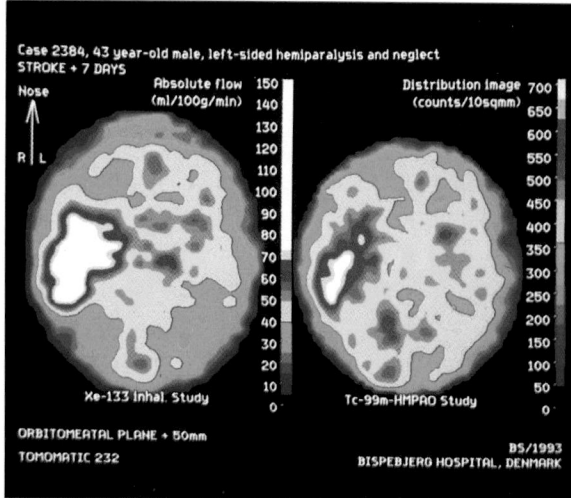

Figure 1 Mild hypofixation of HMPAO relative to ^{133}Xe CBF on day 7 in ischaemic stroke with spontaneous reperfusion. The asymmetry index ratio 0.90 means a HMPAO retention of 10% below the level expected on the basis of [133]Xe

Following reperfusion, the hyperaemia gradually subsides with flow decreasing from high to low values relative to that of the symmetric region in the opposite hemisphere[3,4]. This means that at a certain time point, usually at about day 14 to 20, there is no side-to-side asymmetry. On such HMPAO scans even a large infarct

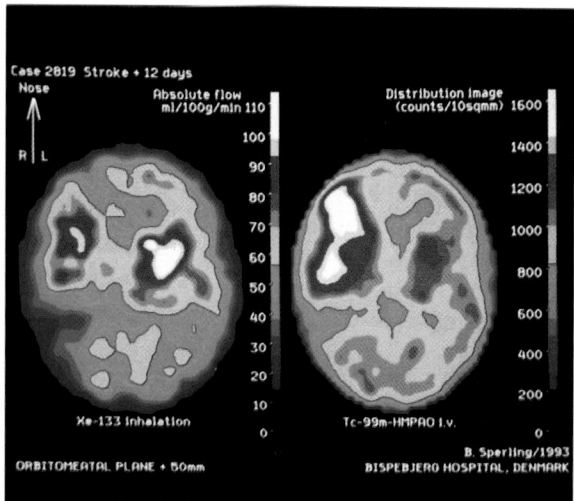

Figure 2 Moderate hyperfixation of HMPAO relative to ^{133}Xe CBF on day 12 in ischaemic stroke with spontaneous reperfusion. The asymmetry index ratio of 1.18 means a HMPAO retention of 18% above the level indicated by measured by [133]Xe

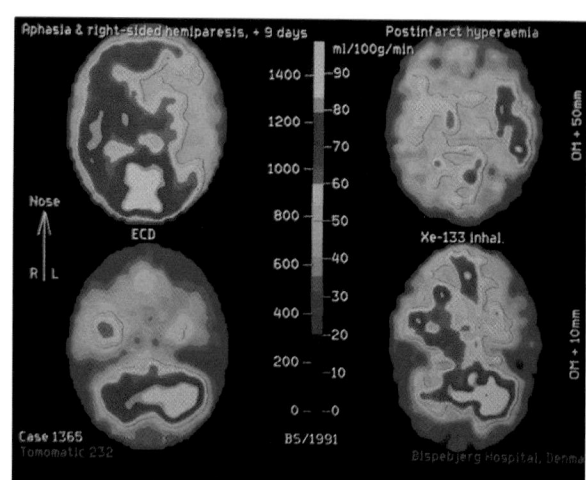

Figure 3 Marked hypofixation of ECD relative to ^{133}Xe CBF on day 9 in ischaemic stroke with spontaneous reperfusion. ECD is not retained in infarct tissue. Note crossed cerebellar diaschisis on lowest cross sections

may be overlooked (Figure 3). Only by careful examination of the images may the infarction be suspected by smaller local hyperaemic or hypoaemic parts (reflow is often not quite uniform) or by cerebellar asymmetry of flow (crossed cerebellar diaschisis). Even so, infarct size may be much underestimated by HMPAO images taken during the second or third week, its full extension may become evident only on a repeated HMPAO scan taken later than one month after onset.

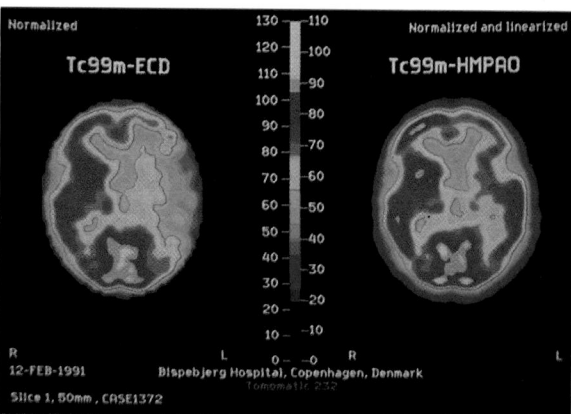

Figure 4 Masking of infarct by HMPAO and not by ECD. In this case of spontaneous reperfusion, CBF was studied in the late subacute phase when 'luxury perfusion' gradually disappears and side-to-side symmetry of HMPAO masks the infarct which is clearly visible using ECD

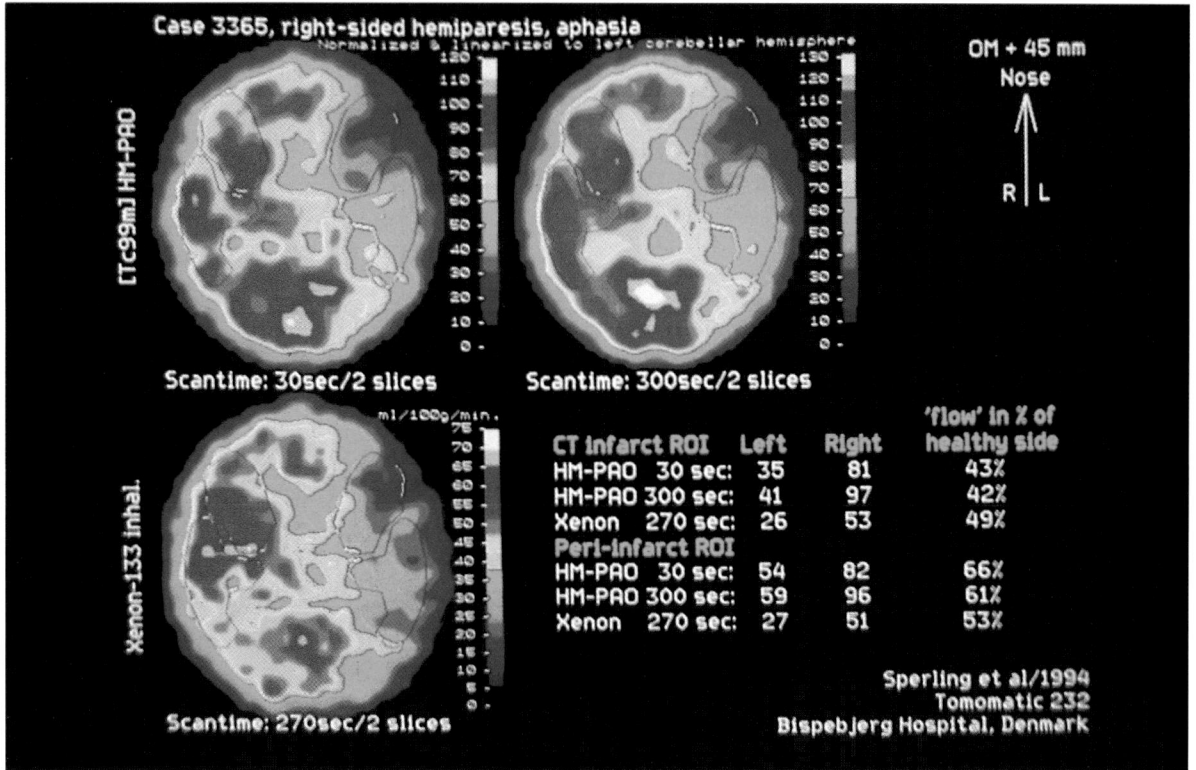

Figure 5 Fast SPECT: HMPAO image recording lasting 30 seconds (upper left) gave practically the same result as 300 seconds (upper right). [133]Xe CBF in the same case (lower left) shows much the same result. The tracer was dose 550 MBq (15 mCi)

A further aspect of HMPAO in acute ischaemic stroke concerns the stability of its retention in the brain. Normally a slow leak of only about 0.5% per hour is seen. In reperfused infarct tissue this leak is increased to levels of perhaps 3% per hour, in particular in the period of hyperfixation. If one delays the recording of the HMPAO image to many hours after tracer injection, then the hyperaemic area with high HMPAO may show up as an area with lower radioactivity than the opposite symmetric area.

ECD

This tracer, ^{99m}Tc labelled ethylenecysteine dimer, has almost the same high retention as HMPAO. The retention mechanism is not the same as ECD and it must be de-esterified enzymatically to become hydrophilic and thereby retained. This de-esterification process is much reduced in infarct tissue so that infarcts show up as low uptake areas by ECD regardless of the level of flow[5]. Due to this marked hypofixation, reflow hyperaemia is not seen after the first few days[6]. For this reason, ECD is considered as a marker of brain metabolism and hence of tissue being intact. This is probably only roughly correct as cases of massive reperfusion may show some degree of ECD uptake, an uptake that might be taken, erroneously, to suggest survival of brain tissue in a typical infarct where all cellular elements are necrotising (Figure 4).

Whether to use HMPAO or ECD to study infarcts in the subacute phase 1 to 3 weeks after onset is a matter of deciding what one wants to look for. If it is infarct blood flow (to decide if reflow has occurred) - then HMPAO must be used. If the aim is to outline the area of the infarct and its surrounding peri-infarct areas, then ECD is best.

Other tracers

CBF measured by ^{133}Xe tomography has the advantage that quantitative data of its ml/100g/min are obtained without the need for arterial sampling. It is well suited for sequential studies spaced with a time interval as little as 30 min. [133]Xe has a low energy primary gamma ray and image resolution is poorer than with HMPAO or ECD. [133]Xe uptake and washout is so rapid that a specialized SPECT instrument designed for this purpose must be used.

CBF can also be measured from the initial brain image of tracers that accumulate in the brain tissue by binding to specific proteins. ^{123}I-isopropylamphetamine IMP and ^{123}I-labelled-iomazenil IMZ are such tracers. IMZ binds to the benzodiazepine receptors on the inhibitory synapses. It is of special interest because the delayed image taken some hours after tracer injection, or, more precisely, the Volume of Distribution image (Vd) obtained by compartmental analysis of early and late scans, is a measure of the intactness of these synapses. Infarcted brain areas show a Vd of IMZ as in the white matter where there are no synapses. With loss of some but not all neurons, as in incompletely infarcted brain areas, Vd is subnormal. In areas of diaschisis, Vd is normal signifying no loss of synapses [7].

Instrumentation

A brain dedicated scanner is preferable as it allows one to see the whole brain with high sensitivity. Two types are available commercially. In some instruments such as in the Headtome (Shimadzu Inc.) or the Ceraspect (Digital Scintigraphic Inc.) only the collimator rotates. In other instruments, the entire camera rotates around the head, e.g. the Neurospect (General Electric Inc.) and the Tomomatic (Medimatic Inc.). The stability of the rotating collimator principle is probably 'bought' at the expense of some loss of sensitivity. Triple-headed all purpose SPECT systems are also highly effective for brain SPECT.

So what is special about performing SPECT in strokes? We prefer to use a collimator with fairly low spatial resolution, in the order of 12 to 15 mm. This boosts sensitivity and allows us to do adequate recording of HMPAO or ECD in a few minutes. In special situations recording times as short as 30 s can be used with little loss in image resolution (Figure 5). Short uptake time is of importance in restless stroke cases as it is in some individuals with neurodegenerative disease. We used a Tomomatic 232 instrument designed for both ^{99m}Tc and ^{133}Xe imaging without the need for changing the collimator.

The first few hours: acute treatment?

Ischaemia means too little blood, i.e. a flow inadequate to sustain the tissue oxygenation required for neuronal function. The threshold of ischaemia lies at about 25 ml/100 g/min, i.e. substantially below the normal cerebral blood flow (CBF) level of 50 to 60 ml/100 g/min. Occlusion of a brain artery leads to ischaemia

as collateral CBF is usually inadequate. However, the residual CBF is probably never zero and its precise level is decisive for the survival time of the cells. Pronounced ischaemia with flow below 15 ml/100 g/min leads to irreversible changes in less than 1 h. Milder ischaemia corresponding to flows between 15 and 25 ml/100 g/min is better tolerated as neuronal function rapidly returns with reperfusion after up to 2 h or even longer. This border zone between pronounced ischaemia and no ischaemia is called the ischaemic penumbra. The duration of reversibility ranging from <1 h to >2 h is called the 'Therapeutic Window', within which thrombolytic therapy can salvage the cells and restitute function. Thus the therapeutic window is not a fixed time limit, as its duration depends on residual flow. Moreover, hypothermia and certain drugs currently being developed for clinical use enhance the nerve cells' tolerance to ischaemia, i.e. prolong the therapeutic window.

This brief overview of ischaemia is meant to serve as a conceptual background for the discussion of CBF measurement in acute ischaemic stroke, specifically for discussing the role of CBF in the context of acute treatment of stroke. If we could measure the residual (collateral) CBF quantitatively, then we might assess the therapeutic window of that area and hence know if effective thrombolysis could be in time or would be too late for salvage of the tissue. The risk of intracranial haemorrhage would seem to preclude indiscriminate use of the therapy in all ischaemic strokes. We must learn to select cases with small risk and good chances of restitution.

Let us assume that we have a stroke patient in whom primary intracerebral haemorrhage has been excluded by a CT scan on admission. With stable neurological signs at, say, 4 h after onset, should we begin tPA (tissue plasminogen activator) therapy or not? This therapeutic dilemma is unresolved as is the additional concern about neuroprotectory measures (Figure 6). We will argue that CBF measured tomographically should be a decisive element in this crucial decision. The basis for this concept is the ischaemic penumbra outlined above.

Optimally, we should be able to exclude haematoma by a CT scan. We were able to measure CBF by CT at the same time. Recording the enhancement of tissue density was by inhalation of about 35% of non-radioactive ('cold') xenon gas. Unfortunately, the enhancement is very small, meaning that the tomography CBF images are noisy. There are other problems too, such as the devastating effect of even the slightest movement of the head during recording. Without going into further details, the limited use of the technique in general and in acute stroke in particular, tells us indirectly about the problems involved. This method has been around for many years and its importance in the context of acute stroke therapy is self-evident. It is not used because it is relatively impractical, inaccurate, and not without risks.

MRI cannot be used for measuring CBF quantitatively in a clinical setting. As it is less effective for detecting a haematoma, it cannot replace CT. Thus, without going into further details we consider SPECT to be the method of choice for measuring CBF in acute stroke. HMPAO or ECD are the easiest tracers to use.

HMPAO may be prepared in about 5 min, while ECD takes about 15 min to prepare. In the time frame of the work-up process of an acute patient, this delay is acceptable as kit preparation may proceed during the time it takes to perform the CT scanning. A short SPECT scanning time is of great importance. This means that one must use a low-resolution, high-sensitivity collimator to keep scanning time to a few minutes.

Current studies on active stroke therapy by thrombolysis give equivocal results. We believe that only cases with larger ischaemic areas of borderline ('penumbral') CBF should be treated. Much work remains to be carried out to define the ischaemic CBF thresholds on SPECT with or without correction for Compton scatter. Controlled clinical trials should then be carried out. Perhaps MR parameters defining the penumbra could be defined[8], so that MR replaces SPECT. No matter how it is accomplished, patient selection is essential, simply because the duration of tolerable ischaemia (the width of the window) varies so markedly.

The first few days: stroke in progression

About 1/3 of stroke patients show a worsening of symptoms over the first few days, often on the first day. The prognosis is rather severe because sudden improvement is not seen: the slow recovery seen in most stroke cases simply proceeds from the new and lower level in such patients. All in all, stroke in progression has a high mortality and a very high morbidity, often resulting in persisting handicap. Little is known about the cause of the progression. Several factors may play be involved e.g. oedema formation, new embolism or microcirculatory clogging by leucocytes or thrombocytes. A reduction in systemic

blood pressure compromising collateral blood flow has been suggested by studies showing that cases with high blood pressure did not show progression.

No systematic studies of CBF and other imaging modalities in stroke-in-progression have been published. Such a study would require serial CBF studies: a study before and after progression and, also if appropriate, after therapeutic intervention. ^{133}Xenon is advantageous for such studies. However the ^{99m}Tc labelled tracers can also be used, e.g. with the split-dose paradigm: first a smaller amount of tracer is used, and prior to the second study the remaining counts from the first study are recorded and subsequently subtracted[9].

Infarction, incomplete infarction and diaschisis

Focal brain ischaemia may give rise to three quite different types of tissue pathology. Primary infarction is a lesion characterised by structureless pannecrosis, i.e. with ischaemic death of all cellular elements, neurons, glia and microvessels. After some days reabsorptive processes become active with scavenger cells such as macrophages and microglia removing cellular debris. Numerous new microvessels form. They lack the tight epithelial junctions constituting the normal blood brain barrier. After some weeks all that remains is a sharply demarcated fluid filled scar. The tissue loss results in localised atrophy with enlarged CSF spaces of the brain surface and of the ventricles.

Secondary incomplete infarction is an area of selective, sometimes laminar neuronal loss due to ischaemic necrosis. The lesion is best known from animal studies, where it is typically seen after brief ischaemia. Since the glia cells, microvessels and neurons are preserved, tissue structure remains intact and the lesion cannot be seen by the naked eye, only by microscopy. The reabsorptive process is inconspicuous, as no macrophages from the blood are involved and no neovascularisation takes place[10,11]. Areas of incomplete infarction are not visible on CT or MR scanning in the acute and subacute phase but after some months a region of local atrophy develops, with some cortical thinning. Incomplete infarction occurs in a narrow zone outside infarcts. Occasionally, it affects larger tissue areas in particular in cases of middle cerebral artery occlusion with borderline (penumbral) collateral flow and with a relatively short lasting period of ischaemia.

Tertiary diaschisis is a condition of disconnection or 'differentiation' of a brain region remote from the ischaemic area. The most well known form is the crossed cerebellar diaschisis typically seen with large hemispheric infarcts, which is due to disruption of the cortico-pontine-cerebellar pathway, a major input to the cerebellum. The blood flow and oxygen uptake is reduced slightly in the cerebellar hemisphere affected by diaschisis, as an expression of the reduced neuronal activity caused by loss of activating input. The inverse phenomenon is also seen, viz. a slight reduction of blood flow in the cortex of the forebrain on the side contralateral to a cerebellar infarct (crossed cerebral diaschisis).

Larger infarcts are initially low flow areas. A broad peri-infarct zone of moderately reduced CBF is seen in most cases. It probably represents mainly the effect of local diaschisis, i.e. reduced neuronal activity due to local disruption of local activating inputs. Smaller deep infarcts cannot be seen by SPECT. However, their presence may often be guessed from a mild reduction of the CBF in the overlying cortex or of contralateral cerebellar regions. Reference has been made repeatedly

to spontaneous reperfusion due to thrombolytic enzymatic activity. This converts the infarct to a zone of high blood flow. The reflow may take some days to reach its maximum, perhaps because new microvessels must form first. The reperfusion gradually subsides and the low level of the chronic state is reached after about 2 months.

Areas of incomplete infarction are also characterised by reduced CBF. Current evidence suggests that it develops in areas of moderate ischaemia of fairly short duration: it appears to be a lesion typical of the ischaemic penumbra occurring with ischaemia duration at the upper limit of the therapeutic window. So far histological evidence has not been obtained except in a few clinical cases[12]. This means that firm conclusions cannot be reached, as the lesion is defined by histological demonstrations of selective neuronal loss. Suggestive evidence in the form of a reduction in benzodiazepine receptor density measured by ^{123}I-iomazenil has been forwarded[7,13].

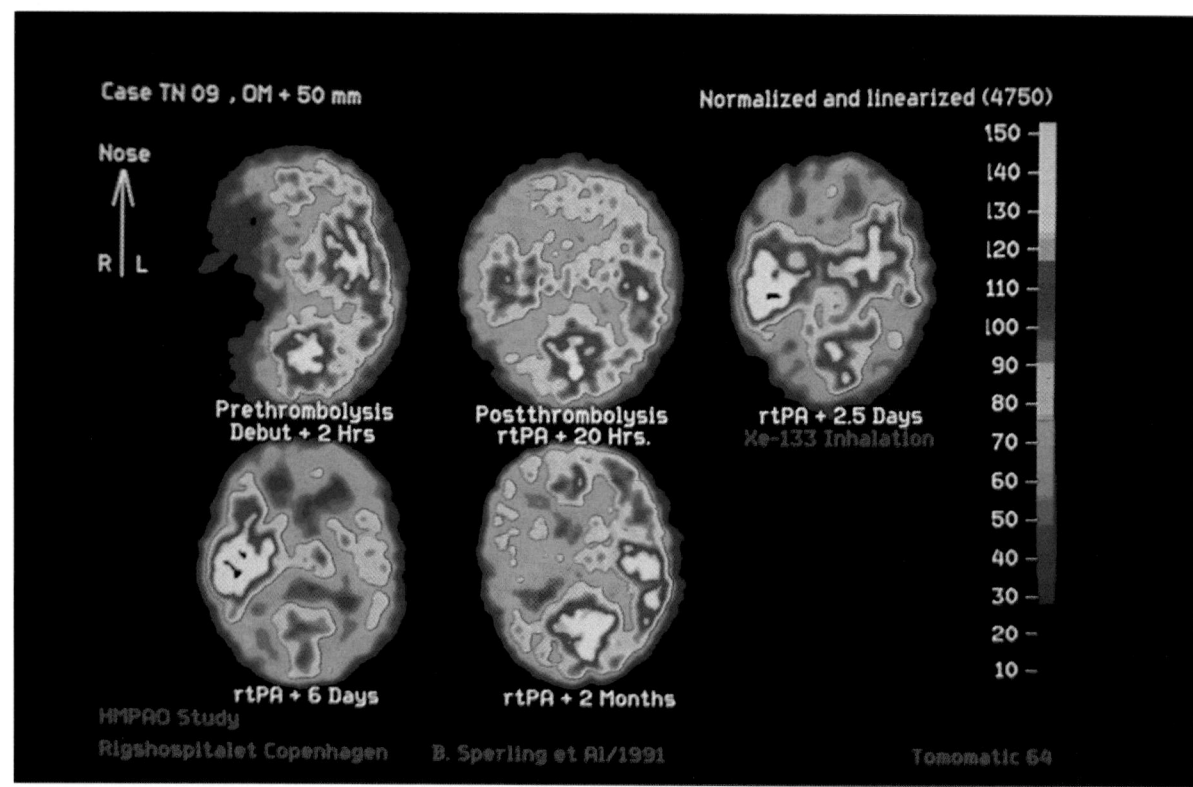

Figure 6 Reperfusion of dense focal ischaemia by plasminogen activator i.v. 2 hours after onset. The massive 'luxury perfusion' on days 2 and 6 reveals that infarction was not avoided. Yet the final image at 2 months shows preserved gyral patterns with moderate CBF reduction anteriorly in the MCA region where CT was normal. A smaller infarction was seen posteriorly. This, combined with exceptionally good and rapid clinical recovery, suggests partial salvage of threatened brain tissue by the rtPA treatment. The tracer used was HMPAO, except on day 2 when Xe-inhalation was used

Routine use of SPECT/CBF in CVD

Cerebrovascular disease covers a wide spectrum of clinical syndromes. Ischaemic stroke is one, transient ischaemic attack is another being separated by an arbitrary time point from a stroke. The delayed ischaemic deficit following severe vasospasm after subarachnoid haemorrhage is a third entity. CVD also comprises chronic progressive syndromes such as vascular dementia as well as primary intracerebral haemorrhage, arterial aneurysms or (arteriovenous)-malformations.

Clinical use of CBF by SPECT can be argued in all these conditions. In our experience, it is particularly useful to obtain a more conclusive diagnosis. In the context of differential diagnosis of acute stroke, many other disease states than those alluded to above are of relevance: epilepsy, migraine, brain tumours. SPECT/CBF is an adjunct to the many other techniques available. Often it contributes decisively. The clinical use of CBF depends on the experience of the user and on the types of cases seen.

On this basis we suggest that CBF/SPECT should be used rather liberally in CVD cases. Were the technique as simple and cheap as a plasma potassium analysis, it would undoubtedly be routine world wide. CBF images and quantitates precisely what stroke is about: a local failure of blood supply. Imaging the key pathogenetic factor makes sense to physician and to patient alike and, as stated, often adds to the diagnostic accuracy. Further detailed analysis of CBF and all ancillary data in a sequential, prospective group of CVD cases is required to enhance diagnostic accuracy.

References

1   Masdeu, J.C. and Brass, L.M. SPECT imaging of stroke. *J. Neuroimaging* 1995, 5 (1), S14

2   Sperling, B. and Lassen, N.A. Hyperfixation of HMPAO in subacute ischemic stroke leading to spuriously high estimates of cerebral blood flow by SPECT. *Stroke* 1993, 24, 193

3   Raynaud, C., Rancurel, G., Tzourio, N. *et al.* SPECT analysis of recent cerebral infarction. *Stroke* 1989, 20, 192

4   Jørgensen, H.S., Sperling, B., Nakayama, H. *et al.* Spontaneous reperfusion of cerebral infarcts in acute stroke patients. Incidence, time course, and clinical outcome: The Copenhagen Stroke Study. *Arch. Neurol.* 1995, in press

5   Lassen, N.A. and Sperling, B.K. [^{99m}]Tc-Bicisate reliably images CBF in chronic brain diseases but fails to show reflow hyperemia in subacute stroke: Report of a multicenter trial of 105 cases comparing [^{133}]Xe and [^{99m}]Tc-Bicisate (ECD, Neurolite) measured by SPECT on same day. *J. Cereb. Blood Flow Metab.* 1994, 14 (1), S44

6   Nakagawara, J., Nakamura, J., Takeda, R. *et al.* Assessment of postischemic reperfusion and diamox activation test in stroke using ^{99m}Tc-ECD SPECT. *J. Cereb. Blood Flow Metab.* 1994, 14 (1), S49

7   Nakagawara, J., Sperling, B., Takeda, R. *et al.* Incomplete brain infarction of early reperfused, CT/MRI intact cortex in embolic stroke: in vivo evidence by ^{123}I-Iomazenil SPECT. *J. Cereb. Blood Flow Metab.* 1995, 15(1), S131

8   Welch, K.M.A., Windham, J., Knight, R.A. *et al.* A model to predict the histopathology of human stroke using diffusion and T_2-weighted magnetic resonance imaging. *Stroke* 1995, 26, 1983

9   Holm, S., Madsen, P.L., Rubin, P. *et al.* ^{99m}Tc-HMPAO activation studies: validation of the split-dose, image subtraction approach. *J. Cereb. Blood Flow Metab.* 1991, 11(2), S766

10 Garcia, J.H., Liu, K.-F. and Ho, K.-L. Neuronal necrosis after middle cerebral artery occlusion in Wistar rats progresses at different time intervals in the caudoputamen and the cortex. *Stroke* 1995, 26, 636

11 Garcia, J.H., Wagner, S., Liu, K.-F. and Hu, X.-J. Neurological deficit and extent of neuronal necrosis attributable to middle cerebral artery occlusion in rats. *Stroke* 1995, 26, 627

12 Lassen, N.A., Losen, T.S., Højgaard, K. and Skriver, E. Incomplete infarction: a CT-negative irreversible ischemic brain lesion. *J. Cereb. Blood Flow Metab.* 1983, 3(1), S602

13 Sette, G., Baron, J.-C., Young, A.R. *et al.* In vivo mapping of brain benzodiazepine receptor changes by positron emission tomography after focal ischemia in the anesthetized baboon. *Stroke* 1993, 24, 2046

SPECT in Neurology and Psychiatry, edited by P.P. De Deyn, R.A. Dierckx, A. Alavi and B.A. Pickut
© 1997 John Libbey & Company Ltd, pp. 307–315

The Cerebrovascular Reserve (CVR): Access by SPECT

Chapter
37

U. Buell, M. Schreckenberger, O. Sabri and U. Cremerius

Introduction

CVR is a well used mechanism for maintaining regional cerebral blood flow (rCBF) within given limits constant by autoregulation. rCBF is, however, governed by the need to offer sufficient metabolic fuel to the cerebral cells. Thus, CVR and metabolic needs (or metabolic reserve) act in close combination. Consequently, multiple factors regulate CVR, including CO_2-tension, perfusion pressure, cerebral blood volume, rheological parameters (e.g. hematocrit), metabolic demands, transneural depression and ageing. The measurement and imaging of CVR by SPECT may be obtained in various ways.

SPECT is, however, only one of the methods employed. SPECT, displaying slices, may be performed by rotating gamma-camera heads, rotating detector assays or a stationary ring crystal[1]. Other nuclear methods are planar probes optimized for ^{133}Xe or PET. Transcranial Doppler sonography is widely used as a non-nuclear method. Xenon enhanced X-ray CT[2] or MRI[3] are still beyond the clinical level.

Parameter employed for CVR

CVR as a function of blood-flow

rCBF may be determined at resting versus stimulated conditions (Table 1). Thus, CVR may be expressed and/or imaged by a flow-ratio (Table 2). The stimuli are: hypercapnia, acetazolamide or motor activation or combinations thereof (see Tables 1 and 3). rCBF may be obtained as a ratio from countrate density in SPECT-slices compared with the contralateral area (Table 2) or with the global CBF. Since extraction rates for ^{99m}Tc compounds are not 100% (e.g. ^{99m}Tc-HMPAO 72%) and they may vary with the conditions used (lower under stimulation because of less contact time), and since there is a high back diffusion especially in high flow areas, stimulated-to-rest rCBF ratios for SPECT are lower than those obtained from the Kety-Schmidt approach (i.e., factor of 2.0, Figure 1, Buell[4]). With ^{133}Xe-DSPECT or with PET, rCBF may be obtained in ml/min/100g (Tables 1 and 2, Figure 3). However, since CVR may be represented by a ratio (Figure 3), absolute flow values are not mandatory.

rCBF at rest is 50 ml/min/100 g. It will be increased by 4% to 61% in normals within SPECT protocols (see Table 4). The stimuli and doses given are shown in Table 3. Pathophysiologically, arterial perfusion pressure is autoregulated in the range of 70-110 Torr. The active increase in rCBF is governed by an increase in diameter of the arterioles. Since the arterioles represent only 5% of the arterial

Department of Nuclear Medicine, Aachen University of Technology, Aachen, Germany

Table 1 Assessment of CVR

Parameter measured	Employing	Resting state versus
rCBFlow, relative	^{133}Xe, ^{123}I-IMP, ^{99m}Tc-HMPAO, ^{99m}Tc-ECD	hypercapnia, acetazolamide motoric movement
rCBFlow, absolute	^{133}Xe, ^{18}FCH$_3$, ^{15}O$_2$	hypercapnia, azetazolamide
rCBVolume	^{99m}Tc RBC	hypercapnia, acetazolamide
rCBV-to-rCBV[a]	^{99m}Tc HMPAO, ECD, RBC	hypercapnia, acetazolamide
	non-nuclear for reference	
blood flow velocity	transcranial Doppler	hypercapnia, acetazolamide

IMP, isopropylamphetamine; HMPAO, hexamethylpropyleneamineoxime; ECD, ethylencysteinedimer; RBC, red blood cell
[a], Resting state ratios already gives access to CVR[4,12,13,15,17,20,25]

cerebral vasculature, such regulated vessel-diameters are somewhat restricted. Moreover, even in an experimental setting (H$_2$ clearance and Laser-Doppler-flowmetry), flow increases observed did not reach the values expected from Hagen-Poiseuille's equation[5]. Hence, passive dilation of other vessels should add to such volume increases.

Protocol

Brain SPECT is performed as a routine[1] using the radiopharmaceuticals listed in Table 1, at resting conditions (injection or inhalation of ^{133}Xe with eyes closed and/or room lights dimmed, ears plugged). For CVR, brain SPECT is repeated after rheological stimulation or by increasing metabolic demand by motoric activation (Table 3). The changes are determined by the parameters listed in Table 2.

The time sequence is of interest: one-day protocols are preferable since physical and psychological conditions could be kept constant. If the physical or biological (^{133}Xe) half-life of the radioactive indicator is short, one-day protocols are available *per se*. However, ^{99m}Tc compounds need special arrangements e.g. split dose for ^{99m}Tc-HMPAO with 185 MBq at rest and 740 MBq after stimulation within 35 min[6] or with a 1:3 ratio[7] or even with an identical dose of 370 MBq each within 45 min[8] (Figure 5). Subtraction (e.g. stimulation minus rest) of images and/or of countrates may be helpful to avoid contaminating radioactivity from the first procedure. However, such mathematical operations may cause increase in statistical error[6]. Other groups[9]

waited 6 to 24 h for reinjection. For ^{123}I-IMP, two day protocols are performed[10].

Stimulation is achieved by using an i.v. injection of acetazolamide, 10 min before injection of the radiopharmaceutical, or adenosine[10] immediately before ^{99m}Tc-HMPAO (Table 3). If CO$_2$ is used for stimulation, endtidal CO$_2$ tension, systemic blood pressure and heart rate should be monitored. Endtidal CO$_2$ should reach a plateau before injection of the radiopharmaceutical.

Table 2 Parameters used for SPECT evaluation

Changes, related to identical area:

- regional increase in ml/min or in ml

- regional increase in % rCBF over baseline or regional ratio stimulation-to-baseline

Changes, related to different areas:

- ratio regional-to-contralateral, i.e. change in symmetry (unilateral pronounced CVD)

- ratio regional-to-total cerebrum

CVR as a function of blood volume

Regional cerebral blood volume (rCBV) is imaged to illustrate the F/V or V/F ratio, correlated to transit time. rCBV (4-5 ml/100 g) is one tenth of rCBF. The regular flow-to-volume ratio is about 10. In CVD, the ratio decreases with decreasing flow and/or increasing volume. Pathophysiologically, cerebral blood volume is located within arteries (11%), arterioles (2%), capillaries (7%), venoles and larger veins (80%)[4]. It may increase in the terminal cerebral circulation passively, by pushing open capillaries and venoles subsequent to actively dilated arterioles. In addition, peripheral cerebral hematocrit increases from 31.8%[11] to 40% (network-Fahraeus-effect to omit autodilution). Thus, rCBV by at least three rheological mechanisms increased to values that can be measured using radioactive labelled blood cells and SPECT.

Protocol

CBV is imaged after labelling of red blood cells with 700 MBq ^{99m}Tc-pertechnetate subsequent to pretinning with a cold pyrophosphate kit[12-14]. After sufficient time for equilibration (10-15 min), SPECT is performed. Since the highest blood volume is in low interest areas (e.g. large veins, sinuses, calvarium and scalp), electronic procedures, available in dedicated nuclear imaging systems must be used to elucidate blood volume within the intracranial vascular supply areas. Absolute quantification may be made by calibration to activity concentration in the blood, and by correcting for the cerebral-to-large vessel hematocrit (ratio for normals of 0.85 used by Sabatini[14]), or ratio of 0.759, determined by Sakai[11]). Total CBV increased by a factor of 1.15 during 5% CO_2 inhalation or by 0.104 ml/mmHg (Sakai[11]). The rCBV or the rCBV-to-CBF ratios show CVR results already at resting conditions[4,12-17].

CVR as a function of flow velocity

Flow velocity within the middle cerebral artery is deter-mined transcranially by Doppler sonography. This velocity correlates to rCBF as long as the diameter of the insonated vessel remains constant. Mean flow velocity is about 60 cm/s. It increases by acetazo-lamide by 30-40%[18,19] and by CO_2 by 76%[19] (Table 4). In addition, velocity may be measured in hypocapnia (hyperventilation), where it decreases.

Protocol

The patient is supine. A TCD transducer is placed over one temporal plane, and the middle cerebral artery is insonated at a depth of 50-55 mm.

Table 3 Stimuli and doses

CO_2 5% (in 20% oxygen and 75% nitrogen gas)	
Acetazolamide	1 g.i.v.
Adenosine	100 µg/kg bodyweight
Angiotensin II	
Motoric activity	various tests (finger tipping, hand grip)

CVR as a function of metabolism

Cellular metabolic need rules the system and CVR is governed by this. On one hand, exhausted CVR is an end-stage indicator, on the other a metabolic reserve exists which protects the neuronal cells subsequent to CVR exhaustion if the basic rCBF becomes critically low[20,21]. Metabolic data (oxygen or glucose consumption under various conditions are obtained exclusively from PET[15,21-23]. Thus, SPECT does as yet give no direct access to the final reserve mechanism. However, increasing the oxygen extraction fraction from 44% (CVR preserved) to 53% (CVR exhausted) and to 61% (hypocapnia) is one of the most important metabolic reserve parameters, which strongly correlates to the CVR[21].

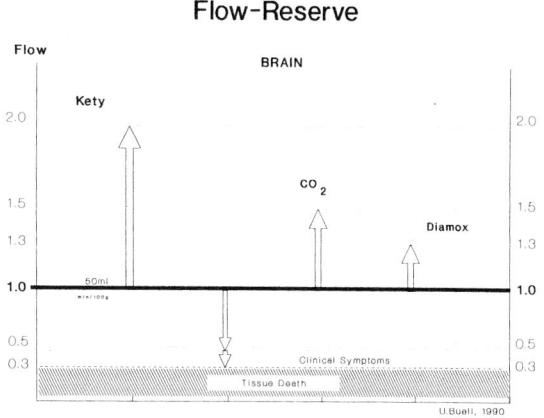

Figure 1 Cerebrovascular reserve (CVR), considered as an increase of rCBF subsequent to stimulation with acetazolamide (Diamox) or CO_2 in normals (performance reserve). In patients with CVD, increase is lower than 1.5 or 1.3. To maintain resting flow normal (1.0), various other factors act as buffer reserve, e.g. increase of blood volume and of hematocrit. Metabolic reserve (e.g. increase of oxygen extraction from 44% to 53%; not displayed) is supposed to compensate ultimately if rCBF at rest decreases below normal. Clinical symptoms are presented if all reserve mechanisms are exhausted

Table 4 Stimulation of regional cerebral blood flow in normals/controls

Reference	Marker - method	Stimulus	+ rCBF increase over baseline
43	^{99m}Tc-HMPAO SPECT	CO_2	1.28
44	^{99m}Tc-HMPAO SPECT	CO_2	1.04
6	^{99m}Tc-HMPAO SPECT	CO_2	1.11
7	^{99m}Tc-HMPAO SPECT	motoric activity	1.15 - 1.22[a]
32	^{123}I-AMP SPECT	acetazolamide	1.50
45	^{18}F CH_3-PET	CO_2	1.61
33	^{133}Xe probes	CO_2	1.25
46	^{133}Xe probe-array	CO_2	1.15 - 1.25[b]
26	^{133}Xe-DSPECT	acetazolamide	1.25
14	^{133}Xe-DSPECT	acetazolamide	1.45
27	^{133}Xe-DSPECT	CO_2 plus acetazol.	1.51
47	^{133}Xe-DSPECT	motoric activity	1.31
19	Transcranial Doppler	CO_2	1.76
19	Transcranial Doppler	acetazolamide	1.50
18	Transcranial Doppler	acetazolamide	1.40
48	Transcranial Doppler	acetazolamide	1.27

[a], primary motor cortex - suppl. motor area; [b], primary motor cortex: elderly - young

Results and discussion

Nuclear medicine is appropriate for imaging applied pathophysiology by evaluation of the global and regional reserves employing emission computerised tomography[20] (SPECT, PET). Pharmacological intervention protocols have been developed to assess flow reserves diagnostically[24].

For clinical demands, there are numerous protocols to determine CVR, only two of which employ SPECT. In contrast to transcranial Doppler, which aims mainly at the middle cerebral artery, SPECT offers regional imaging of rCBF and CVR in all cerebral sections as in various other vascular supply areas, primary motor (PMA) and supplementary motor areas (SMA)[7], or in the basal ganglia[10]. In addition, imaging of regional cerebral blood volume and its relation to rCBF is a complex but clinically validated SPECT (or PET)[15,16] protocol[12,13,17].

Since in chronic cerebrovascular disease, the resting CBF is reduced[12,18,25,26] but the blood flow velocity is not[18], under resting conditions flow velocity and rCBF are not correlated. In addition, there is evidence that transcranial Doppler measurements do not predict rCBF in patients with occlusive carotid disease[27]. However, if vascular supply areas are attached, stimulation yields an increase in both CBF and velocity[8,18,19,26,27].

In normals/controls, it is agreed that the stimulated-to-rest rCBF ratio from ^{99m}Tc compounds is lower than values from ^{133}Xe-DSPECT and lower than CVR from blood flow velocity (Table 4). All data are lower than expected in the maximum. Since algorithms for Xe wash-in/wash-out comprise some corrective assumptions, transcranial Doppler flow velocity is not identical with CBF, and as CVR is not strictly discriminated for grey and white matter, the CVR

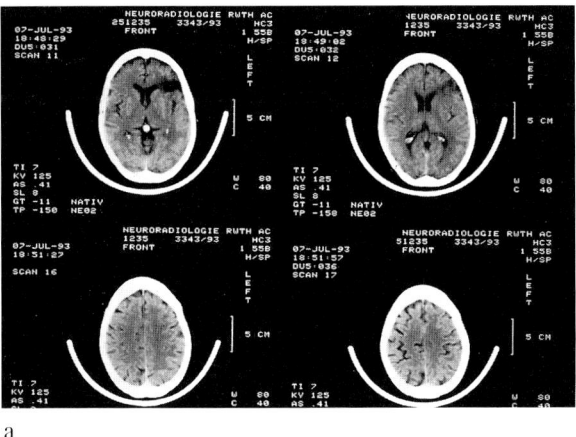

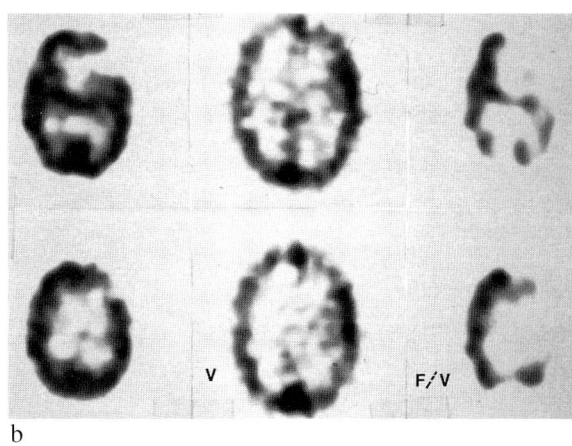

a

b

Figure 2 Male patient (56 years old) with occlusion of left internal carotid artery. Territorial infarction in the anterior supply area of the left middle cerebral artery (MCA) confirmed by CT (a). Congruent finding (arrows) with ^{99m}Tc-HMPAO SPECT (b) (F, left). rCBV SPECT ^{99m}Tc-RBC: V, middle), however, reveals additionally increased CBV within the total MCA supply area of the left hemisphere. Consequently, CVR (F/V; right) is decreased for the total left MCA supply area (normal in CT). Example for a territorial infarction with a large rheological penumbra (exhausted CVR), not revealed by rCBF SPECT but by CVR SPECT only

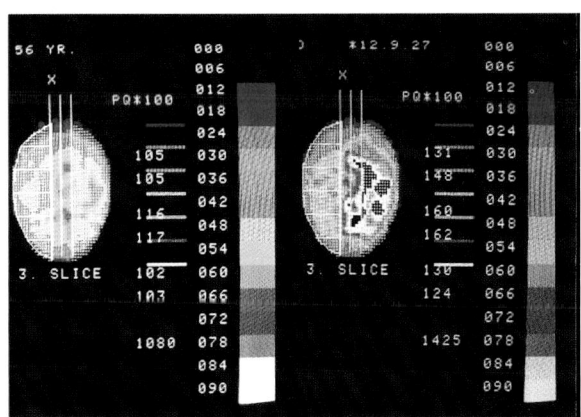

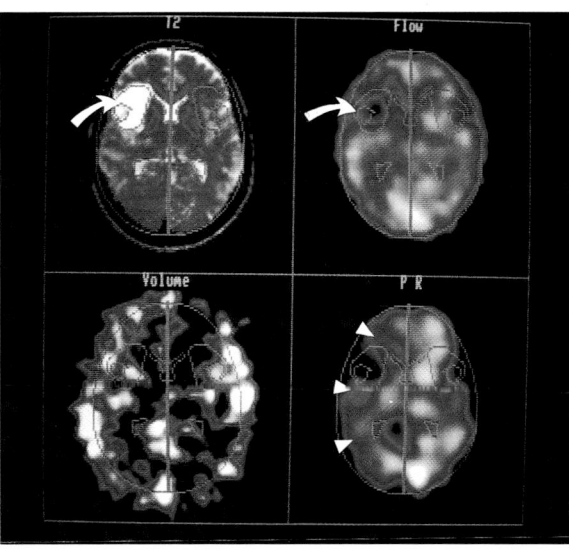

Figure 3 Male patient (56 years old) with occluded left internal carotid artery. Clinical presentation: repetitive transient ischaemic attacks from left hemisphere. ^{133}Xe-DSPECT (Tomomatic 64, 3. (parietal) slice: note: the patient is to be seen from top, left hemisphere is left-sided) at rest (left part) displays reduced rCBF in the left hemisphere and normal in the right one. Right-to-left ratios of rCBF are between 1.02 and 1.16; 1.08 is the global hemispherical ratio at rest. After acetazolamide (right part), rCBF increased much more in the right hemisphere, thus enhancing the ratios to 1.24 to 1.31, the interhemispherical global one to 1.425. Herewith, CVR is represented by an **F** 'assymetry index' before and after stimulation. Note graduation on either vertical bar, illustrating rCBF as ml/min/100 g. Employing these data, CVR will be represented as a rCBF ratio

Figure 4 Female patient (45 years old) with subtotal stenosis of right internal arotid artery. Left-sided paresis of facial nerve, 4 days prior to SPECT. Old territorial infarction (OTI) in the right anterior supply area of the MCA, displayed in MRI (arrow, left-upper quadrant, T_2-weighted). Identical defect in the ^{99m}Tc-HMPAO SPECT (flow, right-upper quadrant). Volume SPECT (left-lower quadrant) displays increased rCBV in either Sylvian area, adjacent to the OTI and in the left hemisphere at rear, yielding two grades of compromised CVR (PR, right-lower quadrant): small area of exhaustion adjacent to the OTI (arrow-heads), additional area of CVR reduction in the rear (posterior supply area of the MCA; arrow). ROIs drawn on the MRI-slice and transferred to the SPECT data-set, help to identify such small additional information from CVR-SPECT

values may be seen as best assumptions. Diffusible SPECT-tracers consisting of large and lipophilic molecules such as HMPAO, ECD or IMP, face the problem of a flow dependent extraction fraction (EF). EF for HMPAO is 72% at normal flow[28] and decreases further during stimulated rCBF. However, exact data on CVR are expected only from SPECT (or PET) as illustrated by Pantano[7] (Table 4). The increasing spatial resolution of the new SPECT machines offers greater scope in the future.

Within the clinical setting, CVR may be employed for three reasons: (i) exclusion of CVD (normal CVR proves an unaffected cerebral vasculature); (ii) monitoring of regional performance (CVR as performance reserve: increase over normal by stimulation in areas dedicated to special tasks (motor cortex, supplementary motor area, visual cortex and/or complex employment of areas during special tasks) (Figure 1); or (iii) detection of CVD by finding CVR already decreased or at work. The latter finding has, however, a most important pathophysiological background: CVR acts as a buffer reserve, since its reduction means that parts of it are used to compensate for reduced perfusion pressure, keeping the basic rCBF constant[15,16]. Imaging of rCBV or CBF-to-CBV ratios illustrates this very clearly (Figure 2). Since the buffer reserve aims at cellular viability, it would be advantageous if flow independent (metabolic) reserves could be imaged by SPECT in addition.

In patients suffering from CVD, CVR is compromised and 'at work'. It is reduced in correlation to the severity of the disease. All working groups present significantly decreased CVR values (end-stage: exhausted (CVR = 1.0)) or changes in rCBF symmetry (Figure 3). Since normal values vary considerably, it is important for each laboratory to establish its dedicated normal values for the method employed (Tables 1 and 4).

For stimulation, complex function sequences[29] may be used. Most simple, however, is the approach to test CVR by primary hypercapnia (CO_2) and/or by acetazolamide (Tables 1 and 3). The latter is an inhibitor of carboanhydrase, potently dilating arterioles in terminal vascular supply areas by activating the adenosine mechanism. Thus, adenosine may be employed directly[30]. Dose response studies for acetazolamide[31] in baboons showed that higher doses are preferable. In man, 500 mg may be too little. Thus, 1 g is used routinely today.

To develop CVR protocols, unilateral occlusive carotid disease has been evaluated[12,25,32,33] since inter-hemispherical comparison could easily be employed. Clinically, however, cerebrovascular disease (CVD) as

part of a common macroangiopathy involves more than this cranial artery. Therefore, since SPECT data could not be quantified sufficiently, interhemispherical comparison (asymmetry) at rest versus stimulation has to be completed by a regional comparison of rest versus stimulation. Thus, differences in severity of vessel involvement may be evaluated from regional CVR imaging which may produce a distinct pattern for either hemisphere and for each vascular supply area corresponding to its involvement (Figures 4 and 5). Twenty-five per cent more patients with CVD were classified correctly using rCBF in combination with rCBV compared with rCBF alone[13]. Burt[9] described 75% more rCBF lesions by acetazolamide-CVR than by resting rCBF. Therefore, multivessel CVD is not a limitation for using CVR and SPECT.

CVR from SPECT procedures proved helpful in classifying patients with subacute or chronic cerebrovascular disease[6,8,9,13,22,34], to look for limited rCVR in early CVD prior to rCBF decrease[4,13,16,35] in reversible clinical deficits[26,36] to outline rheologic penumbra in territorial (Figures 2 and 4) or especially in low-flow infarctions (Figure 5)[8,35], in remote districts (diaschisis[10]) or before and after carotid- or bypass surgery[17,26,37-39] or in subarachnoid haemorrhage[40] or in Moyamoya disease[41] (Table 5).

Table 5 Clinical indications to determine rCVR

CVR in patients assesses

- vasoreactivity, haemodynamic balance, rheologic penumbra

which may be employed to

- detect CVD in early stages

- grade CVD functionally versus morphology

- test the efficiency of collateral pathways

- select for EIAB-surgery

- control effects of carotid endarterectomy or of EIAB

- evaluate subarachnoid haemorrhage

- evaluate Moyamoya disease

or to differentiate

- territorial from low-flow infarctions

- Alzheimer dementia from vascular dementia

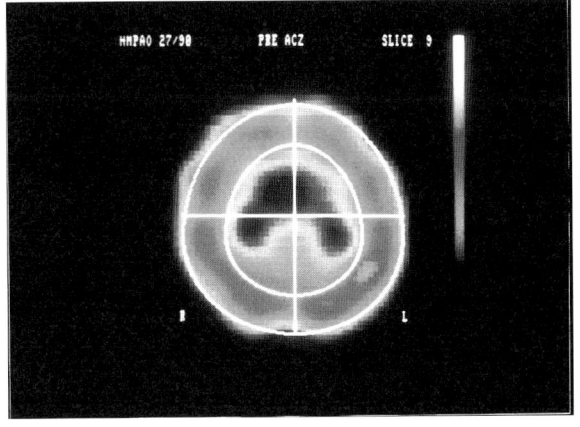 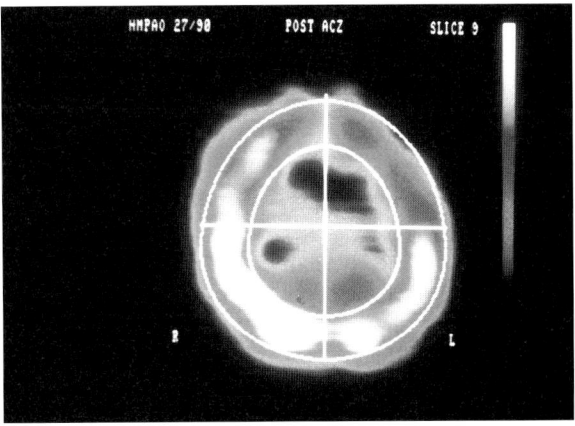

Figure 5 Male patient (60 years old) with occlusion of right common and left carotid and right vertebral arteries, stenosis of left internal carotid artery, suffering from acute right amaurosis fugax. CT scan was normal. Left, pre-acetazolamide; right, post-acetazolamide. Pre-acetazolamide SPECT with ^{99m}Tc-HMPAO (a transaxial + 10 cm OML) revealed symmetrical perfusion, which changed to assymetrical after acetazolamide (b: mind missing flow increase in the supply territories of both aa. cerebrales anteriores and in the anterior and middle branch of the left anterior cerebri media). Right cortex perfusion increased by 26%, left cortex by 10%: exhausted CVR left frontal and parietal. Four weeks after test, the patient developed a low flow infarct in the appropriate area of the left middle cerebral artery. (Courtesy of J. Knop, Duisberg)

Most recently, CVR was found to be impaired in vascular dementia in 78% of the patients studied. In Alzheimer dementia, however, this phenomenon occurred[42] only in 24%. Thus, CVR measurements have been used to differentiate dementia of Alzheimer type from the vascular type. Vascular dementia, however, still requires precise diagnosis (macroangiopathy or microangiopathy; e.g. multi-infarct or Binswanger's disease or a mixture thereof).

In conclusion, CVR by SPECT is a most powerful tool for functional brain imaging, and is already available clinically. CVR is not only a simple parameter of stimulated rCBF, it is a sensitive indicator of both regional performance during stimulation and of regional compensation for low rCBF. In addition, CVR data closely correlate to the amount of oxygen extraction fraction. Thus, CVR imaging is more sensitive in detecting, grading and evaluating cerebrovascular disease than simple CBF imaging. It already reflects metabolic data indirectly. Since competitive protocols are being developed from transcranial Doppler for CBF or functional MRI for rCBV, further progress is needed for SPECT to be used in the study of cellular levels of viability or performance.

References

1   Verhoeff, N.P., Buell, U., Costa, D.C. *et al.* Basics and recommendations for brain SPECT. *Nukl. Med.* 1992, 31, 114

2   Yamashita, T., Hayashi, M., Kashiwagi., S. *et al.* Cerebrovascular reserve capacity in ischemia due to occlusion of a major aterial trunk: studies by xenon-CT and the acetazolamide test. *Comp. Ass. Tomogr.* 1992, 16, 750

3   Rempp, K.A., Brix, G., Wenz, F. *et al.* Quantification of regional cerebral blood flow and volume with dynamic susceptibility contrast-enhanced MR imaging. *Radiology* 1994, 193, 637

4   Buell, U., Reiche, W., Kaiser, H.J. *et al.* Cerebral blood flow to cerebral blood volume relationship as a correlate to cerebral perfusion reserve in 'Stimulated Cerebral Blood Flow', (Eds. P. Schmiedek, K. Einhäupl, C.M. Kirsch), Springer, Berlin, 1992, p.111

5   Haberl, R.L., Heizer, M.L., Marmarou, A. and Ellis E.F. Laser-doppler assessment of brain microcirculation: effect of systemic alterations. *Am. J. Physiol.* 1989, 256, 1247

6   Oku, N., Matsumoto, M., Hashikawa, K. *et al.* Carbon dioxide reactivity by consecutive technetium-^{99m}-HMPAO SPECT in patients with a chronically obstructed major cerebral artery. *J. Nucl. Med.* 1994, 35, 32

7   Pantano, P., Di Peiro, V., Ricci, M. *et al.* Motor stimulation response by ^{99m}Tc-HMPAO split-dose method and SPECT. *Eur. J. Nucl.* 1992, 19, 939

8   Knop, J., Thie, A., Fuchs, C. *et al.* ^{99m}-Tc-HMPAO SPECT with acetazolamide challenge to detect hemodynamic

compromise in occlusive cerebrovascular disease. *Stroke* 1992, 23, 1733

9 Burt, R.W., Witt, R.M., Cikrit, D.F. and Reddy, R.V. Carotid artery disease: evaluation with azetazolamide-enhanced [99m]-Tc HMPAO SPECT. *Radiology* 1992, 182, 461

10 Sakashita, Y., Matsuda, H., Kakuda, K. and Takamori, M. Hypoperfusion and vasoreactivity in the thalamus and cerebellum after stroke. *Stroke* 1993, 24, 84

11 Sakai, F., Nakazawa, K., Tazaki, Y. *et al.* Regional cerebral blood volume and hematocrit measured in normal human volunteers by SPECT. *J. Cereb. Blood Flow Metab.* 1985, 5, 207

12 Buell, U., Stirner, H., Braun, H. *et al.* SPECT with [99m]-Tc-HMPAO and ^{99m}Tc-pertechnetate to assess regional cerebral blood flow (rCBF) and blood volume (rCBV). Preliminary results in cerebrovascular disease and interictal epilepsy. *Nucl. Med. Comm.* 1987, 8, 519

13 Buell, U., Braun, H., Ferbert, A. *et al.* Combined SPECT imaging of regional cerebral blood flow (^{99m}Tc-HMPAO and blood volume ^{99m}Tc RBC) to assess regional cerebral perfusion reserve in patients with cerebrovascular disease. *Nukl. Med.* 1988, 27, 51

14 Sabatini, U., Celsis, P., Viallard, G. *et al.* Quantitative assessment of cerebral blood volume by single-photon emission computd tomography. *Stroke* 1991, 22, 324

15 Gibbs, J.M., Wise, R.J.S., Leenders, K.L. and Jones T. Evaluation of cerebral perfusion reserve in patients with carotid-artery occlusion. *Lancet* 1984, 1, 310

16 Powers, W. Cerebral hemodynamics in ischemic cerebrovascular disease. *Ann. Neurol.* 1991, 29, 231

17 Toyama, H., Takeshita, G., Takeuchi, A. *et al.* Cerebral hemodynamics in patients with chronic obstructive carotid disease by rCBF, rCBV and rCBV/rCBF ratio using SPECT. *J. Nucl. Med.* 1990, 31, 55

18 Piepgras, A., Schmidek, P., Leinsinger, G. *et al.* A simple test to assess cerebrovascular reserve capacity using transcranial Doppler sonography and acetazolamide. *Stroke* 1990, 21, 1306

19 Ringelstein, E.B., Eyck, S.V. and Mertens, I. Evaluation of cerebral vasomotor reactivity by various vasodilating stimul: comparison of CO_2 to acetazolamide. *J. Cereb. Blood Flow Metab.* 1992, 12, 162

20 Buell, U. and Schicha, H. Nuclear medicine to image applied pathophysiology: evaluation of reserves by emission computerized tomography. *Eur. J. Nucl. Med.* 190, 16, 129

21 Kanno, I., Uemura, K., Higano, S. *et al.* Oxygen extraction fraction at maximally vasodilated tissue in the ischemic brain estimated from the regional CO_2 responsiveness measured by PET. *J. Cereb. Blood Flow Metab.* 1988, 8, 227

22 Hirano, T., Menematsu, K., Hasewaga, Y. *et al.* Acetazolamide reactivity on 123I-IMP SPECT in patients with major cerebral artery occlusive disease: correlation with PET parameters. *J. Cereb. Blood Flow Metab.* 1994, 14, 763

23 Pantano, P., Baron, J.C., Lebrun-Grandie, P. *et al.* Regional cerebral blood flow and oxygen consumption in human ageing. *Stroke* 1984, 15, 635

24 Machac, J. and Vallabhajosula, S. Cerebral versus myocardial stress perfusion imaging: role of pharmacological intervention in the diagnostic assessment of flow reserve. *J. Nucl. Med.* 1994, 35, 41

25 Buell, U., Moser, E.A., Schmiedek, P. *et al.* Dynamic SPECT with [133]Xe: regional cerebral blood flow in patients with unilateral cerebrovascular disease. *J. Nucl. Med.* 1984, 25, 441

26 Leinsinger, G., Schmiedek, P., Kreisig, T. *et al.* Bedeutung der zerebrovaskularen Reservekapazität für Diagnostik und Therapie der chronischen zerebralen Ischämie. *Nukl. Med.* 1988, 27, 127

27 Vostrup, S., Zbornikova, V., Sipholm, H. *et al.* CBF and transcranial Doppler sonography during vasodilatory stress tests in patients with common carotid artery occlusion. *Neurol. Res.* 1992, 14, 31

28 Biersack, H.J., Grünwald, F. and Reichmann, K. Zentralnervensystem in 'Nuklearmedizin', (Eds. U Buell, H. Schicha, H.J. Biersack, W.H. Knapp, Ch. Reiners, O. Schober), Thieme, New York, USA, 1994, p.284

29 Tikofsky, R.S. and Hellman, R.S. Brain SPECT: newer activation and interventional studies. *Sem. Nucl. Med.* 1991, 21, 40

30 Ussov, W.W., Vorozhtsova, I.N., Shipulin, V.M. *et al.* Detection of cerebrovascular disease by adenosine ^{99m}Tc-HMPAO SPECT in asymptomatic carotid stenosis. *Eur. J. Nucl.* 1995, 22, 762

31 Dohrmehi, I.C., Oliver, D.W. and Hugo, N. Dose reponse from pharmacological interventions for CBF changes in a baboon model using ^{99m}Tc-HMPAO and SPECT. *Nucl. Med. Comm.* 1993, 14, 573

32 Hashikawa, K., Matsumoto, M., Moriwaki, H. *et al.* Split dose iodine [123]IMP SPECT: sequential quantitative regional cerebral blood flow change with pharmacological intervention. *J. Nucl. Med.* 1994, 35, 1266

33 Keyeux, A., Laterre, C. and Beckers., C.H. Resting and hypercapnic rCBF in patients with unilateral occlusive disease of the internal carotid artery. *J. Nucl. Med.* 1988, 29, 311

34 Weiller, C., Mülges, W., Ringelstein, E.B. *et al.* Patterns of brain infarctions in internal carotid artery dissections. *Neuosurg. Rev.* 1991, 14, 111

35 Weiller, C., Ringelstein, E.B., Reiche, W. and Buell, U. Clinical and hemodynamic aspects of low-flow infarcts. *Stroke* 1991, 22, 117

36 Laloux, P., Richelle, P.F., Meurice, H. and DeCoster, P. Cerebral blood flow and perfusion reserve capacity in hemodynamic carotid transient ischemic attacks due to innominate artery stenosis. *J. Nucl. Med.* 1995, 36, 1268

37 Cikrit, D.F., Burt, R.W., Daising, M.C. *et al.* Acetazolamide enhanced single photon emission computed tomography (SPECT) evaluation of cerebral perfusion before and after endarterectomy. *J. Vasc. Surg.* 1992, 15, 747

38 Kuroda, S., Kamiyama, H., Abe, H. *et al.* Drug-induced hypotension SEP test and acetazolamide test using [133]-Xe SPECT in patients with occlusive carotid disease - selection of candidates for extra-intracranial bypass. *Neurol. Med. Chir. (Tokyo)* 1991, 31, 7

39 Powers, W.J., Grubb, R.L. and Raichle, M.E. Clinical results of extracranial-intracranial bypass surgery in patients with hemodynamic cerebravascular disease. *J. Neurosurg.* 1989, 70, 61

40 Shinoda, J., Kimura, T., Funakoshi, T. *et al.* Acetazolamide reactivity on cerebral blood flow in patients with subarachnoidal haemorrhage. *Acta Neurochir. (Wien)* 1991, 109, 102

41 Hoshi, H., Ohnishi, T., Jinnouchi, S. *et al.* Cerebral blood flow in patients with moyamoya disease evaluated by IMP SPECT. *J. Nucl. Med.* 1994, 35, 44

42 Pavics, L., Grünwald, F., Horn, R. *et al.* rCBF SPECT with ^{99m}Tc-HMPAO and acetazolamide tst in the evaluation of vascular and Alzheimer type of dementia. *Eur. J. Med.* 1995, 22, 772

43 Schmidt, U., Knapp, W.H., Busse, O. *et al.* Veranderung der cerebralen Aufnahme von ^{99m}Tc-HMPAO in Abhängigkeit vom arteriellen CO2-Spiegel. *Nukl. Med.* 1988, 27, A27

44 Choksey, M.S., Costa, D.C., Ianotti, F. *et al.* ^{99m}Tc-HMPAO SPECT and cerebral blood flow: a study of CO^2 reactivity. *Nucl. Med. Comm.* 1989, 10, 609

45 Levine, R.L., Sutherland, J.J, Lagreze, H.L. *et al.* Cerebral perfusion reserve indexes determined by fluoromethane PET. *Stroke* 1988, 19, 19

46 Reich, T. and Rusinek, H. Cerebral cortical and white matter reactivity to carbon dioxide. *Stroke* 1989, 20, 453

47 Guenther, W., Moser, E., Mueller-Spahn, F. *et al.* Pathological cerebral blood flow during motor function in schizophrenic and endogenous depressed patients. *Biol. Psychiatry* 1986, 21, 889

48 Sparigai, E., Speziale, F., Giannoni, M.F. *et al.* Post-carotid endarterectomy hyperperfusion syndrome: preliminary observations for identifying at risk patients by transcranial Doppler sonography and the acetazolamide test. *Eur. J. Vasc. Surg.* 1993, 7, 252

SPECT in Neurology and Psychiatry, edited by P.P. De Deyn, R.A. Dierckx, A. Alavi and B.A. Pickut
© 1997 John Libbey & Company Ltd, pp. 317–322

Clinical Application of Cerebral Perfusion Reserve in Carotid Artery Stenosis

Chapter
38

M. Limburg, D. Legemate, B. Fülesdi[*], C.J. Rehman and
E.A. van Royen

Introduction

Arterial stenosis of the vessels conducting blood to the brain leads to a reduced perfusion pressure. A reduction of the cerebral perfusion pressure leads to vasodilatation. Due to this vasodilatation, adequate tissue oxygenation is maintained. Areas with dilated vessels, an increased oxygen extraction fraction and a reduced blood flow are designated as having a 'misery perfusion'. The responses of the cerebral resistance vessels are part of the cerebral autoregulation. As a result of this autoregulation, the normal cerebral blood flow is maintained within a narrow range. A drop in blood pressure leads to vasodilatation, while an increase leads to vasoconstriction. Eliciting vascular responses may teach us something about the status of the cerebral blood flow. Regions with adequate flow should react in a normal way to stimuli leading to either vasoconstriction or vasodilatation. In areas with a marginal flow, the vessels are maximally dilated and will not vasodilate any further on vasodilatory stimuli. This phenomenon is called diminished or even exhausted cerebrovascular perfusion reserve.

The mechanism by which ischaemic strokes are caused is generally thought to be embolic. Transcranial Doppler (TCD) studies have demonstrated that micro-emboli pass through the large basal intracranial arteries[1], especially during cardiac and carotid surgery, but also in other clinical situations. Given the relatively rare occurrence of cerebral infarction in the presence of frequent micro-emboli, it is likely that the brain vasculature can somehow cope with short term occlusions of the small vessels. It may be that cerebral autoregulation plays a role in this compensating mechanism. On the other hand, some strokes may be directly caused by haemodynamic mechanisms. The anatomy of the circle of Willis is crucial, and may be decisive for the occurrence of large brain infarctions in case cerebral or cerebropetal vessels occlude[2].

In this paper we will first review some of the data on the role of rCBF SPECT in acute ischaemic stroke, and subsequently we will investigate developments that may make rCBF SPECT an important tool guiding treatment of carotid stenoses.

Academic Medical Center,
Amsterdam, Netherlands
[*]Department of Neurology,
University Hospital, Debrecen,
Hungary

rCBF SPECT and acute ischaemic stroke

Brain SPECT imaging of the regional cerebral blood flow has been demonstrated to help in making early diagnosis and prognosis after stroke. rCBF SPECT allows very early detection of cerebral perfusion disturbances before any abnormality will show up on the CT or MRI scan. SPECT imaging detected more cerebral circulatory abnormalities than CT scanning in the first 24 h after stroke onset[3,4]. Most radiopharmaceuticals allow delayed depiction of a 'frozen' image. Very early administration of the radiopharmaceutical captures the situation of that particular moment. In a prospective study in 26 patients with a cerebral infarction, SPECT scanning within 24 h after stroke onset leads to improvements in the ability to predict death within the first week after stroke[5]. Defects above a certain semi-quantitative threshold all lead to early death. Major clinical predictors generally used (such as severity of hemiparesis, depression of consciousness and the presence of conjugate gaze deviation) were less distinctive in this respect than the semi-quantification of the cerebral blood flow defect. SPECT may also be used as a tool to evaluate treatment of brain infarcts with agents such as thrombolytic drugs, e.g. recombinant tissue plasminogen activator (rtPA). Although cerebral angiography is the gold standard technique to investigate vessel occlusions, some important drawbacks hamper its widespread and liberal use in acute ischaemic stroke. The complication rate may be as high as 2% in this vascularly compromised population. Apart from that, an open vessel does not always indicate tissue perfusion, while rCBF SPECT gives a reliable demonstration of this perfusion at the tissue level. An open study on intravenous thrombolysis with rtPA using rCBF SPECT demonstrated restoration of normal flow[6]. However, some caveats must be stressed. Timing of the SPECT after stroke is of major importance for the interpretation of the results. Mechanisms such as hyperperfusion and break-down of the blood-brain barrier in the subacute phase after stroke tend to lead to a diminished size of the perfusion defect, which may lead to false conclusions[7].

At present, rCBF SPECT application in the acute work-up of ischaemic stroke is limited for routine clinical practice. It is, however, an important tool for increasing our insight into the pathophysiology of acute stroke and for the development and evaluation of new treatment strategies. Some new approaches are changing rCBF SPECT from a rather static imaging modality into a more dynamic tool. Eliciting responses from the cerebral autoregulatory system may tell us more on the significance and necessary therapeutic consequences of arterial stenoses. Recognition of brain areas at increased risk for ischaemic infarction may help us in selecting patients who would be most likely to benefit from revascularization procedures.

Cerebral autoregulation

Cerebral autoregulation is the inherent ability of the brain to maintain a constant blood flow over wide ranges of cerebral perfusion pressures. Cerebral autoregulation is possible through the existing vasomotor reactivity of the cerebral resistance vessels (arterioles). Testing of the autoregulation can be performed by measuring changes in the cerebral blood flow through the induction of changes in the blood pressure. The cerebrovascular perfusion reserve gives information about the actual condition of the resistance arterioles, whether they are dilated or constricted. The cerebrovascular resistance increases in cases of higher perfusion pressures and decreases in cases of lower perfusion pressures. Factors playing a role are: transmural pressure changes, pCO_2 changes, nervous activity and endothelial factors. Frequently used vasomotor stimuli that lead to changes of the cerebral blood flow (CBF) and thus may be used for the assessment of the cerebrovascular perfusion reserve are CO_2 inhalation, intravenous administration of acetazolamide, hyperventilation or breath holding.

Carotid endarterectomy for carotid stenosis

Carotid stenosis, strokes and carotid endarterectomy

Recently, two trials have been published reporting that carotid endarterectomy may be effective in cases of symptomatic stenosis exceeding 70%[8,9]. Symptomatic means that the symptoms related to cerebral ischaemia should be attributable to the vascular territory supplied by the affected carotid artery. With a follow up of 3 years, the incidence of ipsilateral stroke in the medically treated group was 8.4%, while addition of surgery to the best available medical treatment leads to 1.1% strokes[8]. This is a relative risk reduction of 87%. Obviously the surgical procedure itself is very effective. However, patients may suffer from surgical complications, strokes in other cerebral regions and may die from e.g. cardiac causes. Taking this into account, the event rate was 21.9% in the medical group after 3 years and 12.3% in the surgically treated group. This implies that approximately 10 patients need to undergo endarterectomy in order to prevent 1 major stroke in 3 years. This measure is usually called 'numbers needed to treat'[10]. All these calculations lead to the conclusion that 9 patients are operated who in fact did not need the operation. A complicating factor is that arterial angiography, which is the gold standard for measuring carotid stenosis, is an invasive procedure with a combined morbidity and mortality rate of about 1 to 2%. Also, it became clear from the results of these trials, that operation of a stenosis of less than 30% was deleterious for the patients, causing more strokes than preventing them. In a later publication the results were presented on the stenoses between 30 and 70%, again no benefit was achieved by prophylactic operation of these patients[11].

Asymptomatic disease

The Asymptomatic Carotid Atherosclerosis Study Executive Committee recently reported results on a total of 1662 patients with asymptomatic carotid artery stenosis of 60% or greater. The median follow-up was 2.7 years. In the surgery group the aggregate estimated risk at 5 years for ipsilateral stroke and any perioperative stroke or death was 5.1% and in the medical group this was 11%12. The perioperative morbidity and mortality were very low with 2.7%, including the risk related to carotid angiography. So, even within these outstanding North-American centres, with extremely low complication rates, about 16 to 19 patients would have to be operated in order to prevent one stroke over 5 years.

Are there ways to recognise patients at an increased risk of stroke, so that we can operate those that have a much higher chance to benefit?

Cerebral perfusion reserve (CPR) in carotid stenosis

Several studies have addressed the issue of whether or not cerebral perfusion reserve is diminished in cases of carotid artery stenosis. Hasegawa et al.[13] investigated 51 patients with a stenosis exceeding 75% or occlusion of the internal carotid arteries. In 20 patients (38%) a reduced cerebral perfusion reserve was present, as measured with ^{123}I-iodoamphetamine (IMP) SPECT after the intravenous administration of acetazolamide. Follow-up acetazolamide testing revealed a normalisation of the test in 5 patients, and progression of stenosis to occlusion in 1 patient. During an average follow-up of 18.5 months, 4 patients died from cardiac causes and no cerebrovascular events happened. Fifteen patients with unilateral stenoses or occlusions of the internal carotid arteries were studied with transcranial Doppler (TCD) after intravenous acetazolamide administration and with ^{99m}Tc hexamethylpropyleneamineoxime (HMPAO) SPECT

by Rosenkranz et al.[14]. All 10 patients with a >80% stenosis showed abnormalities with transcranial Doppler and acetazolamide SPECT compatible with a diminished cerebral perfusion reserve. Fürst et al.[15] examined CO_2 reactivity of the cerebral resistance vessels by means of transcranial Doppler sonography in 91 asymptomatic patients with unilateral high grade carotid artery stenosis and in 37 control subjects. In 65% normal reactivity was present, in 19% a severely diminished ipsilateral reactivity was found, while in 17% the ipsilateral reactivity was supranormal. In this last group there were reduced reactions in the contralateral hemisphere. This may be the result of an interhemispheral steal phenomenon.

Naylor et al.[16] measured the mean cerebral transit time after administration of intravenous [99m]Na pertechnetate. Interhemispherical right-left differences were used as estimations of the cerbrovascular reserve. These authors investigated 104 consecutive patients with symptomatic carotid artery territory disease and ipsilateral internal carotid artery stenosis. The frequency of cerebrovascular reserve impairment increased with the severity of internal carotid artery stenosis. Impairment was present in 0 of 11 patients with <50%stenosis; 4 of 24 with 50-69% stenosis; 14 of 41 with 70 to 89% stenosis and 12 of 28 with 90 to 99% stenosis.

Recently we examined 77 hemispheres in 42 patients (32 symptomatic, 10 asymptomatic) with varying degrees of carotid stenosis[17]. A ^{99m}Tc-HMPAO SPECT was performed before and after intravenous administration of 1 gram of acetazolamide. A significant decrease of the CPR with increasing severity of carotid stenosis was found. Comparable data were found by Sacca et al.[18]. These data are compatible with the concept that carotid artery stenosis leads in a minority of patients (especially those with a more than 80% stenosis) to a decrease in cerebral perfusion reserve and that this decrease correlates with the severity of the stenosis. The fact that various studies used different techniques and standards but still yielded similar results further supports the concept.

Cerebral perfusion reserve changes after carotid endarterectomy

Elimination of haemodynamically significant carotid stenoses leads to improvement in cerebral haemodynamics[9,14,19]. Lord et al.[20] examined 16 patients with haemodynamically significant carotid stenosis. Eight patients demonstrated abnormalities in cerebral perfusion reserve as measured with acetazolamide stress testing and Tc-HMPAO rCBF measurement. After carotid endarterectomy, 7 of these

8 patients showed an improvement. In a study of 25 patients before and after carotid endarterectomy with acetazolamide stimulation and Tc-HMPAO SPECT, Cikrit *et al.*[21] demonstrated a postoperative improvement in vascular reactivity in 21 cases. In the patient group studied by Sacca *et al.*[18] improvement occurred in 20 of 84 cases after endarterectomy (44%). These authors used 'plain' Tc-HMPAO rCBF SPECTs without any form of vascular stimulation. Despite the varying techniques employed and the lack of control observations, it is likely that carotid endarterectomy is followed by improvement of cerebral haemodynamics, as measured with SPECT, in a substantial proportion of patients.

Event prediction by diminished cerebral perfusion reserve

In a retrospective study using Positron Emission Tomography, Powers *et al.*[19] could not establish a relation between significantly impaired cerebral haemodynamics and new cerebrovascular events. They examined 30 patients with symptomatic carotid stenosis of more than 75%. Follow-up at 1 year was available in all patients. In a group of 21 patients with abnormal haemodynamics (increased rCBV/rCBF; CBV = cerebral blood volume), 1 suffered a contralateral stroke and in the 9 patients with normal haemodynamics, 1 suffered an ipsilateral stroke. Obviously this retrospective study does not support the hypothesis that impaired cerebral haemodynamics increase the risk for subsequent ischaemic stroke. However, with 30 patients and only 1 year of follow up, this study lacks the power to exclude this concept. Yamauchi *et al.*[22] performed a similar study. Using PET, they prospectively evaluated 40 patients with symptomatic middle cerebral arterial occlusive disease. Seven patients had an increased oxygen extraction (corresponding to 'misery perfusion') fraction, 4 of whom developed an ipsilateral stroke in the year to follow. In the group of 33 patients with normal oxygen extraction fractions, 2 ipsilateral strokes developed. This is a highly significant difference, even when the results are combined with those of the study of Powers *et al.*[19]. The authors give several explanations for the discrepant findings, from which coincidence is one, and timing differences in PET investigation is another.

In a prospective study Kleiser and Widder[23] investigated 85 patients with occlusions of the internal carotid arteries. They measured cerebral reactivity with transcranial Doppler and CO_2 inhalation. After a mean follow-up of 38 months there were 12 cases with ipsilateral cerebrovascular symptoms in the group of 37 with diminished cerebrovascular perfusion reserve, and in the group with sufficient cerebrovascular perfusion reserve 4 out of 48 patients had ipsilateral cerebrovascular symptoms. Although in a different patient group, this study gives fairly strong support to the hypothesis that patients with diminished cerebrovascular perfusion reserve are at increased risk for future ischaemic events.

Yonas *et al.*[24] performed a retrospective study in which they examined the cerebral perfusion reserve of 68 patients with symptomatic carotid stenoses. They used xenon CT after acetazolamide stimulation. After a mean follow up of 24 months the authors recorded 8 strokes in the group of 22 patients that had a significant reduction of cerebral blood flow; in the group of patients without this severe reduction there were strokes in two out of 46 cases. Also in this retrospective study, a significantly compromised vascular reserve together with a relatively low initial flow correlated with an increased risk for ipsilateral stroke.

Increasing therapeutic effectiveness

The importance of correctly defining indications for surgery can be illustrated as follows. In cases of symptomatic carotid stenosis, about 10 patients have to be operated in order to prevent 1 serious cerebrovascular event from happening in the following 3 years. This implies that on average, 9 out of 10 patients are operated without benefit. In the case of an asymptomatic stenosis the situation is even less favourable. About 16 to 19 patients have to be operated in order to prevent 1 serious stroke from happening in the following 5 years. In this case 15 to 18 patients who do not benefit are in fact operated.

Ways to improve the effectiveness of our clinical interventions should be developed. Using a statistical model, derived from data of the North American carotid surgery trial, Rothwell[9] divided the patients in the European carotid surgery trial into 3 groups: one with <10% risk for cerebrovascular events, one with 10 to 15% and finally, one with >15% risk[25]. This division was based on clinical data at entry. The observed rate of events did in fact match this prediction. In the low risk group carotid endarterectomy produced more harm than benefit. Operation of about 70 patients led to an overall risk of seriously harming 1 patient. In the high risk group, however, 7 patients needed to be operated in order to prevent 1 serious cerebrovascular complication. With this patient selection far fewer patients need to be operated, and fewer patients will be harmed. If this method of patient selection proves to be effective, it might even be more so in the case of asymptomatic stenosis.

If we succeed in proving that cerebral perfusion reserve measurement has a strong predictive power, we can improve our clinical prediction methods. If it will be possible to select those patients that would benefit from these procedures and those that would not, surgery would become much more cost-effective and unnecessary losses of life, functional health and money would be prevented.

Future studies

The data mentioned above are compatible with the theory that a diminished cerebral perfusion reserve, as measured with various methods, is predictive for future ipsilateral ischaemic events. However, with the presently available clinical data there is sufficient room for alternative explanations that range from coincidence to confounding factors. There is a need for firm prospective studies to settle this issue. If patients with a reduced cerebral perfusion reserve are at increased risk for stroke, then an important next step has to be made: does revascularization (e.g. carotid endarterectomy, extracranial-intracranial bypass, angioplasty) improve the prognosis in these patients?

The following clinical problems could be addressed: asymptomatic carotid stenosis, moderate (30-70%) symptomatic stenosis, symptomatic carotid occlusions, and even symptomatic severe (≥70%) stenosis.

The numbers of patients required to participate in such studies are large. If one presumes that 25% of patients with a diminished cerebral perfusion reserve in any of the mentioned clinical circumstances would experience a serious vascular event in the 3 years following inclusion in the study, and that this would be 10% in the group of patients with a normal cerebral perfusion reserve, a group of 110 patients with diminished and a group of 110 patients with normal cerebral perfusion reserve would be needed and followed for 3 years in order to detect this difference.

Comparable sample sizes are needed in order to make the next step: prove that surgical revascularization is effective in this particular group of patients.

A series of studies using different methods and criteria support the idea that measurement of the cerebral perfusion reserve yields information that is not readily available by any other source of information and might be of great value for clinical decision making in carotid artery stenosis. Studies with more clinical power are needed to establish measurement of cerebral perfusion reserve as a powerful tool for better patient management.

References

1 Jansen, C., Vriens, E.M., Eikelboom, B.C. et al. Carotid endarterectomy with transcranial Doppler and Electroencephalography monitoring. A prospective study in 130 patients. Stroke 1993, 24, 665

2 Schomer, D.F., Marks, M.P., Steinberg, G.K. et al. The anatomy of the posterior communicating artery as a risk factor for ischemic cerebral infarction. N. Engl. J. Med. 1994, 330, 1565

3 De Bruïne, F.J., Limburg, M., Van Royen, E.A. et al. SPET brain imaging with Thallium-201-diethyldithiocarbamate in acute ischemic stroke. Eur. J. Nucl. Med. 1990, 17, 248

4 Dierckx, R., Dobbeleir, A., Pickut, B.A. et al. ^{99m}Tc-HMPAO SPECT in acute supratentorial ischaemic infarction, expressing deficits as milliliter zeroperfusion. Eur. J. Nucl. Med. 1995, 22, 427

5 Limburg, M., van Royen, E.A., De Bruïne, J.F. et al. Regional cerebral blood flow single photon emission computed tomography and early death in acute ischemic stroke. Stroke 1990, 21, 1150

6 Herderschee, D., Limburg, M., van Royen, E.A. et al. Thrombolysis with recombinant tissue plasminogen activator in acute ischemic stroke: evaluation with rCBF-SPECT. Acta Neurol. Scand. 1991, 83, 317

7 Limburg, M., van Royen., E.A., Hijdra, A. et al. rCBF-SPECT in acute brain infarction: when does it predict outcome? J. Nucl. Med. 1991, 32, 382

8 European Carotid Surgery Trialists' Collaborative Group MRC European Carotid Surgery Trial (ECST): interim results for symptomatic patients with severe (70-99%) or with mild (1-29%) stenosis. Lancet 1991, 337, 1235

9 North American Symptomatic Carotid Artery Surgery Trial (NASCET) collaborators Beneficial effect of carotid endarterectomy in symptomatic patients with high-grade carotid stenosis. N. Engl. J. Med. 1991, 325, 445

10 Laupacis, A., Naylor, C.D. and Sackett, D.L. How should the results of clinical trials be presented to clinicians? A.C.P.J. Club 1992, A12

11 Anonymous Endarterectomy for moderate symptomatic carotid stenosis: interim results from the MRC European Carotid Surgery Trial. Lancet 1996, 347, 1591

12 Executive Committee for the Asymptomatic Carotid Atherosclerosis Study. Endarterectomy for Asymptomatic Carotid Artery Stenosis. J.A.M.A. 1995, 273, 1421

13 Hasegawa, Y., Yamaguchi, T., Minematsu, K. and Nishimura, T. Sequential change of haemodynamic reserve in patients with major cerebral artery occlusion or severe stenosis. Neuroradiology 1992, 34, 15

14 Rosenkranz, K., Hierholzer, J., Langer, R. et al. Acetazolamide stimulation test in patients with unilateral internal carotid artery obstruction using transcranial Doppler and ^{99m}Tc-HMPAO SPECT. Neurol. Research 1992, 14, 135

15 Fürst, H., Hartl, W.H. and Janssen, I. Patterns of cerebrovascular reactivity in patients with unilateral asymptomatic carotid artery stenosis. *Stroke* 1994, 25, 1193

16 Naylor, A.R., Merrick, M.V., Gillespie, I. *et al.* Prevalence of impaired cerebrovascular reserve in patients with symptomatic carotid artery disease. *British Journal of Surgery* 1994, 81, 45

17 Limburg, M., Rehmann C.J., Legemate D.A. *et al.* Cerebrovascular perfusion reserve in carotid stenosis measured with ^{99m}Tc-HMPAO and acetazolamide provocation. *Acta Neurol. Belgica* 1995, 95, 100

18 Sacca, A., Pedrini, L., Vitacchiano, G. *et al.* Cerebral SPECT with ^{99m}Tc-HMPAO in extracranial carotid pathology: evaluation of changes in the ischemic area after carotid endarterectomy. *Int. Angiol.* 1992, 11, 117

19 Powers, W.J., Tempel, L.W. and Grubb, R.L. Influence of cerebral haemodynamics on stroke risk: one-year follow-up of 30 medically treated patients. *Ann. Neurol.* 1989, 25, 325

20 Lord, R.S.A., Reid, C.V.A., Ramsay, S.C. and Yeates, M.G. Unilateral carotid stenosis and impaired cerebral hemispheric vascular reserve. *Ann. Vasc. Surg.* 1992, 6, 438

21 Cikrit, D.F., Burt, R.W., Dalsing, M.C. *et al.* Acetazolamide enhanced single photon emission computed tomography (SPECT) evaluation of cerebral perfusion before and after carotid endarterectomy. *J. Vasc. Surg.* 1992, 15, 747

22 Yamauchi, H., Fukuyama, H., Nagahama, Y. *et al.* Evidence of misery perfusion and risk for recurrent stroke in major cerebral arterial occlusive diseases from PET. *J.N.N.P.* 1996, 61, 18

23 Kleiser, B. and Widder, B. Course of carotid artery occlusions with impaired cerebrovascular reactivity. *Stroke* 1992, 23, 171

24 Yonas, H., Smith, H.A., Durham, S.R. *et al.* Increased stroke risk predicted by compromised cerebral blood flow reactivity. *J. Neurosurg.* 1993, 79, 483

25 Rothwell, P.M. Can overall results of clinical trials be applied to all patients? *Lancet* 1995, 345, 1616

SPECT in Neurology and Psychiatry, edited by P.P. De Deyn, R.A. Dierckx, A. Alavi and B.A. Pickut
© 1997 John Libbey & Company Ltd, pp. 323–334

SPECT Imaging in Transient Ischaemic Attacks and Subarachnoid Haemorrhage

Chapter
39

P. Laloux

SPECT imaging in transient ischaemic attacks

Transient ischaemic attacks (TIAs) by definition do not leave a neurological deficit beyond 24 h after onset[1]. The duration of focal cerebral hypoperfusion in so-called transient ischaemic attacks is not well known[2-4]. Moreover, a subgroup of TIA patients with infarction on brain computed tomography (CT) has been defined and called 'cerebral infarction with transient signs' (CITS)[5]. For several authors, these TIA patients should be differentiated from those without cerebral infarction due to their differences in aetiological factors, duration and prognosis[6-12]. This categorisation can have important implications for prognosis and therapy. Yet, this differentiation remains controversial[13-16]. Referring to CITS, TIA patients with hypoperfusion on SPECT could be also differentiated from those without hypoperfusion with respect to the duration of TIAs, history of previous TIAs, vascular territory (superficial or deep), risk factors and aetiology. However, the clinical relevance of such a delineation in the therapeutic management of these patients remains unclear.

SPECT sensitivity in transient ischaemic attacks

Several SPECT studies with different methodologies and radiopharmaceuticals have demonstrated regional hypoperfusion in some TIA patients[2-4,17-32]. Recent SPECT studies used the ^{99m}Tc-hexamethylpropyleneamine oxime (HMPAO) tracer, which proved helpful in evaluating the regional cerebral blood flow (rCBF) in patients with cerebrovascular diseases[33]. ^{99m}Tc-ECD (ethyl cysteinate dimer; Neurolite), now available routinely, was also found to be highly sensitive in stroke patients[34]. The long stability *in vitro* makes ^{99m}Tc-ECD easy to use and thus could be very helpful in imaging TIAs.

Because few TIA patients are admitted very early after onset and because the duration of attacks is frequently short (62% lasted less than 60 min in our own series of 76 patients[35], SPECT cannot be easily performed during the ischaemic attack. Moreover, the hospital-based population in many studies may present a selection bias by the fact that the TIA patients with repetitive attacks (47% in our series) are probably more frequently referred to hospital than patients with a single attack.

The prevalence of focal hypoperfusion on SPECT varies greatly according to the series due to their different methodologies and variable admission times. Moreover, a brain CT scan was not always carried out. When the findings of angiograms were not detailed, the sensitivity was 0% to 89% (Table 1)[3,17,19,21,23,24,26]. In patients with normal carotid angiograms, the

Department of Neurology, Mont-Godinne University Hospital, Medical School of the University of Louvain, 5530 Yvoir, Belgium

Table 1 SPECT sensitivity in TIA patients without detailed angiograms

Ref	n	SPECT	Time interval	SPECT sensitivity %	CT sensitivity %
21	7	IMP	?	0	100
3	20	[133]Xe	< 24 hours	60	100
17	13	IMP	?	77	15
24	6	HMPAO	?	33	17
26	7	HMPAO	?	85	43
23	18	HMPAO	< 6 days	89	39
19	30	HMPAO	≤ 4 days	50	17

Table 2 SPECT sensitivity in TIA patients with normal angiograms

Ref	n	SPECT	Time interval	SPECT sensitivity %	CT sensitivity %
27	11	[133]Xe	8-90 days	64	100[a]
29	12	[133]Xe	12 h - 4 yrs	8	-
30	23	[133]Xe	?	48	?
2	12	HMPAO	< 50 hours	33	?

[a],Only 4 patients underwent brain CT

sensitivity varied between 8% and 64% (Table 2)[2,27,29,30]. On the other hand, in selected patients with occlusive carotid disease, several authors[4,18,25,30,31] reported a higher sensitivity ranging from 47% to 100%, except for Russel et al.[28] and Hemmingsen et al.[20] who found a lower sensitivity of 14% and 27%, respectively (Table 3). In our series of 76 non-selected TIA patients, the SPECT sensitivity was significantly higher than that of CT (35% versus 14%; p=0.007[35]. This sensitivity was similar to that found by Bogousslavsky et al.[2] in 12 patients with < 75% stenosis of the internal carotid artery. In 21 patients, Isaka et al.[22] found overall sensitivity rates of 67% in SPECT and 19% in CT.

The low SPECT sensitivity in some studies may be due to deep ischaemic lesions that are not detected by the low spatial resolution of a single-head camera. However, in our series of patients with cortical or deep localization, the sensitivity was not dependent on the vascular territory. The long time interval between the onset and SPECT imaging can decrease the sensitivity[3,19,27]. When SPECT examinations were repeated in the same patients, Hartmann[3] reported sequential changes of rCBF with time. In their 14 patients with blood flow disturbance on day 1, an early and delayed return to normal was found in 4 and 3 patients, respectively. In the aggregate, even if most patients have normal rCBF in the acute or subacute phase, a number of patients may have persisting flow abnormalities as late as 90 days, despite the recovery of their clinical deficits[4,27].

In patients with TIAs in the carotid artery territory, SPECT usually shows a mild perfusion defect which contrasts with the higher degree of hypoperfusion found in cortical carotid infarcts[32]. In our own experience, the mean interhemispheric difference was 14 ± 4% (median, 13%) in TIA patients with prolonged focal hypoperfusion and 27 ± 22% (median, 19%) in stroke patients[33]. In 16 patients with reversible symptoms of cerebrovascular disease (12 TIA and 4 PRIND), Grunwald et al.[36] also found a mild perfusion defect with a tracer accumulation reduced by 13 ± 12% for HMPAO and 8 ± 7% for IMP in the clinically involved hemisphere compared with the contralateral side. Therefore, because the reduction of rCBF is mild in TIAs, combination of visual analysis with semi-quantitative analysis is needed to increase the reliability of SPECT. Indeed, a slight heterogenic SPECT pattern may occasionally be observed in normal individuals.

Clinical relevance of prolonged hypoperfusion in transient ischaemic attacks

In several studies[4,18,30,31,37-39], SPECT showed a focal persisting hypoperfusion in selected patients with occlusive carotid disease and haemodynamic insufficiency. Chollet et al.[18] found in 15 TIA patients an association between the degree and size of hypoperfusion and the presence of severe carotid atherosclerotic lesion. Likewise, Isaka et al.[22] reported in 21 patients larger hypoperfused areas when the patients had intracranial, severe stenotic, multiple, or haemodynamically significant arterial lesions on the ipsilateral side. In non-selected populations, few studies have addressed the issue of whether the duration of attacks, history of previous TIAs, risk factors and aetiology were different in patients with prolonged hypoperfusion. Kassiotis et al.[4] found a possible relationship between the duration of attacks and the presence of hypoperfusion in 4 patients with

Table 3 SPECT sensitivity in TIA patients with carotid occlusive disease

Ref	n	SPECT	Time interval	SPECT sensitivity %	CT sensitivity %
31	14	[133]Xe	2-60 days	64	29[a]
25	12	[133]Xe	> 3 weeks	100	-
	7		< 3 weeks		
4	20	[133]Xe	1-90 days	65	15
18	11	[133]Xe	≤ 10 days	47	33
	4		15-30 days		
28	14	[133]Xe	?	14	100
30	19	[133]Xe	?	79	?
20	31	[133]Xe	days - months	23	16

[a], Only 4 patients underwent brain CT

TIAs due to emboli. Isaka et al.[22] compared the SPECT findings with CT, angiogram, risk factors and clinical findings to determine which factor was most responsible for regional hypoperfusion. They only found significant association with ipsilateral carotid occlusive disease. In 76 patients, we found a persisting perfusion defect more frequently in the patients with attacks lasting more than 120 min, but the difference was not significant. The presence of persisting focal hypoperfusion was not significantly associated with some particular stroke risk and aetiological factors[35]. Besides, a multivariate analysis did not identify any of these factors as an independent variable to discriminate the patients with or without perfusion defect.

Prolonged hypoperfusion and prognosis for stroke recurrence

Some TIA patients have a higher risk of mortality and stroke recurrence. Survival rates range from 70% to 92% at 5 years[40-42] and the incidence of stroke from 0% to 62%[43-45]. Clinical factors such as age, gender, vascular risk factors, aetiology, duration of attacks, treatment, and the presence of relevant infarction on CT can also play an important role in outcome[40,46]. A few studies have been devoted to describing the long-term prognosis of patients with TIA and appropriate cerebral infarction on CT scan. Some have reported a higher risk of death or recurrent stroke when the CT scan showed a relevant brain infarct[8,9], but this was not confirmed by others[14,47]. Similarly, few studies have

addressed the issue of whether persisting regional hypoperfusion on SPECT might be associated with a higher risk of death or stroke recurrence in patients with transient ischaemic attacks. The risk of death has never been evaluated with SPECT studies. In a series of 12 patients, Bogousslavsky et al.[2] reported in 4 of them an association between persisting focal hypoperfusion and early stroke. Yet they selected patients with a < 75% stenosis of the internal carotid artery, a single hemispheric TIA lasting < 1 h and a normal CT 24-36 h after onset. Besides, high interhemispheric differences (> 20 ± 5%) were considered as significant in their semi-quantitative analysis. In 76 consecutive TIA patients without a stroke history (unpublished data), we found that the presence of persisting focal hypoperfusion on SPECT, when considered alone, did not appear to be a significant determinant of ischaemic recurrence. After adjusting for other factors such as the TIA characteristics, stroke risk factors and aetiology, the multivariate analysis identified only the duration of TIA as a significant predictive factor and the presence of hypoperfusion on SPECT was not selected. Given the small number of patients, the same analysis could not be performed for subgroups of patients with a history of TIA, cerebral infarct on CT, large artery disease, cardiac source embolism or unknown aetiology.

Thus, in agreement with the studies on CITS, the presence of prolonged hypoperfusion does not alter the long-term prognosis of non-selected patients with TIAs. However, further larger studies are warranted to confirm the currently available results and more particularly in subgroups of patients.

The confounding SPECT findings in the prediction of outcome are illustrated by the two following case reports. In these TIA patients with a relevant regional hypoperfusion on SPECT, the recurrent stroke could not be related with certainty to the prior perfusion defect. In the first, a 60-year-old patient who experienced two episodes of left hemiparesis and dysarthria lasting 30 min each, SPECT showed a relevant right frontoparietal hypoperfusion (Figure 1a) with normal brain CT. The ischaemic attack and focal hypoperfusion were caused by a haemodynamic insufficiency due to an ipsilateral occlusion of the internal carotid artery associated with a tight stenosis of the contralateral internal carotid artery (Figure 1b). After left carotid endarterectomy, SPECT was unchanged. When the patient presented with a recurrent stroke on the same side 15 months later, SPECT also remained unchanged. A CT scan demonstrated a relevant infarct in the right middle cerebral artery in the previously hypoperfused area (Figure 1c). In the absence of carotid restenosis on Doppler ultra-

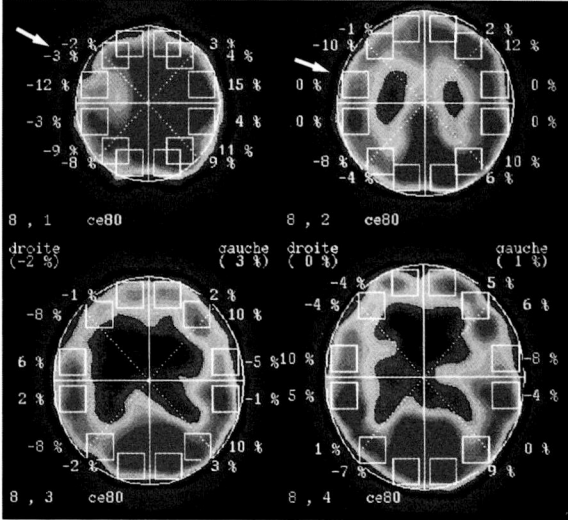

Figure 1a SPECT of right frontoparietal hypoperfusion

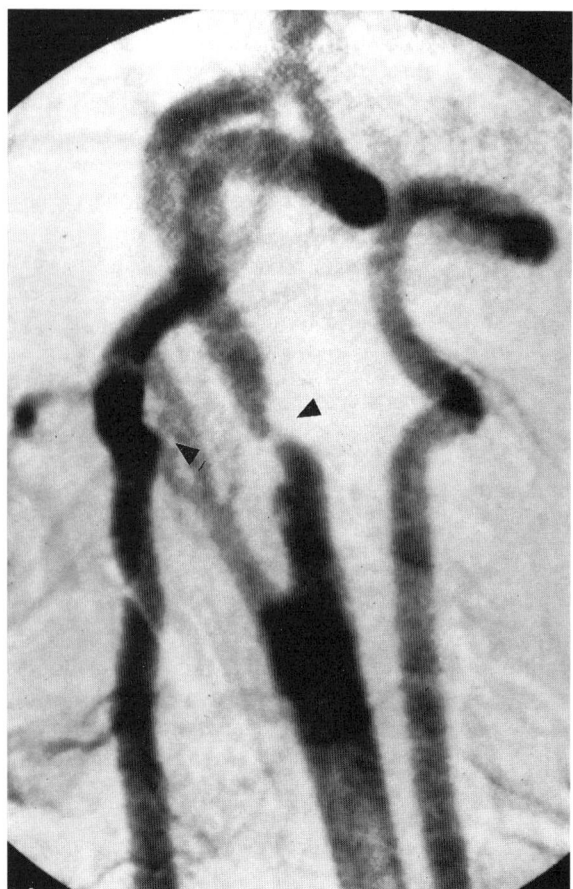

Figure 1b Angiography showing occlusion and tight stenosis of the ipsilateral and contralateral internal carotid artery, respectively

sonography, the likely cause of infarction was carotid source embolism and not transformation of ischaemic region into infarct. In this second case report an 80-year-old patient, who experienced a left hemiparesis lasting 180 min, SPECT showed a relevant right frontoparietal perfusion defect (Figure 2a) with a deep infarct in the right anterior choroidal artery on CT (Figure 2b). The cortical hypoperfusion was due to a mechanism of deafferentation (intrahemispheric cortical diaschisis). Cardiac investigations and Doppler ultrasonography were unremarkable. Hypertensive small vessel disease was the presumed cause of infarction. Twelve months later, the patient complained of persisting weakness in his left leg. Brain CT did not show any recent infarction. Because the hypoperfusion was well correlated with the previous CT-verified infarct, a relationship between the focal perfusion defect and the stroke recurrence could not be ascertained.

Vasoreactivity assessment in transient ischaemic attacks

Several authors reported that acetazolamide, a carbonic anhydrase inhibitor[48,49], or CO_2[50], which both induce dilatation of the cerebral microvasculature, significantly increased SPECT sensitivity for detecting pathological areas in TIA patients with or without occlusive carotid disease[4,18,28,39,51].

Three SPECT studies[4,18,30] have concluded in favour of the usefulness of the vasoreactivity challenge with acetazolamide in the pathophysiological classification of TIAs. The reactivity test could discriminate the TIAs due to thromboemboli from those secondary to a haemodynamically significant carotid occlusive disease[4,30]. SPECT studies with[4,18,30,39,51] or without vasoreactivity[31] test have reported an association between focal hypoperfusion and occlusive disease in the internal carotid artery or the innominate artery[53]. Acetazolamide challenge is a feasible method to detect non-invasively the efficacy of collateral channels and provides additional information for CT, angiographic, and transcranial Doppler findings[52]. Cerebral blood volume measurement with ^{99m}Tc-red blood cells can also be of great value[30,54-56]. In the presence of occlusion or stenosis of the internal carotid artery or middle cerebral artery, SPECT can show decreased rCBF, increased CBV and exhausted cerebrovascular reserve capacity. The hypoperfusion is due to haemodynamic insufficiency, which resolves after endarterectomy[31,37], extracranial-intracranial bypass[38] or angioplasty[53] along with the complete resolution of transient ischaemic attacks. Thus, in this respect, SPECT is a powerful imaging technique to discriminate higher risk TIA patients likely to benefit from vascular surgery or angioplasty.

Pathogenetic origin of asymptomatic focal prolonged hypoperfusion

In patients with cortical infarcts, the rCBF decrease is well correlated with tissue necrosis. In the case of deep-seated infarcts, the chronic cortical flow reduction is probably caused by functional inactivation (diaschisis)[57-60]. However, besides the decrease of the functional input to the cortex, white matter damage can lead to retrograde degeneration and selective cell necrosis in the cortex which may explain the persistence of remote cortical hypoperfusion[61]. On the other hand, in patients without a well-demarcated infarct on CT, the mechanism remains controversial. The role of silent infarcts is possible although uncertain since only thalamic and thalamocapsular infarcts with cognitive impairment may cause ipsilateral cortical hypometabolism and hypoperfusion[62]. The role played by lacunar infarcts undetected on CT cannot be excluded, but a remote hypoperfusion due to small size infarcts is unlikely[63]. Besides diaschisis, a chronic regional haemodynamic insufficiency, more particularly in patients with ispilateral carotid occlusive disease, may explain the persisting hypoperfusion. The extension of cerebral infarct depends in part on the collateral circulation, which can improve the transiently impaired perfusion and prevent tissue necrosis[64-67]. The collateral supply could be adequate to protect the brain tissue against its transformation into completed infarct but not enough to restore a normal rCBF. However, the neuronal function would be preserved without residual neurological deficit because the rCBF remains above the threshold of electrical failure[68] or because the brain oxygen extraction from the blood is increased[69] to maintain

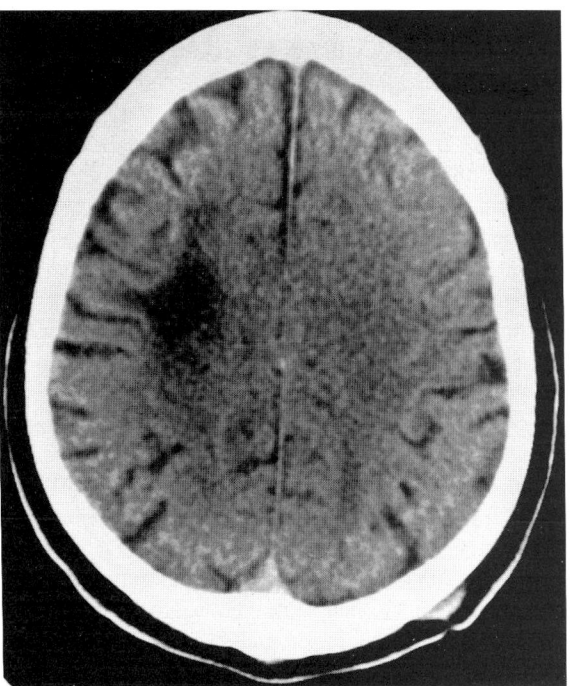

Figure 1c CT scan after stroke recurrence showing subcortical infarct in the right middle cerebral artery territory

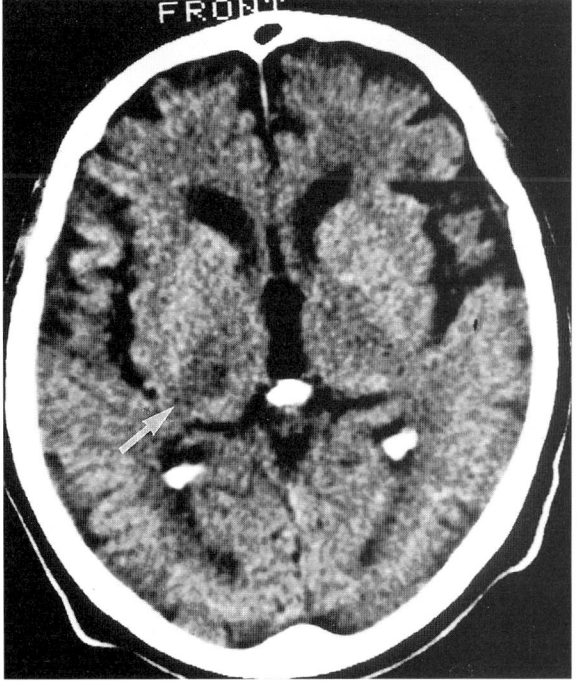

Figure 2b Brain CT of deep infarct in the right anterior choroidal artery territory

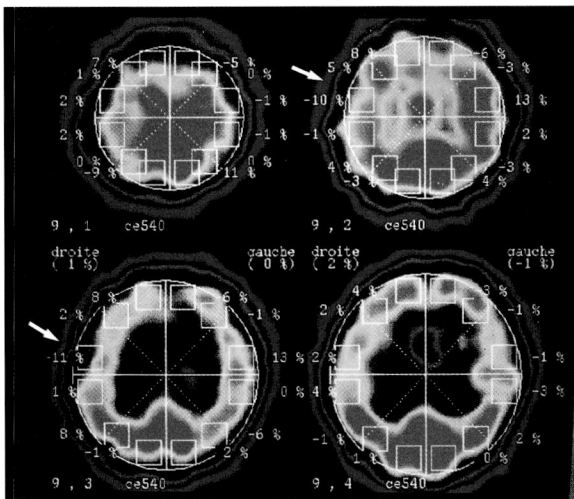

Figure 2a SPECT of right cortical frontoparietal hypoperfusion

adequate cerebral metabolism. Blood flow thresholds can be determined with SPECT using ^{133}Xe and IMP[70], or HMPAO (Laloux *et al.*, unpublished data). These thresholds help to differentiate the infarcted region from the periinfarct area or symptomatic regions without infarction. Yet, this haemodynamic mechanism does not explain why the rCBF is persistently decreased on late SPECT in some patients without carotid occlusive disease. If we assume that the reperfusion process is achieved at the time of SPECT examination, the hypothesis of 'incomplete infarction'[71] should be reconsidered. A state of 'elective emollision', a selective neuronal cell loss, was described by Scholz[72] and observed in regions surrounding areas of complete infarction[73]. A significant correlation was found between reduced blood flow and neuronal loss in the cortex in animal experiments[61,74], the low flow reflecting a lowered metabolic demand. The incomplete infarction may represent a 'transitional state' between TIAs without persisting ischaemic lesion and TIAs with CT-verified infarction. In some patients, the chronic focal hypoperfusion on SPECT is likely to reflect this 'transitional state'. The recent studies in animals[75] and in cerebrovascular dementia[76] give some support to the hypothesis of incomplete infarction, but this concept remains controversial[77-79]. Acetazolamide and CO_2 challenge is useful in discriminating between diaschisis or incomplete infarction and local exhausted cerebrovascular reserve[4,18,80,81]. In case of diaschisis or incomplete infarction, the vasomotor reactivity is expected to be normal. Thus, in the absence of carotid occlusive disease, the vasoreactivity test is needed to determine the underlying mechanism of chronic local hypoperfusion.

Conclusions

SPECT, despite its better sensitivity than CT, does not seem to give additional clinically useful information in non-selected TIA patients regarding their risk factors, aetiology and outcome. Yet, SPECT is a powerful non-invasive imaging technique to delineate TIA patients at high risk for haemodynamic insufficiency in the presence of carotid occlusive disease. In this particular subgroup of patients, the therapeutic decision can depend on the SPECT findings. The current data stress the need for per-forming vasoreactivity assessment because it greatly improves SPECT sensitivity and is useful in differ-entiating the different causes of TIAs. Further studies are still needed to define more precisely the potential role of SPECT in a large population of TIA patients.

SPECT imaging in subarachnoid haemorrhage

Subarachnoid haemorrhage (SAH) accounts for approximately one half of all intracranial haemorrhagic strokes[82]. Vasospasm appears in up to 75% of patients with SAH[83-85] and typically occurs >72 h after the initial bleed with a peak approximately on days 6-10[86]. Vasospasms can yield delayed cerebral ischaemia, manifested as new neurological deficits, in about 30% of SAH patients[86,87], and this is responsible for high morbidity and mortality[86,88]. In addition to cerebral infarction, there is a subset of 'subclinical vasospasm' without CT-verified infarction[84]. Early aggressive hypertensive hypervolaemic therapy[87] combined with calcium antagonists[89,90], free-radicals scavengers or angioplasty[91-94] can greatly improve the outcome of these patients. Therefore, early and accurate differentiation of vasospasm from other causes of neurological deterioration such as oedema, hydrocephalus and electrolyte aberrations is required[87].

Current techniques for early detection of vasospasm

The diagnosis of vasospasm must be made when the patient is still asymptomatic. Angiography is an invasive imaging technique for repeated screening examinations and carries the risk of exacerbation of vasospasm[95,96]. Therefore, transcranial Doppler ultrasonography (TCD) has become the first-choice investigation for detection of vasospasm[97]. It allows serial daily examinations and its reliability is now well accepted[98-101]. However, this technique has important disadvantages, such as the lack of insonation window in some patients and its inability to diagnose distal arterial vasospasm[100,101]. Moreover, these studies only indirectly relate to the risk for cerebral infarction[102]. Indeed, TCD velocities are not reflective of rCBF when autoregulation is intact and especially during conditions of rapidly changing blood flows and blood pressures[84,102]. In the early stages of cerebral vasospasm, when TCD already shows increased velocities, CBF may be still unaffected due to the increased cerebral blood volume (CBV) related to vasodilation of small blood vessels[83,84]. This explains why increased TCD velocities can be found in some SAH patients without neurological deficit. Some authors suggest that there is likely to be a threshold for increased arterial erythocyte velocity at which CBF begins to decrease when homeostatic mechanisms are failing with the occurrence of ischaemic deficits[83,84,101,103]. By contrast, SPECT does not show any regional hypoperfusion when TCD is normal[103]. Thus, TCD and SPECT are useful complementary techniques as these tests respectively evaluate the degree of vessel narrowing and the haemodynamic consequences of vasospasm[84]. The two examinations help to guide the extent of appropriate treatment.

SPECT studies in subarachnoid haemorrhage

A large number of CBF studies, using different methodologies, radiopharmaceuticals and times of examination, have been reported in patients with SAH[25,83-85,103-112]. Stable xenon-enhanced CT has also been used to map hypoperfusion due to vasospasm[113,114]. In some studies, the SPECT findings were correlated with the presence of vasospasm diagnosed on clinical grounds while in others they were correlated with angiography. Table 4 summarizes the different SPECT sensitivities reported in the main studies.

As in PET studies, the CBF reduction can be diffuse or focal[88,115]. Non-tomographic[88,112,116-120] as well as tomographic techniques[83,84,103,110,115] have demonstrated that the regional hypoperfusion correlated well with the presence and severity of delayed ischaemic neurological deficits and with angiographic findings[85,108-112]. Good correlation has also been found with brain CT[83-85,111]. In patients with cerebral infarction, SPECT shows earlier and larger lesions than CT scan abnormalities[106,107,111]. More extensive and severe reduction in rCBF is strongly predictive of cerebral infarct[83,84], particularly when the cerebro-vascular reserve capacity is impaired[106]. Regional CBF measurements with vasoreactivity assessment provide more direct information about the haemodynamic consequences of vasospasms observed with transcranial Doppler[106,107,110]. Moreover, the reactivity tests are useful in differentiating regional hypoperfusion due to haematoma or oedema from local perfusion defects related to vasospasm[110]. The time of occurrence of decreased rCBF in SAH patients has been well documented in different SPECT studies[103,106,110].

SPECT in therapeutic monitoring

Since SPECT studies can detect critical reductions in perfusion before clinical deficits develop, this technique combined with TCD offers the potential to identify candidates for early medical treatment or angioplasty and can be useful in therapeutic monitoring. Two studies have demonstrated the capacity of SPECT to monitor the improvement of cerebral perfusion after medical treatment and angioplasty[84,103]. In patients without neurological deficit, SPECT and TCD should be carried out as soon as possible after surgery (Figure 3). In the case of an abnormal SPECT, a CT scan is needed to document the presence of infarct. On the other hand, in the case of a normal SPECT, serial daily TCD should be performed. Once vasospasm is detected by TCD, SPECT should again be obtained immediately. If TCD is technically impossible or not reliable for any reason, SPECT can also offer an alternative for monitoring.

Limitations of SPECT in subarachnoid haemorrhage

It is important to be aware of some limitations of SPECT in SAH patients. Because SPECT has a lower sensitivity in the deep brain areas, it may overlook the occurrence of small deep infarcts[103]. Besides, some tomographic findings may not be easy to interpret. Indeed, Rosen et al.[109] found, in 9 patients in whom clinical vasospasm did not develop, decreased rCBF near the operative site in 17 of 20 studies. The perfusion defect did not correlate with the patients' neurological condition and was suggestive of postoperative oedema. Therefore, the SPECT data should be interpreted cautiously according to the clinical status, the site of hypoperfusion and the time of investigation. Additionally, some semiquantitative studies have used either corticocerebellar ratios or lesion-to-contralateral-normal ratios. The latter assumes that the contralateral brain is normal for standardization purposes, but this is uncertain in cerebral vasospasm which can involve the two cerebral hemispheres. Thus, Lewis et al.[84] speculated that a

Table 4 SPECT sensitivity in subarachnoid haemorrhage

Ref	n	SPECT	SPECT sensitivity %
111	7	IMP/[133]Xe	100
107	24	HMPAO	67
83	13	HMPAO	100[a]
85	15	HMPAO	90
110	42	IMP + ACZ	77 (grade I, II) 100 (grade III-V)
84	10	HMPAO	100
103	26	HMPAO	69
106	79	IMP + ACZ	71
109	9	HMPAO	85

ACZ: acetazolamide test.

[a], The 7 patients with vasospasm on angiography had hypoperfusion while the remaining 6 without vasospasm were normal

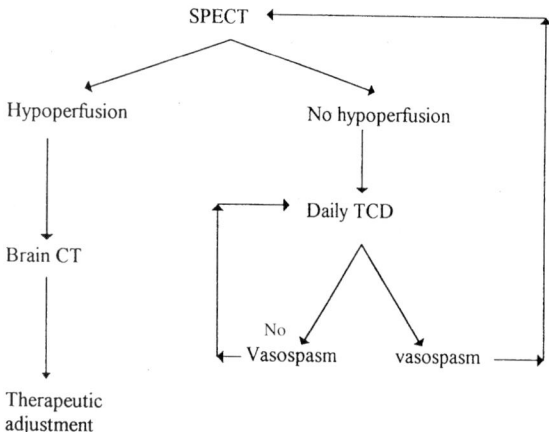

Figure 3 Transcranial Doppler ultrasonography and SPECT studies in the early detection of vasospasm in patients without neurological deficits

cerebral vasospasm which can involve the two cerebral hemispheres. Thus, Lewis *et al.*[84] speculated that a corticocerebellar ratio was the most appropriate method because the cerebellum is more richly supplied with collateral circulation than is the neo-cortex. Lastly, the acetazolamide test can increase the intracranial pressure[122], and should therefore be used with great caution in patients with intracranial hypertension or impaired intracranial compliance[123].

Conclusions

SPECT, despite some limitations, appears to be a powerful non-invasive technique to detect changes in perfusion in SAH patients. In combination with TCD, it allows early diagnosis of vasospasm and thereby helps to guide appropriate treatment in patients at higher risk of cerebral ischaemia.

References

1 NINCDS. Ad Hoc Committee on Cerebrovascular Disease: a classification and outline of cerebrovascular diseases. II. *Stroke* 1975, 6, 565

2 Bogousslavsky, J., Delaloye-Bischof, A., Regli, F. and Delaloye, B. Prolonged hypoperfusion and early stroke after transient ischaemic attack. *Stroke* 1990, 21, 40

3 Hartmann, A. Prolonged disturbances of regional cerebral blood flow in transient ischaemic attacks. *Stroke* 1985, 16, 932

4 Kassiotis, P. and Steinling, M. Le débit sanguin cérébral local et sa réactivité à l'acétazolamide dans les accidents ischémiques transitoires. *Rev. Neurol.* 1987, 143, 806

5 Waxman, S.G. and Toole, J.F. Temporal profile resembling TIA in the setting of cerebral infarction. *Stroke* 1983, 14, 431

6 Bogousslavsky, J. and Regli, F. Cerebral infarct in apparent transient ischaemic attack. *Neurology* 1985, 35, 1501

7 Donnan, G., Tress, B.M. and Bladin, P.F. A prospective study of lacunar infarction using computerized tomography. *Neurology* 1982, 32, 49

8 Evans, G.W., Howard, G., Murros, K.E. *et al.* Cerebral infarction verified by cranial computed tomography and prognosis for survival following transient ischaemic attack. *Stroke* 1991, 22, 431

9 Giroud, M., Gras, P., Milan, C. *et al.* Pronostic des accidents ischémiques transitoires révélant un infarctus. *Rev. Neurol.* 1992, 148, 576

10 Grigg, M.F., Papadakis, K., Nicolaides, A.N. *et al.* The significance of cerebral infarction and atrophy in patients with amaurosis fugax and transient ischaemic attack in relation to internal carotid artery stenosis. *J. Vasc. Surg.* 1980, 2, 215

11 Murros, K.E., Evans, G.W., Toole, J.F. *et al.* Cerebral infarction in patients with transient ischaemic attacks. *J. Neurol.* 1989, 236, 182

12 Zukowski, A.J., Nicolaides, A.N., Lewis, R.T. *et al.* The correlation between the carotid plaque ulceration and cerebral infarction seen on CT scan. *J. Vasc. Surg.* 1984, 1, 782

13 Caplan, L.R. Are terms such as completed stroke or RIND of continued usefulness? *Stroke* 1983, 14, 431

14 Dennis, M., Bamford, J., Sandercock, P. *et al.* Computed tomography in patients with transient ischaemic attacks: when is a transient ischaemic attack not a transient ischaemic attack but a stroke. *J. Neurol.* 1990, 237, 257

15 Koudstaal, P.J., van Gijn, J., Frenken, C.W.G. *et al.* TIA, RIND, minor stroke: a continuum, or different subgroups? *J. Neurol. Neurosurg. Psychiatry* 1992, 55, 95

16 Koudstaal, P.J., van Gijn, J., Lodder, J. *et al.* Transient ischaemic attacks with and without a relevant infarct on computed tomographic scans cannot be distinguished clinically. *Arch. Neurol.* 1991, 48, 916

17 Brott, T.G., Gelfand, M.J., Williams, C.C. *et al.* Frequency and patterns of abnormality detected by iodine-123 amine emission CT after cerebral infarction. *Radiology* 1986, 158, 729

18 Chollet, F., Celsis, P., Clanet, M. *et al.* SPECT study of cerebral blood flow reactivity after acetazolamide in patients with transient ischaemic attacks. *Stroke* 1989, 20, 458

19 De Roo, M., Mortelmans, L., Devos, P. *et al.* Clinical experience with Tc-99m HM-PAO high resolution SPECT of the brain in patients with cerebrovascular accidents. *Eur. J. Nucl. Med.* 1989, 15, 9

20 Hemmingsen, R., Mejsholm, B., Vorstrup, S. *et al.* Carotid surgery, cognitive function, and cerebral blood flow in patients with transient ischaemic attacks. *Ann. Neurol.* 1986, 20, 13

21 Hill, T.C., Holman, B.L., Lovett, R. *et al.* Initial experience with SPECT (Single-photon computerized tomography) of the brain using N-isopropyl I-123 p-iodoamphetamine: concise communication. *J. Nucl. Med.* 1982, 23, 191

22 Isaka, Y., Ashida, K., Liji, O. and Imaizumi, M. Factors causing prolonged hypoperfusion after transient ischaemic attack. *Ann. Nucl. Med.* 1993, 7, 21

23 Just, V.A. and Schröter, J. SPECT des Gehirnes mit ^{99m}Tc-HMPAO bei patienten mit zerebrovaskulärer erkrankung: vergleich mit der CT. *Fortschr. Röntgenstr.* 1989, 151, 611

24 Leonard, J.P., Nowotnik, D.P. and Neirinckx, R.D. ^{99m}Tc-d,l-HMPAO: A new radiopharmaceutical for imaging regional brain perfusion using SPECT: a comparison with iodine-123 HIPDM. *J. Nucl. Med.* 1986, 27, 1819

25 Meyer, J.S., Naritomi, H., Sakai, F. *et al.* Regional cerebral blood flow, diaschisis, and steal after stroke. *Neur. Res.* 1979, 1, 101

26 Podreka, I., Suess, E., Goldenberg, G. *et al.* Initial experience with [99m]Tc- HMPAO brain SPECT. *J. Nucl. Med.* 1987, 28, 1657

27 Rees, J.E., Bull, J.W.D., Ross Russel, R.W. *et al.* Regional cerebral blood-flow in transient ischaemic attacks. *Lancet* 1970, 2, 1210

28 Russel, D., Dybevold, S., Kjartansson, O. *et al.* Cerebral vasoreactivity and blood flow before and 3 months after carotid endarterectomy. *Stroke* 1990, 21, 1029

29 Skinhoj, E., Hoedt-Rasmussen, K., Paulson, O.B. and Lassen, N.A. Regional cerebral blood flow and its autoregulation in patients with transient focal cerebral ischaemic attacks. *Neurology* 1970, 20, 485

30 Toyama, H., Takeshita, G., Takeuchi, A. *et al.* SPECT measurement of cerebral hemodynamics in transient ischaemic attack patients. Evaluation of pathogenesis and detection of misery perfusion. *Jpn J. Nucl. Med.* 1989, 26, 1487

31 Vorstrup, S., Hemmingsen, R., Henriksen, L. *et al.* Regional cerebral blood flow in patients with transient ischaemic attacks studied by Xenon-133 inhalation and emission tomography. *Stroke* 1983, 14, 903

32 Yonekura, M., Austin, G., Poll, N. and Hayward, W. Evaluation of cerebral blood flow in patients with transient ischaemic attacks and minor stroke. *Surg. Neurol.* 1980, 15, 58

33 Laloux, P., Doat, M., Brichant, C. *et al.* Clinical usefulness of [99m]Tc- HMPAO SPECT imaging to map the ischaemic lesion in acute stroke: a reevaluation. *Cerebrovasc. Dis.* 1994, 4, 280

34 Moretti, J.L., Defer, G., Tamgac, F. *et al.* Comparison of brain SPECT using 99m-Tc-ECD (L,LECD) and I-123 IMP in cortical and subcortical strokes. *J. Cereb. Blood Flow Metab.* 1994, 14, S84

35 Laloux, P., Jamart, J., Meurisse, H. *et al.* Persisting perfusion defect in transient ischemic attacks: a new clinically useful subgroup. *Stroke* 1996, 27, 425

36 Grunwald, F., Broich, K., Kropp, J. *et al.* SPECT in reversible symptoms of cerebrovascular disease. *Nuklear Medizin* 1989, 28, 221

37 Cikrit, D.F., Burt, R.W., Dalsing, M.C. *et al.* Acetazolamide enhanced single photon emission computed tomography (SPECT) evaluation of cerebral perfusion before and after carotid endarterectomy. *J. Vasc. Surg.* 1992, 15, 747

38 Piepgras, A., Leinsinger, G., Kirsch, C.M. and Schmiedek, P. STA-MCA bypass in bilateral carotid artery occlusion: clinical results and long-term effect on cerebrovascular reserve capacity. *Neurol. Res.* 1994, 16, 104

39 Vorstrup, S., Engell, H.C., Lindewald, H. and Lassen, N.A. Hemodynamically significant stenosis of the internal carotid artery treated with endarterectomy. *J. Neurosurg.* 1984, 60, 1070

40 Evans, B.A., Sicks, J.D. and Whisnant, J.P. Factors affecting survival and occurrence of stroke in patients with transient ischaemic attacks. *Mayo Clin. Proc.* 1994, 69, 416

41 Muuronen, A. and Kaste, M. Outcome of 314 patients with transient ischaemic attacks. *Stroke* 1982, 13, 24

42 Whisnant, J.P., Matsumoto, N. and Elveback, L.R. Transient cerebral ischaemic attacks in a community: Rochester, Minnesota, 1955 through 1969. *Mayo Clin. Proc.* 1973, 48, 194

43 Brust, J.C.M. Transient ischaemic attacks: natural history and anticoagulation. *Neurology* 1977, 27, 701

44 Ferro, J.M. and Crespo, M. Prognosis after transient ischaemic attack and ischaemic stroke in young adults. *Stroke* 1994, 25, 1611

45 Gautier, J.C., Juillard, J.B.E., Loron, P.L. *et al.* Time interval between transient ischaemic attacks and cerebral infarction. *Stroke* 1987, 18, 298

46 Howard, G., Toole, J.F., Frye-Pierson, J. and Hinshelwood, L.C. Factors influencing the survival of 451 transient ischaemic attack patients. *Stroke* 1987, 18, 552

47 Eliasziw, M., Streifler, J.Y., Spence, J.D. *et al.* Prognosis for patients following a transient ischaemic attack with and without a cerebral infarction on brain CT. *Neurology* 1995, 45, 428

48 Heuser, D., Astrup, J., Lassen, N.A. and Betz, E. Brain carbonic acidosis after acetazolamide. *Acta Physiol. Scand.* 1975, 93, 380

49 Severinghaus, J.W. and Cotev, S. Carbonic acidosis and cerebral vasodilation after diamox. *Scand. J. Clin. Invest.* 1968, 1(102)E

50 Tagaki, Y., Hata, T., Ishitobi, K. and Kitagawa, Y. Cerebral blood flow and CO_2 reactivity before and after carotid endarterectomy. *Acta Neurol. Scand.* 1979, 72, 506

51 Burt, R.W., Witt, R.M., Cikrit, D.F. and Reddy, R.V. Carotid artery disease: evaluation with acetazolamide-enhanced Tc-99m HMPAO SPECT. *Radiology* 1992, 182, 461

52 Knop, J., Thie, A., Fuchs, C. *et al.* 99mTc-HMPAO-SPECT with acetazolamide challenge to detect hemodynamic compromise in occlusive cerebrovascular disease. *Stroke* 1992, 23, 1733

53 Laloux, P., Richelle, F., Meurice, H. and De Coster, P. Cerebral blood flow and perfusion reserve capacity in hemodynamic carotid transient ischaemic attacks due to innominate artery stenosis. *J. Nucl. Med.* 1995, 36, 1268

54 Knapp, W.H., von Kummer, R. and Kübler, W. Imaging of cerebral blood flow-to-volume distribution using SPECT. *J. Nucl. Med.* 1986, 27, 465

55 Powers, W.J. Cerebral hemodynamics in ischaemic cerebrovascular disease. *Ann. Neurol.* 1991, 29, 231

56 Weiller, C., Ringelstein, E.B., Reiche, W. and Buell, U. Clinical and hemodynamic aspects of low-flow infarcts. *Stroke* 1991, 22, 1117

57 Baron, J.C., Bousser, M.G., Comar, D. and Castaigne, P. 'Crossed cerebellar diaschisis' in human supratentorial brain infarction. *Trans. Am. Neurol. Assoc.* 1980, 105, 459

58 Hoedt-Rasmussen, K. and Skinhoj, E. Transneuronal depression of the cerebral hemispheric metabolism in man. *Acta Neurol. Scand.* 1964, 40, 41

59 Kempisky, W.H. Experimental study of distant effects of acute focal brain injury. *Arch. Neurol. Psychiatr.* 1958, 79, 376

60 Lenzi, G.L., Frackowiak, R.S.J. and Jones, T. Regional cerebral blood flow (CBF), oxygen utilization ($CMRO_2$) and oxygen extraction ratio (OER) in acute hemispheric stroke. *J. Cereb. Blood Flow Metab.* 1981, 1, 504

61 Mies, G., Auer, L.M., Ebhardt, G. *et al.* Flow and neuronal density in tissue surrounding chronic infarction. *Stroke* 1983, 14, 22

62 Pappata, S., Mazoyer, B., Tran Dinh, S. *et al.* Effects of capsular or thalamic stroke on metabolism in the cortex and cerebellum: a positron tomography study. *Stroke* 1990, 21, 519

63 Vorstrup, S., Lassen, N.A., Henriksen, L. *et al.* CBF before and after extracranial-intracranial bypass surgery in patients with ischaemic cerebrovascular disease studied with ^{133}Xe-inhalation tomography. *Stroke* 1985, 16, 616

64 Bozzao, L., Fantozzi, L.M., Bastianello, S. *et al.* Early collateral blood supply and late parenchymal brain damage in patients with middle cerebral artery occlusion. *Stroke* 1989, 20, 735

65 Giubilei, F., Lenzi, G.L., Di Piero, V. *et al.* Predictive value of brain perfusion single-photon emission computed tomography in acute ischaemic stroke. *Stroke* 1990, 21, 895

66 Paulson, O.B. Regional cerebral blood flow in apoplexy due to occlusion of the middle cerebral artery. *Neurology* 1970, 20, 63

67 Raynaud, C., Rancurel, G., Samson, Y. *et al.* Pathophysiologic study of chronic infarcts with I-123 isopropyl iodo-amphetamine (IMP): the importance of periinfarct area. *Stroke* 1987, 18, 21

68 Astrup, J., Siesjö, B.K. and Symon, L. Thresholds in cerebral ischaemia - the ischaemic penumbra. *Stroke* 1981, 12, 723

69 Lenzi, G.L., Frackowiak, R.S.J. and Jones, T. Cerebral oxygen metabolism and blood flow in human cerebral ischaemic infarction. *J. Cereb. Blood Flow Metab.* 1982 2, 321

70 Nakano, S., Kinoshita, K., Jinnouchi, S. *et al.* Critical cerebral blood flow thresholds studied by SPECT using xenon-133 and iodine-123 iodoamphetamine. *J. Nucl. Med.* 1989, 30, 337

71 Lassen, N.A. Incomplete cerebral infarction. Focal incomplete ischaemic tissue necrosis not leading to emollision. *Stroke* 1982, 13, 522

72 Scholz, W. Die nicht zur Erweichung führenden unvollständigen Gewebsnekrosen. (Elektive Parenchyümnekrose) in 'Handbuch der speziellen patologischen Anatomie und Histologie XIII', (Eds. B. Bandteil, O. Lubarsch, F. Henke, R. Rössle, W. Scholz), Springer Verlag, Berlin, 1957, p.1284

73 Lassen, N.A., Olsen, T.S. and Hogaard, K. Incomplete infarction. A CT-negative irreversible ischaemic brain lesion. *J. Cereb. Blood Flow Metab.* 1983, 3, 602

74 Marcoux, F.W., Morawetz, R.B., Crowell, R.M. *et al.* Differential regional vulnerability in transient focal ischaemia. *Stroke* 1982, 13, 339

75 Garcia, J.H., Wagner, S., Liu, K.F. *et al.* Neurological deficit and extent of neuronal necrosis attributable to middle cerebral artery occlusion in rats: statistical validation. *Stroke* 1995, 26, 627

76 Brun, A. Pathology and pathophysiology of cerebrovascular dementia: pure subgroups of obstructive and hypoperfusive etiology. *Dementia* 1994, 5, 145

77 Frackowiak, R.S.J. The pathophysiology of human cerebral ischaemia: a new perspective obtained with positron tomography. *Q. J. Med.* 1985, 57, 713

78 Nedergaard, M., Astrup, J. and Klinken, L. Cell density and cortex thickness in the border zone surrounding old infarcts in the human brain. *Stroke* 1984, 15, 1033

79 Torvick, A. and Svindland, A. Is there a transitional zone between brain infarcts and the surrounding brain? A histological study. *Acta Neurol. Scand.* 1986, 74, 365

80 Holl, K., Heissler, H.E., Nemati, M. *et al.* Die Wirkung der Acetazolamin-induzierten, endogenen Volumenbelastung des zerebrospinalen Systems auf den intrakraniellen Druck. Diamox,-Wirkung auf den intra kraniellen Druck (ICP). *Neurochirurgia* 1990, 33, 29

81 Rancurel, G., Raynaud, C., Cabanis, E. *et al.* Résultats obtenus dans dix cas d'infarctus cérébraux sylviens récents par l'I 123 isopropyl-iodoamphetamine avec la gammatomographie à haute sensibilité: essai d'exploration de l'aire peri-infarctus et de la pénombre ischémique in 'Current Problems in Neurology - Pénombre et ischémie cérébrale', John Libbey, Paris, 1986, p.63

82 Sacco, R.L. Current epidemiology of stroke in 'Current re view of cerebrovascular disease', (Eds. M. Fisher, J. Bogousslavsky), Current Medicine, Philadelphia, 1993, p.3

83 Davis, S., Andrews, J., Lichtenstein, M. *et al.* A single-photon emission computed tomography study of hypoperfusion after subarachnoid haemorrhage. *Stroke* 1990, 21, 252

84 Lewis, D.H., Eskridge, J.M., Newell, D.W. *et al.* Brain SPECT and the effect of cerebral angioplasty in delayed ischaemia due to vasospasm. *J. Nucl. Med.* 1992, 33, 1789

85 Soucy, I.P., McNamara, D., Mohr, G. *et al.* Evaluation of vasospasm secondary to subarachnoid haemorrhage with ^{99m}Tc-hexamethyl-propyleneamine oxime (HMPAO) tomoscintigraphy. *J. Nucl. Med.* 1990, 31, 972

86 Barker, F.G. II. and Heros, R.C. Clinical aspects of vasospasm. *Neurosurg. Clin. N. Am.* 1990, 1, 277

87 Biller, J., Godersky, J.C. and Adams, H.P. Jr. Management of aneurysmal subarachnoid haemorrhage. *Curr. Concepts Cerebrovas. Dis. Stroke* 1988, 23, 13

88 Voldby, B. Alterations in vasomotor reactivity in subarachnoid haemorrhage in 'Cerebral blood flow', (Ed. J. H. Wood), McGraw-Hill, New York, 1987, p.402

89 Flamm, E.S., Adams, H.P. Jr., Beck, D.W. *et al.* Dose-escalation study of intravenous nicardipine in patients with aneurysmal subarachnoid haemorrhage. *J. Neurosurg.* 1988, 68, 393

90 Pickard, J.D., Murray, G.D., Illingworth, R. *et al.* Effect of oral nimodipine on cerebral infarction and outcome after subarachnoid haemorrhage: British aneurysm nimodipine trial. *Br. Med. J.* 1989, 298, 636

91 Eskridge, J.M., Newell, D.W. and Pendleton, G.A. Transluminal angioplasty for treatment of vasospasm. *Neurosurg. Clin. N. Am.* 1990, 1, 387

92 Higashida, R.T., Halbach, V.V., Cahan, L.D. *et al.* Transluminal angioplasty for treatment of intracranial arterial vasospasm. *J. Neurosurg.* 1989, 71, 648

93 Newell, D.W., Eskridge, J.M., Mayberg, M.R. *et al.* Angioplasty for the treatment of symptomatic vasospasm following subarachnoid haemorrhage. *J. Neurosurg.* 1989, 71, 654

94 Zubkov, Y.N., Nikiforov, B.M. and Shustin, V.A. Balloon catheter technique for dilatation of constricted cerebral arteries after aneurysmal subarachnoid haemorrhage. *Acta Neurochir.* 1984, 70, 65

95 Mani, R.L. and Eisenberg, R.L. Complication of catheter cerebral arteriography: analysis of 5,000 procedures. II. Relation of complication rates to clinical and arteriographic diagnoses. *A. J. R.* 1978, 131, 867

96 Perret, G. and Nishioka, H. Report on the cooperative study of intracranial aneurysms and subarachnoid haemorrhage. Section IV. Cerebral angiography. An analysis of the diagnostic value and complications of carotid and vertebral angiography in 5,484 patients. *J. Neurosurg.* 1966, 25, 98

97 Caplan, L.R., Brass, L.M., De Witt, L.D. *et al.* Transcranial Doppler ultrasound. Present status. *Neurology* 1990, 40, 696

98 Aaslid, R., Huber, P. and Nornes, H. Evaluation of cerebrovascular spasm with transcranial Doppler ultrasound. *J. Neurosurg.* 1984, 60, 37

99 Harders, A.G. and Gilsbach, J.M. Time course of blood velocity changes related to vasospasm in the circle of Willis measured by transcranial Doppler ultrasound. *J. Neurosurg.* 1987, 66, 718

100 Seiler, R.W., Grolimund, P., Aaslid, R. *et al.* Cerebral vasospasm evaluated by transcranial ultrasound correlated with clinical grade and CT-visualized subarachnoid haemorrhage. *J. Neurosurg.* 1986, 64, 594

101 Sekhar, L.N., Weschsler, L.R., Yonas, H. *et al.* Value of transcranial Doppler examination in the diagnosis of cerebral vasospasm after subarachnoid haemorrhage. *Neurosurgery* 1988, 22, 813

102 Kontos, H.A. Validity of cerebral arterial blood flow calculations from velocity measurements (editorial). *Stroke* 1989, 20, 1

103 Tranquart, F., Ades, P.E., Groussin, P. *et al.* Postoperative assessment of cerebral blood flow in subarachnoid haemorrhage by means of (99m)Tc-HMPAO tomography. *Eur. J. Neurol. Med.* 1993, 20, 53

104 Ades, P.E., Groussin, P., Arbeille, P. and Rieant, J.F. Apport de la tomoscintigraphie à l' HMPAO Tc99 dans la surveillance des ischémies post-hémorragies méningées. *Circ. Métab. Cerveau* 1989, 6, 262

105 Hellman, R.S. and Tikofsky, R.S. An overview of the contribution of regional cerebral blood flow studies in cerebrovascular disease: is there a role for single photon emission computed tomography? *Semin. Nucl. Med.* 1990, 10, 303

106 Kimura, T., Shinoda, J. and Funakoshi, T. Prediction of cerebral infarction due to vasospasm following aneurysmal subarachnoid haemorrhage using acetazolamide-activated (123)I-IMP SPECT. *Acta Neurochir.* 1993, 123, 125

107 Maini, C.L., Castellano, G., Benech, F. *et al.* (99)Tc(m)-HMPAO brain SPECT in subarachnoid haemorrhage. *Nucl. Med. Commun.* 1990, 11, 491

108 Rawluk, D., Smith, F.W., Deans, H.E. *et al.* Technetium 99m HMPAO scanning in patients with subarachnoid haemorrhage: a preliminary study. *Br. J. Radiol.* 1988, 61, 26

109 Rosen, J.M., Butala, A.V., Oropello, J.M. *et al.* Postoperative changes on brain SPECT imaging after aneurysmal subarachnoid haemorrhage: a potential pitfall in the evaluation of vasospasm. *Clin. Nucl. Med.* 1994, 19, 595

110 Shinoda, J., Kimura, T., Funakoshi, T. *et al.* Acetazolamide reactivity on cerebral blood flow in patients with subarachnoid haemorrhage. *Acta Neurochir.* 1991, 109, 102

111 Ueda, T., Kinoshita, K. and Watanabe, K. Local cerebral blood flow measurement using (123)I-IMP SPECT in patients with cerebrovascular diseases. *Neurol. Med. Chir.* 1987, 27, 415

112 Yamakami, I., Isobe, K., Yamaura, T. and Makino, H. Vasospasm and regional cerebral blood flow (rCBF) in patients with ruptured intracranial aneurysm: serial rCBF studies with the Xenon-133 inhalation method. *Neurosurgery* 1983, 13, 394

113 Yonas, H., Good, W.F., Gur, D. *et al.* Mapping cerebral blood flow by xenon-enhanced computed tomography: clinical experience. *Radiology* 1984, 152, 435

114 Yonas, H., Wolfson, S.K. Jr., Gur, D. *et al.* Clinical experience with the use of xenon-enhanced CT blood flow mapping in cerebral vascular disease. *Stroke* 1984, 15, 443

115 Mickey, B., Vorstrup, S., Voldby, B. *et al.* Serial measurement of regional cerebral blood flow in patients with SAH using 133Xe inhalation and emission computerized tomography. *J. Neurosurg.* 1984, 60, 916

116 Geraud, G., Tremoulet, M., Guell, A. and Bes, A. The prognostic value of noninvasive CBF measurement in subarachnoid haemorrhage. *Stroke* 1984, 15, 301

117 Hayashi, M., Kobayashi, H., Kawano, H. *et al.* Cerebral blood flow and ICP patterns in patients with communicating hydrocephalus after aneurysm rupture. *J. Neurosurg.* 1984, 61, 30

118 Knuckey, N.W., Fox, R.A., Surveyor, I. and Stokes, B.A.R. Early cerebral blood flow and computerized tomography in predicting ischaemia after aneurysm rupture. *J. Neurosurg.* 1985, 62, 850

119 Merory, J., Thomas, D.J., Humphrey, P.R.D. *et al.* Cerebral blood flow after surgery for recent subarachnoid haemorrhage. *J. Neurol. Neurosurg. Psychiatry* 1980, 43, 214

120 Meyer, C.H., Lowe, D., Meyer, M. *et al.* Progressive change in cerebral blood flow during the first three weeks after subarachnoid haemorrhage. *Neurosurgery* 1983, 12, 58

121 Rosenstein, J., Wang, A.D.-J., Symon, L. and Susuki, M. Relationship between hemispheric cerebral blood flow, central conduction time and clinical grade in aneurysmal subarachnoid haemorrhage. *J. Neurosurg.* 1985, 62, 25

122 Holl, K., Nemati, N., Heissler, H. et al. Chronic cerebrovascular insufficiency on the xenon CT scan. *Neurosurg. Rev.* 1989, 12, 205

123 Wilkinson, H.A. Cerebral blood flow response to acetazolamide. *J. Neurosurg.* 1989, 70, 15

SPECT in Neurology and Psychiatry, edited by P.P. De Deyn, R.A. Dierckx, A. Alavi and B.A. Pickut
© 1997 John Libbey & Company Ltd, pp. 335–346

Applications of rCBF Brain SPECT and NMR Imaging in the Evaluation of Stroke: Implications in Rehabilitation Prognosis

Chapter

40

J.M. Mountz, G. Deutsch, H.P. Hetherington, C. Inampudi,
E. San Pedro, H.-G. Liu, J.W. Pan, G.F. Mason,
M. Mennemeier, J.S. Richards, G.M. Pohost

Introduction

In general, two competing but not necessarily mutually exclusive models can explain the mechanisms underlying the often observed recovery of classic neurological and cognitive function (e.g., limb movement, speech production, language comprehension, perceptual skills) after stroke. One model is that recovery essentially reflects resolution of a temporary cessation of function in brain tissue not directly destroyed by the stroke but nevertheless affected via deafferentation and a consequent 'diaschisis'. The second model is that recovery involves spared brain taking on functions previously performed by damaged brain tissue. Thus, the first model emphasises changes associated with temporarily affected brain, whereas the second accentuates reorganisation in non-involved brain.

Specific aims

The goal of this project is to identify the recoverable component of the stroke penumbra (peri-infarction region) by separating anatomic, vascular, and metabolic defects in post acute stroke using the techniques of rCBF brain SPECT, MRI, and MRSI. To achieve this characterisation of the stroke region, four types of measurements were performed, as follows:

1. Quantification of the extent of structural versus blood flow impairment in post-stroke patients via high resolution MRI and ^{99m}Tc-HMPAO SPECT brain studies.
2. Use of cerebrovascular (CV) reactivity testing with rest/stress SPECT brain scans in stroke patients for the purpose of assessing vascular reserve and specifically identifying the presence or absence of a vascular constraint component to any rCBF reduction seen outside the region of cerebral infarction.
3. Performance of ^{1}H magnetic resonance spectroscopic imaging (MRSI) studies in stroke patients for the purpose of providing metabolic evidence of the presence or absence of an ischaemic component to any rCBF reduction seen outside the infarction zone, and to permit assessment of the presence of selective neuronal loss in regions defined as diaschisis by the SPECT.
4. Comparison of the SPECT rCBF reactivity findings in the peri-infarction region with the MRSI results.

Division of Nuclear Medicine,
University of Alabama at
Birmingham Medical Center, 619
19th Street South, Birmingham,
AL 35233, USA

Hypothesis and significance

It is proposed that the physiological basis for the initial neurological and cognitive impairment associated with stroke is due to the combined effects of absent tissue (infarction) and reduced neurometabolic activity outside of the infarction.

Since the amount of neural tissue with diaschisis identifies the amount of affected brain that has the potential for recovery, it is hypothesised that quantification of the diaschisis volume is highly correlated with stroke recovery[1]. Identification of diaschisis can be achieved in two ways:

1. By determining the volume of brain with reduced regional cerebral blood flow (rCBF) but with good CV reactivity using resting state rCBF brain SPECT compared with stress rCBF brain SPECT measurements.
2. By determining the metabolic abnormalities in the regions with presumed diaschisis by ^{1}H magnetic resonance spectroscopic imaging (MRSI).

SPECT

To characterise the vascular state of the penumbra defect volume, cerebrovascular reactivity to acetazolamide was used. It is hypothesised that CV reactivity (using intravenous acetazolamide) identifies the presence or absence of vascular constraints and can be used in assessing the nature of rCBF reductions observed in resting state rCBF brain SPECT studies. Good rCBF reactivity to acetazolamide stress in a region with low baseline rCBF indicates vascular adequacy. These studies therefore provide a method of discriminating between diaschisis and ischaemic regions since low baseline rCBF due to neuronal diaschisis or selective neuronal loss will become more normal at stress.

It is hypothesised that the defect volume seen on functional SPECT imaging in excess of the defect volume seen on morphologic structure MRI indicates impaired, viable, and potentially recoverable brain tissue[2]. By converting rCBF defect volume and anatomic defect volume to common comparable units (i.e. cc), a SPECT/MRI defect volume ratio can be calculated that has predictive value concerning stroke recovery potential.

MRSI

It is hypothesised that MRSI lactate measurements can provide an essential complementary assessment of an ischaemic versus a diaschiatic cause for reduced metabolism and rCBF in the peri-infarction region by indicating the presence or absence of anaerobic glycolysis. Lactate measurements may be elevated at the rim of the infarction due to leukocyte infiltration. However, elevation of lactate in the stroke penumbra distant to the rim provides evidence of ischaemia as a result of its production during the anaerobic glycolysis accompanying oxygen deprivation (lactate accumulates because it is removed less efficiently due to low perfusion).

In regions of 'pure' diaschisis, steady state ^{1}H MRSI regional measurements of N-acetyl aspartate (NAA), creatine (CR), choline (CH), and lactate (LAC) are all expected to be normal since the reduced metabolism is presumed to be due solely to deafferentation of normal stimulatory input to the region and not to any real rCBF or metabolite constraints. However, if selective neuronal loss is contributing to the low rCBF, NAA will be reduced. NAA appears to be a neuronal marker and is expected to be low in regions with neuronal loss (as well as in the chronic ischaemic conditions described above). Choline, as an indicator of increased membrane breakdown, may be increased in areas of neuronal loss (as well as in the ischaemic conditions described above) but should be normal in 'pure' diaschisis. Creatine is an intracellular compound which serves as a marker for cell integrity. Creatine is reduced where cells are dead, but can be elevated in gliosis.

Stroke rehabilitation

Presently, rehabilitation of stroke patients is composed of varying combinations of compensatory and facilitatory techniques. Compensatory training techniques emphasise attention to unaffected neuro-muscular components to improve functional status. Facilitatory techniques attempt to promote or hasten the recovery of affected extremities to a normal movement pattern[3-5]. Since the resolution of diaschisis is one mechanism of neurological recovery from stroke, by being able to document diaschisis, and by showing an association between neurological and functional recovery with the resolution of diaschisis, a better understanding of the stroke recovery process will be realised. This understanding should foster the ability to better design rehabilitation strategies that can be tailored to the individual patient's neurological deficits.

Methods

Subject selection criteria

Three major categories of cerebrovascular disease from 11 patients, based on clinical neurological work up including standard CT or MRI, duplex carotid ultrasound, carotid angiography, and transcranial Doppler (TCD) were studied.

1. Unilateral stroke without haemodynamic abnormality.
2. Unilateral stroke with cerebral haemodynamic insufficiency.
3. Unilateral cerebral haemodynamic insufficiency (without stroke), as control for condition B.

SPECT methods

During rest studies subjects received an intravenous injection of approximately 25 mCi ^{99m}Tc-HMPAO, where ambient light and noise were reduced as much as possible. During vasoreactive stress tests, Diamox rCBF brain SPECT was performed by acquiring two ^{99m}Tc-HMPAO brain SPECT scan acquisitions back-to-back. During the first scan at rest 8 mCi ^{99m}Tc-HMPAO was injected. This scan was immediately followed by an i.v. injection of 1 gram Diamox. After 15 min, 32 mCi ^{99m}Tc-HMPAO was injected and the second rCBF brain SPECT scan was performed.

SPECT image acquisition was performed by the ADAC dual head SPECT gamma camera with the following acquisition parameters: 64 equal angular stops for each head (128 total views) at 30 sec/stop acquiring 90,000 counts/stop over 360°. The camera was equipped with low energy, high resolution collimators. The camera extrinsic resolution for a 25 cm field of view using a 128x128 matrix in air was approximately 8.5 mm FWHM (normal tracer dose) at an object radius of 11 cm for an average brain acquisition rotation radius of 13 cm. Data were stored and processed on an ADAC Pegasys workstation and analysis system in a 128 by 128 digital matrix using reconstruction filters optimised to the count activity per pixel[6].

SPECT semiquantitative analysis method

Annular cortical regions-of-interest (ROIs) were defined on the brain SPECT scan section of interest using a semi-automated ROI method yielding the values of maximum and average counts per pixel in 15° or 30° sectors progressing circumferentially around the brain; clockwise from the 12 o'clock position. The outer border is defined by the location of the pixels having counts per pixel values at 50% of the mean counts per pixel in the section under analysis. The inner border is defined at an equal-angular distance of 8 pixels (1.56 cm) directed radially inward from the outer boundary. This circumferential cortical ROI generator algorithm is standard at the University

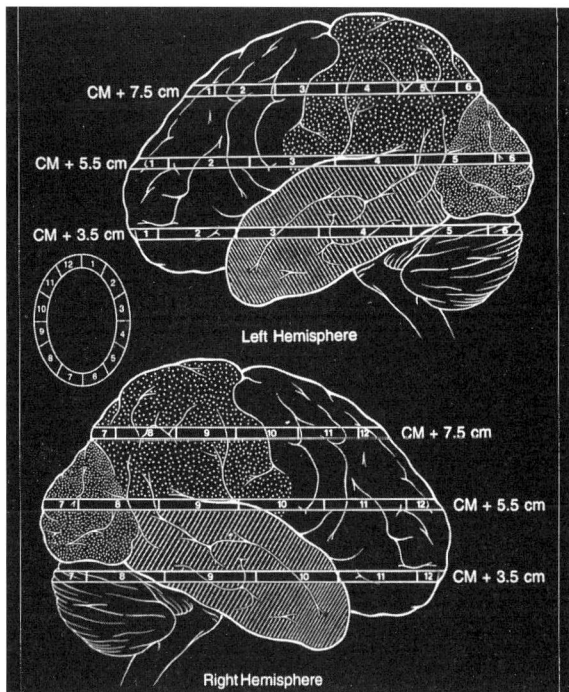

Figure 1a Illustration of the lateral view of the left and right hemispheres of the brain. Drawn on the hemispheres are the positions of the sections typically sampled for semi-quantitative analysis. Three levels positioned at canthomeatal (CM) +3.5cm, CM+5.5cm, and CM+7.5cm. Also shown on the diagram is an oval illustrating the positions of the regions of interest progressing from the anterior left hemisphere (region 1) clockwise to the anterior right hemisphere (region 12). (From reference 8, with permission)

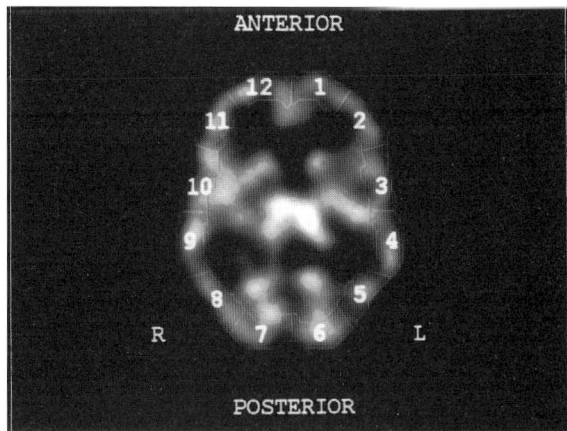

Figure 1b Actual SPECT scan section demonstrating the outer border, inner border, and the subdivisions for each cortical region of interest for equal angular 30° sectors. Using these regions of interest one obtains 12 cortical sampling areas from the frontal, lateral, and posterior portions of the brain

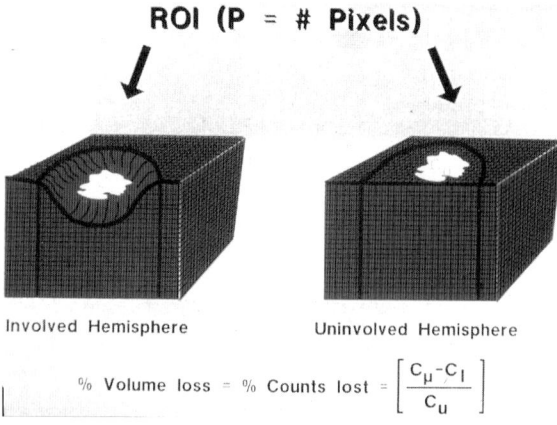

Figure 2 Illustration of the relationship between the percentage count loss and the percentage volume loss for the involved (stroke) and uninvolved hemispheres of the brain. To properly draw the regions of interest one must completely circumscribe the stroke defect. In addition, there should be normal cerebral perfusion to the uninvolved hemisphere (i.e. the hemisphere contralateral to the stroke). (From reference 9, with permission)

of Alabama at Birmingham[7,8], and is illustrated in Figure 1. The ROI count value is the average of the top 10% of counts per pixel within that ROI. Maximum counts per pixel values were also used.

The method to measure SPECT defect size in unilateral cerebrovascular disease patients has been described in detail in prior reports[9]. The method provides a SPECT volume defect in cubic centimetres as illustrated in Figure 2, and is expressed by the formula:

$$V_T = V_P \times \sum_{i=1}^{n} [(Mi-Si)/Mi] \times Pi$$

where V_T is the total SPECT volume defect of the lesion, V_P is the volume (cc) of the individual pixel, Si represents the counts within the entire stroke region on the ith section, Mi represents the counts within the mirrored region in the uninvolved hemisphere on the same section, and Pi is the number of pixels in the region of interest; the sum on i is taken overall scan sections that have an rCBF SPECT defect.

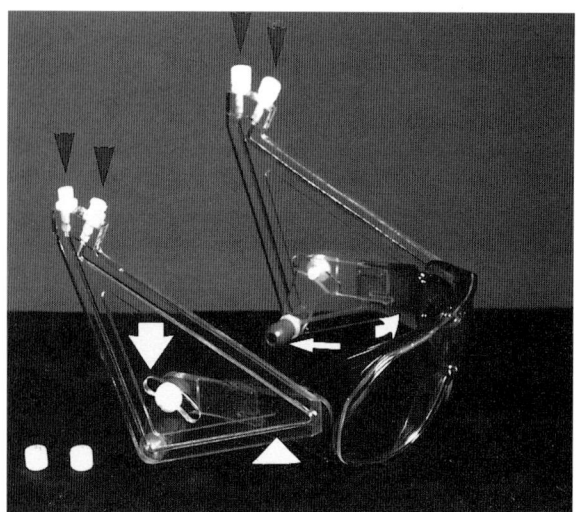

Figure 3a Picture of the reference system. The earplugs (white thin arrow) provide a stable anchor in the external auditory meatus. The adjustable locking slots (white curved arrow) fit the supporting glasses frame firmly to the head. The triangles are pivoted in the plastic slot (white thick arrows) to provide consistent alignment of the baseline (white arrowhead) to the canthomeatal (CM) line. The tubing filling ports (black arrowheads) are easily filled with liquid contrast or tracer by a standard syringe. (From reference 12, with permission)

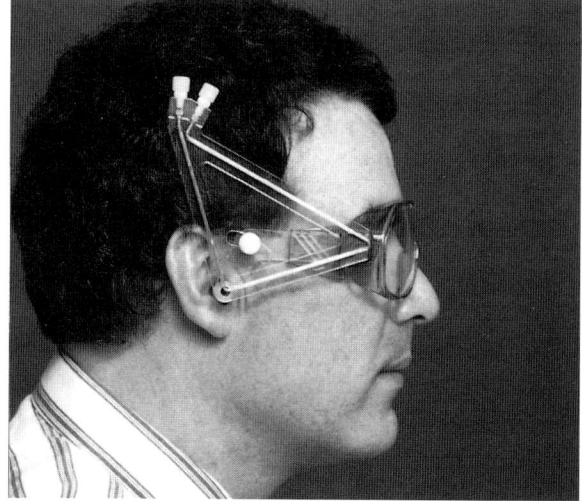

Figure 3b Picture of the reference system properly positioned on a subject. The reference system is placed on each subject with similar ease as putting on one's own glasses. Once the glasses frame is firmly in place, the triangles are independently rotated parallel to the subjects CM line. (From reference 12, with permission)

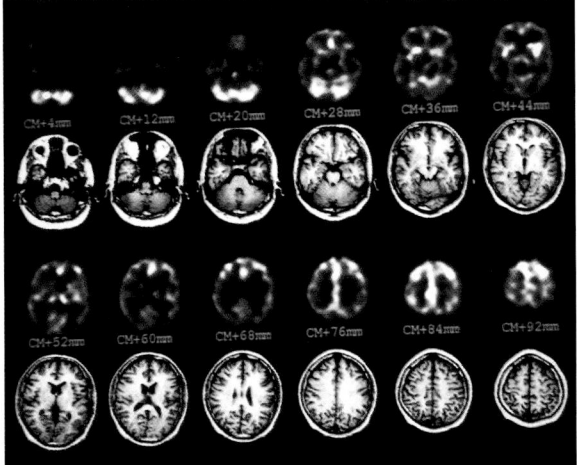
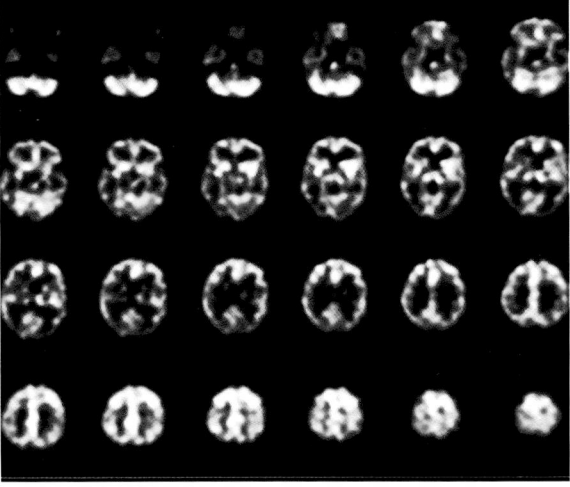

Figure 4a Example of a normal subject. The SPECT brain scan has been precisely co-registered with the MRI scan and sections are displayed parallel to and serially above the canthomeatal line at levels indicated on the figure. Comparison of normal brain SPECT scan perfusion can be correlated with the corresponding anatomic structure on the MRI scan section positioned below each brain SPECT scan section. (From reference 13, with permission)

Figure 4c By use of the reference system device and co-registration software, the SPECT scan is sectioned and oriented exactly to match the MRI scan sections shown in Figure 4b

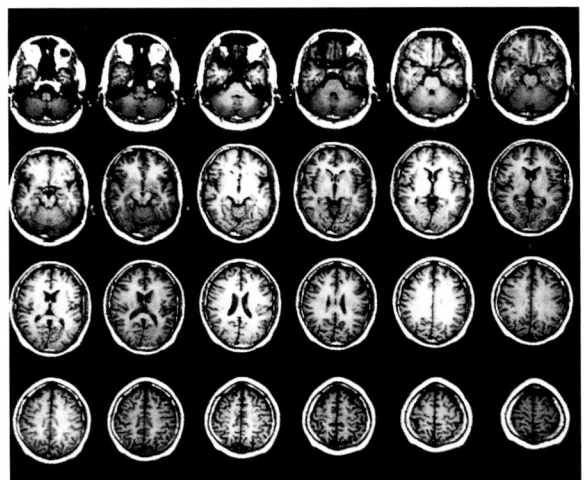
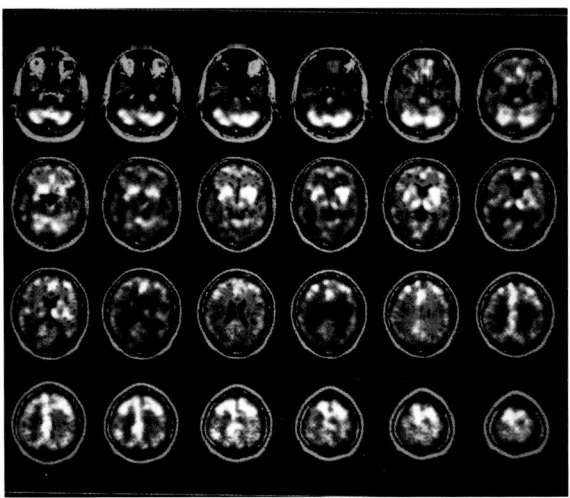

Figure 4b T1 weighted sections of an MRI scan with section thickness of approximately 4mm. The scan is orientated parallel to the canthomeatal line

Figure 4d Images obtained by combining the MRI and SPECT images shown in figures 4b and 4c to obtain 'fusion images' in which the observer can see structure and function simultaneously

Since it is well known that the rCBF in the stroke zone is never absolutely zero[10], and is bevelled at the edges due to the inherent relatively low resolution of SPECT as compared with CT or MRI, this equation is of great utility since it allows accurate calculation of a 'hypothetical volume of zero perfusion' by comparing the stroke hemisphere with the 'uninvolved' brain hemisphere. This index provides an objective method to quantify the rCBF SPECT defect size volume (in cc) relative to the volume of necrotic tissue easily measured on the CT or MRI scans (in cc). The MRI defect size is defined by the sum of all areas of low signal intensity (infarcted tissue) visualised on contiguous T1 weighted MRI sections. The use of this measurement has been successfully implemented both in the evaluation of stroke outcome prognosis, and comparison of the stroke induced rCBF defect size with other stroke parameters[2,11]. SPECT and MRI images were accurately co-aligned using a reference system technique standard at the University of Alabama at Birmingham[12,13] as illustrated in Figure 3. Figure 4 shows the accuracy of co-registration by illustrating a series of MRI images, accurately co-aligned [99mTc]-HMPAO brain SPECT, and fusion images composed of combining the MRI and co-aligned SPECT images.

T [1]H-SI methods

Contributions from extra-cerebral lipids were suppressed using an adiabatic inversion pulse followed by dephasing gradients and an inversion recovery delay optimised to suppress lipids as shown in Figure 5. Water suppression was accomplished using a broad band semi-selective refocussing pulse.

SI data were acquired using TR/TIR/TE of (2000/265/50). The spectroscopic image was acquired using a FOV of 240x240mm utilising 32x32 phase encodes with a slice thickness of 1cm. The spectral domain was processed using a convolution difference of 50Hz to eliminate broad water components followed by 3Hz of exponential broadening. Two spatial and one spectral Fourier transforms were performed to generate the 2D SI data[14-17].

All voxels within the ROI were analysed using NMR1 and the line width, resonance area, and chemical shift were determined. From these data the CR/NAA, CH/NAA, and LAC/NAA ratios were determined for all pixels.

A database of metabolite ratios from 10 healthy volunteers for grey and white matter volumes for structures within the parietal, occipital, frontal, and temporal lobes was used for comparison. To visualise those regions in patients that show significant differences from normal data, all voxels within the

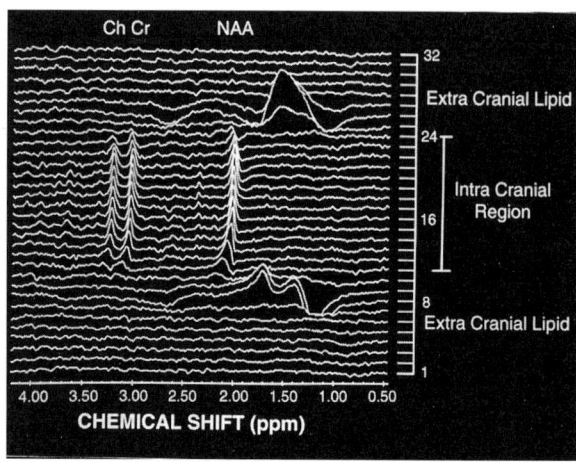

Figure 5 [1]H-SI stacked plot demonstration the ability to suppress intracranial lipid contamination from the scalp, and the absence of intracranial lactate (which would appear at 1.35 ppm if present) in a normal subject. (From reference 7, with permission)

selected ROI were compared with the normal data using a highlighted colour scale to demonstrate those ratios which were greater than four standard deviations for normal white matter and two standard deviations for normal grey matter.

Results

Limited peri-infarction region

Figure 6a shows MRI, SPECT, and SPECT-MRI fusion images of a 46 year old man who suffered a right MCA territory stroke with resulting left hemiparesis. Figure 6b shows that there is no significant diaschisis volume or ischaemic residual associated with the stroke. The calculated right MCA territory defect volume from the anatomic scan (Figure 6a) was 57.9 cc. The rest and Diamox SPECT (Figure 6b) have essentially equal defect volumes of hypothetical zero perfusion (67.4 cc, and 63.3 cc, respectively). The cortical circumferential profile plots (Figure 6c) are virtually identical comparing the rest with the stress condition. The NAA image (Figure 6d) shows essentially no metabolic signal from the anatomic region of the stroke. Spectra taken from positions A, B, and C (labelled on Figure 6d) demonstrate normal metabolite concentrations in normal cerebral tissue contralateral to the stroke (A), and characteristic abnormal levels in the centre of the infarction (B) and at the stroke rim (C). Spectra from the normal region (A) have normal ratios of Cr/NAA and Ch/NAA. Spectra from infarcted tissue (region B)

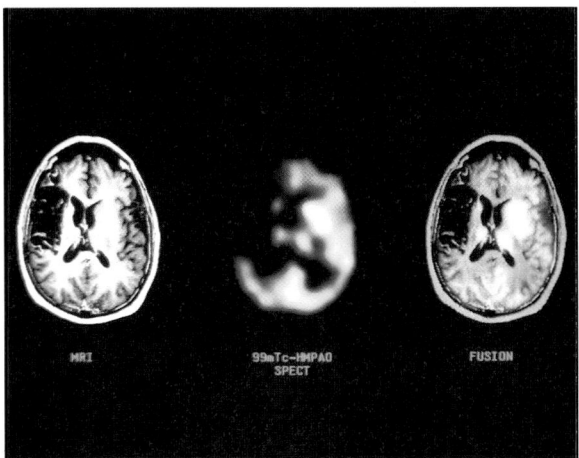

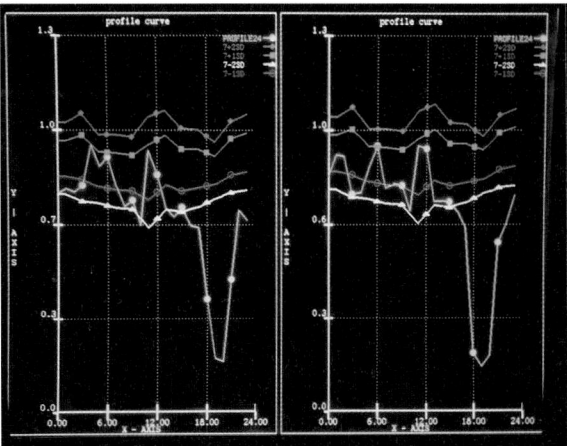

Figure 6a Images of the MRI (left), rCBF brain SPECT (middle), and rCBF brain SPECT/MRI fusion image (right) are shown of a 46 year old patient who had a right MCA territory infarction seven weeks prior to these scans. The MRI scan (left) shows the anatomy of the infarction. The co-registered ^{99m}Tc-HMPAO brain SPECT scan section (middle) shows that the stroke involves areas of hypoperfusion not only of the cortex as seen on the MRI but also in the surrounding brain, particularly the subcortical nuclei (caudate and thalamus). The fusion image (right) allows one to simultaneously visualise the blood flow and anatomical deficits. (From reference 13, with permission)

Figure 6c The graph on the left is a plot of the circumferential rCBF profile (light blue line) from the patient shown in Figure 6a at rest. The other four lines represent the ±1 and ±2 s.d. for normal controls. The semiquantitative cortical ROI values show the large perfusion defect in the right hemisphere corresponding to the infarction (position 20 on the x-axis). The graph on the right is the circumferential rCBF profile post-Diamox, which is virtually identical to the pre-Diamox profile. (From reference 8, with permission)

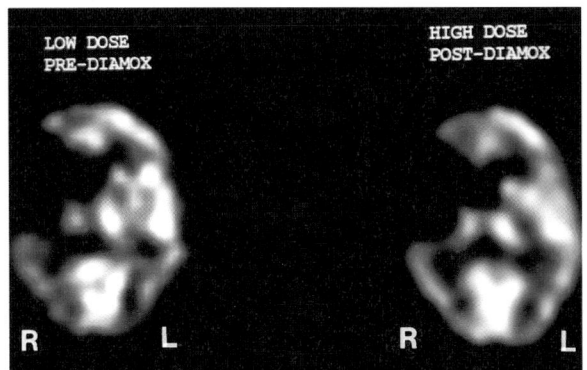

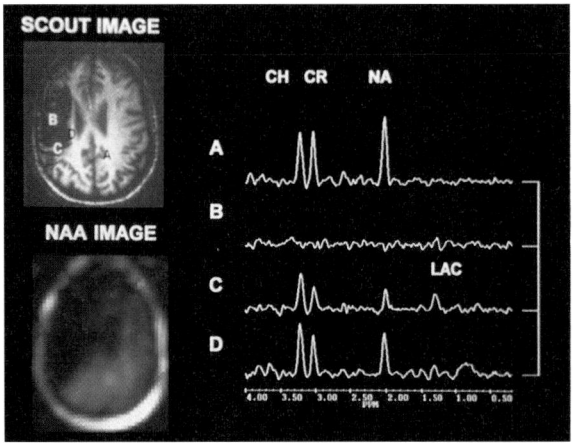

Figure 6b Sections from the pre-Diamox (left) and post-Diamox (right) ^{99m}Tc-HMPAO brain SPECT scans illustrating that there are nearly equal defect volumes of zero hypothetical perfusion (67.4 cc, and 63.3 cc, respectively). (From reference 7, with permission)

Figure 6d MRI scout image (top), and NAA image (bottom) of the patient described in Figure 6a. Spectra shown to the right are taken from a normal brain region (A), infarcted brain region (B), and stroke rim region (C) demonstrate complete absence of metabolite signal. Spectra from the stroke rim (region C) show decreases in Cr/NAA, Ch/NAA and increased LAC/NAA.

Thresholded ratio images of CR/NAA and LAC/NAA were calculated. All pixels within the measured region were analysed using NMR1, and the resonance areas, line widths and peak positions of NAA, CR, CH, and LAC were determined. The pixels in the CR/NAA image representing pixels which had CR/NAA ratios greater than 0.9 (four standard deviations higher than that observed in normal parietal white matter and two standard deviations higher than that observed in normal parietal grey matter in healthy controls) were superimposed on the scout MRI and highlighted. A colour scale on each image displayed the relationship between the highlighted colour and the measured metabolite ratio. Pixels displaying ratios greater than the highest ratio listed were highlighted with the brightest colour of the scale.

Ischaemia

An example of vascular compromise is demonstrated by a Diamox stress test using the split dose method in a 58 year old male patient with chronic cerebral ischaemia who was admitted with transient right lower extremity sensory loss. A cerebral angiogram showed an old occlusion of the right ICA and a new occlusion of the left ICA. The MRI brain scan showed only a small region of white matter ischaemic disease in the left centrum semi-ovale (Figure 7a). The low dose

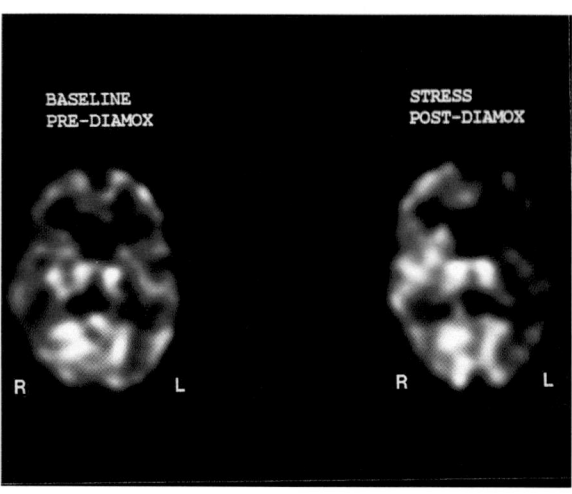

Figure 7b The low dose pre-Diamox ^{99m}Tc-HMPAO brain SPECT scan section shows no significant defects in perfusion (left). High dose post-Diamox 'stress' ^{99m}Tc-HMPAO brain SPECT scan (right) demonstrates a large region of decreased rCBF to the left frontal, temporal, and parietal lobes. (From reference 7, with permission)

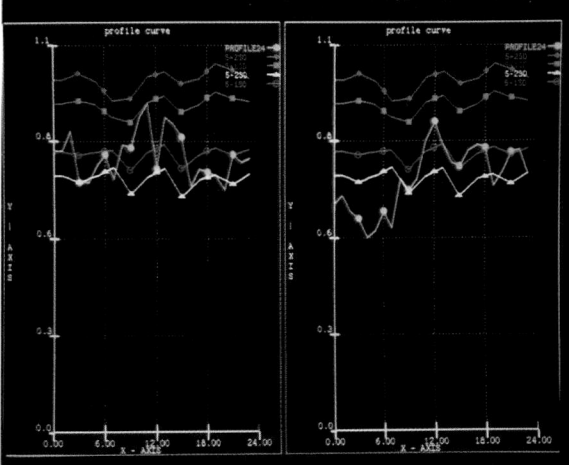

Figure 7c The graph (left) is a plot of the circumferential rCBF profile comparing the pre-Diamox SPECT scan from the patient shown in Figure 7b with age matched normal controls. The semiquantitative cortical ROI values for this 'non-stress' scan is within normal range. The graph (right) is a plot of the circumferential rCBF profile comparing the post-Diamox SPECT scan for the same patient with age matched normal controls. The semiquantitative cortical ROI values for the 'stress' scan shows marked reduction of rCBF to the territory of the left internal carotid artery. (From reference 7, with permission)

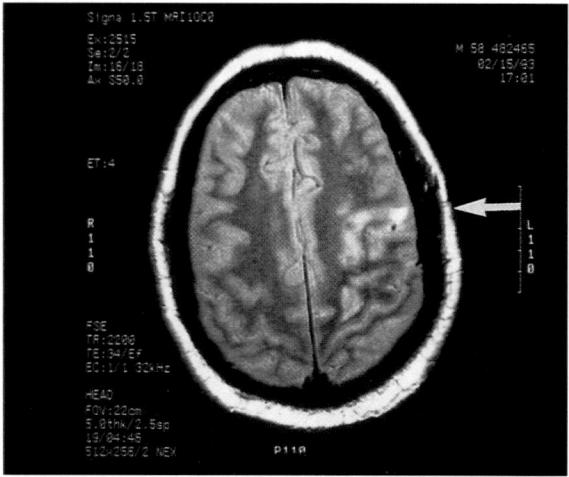

Figure 7a The MRI scan of a 58 year old male with transient ischaemic attacks. Note the small area of high signal intensity due to neuronal loss secondary to chronic cerebral ischaemia (arrow)

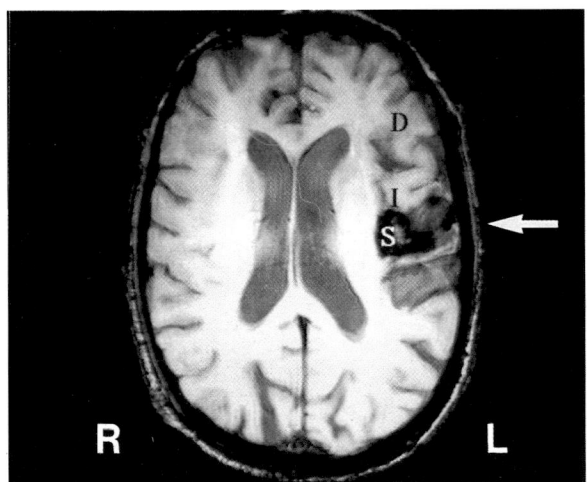

Figure 8a The MRI scan demonstrates low signal intensity in the left temporal and parietal lobe representing the cerebral infarction (arrow)

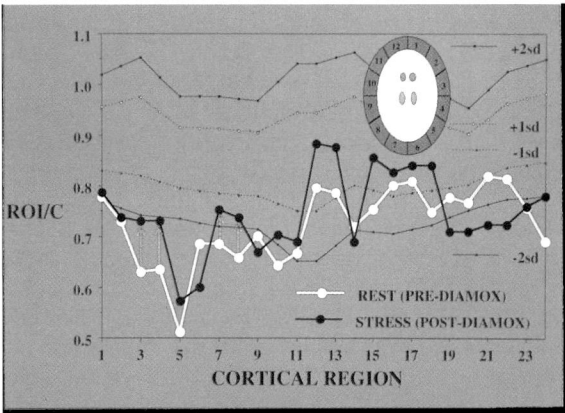

Figure 8c Graph of the 24 ROI circumferential rCBF profile illustrating the relative reduction (up arrows on graph) of the rCBF defect size post Diamox, compared with the pre-Diamox study. The ±1s.d. and ±2s.d. for the normal rCBF profiles at the same level are also illustrated. (From reference 8, with permission)

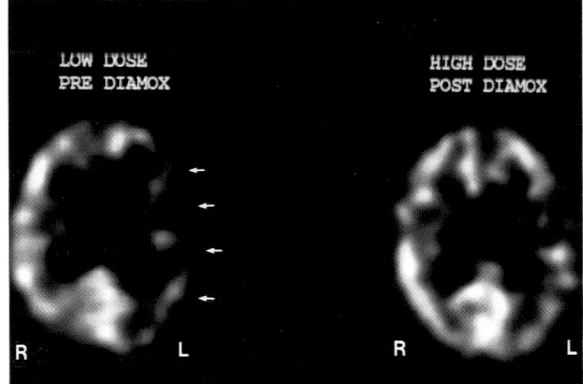

Figure 8b The low-dose, pre-Diamox, rest ^{99m}Tc-HMPAO brain SPECT scan section (left) demonstrates a relatively large area of hypoperfusion involving essentially the entire territory of the left middle cerebral artery (arrows). The high dose, post-Diamox, stress ^{99m}Tc-HMPAO brain SPECT scan (right) shows a reduction in the size of the perfusion defect, which more nearly equals the defect size observed on MRI (Figure 8a). (From reference 8, with permission)

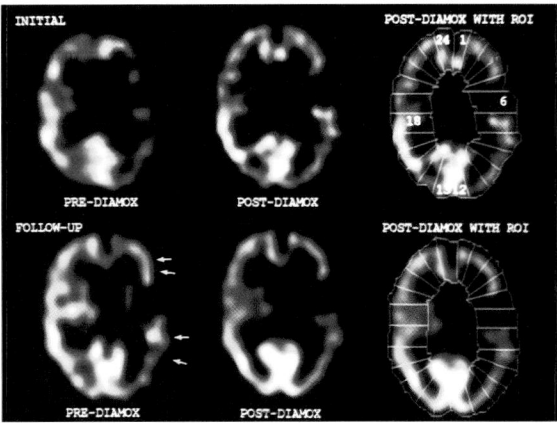

Figure 8d One year follow-up rest/stress scan sections for the same patient described in Figure 8a. Top row shows the pre and post Diamox sections from the initial evaluation, and the regions of interest used in the calculation of the SPECT defect volume. The bottom row shows the pre and post Diamox sections from the follow-up evaluation. Note the recovery of rCBF to the areas of diaschisis detected on the initial evaluation (arrows)

99mTc-HMPAO pre-Diamox brain SPECT scan showed no significant defects in perfusion (Figure 7b, left). However the post-Diamox 'stress' scan showed a large region of decreased rCBF in the left frontal, temporal, and parietal lobes representing severe rCBF compromise in the entire distribution of the left internal carotid artery (Figure 7b, right). Figure 7c shows the rest/stress circumferential profile curves. The effective volume of zero perfusion on the post-Diamox 'stress' 99mTc-HMPAO brain SPECT scan was calculated to be 75.1 cc. This case exemplifies the ability of the brain to provide effective vascular collateral supplies to the territory of a major arterial blockade. The cerebrovascular stress test, however, clearly revealed the limitations of such collateral circulation. In this patient there was a significant reduction of relative rCBF involving the entire territory of the left internal carotid artery observed on the post Diamox challenge rCBF brain SPECT scan. It remains to be seen whether such viable but vascularly constrained territories would benefit from neurosurgical intervention such as carotid endarterectomy or revascularisation procedures.

Diaschisis

What at first appears to be 'paradoxical' cerebrovascular reactivity is illustrated in the case of a 77 year old male who presented with marked right upper and lower extremity sensory and motor deficits one month prior to brain imaging. Sensory evaluation was difficult to assess due to the patient's severe receptive and expressive aphasic deficits. The patient demonstrated much better than average functional recovery of his neurological and cognitive deficits. The MRI scan showed an area of low signal intensity in the

left temporal and parietal lobe representing this patient's infarction (Figure 8a). The resting state, low-dose 99mTc-HMPAO brain SPECT scan demonstrated a relatively large area of hypoperfusion involving essentially the entire distribution of the left middle cerebral artery (Figure 8b, left). The effective volume of zero perfusion

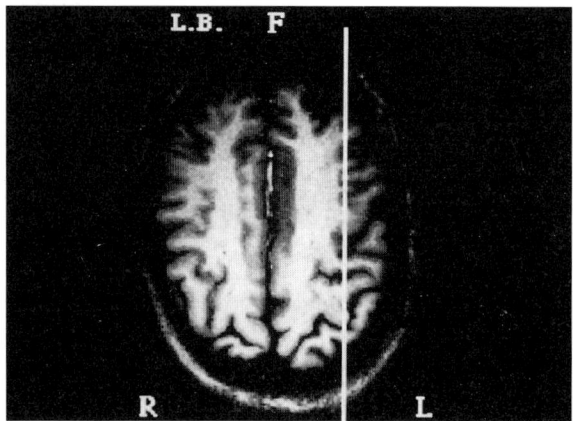

Figure 9b The MRI section selected for spectroscopic analysis from the same patient shown in Figure 9a. (From reference 7, with permission)

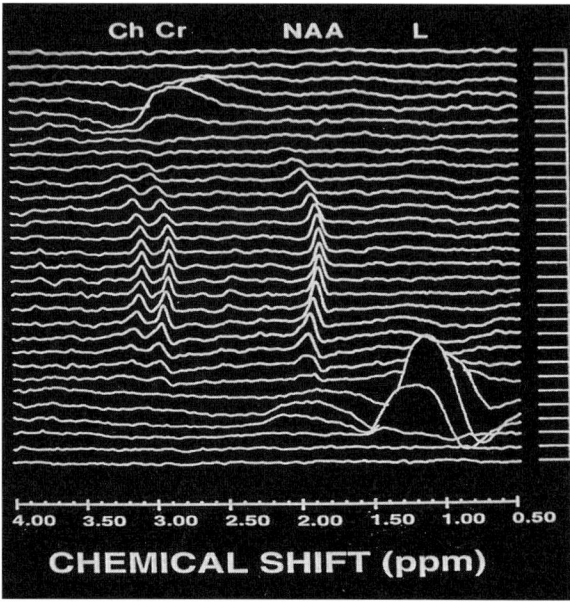

Figure 9c A stacked plot of the 1H spectra (posterior to anterior along the vertical line shown in Figure 9b. In the zone of diaschisis identified on the rCBF brain SPECT (Figure 9a) there is normal lactate, with normal Ch and Cr to NAA ratios. (From reference 7, with permission)

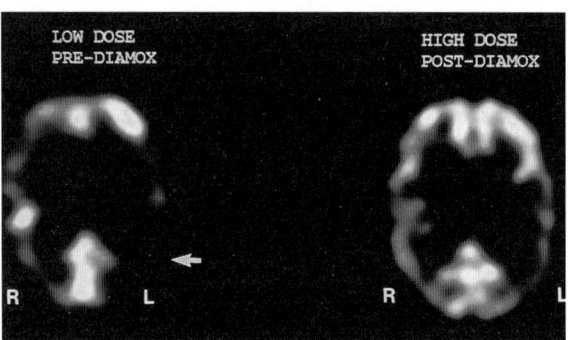

Figure 9a The rCBF SPECT scan shows increased perfusion 'reverse Diamox effect' in the left posterior parietal region (arrow) as evidenced by a relative increase in rCBF post Diamox in a patient with a white matter infarction positioned inferior to this brain level resulting in disconnectivity and associated diaschisis. (From reference 7, with permission)

on the rest SPECT scan was calculated to be 68.1 cc. The post-Diamox, high dose [99mTc]-HMPAO brain SPECT scan (Figure 8b, right), however, demonstrated a large reduction of the perfusion defect (effective volume of zero perfusion was reduced to 14.3 cc), with more sharply delineated borders, and more closely corresponding to the size of the defect volume measured from the MRI anatomic scan (13.7 cm).

The patient's semiquantitative rCBF circumferential profile at 7.5 cm above the CM line is shown in Figure 8c, illustrating the relative reduction of the rCBF defect size post-Diamox, compared with the resting pre-Diamox study. This case illustrates the lack of vascular constraints in this patient's stroke penumbra region, suggesting that the decreased perfusion at rest is due to reduced metabolism - presumably due to diaschisis or, in part, selective neuronal loss or 'incomplete infarction'. The 'hyper-reactivity' to vasodilators in such low neuronal activity regions reflects a non-linearity of rCBF response in maximally constricted but uncompromised vessels. The use of this test and the 'reverse-Diamox effect' may provide an indication of a good recovery status, as was observed in this patient. For this patient, at one year follow-up the effective volume of zero perfusion on the rest SPECT scan was calculated to be 16.8 cc, while the defect volume on the Diamox challenge scan was calculated to be 14.5 cc. The significant reduction in the rest volume defect indicates neuro-metabolic recovery of brain function over the follow-up time period. The patient experienced very substantial cognitive and neurological recovery of the stroke induced deficits on the one year post-stroke follow-up neurological evaluation which, in retrospect, could have been

predicted based on the substantial volume of diaschisis found on his initial rest/stress rCBF brain SPECT studies. The follow-up rest/stress scan (Figure 8d) demonstrated restoration of rCBF to the areas of significant diaschisis seen on the initial resting scan. Another example of pure cortical diaschisis is illustrated in Figures 9a-9c. These images show data from another patient presenting with right-sided neurological deficits. The rCBF brain SPECT scan showed increased perfusion, or 'paradoxical Diamox effect' in the left posterior parietal region as shown by relatively increased rCBF post Diamox (Figure 9a). The patient suffered a white matter stroke inferior to the MRI section (Figure 9b) selected for spectroscopic analysis. A stacked plot of the ^{1}H spectra (posterior to anterior along the vertical line shown in Figure 9a), in the zone of diaschisis found on rCBF brain SPECT, shows normal lactate and normal Ch and Cr to NAA ratios (Figure 9c). The normal metabolite ratios and absence of lactate in this region help validate our conclusion, based on rCBF brain SPECT reactivity, that the low baseline rCBF is a secondary consequence of diaschisis rather than a result of vascular constraints.

Discussion

rCBF SPECT, MRI, and MRSI complementary measures hypothesis

While it is suggested that SPECT measurements of rCBF, rCBF reactivity, and MRSI measurements of metabolism can separately provide sufficient information to determine the presence of both haemodynamic insufficiency and non-haemodynamically constrained reduction in neuro-metabolic activity, both techniques were employed for the following reasons.

1. SPECT directly measures vascular status, MRSI directly measures metabolic status.
2. Proposing that SPECT measurements of vascular reactivity and MRSI measurements of lactate can identify ischaemia relies on different assumptions. Mutual agreement would validate these assumptions.
3. Truly complimentary information is provided by the two techniques in attempting to determine the nature of primary neurometabolic activity reductions (i.e., those not due to vascular constraints).

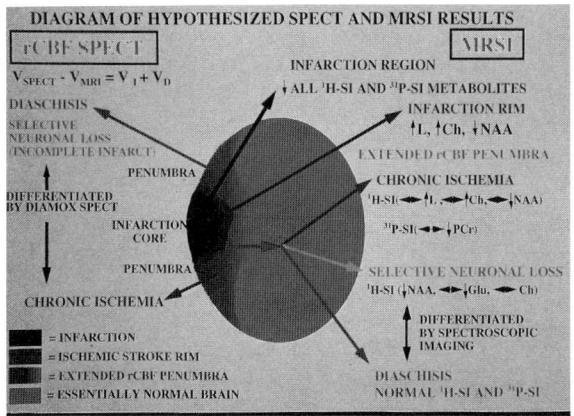

Figure 10 Illustration of the expected abnormalities for the separate components of the stroke 'penumbra' (ischaemia, diaschisis, and selective neuronal loss) as measured by rest/stress rCBF SPECT, MRI, and ^{1}H and ^{31}P SI

The presence of diaschisis is suggested if the rCBF SPECT defect volume is greater than the MRI defect volume, and can be substantiated and quantified if ischaemia is ruled out by either good Diamox reactivity on rCBF SPECT or normal metabolite levels on MRSI. Selective neuronal loss can be evaluated by a combination of rCBF SPECT reactivity with Diamox and ^{1}H-SI. SPECT reactivity measurements can separate the chronic ischaemic subjects from the diaschisis/selective neuronal loss group. The ^{1}H-SI will then separate the patients with diaschisis from those with selective neuronal loss.

Figure 10 shows an illustration of the expected abnormalities for the separate components of the stroke 'penumbra' (ischaemia, diaschisis, and selective neuronal loss) as measured by rest/stress rCBF SPECT, MRI and ^{1}H-SI. This figure also illustrates several hypotheses concerning ^{31}P-SI findings in the stroke penumbra. These combined measures will permit a temporal characterisation of all major components of the stroke induced 'extended rCBF penumbra region', and allow an analysis of how each component evolves and contributes to the neurological deficits as well as the prognosis for recovery from the stroke.

Acknowledgement

This work was supported, in part, by a grant from the NICHD (1RO1HD32100-01-A1) to the Principal Author (J.M.M.).

References

1   Von Monakow, C. Diaschisis (1914 article, Harris G [trans]), in ' Brain and Behaviour I: Mood States and Mind'. (Ed. K.H. Pribram), Penguin, Baltimore, 1969, 27

2   Mountz, J.M., Modell, J.G., Foster, N.L *et al*. Prognostication of recovery following stroke using the comparison of CT and technetium-99m HMPAO SPECT. *J. Nucl. Med.* 1990, 31, 61

3   Sawner, K. and LaVigne, J. (Eds.) in 'Brunnstrom's movement therapy in hemiplegia: a neurophysiological approach', Lippincott, Philadelphia, USA, 1992

4   Bobath, B. in 'Adult hemiplegia evaluation and treatment', Heinemann Medical Books, Oxford, UK, 1990

5   Voss, D.E., Ionta, M.K. and Myers, B.J. in 'Proprioceptive neuromuscular facilitation', Harper & Row, Philadelphia, USA, 1985

6   Liu, H.G., Harris, J.M., Inampudi, C.S. and Mountz, J.M. Optimal Reconstruction Filter Parameters for Multi-headed Brain SPECT: Dependence on Count Activity. *J. Nucl. Med. Technol.* 1995, 23, 251

7   Mountz, J.M., Deutsch, G., Kuzniecky, R. and Rosenfeld, S.S. Brain SPECT: 1994 Update in 'Nuclear Medicine Annual 1994', (Ed. L.M.Freeman), Raven Press, New York, USA, 1994, 1

8   Mountz, J.M., Deutsch, G. and Khan, S.H. Regional cerebral blood flow changes in stroke imaged by ^{99m}Tc HMPAO SPECT with corresponding anatomic image comparison. *Clin. Nucl. Med.* 1993, 18, 1067

9   Mountz, J.M. A method of analysis of SPECT blood flow image data for comparison with computed tomography. *Clin. Nucl. Med.* 1989, 14, 192

10   Lassen, N.A. Imaging brain infarcts by single photon emission tomography with new tracers. *Eur. J. Nucl. Med.* 1994, 21, 189

11   Dierckx, R.A., Dobbeleir, A., Pickut, B.A., *et al*. Technetium-99m HMPAO SPET in acute supratentorial ischaemic infarction, expressing deficits as millilitre of zero perfusion. *Eur. J. Nucl. Med.*1995, 22, 427

12   Mountz, J.M., Wilson, M.W., Wolff, C.G.*et al.* Validation of a reference method for correlation of anatomic and functional brain images. *Computerized Medical Imaging and Graphics* 1994, 18, 163

13   Mountz, J.M., Zhang, B., Liu, H,G. and Inampudi, C. A reference method for correlation of anatomic and functional brain images: validation and clinical application. *Seminars in Nuclear Medicine* 1994, 24, 256

14   Hetherington, H.P., Vaughan, J.T., Pan, J.W. *et al*. High Resolution Neuroimaging at 4.1T . *Proc. Soc. Magn. Reson. Imaging* 1993, 313

15   Geen, H. and Freeman, R. Band selective excitation for multidimensional NMR spectroscopy. *J. Magn. Reson.* 1990, 87, 415

16   Hetherington, H.P., Pan, J.W., Mason, G.F. *et al*. 2D 1H Spectroscopic imaging of the human brain at 4.1T. *Mag. Reson. in Med.* 1994, 32, 530

17   Hetherington, H.P., Kuzniecky, R., Pan, J.W. *et al*. Identification of the Epileptic Focus in Temporal Lobe Epilepsy by High Resolution Spectroscopic Imaging at 4.1T. *Proc. Soc. Magn. Reson.* 1995, 396

SPECT in Neurology and Psychiatry, edited by P.P. De Deyn, R.A. Dierckx, A. Alavi and B.A. Pickut
© 1997 John Libbey & Company Ltd, pp. 347–350

SPECT and Stroke with Particular Regard to Functional Recovery

Chapter
41

P. Pantano, G.L. Lenzi and C. Fieschi

Introduction

In acute stroke, the clinical outcome may be only partially predicted by the evaluation of some clinical parameters[1]. It has been also observed that, when a CT scan is performed during a very early phase of supratentorial ischaemic stroke, positive early CT findings, such as an early hypodensity and/or sulcal effacement, can predict the final brain damage[2]. The study of cerebral blood flow (CBF) in patients with stroke may provide useful data for clinical management especially in the acute phase of stroke[3].

Furthermore, the degree of CBF decrease in the very acute stages of stroke, especially if considered along with the severity of the clinical status, seems to represent a good predictor of long-term clinical outcome. In a SPECT study[4], we have identified three different patterns: 1) a CBF decrease in the affected hemisphere >40% with respect to the contralateral side, associated with a severe clinical status, which indicated a poor outcome; 2) a mild CBF reduction (<40% of the contralateral side) associated with less compromised clinical conditions, which indicated a good outcome; 3) a mismatching between the CBF decrease and the clinical severity, which indicated a variable prognosis (Table 1).

The value of CBF assessment in the acute phase of stroke has been confirmed more recently by a PET study that has identified the same three patterns, on the basis of the degree of impairment of both CBF and oxygen metabolism (in spite of clinical conditions)[5]. SPECT in acute stroke may be used not only to select patients for therapeutical trials but also to evaluate the effects on CBF due to specific therapies. However, functional neuroimaging may also provide useful information after the acute phase of stroke.

Population studies indicate that the incidence of stroke is 1-2 per 1,000 persons annually and mortality is about 30% (20% if only ischaemic stroke is considered). The outcome of survivors may be evaluated as follows: 10% without disability; 40% with a mild disability; 40% with a severe disability; 10% requiring institutionalisation[6]. Many patients therefore show post-stroke neurological deficits that could be improved with rehabilitative treatments. On the other hand, the social and economic impact of stroke is represented not only by the cost of the acute care and loss of income, but also by the costs due to rehabilitation and long-term institutionalisation. It is general opinion that intensive rehabilitation may only be effective in a select group of patients. Therefore it is important to develop criteria that allow an early selection of patients for rehabilitation.

Department of Neurological Sciences, University of Rome 'La Sapienza', Viale dell'Universita30, 00185 Rome, Italy

Theoretically, clinical recovery may be due to regression of functional phenomena, such as diaschisis, and/or to brain reorganisation leading to the 'taking-over' of functions of the damaged tissue by other neuronal groups. Attentional and intentional processes may also contribute. Recently, advances in neuroimaging techniques have offered new insights into this problem. It is a common experience that the area of hypoperfusion is larger than the structural lesion even in patients with chronic stroke[7]. The peripheral area of hypoperfusion that can correspond to apparently intact tissue is probably due to different factors, such as ischaemic penumbra[8], incomplete infarction[9], and diaschisis[10]. To understand which of these factors plays a principal role in individual patients is important for prognosis. The potential reversibility of both ischaemic penumbra and diaschisis, although with different pathophysiological mechanisms, contrasts with the irreversible selective neuronal damage of the incomplete infarction. The recent use of ^{123}I-iomazenil in stroke patients[11], on the basis of experimental results[12], may help in this regard.

Diaschisis is a frequent finding in stroke patients[10]. It represents a cerebral region with reduced CBF and metabolism, despite of the structural integrity of the tissue and is a consequence of the loss of excitatory (or inhibitory) afferents caused by the ishaemic (or haemorrhagic) lesion. Decreased values of CBF and metabolism have been reported in the cerebellar hemisphere contralateral to the side of a supratentorial infarct. This finding, termed crossed cerebellar diaschisis[13], is well identified by SPECT[14,15] and seems to occur at least in 50% of patients suffering from supratentorial stroke. Similarly, a functional hypoactivity of the cerebral cortex ipsilateral to a subcortical lesion has been reported by both PET and SPECT studies[16-18].

Cortical diaschisis seems to correlate with neuropsychological deficits. In a SPECT study with ^{123}I-HIPDM, Perani et al.[20] found that patients with neglect or aphasia following a subcortical lesion had significantly greater reduction of cortical perfusion than patients without neuropsychological defects. Furthermore, the recovery from aphasia and neglect some months after a subcortical stroke was found to be associated with a significant improvement of cortical perfusion[20]. On the other hand, the clinical expression, if any, of cerebellar diaschisis is still controversial.

In a SPECT study on 27 stroke patients, we reported that crossed cerebellar diaschisis was more frequent and severe in patients with a prolonged muscular flaccidity (PMF) of the hemiparetic limbs than in patients with spastic hemiplegia, regardless of motor deficit severity, time elapsed since stroke and lesion size[21]. Since hypotonia is a classical symptom of cerebellar disease in humans, we hypothesised that the persistence of flaccidity could be the clinical expression of a cerebellar dysfunction due to diaschisis.

However, the cause of PMF in stroke patients appears to be more complex. Following stroke, muscular flaccidity of the affected limbs may persist for a varying period of time. It is unknown why flaccidity rapidly disappears evolving into spasticity in most patients but persists in others. From a clinical point of view it would be important to understand the causes of these two different functional outcomes since PMF represents a negative factor for both motor recovery and rehabilitation.

In a more recent SPECT study[22] we correlated CT/MR and ^{99m}Tc-HMPAO SPECT with clinical findings in 42 patients at a mean time interval of 3 months after stroke. The patients were divided into two cohorts with either flaccid (PMF) or spastic (MSp) hemiparesis. Although patients with PMF had a greater motor deficit, the mean structural volume of the ischaemic lesion was similar to that of the MSp cohort. There was a significantly higher prevalence of the structural involvement of the lentiform nucleus in PMF cases. Furthermore, SPECT showed that relative perfusion in the lentiform nucleus, thalamus and contralateral cerebellar hemisphere was significantly lower in PMF than in MSp patients. A subgroup of patients with only subcortical structural lesions also showed significantly lower relative perfusion in the ipsilateral frontal association areas.

A primary involvement of the lentiform nucleus by the structural lesion was supposed to be crucial for the persistence of flaccidity after stroke. However, CBF changes in other structurally intact regions indicated their additional role. We concluded that both subcortical-cortical loops involved in motor control, i.e. cortex-basal ganglia-thalamus-cortex and cortex-pons-cerebellum-thalamus-cortex, are more widely and more severely affected in patients with PMF. It remains to be seen whether the regression of the hypoperfusion in the above-mentioned intact brain areas is associated with the evolution from flaccidity into spasticity.

An important role in the study of the recovery of neurological functions is played by activation studies using PET or SPECT. Activation studies are used to investigate which cerebral areas are involved during the execution of a specific task both in physiological and pathological conditions. While studies in normal subjects are useful to investigate the physiology of complex systems, such as language and memory, and the cerebral areas involved in a neural network, studies on patients are mainly aimed at investigating the mechanisms responsible for recovery. The recovery of motor function has been more thoroughly investigated and has represented the basis for the study of the recovery of more complex cerebral functions.

Two factors of cerebral plasticity have been identified by PET as important in determining motor recovery: when patients are required to move their previously paretic hand, a CBF increase may be observed in cerebral areas of both the affected (anatomical extension of specialised motor areas) and the unaffected hemisphere (recruitment of ipsilateral motor pathways), as documented previously[23,24].

Activation studies may also be performed by using SPECT. Although the ^{133}Xe inhalation method is the most suitable for this purpose, the ^{99m}Tc-HMPAO split-dose method[25] may be used as an alternative. Di Piero et al.[26] studied CBF changes induced by finger movements of the normal and the previously paretic hand in 14 patients who had recovered from a stroke. They found a different pattern of activation of the

cerebral motor area. While the movements of the normal hand showed the activation of the contralateral motor regions (as it occurs in controls), the performance of the same motor task by the previously paretic hand was associated with a CBF increase of the motor areas of the unaffected ipsilateral hemisphere (Table 2). Individual analysis showed differences in the degree of the CBF increase and in the number and location of activated areas among patients, suggesting that the restoration of the motor function is a complex phenomenon which also depends on individual factors such as the location and the extent of the lesion and the residual neuronal viability in damaged brain structures.

Another important factor influencing the clinical recovery is the patient's age. Recovery of function is remarkable when the brain is damaged early in life, as in a young patient we described[27] who showed no motor deficits despite a large right cortico-subcortical lesion. In this patient, SPECT motor activation study showed CBF increase in the left premotor and sensorimotor cortices irrespective of the hand he was moving. This study strongly supports the potential role of the ipsilateral corticospinal tract in subserving hand movements after early brain damage.

In conclusion, SPECT is a reliable and useful tool to study stroke patients both in the acute and chronic phase. It may be used, along with the evaluation of both the clinical status and the morphological characteristics of the lesion, to better understand mechanisms of clinical recovery, to select patients to be submitted to specific therapies (acute therapeutical trials and rehabilitation) and to evaluate the therapeutic effects by CBF.

Table 1 Patterns of clinical outcome in 32 stroke patients studied with perfsuion SPECT within 6 h from clinical onset (Giubilei et al.[4])

	CBF decrease	Early clinical status	Clinical outcome (1 month)
I	Severe (AI>40%)	Severe (CNS<6.5)	Poor
II	Mild (AI<40%)	Mild (CNS>6.5)	Good
III	Severe (AI>40%)	Mild (CNS>6.5)	Variable
	Mild (AI<40%)	Severe (CNS<6.5)	

AI= Count asymmetry index; CNS= Canadian neurological scale

Table 2 Significant CBF changes during normal and previous paretic hand motor activations (finger opposition) with respect to the resting state in 14 stroke patients (Di Piero et al.[26])

Regions	Normal hand		Previously paretic hand	
	unaffected hemisphere	affected hemisphere	unaffected hemisphere	affected hemisphere
Primary motor cortex	+17%	ns	+16%	+18%
Supplementary motor cortex	+12%	ns	+11%	ns
Premotor cortex	+13%	ns	+21%	ns

References

1 Fiorelli, M., Alpérovitch, A., Argentino, C. et al. Prediction of death or disablement at four months based on clinical characteristics identified in the early hours of acute ischemic stroke. Arch. Neurol. 1995, 52, 250

2 Bozzao, L., Bastianello, S., Fantozzi, L.M. et al. Correlation of angiographic and sequential CT findings in patients with evolving cerebral infarction. A. J. N. R. 1989, 10, 1215

3 Lenzi, G.L., Frackowiak, R.S.J. and Jones, T. Cerebral oxygen metabolism and blood flow in human cerebral infarction. J. Cereb. Blood Flow Metab. 1982, 2, 321

4 Giubilei, F., Lenzi, G.L., Di Piero, V. et al. Predictive value of brain perfusion single photon emission computed tomography in acute ischemic stroke. Stroke 1990, 21, 895

5 Marchal, G., Serrati, C., Rioux, P. et al. PET imaging of cerebral perfusion and oxygen consumption in acute ischaemic stroke: relation to outcome. Lancet 1993, 341 (8850), 925

6   Stallones, R.A., Dyken, M.L., Fang, H.C.H. *et al.* Epidemiology for stroke facilities planning. *Stroke* 1972, 3, 360

7   Raynaud, C., Rancurel, G., Samson, Y. *et al.* Pathophysiological study of chronic infarcts with I-123 isopropyl iodoamphetamine (IMP): The importance of the periinfarct area. *Stroke* 1987, 18, 21

8   Astrup, J., Siesjo, B.K. and Symon, L. Threshold in cerebral ischemia; the ischemic penumbra. *Stroke* 1982, 12, 723

9   Lassen, N.L., Olsen, T.S., Hojgaard, K. and Skriver, E. Incomplete infarction: a CT-negative irreversible ischemic brain lesion. *J. Cereb. Blood Flow Metab.* 1983, 3(1), S602

10 Feeney, M.D. and Baron, J.C. Diaschisis. *Stroke* 1986, 17, 817

11 Nakagawara, J., Sperling, B., Takeda, R. *et al.* Incomplete brain infarction of early reperfused, CT/MRI intact cortex in embolic stroke: in vivo evidence by 123-I-Iomazenil SPECT. *J. Cereb. Blood Flow Metab.* 1995, 15(1), S131

12 Sette, G., Baron, J.C., Young, A.R. *et al.* In vivo mapping of brain benzodiazepine receptor changes by positron emission tomography after focal ischemia in the anesthetized baboon. *Stroke* 1993, 24, 2046

13 Baron, J.C., Bousser, M.G., Comar, D. and Castaigne, P. Crossed cerebellar diaschisis in human supratentorial brain infarction (abstract). *Ann. Neurol.* 1980, 8, 128

14 Meneghetti, G., Vorstrup, S., Mickey, B. *et al.* Crossed cerebellar diaschisis in ischemic stroke: a study of regional cerebral blood flow by 133- Xe inhalation and single photon emission computerized tomography. *J. Cereb. Blood Flow Metab.* 1984, 4, 235

15 Pantano, P., Lenzi, G.L., Guidetti, B. *et al.* Crossed cerebellar diaschisis in patients with cerebral ischemia assessed by SPECT and I-123 HIPDM. *Europ. Neurol.* 1987, 27, 142

16 Baron, J.C., D'Antona, R., Pantano, P. *et al.* Effects of thalamic stroke on energy metabolism of the cerebral cortex. *Brain* 1986, 109, 1243

17 Metter, E.J., Kempler, D., Jackson, C.A. *et al.* Cerebellar glucose metabolism in chronic aphasia. *Neurology* 1987, 37, 1599

18 Perani, D., Di Piero, V., Lucignani, G. *et al.* Remote effects of subcortical cerebrovascular lesions: a SPECT cerebral perfusion study. *J. Cereb. Blood Flow Metab.* 1988, 8, 560

19 Perani, D., Vallar, G., Cappa, S. *et al.* Aphasia and neglect after subcortical stroke. *Brain* 1987, 110, 1211

20 Vallar, G., Perani, D., Cappa, S. *et al.* Recovery from aphasia and neglect after subcortical stroke: neuropsychological and cerebral perfusion study. *J. Neurol. Neurosurg. Psych.* 1988, 51, 1269

21 Pantano, P., Formisano, R., Ricci, M. *et al.* Prolonged muscular flaccidity in stroke patients is associated with crossed cerebellar diaschisis. *Cerebrovasc. Dis.* 1993, 3, 80

22 Pantano, P., Formisano, R., Ricci, M. *et al.* Prolonged muscular flaccidity after stroke: morphological and functional brain alterations. *Brain* 1995, 118, 1329

23 Chollet, F., Di Piero, V., Wise, R.J.S. *et al.* The functional anatomy of motor recovery after stroke in humans: a study with positron emission tomography. *Ann. Neurol.* 1991, 29, 63

24 Weiller, C., Chollet, F., Friston, K.J. *et al.* Functional reorganization of the brain in recovery from striatocapsular infarction in man. *Ann. Neurol.* 1992, 31, 463

25 Pantano, P., Di Piero, V., Ricci, M. *et al.* Motor stimulation response by technetium-99m hexamethylpropylene amine oxime split-dose method and single photon emission tomography. *Eur. J. Nucl. Med.* 1992, 19, 939

26 Di Piero, V., Ricci, M., Toni, D. *et al.* Functional recovery after stroke: a motor activation SPECT study. *J. Cereb. Blood Flow Metab.* 1993, 13(1), S802

27 Sabatini, U., Toni, D., Pantano, P. *et al.* Motor recovery after early brain damage: a case of brain plasticity. *Stroke* 1994, 25, 514

SPECT in Neurology and Psychiatry, edited by P.P. De Deyn, R.A. Dierckx, A. Alavi and B.A. Pickut

SPECT Control of Cerebral Perfusion Reserve in Carotid Artery Disease Treated Rheotherapeutically

Chapter
42

W.Y.Ussov, B.N. Kozlov*, I.Y. Shvera, M.P. Plotnikov, S.P. Yaroshevsky and V.M. Shipulin

Introduction

In addition to atherosclerotic stenoses of the internal carotid artery[1] and arterial hypertension, the rheology of blood has been shown to influence the incidence and clinical course of cerebrovascular disorders[2]. The high incidence of strokes in polycythaemia vera is a well-known fact[3]. However, anaemic patients show less common disorders of cerebral blood flow than in the general population[4,5]. Rheological therapy with haemodilution using dextranes with molecular weight >80 000 was therefore introduced as a pathophysiologically based technique aimed at improving the collateral and residual blood flow in patients with ischaemic stroke[6]. Some authors advocate high-volume haemodilution and decreasing the hematocrit extensively as a technique for stimulating cerebral blood flow[7] and improving clinical results[8] in stroke, although multicentre trials have not given conclusive evidence for this[9].

Nevertheless, rheological therapy has never been employed for the prevention, either primary or secondary, of stroke in patients with cerebrovascular disease due to atherosclerotic stenosis of internal carotid artery. Plasmapheresis, which comprises stepwise withdrawal of extensive, >2000 ml, volumes of plasma and substitution with dextranes or albumin solution was introduced to clinical therapy of chronic atherosclerotic disorders[10,11], and recent results are favourable for its effectiveness in the secondary prevention of stroke in patients who have already undergone single or multiple PRIND[12]. The pathophysiological mechanisms of the clinical effect remain unclear.

The perfusion reserve of a particular cerebral vascular region has been widely shown to be one of the factors definitively determining the probability of stroke or TIAs in the region[13]. Both the measurement of the perfusion reserve using CO_2[14] or the acetazolamide test[15], and quantification of perfusion reserve as the ratio {rCBV/rCBF} [13] have shown definitive predictive value.

We have undertaken a pilot study aimed at the quantification of cerebral blood flow (CBF), blood volume (CBV) and CBV/CBF ratio in the course of the plasmapheretic rheotherapeutical treatment of neurologically low or asymptomatic patients with atherosclerotic stenoses of the internal carotid artery.

Tomsk Institute of Cardiology, Kievskaya 111, Tomsk, Siberia, Russia
*Siberian Medical University, Moscowsky tract 2, Tomsk 634 050, Siberia, Russia

Materials and methods

Clinical characteristics of patients

Eight patients were referred for the study; all with isolated unilateral stenosis of internal carotid artery (exceeding 70% of the vascular lumen). In each patient the location and severity of stenosis was diagnosed using digital subtraction angiography with non-ionic contrasts (angiographic system 'Angioscop D-33', by Siemens Medical). Quantification of stenosis was performed by using a planimetric technique such as that described by Alexandrov et al.[16]. Four patients underwent single transient ischaemic attacks during the previous six months, and did not demonstrate any evidence for neurological deficit at the point of study. Four were asymptomatic when examined by the neurologist and were referred by the district cardiologist because of carotid artery bruit. In all patients, coronary heart disease of angina severity classes II-III was diagnosed clinically, and then verified by coronary angiography.

In all patients rCBV and rCBF SPECT studies were performed before and four days after completion of the plasmapheresis treatment. In each patient, an informed consent was obtained. The study was approved by the Ethical Committee of the Tomsk Medical Research Centre.

Technique of plasmapheresis therapy

All patients underwent serial plasmapheresis treatment with extensive extraction of plasma. Plasmapheresis was performed using RK-05 plasmaseparator (Institute of Medical Technics, Moscow). Heparin (100 units/kg of body weight) was used as anticoagulant and stabiliser. Blood withdrawal, substitution of blood volume with dextranes and return of erythromass were performed through routine venous access via vena cubitalis. Blood was withdrawn as quickly as 40 ml per min, the total volume withdrawn per session was 650-700 ml. At the same time, a solution of high-molecular dextran was re-infused into the patient at the same rate. Blood plasma was then separated and decanted. The volume of red blood cells was anticoagulated and reinfused to the patient immediately. In total every patient underwent four sessions, so that the total volume of plasma withdrawn was over 1800 ml in each patient. In all patients, blood samples were taken for everyday control of blood cell count, biochemistry and coagulogram.

Medical therapy was stopped completely five days before the start of the plasmapheretic session, except that nitroglycerin was taken sublingually for angina attacks. No additional anticoagulant therapy was administered during this time.

SPECT quantification of regional cerebral blood volume (rCBV) and cerebral blood flow (rCBF)

The perfusion reserve was quantified as the ratio rCBV/rCBF, which has units of mean transit time (s). rCBV and rCBF were studied using ^{99m}Tc -labelled red blood cells (RBC) and ^{99m}Tc - HMPAO, respectively.

Cerebral blood volume study using SPECT with ^{99m}Tc -labelled red blood cells

rCBV values were quantified using the technique proposed by Kuhl et al.[17] with technical adjustment to the equipment currently in use at the Institute of Cardiology. For in vivo labelling of red blood cells with ^{99m}Tc an 100 mg aliquot of $Sn(II)Cl_2$ pyrophosphate solution in saline, taken from a vial of PyrphoTech commercial kit (by Diamed Ltd, Moscow) was injected into the patient intravenously. In approximately 20 min, the patient was given with an intravenous bolus of 740 MBq of fresh ^{99m}Tc eluate obtained from a commercial ^{99}Mo generator. After four or five minutes, a SPECT study of rCBV was performed using a rotating SPECT single-head gamma-camera ('Omega 500', Technicare Corporation, Ohio) supplied with a high resolution low energy collimator and interfaced with dedicated computer system for scintigraphic data processing (SCINTI 3.3, by Gelmos Ltd, Moscow). Sixty projections of the head, in 64x64 matrix, of 20 s each, were acquired over 360°. The total count was over 3 000 000 in each study. The spatial resolution (as full width at the half maximum) was 18-20 mm at the centre of the field of view. Tomographic sections were obtained by filtered backprojection (Butterworth filter of order 4 with cut-off frequency 0.4) as a set of transversal slices. A 5 ml blood sample was taken from the cubital vein of the intact arm immediately after rCBV SPECT acquisition. rCBV was then calculated from a comparison of local counts per voxel in cortical regions of rCBV SPECT with the blood sample radioactivity measured in front of a gamma camera. rCBV values were separately obtained for perfusion regions of the anterior, middle and posterior cerebral arteries in each hemisphere.

Cerebral perfusion SPECT and rCBF quantification with ^{99m}Tc-HMPAO

All patients were studied 24 h after the rCBV study by using brain SPECT with ^{99m}Tc - HMPAO[18] (obtained from Diamed Ltd, Moscow, prepared with 740 MBq of fresh ^{99m}Tc eluate). The first pass of radioactive bolus was recorded as a set of 1 s frames for as long as 1 min, followed by 10 s frames for a further 5 min. Simultaneously, arterialised venous blood samples were taken from vena cubitalis contralateral to the injection side, for quantification of blood clearance of radioactivity. Brain SPECT studies were performed 10-12 min after the bolus injection of [99mTc]-HMPAO by using the same hardware as in the rCBV studies. Again, 60 projections in a 64x64 matrix, of 20 s each, were acquired over 360° with a total count of over 5 500 000 per study. SPECT sections were obtained by filtered backprojection (Butterworth filter of order 4 with cutoff frequency 0.4) and corrected by Chung algorithm.

rCBF values were then calculated by the O. Nickel technique[19] for brain regions supplied by a. cerebri anterior, media, and posterior, for both hemispheres. Scintigraphic regions of interest were placed exactly as in the rCBV SPECT study . Additionally, the volume of cerebral tissue at zero perfusion was quantified using a modified J. Mountz technique[20]. In particular, the normal file of [99mTc]-HMPAO uptake in various regions of the brain was previously obtained from 12 control subjects as counts per voxel normalised to the injected dose, as proposed by Podreka et al.[21].

The factor {mean uptake per voxel in normals -2* (s.d.)} was assumed as a reference border for discovering hypoperfusion in any particular region. The zero per-fusion volume, called the volume of cerebral damage (VCD) was then calculated as $\int [(RU-U)/RU] \, dV$, where RU is the reference normal uptake per voxel in the region and U is the actual uptake there. The integral was taken over all voxels with decreased uptake.

Results

Visual reporting of cerebral perfusion SPECT studies revealed in all patients an obvious improvement in cerebral blood flow on the stenosis-dependent side, induced by plasmapheresis. A typical example of rCBF SPECT changes is presented in Figure 1. Quantitative studies verified the visual impression.

The results of rCBF and rCBV follow-up in the course of plasmapheretic therapy are presented in Table 1. rCBV, obviously increased in regions supplied by stenotic ICA before plasmapheresis, did decrease after this procedure, so that essentially no interhemispheric difference was observed and the rCBV values were returned to normal ranges. rCBF in stenosis-dependent cerebral regions, contradictory to rCBV, increased significantly after plasmapheresis. Of specific interest is the fact that not only poststenotic, but also intact hemispheres did demonstrate an increase in cerebral blood flow as a result of plasmapheresis.

Values of rCBV, rCBF and the rCBV/rCBF ratio remained essentially unchanged in the a. cerebri posterior – dependent perfusion region. In fact,

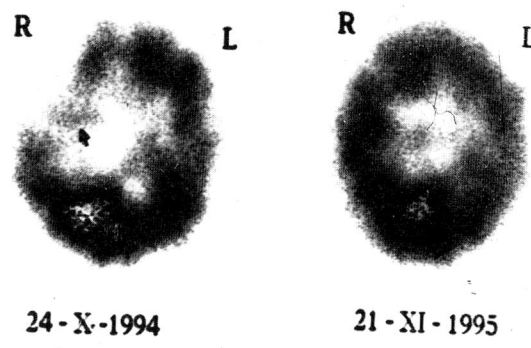

24 - X - 1994   21 - XI - 1995

Figure 1 Cerebral perfusion SPECT with [99mTc]-HMPAO in a patient with 78% stenosis of the right internal carotid artery before and after plasmapheresis treatment. There is disappearance of interhemispheric rCBF asymmetry owing to an improvement in the stenosis-dependent region

preplasmapheresis values on both intact and stenotic sides did not differ from each other and were in the normal range.

Six patients in whom the rCBV/rCBF decreased after plasmapheresis treatment of <5.1s, did not demonstrate any neurological symptoms six months after the study. Two patients, in whom the rCBV/rCBF values were higher, had TIAs in three and four months after stopping of plasmapheresis. VCD decreased significantly after plasmapheresis treatment in the group. In two patients who had VCD values as much as 28 and 23 cm^3 before treatment, this diminished to almost zero.

The clinical parameters presented in Table 2 underwent significant changes in most of the blood count as well as in the blood biochemical and blood lipid parameters, which are essential in determining blood rheology[22]. When applying a correlation analysis for quantification of relationships between blood parameters and rCBV, rCBF and rCBV/rCBF values, we have not obtained any significant single or multiple correlation.

Discussion

Disappearance of the deficit of cerebrovascular perfusion reserve after successful surgical correction of carotid stenosis is a well-known occurrence[23]. The facility for rheotherapeutical procedures, in particular plasmapheresis, to make beneficial changes to the cerebral circulation similar to the effects of carotid surgery is unexpected since no improvements in vascular anatomy are induced by this kind of treatment.

Table 1 Indices of SPECT blood flow and blood volume in the course of rheotherapeutical treatment of cerebrovascular disease

| Vascular region | Index | Control subjects (n = 8) | | Patients with unilateral cerebrovascular disease (n = 8) | | | |
| | | | | Before plasmapheresis (n = 8) | | 4 days after plasmapheresis (n = 8) | |
		Left hemisphera	Right hemisphera	Intact hemisphera	Involved hemisphera	Intact hemisphera	Intact hemisphera
A.cerebri anterior	rCBF ml/mim/100cm^3	55.6 (s.d. 2.8)	55.5 (s.d. 3.1)	55.7 (s.d. 2.4)	50.5 (s.d. 3.4)	54.3 (s.d. 3.6)	51.7 (s.d. 2.9)
	rCBV ml/100cm^3	4.2 (s.d. 0.2)	4.1 (s.d. 0.2)	4.2 (s.d. 0.2)	4.4 (s.d. 0.2)	4.0 (s.d. 0.1)	4.3 (s.d. 0.2)
	rCBV/rCBF, sec	4.3 (s.d. 0.2)	4.4 (s.d. 0.3)	4.6 (s.d. 0.2)	5.2 (s.d. 0.2)	4.4 (s.d. 0.1)	4.9 (s.d. 0.1) [a]
A.cerebri media	rCBF ml/min/100cm^3	51.8 (s.d. 2.3)	52.4 (s.d. 2.2)	49.9 (s.d. 2.0)	44.7 (s.d. 3.1)	53.1 (s.d. 1.9) [a]	53.0 (s.d. 3.1) [b]
	rCBV ml/100cm^3	4.4 (s.d. 0.2)	4.5 (s.d. 0.1)	4.7 (s.d. 0.1)	5.4 (s.d. 0.2)	4.3 (s.d. 0.3) [a]	4.8 (s.d. 0.2) [b]
	rCBV/rCBF, sec	4.9 (s.d. 0.2)	4.9 (s.d. 0.2)	5.3 (s.d. 0.2)	7.2 (s.d. 0.2)	4.9 (s.d. 0.3) [a]	5.4 (s.d. 0.2) [b]
A.cerebri posterior	rCBF ml/min/100cm^3	56.7 (s.d. 3.1)	57.3 (s.d. 2.9)	58.7 (s.d. 3.0)	56.9 (s.d. 2.7)	57.3 (s.d. 2.8)	56.7 (s.d. 4.2)
	rCBV ml/100cm^3	5.4 (s.d. 0.3)	5.5 (s.d. 0.3)	5.9 (s.d. 0.3)	5.1 (s.d. 0.3)	5.1 (s.d. 0.2)	5.0 (s.d. 0.3)
	rCBV/rCBF, sec	5.3 (s.d. 0.2)	5.2 (s.d. 0.1)	5.3 (s.d. 0.2)	5.4 (s.d. 0.1)	5.3 (s.d. 0.1)	5.3 (s.d. 0.2)

[a], $p < 0.05$; [b], $p < 0.001$, as compared with pre-treatment values

Table 2 Changes in rheologically relevant blood indices induced by plasmapheresis therapy in patients with cerebrovascular disease (n = 8)

Index	before plasmapheresis (n = 8)	2-4 days after plasmapharesis (n = 8)	p[a]
Haemoglobin g/l	167.7 s.d. 3.35	163.0 s.d. 2.8	> 0.05
Red blood cells x 10^{12}/l	4.63 s.d. 1.42	4.55 s.d. 1.61	< 0.01
Platelets x 10^9/l	315 s.d. 15.4	275.4 s.d. 14.6	< 0.01
Hematocrit, %	47.1 s.d. 1.1	41.0 s.d. 0.8	< 0.01
Sedimentation rate, mm/h	4.0 s.d. 0.2	13.3 s.d. 0.4	< 0.01
Total blood protein, g/l	7.82 s.d. 1.2	6.8 s.d. 1.6	< 0.05
Albumin, %	52.7 s.d. 1.3	60.2 s.d. 1.7	< 0.01
Globulins, %			
α	3.7 s.d. 0.3	3.6 s.d. 0.3	> 0.05
α	8.2 s.d. 0.5	6.8 s.d. 0.2	< 0.01
β	12.8 s.d. 0.7	10.1 s.d. 0.8	< 0.05
γ	21.5 s.d. 1.8	17.4 s.d. 1.6	< 0.05
Fibrinogen, g/l	4.4 s.d. 0.3	3.1 s.d. 0.1	< 0.05
Fibrinogen B, g/l	1.2 s.d. 0.3	0.2 s.d. 0.1	< 0.005
Total fibrinolytic activity, %	5.83 s.d. 0.61	4.84 s.d. 0.2	< 0.05
Cholestin, mM/l	6.9 s.d. 0.3	5.3 s.d. 0.3	< 0.01
β-lipoproteins, IU	119.7 s.d. 5.9	66.8 s.d. 4.8	< 0.01
Triglycerides, mM/l	2.03 s.d. 0.07	1.51 s.d. 0.16	< 0.01

[a], p are given as compared with pre-treatment values

Much of the effect can be ascribed to an improvement in blood rheology due to the procedure.

The essential role of rheological factors in the pathogenesis of stroke, in particular their influence on cerebrovascular reserve, has been stressed by numerous authors[2,5,6,8,24]. Quantitative rCBV and rCBF data observed in our patients before the start of the treatment are quite consistent with the conception of the compensatory role of the cerebral vasodilatory mechanisms in carotid stenosis[25]. A decrease in perfusion pressure in the artery supplying the post-stenotic area of the brain induces extensive vasodilatation through adenosine-dependent mechanisms, and can preserve rCBF for supplying the oxygen demand of the brain[14,24,25]. At the same time, these compensatory mechanisms also promote a slowing of capillary transit and an increase in endothelial adhesiveness of platelets and red blood cells[2,26]. Further, deterioration of blood cells and plasma rheology reduce the beneficial effects of cerebral vasodilatation, so the rCBF tends to decrease[2,24]. All these effects cause the simultaneous rise of rCBV and diminution of rCBF and reduction in rCBV/rCBF ratio in the patients.

It has been shown by some authors that haemodilution therapy increases cerebral blood flow especially in cerebral ischaemic conditions[8,27,28]. Improving the blood rheology serves as an essential mechanism for this[29,30], because it provides greater blood flow at the same arteriolar perfusion pressure. In acute stroke, this effect does not provide any real clinical effect, as after several hours of severe critical ischaemia, the treatment may be not in a position to reverse profound cellular damage.

Previous studies have demonstrated prominent improvement in both blood cells and plasma rheological factors by plasmapheresis, in particular when extensive amounts of plasma are withdrawn and substituted with either human albumin or high molecular dextrane[12]. We can ascribe the beneficial changes of cerebral blood flow and improvement of cerebral perfusion reserve to this rheotherapeutical effect of plasmapheresis. Data on changes in clinical parameters of the patients presented in Table 2 argue in favour of this hypothesis, although no definitive correlation was observed in this restricted number of patients. Improvement in endothelial functions due to plasmapheresis, although not evaluated in this study, can play an essential role in improving the cerebrovascular perfusion reserve as well.

When discussing the pathophysiological mechanisms involved in the effects of plasmapheresis on cerebral circulation, we should also mention a significant decrease in the hematocrit. This mechanism probably contributes to the improvement of rCBF, in particular in regions that had normal rCBF and rCBV values before plasmapheresis, as it does in anaemic patients[5]. Nevertheless, the decrease in blood haemoglobin was not as prominent, so oxygen blood transport capacities remained essentially in the normal ranges. In this restricted number of patients, no single or multiple correlation of blood rheological factors with parameters of cerebral circulation was significant. More extensive groups will probably make such relationships more clear.

We referred the patients for this study carefully, so that those recruited had not undergone stroke with irreversible ischaemic deficit before. In each patient, no neurological deficit was present at the moment of study. Bearing in mind that in every patient the degree of ICA stenosis exceeded 70% of the lumen and was definitively significant haemodynamically, we can suggest that such patients possessed an extensive amount of cerebral tissue with entirely preserved viability, but decreased perfusion reserve. The haemodynamic condition of such regions can be improved by rheotherapy, as has been shown in studies with hypervolaemic haemodilution[8,31].

Although more extensive studies are necessary for defining which groups of patients can benefit most from plasmapheresis, we can suggest plasmapheresis as a technique for the short-term prevention of stroke in patients in whom surgical correction of ICA stenosis cannot be performed due to temporary contraindications. Regular (three or four times per year) use of plasmapheresis can be proposed in carotid disease patients in whom surgical correction can not be performed technically.

This study was the first stage of an extensive evaluation of the long-term effects of plasmapheresis on cerebral perfusion. As we have mentioned above, patients remained clinically unchanged and did not demonstrate TIAs, PRIND or stroke events, if the rCBV/rCBF ratio in the stenosis-dependent region did decrease below 5.1s after plasmapheresis. This value is now assumed as the target for plasmapheresis correction of carotid disease. Further studies are now in progress, which aim to clear the prognostic role of rCBV/rCBF ratio in rheotherapeutical treatment. Plasmapheresis treatment needs to be studied more extensively as a technique for stroke prevention using a clinical randomised trial. It would also be useful to study how long the beneficial changes of rCBV and rCBF are preserved. If proven effective, plasmapheretic rheotherapy could provide definitive treatment for patients with technically inaccessible stenoses of cerebral arteries and high risk of stroke, or could be employed as an adjuvant treatment in patients with severe bilateral atherosclerosis when preparing the patient for carotid surgery.

Conclusion

The results of the study presented here, although based on data from a carefully selected group of neurologically intact patients, are of pilot nature because of the relatively small number of persons studied here. Nevertheless, we can conclude that SPECT studies of cerebral perfusion and blood volume already give evidence for improvement in the cerebral perfusion reserve by plasmapheresis. It has been shown before that the rheological and biochemical effects of plasmapheresis last as long as 3 - 5 months. If plasmapheresis-induced improvement of the perfusion reserve does last as long as changes in biochemistry, the technique can be employed for the routine prevention of cerebral ischaemia in high risk patients. This study is currently in progress.

References

1   Schroeder, T. Hemodynamic significance of internal carotid artery disease. *Acta Neurol. Scand.* 1988, 77, 353

2   Schmid-Schoenbein, H., Driesen, G. and Gallasch, H. Hemorheology and cerebral infarction : on the role of pathological blood tixotropy in the pathogenesis of and therapy for states of acute cerebral hypoperfusion in 'Cerebral ischemia and hemorheology', (Eds. A. Hartmann, W. Kuchinsky), Springer Verlag, Berlin, Germany, 1987, p.27

3   Chievitz, E. and Thiede, T. Complications and causes of death in polycythaemia. *Acta Med. Scand.* 1962, 172, 513

4   Elwood, P., Waters, W., Benjamin, I. and Sweetman, P. Mortality and anaemia in woman. *Lancet* 1974, 1, 891

5   Thomas, D.J. The influence of haematocrit on the cerebral circulation *Acta Neurol. Scand.* 1989, 127, 56

6   Hartmann, A. and Kuchinsky, W. (Eds.) in 'Cerebral ischemia and hemorheology', Springer Verlag, Berlin, Germany, 1987

7   Agnoli, A. and De-Marinis, M. Presupposti fisiopatologici alla terapia con emodiluzione nell'infarto cerebrale acuto *Res. Clin. Lab* . 1989, 19, 59

8   Hartmann, A. Effect of hemodilution on regional cerebral blood flow. *Acta Neurol. Scand.* 1989, 127, 36

9   Scandinavian Study Group, Multicenter trial of hemodilution in acute ischemic stroke. I.Results in the total patient population. *Stroke* 1987, 18, 691

10 Lopukhin, Yu.M. and Molodenkov, B.M. in 'Haemosorption' , Meditsina, Moscow, 1978, p.167

11 Lopukhin, Yu.M. New approaches to prophylaxis and treatment of atherosclerosis. *Cardiologia* 1986, 5

12 Kozlov, B.N. Application of plasmapheresis in complex angiosurgical treatment of carotid atherosclerotic disease. *Ph. D. Thesis* Tomsk , 1992, p. 84

13 Buell, U. and Schicta, H. Tomographische Funktionsdiagnostik in der Nuklearmedizin : Erfassung Regionaler Reserven und Bilanzen. *Nuklear Med.* 1989, 28, 45

14 Gibbs, J.M., Wise, R.J.S., Leenders, K.L. and Jones, T. Evaluation of cerebral perfusion reserve in patients with carotid artery occlusion. *Lancet* 1984, 1, 310

15 Leinsinger, G., Schmiedek, P., Kreisig, T. *et al.* 133-Xe-DSPECT: Bedeuting der Zerebrovaskulaeren Reservekapazitaet fuer Diagnostik und Therapie der chronischen zerebralen Ischaemie. *Nuklearmedizin* 1988, 27, 127

16 Alexandrov, A.V., Bladin, C.F., Maggisano, R. and Norris, J.W. Measuring carotid stenosis. *Stroke* 1993, 24, 1292

17 Kuhl, D.E., Martin, R., Alavi, A. *et al.* Local cerebral blood volume determined by three dimensional reconstruction of radionuclide data *Circulat. Res.* 1975, 36, 610

18 Andersen, A.R., Friberg, H., Lassen, N.A. *et al.* Serial studies of cerebral blood flow using [99mTc]-HMPAO: a comparison with [133Xe]. *Nucl. Med. Communicat.* 1987, 8, 549

19 Nickel, O., Ulrich, P., Naegele-Woerle, B. *et al.* rCBF quantification with 99mTc-HMPAO SPECT and 195mAu : theory and first results in 'Nuklearmedizin : New trends and possibilities in Nuclear Medicine', *Proc. Eur. Nucl. Med. Congr.* Budapest 24 - 28 August 1987, p.289

20 Mountz, J.M. A method of analysis of SPECT blood flow image data for comparison with computed tomography *Clin. Nucl. Med.* 1989, 14, 192

21 Podreka, I., Hoell, K., Dal-Bianco, P. and Goldenberg, G. Klinische und technische Aspekte der SPECT-Hirnszintigraphie mit 123-I-N-Isopropyl-Amphetamin. *Nuc. Compact.* 1984, 15, 305

22 Begg, T.B. and Hearns, J.B. Components in blood viscosity. The relative contribution of haematocrit, plasma fibrinogen and other proteins. *Clin. Sci.* 1966, 31, 87

23 Ramsay, S.C., Yeates, M.G., Lord, R.S. *et al.* Use of Technetium-HMPAO to demonstrate changes in cerebral blood flow reserve following carotid endarterectomy. *J. Nucl. Med.* 1991, 32, 1382

24 Tomita, M. Significance of cerebral blood volume in 'Cerebral Hyperemia and Ischemia : from the Standpoint of Cerebral Blood Volume', Elsevier Science, Osaka, Japan, 1988

25 Toyama, H., Takeshita, G., Takeuchi, A. *et al.* Cerebral hemodynamics in patients with chronic obstructive carotid disease by rCBF, rCBV and rCBV/rCBF ratio using SPECT. *J. Nucl. Med.* 1990, 31, 55

26 Karaganov, Ya .L., Kerdivarenko, N.V. and Levin, B.N. in 'Microangiology', Scientia, Kishinev, 1982, p.210

27 Heros, R.C. and Korosue, K. Haemodilution for cerebral ishemia. *Stroke* 1989, 20, 423

28 Korosue, K and Heros, R.C. Mechanisms of cerebral blood flow augmentation by hemodilution in rabbits. *Stroke* 1992, 23, 1487

29 Henriksen, L., Paulson, O.B. and Smith, R.J. Cerebral blood flow following normovolaemic haemodilution in patients with high hematocrit. *Ann. Neurol.* 1981, 9, 454

30 Humphrey, P.R.D., duBoulay, G.H., Marshall, J. *et al.* Cerebral blood flow and viscosity in relative polycythaemia. *Lancet* 1979, 2, 873

31 Kee, D.B. and Wood, J.H. Rheology of the cerebral circulation . *Neurosurgery* 1984, 15, 125

SPECT in Neurology and Psychiatry, edited by P.P. De Deyn, R.A. Dierckx, A. Alavi and B.A. Pickut
© 1997 John Libbey & Company Ltd, pp. 359–363

Assessment of Cerebral Perfusion in Acute Intracerebral Haematoma by Means of ^{99m}Tc-ECD perfusion SPECT

Chapter

43

B. Pfausler, G. Grubwieser, U. Sailer,
E. Donnemiller, G. Riccabona and E. Schmutzhard

Introduction

Cerebral CT scans are essential in the diagnosis of spontaneous intracerebral haematoma as a cause of sudden focal neurological deficits [1,2]. The clinical course in patients with intracerebral haematoma is highly variable: some deteriorate and others do not, deterioration sometimes being delayed for several days. Focal neurological signs such as hemiparesis, hemihypesthesia, hemianopia, aphasia and neglect syndrome are usually caused by cortical lesions in the brain. A combination of these signs and symptoms can be found in strictly subcortical haemorrhagic striatocapsular infarctions as well as in strictly basal ganglia haemorrhage [3]. In patients with striatocapsular ischaemic infarctions, hypoperfusion in the corresponding cortex has been described previously [2]. Similar mechanisms are thought to exist in spontaneous intracerebral haematoma of a hypertensive nature, although no perfusion studies in such patients have been carried out so far. Functional cerebral imaging with SPECT shows not only irreversible cerebral lesions of the brain within the area of the haemorrhage (cold spot) as seen in cerebral computerised tomography, but also zones of reversible haemodynamic dysbalance ('penumbra zone') which correspond to brain tissue with possible reversible hypoperfusion around the irreversibly damaged region of the haematoma [4-6].

This study aims to explain the existence of a 'penumbra zone', i.e. hypoperfused area surrounding spontaneous hypertensive intracerebral (basal ganglia) haematoma. Possible new treatment strategies for such acute intracerebral haemorrhages, aiming at the restoration of adequate perfusion in the 'penumbra zones', and thus limiting the extent of permanent damage, will be discussed.

Patients and methods

Ten patients with spontaneous intracerebral haemorrhage located within the basal ganglia on initial CT scan as cause of a first ever stroke were enrolled. All patients underwent CT scan and SPECT scanning under intensive care monitoring conditions within 8 h of admission to the Neurological Intensive Care Unit of the University Hospital Innsbruck, Austria. The CT scans were obtained with a Somatom Plus scanner (Siemens), equipped with software that allowed volumetric assessment. The size of each haemorrhage was measured on any section showing the lesion, the margins of haemorrhage were traced on the monitor screen with a cursor and the volume was then calculated using the computerised program. ^{99m}Tc-ECD 555-740 MBq (ethyl cysteinate dimer) was administered intravenously in a quiet room. Data acquisition was started 15 min after tracer application. Patients were placed in a supine position with covered

University Hospital, Arichstrasse 35, A-6020, Innsbruck, Austria eyes, their head fixed in an appropriate head holder. SPECT studies were performed with a single head rotating Anger camera (Siemens Orbiter ZLC 3700) equipped with LEAP collimator (low energy, all purpose), which yielded an image resolution of approximately 2.3 cm in a distance of 20 cm rotation radius (FWHM). In one angular sampling interval, 64 projections were acquired in 360°. The acquisition time per projection was 25 s. The matrix size was 64x64, pixel size 6.25x6.25. The energy window was set at 15% for 150 keV. Transversal, sagittal and coronal slices were reconstructed using Ramp and Butterworth filters (cutoff 0.5). Attenuation was corrected using Soerenson's method, with an attenuation coefficient of 0.14 cm. Quality control procedures were made once a month with a high count flood source with 120M counts in matrix size 128x128, and every 3 months at the centre of rotation. After acquisition, data were transferred from Max Delta to NUD (Nuclear Diagnostics) and SPECT reconstruction using Wiener 24-filter type was made. Analysis of the SPECT studies was performed on a Sun Spark 10/40 computer equipped with the operating system Solaris 2.3 and software from NUD with the program Hermes. For volume measurement, we used the program MultiModality - region growing, which uses thresholding criteria without edge functions. By selecting the speed and limit (minimum 0-30, maximum 40 +/-5) within the given manual ROI, the region growing is limited to a particular volume of the scan[7,8]. SPECT and CT scans were compared visually with respect to volume, diameter, additional cortical cold areas, and a differentiation quotient was calculated. In 3 patients, CT and SPECT scans were repeated after four weeks.

Results

The demographic data of 10 patients (four males, 6 females, median age 61.5 years, range 41-75 years) as well as the neurological signs and symptoms and possible additional aetiological factors are listed in Table 1. Table 2 shows the cerebral CT and SPECT volumetric data of all 10 patients. In all patients the perfusion deficit measured by SPECT was significantly larger than the volme of intracranial haemorrhage measured on CT scan. The differences ranged from factors of 1.6 to 12.2, i.e. SPECT measured volumes on average 4.3 times larger than CT volumes. Figure 1a shows a typical haematoma in a cerebral CT scan. Figure 1b shows the corresponding SPECT of the same patient, clearly exhibiting the large cold spot with the similar volume size (compared with CT) and the surrounding hypoperfused area ('penumbra zone').

Discussion

Spontaneous intracerebral haemorrhages caused by arterial hypertension will have a poor prognosis with mortality rates ranging from 10-20%[9]. In most instances, hypertensive intracerebral haemorrhage is located within the basal ganglia. Nevertheless, the neurological focal signs and symptoms are frequently much more serious and intense than the hyperdense area in the cerebral CT scan would implicate. Within a few days, a hypodense ringlike area usually surrounds the intracranial (basal ganglia) haematoma, indicating oedema and/or possibly ischaemic lesions due to hypoperfusion[10]. In our series of 10 consecutive patients with hypertensive basal ganglia haematoma confirmed by cerebral CT scan, a perfusion SPECT with Neurolite® was performed within 8 h of onset of focal neurological signs and symptoms. A perfusion deficit, on average 4.3 times larger than the CT measured haematoma and, thus, reaching far beyond the cold spot of the haematoma could be found regularly with this method, which excedes the findings in post traumatic intracerebral haemorrhage[11]. This indicates that, at least partially, the clinical/ neurological focal deficit is caused not only by the destruction of brain tissue due to the haemorrhage but also by hypoperfusion of the surrounding area, the so called 'penumbra'. The aetiology of this hypoperfused penumbra is most likely to be due to locally increased intracranial pressure caused by haemorrhage. Autoregulation mechanisms seem to be of limited efficacy in these patients with longstanding arterial hypertension. Given the risk of either rebleeding or deterioration of the initial haemorrhage in these patients, therapy aims at controlling blood pressure[9,10,12]. Such a well meant therapeutic step might be deleterious in view of our findings. In patients with cerebral ischaemia, it is well know that initial elevated blood pressure values (if not extremely high) should not be lowered too quickly to avoid aggravation of the ischaemia[11]. Our findings suggest that a similar approach should be employed in patients with spontaneous hypertensive intracerebral haemorrhage, thus saving parts of the hypoperfused 'penumbra' area which frequently involves essential parts of the cortex or the internal capsule. Therefore, severe longstanding neurological deficit and sequelae respectively, e.g. hemiplegia, aphasia, could possibly, and at least partially, be prevented. The hypoperfusion of the 'penumbra' is reversible as indicated in 3 of our patients in whom follow up CT and SPECT scans could be made, confirming the therapeutic implications discussed above.

Table 1 Clinical signs, symptoms and aetiology in 10 consecutive patients with spontaneous intracerebral haematoma

Patient number	Sex	Age	Clinical signs and symptoms	Aetiology
1	m	51	hemiparesis left, hemihypaesthesia left, homonymic hemianopia to the left side, hemineglect for the left side	hypertension
2	m	65	hemiparesis left, hemihypaesthesia left, homonymic hemianopia to the left side	hypertension diabetes mellitus
3	f	50	hemiparesis right, hemihypaesthesia right, Korsakow-syndrome	latent hypertension
4	m	75	hemiparesis right, hemihypaesthesia right, global aphasia	hypertension
5	f	67	hemiparesis right, hemihypaesthesia right, expressive aphasia	hypertension
6	f	41	hemiparesis right (slight)	hypertension
7	f	58	hemiparesis right, hemihypaesthesia right, global aphasia, homonymic hemianopia to the left side	hypertension diabetes mellitus thrombopenia
8	f	55	hemiparesis left, hemihypaesthesia left, homonymic hemianopia to the left side	hypertension
9	m	75	hemiparesis right (slight), 'thalamic' aphasia	hypertension
10	f	71	spastic hemiparesis left	hypertension

Table 2 Volumes of intracerebral haematoma measured by CT and perfusion deficits in patients with intracerebral haematoma measured by SPECT

Patient number	CT volume	SPECT volume
1	66.2	104.9
2	5.5	16.7
3	4.4	37.9
4	18.7	72.1
5	6.4	80.5
6	2.0	7.3
7	58.3	128.2
8	27.2	57.4
9	6.8	22.1
10	6.8	17.0

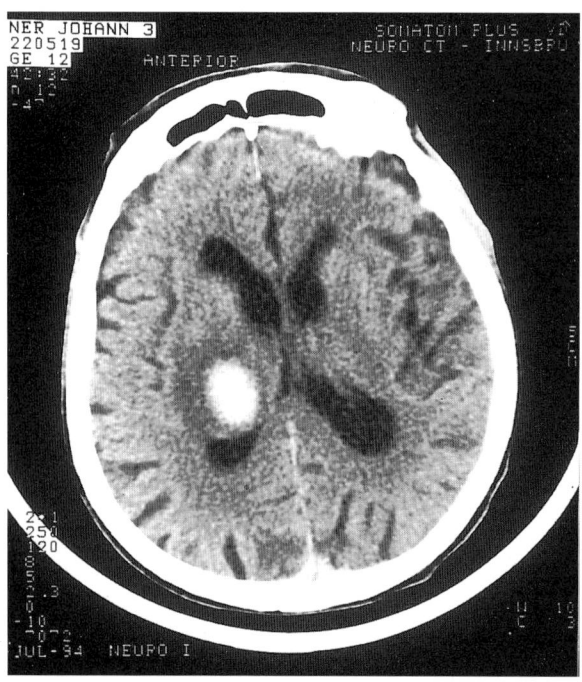

Figure 1a Typical CT appearance of a hypertensive intracerebral haematoma

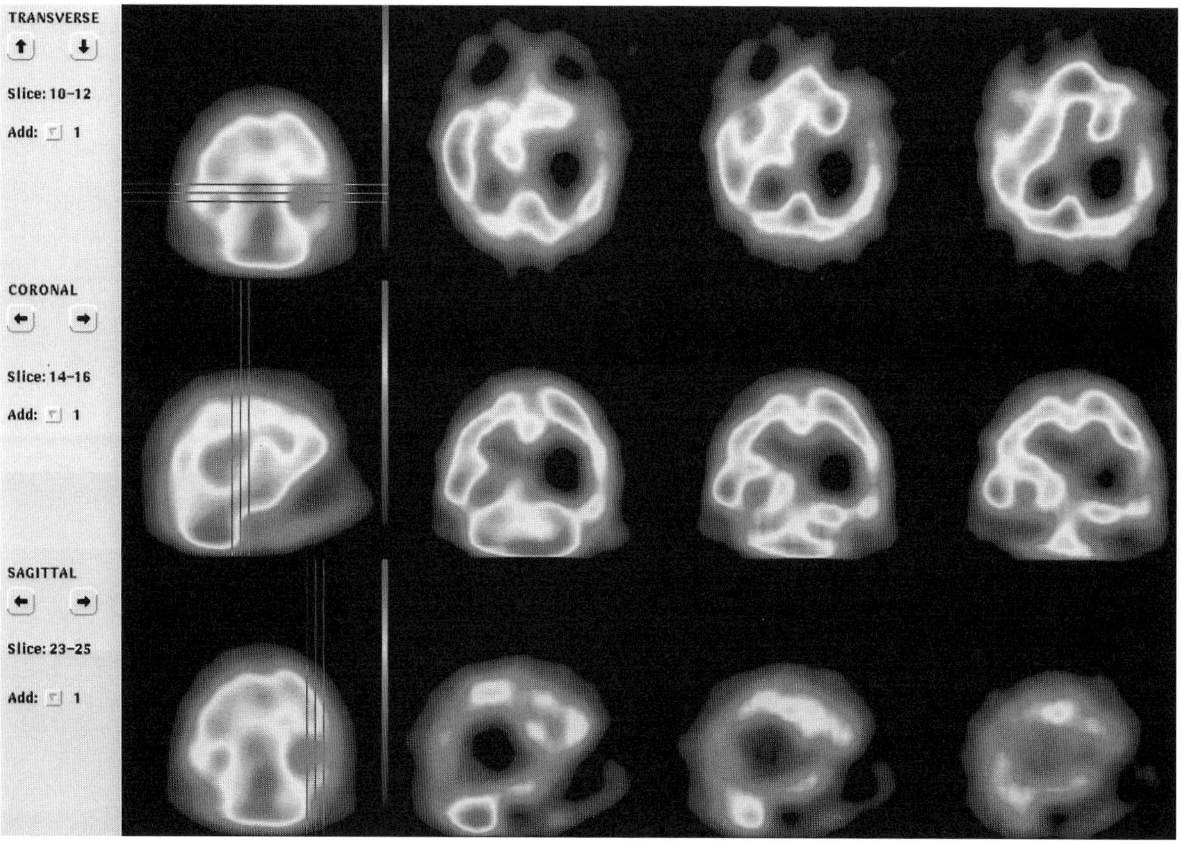

Figure 1b ^{99m}Tc-ECD perfusion SPECT in the same patient with intracerebral haematoma; note cold spot and 'penumbra'

References

1   Bryan, R.N. Imaging in acute stroke. *Radiology* 1990, 177, 615

2   Ghika, J., Bogousslavsky, J. and Regli, F. Infarcts in the territory of the deep perforators from the carotid system. *Neurology* 1989, 39, 507

3   Bamford, J. Clinical examination in the diagnosis and subclassification of stroke. *Lancet* 1992, 339, 400

4   Giubilei, F., Lenzi,G.K., Di Peiro, V. *et al.* Predictive value of brain perfusion single-photon emission computed tomography in acute cerebral ischaemia. *Stroke* 1990, 21, 895

5   Hellman, R.S. and Tikofsky, R.S. An overview of the contributions of regional cerebral blood flow studies in cerebrovascular disease: is there a role for single photon emission computed tomography? *Semin. Nucl. Med.* 1990, 20, 303

6   Holman, B.L., Hellman, R.S., Goldsmith, S.J. *et al.* Biodistribution, dosimetry, and clinical evaluation of technetium-^{99m} ethyl cysteinate dimer in normal subjects and in patients with chronic cerebral infarction. *J. Nucl. Med.* 1989, 30, 1018

7   Murase, K., Tanada, S, Yasuhara, Y. *et al.* SPECT volume measurement using an automatic threshold selection method combined with a V filter. *Eur. J. Nucl. Med.* 1989, 15, 21

8   Savolainen, S., Pohjonen, H., Sipila, O. and Liewandahl, K. Segmentation methods for volume determination ^{111}In ^{99m}Tc SPECT. *Nucl. Med. Commun.* 1995, 16, 370

9   Batjer, H.H., Reisch, J.S., Allen, B.C. *et al.* Failure of surgery to improve outcome in hypertensive putaminal haemorrhage. *Arch. Neurol.* 1990, 47, 1103

10 Ropper, A.H., Schütz, H.G. Spontaneous Intracerebral Haemorrhage in 'Neuro Critical Care', (Ed. W. Hacke), Springer Verlag, Berlin, Germany, 1994, p.621

11 Brass, L.M., Walovitch, R.C. and Joseph, J.L. The role of single photon emission computed tomography brain imaging with ^{99m}Tc-bicisate in the localization and definition of mechanism of ischemic stroke. *J. Cereb. Blood Flow Metab.* 1994, 14(1), 91

12 Kase, C.S., Mohr, J. and Caplan, L.R. Intracerebral haemorrhage in 'Stroke pathophysiology, diagnosis and management', (Eds. H.J.M. Barnett, J.P., Mohr, B.M. Stein, F.M. Yatsu), Churchill Livingstone, New York, USA, 1992, p.561

13 Choskey, M.S., Costa, D.C., Jannotti, F. *et al.* ^{99m}Tc-HMPAO SPECT studies in traumatic intracerebral haematoma. *J. Neurol. Neurosurg. Psychiatry* 1991, 54, 6

SPECT in Neurology and Psychiatry, edited by P.P. De Deyn, R.A. Dierckx, A. Alavi and B.A. Pickut

Prognostic Significance of Perfusion Defect in the Periinfarct Area

Chapter
44

P. Laloux, E.C. Laterre, P. De Coster and J. Jamart

Introduction

Although functional status is actually the most important goal of therapeutic strategy for each individual patient, prediction of infarct size and determination of cerebral blood flow (CBF) threshold values for the survival of brain tissue may have some important implications as well. The ischaemic threshold concept is currently the cornerstone in the management of cerebral infarction in clinical or therapeutic trials. For example, thrombolytic agents aim to restore CBF in oligemic brain tissue in order to normalise the imbalance between blood supply and metabolism. However, determination of the ischaemic threshold has been dependent on data from experimental studies of uniform occlusion models or from clinical investigations of patients with subacute or chronic cerebral infarction studied by positron emission computed tomography (PET)[1-5]. Until now, it has been difficult to estimate the ischaemic flow threshold in the acute stage of cerebral ischaemia in a clinical setting. However, semiquantitative evaluation has been made possible by SPECT imaging, which can be performed easily in an emergency.

Many studies have shown that the area of ischaemia extended beyond the region of overt structural change[5-15]. In the chronic phase, the blood flow was decreased not only in the infarct area, defined by the hypodense image on the CT scan, but also in most cases in extensive periinfarct areas, defined by the regions surrounding the infarct area.

Thus, the goals of this SPECT study were: (1) to assess the value of SPECT indices such as the degree and size of hypoperfusion, crossed cerebellar diaschisis, and the presence of periinfarct area as a predictor of infarct size; (2) to determine the ischaemic CBF threshold defined as the critical value for the morphological changes with referring CT images; (3) to correlate the periinfarct area with the clinical outcome evaluated at 1 month.

Patients and methods

Patients

We selected from our Stroke Data Bank 55 consecutive patients, each without a stroke history, who presented with acute ischaemia (< 12 h) in the carotid artery territory. All patients underwent ^{99m}Tc-HMPAO SPECT within the first 36 h. Patients with transient ischaemic attacks were excluded. Because of the low spatial resolution of SPECT, using in this study a single-head camera, the subcortical regions could not be studied directly by drawing regions of interest

Mont-Godinne University Hospital, Medical School of the University of Louvain, 5530 Yvoir, Belgium

in the deep areas. We selected 21 patients (16 men, 5 women) aged 49 - 88 (mean, 71 ± 9; median, 73) years with ischaemia in the cortical middle (MCA) or anterior (ACA) cerebral artery territory in 19 and 2 patients, respectively. Patients with subcortical infarcts were retrospectively excluded by the findings on follow-up CT. In patients with normal CT, cortical carotid lesion was defined clinically by the presence of signs compatible with cortical localisation (hemiplegia with predominant brachiofacial involvement, monoplegia, neuropsychological impairment). The time of onset was recorded and 04.00 a.m. was arbitrarily chosen when the patient awoke with deficit.

All patients underwent Doppler ultrasonography of the extracranial cerebral arteries. Intra-arterial angiography was performed in 10 (48%) of 21 patients in whom ultrasonography had indicated atherosclerotic carotid disease. All patients received standard treatment including haemodilution when the hematocrit level was > 45% and anticoagulant in case a stroke was in progression or there were cardiac emboli.

Method of brain CT

An initial brain CT without contrast (Siemens DRH) was performed in all patients in order to rule out intracranial haemorrhage. Follow-up CT scanning with contrast was obtained in all patients between day 2 and day 9 with a mean time interval of 5 days. This time of CT scanning precluded some potential bias due to the 'fogging effect'. Contiguous axial slices (matrix of 512 pixels) were obtained parallel to the canthomeatal line. The slice thickness was 4 mm (scan time, 7 seconds per slice) in the posterior fossa and 8 mm (scan time, 5 seconds per slice) in the cerebral hemispheres. Acute or subacute cerebral infarct was defined by the presence of at least one of the following CT characteristics: focal hypodensity, mass effect on adjacent ventricles and cerebral sulci and fissures, and peripheral contrast enhancement[16]. Topography of infarcts was classified according to the vascular anatomic territory[17]. The definition of cortical or subcortical infarcts was the same as that used in a previous study[18]. Special attention was paid to record the presence of silent chronic cerebral infarcts according to the following CT characteristics: well-defined low attenuation area (10-25 HU or isodense with the cerebrospinal fluid), sharply demarcated margins, no oedema, no contrast enhancement, no expansive features, possible enlargement of adjacent ventricles and cerebral sulci and fissures[16,19].

The extent of infarcts was evaluated on follow-up scans. Infarcts were categorised according to the maximum diameter of hypodense lesion (≤3 cm or

> 3 cm)[11]. Using follow-up CT on morphological damages, the patients were classified into two groups[15]: (1) an infarct group that included the patients with completed infarction associated with neurological deficits; (2) a non-infarct group that included the patients with neurological deficits on admission who showed no structural changes on follow-up CT.

Method of SPECT

Regional cerebral blood flow was measured by brain SPECT after the intravenous injection of 20 mCi (740 MBq) ^{99m}Tc-HMPAO (Ceretec, Amersham) to the patient under resting conditions with eyes open in a dim, quiet room. Acquisition was carried out 10 to 30 min after injection of the tracer with a single-head rotating gamma camera (General Electric; 64 projections of 30 s each; spatial resolution of 12 mm FWHM). Filtered backprojection with linearisation was performed for data reconstruction using a Sheeplogan filter (with Hanning window) which is a modified version of the Ramp filter. Correction of scatter and attenuation were removed with the aim of improving the processing time. In a semi-quantitative analysis comparing symmetrical cortical areas at equivalent depths, ratios of counts are not affected by such a method of correction. A correction factor to limit hyperfixation error in patients evaluated in the subacute phase[20] had not yet been implemented routinely at the time of this study. The raw data were first compressed to allow reconstruction of consecutive parallel axial slices every 12 mm parallel to and above the orbitomeatal line (OM). The plane for SPECT imaging was adjusted to be parallel to the orbito-meatal line in order to match the CT plane.

SPECT findings were evaluated blindly by the department of Nuclear Medicine without knowledge of the clinical data. For quantification, with a computerised program developed in our laboratory, 16 symmetrical regions of interest (ROIs of 3 x 3 pixels; pixel size, 6 mm) were located automatically, 6 along the cortical ribbon over each cerebral hemisphere and 2 over each cerebellar hemisphere. The cerebral ROIs covered the prefrontal, frontal, frontoparietal, parietal, temporal, parieto-occipital and occipital regions. The images in the inferior anterior temporal and high vertex cortical regions were excluded because of greater side-to-side variability. Thus, for each patient, semi-quantitative analysis was performed in 4 selected axial slices ranging from OM + 12 mm to OM + 60 mm. In each ROI, the difference in total count was expressed as a percentage of the value from the contralateral asymptomatic hemisphere with a normal cerebral blood flow. An interhemispheric difference of at least 10% was considered to be

Table 1 Demographic data and imaging findings

Cases	Doppler / angiogram[a]	Degree	SPECT Size	CCD[b]	Periinfarct area	CT
1/M/72	N	5%	0	0	0	0
2/M/63	N	14%	2	0	0	0
3/F/88	N	13%	1	0	+	+
4/F/69	N	45%	9	0	+	+
5/M/61	N	69%	9	1	+	+
6/M/79	N	32%	13	0	+	+
7/M/72	N	35%	9	0	+	+
8/M/57	occl. ipsilateral	52%	9	0	+	+
9/F/77	occl. ipsilateral 50% contralateral	62%	17	1	+	+
10/M/64	N	19%	3	0	0	0
11/M/78	N	28%	7	1	+	+
12/F/73	70% contralateral	9%	0	0	0	0
13/M/81	80% ipsilateral	53%	4	1	0	+
14/M/79	occl. ipsilateral	28%	8	0	+	+
15/M/82	N	59%	6	1	0	+
16/M/49	N	5%	0	0	0	0
17/F/57	occl. ipsilateral	18%	2	0	+	+
18/M/75	occl. ipsilateral	56%	3	1	+	+
19/M/76	70% bilateral	31%	3	1	+	+
20/M/71	N	10%	1	0	0	+
21/M/74	<90% ipsilateral 50% contralateral	32%	5	0	+	+

[a], N, normal; [b], CCD, crossed cerebellar diaschisis

significant[21,22]. This level of significance was also found in 9 control patients (3 men, 6 women) aged 30 to 62 (mean, 40 ± 10) years, suffering from tension-type headache, in whom a CT scan was normal (unpublished data). The average of the interhemispheric differences was 1.01 ± 0.04 and 1.00 ± 0.04 for the right and left cerebral ROIs, respectively. For each patient, the degree of hypoperfusion was defined by the highest interhemispheric difference. We determined the size of hypoperfusion by the number of regions of interest with an interhemispheric difference

of at least 10% in the hemispheric slices selected by our methodology. Crossed cerebellar diaschisis (CCD) was defined by the presence of at least 5% hypoperfusion in the cerebellar hemisphere contralateral to the hemispheric hypoperfusion[23,24]. In the infarct group, the infarct area and periinfarct area were defined as the area of abnormal perfusion corresponding to the low density area on follow-up CT and the surrounding regions, respectively. In order to study the flow threshold for the survival of brain tissue, we tried to discriminate between the periinfarct area and infarct area according to the average of the lowest and highest degree of hypoperfusion in each region. In the non-infarct group, the clinically relevant area of abnormal perfusion without structural change on follow-up CT was considered for analysis.

The mean time interval of SPECT examinations was 14 h 51 min (range, 3 h 7 min to 35 h 38 min). SPECT was obtained within the first 24 h in 17 (81%) patients.

Clinical and outcome evaluations

Outcome evaluations were performed by neurologists blinded to SPECT data. Clinical short-term outcome was evaluated 1 month after the onset by the Rankin Scale[25] from which the functional status was derived, classifying patients with good (score of 1 to 3) or poor (score of 4 to 6) outcome. The presence of periinfarct area and the average of its highest degree of hypo-perfusion were used as parameters to discriminate between patients with poor or good outcome. Furthermore, the infarct size (≤3 cm or > 3 cm) on follow-up CT scans was considered. We studied which SPECT indices were associated with large or small infarcts.

Statistical analysis

Numerical parameters were expressed as mean ± s.d. and medians, and were compared using Wilcoxon rank sum test. Frequencies were compared by Fisher exact test. All the tests were two-tailed.

Results

Clinical data and imaging findings

All demographic data as well as the SPECT, CT and angiographic findings are shown in Table 1. At 1 month, the clinical outcome was considered good in 16 patients and poor in 5 patients. Two patients died of transtentorial herniation and heart failure, respectively.

Follow-up CT showed a cortical infarct in 16 (76%) patients localised in the MCA territory in 14 and ACA territory in 2. The size of infarct was ≤ 3 cm in 4 (25%) patients and > 3 cm in 12 (75%). The non-infarct group consisted of 5 patients with neurological signs on admission compatible with cortical MCA involvement.

SPECT showed a clinically relevant perfusion defect in 18 (86%) patients (Table 1). The mean degree and size of hypoperfusion were 36 ± 18% (median, 32%; range, 10-69%) and 6 ± 6 (median, 4; range, 1-26), res-pectively. We found a crossed cerebellar diaschisis in 7 (39%) patients with a mean degree of hypoperfusion

of 15 ± 7% (median, 12%; range, 6-25%). In the infarct group, all patients had a significant hypoperfusion. The size of hypoperfusion was higher than that of the CT hypodense area in 13 (81%) patients who therefore exhibited an abnormal blood flow in the periinfarct area (Table 1). In the remaining three patients, the infarct size was similar to that of hypoperfusion. The extent of the periinfarct areas paralleled the distribution of the affected vascular territory of the completed infarcts. In the non-infarct group, SPECT showed a focal hypoperfusion in 2 of the 5 patients with no structural damage on follow-up CT (Table 1).

Eight (38%) patients had an atherosclerotic stenosis or occlusion in the internal carotid artery ipsilateral to the ischaemic lesion. The mean degree of hypoperfusion in the ischaemic territory was higher in patients with (42 ± 15%; median, 42%) than in those without carotid artery disease (26 ± 20%; median, 19%), but without reaching statistical significance (Table 2). The mean size of hypoperfusion was similar for each of the two groups. Carotid artery disease was more frequently associated with the presence of periinfarct area (87% versus 46%), but the difference was not statistically significant.

Prediction of infarct size and determination of flow threshold for the survival of brain tissue

A higher degree and size of hypoperfusion were associated with a large infarct (Table 3). The presence of crossed cerebellar diaschisis and perfusion defect in the periinfarct area were more frequent in the patients with a large infarct, however the difference was not statistically significant.

Table 2 SPECT findings in patients with carotid artery disease

SPECT	Carotid artery disease	
	Present n = 8	Absent n = 13
Mean degree of hypoperfusion	42 ± 15%[a] (42%)	26 ± 20% (19%)
Mean size of hypoperfusion	8 ± 8 (4)	5 ± 4 (3)
Periinfarct area present	7 (87%)	6 (46%)
absent	1 (13%)	7 (54%)

[a], p=0.096 (Wilcoxon rank sum test)
Median values and percentages are shown in parentheses for the mean degree and size of hypoperfusion and periinfarct area, respectively

Table 3 SPECT indices according to computed tomographic findings

SPECT indices		N	None or ≤ 3 cm hypodensity n = 9	> 3 cm hypodensity n = 12
Mean degree			13 ± 7% (13%)	46 ± 14% (48%)[a]
Mean size			2 ± 2 (1)	9 ± 6 (8)[a]
Crossed cerebellar	present	7	1	6
diaschisis	absent	14	8	6
Periinfarct	present	15	5	10
area	absent	6	4	2

[a], p<0.001 (Wilcoxon rank sum test)
Median values are shown in parentheses

The mean degree and size of hypoperfusion is calculated in the hemispheric region including the periinfarct and infarct area; the periinfarct area is defined by the presence of hypoperfusion in the region surrounding the CT infarct and in patients with normal CT

Table 4 Degree of hypoperfusion in the periinfarct area and infarct area

Cases	Periinfarct area		Infarct area	
	Lowest degree (%)	Highest degree (%)	Lowest degree (%)	Highest degree (%)
3	7	11	13	13
4	6	16	21	45
5	6	15	34	69
6	11	22	24	32
7	8	16	20	35
8	11	16	17	52
9	4	14	20	62
11	9	17	15	28
13	-	-	13	53
14	7	16	22	28
15	-	-	19	59
17	5	7	11	18
18	10	17	25	56
19	7	15	23	31
20	-	-	11	11
21	16	16	17	32
Mean	8	15	19	39

No periinfarct was found in 3 patients

Table 5 Severity of hypoperfusion in the periinfarct area and infarct area

Averaged degree of hypoperfusion	Infarct group	
	Periinfarct area n = 13	Infarct area n = 16
Lowest degree	8 ± 3% (7)	19 ± 6% (20)[a]
Highest degree	15 ± 3% (16)	39 ± 17% (34)[b]
Highest - lowest	7 ± 3% (8)	20 ± 15% (15)[c]

[a], $p<0.0001$; [b], $p<0.001$; [c], $p=0.033$ (Wilcoxon rank sum test)
Median values are shown in parentheses

The lowest and highest degree of hypoperfusion in the periinfarct area and infarct area for each patient are given in Table 4. In the infarct group, the average of the lowest and highest degree of hypoperfusion was significantly different between the infarct area and periinfarct area (Table 5). Both areas were also significantly differentiated by the difference between the lowest and highest degree of hypoperfusion. In the small non-infarct group of 2 patients, the lowest (4% and 10%) and highest (14% and 19%) degree of hypoperfusion were close to those of the periinfarct area in the infarct group. Since the periinfarct area is characterised by perfusion defect without structural damage on CT, the flow threshold value for the viability of brain tissue should be between the lowest degree of hypoperfusion in the infarct area (mean, 19 ± 6%) and the highest degree in the periinfarct area (mean, 15 ± 3%). The range of overlap, found in 5 patients, between the infarct area (lowest degree) and periinfarct area (highest degree) was from 11% to 22%.

Clinical significance of periinfarct area with reference to outcome

A periinfarct area was found more frequently in the patients with good outcome than in those with poor outcome, but the difference was not significant (Table 6). Three patients exhibited an infarct without hypoperfusion in the periinfarct area. In one of them, the degree (10%) and size (1) of hypoperfusion in the infarct area were low and the outcome was excellent (Rankin scale 1). In the other 2 patients, the degree (53% and 59%) and size (4 and 6) of hypoperfusion were high. One of them died and the second remained disabled but independent of others (Rankin scale 6 and 3). The average of the highest degree of hypoperfusion in the periinfarct area was not significantly different between the patients with poor (16 ± 1%; median 16%) or good (15 ± 4%; median 16%) outcome.

Illustrative case reports

Case 1. A 79 year old man was admitted for paresis in the left arm and leg. Neurological examination showed, on admission, a left hemiparesis, brachial hypesthesia, hemineglect, hemianosognosia, somnolence and dysarthria (Canadian Neurological Scale: score 2). Brain CT, on day 9, showed a large complete (> 3cm) infarction in the right middle cerebral artery territory (Figure 1a). SPECT, performed 23 h after onset, demonstrated a right frontoparietal hypoperfusion in the infarct area (asymmetry index from -22% to -28%) and in the periinfarct area (from -7% to -16%) (Figure 1b). Selective arterial angiography showed an occlusion of the right internal carotid artery. The patient remained disabled and dependent on others (Rankin Scale: score 4).

Case 2. A 82 year old man was admitted because he suddenly experienced a right hemiplegia with aphasia. On admission, neurological examination showed a dense right hemiplegia, hemihypesthesia and motor aphasia (Canadian Neurological Scale: score 3). Brain CT, carried out on day 5, demonstrated a large (> 3 cm) infarction in the anterior and posterior border zone of the middle cerebral artery territory (Figure 2a). Five hours after onset, SPECT showed a left frontal and parieto-occipital hypoperfusion (asymmetry index from -19% to -59%) in the infarct area (Figure 2b). The regional perfusion was normal in the periinfarct area. Selective arterial angiography was normal. The patient remained in part dependent on others, but the outcome was considered as good with a significant improvement of the neurological examination (Rankin Scale: score 3).

Discussion

Our study included only patients with cortical carotid ischaemia with a high SPECT sensitivity, as demonstrated previously[18]. Subcortical infarcts were excluded because regions of interest could not be placed in deep areas with our SPECT methodology. As with Raynaud's study[14] (17 cases) and that of Shimosegawa et al.[15] (31 cases), our population is characterised by a small number of patients (21 cases), so that our results must be interpreted carefully.

Table 6 Hypoperfusion in the periinfarct area and outcome

Periinfarct Area	N	Outcome	
		Good n=16	Poor n=8
Present	13	9 (69%)	4 (31%)
Absent	8	2 (25%)	6 (75%)

Periinfarct area

SPECT performed in the early hours after onset showed a high sensitivity (86%), as expected, whereas the CT sensitivity after 48 h was 76%. We found a periinfarct area in 13 (81%) of 16 patients with CT proved cortical infarct. This prevalence is similar to that found in the series of Shimosegawa et al.[15] (83%). The precise nature of periinfarct hypoperfusion remains unclear. It might be caused by either the direct haemodynamic effects of vessel occlusion or by disconnection and deactivation of the cortex surrounding the infarct[5,9,11,12,14]. Another suggested mechanism was selective neuronal loss without frank infarct ion[26,27], but this was not confirmed completely by a neuropathological study[28]. As compared with other studies[14,15], the periinfarct areas paralleled the vascular distribution of the completed infarcts. We did not note any extension of the perfusion defect in the occipital regions. This vascular distribution indicates that the hypoperfusion in the periinfarct area maybe mainly due to direct alterations of blood flow in brain tissue with good collateral circulation, although the effect of deafferentation cannot be entirely excluded[15]. Deafferentation has been described mainly for the cerebellum and crossed cerebellar diaschisis[29]. The serial ^{123}I-IMP SPECT study of Raynaud et al.[14] performed first at 10 min and then at 2 h showed a persistent hypofixation in the periinfarct area, while the crossed cerebellar diaschisis had disappeared at the second examination. Thus, even if an intrahemispheric diaschisis cannot be ruled out, it does not seem to be the main mechanism. In the same study, PET examinations have also been performed to evaluate the cerebral metabolism in the periinfarct area. The results showed that the perfusion in the peripheral area was only mildly reduced and was sufficient for adequate metabolism. This suggests a satisfactory restoration of local blood flow by development of collateral circulation that prevents transformation into an infarct[14]. Such collateral blood flow following occlusion of the internal carotid artery has been well described[30,31]. Several reports have shown that a good collateral blood supply during the first few hours after an ischaemic stroke reduced the volume of final parenchymal brain damage[31-33]. In our series, which included a small number of patients, a severe atherosclerotic disease in the internal carotid artery, with potential cerebral haemodynamic effects, was more frequently but not significantly associated with the presence of periinfarct area. Even though the total size of perfusion deficit has been shown to be higher in patients with carotid occlusion than in those with no detectable arterial occlusion[31,33] our data show that the presence of periinfarct area does not seem to

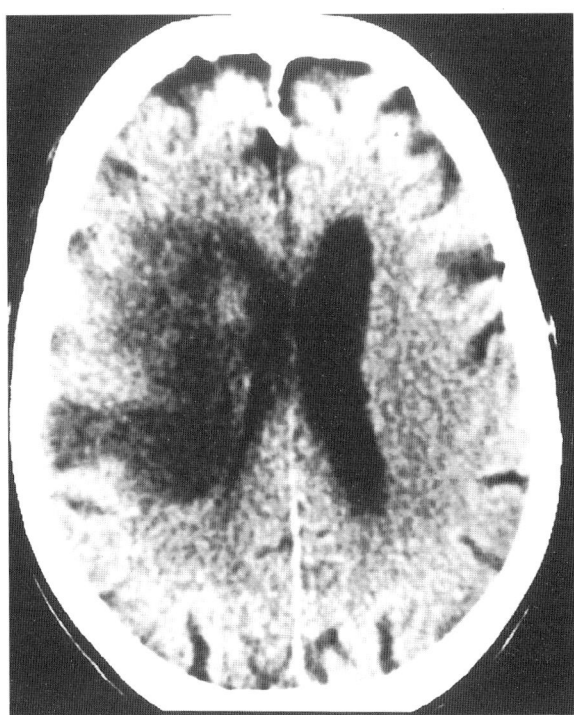

Figure 1a Brain CT on day 9, right MCA infarct

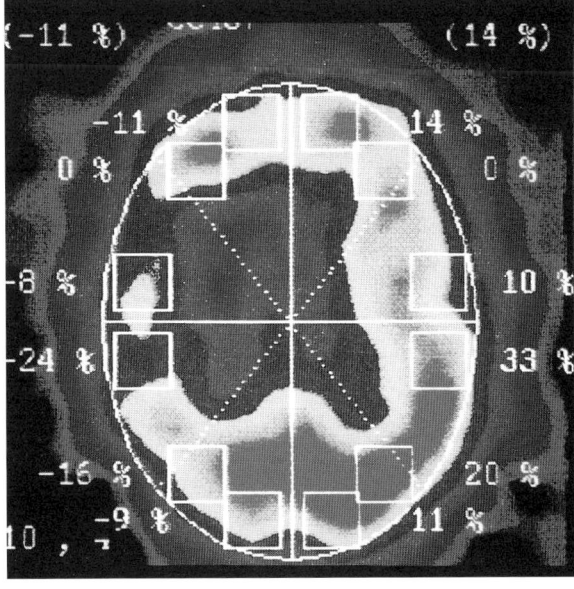

Figure 1b SPECT < 24 h : right hypoperfusion in the infarct and periinfarct area

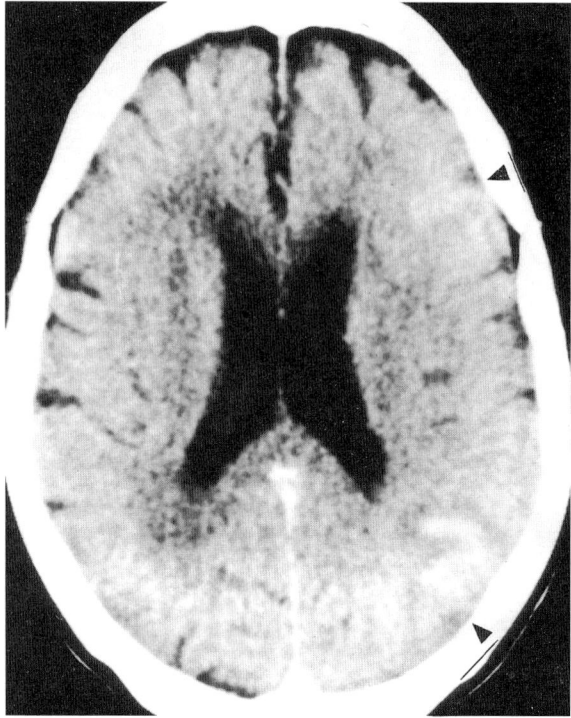

Figure 2a Brain CT on day 5, left cortical MCA infarct

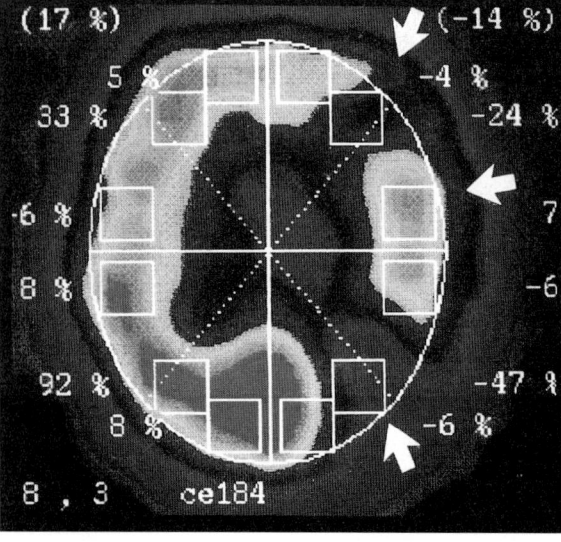

Figure 2b SPECT < 24 h : left hypoperfusion in the infarct area and no hypoperfusion in the periinfarct area

be related to the cause of ischaemia *per se* but depends much more on the development of collateral circulation.

Prediction of infarct size

In agreement with Giubilei *et al.*[31], we observed an early severe impairment of regional cerebral blood flow with higher degree and size of hypoperfusion in patients with a large hypodense area on follow-up CT scan. Given that a perfusion deficit appears on SPECT before morphologic abnormalities appear on CT[18,31,34-39], our data support the possibility that a SPECT study can predict morphologic damage in the first hours after the onset of stroke.

Determination of flow threshold for the survival of brain tissue

The present study demonstrates on follow-up CT scans that an area of extremely low perfusion consistent with the completed infarct (the infarct core area) is surrounded in 81% of patients by a region of moderate hypoperfusion in the adjacent normal tissue (the periinfarct area). Both areas could be easily differentiated by the degree of hypoperfusion. Since development of cerebral infarction depends on the duration and severity of ischaemia, determination of flow threshold for the viability of brain tissue might be useful when therapeutic intervention is under consideration. Although SPECT measurements of cerebral blood flow alone cannot differentiate metabolic inactivity from normal tissue function[40], we tried to determine an ischaemic threshold of morphological damage. Like Shimosegawa *et al.*[15], we were able to set an ischaemic threshold which was between the highest degree of hypoperfusion in the periinfarct area (15% ± 3) and the lowest degree of hypoperfusion in the infarct area (19% ± 6). However, our results may be biased by the time of SPECT investigation. Indeed, as SPECT was performed within 36 h, the degree of hypoperfusion in the infarct area can be influenced by relatively hyperaemic lesions, so measurement of cerebral metabolism by PET study is necessary for the accurate determination of an ischaemic threshold. Yet, despite this limitation, our findings suggest that SPECT, a technique that is easily available in the clinical setting, can offer an alternative method for predicting the viability of brain tissue. In practice, patients with a severe impairment of perfusion above 20% and without a periinfarct area are not likely to benefit from therapeutic reperfusion such as thrombolysis. This point has been emphasised by several authors[41-44], who have reported poor prognosis and early death from transtentorial herniation in patients with severe perfusion defect. By contrast, patients with mild hypoperfusion or with a periinfarct area reflecting the collateral circulation supply were more likely to benefit from thrombolysis in the acute phase[32,41-43].

Periinfarct area and clinical outcome

According to our findings, we tried to determine whether the presence of a periinfarct area could be associated with a better prognosis. Although most of the patients with good outcome had a periinfarct area, we found no significant association between the clinical outcome at 1 month and either the presence of periinfarct area or the degree of hypoperfusion in this region. The lack of significance might be due to the small number of patients in our series and the short-term evaluation of outcome at 1 month. Raynaud et al.[14] also reported no correlation between the IMP uptake decrease in the peripheral area and the status of the patients. However, the volume of the peripheral area correlated well with the neurological status. Our SPECT methodology did not allow us to measure the volume of the periinfarct area in order to corroborate this assertion.

Conclusions

SPECT, despite some limitations, can predict infarct size in the early hours after stroke onset. Determination of an ischaemic blood flow threshold is possible on SPECT scans. The periinfarct area, reflecting the collateral circulation supply, plays an important role in clarifying which patients are likely to benefit from early therapeutic reperfusion. Further large scale studies are needed to confirm these findings.

References

1 Jafar, J.J. and Cromwell, R.M. Focal ischemic thresholds in 'Cerebral Blood Flow: physiologic and clinical aspects', (Ed. J.H. Wood), McGraw-Hill, New York, USA, 1987, p.449

2 Jones, T.H., Morawetz, R.B., Cromwell, R.M. et al. Thresholds of focal cerebral ischemia in awake monkeys. J. Neurosurg. 1981, 54, 773

3 Lenzi, G.L., Frackowiak, R.S.J and Jones, T. Cerebral oxygen metabolism and blood flow in human cerebral ischemic infarction. J. Cereb. Blood Flow Metab. 1982, 2, 321

4 Mies, G., Auer, L.M, Ebhardt, G. et al. Flow and neuronal density in tissues surrounding chronic infarction. Stroke 1983, 14, 22

5 Raynaud, C., Rancurel, G., Tzourio, N. et al. SPECT analysis of recent cerebral infarction. Stroke 1989, 20, 192

6 Devous, M.D., Lewis, S.E., Kulkarni, P.V. and Bonte, F.J. A comparison of regional cerebral blood flow measured with I-123-labelled diamine or amphetamine and radioactive tracer microspheres. J. Nucl. Med. 1983, 24, 6

7 Kuhl, D.E, Wu, J.L, Lin, T.H. et al. Mapping local cerebral blood flow by means of emission computed tomography of N-isopropyl-p-^{123}I-iodoamphetamine (IMP) tomography. J. Nucl. Med. 1981, 22, 16

8 Kuhl, D.E., Barrio, J.R., Huang, S.C. et al. Quantifying local cerebral blood flow with N-isopropyl-p-I-123 iodoamphetamine (IMP) tomography. J. Nucl. Med. 1982, 23, 196

9 Kuhl, D.E., Phelps, M.E., Kowell, A.P. et al. Effects of stroke on local cerebral metabolism and perfusion: mapping by emission computed tomography of [18]FDG and [13]NH$_3$. Ann. Neurol. 1980, 8, 40

10 Moretti, J.L., Askienazy, S., Cesaro, P. et al. I-123 N-isopropyl amphetamine (I-123) IMP SPECT in epilepsy and cerebral ischemia. J. Nucl. Med. 1983, I, 108

11 Olsen, S.T., Larsen, B., Skriver, E.B. et al. Focal cerebral hyperemia in acute stroke: incidence, pathophysiology and clinical significance. Stroke 1981, 12, 598

12 Olsen, T.S., Larsen, B., Herning. et al. Blood flow and vascular reactivity in collaterally perfused brain tissue. Evidence of an ischaemic penumbra in patients with acute stroke. Stroke 1983, 14, 332

13 Rapin, J.R., Duterte, D., Lageron, A. and Le Poncin-Lafitte, M. Etude autoradiographique du debit sanguin cerebral a l'aide de l'isopropyl iodoamphetamine. Circul. Metab. Cerveau. 1983, 1, 81

14 Raynaud, C., Rancurel, G., Samson, Y. et al. Pathophysiologic study of chronic infarcts with I-123 isopropyl iodo-amphetamine (IMP): the importance of periinfarct area. Stroke 1987, 18, 21

15 Shimosegawa, E., Hatazawa, J., Inugami, A. et al. Cerebral infarction within six hours of onset: prediction of completed infarction with technetium-99m-HMPAO SPECT. J. Nucl. Med. 1994, 35, 1097

16 Haughton, V.M. Vascular diseases in 'Cranial computed tomography: a comprehensive text', (Eds. A.L.Williams, V.M. Haughton), C.V. Mosby Co., St Louis, USA, 1985, p. 88

17 Damasio, H. A computed tomographic guide to the identification of cerebral vascular territories. Arch. Neurol. 1983, 40, 138

18 Laloux, P., Doat, M., Brichant, C. et al. Clinical usefulness of Technetium-99m HMPAO SPECT imaging to map the ischemic lesion in acute stroke: a reevaluation. Cerebrovasc. Dis. 1994, 4, 280

19 Laloux, P., Ossemann, M. and Jamart, J. Stroke subtypes and risk factors associated with silent infarctions in patients with first-ever ischemic stroke or transient ischemic attack. Acta Neurol. Belg. 1994, 94, 17

20 Sperling, B. and Lassen, N.A. Hyperfixation of HMPAO in subacute ischemic stroke leading to spuriously high estimates of cerebral blood flow by SPECT. Stroke 1993, 24, 193

21 Moretti, J.L., Defer, G., Cinotti, L. *et al.* 'Luxury perfusion' with 99mTc-HMPAO and 123I-IMP SPECT imaging during the subacute phase of stroke. *Eur. J. Nucl. Med.* 1990, 16, 17

22 Podreka, I., Suess, E., Goldenberg, G. *et al.* Initial experience with technetium-99m HMPAO brain SPECT. *J. Nucl. Med.* 1987, VOL,

23 Meneghetti, S., Vorstrup, B., Mickey, B. *et al.* Crossed cerebellar diaschisis in ischemic stroke: a study of regional cerebral blood flow by ^{133}Xe inhalation and single photon emission computerized tomography. *J. Cereb. Blood Flow Metab.* 1984, 4, 235

24 Steinling, M., Mazingue, A., Kassiotis, Ph. *et al.* Le HmPaO Tc comme indicateur du debit sanguin cerebral local: etude quantifiee comparee a la methode par inhalation au Xenon 133. *Ann. Radiol.* 1988, 31, 229

25 Rankin, J. Cerebral vascular events in patients over the age of 60. 2. Prognosis. *Scott. Med. J.* 1957, 2, 200

26 Lassen, N.A., Henriksen, L., Holm, S. *et al.* Cerebral blood flow tomography: xenon-133 compared with isopropyl-amphetamine-iodine-123: concise communication. *J. Nucl. Med.* 1983, 24, 17

27 Nakano, S., Kinoshita, K., Jinnouchi, S. *et al.* Critical cerebral blood flow thresholds studied by SPECT using xenon-133 and iodine-123 iodoamphetamine. *J. Nucl. Med.* 1989, 30, 337

28 Nedergaard, M., Astrup, J. and Klinken, L. Cell density and cortex thickness in the border zone surrounding old infarcts in human brain. *Stroke* 1984, 6, 1033

29 Baron, J.C., Bousser, M.G., Comar, D. and Castaigne, P. Crossed cerebellar diaschisis in human supratentorial brain infarction. *Trans. Am. Neurol. Assoc.* 1980, 105, 459

30 De Ley, G., Nshimyumremyi, J.B. and Leusen, I. Hemispheric blood flow in the rat after unilateral common carotid occlusion: evolution with time. *Stroke* 1985, 16, 69

31 Giubilei, F., Lenzi, G.L., Di Piero, V. *et al.* Predictive value of brain perfusion single-photon emission computed tomography in acute ischemic stroke. *Stroke* 1990, 21, 895

32 Bozzao, L., Fantozzi, L.M., Bastianello, S. *et al.* Early collateral blood supply and late parenchymal brain damage in patients with middle cerebral artery occlusion. *Stroke* 1989, 20, 735

33 Paulson, O.B. Regional cerebral blood flow in apoplexy due to occlusion of the middle cerebral artery. *Neurology* 1970, 20, 63

34 Feldman, M., Voth, E., Dressler, D. *et al.* [99mTc]-hexamethylpropylene amine oxime SPECT and X-ray CT in acute ischaemia. *J. Neurol.* 1990, 237, 475

35 Hayman, L.A., Taber, K.H., Jhingran, S.G. *et al.* Cerebral infarction: Diagnosis and assessment of prognosis by using [123]IMP-SPECT and CT. *A. J. N. R.* 1989, 10, 557

36 Holman, B.L., Hill, T.C., Polak, J.F. *et al.* Cerebral perfusion imaging with iodine 123-labeled amines. *Arch. Neurol.* 1984, 41, 1060

37 Inoue, Y., Takemoto, K., Miyamoto, T. *et al.* Sequential computed tomography scans in acute cerebral infarction. *Radiology* 1980, 135, 655

38 Kobayashi, H., Hayashi, M., Kawano, H. *et al.* Cerebral blood flow studies using N-iospropyl I-123-p-iodoamphetamine. *Stroke.* 1985, 16, 293

39 Lee, R.G.L., Hill, T.C., Holman, B.L. and Clouse, M.E.N. Isopropyl (I-123)p-iodoamphetamine brain scans with single photon emission computed tomography: discordance with transmission computed tomography. *Radiology* 1982, 145, 795

40 Wise, R.J.S., Bernardi, S., Frackowiak, R.S.J. *et al.* Serial observations on the pathophysiology of acute stroke. *Brain* 1983, 106, 197

41 Hanson, S.K., Grotta, J.C., Rhoades, H. *et al.* Value of single photon emission computed tomography in acute stroke therapeutic trials. *Stroke* 1993, 24, 1322

42 Herderschee, D., Limburg, M., Hijdra, A. *et al.* Treatment of acute ischemic stroke with recombinant tissue plasminogen activator: evaluation with regional cerebral blood flow single photon emission computed tomography in Thrombolytic therapy in acute ischemic stroke', (Eds. W. Hacke, G. J. del Zoppo, M. Hirschberg), Springer-Verlag, Berlin, Germany, 1991, p. 244

43 Marchal, G., Serrati, C., Rioux, P. *et al.* PET imaging of cerebral perfusion and oxygen consumption in acute ischaemic stroke: relation to outcome. *Lancet* 1993, 341, 925

44 Ringelstein, E.B., Biniek, R., Weiller, C. *et al.* Type and extent of hemispheric brain infarction and clinical outcome in early and delayed middle cerebral artery recanalization. *Neurology* 1992, 42, 289

Section

8

Tumours

SPECT in Neurology and Psychiatry, edited by P.P. De Deyn, R.A. Dierckx, A. Alavi and B.A. Pickut
© 1997 John Libbey & Company Ltd, pp. 377–385

[201]Thallium SPECT in Neuro-Oncology

Chapter
45

R.A.Dierckx[*#], A.B. Newberg, B.A. Pickut[**], I.M. Dierckx[**],
A. Dobbeleir[**], K. Audenaert[*], A. Alavi and P.P. De Deyn[**#]

Tumour imaging

In the early 1970s, the introduction of X-ray computed tomography (CT) scans, and later on, magnetic resonance imaging (MRI), enabling tomographic anatomical information obtained with high spatial resolution, led to a decrease in the use of radionuclide imaging in the management of brain tumours. However, using the morphological imaging techniques of CT and MRI several limitations remain, such as difficulties in distinguishing oedema and gliosis, under- and over-estimation of tumour extention, and lack of metabolic information[1-3]. Using adequate tracers, the functional imaging techniques of positron emission tomography (PET) and single photon emission computed tomography (SPECT) offer several advantages over the anatomical imaging modalities.

Functional imaging helps in the early (differential) diagnosis of structural lesions, provides prognostic information and helps in the follow-up after therapeutic intervention. The latter is particularly the case in terms of differentiating recurrent tumour from necrosis secondary to radiation or chemotherapy.

Radiopharmaceuticals used for nuclear diagnostic imaging in oncology may be classified into various groups according to their working mechanism. Radiotracers may help delineate non-specific alterations of function and metabolism. For example,[99m]Tc-DTPA has been used in order to identify areas of disruption in the blood-brain-barrier (BBB), which is commonly seen in various central nervous system disorders. The introduction of labelled hexamethylpropyleneamine oxime (HMPAO) was a breakthrough, providing a ^{99m}Tc tracer capable of passing the intact BBB and to remain fixed long enough to allow SPECT imaging. ^{99m}Tc-HMPAO SPECT studies have been used in order to measure changes in cerebral blood flow (CBF) in several central nervous system disorders including brain tumours[4-8]. While perfusion studies may be performed as well, PET studies have mainy utilised ^{18}F labelled fluorodeoxyglucose to measure cerebral and tumoral metabolism[4,9,10].

For brain tumours, however, expectations of a functional parameter similar to FDG-PET were not met using perfusion SPECT[11,12]. Perfusion tracers such as ^{99m}Tc-HMPAO primarily reflect regional cerebral blood flow and only by inference local brain metabolism[13-17]. Moreover, uptake in brain tumours may be determined on the one hand by dynamic variables, such as the state of the BBB, neovascularisation, cellular differentiation and treatment of the tumour studied, and on the other hand by characteristics specific to the perfusion tracers used[5]. In the case of ^{123}I-iodoamphetamine (IMP), accumulation may be dependent on

Division of Nuclear Medicine, Department of Radiology, Hospital of the University of Pennsylvania, USA
[*]Division of Nuclear Medicine, University Hospital Ghent, Belgium
[**]Departments of Neurology, Radiology and Nuclear Medicine, Middelheim Hospital, Belgium
[#]Born Bung Foundation U.I.A.,University of Antwerp, Belgium

the presence of the non-specific amine receptors, while for [99mTc]-HMPAO a statistically significant correlation has been reported between uptake and gluthatione content of brain tumour[18,19]. This has led to the exploration of more suitable metabolic SPECT tracers from which [201Tl] emerged[20-22].

Also, indications for perfusion SPECT in brain tumours have been reconsidered and presently include : acquisition of information of therapeutic efficacy; evaluation of additional functional involvement and coregistration with [201Tl] for orientation (Figure 1) and to enhance ability to distinguish glioma from radionecrosis[24-31].

The mitochondrial uptake mechanism and the advantages of [99mTc] labelling have already led to the preliminary use of methoxyisobutylisonitrile (MIBI) as an alternative to [201Tl] for the same clinical indications[32,33]. Another tracer under investigation, but based on a more specific uptake mechanism, is the [123I] labelled aminoacid analogue alpha-methyl-tyrosine[34,35]. A number of radionuclides and radiopharmaceuticals have been used both for PET and SPECT imaging to study specific receptor characteristics of brain tumours. For SPECT,

preparations such as [123I]-iodobenzamide and [111I]-octreotide have been tried to measure whether brain tumours express various receptor sites[36-39]. Radio-immunoscintigraphy has been used to determine whether brain tumour cells express any particular antigens[40]. However, the latter examinations are experimental and focus on specific questions with possible therapeutic implications.

History of [201Tl] imaging

[201Tl] is generally considered to be a metabolic tracer since it behaves in a manner that is biologically similar to potassium. [201Tl] was first used in the 1970s to obtain myocardial images, and it is still widely used today as a myocardial perfusion and viability tracer. With regard to tumours, as early as 1965, Charkes *et al.*[41] noted that there was an accumulation of a potassium analogue, [131Cs]. Around 1980, using planar imaging, Ancri *et al.*[42,43] compared the physically more favourable potassium analogue [201Tl] with pertechnetate in brain tumours. They found that [201Tl] yielded better definition in approximately two-thirds of patients and that small metastases which were invisible with pertechnetate could be demonstrated with [201Tl].

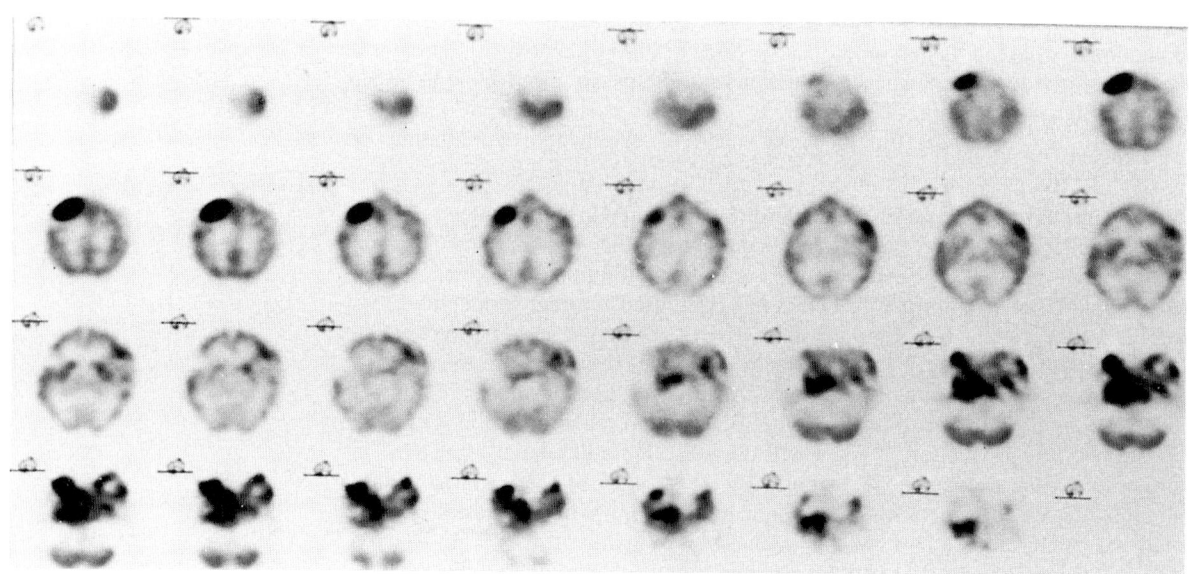

Figure 1 SPECT examination of a 59-year-old woman suffering from two meningiomata. One of the meningiomata was an 'en plaque' meningeoma of the lesser wing with extension in the nasopharynx and both orbitae. A second globoid meningeoma localisation was shown in the right frontal lobe. Transaxial slices of combined [99mTc] HMPAO SPECT and [201Tl] SPECT images were superimposed on a Sun workstation and time was allowed for orientation of the focal [201Tl] accumulations. [201Tl] SPECT images were obtained 15 min after intravenous administration of 4 mCi [201Tl] using a rotating three head SPECT system equipped with parallel hole collimators. Projection data were accumulated in a 128x64 matrix, 60 sec/angle, 40 angles for each detector (3° steps, 120° rotation). Projection images were smoothed and reconstructed in a 64x64 matrix, using Butterworth filtered backprojection. The tumour to non-tumour ratio (homologous contralateral region of interest) varied between 7 and 9

In 1987, Kaplan et al.[44] studied 29 patients with grade III and IV gliomas after radiation therapy using ^{201}Tl followed by ^{99m}Tc-glucoheptonate and ^{67}Ga scans to see if functional imaging reflected clinical status better than did CT scanning. Since seven patients died shortly afterwards it was possible to show using neuropathological verification that ^{201}Tl imaging was better at distinguishing viable tumour burden compared with CT scans, ^{99m}Tc-glucoheptonate, or ^{67}Ga scans. [67]Ga gave similar results, unless patients were receiving steroids. Interestingly, ^{201}Tl uptake was minimally affected by the concommitant use of steroids. This study by Kaplan et al. boosted a large number of clinical ^{201}Tl SPECT studies.

Physical and uptake characteristics

There are a number of characteristics of ^{201}Tl imaging that make such techniques of use in the study of brain tumours. However, as with any imaging modality there are also limitations. Thus, we must consider the pharmacokinetics and other characteristics of ^{201}Tl imaging in order to evaluate its contribution, both present and future, for the diagnosis and management of brain tumours.

[201]Tl is a cyclotron product with a half-life of 73 h, and peak energies of 69-83, 135 and 167 keV. For an adult dose of 111 MBq (3mCi) the EDE = (0.3766) x (111) = 41.8 mSv (4.19 rem)[45].

In tumour-bearing animals, ^{201}Tl has been shown to accumulate in viable tumour tissue more than in connective tissue, especially in inflammatory cells, and it is barely detectable in necrotic tumour tissue[46]. With regard to contrast ^{201}Tl has the advantage to rapidly (approximately 5 min for 91.5% of radioactivity) disappear from the blood in a bi-exponential mode[42].

In the brain, tumour cells have a much higher affinity for ^{201}Tl than either white or grey matter, which show respectively little or no ^{201}Tl uptake and showing low affinity[47]. Also, the disruption of the BBB around tumours allows for a greater uptake of ^{201}Tl in tumours than in the normal tissue with an intact BBB. The list of possible factors influencing ^{201}Tl uptake by tumours include blood flow, state of the BBB, tissue viability, tumour type, function of the sodium-potassium pump system, cotransport system, calcium ion channel system, vascular immaturity with leakage and an increased cellular membrane permeability[48,49]. Sequential studies have shown that the first 5 min acquisition, that is the first extraction of ^{201}Tl, depends on regional blood flow, blood volume and permeability of the BBB, while the later acquisition depends on active transport by the membrane pump of the tumour cell[50].

More specifically, the cellular component of ^{201}Tl uptake has been demonstrated by several studies. Increased ^{201}Tl uptake is associated with higher grade gliomas[51]. It has also been demonstrated that BBB disruption can occur without ^{201}Tl accumulation, which has been observed in radiation necrosis and resolving haematoma[44,51]. Furthermore, a study utilising a microsphere model showed that the relative contribution of the sodium-potassium ATPase activity has been shown to account for ten times more ^{201}Tl uptake than tumour blood flow[48].

Methodological aspects

In terms of the clinical application of ^{201}Tl imaging in brain tumours, there are several strengths to the technique. The results are reproducible with minimal intraobserver and interobserver variability[52].

Therefore, there is good reliability of ^{201}Tl imaging. [201]Tl provides a clinically useful objective parameter of proliferative tumour activity[53].

The most widely used approaches for semi-quantification are tumour to cardiac uptake ratios using planar scans and the use of mean tumoral region of interest (ROI) counts normalised to homologous contralateral brain activity using SPECT[51,52,54]. Miscellaneous methods have included e.g. the use of peak pixel values, the use of the contralateral scalp or contralateral hemispheric activity as a reference, and the use of volume indices[55,56].

Clinical indications

With regard to differential diagnosis of brain lesions, Black et al.[51] reported that gliomas of high and low grade could be distinguished with 89% accuracy using a cut off value of 1.5 for the tumour-to-cardiac ratio. Thus, high grade tumours have high ratios and low grade tumours have lower values[57,58]. Since brain tumours may be heterogeneous with intermixed portions of low and high grade malignancy and since the therapeutic strategy is determined based upon the recognition of the most malignant portion, ^{201}Tl SPECT may be useful in helping with the management of brain tumours. As an example thallium SPECT may serve to guide biopsy and as a control for sampling and/or interpretation errors[59].

In patients with structural brain lesions and acquired immunodeficiency syndrome, ^{201}Tl SPECT can help distinguish lymphoma lesions from infections such as toxoplasmosis or progressive multifocal leuko-encephalopathy[60-62].

Dierckx et al.[63] reviewed 90 records of patients in whom SPECT was performed because of clinical or radiological suspicion of tumoral invasion, including relapse, and in whom a definitive diagnosis was obtained histologically. Indications consisted of non-contrast enhancing CT scan lesions, viable tumours after surgical resection and/or radiation therapy, or a history of primary neoplasm accompanied by an atypical symptomatology or atypical radiological findings. The different pathologies finally evaluated with the number in parenthesis include astrocytoma (number, n = 14) glioblastoma multiforme (14), oligodendroglioma (3), pituitary adenoma (2), lymphoma (3), meningeoma (3), metastasis (14), gliosis (3), ischaemic infarction (15), haemorrhagic infarction (5), intracranial haemorrhage (6) and miscellaneous (18).

It was shown in a problem-solving context that for identifying viable tumour, the sensitivity of ^{201}Tl SPECT was 68.7% and the specificity was 80.9%. ^{201}Tl SPECT proved to be a particularly good parameter for detection of viable tumour.

Other studies, including comparisons with other imaging modalities, have agreed with these findings that ^{201}Tl SPECT is useful in discriminating cerebral radiation necrosis from recurrent tumour, estimating residual tumour burden and detecting tumour regrowth earlier in postoperative patients[54,64-69].

At present, it is accurate to state that ^{201}Tl is useful for differentiating benign lesions (i.e. gliosis) from viable tumours. Furthermore, in general, higher ^{201}Tl uptake is associated with higher grade malignancies. However, overlap exists between various types of brain tumours. For example, meningeomas have a high ^{201}Tl uptake[66]. Given the above mentioned limitations, several groups have found improved specificity by using sequential studies with e.g. early (15 min post ^{201}Tl injection), delayed (4-6 h), and 'superdelayed' (24-96 h) studies[50,70,72].

Ueda et al.[50] showed that rapid and high accumulation with prolonged uptake and retention of ^{201}Tl may indicate the degree of tumour malignancy. Jinnouchi et al.[70] showed that while an early high ^{201}Tl uptake may be found in all types of meningeomas, a high retention index seems to be predictive of the malignant potential of a meningeoma. Another study by Kojima et al.[71] suggested that ^{201}Tl SPECT might be useful in differentiating meningeomas and malignant gliomas from cerebral metastases. Meningeomas and malignant gliomas tend to have a higher retention of ^{201}Tl after 96 h.

^{201}Tl SPECT imaging also can yield false positive results in patients with tuberculosis, candidiasis, and bacterial abscesses[73,74]. However, it should be mentioned that there may be an alternative diagnosis and other radionuclide imaging techniques may be useful such as labelled white blood cell scans[75,76]. Haemorrhagic infarction has also been found to have increased ^{201}Tl uptake after a free minimal interval of 5 days, but decreased activity is to be expected on repeat scans[63].

Determining prognosis is an important aspect to the management of patients with brain tumours. Patients with anaplastic astrocytoma have a median survival of two years compared with patients with glioblastoma multiforme, which carries a median survival of eight months. Patients with low grade astrocytomas have survival rates of 71% at two years, 55% at five years, and 43% at ten years[77]. In terms of prognosis, Kosuda et al. recently showed that ^{201}Tl SPECT may be useful for predicting survival of patients with suspected recurrent brain tumour[78].

Vertosick et al.[79] demonstrated a significant negative correlation of the ^{201}Tl index at the point of treatment failure and the survival in patients with glioblastoma multiforme. A related study showed that the ^{201}Tl index correlated with the degree of malignancy based on the proliferating cell nuclear antigen which has been used to assess tumour proliferation.

However, the ^{201}Tl index did not correlate with another marker for tumour proliferation[80]. Therefore, it remains to be studied how closely ^{201}Tl imaging compared with the expression of various tumour antigen markers.

Another interesting area of study is in patients who have malignant degeneration of low grade astrocytoma. This malignant degeneration occurs in 13 to 50% of patients.

Oriuchi al.[53] showed a change of the ^{201}Tl index in follow-up studies of several patients with low grade astrocytomas. Thus, these preliminary data suggest that ^{201}Tl SPECT may be useful in the follow-up and management of patients with low grade astrocytomas with those patients with increased ^{201}Tl uptake receiving more aggressive treatment

Brain tumours in children

Despite the apparent usefulness of ^{201}Tl SPECT in adults with cerebral gliomas, the indications for SPECT in paediatric brain tumour patients are not well defined. They have also been studied less extensively until now[28,81-84].

A study by Rollins et al.[84] compared ^{201}Tl SPECT with gadolinium-enchanced MR (Gd-MRI) to determine whether SPECT provides additional information that cannot be derived from Gd-MRI. The tumours included in this study with the number in parentheses were pilocytic astrocytoma (7), medulloblastoma (5), brainstem glioma or glioblastoma (4), germinoma (3), optic glioma (2), mixed glioma (1), primitive neuroectodermal tumour (1), and choroid plexus carcinoma (1). The results indicated that ^{201}Tl SPECT underestimated tumour burden since non-enhancing regions of the tumours on Gd-MRI did not show marked ^{201}Tl uptake. Further, ^{201}Tl indices were not found to correlate with histological grade, biological aggressiveness, or tumour type. The fact that ^{201}Tl SPECT was not as useful in paediatric tumours in this study may have been related to the variety of tumour types studied. In adults also, ^{201}Tl SPECT has been shown to be useful in particular tumours such as gliomas. Therefore, additional studies will be necessary in order to determine the usefulness of ^{201}Tl SPECT in the study and management of paediatric brain tumours.

[201]Tl SPECT versus MRI and PET

[201]Tl SPECT has been shown to be of particular value in following patients after tumour therapy. Yoshii et al.[85] showed that ^{201}Tl SPECT was superior to MRI in the differential diagnosis between radiation necrosis and recurrent tumour. This may partly result from the overestimation of viability with gadolinium enhanced MRI. However, other studies have shown some limitations with ^{201}Tl SPECT imaging in the differentiation of recurrent tumour from radiation necrosis[25,30].

A prospective evaluation of 34 patients with brain tumours after surgical resection, radiation therapy, or chemotherapy, by Lorberboym et al.[67] found that ^{201}Tl SPECT was more reliable than CT scans in identifying progression, improvement, or no change in brain tumour burden.

Several studies have been performed comparing ^{201}Tl SPECT to PET imaging. PET scans using ^{18}F-fluorodeoxyglucose have been performed for studies similar to those made with SPECT.

Specifically, FDG-PET scans have been used for preoperative grading, follow-up after treatment, diagnosis of tumour recurrence and prognosis. The question is how SPECT compares with PET. Also, the question is whether absolute quantification is necessary in the study and clinical management of brain tumours.

Kahn et al.[86] reported that no statistically significant difference was found in the sensitivity or specificity between ^{201}Tl SPECT and FDG-PET scans. One of the contributing factors may be that the lower resolution of SPECT is compensated by the higher contrast as compared with FDG-PET in which uptake also occurs in normal brain tissue. Black et al.[87] also reported that ^{201}Tl SPECT and FDG-PET are equal predictors of glioma grade and recurrence.

Buchpiguel et al.[88] showed that while SPECT might be better than PET in detecting recurrent tumour, it is not as specific as PET in detecting radiation necrosis. They compared the ability of FDG-PET and ^{201}Tl SPECT in differentiating recurrent brain tumour from radiation necrosis[88,89]. Thirteen patients were studied who had all undergone radiation therapy and were considered to have a high pre-test probability for tumour recurrence. In these patients, fourteen lesions were identified by gadolinium enhanced MRI. Nine of the lesions were confirmed by histopathology and the other five were confirmed by clinical outcome. The results indicated that PET had only a 64% sensitivity for detecting recurrent tumour, compared with a 100% sensitivity of ^{201}Tl SPECT. However, SPECT had only a 33% specificity for detecting radiation necrosis compared with 100% specificity for PET. Further, both imaging modalities yielded reliable and reproducible results. This study suggested that PET is the most specific test for radiation necrosis despite its relatively low sensitivity for recurrent tumour. On the other hand, ^{201}Tl SPECT may have limited specificity for detecting radiation necrosis, however, its high sensitivity for tumour recurrence strengthens its clinical application in brain tumours for which magnetic resonance imaging or PET are negative or inconclusive.

SPECT perspectives

In the context of ^{201}Tl SPECT, the present alternative to SPECT using ^{99m}Tc-labelled methoxyisobutylisonitrile (MIBI) should be mentioned. The cellular uptake mechanism and advantages of ^{99m}Tc labelling have led to the tentative use of ^{99m}Tc MIBI in brain tumours[90]. It has been proposed that malignant tumours maintain higher (more negative) mitochondrial and plasma transmembrane potentials secondary to their increased metabolic requirements, which could promote increased accumulation of ^{99m}Tc MIBI within these tissues[32,33]. Preliminary experience and comparison with ^{201}Tl accumulation in malignant tumours in general suggest a sensitivity in the same order of magnitude[91]. In 23 patients with suspected recurrent brain tumours, Macapinlac et al.[92] found both ^{201}Tl and ^{99m}Tc MIBI useful for detecting supratentorial tumours, but suggested that there may be lower uptake of ^{99m}Tc MIBI than of ^{201}Tl in low-grade tumours. In a within subject comparison in childhood brain tumours

O'Tuama[93] showed that clearer identification of boundaries using ^{99m}Tc MIBI versus ^{201}Tl SPECT may be an advantage in applications e.g. radiotherapy port planning.

Another upcoming tracer with different pharmacokinetic characteristics detailed by Langen *et al.*[34,35], is ^{123}I labelled alpha-methyltyrosine. This tracer appears to be a suitable SPECT tracer of amino acid uptake, although it is not incorporated into protein.

Conclusion

In conclusion, ^{201}Tl SPECT imaging has been found to have several useful applications with regard to the study and management of brain tumours. ^{201}Tl SPECT has been shown to be useful in the differentiation of recurrent tumour from radiation necrosis, in determining the degree of tumour malignancy, and in predicting overall prognosis. Future studies will be needed to explore the use of ^{201}Tl in the study of other types of brain tumours, especially in the paediatric population. Further, a more definitive role of ^{201}Tl SPECT in the evaluation of brain tumours, in conjunction with other functional and anatomical imaging techniques needs to be explored.

References

1 Burger, P.C., Heinz, E.R., Shibata, T. and Kleihaus, P. Topographic anatomy and CT correlations in the untreated glioblastoma multiforme. *J. Neurosurg.* 1988, 68, 698

2 Cairncross, J.G., Macdonald, D.R., Pexman, J.H.W. and Ives, F.J. Steroid-induced CT-changes in patients with recurrent malignant glioma. *Neurol.* 1988, 38, 724

3 Chamberlain, M.C., Murovic, J.A. and Levin, V.A. Absence of contrast enhancement on CT brain scans with supratentorial malignant gliomas. *Neurol.* 1988, 38, 1371

4 Alavi, J.B., Alavi, A., Chawluk, J. *et al.* Positron emission tomography in patients with glioma : a predictor of prognosis. *Cancer* 1988, 62, 1074

5 Biersack, H.J., Grünwald, F., Reichmann, K. *et al.* Functional brain imaging with single photon emission computerized tomography using Tc-99m labelled HMPAO in 'Nuclear Medicine Ann.', (Ed. L.M. Freeman), Raven Press, New York, p. 59

6 Ell, P. and Costa, D.C. The role of nuclear medicine in neurology and psychiatry. *Curr. Opinions. Neurol. Psychiatry* 1992, 5, 863

7 Langen, K-J., Herzog, H., Rota, E. *et al.* Tomographic studies of rCBF with Tc-99m HMPAO SPECT in comparison with PET in patients with primary brain tumours. *Neurosurg. Rev.* 1987, 10, 23

8 Langen, K-J., Herzog, H., Kuwert, T. *et al.* Tomographic studies of rCBF with Tc-99m HMPAO SPECT in patients with brain tumours : comparison with C-1502 continuous inhalation technique and PET. *J. Cereb. Blood Flow Metab.* 1988, 8, S90

9 Alavi, A. and Hirsch, L.J. Studies of central nervous system disorders with single photon emission computerized tomography and positron emission tomography : evolution over the past 2 decades. *Semin. Nucl. Med.* 1991, 21, 58

10 Rozenthal, J.M. Positron emission tomography (PET) and single photon emission computed tomography of brain tumours. *Neurologic Clinics* 1991, 9, 287

11 Brooks, D.J., Beaney, R.P. and Thomas, D.G. The role of positron emission tomography in the study of cerebral tumours. *Semin. Oncol.* 1986, 13, 83

12 Coleman, R.E., Hoffman, J.M., Hanson, M.W. *et al.* Clinical application of PET for the evaluation of brain tumours. *J. Nucl. Med.* 1991, 32, 616

13 Kuschinsky, W. Coupling between functional activity, metabolism and blood flow in the brain. *Microcirculation* 1982, 2, 357

14 Lequin, M.H., Blok, D., Pauwels and E.K.J. Radiopharmaceuticals for functional brain imaging with SPECT in 'Nuclear Medicine Ann.', (Ed. L.M. Freeman), Raven Press, New York, p. 37

15 Neirinckx, R.D., Canning, L.R., Piper, I.M. *et al.* Technetium-99m d,1-HMPAO. A new radiopharmaceutical for SPECT imaging of regional cerebral blood perfusion. *J. Nucl. Med.* 1987, 28, 191

16 Reba, R.C. and Holman, B.L. Brain perfusion radiotracers in 'Radiopharmaceuticals and brain pathology studied with PET and SPECT', (Eds. M. Diksic, R.C. Reba), CRC Press, Boston, 1991, p. 35

17 Roy, C.S. and Sherrington, C.S. On the regulation of the blood supply of the brain. *J. Physiol.* 1980, 11, 37

18 Suess, E., Malessa, S., Ungersböck, K. *et al.* Technetium-99m-d,1-hexamethylpropylene amine oxime (HMPAO) uptake and gluthatione content in brain tumours. *J. Nucl. Med.* 1991, 32, 1675

19 Winchell, H.S., Horst, W.D., Braun, W.H. *et al.* N-isopropyl-(I123)p-iodoamphetamine:single-pass brain uptake and wash-out;binding to brain synaptosomes and localization in dog and monkey brain. *J. Nucl. Med.* 1980, 21, 947

20 Biersack, H.J., Grünwald, F. and Kropp, J. Single photon emission computerized tomography imaging of brain tumours. *Semin. Nucl. Med.* 1991, 21, 2

21 Elgazzar, A.H., Fernandez-Ulloa, M. and Silberstein, E.B. ^{201}Tl as a tumour localizing agent: current status and future considerations. *Nucl. Med. Comm.* 1993, 14, 96

22 Holman, B.L. and Abdel-Dayem, H. The clinical role of SPECT in patients with brain tumours. *J. Neuroimaging* 1995, 5, S34

23 Prat Acin, R., Diaz Vincente, J., Banzo, J. *et al.* The use of SPECT with ²⁰¹Tl in the evaluation of brain tumours. *Rev. Neurol.* 1996, 24, 909

24 Babich, J.W., Keeling, F., Flower, M.A. *et al.* Initial experience with Tc-99m HMPAO in the study of brain tumours. *Eur. J. Nucl. Med.* 1988, 14, 39

25 Carvalho, P.A., Schwartz, R.B., Alexander, E. *et al.* Detection of recurrent gliomas with quantitative thallium-201/technetium-99m HMPAO single photon emission computerized tomography. *J. Neurosurg.* 1992, 77, 565

26 Langen, K-J., Roosen, N., Herzog, H. *et al.* Investigation of brain tumours with Tc-99mm HMPAO SPECT. *Nucl. Med. Comm.* 1989, 10, 325

27 Lindegaard, M.W., Skretting, A., Hager, B. *et al.* Cerebral and cerebellar uptake of Tc-99m-(d,1)-hexamethyl-propyleneamine oxime (HMPAO) in patients with brain tumour studied by singe photon emission computerized tomography. *Eur. J. Nucl. Med.* 1986, 12, 417

28 O'Tuama, L.A., Janicek, M., Barnes, P.D. *et al.* Tl-201/Tc-99m HMPAO SPECT imaging of treated childhood brain tumours. *Pediatr. Neurol.* 1991, 7, 249

29 Rodrigues, M., Fonseca, A.T., Salgado, D. and Vieira, M.R. Tc-99m HMPAO brain SPECT in the evaluation of prognosis after surgical resection of astrocytoma. Comparison with other noninvasive imaging techniques (CT, MRI and ²⁰¹Tl SPECT). *Nucl. Med. Comm.* 1993, 14, 1050

30 Schwartz, R.B., Carvalho, P.A., Alexander, E. *et al.* Radiation necrosis vs high-grade recurrent glioma : differentiation by using dual-isotope SPECT with ²⁰¹Tl and Tc-99m HMPAO. *Am. J. Neuroradiol.* 1991, 1, 1187

31 Zhang, J.J., Park, Ch., Kim, S.M. *et al.* Dual isotope SPECT in the evaluation of recurrent brain tumour. *Clin. Nucl. Med.* 1992, 17, 663

32 Piwnica-Worms, D. and Holman, B.L. Editorial : Noncardiac applications of hexakis (alkylisontrile) Technetium-99m complexes. *J. Nucl. Med.* 1990, 31, 1166

33 Piwnica-Worms, D., Kronauge, J.F. and Chiu, M.L. Uptake and retention of hexakis (2-methoxyisobutyl isontrile) technetium (I) in cultured chick myocardial cells. Mitochondrial and plasma membrane potential dependence. *Circulation* 1990, 82, 1836

34 Langen, K-J., Coenen, H.H., Roosen, N. *et al.* SPECT studies of brain tumours with 3-I123 iodo-alpha-methyl tyrosine : comparison with PET, I-124 IMT and first clinical results. *J. Nucl. Med.* 1990, 31, 281

35 Langen, K-J., Roosen, N., Coenen, H.H. *et al.* Brain and brain tumour uptake of L-3-I123 iodo-alpha-methyl tyrosine: competition with natural L-amino acids. *J. Nucl. Med.* 1991, 32, 1225

36 Bohuslavizki, K.H., Brenner, W., Braunsdorf, W.E. *et al.* Somatostatin receptor scintigraphy in the differential diagnosis of meningeoma. *Nucl. Med. Comm.* 1996, 17, 302

37 Haldemann, A.R., Rosler, H., Barth, A. *et al.* Somatostatin receptor scintigraphy in central nervous system tumours : role of blood-brain barrier permeability. *J. Nucl. Med.* 1995, 36, 403

38 Lee, J.D., Kim, D.J., Lee, J.T. *et al.* Indium-111 pentetreotide imaging in intra-axial brain tumours : comparison with ²⁰¹Tl and MRI. *J. Nucl. Med.* 1995, 36, 537

39 Verhoeff, N.P.L.G., Bemelman, F.J., Wiersinga, W. *et al.* Imaging of dopamine D2 and somatostatine receptors in vivo using single photonemission tomography in a patient with a TSH/PRL producing pituitary adenoma. *Eur. J. Nucl. Med.* 1993, 20, 555

40 Lastoria, S., Castelli, L., Vergara, E. *et al.* Human gliomas radioimmunoimaging with I-131 BC-2 murine IgG: preliminary report. *J. Nucl. Med. Allied Sci.* 1990, 34, 173

41 Charkes, N.D., Sklaroff, D.M. and Gersohn, C.J. Tumour scanning with radioactive 131-Cesium. *J. Nucl. Med.* 1985, 6, 300

42 Ancri, D., Basset, J.Y., Longchampt, M.F. and Etavard, Ch. Diagnosis of cerebral lesions by ²⁰¹Tl. *Radiol.* 1978, 128, 417

43 Ancri, D. and Basset, J.Y. Diagnosis of cerebral metastases by Thallium 201. *Brit. J. Rad.* 1980, 53, 443

44 Kaplan, W.D., Takvorian, T., Morris, J.H. *et al.* ²⁰¹Tl brain tumour imaging : a comparative study with pathologic correlation. *J. Nucl. Med.* 1987, 28, 47

45 Castronovo, F.P. ²⁰¹Tl labelled TlCl dosimetry revisited. *Nucl. Med. Comm.* 1993, 14, 104

46 Ando, A., Ando, I., Katayama, M. *et al.* Biodistribution of ²⁰¹Tl in tumour bearing animals and inflammatory lesions induced animals. *Eur. J. Nucl. Med.* 1987, 12, 567

47 Rubertone, J.A., Woo, D.V., Emrich, J.G. and Brady, L.W. Brain uptake of ²⁰¹Tl from the cerebrospinal fluid compartment. *J. Nucl. Med.* 1993, 34, 99

48 Sehweil, A.M., McKillop, J.H., Milroy, R. *et al.* Mechanism of ²⁰¹Tl uptake in tumours. *Eur. J. Nucl. Med* 1989, 15, 376

49 Waxman, A.D. ²⁰¹Tl in nuclear oncology in 'Nuclear Medicine Ann.', (Ed. L.M. Freeman), Raven Press, New York, 1991, p.193

50 Ueda, T., Kaji, Y., Wakisaka, S. *et al.* Time sequential single photon emission computed tomography studies in brain tumour using ²⁰¹Tl. *Eur. J. Nucl. Med.* 1993, 20, 138

51 Black, K.L., Hawkins, R.A., Kim, K.T. *et al.* Use of ²⁰¹Tl SPECT to quantitate malignancy grade of gliomas. *J. Neurosurg.* 1989, 71, 342

52 Kim, K.T., Black, K.l., Marciano, D. *et al.* ²⁰¹Tl SPECT imaging of brain tumours : methods and results. *J. Nucl. Med.* 1990, 31, 965

53 Oriuchi, N., Tamura, M., Shibazaki, T. *et al.* Clinical evaluation of ²⁰¹Tl SPECT in supratentorial gliomas: relationship to histologic grade, prognosis and proliferative activity. *J. Nucl. Med.* 1993, 34, 2085

54 Mountz, J.M., Stafford-Schuck, K., McKeever, P.E. *et al.* ²⁰¹Tl tumour/cardiac ratio estimation of residual astrocytoma. *J. Neurosurg.* 1988, 68, 705

55 Rubinstein, R., Karger, H., Pietrzyk, U. *et al.* Use of Thallium brain SPECT, image registration and semiquantitative analysis in the follow-up of brain tumours. *Eur. J. Radiol.* 1996, 21, 188

56 Togawa, T., Yui, N., Kinoshita, F. and Namba, H. A study on thallium-201 SPECT in brain metastases of lung cancer: with special reference to tumor size and tumor to normal brain thallium uptake ratio. *Kaku-Igaku* 1995, 32, 217

57 Sjoholm, H., Elmqvist, D., Rehncrona, S. *et al.* SPECT imaging of gliomas with ^{201}Tl and Tc-99m HMPAO. *Acta Neurol. Scand.* 1995, 91, 66

58 Slizofski, W.J., Krishna, L., Katsetos, C.D. *et al.* Thallium imaging for brain tumours with results measured by a semiquantitative index and correlated with histopathology. *Cancer* 1994, 74, 3190

59 Burkard, R., Kaiser, K.P., Wieler, H. *et al.* Contribution of ^{201}Tl SPECT to the grading of tumourous alterations of the brain. *Neurosurg. Rev.* 1992, 15, 265

60 Ruiz, A., Ganz, W.I., Post, M.J. *et al.* Use of ^{201}Tl brain SPECT to differentiate cerebral lymphoma from toxoplasma encephalitis in AIDS patients. *Am. J. Neuroradiol.* 1994, 15, 1885

61 O'Malley, J.P., Ziessman, H.A., Kumar, P.N. *et al.* Diagnosis of intracranial lymphoma in patients with AIDS : value of Tl-201 single photon emission computed tomography. *Am. J. Roentgenol.* 1994, 163, 417

62 Berry, I., Gaillard, J.F., Guo, Z. *et al.* Cerebral lesions in AIDS : What can be expected from scintigraphy? Cerebral tomographic scintigraphy using [201]Tl : a contribution to the differential diagnosis of lymphomas and infectious lesions. *J. Neuroradiol.* 1995, 22, 218

63 Dierckx, R.A., Martin, J.J., Dobbeleir, A. *et al.* Sensitivity and specificity of ^{201}Tl single photon emission tomography in the functional detection and differential diagnosis of brain tumours. *Eur. J. Nucl. Med.* 1994, 21, 621

64 Alexander, E. 3rd, Loeffler, J.S., Schwarz, R.B. *et al.* [201]Tl technetium-99m HMPAO single photon emission computed tomography (SPECT) imaging for guiding stereotactic craniotomy in heavily irradiated malignant glioma patients. *Acta Neurochir. Wien* 1993, 122, 215

65 Barzen, G., Schubert, C., Richter, W. *et al.*Brain scintigraphy (SPECT) with ^{201}Tl in primary brain tumours. *Stralenther. Onkol.* 1992, 168, 732

66 Kosuda, S., Fujii, I.I., Suzuki, K. *et al.* Reassessment of quantitative ^{201}Tl brain SPECT for miscellaneous brain tumours. *Ann. Nucl. Med.* 1993, 7, 257

67 Lorberboym, M., Baram, J., Feibel, M. *et al.* A prospective evaluation of ^{201}Tl single photon emission computerized tomography for brain tumour burden. *Int. J. Rad. Oncol. Biol. Phys.* 1995, 32, 249

68 Moestafa, H.M., Omar, W.M., Ezzat, I. *et al.* [201]Tl single photon emission tomography in the evaluation of residual and recurrent astrocytoma. *Nucl. Med. Comm.* 1994, 15, 140

69 Tomura, N., Kobayashi, M., Oyama, Y. *et al.* [201]Tl single photon emission computed tomography in the evaluation of therapeutic response for brain tumours. *Kaku-Igaku* 1994, 31, 951

70 Jinnouchi, S., Hoshi, H., Ohnishi, T. *et al.* [201]Tl SPECT for predicting histological types of meningeomas. *J. Nucl. Med.* 1993, 34, 2091

71 Kojima, Y., Kuwana, N., Noji, M. and Tosa, J. Differentiation of malignant glioma and metastatic brain tumour by ^{201}Tl single photon emission computed tomography. *Neurologia Medico-Chirurgica* 1994, 34, 588

72 Komatani, A., Akutsu, T. and Yamaguchi, K. The most suitable parameter to distinguish brain tumour using ^{201}Tl chloride and SPECT. *Kaku Igaku* 1993, 30, 1393

73 Krishna, I., Slizofski, W.J., Katsetos, C.D. *et al.* Abnormal intracerebral thallium localization in a bacterial brain abscess. *J. Nucl. Med.* 1992, 33, 2017

74 Tonami, N., Matsuda, H., Ooba, H. *et al.* [201]Tl accumulation in cerebral candidiasis : unexpected finding on SPECT. *Clin. Nucl. Med.* 1990, 15, 397

75 Palestro, C.J., Swyer, A.J., Kim, C.K. *et al.* Role of In-111 labelled leukocyte scintigraphy in the diagnosis of intracerebral lesions. *Clin. Nucl. Med.* 1991, 16, 305

76 Schmidt, K.G., Rasmussen, J.W., Frederiksen P.B *et al.* Indium-111-granulocyte scintigraphy in brain abscess diagnosis: limitations and pitfalls. *J. Nucl. Med.* 1990, 31, 1121

77 North, C.A., North, R.B., Epstein J.A. *et al.* Low-grade cerebral astrocytomas. Survival and quality of life after radiation therapy. *Cancer* 1990, 66, 6

78 Kosuda, S., Fujii, H., Aoki, S. *et al.* Prediction of survival in patients with suspected recurrent cerebral tumours by quantitative ^{201}Tl single photon emission computed tomography. *Int. J. Radiat. Oncol. Biol. Phys.* 1994, 30, 1201

79 Vertosick, F.T., Selker, R.G., Grossman, S.J. and Joyce, J.M. Correlation of ^{201}Tl single photon emission computed tomography and survival after treatment failure in patients with glioblastoma multiforme. *Neurosurg.* 1994, 34, 396

80 Ishibashi, M., Taguchi, A., Sugita, Y .*et al.* [201]Tl in brain tumours : relationship between tumour cell activity in astrocytic tumour and proliferating cell nuclear antigen. *J. Nucl. Med.* 1995, 36, 2201

81 Bhargava, S., Coel, M. and Wilkinson, R. Thallium-201 single photon emission computed tomography imaging in pediatric brain tumor. *Pediatr. Nurosurg.* 1991/2, 17, 95

82 Maria, B.L., Drane, W.E., Quisling, R.G. *et al.* Value of ^{201}Tl SPECT imaging in childhood brain tumours. *Pediatr. Neurosurg.* 1994, 20, 11

83 Nadel, H.R. [201]Tl for oncological imaging in children. *Sem. Nucl. Med.* 1993, 23, 243

84 Rollins, N.K., Lowry, P.A. and Shapiro, K.N. Comparison of gadolinium-enhanced MR and ^{201}Tl single photon emission computed tomography in pediatric brain tumours. *Pediatr. Neurosurg.* 1995, 22, 8

85 Yoshii, Y., Satou, M., Yamamoto, T. *et al.* The role of ^{201}Tl single photon emission computed tomography in the investigation and characterization of brain tumours in man and their response to treatment. *Eur. J. Nucl. Med.* 1993, 20, 39

86 Kahnn, D., Follett, K.A., Bushnell, D.L. *et al.* Diagnosis of recurrent brain tumour : value of ^{201}Tl versus F-18 Fluoro-deoxyglucose PET. *Am. J. Roentgenol.* 1994, 163, 1459

87 Black, K.L., Emerick, T., Hoh, C. *et al.* [201]Tl SPECT and positron emission tomography equal predictors of glioma grade and recurrence. *Neurol. Res.* 1994, 16, 93

88 Buchpiguel, C.A., Alavi, K.B., Alavi, A. and Kenyon, L.C. PET versus SPECT in distinguishing radiation necrosis from tumour recurrence. *J. Nucl. Med.* 1995, 36, 159

89 Buchpiguel, C.A., Alavi, K.B., Alavi, A. and Payer, F. Post radiation therapy-surgery evaluation of brain tumors. A critical comparison between FDG-PET and ^{201}Tl SPECT imaging (1996, unpublished data)

90 O'Tuama, L.A., Packard, A.B. and Treves, S.T. SPECT imaging of pediatric brain tumour with hexakis (methoxyisobutylisontrile) technetium (I). *J. Nucl. Med.* 1990, 31, 2040

91 Aktolun, C., Bayhan, H. and Kir, M. Clinical experience with Tc-99m MIBI imaging in patients with malignant tumours. Preliminary results and comparison with [201]Tl. *Clin. Nucl. Med.* 1992, 17, 171

92 Macapinlac, H.A., Scott, A., Caluser, C. *et al.* Comparison of ^{201}Tl and Tc-99m methoxyisobutylisontrile (MIBI) with MRI in the evaluation of recurrent brain tumours (abstract). *J. Nucl. Med.* 1992, 33, 867

93 O'Tuama, L.A., Treves, S.T., Larar, J.N. *et al.* [201]Tl versus technetium-99m MIBI SPECT in evaluation of childhood brain tumours : a within-subject comparison. *J. Nucl. Med.* 1993, 34, 1054

SPECT in Neurology and Psychiatry, edited by P.P. De Deyn, R.A. Dierckx, A. Alavi and B.A. Pickut
© 1997 John Libbey & Company Ltd, pp. 387–391

Evaluation of ^{123}I-α-L-Methyltyrosine as a SPECT Tracer of Amino Acid uptake in Brain Tumours

Chapter
46

K.-J. Langen

Introduction

The diagnostic workup of brain tumour has made rapid progress with the development of cranial computed tomography (CCT) and magnetic resonance imaging (MRI). Today these methods are unsurpassed diagnostic modalities for the detection of cerebral lesions. The differentiation of tumour tissue from oedematous, necrotic and fibromatous tissue, however, is sometimes not optimal. Among the many radiolabelled substrates used to investigate the biological behaviour of intracranial tumours, radiolabelled amino acids is one group which holds great promise for the differentiation of intracerebral tumour spread, especially in the case of intracerebral gliomas[1-10]. In a case study by Bergström *et al.*[1] the results of CT ^{11}C-L-methionine PET, ^{11}C-glucose PET and ^{68}Ga-EDTA PET in a patient with a glioma were compared. As the patient died a few days after the investigations, these results could be compared with the histopathological specimen and it could be shown that the extent of the amino acid study correlated exactly with histological tumour spread while the other methods underestimated tumour extent. Meanwhile, various PET studies have shown that the accumulation of ^{11}C-methyl-L-methionine (MET) spreads beyond the tumour margin as defined by CT and MRI and correlates with histological tumour spread[4,6,7,10,11]. The diagnostic potential of amino acid accumulation in gliomas for tumour grading prognosis, detection of recurrence and therapeutic response is still under investigation. The underlying mechanism of increased accumulation of large neutral amino acids in cerebral gliomas has not yet been explained. On one hand it is assumed that increased protein synthesis is the driving force, but on the other hand a number of studies have given rise to the assumption that transmembranous transport phenomena play a major role in the uptake process[2,3,12-14]. While brain imaging of amino acid uptake is easy to carry out with ^{11}C-labelling and PET, tracers for single photon emission computer tomography (SPECT) are rarely available. Amino acids labelled with γ-emitters, however, would offer a more widespread application of amino acid studies, as SPECT is generally available and relatively inexpensive. L-3-[^{123}I]-Iodo-α-methyl-tyrosine (IMT) is an amino acid analogue initially tested for pancreas imaging and melanoma detection[15,16]. Recently, a number of studies have been undertaken to evaluate the applicability of IMT as a tracer of amino acid uptake in brain tumours[17-24].

In this chapter, current understanding about the biological behaviour of IMT and the present state of clinical evaluation are summarised.

Institute of Medicine,
Research Center Jülich,
P. O. Box 1913, 52425 Julich,
Germany

Radiosynthesis, whole-body kinetics and dosimetry

Synthesis of L-3-[^{123}I]-iodo-α-methyl-tyrosine is usually performed by direct electrophilic iodination starting with no carrier added ^{123}I and 1 µg of carrier $k_i^{15,16}$. The methods of labelling and of high performance liquid chromatography (HPLC) for isolation and purification of the radiopharmaceutical have been described. The radiochemical yield of the procedure is between 60 and 80%. High no carrier added radioiodination yields (>80%) have been described recently using Iodo-gen[tm] in a heterogenous aqueous system[25]. The specific activity is >167 GBq/mmol (4500 Ci/mmol).

The whole-body kinetics of IMT has been evaluated in five male patients with cerebral gliomas up to 5 h after injection of IMT[26]. IMT was eliminated rapidly by the kidneys (57 ± 6% at 1.5 h, 70 ± 4% at 3 h and 79 ± 4% at 5 h. The effective dose according to ICRP 60 was 7.67 mSv/MBq. At a recommended dose of 550 MBq IMT for brain SPECT, the effective dose is 4.2 mSv and thus in the range of routine nuclear medicine investigations.

Experimental studies

The metabolic behaviour of IMT in the brain has been evaluated in NMRI of mice[18]. Analysis of the brain homogenate after 40 min incorporation time and discontinuous gel electrophoresis of the protein pellet revealed that all radioactivity can be eluted as a monomolecular mass fraction of low molecular weight, indicating that there is no incorporation of IMT into protein. Furthermore, high preformance liquid chromatography showed that 40 min after injection >95% of the radioactivity in the brain is still present as intact IMT i.e. no significant amounts of metabolites of IMT are formed in the brain or taken up from the plasma within one hour of injection. Analysis of the patient´s plasma after IMT injection exhibits a decrease of radioactivity in the form of the administered tracer to 30% of total plasma activity at 90 min post injection[18]. Free radioactive iodide in plasma increases slowly from 0.5% at 4 min to 4% of total plasma activity at 90 min post injection so that the signal from free radioactive iodide appears to be negligible during the period of SPECT studies (0-60 min). Another experimental study[21] demonstrated that IMT transport across the blood brain barrier is similar to L-tyrosine, saturable and cross inhibitable by L-tyrosine. Analysis of the brain homogenates confirmed the results of >80% of the radioactivity as unaltered IMT with a lack of participation in protein synthesis or other metabolic pathways.

In a recent study[22], IMT uptake in a human glioma cell line was compared with other tracers at exponential growth phase and after reaching a plateau phase. The proliferation activity of the cells was confirmed by incubation with the DNA precursor ^{3}H-thymidine. In the rapidly proliferating cells IMT uptake was increased by a factor 4.4 ± 1.3 in relation to the slowly proliferating cells, methionine uptake by a factor 3.6 ± 0.8, leucine (3.8 ± 0.8) and to deoxyglucose (3.6 ± 0.8). These results indicate that the uptake of the non-metabolisable amino acid analogue IMT is increased in rapidly proliferating glioma cells to the same extent as methionine or leucine, which indicates an activation of transport mechanisms for large neutral amino acids in proliferating glioma cells. As IMT is assumed to be transported by the L-carrier system like other large neutral amino acids[19,27], the experiments for IMT were repeated during inhibition of the L-carrier by 2-amino-2-norbornane-carboxylic acid (BCH). This led to reduction of IMT uptake to 20% of the uptake without BCH inhibition, which indicates that the uptake of IMT is mediated by the L-1-amino acid carrier system (Langen, unpublished observation).

IMT studies in humans

The first IMT SPECT studies of cerebral gliomas began in the late eighties[17,18]. In the latter study the intracerebral kinetics of IMT was investigated in two patients using IMT labelled with the positron emitting iodine isotope 124I, which allowed investigation of the intracerebral kinetics by positron emission tomography. In that study it could be shown that IMT concentration in the brain and brain tumours reaches a maximum after about 15 min followed by a slow washout. Therefore the optimal time for IMT brain SPECT is between 15 and 60 min post injection. The specificity of IMT uptake in the human brain and brain tumours was investigated by a competition study in 10 patients with brain tumours19. SPECT studies were made repeatedly before and after infusion of natural L-amino acids. In that study it could be shown that by the infusion of natural L-amino acids, IMT uptake decreased by 45.6 ± 15.4% in the normal brain (n = 10, p<0.001) and by 53.2% ± 14.1% for gliomas (n = 5, p<0.01). In two meningeomas and a metastasis, no major change of uptake under infusion was observed. These data proved that IMT competes with naturally occurring L-amino acids for transport into normal brain and gliomas. The competitive effects in gliomas and normal brain tissue were similar, so that the tumour/brain ratios were independent from the amino acid plasma levels. This simplifies the comparability of follow-up SPECT studies in gliomas because the dietary status does not need to be identical.

Nevertheless, it is advisable to study patients under fasting conditions because brain and brain tumour uptake is higher and gives better count rates in the SPECT study and thus provides better delineation of gliomas. Moreover, the washout of IMT from the brain was slower under fasting conditions. In brain metastases and meningeomas, however, there was a considerable influence of the dietary status on the tumour/brain ratios (changes up to 70%). Therefore, in the case of brain tumours originating from tissues external to the brain, a constant dietary status is needed in follow-up studies.

In order to further validate IMT as a SPECT tracer of amino acid uptake in brain tumours a comparative study was undertaken of PET using ^{11}C-L-methionine and IMT SPECT[20]. In 14 patients with cerebral gliomas, both investigations were carried out on the same day and under fasting conditions. All gliomas showed increased uptake for both tracers in relation to normal brain. The tumour/cortex ratios between 15 and 60 min p.i. were slightly lower for IMT (1.77 ± 0.32) as for methionine (2.24 ± 0.45, n = 14, p<0.02). This could be explained partially by the higher influence of scattering in the SPECT studies and the higher washout of IMT. The visual comparison of the scans yielded no differences in tumour size and shape with methionine PET and IMT SPECT. An example is shown in Figure 1. The tumour/cortex ratios of IMT SPECT and

methionine PET, however, showed only a low correlation (r = 0.53, n = 14, p<0.05) and differences in tumour uptake for IMT and methionine were noted in individual gliomas, i.e., higher uptake for methionine but also for IMT. Tracer kinetics were compared using dynamic SPECT using a triple-headed system and dynamic PET acquisitions, and showed that these differences were caused mainly by differences in the initial transport process. IMT showed a maximal tracer uptake in brain and brain tumours about 15 min post injection (Figure 2), which was followed by a tracer washout of $44 \pm 13.5\%$ in gliomas (p = 0.001, n = 10) and $35.3 \pm 5.4\%$ in normal brain (p = 0.001, n = 10) at 60 min post injection. For methionine, there was no significant change in tracer concentration in tumour tissue or brain tissue between 15 and 16 min post injection and tumour to cortex ratios remained constant. The tumour/cortex ratios for IMT decreased significantly from 15 to 60 min post injection (1.96 ± 0.42 versus 1.61 ± 0.29, n = 10, p<0.05), while there was no change for methionine (2.34 ± 0.44 versus 2.30 ± 0.55, n = 10). The loss of IMT from the tissue between 15 and 60 min post injection can be explained by a low intracellular binding of IMT, and confirmed the experimental studies that IMT is not incorporated into protein. The lack of significant intracellular binding was also confirmed by the kinetic analysis of the IMT data. Non-linear regression analysis using a two compartment model yielded satisfactory fits to the

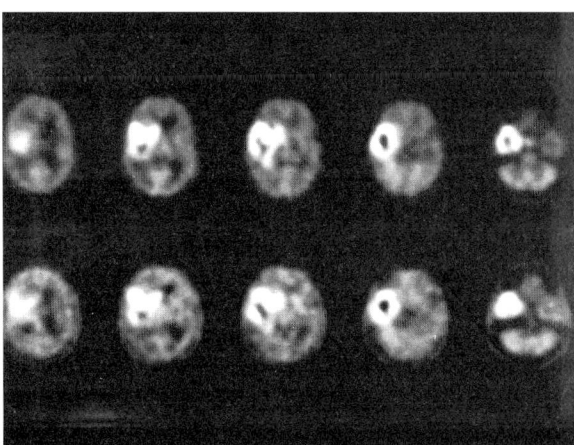

Figure 1a Comparison of IMT SPECT scans (upper row) and MET PET scans (lower row) added up from 15 to 60 min post injection of patient with a glioblastoma. The MET PET scans are smoothed to the resolution of the SPECT scans. The extent of the tumour area with increased tracer uptake appears to be identical for IMT and MET

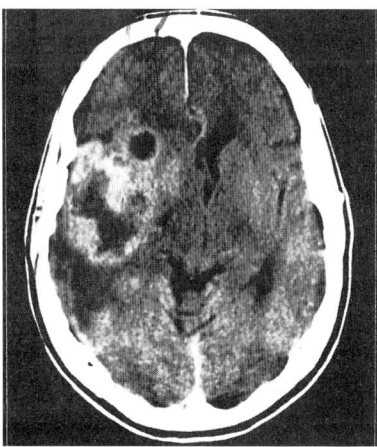

Figure 1b The contrast enhanced CT scan of the same patient

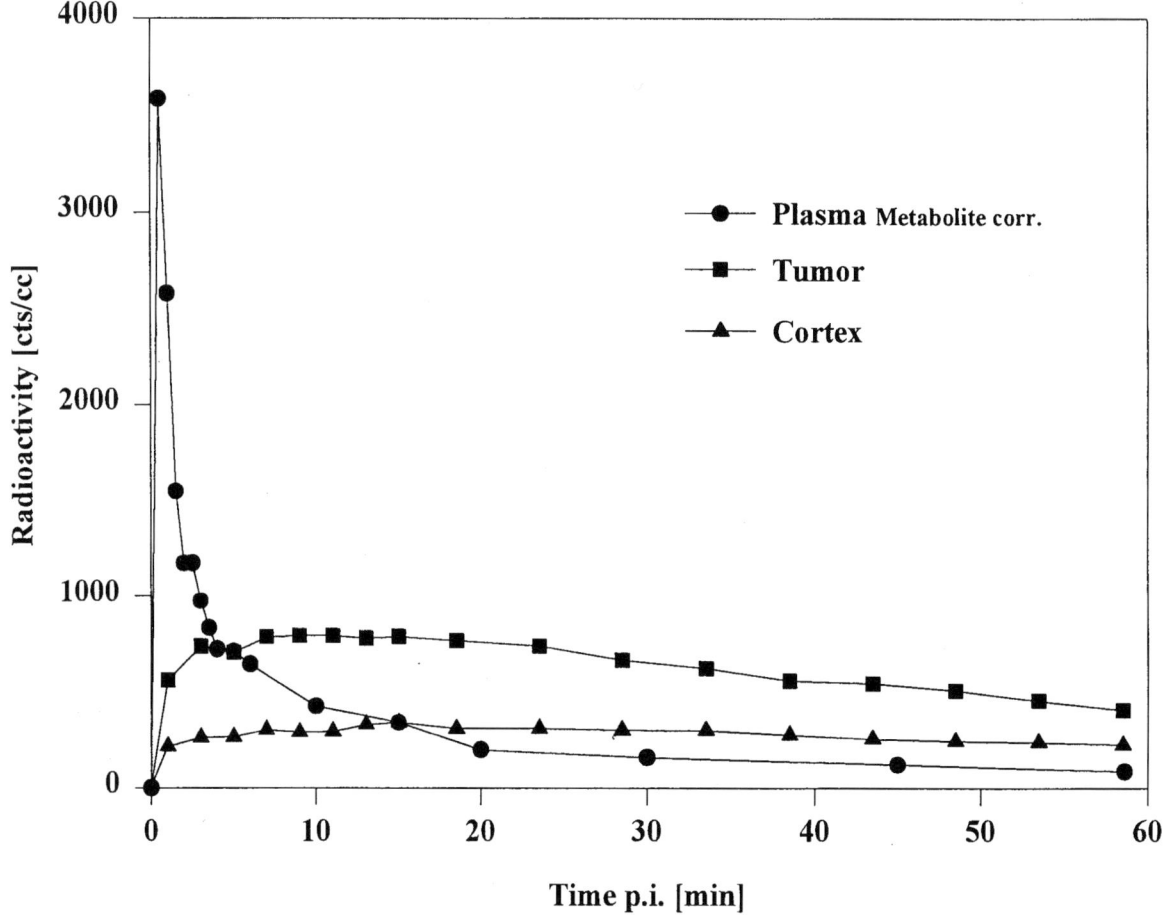

Figure 2 Kinetics of ^{123}I- α -methyltyrosine in tumour, cortex and plasma. The plasma curve is corrected for non-^{123}I- α - methyltyrosine radioactivity. Radioactivity in tumour and brain reaches a maximum after about 15 min followed by a slow washout process which is slightly faster for the tumour than for cortex indicating low intracellular binding. The optimal time for SPECT acquisition is within 15 to 60 min post injection

data and addition of k3 to the fit procedure yielded small values for k3 without a remarkable improvement in the fit.

The most important result of this comparative study remains that imaging of intracerebral tumour infiltration of gliomas is similar for both methods, and that IMT SPECT offers a considerable part of the diagnostic potential attainable with MET and PET.

Clinical studies

The clinical role of IMT SPECT for the diagnosis of cerebral gliomas is still under clinical evaluation. A dependency of IMT uptake on histological tumour grade has been reported[18,28]. A clear separation in in-dividual cases, however, remains difficult because there are large zones of overlap. IMT SPECT appears to be

helpful to differentiate unclear intracerebral space occupying lesions and to detect tumour recurrency[28]. On the other hand, increased IMT uptake has been shown shortly after surgical intervention without the presence of glioma tissue[29]. Initial evaluations of chemotherapy effects in gliomas by IMT SPECT showed that patients with stable clinical course and reduction of tumour volume showed a decrease or a stable IMT uptake ratio, while non-responders showed an increase in the tumour to cortex ratio[23]. Follow-up studies of IMT uptake in brain tumours during radiotherapy in 20 patients with brain tumours showed measurable changes in amino acid transport in astrocytomas and glioblastomas. One patient with increasing tumour brain/ratio survived<4 weeks[24]. These results indicate that IMT SPECT may help to guide therapeutic strategy in patients with gliomas.

In conclusion, clinical experiences with IMT SPECT in the management of patients with cerebral gliomas are still limited but the results reported are similar to those of MET and PET. The biological meaning of the signal obtained by amino acid uptake studies, for IMT SPECT as well as for PET using any other amino acid, has still to be elucidated.

References

1   Bergström, M., Collins, V.P., Ehrin, E. *et al.* Discrepancies in brain tumour extent as shown by computed tomography and positron tomography using ^{68}Ga-EDTA, ^{11}C-glucose and ^{11}C-methionine. *J. Comput. Assist. Tomogr.* 1983, 7, 1062

2   Bergström, M., Lundquist, H., Ericson, K. *et al.* Comparison of the accumulation kinetics of L-(methyl-^{11}C)-methionine and D-(methyl-^{11}C)-methionine in brain tumours studied with positron emission tomography. *Acta Radiologica* 1987, 28, 225

3   Bergström, M., Ericson, K., Hagenfeldt, L. *et al.* PET study of methionine accumulation in glioma and normal brain tissue: competition with branched chain amino acids. *J. Comput. Assist. Tomogr.* 1987, 11, 208

4   Ericson, K., Lilja, A., Bergström, M. *et al.* Positron emission tomography with (^{11}C]methyl)-L-methionine, ^{11}C]D-glucose, and ^{68}Ga]EDTA in supratentorial tumours. *J. Comput. Assist. Tomogr.* 1985, 9, 683

5   Ericson, K., Blomqvist, G., Bergström, M. *et al.* Application of a kinetic model on the methionine accumulation in intracranial tumours studied with positron emission tomography. *Acta Radiol.* 1987, 28, 505

6   Mosskin, M., von Holst, H., Bergström, M. *et al.* Positron emission tomography with ^{11}C-L-methionine and X-ray computed tomography of intracranial tumours compared with histopathologic examination of multiple biopsies. *Acta Radiologica* 1987, 28, 673

7   Mosskin, M., Ericson, K., Hindmarsh, T. *et al.* Positron emission tomography compared with MRI and CT in supratentorial gliomas using multiple stereotactic biopsies as reference. *Acta Radiologica* 1989, 30, 225

8   Derlon, J.M., Boudet, C., Bustany, P. *et al.* [11]C]-L-methionine uptake in gliomas. *Neurosurgery* 1989, 25, 720

9   Hatazawa, J., Ishiwata, K, Itoh, M. *et al.* Quantitative evaluation of L-[methyl-C-11]methionine uptake in tumour using positron emission tomography. *J. Nucl. Med.* 1989, 30, 1809

10 Ogawa, T., Shishido, F, Kanno, I. *et al.* Cerebral glioma: evaluation with methionine PET. *Radiology* 1993, 186, 45

11 Csaplár, K., Langen, K.-J., Mühlensiepen, H. *et al.* 3H-L-Methionine and 14C-deoxyglucose autoradiography: comparison with histological tumour spread in a rat glioma model. *Eur. J. Nucl. Med* 1995, 22, 866

12 Schober, O., Meyer, G.-J., Stolke, D. and Hundeshagen, H. Brain tumour imaging using C-11-labelled L-methionine and D-methionine. *J. Nucl. Med.* 1985, 26, 98

13 Wienhard, K., Herholz, K., Coenen, H.H. *et al.* Increased amino acid transport into brain tumours measured by PET of L-[2-^{18}F]fluoro-tyrosine. *J. Nucl. Med.* 1991, 32, 1338

14 Ishiwata, K., Kubota, K., Murakami, M. *et al.* Re-evaluation of amino acid PET studies: can the protein synthesis rates in brain and tumour tissues be measured in vivo? *J. Nucl. Med.* 1993, 34, 1936

15 Tisljar, U., Kloster, G., Ritzl, F. and Stöcklin, G. Accumulation of radioiodinated L-α-methyltyrosine in pancreas of mice: concise communication. *J. Nucl. Med.* 1979, 20, 973

16 Kloster, G. and Bockslaff, H. L-3-^{123}I-α-methyltyrosine for melanoma detection: a comparative evaluation. *Int. J. Nucl. Med. Biol.* 1982, 9, 259

17 Biersack, H.J., Coenen, H.H., Stöcklin, G. *et al.* Imaging of brain tumours with L-3-[^{123}I]iodo-α-methyl tyrosine and SPECT. *J. Nucl. Med.* 1989, 30, 110

18 Langen, K.-J., Coenen, H.H,. Roosen, N. *et al.* SPECT studies of brain tumours with L-3-[^{123}I]iodo-α-methyl tyrosine: comparison with PET, [124]IMT and first clinical results. *J. Nucl. Med.* 1990, 31, 281

19 Langen, K.-J., Roosen, N., Coenen, H.H. *et al.*Brain and brain tumour uptake of L-3-[^{123}I]iodo-α-methyl tyrosine: competition with natural L-amino acids. *J. Nucl. Med.* 1991, 32, 1225

20 Langen, K.-J., Ziemons, K., Kiwit, J.P.W. *et al.* 3-[^{123}I-α-Methyl-Tyrosin] and [Methyl-^{11}C]-L-Methionine uptake in cerebral gliomas: a comparative study using SPECT and PET. *J. Nucl. Med.* 1997, 38, 517

21 Kawai, K., Fujibayashi, Y., Saji, H. *et al.* A strategy for the study of cerebral amino acid transport using iodine-123-labeled amino acid radiopharmaceutical: 3-Iodo-alpha-methyl-L-tyrosine. *J. Nucl. Med.* 1991, 32, 819

22 Csaplár, K., Langen, K.-J., Mühlensiepen, H. *et al.* Investigation of ^{123}I-α-methyl-tyrosine and ^{125}I-o-methyl-α-methyl-tyrosine uptake in glioma cell cultures. *Eur. J. Nucl. Med.* 1995, 22, 866

23 Wunderlich, G., Schmidt, D., Langen, K.-J *et al.* Evaluation of chemotherapy in gliomas by I-123-α-methyl-I-tyrosine SPECT: first results. *Eur. J. Nucl. Med.* 1995, 8, 796

24 Otto, L., Dannenberg, C., Feyer, P. *et al.* ^{123}I-α–Methyl-tyrosine uptake of brain tumours - influence of radiotherapy. *Eur. J. Nucl. Med.* 1995, 22, 796

25 Krummeich, C., Holschbach, M. and Stöcklin, G. Direct electrophilic radioiodination of tyrosine analogues: their in-vivo stability and brain uptake in mice. *Appl. Rad. Isot.* 1994, 45, 929

26 Schmidt, D., Langen, K.-J., Herzog, H. *et al.* Whole-body kinetics and dosimetry of ^{123}I-α-methyl-tyrosine. *J. Nucl. Med.* 1995, 36, 97

27 Oldendorf, W.H. Saturation of amino acid uptake by human brain tumour demonstrated by SPECT (Editorial). *J. Nucl. Med.* 1991, 32, 1229

28 Schober, O., Assmann S. , Wagner W. *et al.* The assessment of ^{123}I-α-methyltyrosine (IMT) in the follow up of primary brain tumours. *Eur. J. Nucl. Med.* 1994, 21, 789

29 McGarvie, J., Patterson, J., Wyper, D *et al.* Does neurosurgical resection cause uptake of ^{201}Tl and ^{123}I-α-methyl-I-tyrosine in the brain? *Eur. J. Nucl. Med.* 1995, 22, 866

SPECT in Neurology and Psychiatry, edited by P.P. De Deyn, R.A. Dierckx, A. Alavi and B.A. Pickut
© 1997 John Libbey & Company Ltd, pp. 393–401

SPECT Receptor Binding Studies in Brain Oncology with particular attention to Somatostatin-Receptor Scintigraphy (SRS) in Differential Diagnosis of Meningeoma

Chapter
47

K.H. Bohuslavizki, W. Brenner, W.E.K. Braunsdorf[*],
A. Behnke[*], N. Jahn, S. Tinnemeyer, H.-H. Hugo[*], H. Wolf,
C. Sippel, G. Tönshoff, M. Clausen, H.M. Mehdorn[*] and
E. Henze

Introduction

Somatostatin receptors have been described on the surface of various cell types both *in vitro* and *in vivo*[1-12]. The main clinical benefit of functional imaging using radiolabelled somatostatin analogues has been shown in gastroentero-pancreatic tumours[13-20]. Scintigraph of small cell lung cancer[17,21-23], endocrine ophthalmopathy[24-26], malignant lymphoma[11], and meningeoma[27-36] using ^{111}In-octreotide is currently under discussion. In meningeoma, somatostatin receptor expression was shown to be near 100%, both in scintigraphy[27-36] and in cell culture studies[3,6-9]. Therefore, SRS was suggested by various authors for differential diagnosis of neurinoma versus meningeoma[29,31,33,35]. However, we observed negative scintigrams in some patients with histologically proven meningeoma. In consequence, the exclusion of meningeoma by a lack of tracer uptake seems questionable. Therefore, the aim of this study was to reassess the clinical impact of SRS in patients with suspected meningeoma.

Methods

Patients

In total, 78 patients with suspected meningeoma were referred for SRS between November 1993 and July 1995. Out of the total, 59 with surgical treatment and subsequent histological evaluation were included in the study. There were 18 male and 41 female subjects. Their median age was 59 years, ranging from 26 to 83 years. Tumour volumes were calculated from MRI images under assumption of a rotational ellipsoid, and ranged from 0.3 to 112.8 ml. Details of patients' characteristics are given in Table 1.

Clinic of Nuclear Medicine,
Christian-Albrechts-University of
Kiel, Arnold-Heller-Str. 9,
D-24105 Kiel, Germany
*Clinic of Neurosurgery,
Christian-Albrechts-University of
Kiel, Weimarer Str. 8, D-24106
Kiel, Germany

Table 1 Clinical data of patients showing size and location of the tumour, histological results and evaluation of somatostatin receptor scintigraphy (SRS) with respect to true positive (TP), true negative (TN), false positive (FP), and false negative (FN). CPA: cerebello pontine angle

Patient	Location	Size [cm]	Histology	SRS	Evaluation
f / 50	Right petrous	6.4•4.0•3.0	Psammomatous	pos	TP
f / 60	Left petrous	5.1•5.5•3.2	Transitional cell	pos	TP
m / 27	Right petrous	1.0•2.5•1.5	Meningotheliomatous	pos	TP
f / 83	Base of skull	2.5•1.8•1.5	Meningotheliomatous	pos	TP
f / 80	Left parietal	3.5•2.0•3.0	Meningotheliomatous	pos	TP
f / 64	Cavernous sinus	2.8•2.0•1.8	Meningotheliomatous	pos	TP
m / 42	Left parietal	5.4•5.2•5.3	Meningotheliomatous	pos	TP
f / 56	Cervical 2/3	1.2•0.7•2.5	Meningotheliomatous	pos	TP
f / 80	Falx cerebri	2.5•3.0•2.0	Transitional cell	pos	TP
f / 61	Clival	3.5•3.0•2.6	Secretory	pos	TP
m / 81	Left parietal	4.0•2.5•3.0	Meningotheliomatous	pos	TP
m / 67	Left temporal	3.6•1.5•2.4	Transitional cell	pos	TP
f / 73	Clival	2.0•1.1•2.1	Menigotheliomatous	pos	TP
f / 49	Cavernous sinus	2.2•2.2•1.7	Meningotheliomatous	pos	TP
f / 61	Left parasagittal	2.5•3.1•2.7	Transitional cell	pos	TP
f / 75	Right frontal	2.5•2.9•2.0	Meningotheliomatous	pos	TP
f / 51	Right frontal	5.2•4.4•4.9	Meningotheliomatous	pos	TP
m / 70	Left parasagittal	6.0•5.0•5.5	Meningotheliomatous	pos	TP
f / 59	Thoracal 1/2	0.7•1.2•3.0	Meningotheliomatous	pos	TP
f / 63	Cavernous sinus	2.5•1.6•3.1	Meningotheliomatous	pos	TP
f / 68	Right petrous	1.7•2.1•2.4	Meningotheliomatous	pos	TP
m / 70	Left petrous	4.0•4.0•4.5	Meningotheliomatous	pos	TP
f / 54	Cavernous sinus	3.5•4.0•3.0	Transitional cell	pos	TP
f / 38	Left petrous	3.0•1.5•3.0	Meningotheliomatous	pos	TP
m / 69	Falx cerebri	2.5•2.5•3.0	Meningotheliomatous	pos	TP
m / 53	Tentorium cerebelli	4.0•3.8•3.0	Fibroblastic	pos	TP
m / 52	Right frontal	7.5•5.9•5.1	Meningotheliomatous	pos	TP
f / 69	Left sagittal	0.8•0.8•1.3	Malignant	pos	TP
f / 69	Right sagittal	2.0•2.1•1.2	Malignant	pos	TP
f / 69	Left parietal	1.4•1.6•2.2	Malignant	pos	TP
f / 69	Right occipital	2.6•3.1•2.3	Malignant	pos	TP
f / 39	Left lateral ventricle	4.1•4.0•4.7	Fibroblastic	pos	TP

Table 1 continued

Patient	Location	Size [cm]	Histology	SRS	Evaluation
f / 52	Olfactory nerve	3.8•3.8•2.5	Meningotheliomatous	pos	TP
m / 74	Clival	2.5•1.7•2.3	Meningotheliomatous	pos	TP
f / 54	Right petrosal sinus	3.0•2.5•2.8	Fibrobalstic	pos	TP
f / 71	Right retroorbital	2.5•2.0•2.7	Fibrobalstic	pos	TP
f / 64	Right CPA	3.2•2.8•3.0	Glomus jugulare tumour	pos	FP
f / 29	Hypophysis	1.5•2.5•2.0	Inactive adenoma	pos	FP
f / 73	Right petrous	4.5•4.5•3.0	Inflammation	pos	FP
m / 32	Hypophysis	2.5•2.8•2.8	Active adenoma	pos	FP
f / 73	Left retroorbital	1.0•1.3•1.0	Fibroblastic	neg	FN
f / 51	Thoracal 1	1.5•1.2•1.4	Transitional cell	neg	FN
f / 32	Right petrous bone	1.3•1.0•1.5	Microcystic	neg	FN
f / 38	Left petrous bone	3.0•1.5•3.0	Meningotheliomatous	neg	FN
f / 69	Neck	2.5•1.5•2.6	Malignant	neg	FN
f / 73	Foramen magnum	1.4•1.4•1.4	Atypical	neg	FN
f / 72	Cervical 3	1.2•1.4•2.0	Transitional cell	neg	FN
f / 26	Thoracal 12	1.7•1.8•6.0	Ependymoma	neg	TN
m / 33	Right CPA	2.0•1.8•1.5	Dermoid cyst	neg	TN
f / 54	Hypophysis	2.0•1.6•1.9	Active adenoma	neg	TN
m / 29	Bulb of jugular vein	2.0•2.0•1.5	Carcinoma	neg	TN
m / 42	Hypophysis	1.5•1.8•1.8	Active adenoma	neg	TN
f / 56	Hypophysis	1.0•1.5•0.7	Inactive adenoma	neg	TN
m / 56	Hypophysis	0.8•0.8•0.8	Active adenoma	neg	TN
f / 46	Right CPA	3.1•1.9•1.8	Neurinoma	neg	TN
f / 73	Left parietal	2.0•1.9•2.0	Breast cancer metastasis	neg	TN
f / 61	Falx cerebri	2.5•1.9•2.3	Ø	neg	TN
f / 72	Lumbar 3/4	2.5•3.0•2.5	Neurinoma	neg	TN
m / 39	Right parietal	2.9•3.6•2.5	Glioblastoma	neg	TN

Histological staining

Surgical specimens were fixed in 4% formaldehyde and embedded in paraffin for histopathological examination. Sections of 4 µm thickness were stained both with Hematoxylin-Eosin (HE) and Elastica van Gieson (EvG).

Imaging protocol

After an intravenous injection of 200 MBq ^{111}In-octreotide (Mallinckrodt, Petten, The Netherlands) digital whole-body acquisition in anterior and posterior projection was obtained at 10 min, 1, 4, and 24 h with a scan speed of 10 cm/min. The large-field-of-view gamma-camera (Bodyscan, Siemens, Erlangen, Germany) was equipped with a medium-energy parallel hole collimator, the energy window was adjusted to both [111]In- peaks at 173 and 247 keV with a symmetric 20% window.

In addition, single photon emission computed tomography (SPECT) was performed at 4 and 24 h with a single head large-field-of-view camera (Diacam, Siemens, Erlangen, Germany). Data were acquired over 360° for 64 angles in a step-and-shoot mode, and projections were stored in a 128 matrix.

MRI was performed either on a 1.5T Magnetom Vision (Siemens, Erlangen, Germany) or a 1.0T Magnetom Expert (Siemens, Erlangen, Germany). Both T1-weighted (TR=500 ms, TE=12 ms) and T2-weighted spin-echo sequences (TR=3600 ms, TE=98 ms) were acquired with a slice thickness of 6–8 mm. Gadolinium-DTPA (Schering, Berlin, Germany) was administered intravenously at a dosage of 0.1 mmol/kg body weight for contrast enhanced image acquisition.

Quantification

Quantitative evaluation of regional uptake was performed by placing a circular ROI over the lesion and a background area located contralaterally or directly beneath the lesion, allowing the calculation of a target-to-background ratio (T/B). Relative percentage tumour uptake was measured by relating the activity within the lesion ROI to whole body activity after

Table 2 Tumour-to-background ratio of somatostatin receptor scintigraphy with respect to histological evaluation at different time post injection of ^{111}In-octreotide. Data represent mean ± one standard deviation

Time p.i.	T/B ratio [ ]			
	True positive n=36	False positive n=4	False negative n=7	True negative n=12
10 min	1.97 ± 0.85	2.53 ± 1.34	1.15 ± 0.48	1.29 ± 0.27
1 h	2.10 ± 0.64	3.24 ± 1.88	1.27 ± 0.45	1.34 ± 0.34
4 h	2.61 ± 0.90	5.09 ± 4.04	1.13 ± 0.55	1.31 ± 0.32
24 h	3.58 ± 1.96	7.01 ± 6.00	1.29 ± 0.38	1.42 ± 0.33

correction for background activity. All quantifications were calculated as geometric means of the anterior and posterior projections. The results are given as mean ± one standard deviation. Two-tailed students t-test for unpaired data was used to evaluate statistical differences, with $p < 0.05$ considered to be statistically significant[37].

Sensitivity and specificity were calculated for SRS uptake versus presence of meningeoma.

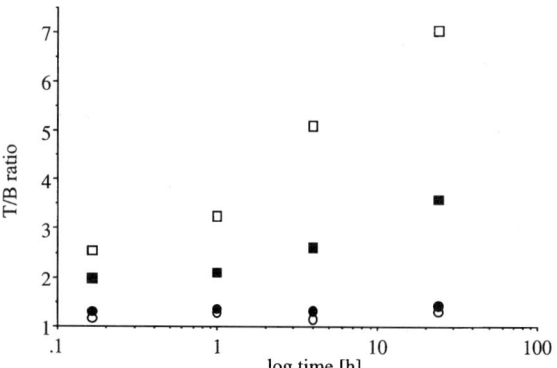

Figure 1 Geometric mean of tumour-to-background ratio derived from anterior and posterior projection of somatostatin receptor scintigraphy in 59 patients with suspected meningeoma versus logarithm of time post injection in hours. Filled squares: 36 true positive; open squares: 4 false positive; open circles: 7 false negative; filled circles: 12 true negative. For standard deviation see Table 2

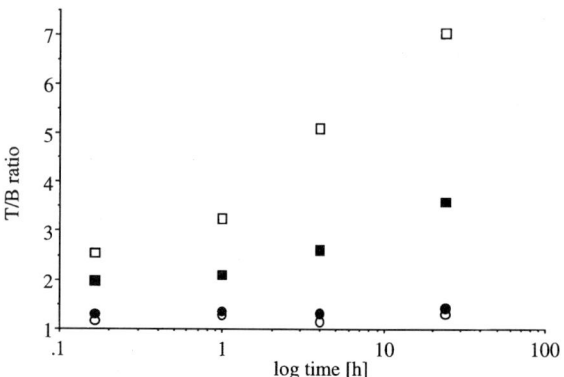

Figure 2 Geometric mean of uptake in per cent of whole body activity derived from anterior and posterior projection of somatostatin receptor scintigraphy in 59 patients with suspected meningeoma versus logarithm of time post injection in hours. Filled squares: 36 true positive; open squares: 4 false positive; open circles: 7 false negative; filled circles: 12 true negative. For standard deviation see Table 3

Results

Evaluation of SRS with respect to histological diagnosis, tumour volume, and location of tumours are given in detail in Table 1. There was no correlation between detailed histological analysis, scintigraphic result and anatomical location. Therefore, only pooled data were given. Mean values of both tumour-to-background ratio versus time and uptake versus time regarding all patients are shown in Figures 1 and 2, respectively. Corresponding scatter data are given in detail in Tables 2 and 3. A statistical evaluation for all 59 patients is given in detail in Table 4. Data were stratified for different tumour volumes.

As expected, no additional benefit was yielded by SRS in 4 patients with false positive results (cf. Table 1). These were patients suffering from a jugular glomus tumour located at the right cerebello pontine angle, an inflammatory process of the right petrous bone, a hormonally inactive pituitary adenoma, and a hormonally active pituitary adenoma. The latter exhibited the most intense uptake and maximum T/B ratio of all patients investigated. A coronal Gd-DTPA enhanced T1-weighted slice, the respective coronal

Table 3 Uptake of somatostatin receptor scintigraphy in percentage of whole body activity with respect to histological evaluation at different time post injection of ^{111}In-octreotide. Data represent mean ± one standard deviation

| Time p.i. | Uptake [% WB] | | | |
	True positive n=36	False positive n=4	False negative n=7	True negative n=12
10 min	0.24 ± 0.24	0.38 ± 0.44	0.12 ± 0.14	0.06 ± 0.03
1 h	0.23 ± 0.17	0.43 ± 0.47	0.10 ± 0.08	0.06 ± 0.06
4 h	0.33 ± 0.26	0.71 ± 0.90	0.08 ± 0.04	0.06 ± 0.04
24 h	0.44 ± 0.49	1.32 ± 1.89	0.05 ± 0.04	0.05 ± 0.07

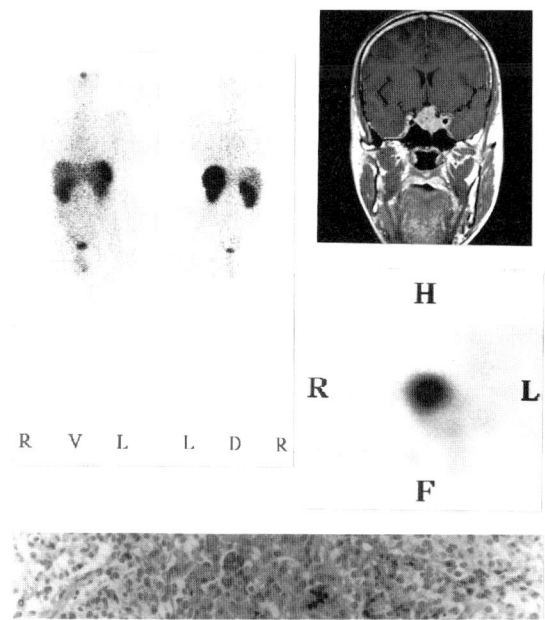

Figure 3 Example of a false positive patient (m/32). Planar somatostatin receptor scintigraphy 4 h post injection in anterior and posterior projection, coronal Gd-DTPA enhanced T1-weighted MRI slice, corresponding coronal SPECT slice, and histology of a hormonally active pituitary adenoma (EvG, magnification: 50 times). Note, cranial displacement of the sellar diaphragm

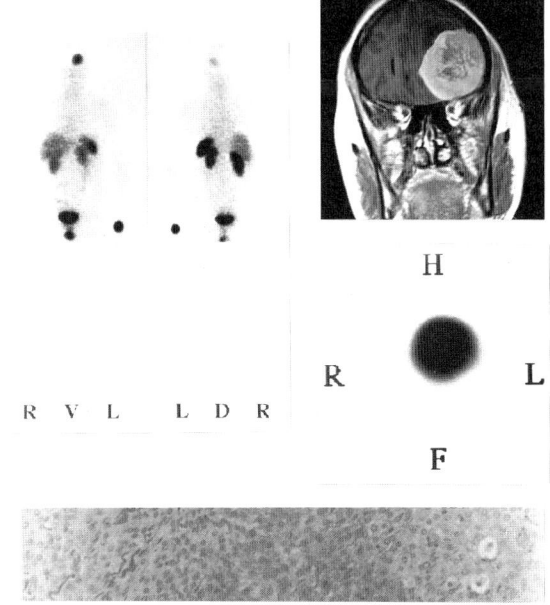

Figure 4 Example of a true positive patient (f/51). Planar somatostatin receptor scintigraphy 4 h post injection in anterior and posterior projection, coronal Gd-DTPA enhanced T1-weighted MRI slice, corresponding coronal SPECT slice, and histology of meningotheliomatous meningeoma (EvG, magnification: 50 times). There are cystic necrotic areas inside the meningeoma, complete compression of frontal horn of the left lateral ventricle, and displacement of midline structures to the right side

Table 4 Results of somatostatin receptor scintigraphy (SRS+/SRS-) with respect to histological evaluation (men+/-) according to different tumour volume

	All patients		< 10 ml		> 10 ml	
	SRS+	SRS–	SRS+	SRS–	SRS+	SRS–
Men+	36	7	13	7	23	0
Men–	4	12	0	2	4	10

Table 5 Stratification of somatostatin receptor scintigraphy according to different tumour volume

Volume	N	Sensitivity	Specificity	PPV	NPV
All	59	83.7%	75.0%	90.0%	63.2%
< 10 ml	32	65.0%	100.0%	100.0%	22.2 %
> 10 ml	27	100.0%	71.4%	85.2%	100.0%

SPECT slice, planar SRS in anterior and posterior projection, and histology are shown in Figure 3.

In 13 patients with a tumour volume of <10 ml and in 23 patients with a tumour volume of >10 ml, true positive somatostatin receptor scintigrams could be shown in planar images (cf. Table 1-3). Both an increasing T/B-ratio and an increasing uptake of ^{111}In-octreotide were observed. This is shown in Figures 1 and 2 (filled squares). In 5 out of these 36 patients, localisation could be clarified by SPECT images only as compared with planar SRS. In another 5 of these 36 patients significant information could be added by somatostatin receptor imaging as compared with MRI. One of these patients is shown in Figure 4, in which MRI does not yield sufficient information on whether meningeoma or neurinoma is the underlying process. However, SRS clearly demonstrates marked tracer uptake in planar projections as well as in transverse SPECT slices. Meningotheliomatous meningeoma was proven histologically.

A lack of somatostatin receptors could be demonstrated correctly negative in 12 patients. The corresponding lack of an increase of T/B ratio and uptake is shown in Figures 1 and 2 (filled circles), respectively. Tumour volume was >10 ml in 10 patients. Significant clinical information could be added in 4 of these patients by SRS. One of them showed a mass located at the right cerebello pontine angle with criteria of both neurinoma and meningeoma in MRI (Figure 5) and thus, MRI was not decisive. However, SRS clearly demonstrated a lack of somatostatin receptors in the right cerebello pontine angle, and histological examination confirmed the presence of a neurinoma.

In 7 patients with histologically proven meningeoma, SRS yielded false negative results. Consequently, T/B ratio and uptake values did not increase with time as shown in Figures 1 and 2 (open circles). While there was neither correlation with location nor with histological type of the meningeoma, tumour volume was <10 ml in all patients (cf. Table 2). One of these patients is shown in Figure 6. The sagittal T1-weighted Gd-DTPA enhanced MRI slice demonstrates a tumour mass in the right neck that was proven to be a malignant meningeoma. However, somatostatin receptors could not be demonstrated on planar images or in SPECT images.

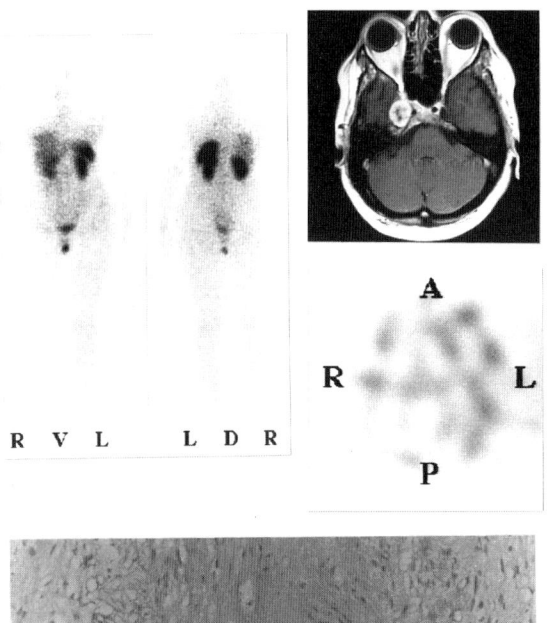

Figure 5 Example of a true negative patient (f/46). Planar somatostatin receptor scintigraphy 4 h post injection in anterior and posterior projection, transverse Gd-DTPA enhanced T1-weighted MRI slice, corresponding transverse SPECT slice, and histology of neurinoma (EvG, magnification: 50 times) located at the right cerebello pontine angle. The tumour that is clearly visible by MRI is not detectable on SRS, thus demonstrating a lack of somatostatin receptors

Discussion

While meningeoma and neurinoma are tumours that have similar sites, e.g. cerebello pontine angle or spine, surgical treatment may require different strategies due

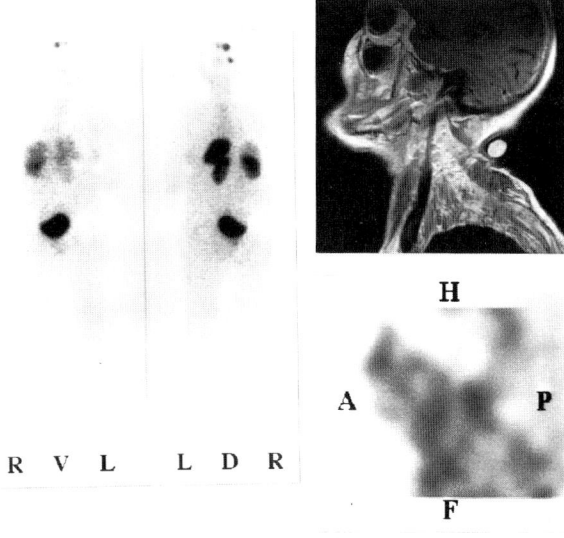

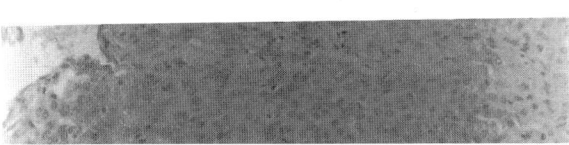

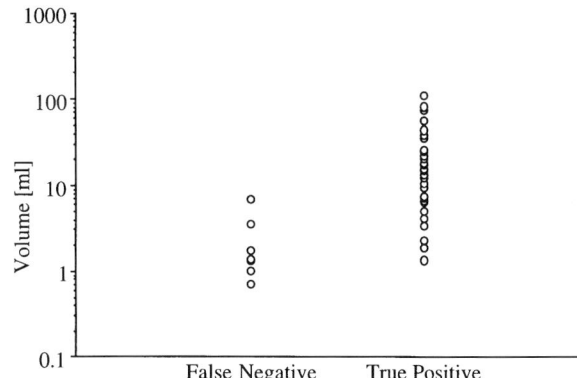

Figure 7 Tumour volume of patients with false negative and true positive somatostatin receptor scintigraphy. All patients with false negative somatostatin receptor scintigraphy have tumour volumes of <10 ml

Figure 6 Example of a false negative patient (f/69). Planar somatostatin receptor scintigraphy 4 h post injection in anterior and posterior projection, sagittal Gd-DTPA enhanced T1-weighted MRI slice, corresponding sagittal SPECT slice, and histology of malignant meningeoma (EvG, magnification: 50 times). The metastasis in the nuchal area is clearly visible by MRI but not detectable on SRS. However, four further localizations can be visualized on planar SRS in anterior and posterior projection (corresponding MRI and SPECT slices not shown)

to their different biological behaviour. Therefore, preoperative discrimination is required by the neurosurgeon. Usually, meningeoma and neurinoma can be discriminated sucessfully by MRI[38-40], but not in all patients.

Somatostatin receptors are expressed by meningeoma in near 100% both in cell cultures[3,6-9] and *in vivo* by scintigraphic imaging using ^{111}In-octreotide[27-36]. On the other hand, it is known from autoradiographic studies[9,41] that neurinoma do not express somatostatin receptors on their surface. Consequently, our three cases with neurinoma exhibited true negative somatostatin receptor scintigrams in accordance with the literature[31-33]. Functional imaging using ^{111}In-octreotide was suggested to clearly discriminate meningeoma and neurinoma[29,31,33,35]. This was shown successfully in 4 patients suffering from both multiple meningeoma and neurinoma on the basis of neurofibromatosis[33].

In conflict with the literature[3,6-9] we found false negative SRS in 7 patients with histologically proven meningeoma. Neither histological type nor localisation of the meningeoma correlated with their negative tracer uptake (cf. Table 1). Therefore, exclusion of meningeoma by a negative somatostatin receptor scintigram is no longer permitted. However, this undesired result might have a positive outcome: in a larger series of patients, varying expression of somatostatin receptors should be tested for any differences in biological behaviour.

In contrast to histology and localisation, tumour volume was associated with tracer uptake. While all meningeoma of more than 10 ml in volume could be imaged positively, SRS was positive in meningeoma below 10 ml in 65% only (Figure 7). Thus, the known sensitivity of near 100%[27-36] needs to be qualified with respect to tumour size. Our data are consistent with the literature[27-36] for large meningeoma.

False positive SRS was observed in four patients with various diseases. Their final diagnosis could be established by MRI alone (Table 1): two pituitary adenoma, an inflammatory process of the petrous bone and a jugular glomus tumour. Tracer uptake in these tumours is known to be variable[16,20,35]. Accordingly, for these patients there is no need for SRS.

The clinical benefit of SRS in preoperative work-up of patients with suspected meningeoma has to be defined carefully. MRI is mandatory during clinical work-up. In most tumours final diagnosis can be established by MRI alone. This holds for 39 out of 48 patients in our study. However, in some cases MRI alone is not decisive and yields two possible differential diagnoses. When these two tumours under consideration have a different expression of somatostatin receptors, they can be discriminated by functional imaging using SRS. In our study this holds for 9/48 patients. In five out of these SRS could correctly diagnose meningeoma. In 4 patients with large tumours, a lack of somatostatin receptors enabled exclusion of meningeoma. Histologically, neurinoma and ependymoma were found, which both fail to express somatostatin receptors on their surface[3,6-9,27,31,33,41]. In our study all patients who benefitted from SRS had a tumour size of >10 ml. This equals a diameter of 2.7 cm assuming a rotational ellipsoid.

It is conceivable that in a larger series, patients with lower tumour volumes may benefit as well. With preselection by MRI, as mentioned above, positive SRS will confirm meningeoma independent of tumour size. With small tumours, negative SRS will carry no clinically useful information.

The main clinical result of this study is based on the lack of somatostatin receptors in neurinoma. It remains to be seen whether this holds true for chordoma and ganglion Gasseri tumours as well. These tumours are located at the skull base and are difficult to diagnose by MRI alone. Furthermore, scar tissue should be easily distinguished from meningeoma by SRS. This was observed in a single patient in which MRI could not discriminate between recurrent meningeoma and scar tissue. Tracer uptake in SRS correctly identified tumour recurrency and, thus, assisted in clinical decision-making.

Conclusions

Functional imaging by somatostatin receptor scintigraphy has a significant impact in the differential diagnosis of patients with suspected meningeoma. Large meningeoma can be excluded by scintigraphy alone, while meningeoma of any size may be confirmed in combination with specific MRI results only.

Acknowledgement

We thank C. Bahr, A. Bauer, R. Bradtke, C. Fock, I. Hamann, D. Hundt, W. Latendorf, G. Mester, S. Ossowski, M. Reymann and E. Schmidt for technical assistance.

References

1 Bakker, W.H., Albert, R., Bruns, C. et al. [^{111}In-DTPA-D-Phe[1]]-octreotide, a potential radiopharmaceutical for imaging of somatostatin receptor-positive tumors: synthesis, radiolabeling and in vitro validation. *Life Sci.* 1991, 49, 1583

2 Bakker, W.H., Krenning, E.P., Reubi, J.C. et al. In vivo application of [^{111}In-DTPA-D-Phe[1]]-octreotide for detection of somatostatin receptor-positive tumors in rats. *Life Sci.*1991, 49, 1593

3 Koper, J.W., Markstein, R., Kohler, C. et al. Somatostatin inhibits the activity of adenylate cyclase in cultured human meningioma cells and stimulates their growth. *J. Clin. Endocr. Metab.* 1992, 74, 543

4 Lamberts, S.W.J., Hofland, L.J., van Koetsveld, P.M. et al. Parallel in vivo and in vitro detection of functional somatostatin receptors in human endocrine pancreatic tumors: consequences with regard to diagnosis, localization, and therapy. *J. Clin. Endocr. Metab.* 1990, 72, 566

5 O´Byrne, K.J., Halmos, G., Pinski, J. et al. Somatostatin receptor expression in lung cancer. *Eur. J. Cancer* 1994, 30A, 1682

6 Reubi, J.C., Krenning, E.P., Lamberts, S.W.J. and Kvols, L. In vitro detection of somatostatin receptors in human tumors. *Digestion* 1993, 54, 76

7 Reubi, J.C., Kvols, L., Krenning, E.P. and Lamberts, S.W.J. In vitro and in vivo detection of somatostatin receptors in human malignant tissue. *Acta Oncol.* 1991, 30, 463

8 Reubi, J.C., Laissue, J., Krenning, E.P. and Lamberts, S.W.J. Somatostatin receptors in human cancer: incidence, characteristics, functional correlates and clinical implications. *J. Steroid. Biochim. Molec. Biol.* 1992, 43, 27

9 Reubi, J.C., Maurer, R., Klijn, J.G.M. et al. High incidence of somatostatin receptors in human meningiomas: biochemical characterization. *J. Clin. Endocrinol. Metab.* 1986, 63, 433

10 Reubi, J.C., Waser, B., Sheppard, M. and Macaulay, V. Somatostatin receptors are present in small-cell but not in non-small cell primary lung carcinomas: relationship to EGF-receptors. *Int. J. Cancer* 1990, 45, 269

11 Reubi, J.C., Waser, B., van Hagen, M. et al. In vitro and in vivo detection of somatostatin receptors in human malignant lymphomas. *Int. J. Cancer* 1992, 50, 895

12 Taylor, J.E., Coy, D.H. and Moreau, J.P. High affinity binding of [^{125}I-Tyr[11]]somatostatin-14 to human small cell lung carcinoma (NCI-H69). *Life Sci.* 1988, 43, 421

13 Krenning, E.P., Breemann, W.A.P., Kooij, P.P.M. et al. Localisation of endocrine-related tumors with radioiodinated analogue of somatostatin. *Lancet* 1989, 333, 242

14 Krenning, E.P., Kwekkeboom, D.J., Oie, H.Y. et al. Somatostatin receptor imaging of endocrine gastrointestinal tumors. *Schweiz. Med. Wschr.* 1992, 122, 634

15 Krenning, E.P., Kwekkeboom, D.J., Reubi, J.C. et al. ^{111}In-octreotide scintigraphy in oncology. *Metabolism* 1992, 9, 83

16 Krenning, E.P., Kwekkeboom, D.J., Bakker, W.H. *et al.* Somatostatin receptor scintigraphy with [^{111}In-DTPA-D-Phe^1]- and [^{123}Tyr^3]-octreotide: the Rotterdam experience with more than 1000 patients. *Eur. J. Nucl. Med.* 1993, 20, 716

17 Kwekkeboom, D.J., Krenning, E.P., Bakker, W.H. *et al.* Radioiodinated somatostatin analog scintigraphy in small-cell lung cancer. *J. Nucl. Med.* 1991, 32, 1845

18 Lamberts, S.W.J., Bakker, W.H., Reubi, J.C. and Krenning, E.P. Somatostatin-receptor imaging in the localization of endocrine tumors. *New Eng. J. Med.* 1990, 323, 1246

19 Lamberts, S.W.J., Krenning, E.P. and Reubi, J.C. The role of somatostatin and its analogs in the diagnosis and treatment of tumors. *Endocrine Reviews* 1991, 12, 450

20 von Werder, K. and Faglia, G. Potential indications for octreotide in endocrinology. *Metabolism* 1992, 9, 91

21 Kwekkeboom, D.J., Siang Kho, G., Lamberts, S.W.J. *et al.* The value of octreotide scintigraphy in patients with lung cancer. *Eur. J. Nucl. Med.* 1994, 21, 1106

22 Macaulay, V.M., Smith, I.E., Everard, M.J. *et al.* Experimental and clinical studies with somatostatin analogue octreotide in small cell lung cancer. *Br. J. Cancer* 1994, 69, 451

23 Maini, C.L., Tofani, A., Venturo, I. *et al.* Somatostatin receptor imaging in small cell lung cancer using *111*In-DTPA-octreotide: a preliminary study. *Nucl. Med. Commun.* 1993, 14, 962

24 Bohuslavizki, K.H., Oberwöhrmann, S., Brenner, W. *et al.* ^{111}In-octreotide imaging in patients with long-acting Graves´ ophthalmopathy. *Nucl. Med. Commun.* 1995, in press

25 Kahaly, G., Diaz, M., Beyer, J. and Bockisch, A. Indium-111-pentetreotide scintigraphy in Graves´ ophthalmopathy. *J. Nucl. Med.* 1995, 36, 550

26 Postema, P.T., Krenning, E.P., Wijngaarde, R. *et al.* [^{123}In-DTPA-D-Phe^1]-octreotide scintigraphy in thyroidal and orbital Graves´ disease: a parameter for disease activity? *J. Clin. Endocrinol. Metab.*1994, 79, 1845

27 Haldemann, A.R., Rösler, H., Barth, A. *et al.* Somatostatin receptor scintigraphy in central nervous system tumors: role of blood-brain barrier permeability. *J. Nucl. Med.* 1995, 36, 403

28 Hildebrandt, G., Scheidhauer, K., Luyken, C. *et al.* High sensitivity of the in vivo detection of somatostatin receptors by ^{111}Indium-[DTPA-octreotide]-scintigraphy in meningeoma patients. *Acta Neurochir. Wien.* 1994, 126, 63

29 Jochens, R., Cordes, M., Wolters, A. *et al.* Untersuchungen von Hirntumoren und Hirnmetastasen mit [^{111}In-DTPA-D-Phe^1]-Octreotide-SPECT. *Klin. Neurorad.* 1995, 5, 1

30 Lee, J.D., Kim, D.I., Lee, J.T. *et al.* Indium-111-pentetreotide imaging in intra-axial brain tumors: comparison with Thallium-201 SPECT and MRI. *J. Nucl. Med.* 1995, 36, 537

31 Luyken, C., Hildebrandt, G., Scheidhauer, K. and Krisch, B. Diagnostic value of somatostatin-receptor-scintigraphy in patients with intracranial tumours. *Nuklearmediziner* 1993, 16, 317

32 Luyken, C., Scheidhauer, K., Schomäcker, K. *et al.* Erste Erfahrungen mit der Somatostatin-Rezeptor-Szintigraphie bei 71 Patienten mit intracraniellen Tumoren [abstract]. *Nucl. Med.* 1993, 32, A21

33 Maini, C.L., Cioffi, R.P., Tofani, A. *et al.* ^{111}In-octreotide scintigraphy in neurofibromatosis. *Eur. J. Nucl. Med.* 1995, 22, 201

34 Maini, C.L., Tofani, A., Sciuto, R. *et al.* Scintigraphy visualization of somatostatin receptors in human meningiomas using 111-indium-DTPA-D-Phe-1-octreotide. *Nucl. Med. Commun.* 1993, 14, 505

35 Scheidhauer, K., Hildebrand, G., Luyken, C. *et al.* Somatostatin receptor scintigraphy in brain tumors and pituitary tumors: first experiences. *Horm. Metab. Res.* 1993, 27, 59

36 Scheidhauer, K., Hildebrandt, G., Luyken, C. *et al.* Receptor imaging using ^{111}In-pentetreotide in pituitary tumors and meningeomas [abstract]. *Eur. J. Nucl. Med.* 1992, 19, 735

37 Sachs, L. in 'Applied statistics. A handbook of techniques', Springer, Berlin, 1984

38 Bydder, G.M., Kingsley, P.E., Brown, J. *et al.* MR imaging of meningeomas including studies with and without gadolinium-DTPA. *J. Comput. Assist. Tomogr.* 1985, 9, 690

39 Huk, W.J., Gademann, G. and Friedmann, G. in 'Magnetic resonance imaging of central nervous system disease', Springer, 1990

40 McConachie, N.S., Worthington, B.S., Cornford, E.J. *et al.* Review article: Computed tomography and magnetic resonance in the diagnosis of intraventricular cerebral masses. *Br. J. Rad.* 1994, 67, 223

41 Reubi, J.C., Lang, W., Maurer, R. *et al.* Distribution and biochemical characterization of somatostatin receptors in tumors of the human central nervous system. *Cancer Res.* 1987, 47, 575

SPECT in Neurology and Psychiatry, edited by P.P. De Deyn, R.A. Dierckx, A. Alavi and B.A. Pickut

Sestamibi Kinetic Parameters in Recurrent Brain Tumours Estimated by Dynamic SPECT Scanning and Two-Compartmental Modelling

Chapter
48

S. Raja

Introduction

[99m]Tc sestamibi (MIBI), the widely used myocardial perfusion agent, has been reported to be taken up by various malignant tumours. Hassen *et al.*[1] initially demonstrated its utility in differentiating malignant from benign lung lesions[2]. Subsequently, enhanced accumulation of MIBI was seen in osteosarcoma[3]. Using MIBI and ^{201}Tl, comparable sensitivity and specificity for detection of primary brain tumours in children[4] and recurrent brain tumours in adults[5] has been demonstrated by semiquantitative (tumour to normal brain ratios) analysis.

Abdel Dayem *et al.*[6] postulated that delayed ^{201}Tl imaging at 2-3 h compared with early imaging at 30 min may help in differentiating neovascular/granulating tissue from recurrent tumour in patients treated with radiotherapy/chemotherapy. This has been attributed to the fact that ^{201}Tl washes out more rapidly from vascular/granulating tissue relative to tumour. We postulated that the kinetic behaviour of MIBI may be similar to ^{201}Tl in differentiating recurrent brain tumours from radiation necrosis. We evaluated the utility of obtaining MIBI kinetic parameters, by dynamic SPECT brain scanning and two compartment modelling in patients with suspected recurrent brain tumours (TU).

Methods

Thirteen consecutive patients with suspected recurrent brain TU (11 glioblastoma multiforme (GBM) and 2 pituitary PITTU) underwent sequential SPECT scanning (framing rate 10 s x 12, 30 s x 6, 60 s x 5, 300 s x 5; for a total of 28 frames in 35 min) on a 3-headed gamma camera (Trionix), after 20 mCi of ^{99m}Tc sestamibi i.v. (Figure 1). The projection data were acquired on a 64 x 64 matrix in a continuous acquisition mode. The sequential SPECT projection data were reconstructed by routine backprojection algorithms, using Butterworth filter-cut off = 0.5 and roll off = 5.

Time activity profiles were obtained by flagging 6 x 6 pixel ROIs over the following areas: suspected tumours, contralateral normal brain, choroid plexus, pituitary (normal/tumour), cranial vault/scalp contralateral to the tumour. The kinetic parameters k1, k2 and V were obtained by supplying the sagittal sinus time activity curve along with its intergral and the tissue (tumour) activity profile as independent variables in a multiple linear regression fitting of the tissue activity.

Five of the GMB showed focal enhanced accumulation of sestamibi and FDG. Further analysis was made on these 5 patients and 2 with PITTU.

Department of Nuclear Medicine,
The Cleveland Clinic Foundation,
9500 Euclid Avenue, Cleveland,
Ohio 44195, USA

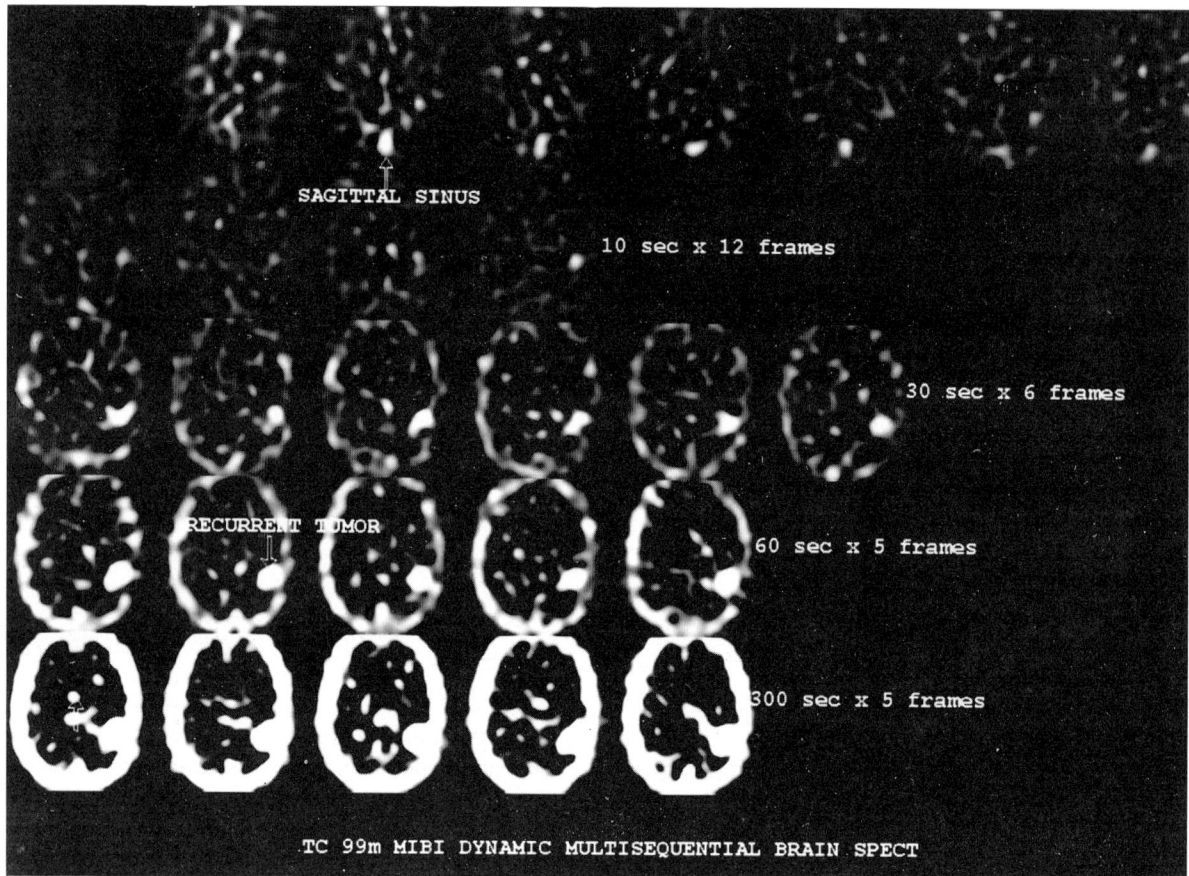

Figure 1 Middle aged woman with history of status post resection left parietal glioblastoma multiforme. Follow-up MRI scan showed enlarging and contrast enhancing lesion in the left parietal region. [18]F FDG PET scan demonstrated intense focal uptake, concordant with MRI abnormality. [99m]Tc MIBI scan also demonstrated enhanced uptake concordant to the FDG PET scan. The estimated kinetic parameters of the tumour were: k1 = 0.026 min^{-1}; k2 = 0.010 min^{-1}; V = 0.175 ml

Results

Of the 13 patients, 5 showed enhanced accumulation of FDG, corresponding to the contrast enhancement of MRI. Further compartmental analyses were obtained for these 5 patients.

The kinetic parameters obtained in one patient with positive biopsy for pituitary tumour had high k1, and low k2 (0.533 and 0.015, respectively), and decreased V (0.011). However, in the second patient with complete removal of pituitary tumour, the k1 (0.764), and k2 (0.206) and V (0.88) were relatively high.

	k1 min^{-1}		k2 min^{-1}		V ml	
	mean	std	mean	std	mean	std
TU	0.223	0.181	0.077	0.117	0.052	0.025
PIT	0.323	0.074	0.015	0.005	0.493	0.093
CP	0.232	0.067	0.024	0.028	0.14	0.048
NB	0.051	0.053	0.193	0.143	0.101	0.070
BM	0.126	0.080	0.028	0.017	0.106	0.067

Discussion

Early diagnosis and differentiation of recurrent brain tumours may have important therapeutic and prognostic implications. Although contrast enhancement on follow-up CT/MRI suggests tumour recurrence, it is non-specific. Contrast enhancement does not reliably distinguish recurrent tumour from tumour necrosis and radiation fibrosis. Metabolic imaging with fluorodeoxyglucose and positron emission tomography has been shown to be accurate for the evaluation of suspected recurrent brain tumours[6]; however, it is expensive and limited in its availability.

The mechanism of MIBI uptake in tumours, along with the optimal physical properties of ^{99m}Tc for imaging, has led to the use of ^{99m}Tc MIBI in brain tumours[7,8]. Utilising tumour versus contralateral normal brain ratios, in 23 patients, with progressive symptoms and contrast enhanced lesions on MRI, Macapinlac[9] demonstrated that a ratio of 1.5 or greater was sensitive enough to differentiate recurrent tumour from radiation necrosis. However, in two patients with lesions adjacent to the choroid plexus, the tumour uptake could not be separated from normal choroid plexus astrocytoma, the MIBI SPECT was falsely negative.

It has been suggested that semiquantitative analysis such as tumour to non-tumour, tumour to calvarium, and tumour to cardiac ratios of ^{201}Tl is superior to visual analysis[6] in the detection of primary and recurrent brain tumours[10]. Abdel-Dayem et al.[5] suggest that ratio analysis along with early and delayed tumour imaging may be more helpful. As neoplastic tissues demonstrate high uptake with prolonged retention as opposed to poor uptake and rapid washout in vascular/granulating tissue, we postulated that the estimation of MIBI kinetic parameters (washin, washout and vascular distribution volumes) may help in differentiating viable tumour from normal and/or necrotic tissue. We have attempted to obtain the kinetic parameters non-invasively, without arterial sampling for the input function. As shown by Hubner et al.[11] with ^{11}C ACBC PET scanning of brain tumours, the input function obtained by sampling the sagittal sinus may suffice in case of tracers not actively taken up by normal brain.

Our study demonstrates the feasibility of imaging MIBI kinetic parameters by dynamic SPECT scanning and two compartment modelling. Estimation of kinetic parameters allows differentiation of abnormal from normal tissue. For example, separation of tumour from choroid plexus activity is possible using V, the vascular distribution volume - 0.052 versus 0.14 and k2 - 0.077 min^{-1} versus 0.024 min^{-1}, even though k1 was not

significantly different, 0.223 versus 0.232 respectively. Normal brain had relatively slow washin (k1=0.051) and the highest washout rate (k2=0.193) compared with tumour, which had fast washin and slow washout. The pituitary gland demonstrated the highest washin with poor washout rates along with high vascular volume. Calvarial activity (bone marrow + scalp) had kinetic parameter values between normal brain and tumour.

The kinetic parameters in one patient with positive biopsy for recurrent pituitary tumour had rapid washin with slow washout and decreased vascular volume, suggesting a solid but relatively avascular tumour. The second patient, in whom the tumour had been completely removed, had rapid washin and washout with very high vascular volume, suggesting vascular/granulating tissue.

Conclusion

This pilot study demonstrates the feasibility of imaging sestamibi kinetic behaviour, and its ability to differentiate tumours from normal and abnormal intracranial tissues. Further studies are necessary to define more precisely the kinetic parameters in normal and neoplastic tissues. We believe this technique may be useful in differentiating: benign from malignant tissue; recurrent tumour from necrosis; response to therapy and multi drug resistence.

References

1   Hassen, I.M., Schwell, A., Constantinindes, C. et al. Uptake and kinetics of Tc-99m-haxakis 2-methoxyisobutyl isonitrile in benign and malignant lesions in the lungs. Clin. Nucl. Med. 1984, 14, 333

2   Muller, S.P., Reiners, C., Pass, M. et al. Tc-99m MIBI and Tl-201 uptake in bronchial carcinoma. J. Nucl. Med. 1989, 30, 845

3   Caner, B., Kitapci, M. and Aras, T. Increased accummulation of haxakis (2-methoxyisobutyl isontrile) technetium (I) in osteosarcoma and its metastatic lymph nodes. J. Nucl. Med. 1991, 32, 10

4   Lorcan, A., O'Tuama, L.A., Treves, S.T. et al. Thallium-201 versus technetium 99m MIBI SPECT in evaluation of childhood brain tumours; a within subject comparison. J. Nucl. Med. 1993, 34, 1045

5   Abdel-Dayem, H.M., Scott, A.M. and Macapinlac, H.A. Role of TI-201 chloride and Tc-99m Sestamibi in tumour imaging. Nucl. Med. Ann. 1989, 181, 234

6   Coleman, R.E., Hoffman, J.M., Janson, M.W. et al. Clinical Applications of PET for the evaluation of brain tumours. J. Nucl. Med. 1991, 32, 616

Trauma Capitis

SPECT in Neurology and Psychiatry, edited by P.P. De Deyn, R.A. Dierckx, A. Alavi and B.A. Pickut
© 1997 John Libbey & Company Ltd, pp. 409–414

Neuroimaging in Patients with Head Trauma

Chapter
49

A.B. Newberg and A. Alavi

Introduction

Head trauma is a neurological disorder that affects as many as several hundred thousand individuals every year. It has been estimated that seventy-five thousand brain injuries each year result in long-term disability in the US[1]. Motor vehicle accidents cause a large proportion of these head injuries, particularly in the young male population. However, people of all ages can suffer from various forms of head trauma. Thus, the overall incidence of traumatic brain injury is similar to the incidence of stroke. Mortality associated with head injury is the highest during the first 48 h post-trauma[2]. Since appropriate medical and neurological evaluation of these patients plays an important role in initiating the required therapies and determining prognosis, various neuroimaging methods have been employed to determine the extent and nature of brain injuries. The neuroimaging techniques most widely used include X-ray computed tomography (CT), magnetic resonance imaging (MRI), positron emission tomography (PET), and single photon emission computed tomography (SPECT).

X-ray (CT) and MRI

The development of modern tomographic anatomical imaging has led to a major impact on the diagnosis and management of head trauma. MRI is more sensitive and accurate in diagnosing cerebral pathology[3,4], but CT is considered the first-line imaging technique for the management of head injured patients in the acute setting[5,6]. One study[7] indicated that CT is the procedure of choice for moderate to high risk head injury patients. Low risk patients can be observed without performing imaging studies at all. CT is superior to MRI in detecting bone fractures of the skull as well as for detecting subarachnoid haemorrhage[7,8]. CT is an excellent imaging technique for distinguishing parenchymal haemorrhage from oedema. Another reason for the success of CT in acute head trauma is that it is more available and more cost effective than MRI, and CT scans can be completed in a short period of time. A retrospective study by Reinus *et al.*[9] indicated that patients with evidence of alcohol intoxication, a history of amnesia, or focal neurological deficits would benefit most from CT evaluation.

CT also has several limitations as an imaging technique. CT often underestimates non-haemorrhagic parenchymal injury and the extent of the lesions detected by CT does not correlate well with the neurolgical deficit, the level of consciousness, or the clinical prognosis. Levin *et al.*[4] showed no correlation between the degree of parenchymal lesions seen by CT and the initial

Division of Nuclear Medicine,
117 Donner Building, H.U.P.,
3400 Spruce Street, Philadelphia,
PA 19104, USA

Glasgow Coma Scale (GCS) score while there was a significant correlation between the size of extra-parenchymal lesions and the GCS score. Similarly, Ruff et al.[10] found no correlation between CT scan abnormalities and neuro-psychological test results.

MRI has been found to be superior to CT at 48 to 72 h after trauma. Even in minor head trauma, one study[11] reported that 10% of patients had lesions on MRI. Yealy et al.[7] suggested that MRI is indicated after CT is obtained if subtle acute non-haemorrhagic and subacute haemorrhagic lesions are suspected. MRI is also very sensitive for detecting intracranial lesions[3-6,12-16]. Ogawa et al.[3] found that MRI was significantly more sensitive in detecting intraaxial lesions in patients with acute or chronic head injury compared with CT images. However, no study had determined the clinical significance of the large number of lesions found on MRI in head trauma patients as many of the lesions do not have corresponding clinical deficits.

One study showed that MRI could characterise lesions as diffuse axonal injury (DAI), cortical contusion, subcortical grey-matter injury, and brain stem injury. DAI refers to the shearing injury of white matter and appears pathologically as small haemorrhages in the corpus callosum and dorsolateral brain stem in addition to diffuse damage to the axons[17]. MRI also has advantages in distinguishing haemorrhagic contusion from surrounding oedema, for detecting subdural haematomas, and detecting shearing injuries that are seen as zones of high intensive oedema on T_2 weighted images. CT is not often able to detect such lesions due to volume averaging effects and interference from bony structures[14]. It is hoped that further studies will demonstrate that MRI can determine the prognosis of patients with head trauma better than CT, since the latter has been shown to be a poor predictor of clinical outcome[18]. Preliminary studies have not found a relationship between MRI results and neuro-psychological testing[10].

One study examined the role of gadolinium enhanced MRI in evaluating patients with head trauma[19]. The results indicated that gadolinium enhanced MRI was no better than non-enhanced techniques in detecting lesions resulting from head injury. The use of magnetic resonance angiography (MRA) may be valuable for detecting vascular abnormalities[6] such as arterial occlusions, arteriovenous fistulae, dissecting aneurysms and venous sinus thrombosis in patients with head trauma. Functional MRI may also play a role in investigating deficits in various structures by measuring changes in cerebral activity during activation tasks. Thus, functional MRI may be useful in evaluating rehabilitation potential in head injury

patients[20-22]. Nuclear magnetic resonance spectroscopy (MRS) has been shown to reveal certain metabolic abnormalities during the acute phases of head trauma[23,24]. It has been suggested that MRS may be a helpful adjunct to MRI in the diagnosis of patients with head trauma[23].

Positron Emission Tomography (PET)

A limited number of studies using PET for the evaluation of patients with head trauma have been reported. By now, it is well documented that PET cannot distinguish between functional abnormalities related to structural damage and those without such findings[25]. Thus, it is essential that one compares PET images with the corresponding anatomical images obtained by MRI or CT. In general, cerebral dysfunction can extend far beyond the boundary of anatomical lesions[25,26] and may even appear in remote locations from the trauma. Alavi et al.[27] showed that approximately 33% of anatomical lesions were associated with larger and more widespread metabolic abnormalities. Also, as much as 42% of PET abnormalities were not associated with any anatomical lesions. One other finding was that patients suffering from severe axonal injury were found to have significantly reduced glucose metabolism in the occipital and visual cortices as compared with the rest of the brain. This reduction was transient in most patients and the cause for this hypometabolism is not known[27,28].

Cortical contusions, intracranial haematoma, and resultant encephalomalacia have metabolic effects that are confined primarily to the site of the injury as determined by PET imaging. However, subdural and epidural haematomas often cause widespread hypometabolism and may even affect the contralateral hemisphere[29]. Another entity, diffuse axonal injury, has been found to cause diffuse cortical hypometabolism, and there is a marked decrease in metabolism in the parieto-occipital cortex[27]. This is particularly true in the visual cortex of patients with DAI when compared with normal subjects and patients with other types of head injuries. The cause of this visual cortex hypometabolism is unknown. However, it is believed that it may be caused by the disruption of callosal input to the visual cortex or by disruption of the primary visual inupt as the result of shearing axonal injuries of the optic and geniculo-calcarine tracts[27].

Crossed cerebellar diaschisis, as well as ipsilateral cerebellar hypometabolism, has been reported in head injury patients with supratentorial lesions[30]. The association of suptratentorial lesions with the presence and laterality of cerebellar hypometabolism was determined for both diffuse and focal lesions.

Forty-five per cent of diffuse lesions observed in the head trauma patients were associated with right sided cerebellar hypometabolism, while only 9% were associated with the left sided cerebellar hypometabolism. Forty-six per cent of focal unilateral lesions were associated with contralateral cerebellar hypometabolism. This was significantly greater than the 24% of the focal unilateral lesions associated with ipsilateral cerebellar hypometabolism. Similar results were found when comparing other types of head injury such as cortical contusions, hemispheric penetration injuries, intracerebral haematomas, basal ganglia haemorrhages, and extraparenchymal lesions. Interestingly, the most pronounced difference for all categories of focal lesions was noted for those lesions ranked by a neurosurgeon as the patient's most severe injury.

Of patients with focal injuries alone, virtually all had contralateral and none had ipsilateral cerebellar hypometabolism to the most severe lesion. Interestingly, patients with both focal and diffuse injuries did not show any predilection for the laterality of cerebellar hypometabolism. The results obtained from patients with serial PET scans showed that the cerebellar hypometabolism is not consistent with time. This may be due either to the reversibility of cerebellar diaschisis resulting from acute brain injury or it may be related to the competing effects of multiple lesions in the same patient.

Alavi et al.[27] found a good correlation between the severity of head trauma as measured by the Glasgow Coma Scale (GCS) and the extent of the whole brain hypometabolism as measured by FDG-PET (the GCS scores range from 1 to 15 with 15 representing normal consciousness and 1 being totally unresponsive). No significant differences in cerebral metabolism were observed in head trauma patients with a GCS of 14 or 15, compared with normal controls. Head trauma patients with GCS scores of 13 or lower did have significantly decreased cortical metabolism compared with controls. Thus, cerebral metabolism is believed to be a good indicator of functional activity in patients with head trauma. Other studies have shown that the hypometabolism shown in PET images correlates with neuropsychological and language testing. Thus, PET imaging may have important implications for the rehabilitation potential of head injury patients[31,32]. Further, global and regional metabolic rates have been found to improve as patients recover from head trauma[26,29].

Several studies have attempted to relate neuropsychological tests to lesions found on PET images. Ruff et al.[10] presented a study of six head trauma patients. Five of the six patients had decreased anterior frontal metablolism as measured by PET. The

authors further suggested that this hypometabolism correlated well with the generalised cognitive dysfunction and behavioural changes in these patients as measured by neuropsychological testing. Unfortunately, there were not enough subjects to use statistical analysis in determining the correlation between PET imaging and neuropsychological testing. Furthermore, with the use of quantitative PET, more accurate correlations might be found.

SPECT

SPECT studies have yielded results similar to those found with PET in head trauma patients. SPECT can detect abnormalities in cerebral blood flow indicating areas of dysfunction secondary to brain injury. It is well established that blood flow and metabolism are coupled in most diseased states. However, in acute states such as soon after a head injury or cerebrovascular accident, dissociation occurs between blood flow and metabolism. Therefore, the value of SPECT flow studies in the acute phase of head trauma is limited because of this uncoupling phenomena.

SPECT has been shown to be more sensitive than CT for detecting lesions in patients with head injury. Investigators have found a greater number of abnormalities that were also noted to be detected earlier on HMPAO SPECT scans compared with CT scans[33-36]. Gray et al.[37] found that 80% of head injury patients had cerebral blood flow deficits on SPECT of which only 55% were found to have abnormalities on CT scans. The lesions found on SPECT have generally been larger in size than those detected using CT. As indicated above, SPECT studies have found a higher number of defects when compared with CT images. However, Roper et al.[38] found that while 39% of lesions in head injury patients on SPECT were not seen with CT, 27% of lesions found on CT were not found on SPECT. The results from this study led the authors to the conclusion that some types of cerebral contusions are associated with decreased blood flow while others are not, SPECT studies have also shown that blood flow to injured areas was similar to that in the non-injured brain areas[38]. This may have resulted from luxury perfusion to these areas with the subsequent uncoupling of cerebral flow with the cerebral metabolism. Similar findings were reported by Fumeya et al.[39], who found that lesions detected with CT were found to range from hyperperfused to hypoperfused on SPECT. However, lesions not detected with CT were found to be only hypometabolic on SPECT.

SPECT has been reported to be better than CT in distinguishing lesions with a poor prognosis from those with a favourable prognosis. Patients with larger lesions, multiple defects and lesions involving the brain stem on SPECT images tend to have a poorer prognosis compared with patients with smaller, non-focal lesions[34,40]. Another study indicated that a negative initial SPECT scan after trauma is a good predictor for a favourable clinical outcome[41]. In a similar study, patients with the greatest disability were found to have the greatest number of lesions and the lowest cerebral blood flow as determined by SPECT[35]. Further, there was a strong correlation between the GCS and the global cerebral blood flow. Another study indicated that SPECT might be able to determine whether patients will develop symptoms such as post-traumatic headache[33].

Gray et al.[37] studied patients with a remote history of head trauma. They found that 80% of head injury patients had deficits of regional cerebral blood flow. By comparison only 55% of those same patients were found to have lesions on CT. This difference was similar for patients with both minor and severe head injuries. Patients with minor injuries were found to have deficits on SPECT in 60% of the cases, while CT detected lesions in only 25% of the cases. However, this report did not indicate that there was any correlation between clinical deficits utilising neuropsychiatric testing and regional cerebral blood flow.

Paediatric head injury

As in adult head injury, the initial diagnostic test in the paediatric patient with a head injury is X-ray CT. However, several studies have found that MRI may play a complimentary role in the evaluation of these patients[6,42,43]. Bernardi et al.[42] showed that MRI is better able to determine the extent and location of haemorrhagic and non-haemorrhagic lesions than CT. Levin et al.[43] showed that MR images can demonstrate a relationship between cognitive dysfunction secondary to head injury and the severity of that injury. Another group found that children with frontal lobe lesions were more frequently disabled than those who sustained diffuse injury[44]. Furthermore, the frontal lobe was found to be the most frequent site of injury. Yealy et al.[7] indicated that MRI might be useful in evaluating children who are suspected to be victims of child abuse, since they might suffer from small haemorrhagic and non-haemorrhagic lesions that might be undetectable with CT.

PET studies of paediatric brain trauma have revealed findings similar to those in adults. Worley et al.[45] showed that PET images taken within 12 weeks of the injury correlated well with outcome, while PET images after 12 weeks did not. While only a few patients were followed longitudinally, there was no correlation found between PET images and improvement in clinical symptoms.

Conclusion

As discussed above, neuroimaging is an important technique in the evaluation and management of head trauma. CT is considered the imaging modality of choice for the management of acute head injury since it provides rapid assessment of major brain injuries, is readily available in most medical institutions, and is of relatively little cost. Specifically, it provides information regarding intracranial bleeding and possibly mass effect, which may require immediate intervention. It is also the most useful technique for detecting skull fractures. However, CT does not have the resolution offered by MRI. Although MRI is more expensive, it is becoming widely available and can provide better sensitivity for detecting intracranial lesions and haemorrhage than that of CT. Despite the extensive use of these anatomical imaging techniques in the evaluation of patients with acute head trauma, at this time, it has yet to be determined whether the lesions seen on CT or MRI correlate well with cognitive dysfunction and overall prognosis. In fact, studies to date show that this poor correlation may be the major limitation of MRI and CT.

The functional imaging techniques with PET and SPECT provide several advantages over anatomical imaging. PET and SPECT can often reveal areas of hypometabolism or hypoperfusion that are not detectable by MRI or CT. PET and SPECT can also find more lesions than CT. However, it has not yet been shown that PET and SPECT can find more lesions than MRI, especially since MRI can detect very small lesions because of its high resolution. PET and SPECT do not have the resolution of MRI, but their ability to measure function may be a more important technique for evaluating head injury. PET and SPECT seem to correlate better with prognosis and cognitive dysfunction than either MRI or CT. This may have particular value in the long term management of head trauma patients. Currently, PET is not widely available for use in most medical centres and therefore is limited in its use for acute head trauma patients. SPECT is more available and less costly than PET, and thus is more practical than PET for the routine evaluation of head injury. SPECT is limited by its poorer resolution and difficulty in quantification compared with PET. Further, in order for SPECT to match the characteristics of PET significantly increases the cost.

In summary, CT is likely to be the main neuroimaging technique in the evaluation of the acute head trauma patient. However, for additional evaluation and information, as well as long term follow-up, MRI, PET, and SPECT each offer special facilities in the care of head trauma patients. As technologies improve and more studies are performed, there will be a need for a continued evaluation of the neuroimaging techniques and their use in head trauma.

References

1   Kraus, J.F. Epidemiology of brain injury, in 'Head Injury', (Ed. P.R. Cooper) Williams and Wilkins, Baltimore, USA, 1993, p.1

2   Langfitt, T.W. and Gennarelli, T.A. Can the outcome from head injury be improved? *Neurosurg.* 1982, 56, 19

3   Ogawa, T., Sekino, H., Uzura, M. *et al.* Comparative study of magnetic resonance and CT scan imaging in case of severe head injury. *Acta Neurochir. Suppl.* 1992, 55, 8

4   Levin, H.S., Williams, D.H., Eisenberg, H.M. *et al.* Serial MRI and neurobehavioural findings after mild to moderate closed head injury. *J. Neurol. Neurosurg. Psychiatry* 1992, 55, 255

5   Kelly, A.B., Zimmerman, R.D., Snow, R.B. *et al.* Head trauma. Comparison of MRI and CT-experience in 100 patients. *A.J.N.R.* 1988, 9, 699

6   Sklar, E.M., Quencer, R.M., Bowen, B.C. *et al.* Magnetic resonsance applications in cerebral injury. *Radiol. Clin. North America.* 1992, 30. 353

7   Yealy, D.M. and Hogan, D.E. Imaging after head trauma, who needs what? *Emerg. Med. Clin. N. Am.* 1991, 9, 707

8   Jennett, B. Diagnosis and management of head trauma. *J. Neurotrauma* 1991, 8, S15

9   Reinus, W.R., Wippold, F.J. and Erickson, K.K. Practical selection criteria for noncontrast cranial computed tomography in patients with head trauma. *Ann. Emerg. Med.* 1993, 22, 1148

10 Ruff, R.M., Buchsbaum, M.S., Troster, A.L. *et al.* Computerized tomography, neuropsychology, and positron emission tomography in the evaluation of head injury. *Neuropsych. Neuropsychol. Behav. Neurol.* 1989, 2, 103

11 Doezema, D., King, J.N., Tandberg, D. *et al.* Magnetic resonance imaging in minory head injury. *Ann. Emerg. Med.* 1991, 20, 1281

12 Levin, H.S., Amparo, E., Eisenberg, H.M. *et al.* Magnetic resonance imaging and computerized tomography in relation to the neurobehavioural sequelae of mild and moderate head injuries. *J. Neurosurg.* 1987, 66, 706

13 Gentry, L.R., Godersky, J.C., Thompson, B. *et al.* Prospective comparative study of intermediate-field MRI and CT in the evaluation of closed head trauma. *Am. J. Roentgenol.* 1988, 150, 673

14 Zimmerman, R.A., Bilaniuk, L.T., Hackney, D.B. *et al.* Head injury, early results comparing CT and high-field MR *Am. J. Roentgenol.* 1986, 147, 1215

15 Gentry, L.R., Godersky, J.C. and Thompson B. MR imaging of head trauma, review of the distribution and radiopathologic features of traumatic lesions. *Am. J. Roentgenol.* 1988, 150, 663

16 Yokota, H., Kurokawa, A., Otsuka, T. *et al.* Significance of magnetic resonance imaging in acute head injury. *J. Trauma* 1991, 31, 351

17 Gennarelli, T.A., Adams, J. H. and Graham, D.I. Diffuse axonal injury - a new conceptual approach to an old problem, in 'Mechanisms of secondary brain damage,' (Eds. A. Baethmann, K.G. Go, A. Unterberg) Plenum Press, Boston, USA, 1986, p.15

18 Crow, W. Aspects of neuroradiology of head injury. *Neurosurg. Clin. N. Am.* 1991, 2, 321

19 Lang, D.A., Hadley, D.M., Teasdale, G.M. *et al.* Gadolinium enhanced magnetic resonance imaging in acute head injury. *Acta. Neurochir.* 1991, 109, 5

20 Ellis, S.J. Functional magnetic resonance, neurological enlightenment? *Lancet* 1993, 342, 882

21 Frahm, J., Merboldt, K.D. and Hanicke, W. Functional MRI of human brain activations at high spatial resolution. *Magn. Reson. Med.* 1993, 29, 139

22 Le Bihan, D. Functional magnetic imaging of the brain. *Ann. Int. Med.* 1995, 122, 296

23 Moats, R.A., Watson, L., Shonk, T. *et al.* Added value of automated clinical proton MRI spectroscopy of the brain. *J. Comp. Assist. Tomogr.* 1995, 19, 480

24 Sutton, L.N., Wang, Z., Duhaime, A.C. *et al.* Tissue lactate in paediatric head trauma, a clinical study using 1H NMR spectroscopy. *Paediatr. Neurosurg.* 1995, 22, 81

25 Langfitt, T.W., Obrist, W.D., Alavi, A. *et al.* Computerized tomography, magnetic resonance imaging, and positron emission tomography in the study of brain trauma. Preliminary observations. *J. Neurosurg.* 1986, 64, 760

26 Alavi, A., Fazekas, T., Alves, W. *et al.* Positron emission tomography in the evaluation of head injury. *J. Cereb. Blood Flow Metab.* 1987, 7, S646

27 Alavi, A. Functional and anatomical studies of head injury. *J. Neuropsychiatry* 1989, 1, S45

28 Wegener, W.A. and Alavi, A. Positron-emission tomography in neuropsychiatric disorder. *Curr. Op. Radiol.* 1989, 1, 475

29 George, J.K., Alavi, A., Zimmerman, R.A. *et al.* Metabolic (PET) correlates of anatomic lesions (CT/MRI) produced by head trauma. *J. Nucl. Med.* 1989, 30, 802

30 Alavi, A., Gosfield, T., Cho, W. *et al.* Unusual patterns of cerebellar hypometabolism in head trauma (HT). *J. Nucl. Med.* 1990, 31, 741

31 Rao, N., Turski, P.A., Polcyn, R.E. *et al.* 18F positron emission computed tomography in closed head injury. *Arch. Phys. Med. Rehab.* 1984, 65, 780

32 Souder, E., Alavi, A., Uzell, B. *et al.* Correlation of FDG-PET and neuropsychological findings in head injured patients preliminary data. *J. Nucl. Med.* 1990, 31, 876

33 Abdel-Dayem, H.M., Sadek, S.A. and Kouris, K. Changes in cerebral perfusion after acute head injury, comparison of CT with Tc-99m HMPAO SPECT. *Radiology* 1987, 165, 221

34 Reid, R.H., Gulenchyn, K.Y., Ballinger, J.R. *et al.* Cerebral perfusion imaging with technetium-99m HMPAO following cerebral trauma, initial experience. *Clin. Nucl. Med.* 1990, 15, 383

35 Newton, M.R., Greenwood, R.J., Britton, K.E. *et al.* A study comparing SPECT with CT and MRI after closed head injury. *J. Neurol. Neurosurg. Psychiatry* 1992, 55, 92

36 Masdeu, J.C., Van Heertum, R.L., Kleiman, A. *et al.* Early single photon emission computed tomography in mild head trauma. A controlled study. *J. Neuroimaging* 1994, 4, 177

37 Gray, B.G., Ichise, M., Chung, D-G. *et al.* Technetium-99m-HMPAO SPECT in the evaluation of patients with a remote history of traumatic brain injury, a comparison with X-ray computed tomography. *J. Nucl. Med.* 1992, 33, 52

38 Roper, S.N., Ismael, M.I., King, W.A. *et al.* An analysis of cerebral blood flow in acute closed-head injury using Tc-99m-HMPAO SPECT in computed tomography. *J. Nucl. Med.* 1991, 32, 684

39 Fumeya, H., Ito, K., Yamagiwa, O. *et al.* Analysis of MRI and SPECT in patients with acute head injury. *Acta Neuochir. Suppl* 1990, 51, 283

40 Holman, B.L. and Devous, M.D. Functional brain SPECT, the emergence of a powerful clinical method. *J. Nucl. Med.* 1992, 33, 1888

41 Jacobs, A., Put, E., Ingels, M. and Bossuyt, A. Prospective evaluation of technetium-99m-HMPAO SPECT in mild and moderate traumatic brain injury. *J. Nucl. Med.* 1994, 35, 942

42 Bernardi, B., Zimmerman, R.A. and Bilaniuk, L.T. Neuroradiologic evaluation of paediatric craniocerebral trauma. *Top. Magn. Reson. Imaging* 1993, 5, 161

43 Levin, H.S., Culhane, K.A., Mendelsohn, D. *et al.* Cognition in relation to magnetic resonance imaging in head-injured children and adolescents. *Arch. Neurol.* 1993, 50, 897

44 Mendelsohn, D., Levin, H.S., Lilly, M. *et al.* Late MRI after head injury in children, relationship to clinical features and outcome. *Childs. Nerv. Syst.* 1992, 8, 445

45 Worley, G., Hoffman, J.M., Paine, S.S. *et al.* 18-Fluorodeoxyglucose positron emission tomography in children and adolescents with traumatic brain injury. *Develop. Med. Child. Neurol.* 1995, 37, 213

SPECT in Neurology and Psychiatry, edited by P.P. De Deyn, R.A. Dierckx, A. Alavi and B.A. Pickut

Regional Cerebral Blood Flow SPECT in Mild and Moderate Head Injury

Chapter
50

A. Jacobs, E. Put, M. Ingels, T. Put[*] and A. Bossuyt[**]

Introduction

Mild and moderate traumatic brain injury are disorders with a high incidence. In particular for mild head injury, the reported incidences obtained from epidemiological studies in the US and Europe vary considerably, but the estimated incidence rates are mostly in the range of 200 to 250 cases per 100,000 population per year[1]. Mild head injuries represent ± 50 to 80% of all head injury cases in the United States[2]. Although only a small percentage of patients (up to 3%) show early serious complications requiring neurosurgical intervention[3], in some cases important neurobehavioural sequelae may develop[4]. The socio-economic impact of mild head injury, in particular on employment, is well documented[5,6].

The role of morphological techniques (especially CT) in minor forms of head injury is probably limited. Indeed, whereas CT plays an important role in the detection of intracranial lesions which may require neurosurgical intervention, CT performed in the acute stage of mild head trauma is positive in only 3-18% of cases[7]. Moreover, the predictive value (positive and negative) of CT is poor[8]. In the chronic stages, there is a lack of correlation between anatomical and clinical findings[9].

A number of studies on patients with head injury have already demonstrated that brain perfusion SPECT is more sensitive than CT in the detection of cerebral abnormalities. Abdel-Dayem *et al.*[10] showed, in a group of patients who were all in a state of diminished consciousness after chiefly severe head trauma, that SPECT performed within 72 h post injury allows the earlier detection of a larger number of lesions that CT, and that SPECT lesions appeared to be larger than the corresponding CT abnormalities. Moreover, certain SPECT patterns seemed to be predictive for prognosis. In another comparative study of SPECT and CT in acute closed head injury with a variable degree of severity, Roper *et al.*[11] found SPECT to be most useful in the detection of focal, rather than diffuse, disturbances of cerebral blood flow; these authors also observed that two types of traumatic contusions can be distinguished: a first type characterised by a diminished blood flow, detectable with SPECT, and a second type with a normal blood flow. Ichise *et al.*[12] studied the correlation of SPECT, CT and MRI with neuropsychological performance in chronic traumatic brain injury; these researchers found that SPECT could demonstrate brain dysfunction in morphologically intact brain regions and therefore provide objective evidence for some of the impaired neuropsychological performance.

Department of Nuclear Medicine, Virga Jesse Hospital, Hasselt, Belgium
[*]Department of Neurosurgery, St.-Franciskus Hospital, Heusden-Zolder, Belgium
[**]Department of Nuclear Medicine, University Hospital, Free University of Brussels (VUB), Jette, Belgium

The observation that rCBF SPECT can depict lesions that are larger or more numerous than on CT does not by itself indicate SPECT as the imaging modality of choice in traumatic brain injury. Therefore the clinical significance of regional changes identified by rCBF SPECT still needs to be better established.

We reported previously[13] that a normal early post injury SPECT is a reliable predictor of a favourable clinical outcome. However, an abnormal initial SPECT appeared to be insufficient as a prognosticator of the outcome and a large fraction of patients (24%) with a positive control SPECT at 3 months post injury were completely free of symptoms. These findings indicate the need for longer follow-up data, in order to assess the further evolution of SPECT changes in relation to clinical data.

In the present study, SPECT data were correlated with clinical parameters in the early post-traumatic stage of mild and moderate head injury patients, providing a basal reference examination, and, in cases of persisting rCBF disturbances, during a follow-up of 1 year.

Materials and methods

Patient population

Patients (168) were initially enrolled and underwent at least an early post-traumatic rCBF SPECT and a CT. Nineteen of these patients did not have the premised follow-up. The remaining 149 patients (92 male and 57 female, with a mean age of 36 years and an age range of 11 to 71 years), all having sustained a closed-cranial trauma, were then included for data analysis. In 92% of these cases the trauma was caused by a car, motorcycle or bicycle accident; the remaining patients were injured by a fall, an assault or a blow to the head during professional activity or sports practice. Exclusion criteria consisted of: previous cranial trauma, epilepsy or other neurological disorders known before the trauma, psychiatric diseases, drug or alcohol abuse, CT showing important cortical atrophy or focal lesions (such as arachnoid cysts) unrelated to the trauma, and an unreliable anamnesis concerning the trauma.

Two subgroups were considered according to the severity of the trauma. A first subgroup of moderate trauma (ModTr) was composed of 90 patients who had presented a coma, with an admission score of ≥11 on the Glasgow Coma Scale, a retrograde amnesia (<24 h) and/or an abnormal CT (related to the trauma). The second subgroup, comprising the remaining 59 subjects, consisted of mild trauma (MilTr) cases, defined as patients who were referred for minor neurological complaints after a head trauma, but who

had no loss of consciousness or retrograde amnesia and had a normal CT.

Study design

The study set-up is shown in Figure 1.

Early post-traumatic evaluation. All 149 patients underwent an initial ^{99m}Tc-HMPAO brain SPECT study (SPECT0) and a CT within 4 weeks after the trauma (75/149 within 3 days, 49/149 between 4 and 7 days, 14/149 during the 2nd week and 11/149 between 2 and 4 weeks after the trauma). All SPECT studies were performed at most 4 days after the CT scan.

Follow-up. The first re-evaluation (T3mo) took place after a mean time interval of 3.3 months (range 2.9 - 3.4 months) from the time of SPECT0, the second (T6mo) at 6.2 months (range 5.8 - 6.4 months) and the third (T12mo) at 12.3 months (range 11.9 - 12.7 months). In order to avoid unjustified radiation exposure, the study was designed so that patients with a normal previous SPECT were not submitted to a repeat SPECT, unless a deterioration of their clinical status had been observed.

According to their SPECT0 result, either normal or abnormal, two patient groups can be considered. At T3mo, all patients with a normal SPECT0 were re-evaluated clinically (CLIN3mo) but had no repeat SPECT; only in case of persisting symptoms at T3mo, a further clinical re-evaluation took place at T6mo (CLIN6mo) and, in case of clinical abnormalities at T6mo, at T12mo (CLIN12mo) as well.

At T3mo, patients with an abnormal SPECT0, had a repeat SPECT (SPECT3mo) and were re-evaluated clinically (CLIN3mo), yielding 4 possible combinations of SPECT result (SPECT3mo+ or -) and clinical evaluation (CLIN3mo+ or -). For patients with the combination of SPECT3mo- and CLIN3mo- the follow-up was ended. Patients presenting with the combination of SPECT 3mo- and CLIN3mo+ were re-evaluated only clinically, at T6mo (CLIN6mo).

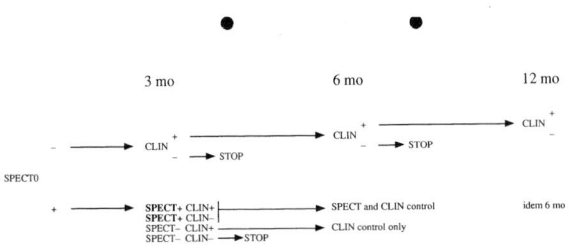

Figure 1 Study set-up. SPECT0 = early post-traumatic SPECT (within 1 month after the trauma); CLIN = clinical evaluation

Patients showing one of the remaining combinations (SPECT3mo+ and CLIN3mo+ or SPECT3mo+ and CLIN3mo-) underwent a repeat SPECT at T6mo (SPECT6mo) as well as a clinical evaluation (CLIN6mo). Exactly the same scheme of re-evaluation as at T6mo was then used at T12mo, according to the combination of the SPECT6mo and CLIN6mo results.

During this follow-up, patients were not included in head trauma rehabilitation programmes.

Clinical evaluation

All patients underwent a complete neurological examination and an explicit questioning concerning postconcussive symptoms, based on the list of symptomatology given by Rutherford et al.[14]. Each subject also had to perform a memory and concentration test. Only if no signs and no symptoms were recorded, was a patient considered as being 'clinically negative' (CLIN-). The presence of 1 symptom or sign was considered sufficient for classifying the patient as being 'clinically positive' (CLIN+).

SPECT imaging

SPECT imaging was performed after intravenous injection of 740 MBq of ^{99m}Tc-HMPAO (Ceretec, Amersham, UK). Patients were injected in a quiet and dimly lit room. Imaging started 15-30 min after injection.

Tomographic images were obtained using a single-head rotating gamma camera (Toshiba GCA-901A) equipped with a low energy high resolution collimator. Data were collected from 60 projections in the 140 keV photopeak (20% window) over 360° in 64x64 matrices, with an acquisition time of 30 sec/view. A zoom factor of 1.5 was used. Orthogonal transverse, coronal and sagittal planes were generated by filtered back-projection using a Butterworth filter (cutoff 0.4 cm^{-1}; order 7), followed by orbitomeatal reorientation of the reconstructed volume. The final data set used for interpretation consisted of 2-pixel thick (5.6 mm/pixel) transaxial, coronal and sagittal slices. Each set of images was normalised to its maximal pixel count and a lower threshold of 15% was set on a 256 'spectrum' colour scale.

Data analysis

All HMPAO SPECT studies were first visually graded independently by three experienced observers adjudging a score of 0 (no lesions) to 4, without knowledge of the clinical data. Each lesion was scored

from 1 to 3 according to the volume and the severity of the hypoperfusion: 1 = small (5.6 - 11.2 cm^3) lesion with moderately decreased perfusion (tracer uptake reduced with 10-20% compared with contralateral side or to 55-70% of maximum); 2 = large (>11.2 cm^3 lesion with moderately decreased perfusion or small lesion with markedly decreased perfusion (tracer uptake reduced with >20% compared with contralateral side or to <55% of maximum); 3 = large lesion with markedly decreased perfusion. In patients with multiple lesions the scores were added up to a maximum of 4. Each study was then graded by agreement of all three observers. The localisation of all SPECT lesions was noted.

The Wilcoxon signed rank test was used for evaluating the evolution of the SPECT abnormality score in patients who kept showing a positive SPECT at subsequent times of examination (T0 - T3mo, T3mo - T6mo and T6mo - T12mo). In order to show the global trend in the evolution of SPECT and clinical results, the fraction of patients with persistently positive SPECT and clinical findings at subsequent times of control was expressed in relation to the total number of patients who underwent the initial evaluation at T0.

Results

Subgroup of moderate trauma (ModTr) (n=90)

An overview of the results obtained in this subgroup is given in Figure 2.

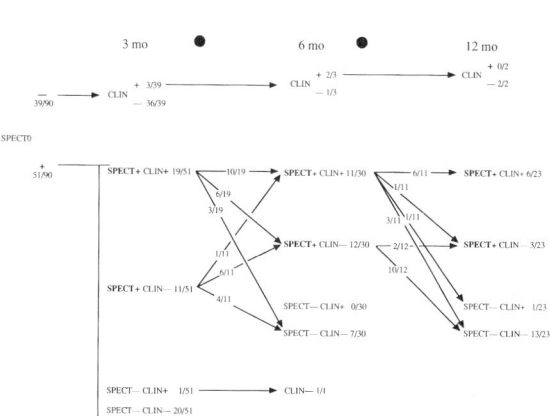

Figure 2 Subgroup of moderate trauma. Overview of SPECT and CLIN results at the different times of evaluation: at the early post-traumatic stage (SPECT0) and during follow-up at 3 mo, 6 mo and 12 mo post injury

Initial SPECT and CT findings

The initial SPECT (SPECT0) was positive in 51/90 (57%) patients, with a mean score of abnormality of 1.9 (s.d. 0.6). In 10/51 of these cases, the initially performed CT scan showed lesions of the following kind: 3/10 were thin subdural haematomas; 3/10 haemorrhagic contusions; 3/10 non-haemorrhagic contusions and 1/10 corresponded to a cerebellar infarction. SPECT0 was normal in 39/90 (43%) patients, with a positive concomitant CT in 3/39 cases; in all 3 patients CT lesion size was <0.5 cm and it concerned a white matter infarction in one patient, a cortical infarction in another and a haemorrhagic contusion in a third one.

The power of SPECT0 in predicting the clinical outcome at T3mo was determined as follows. The negative predictive value (NPV) of SPECT0, given as P (CLIN3mo-/SPECT0-), was 36/39 (92%). Of the remaining 3 patients with the combination (CLIN3mo+ / SPECT0-), 2/3 still presented clinical signs at T6mo, but both were CLIN- at T12mo. The positive predictive value (PPV), given as P (CLIN3mo+ / SPECT0+), was 20/51 (39%); it must be noted that a significantly larger (p=0.04) SPECT0+ score was found in the CLIN3mo+ group (mean SPECT0 score = 2.0), compared with the CLIN3mo- group (mean SPECT0 score = 1.5).

Follow-up

A gradual decrease in the fraction of SPECT+ patients was observed at subsequent times, but clinical normalisation occurred earlier than normalisation of SPECT studies (Table 1).

Of all patients with a positive inital SPECT, 20/51 (39%) had completely negative clinical as well as SPECT findings at 3 months post injury and did not have to be re-evaluated afterwards. Only 1/11 patients presenting with the combination of SPECT+CLIN- at T3mo, had to be categorised as SPECT+CLIN+ at T6mo. The fraction of patients showing the

Table 2 ModTr subgroup. Evolution of mean SPECT+ scores during follow-up. Only those patients with a persistently positive SPECT at subsequent times of evaluation were considered

Time interval	Number of patients	Evolution of SPECT scores
0-3 mo	30	1.9 - 1.6 (p=0.01)
3-6 mo	23	1.7 - 1.3 (p=0.001)
6-12 mo	9	1.9 - 1.7 (p=0.05)

combination of SPECT- and CLIN+ ('false negative fraction') at T3mo was only 1/51 (2%); at T6mo none of the patients showed this combination and at T12mo it was noted in 1/23 (4%).

A clear evolution in the 'false positive fraction' (SPECT+CLIN-) was observed. At T3mo this combination occurred in 11/51 (22%) patients; at T6mo in 12/30 (40%) cases. But at T12mo post injury this fraction had decreased to 3/23 (13%). The number of patients showing the combination of SPECT+ and CLIN+ decreased from 19/51 (37%) at T3mo to 6/23 (26%) at T12mo. Concerning the severity of SPECT lesions, a significant decrease in SPECT+ score was observed for all considered time intervals (Table 2).

Evaluation of patients with an abnormal initial CT:

In SPECT0+ patients (n = 10): 5/10 patients were CLIN- and had a negative control SPECT as well as a negative CT at T3mo. The remaining 5/10 patients presented the combination of CLIN+ and SPECT+ at T3mo and 3/5 still showed CT abnormalities. At T6mo all 5/5 patients showed the same findings as at T3mo. At T12mo, however, only 1/5 still presented with clinical symptoms and SPECT as well as CT lesions; 3/5 were CLIN- and SPECT- with 1/3 still showing a CT lesion; in the remaining case SPECT and CT had

Table 1 ModTr subgroup. Fraction of CLIN+ and SPECT+ patients at 3, 6 and 12 months post injury

	CLIN+	SPECT+
3 mo	23/90 (26%)	30/90 (33%)
6 mo	13/90 (14%)	23/90 (26%)
12 mo	7/90 (8%)	9/90 (10%)

CLIN+ = positive clinical evaluation; SPECT+ = positive SPECT result

Table 3 MilTr subgroup. Fraction of CLIN+ and SPECT+ patients at 3, 6 and 12 months post injury

	CLIN+	SPECT+
3 mo	19/59 (32%)	20/59 (34%)
6 mo	10/59 (17%)	11/59 (19%)
12 mo	4/59 (7%)	4/59 (7%)

CLIN+ = positive clinical evaluation; SPECT+ = positive SPECT result

Table 4 MilTr subgroup. Evolution of mean SPECT+ scores during follow-up. Only those patients with a persistently positive SPECT at subsequent times of evaluation were considered

Time interval	Number of patients	Evolution of SPECT scores
0-3 mo	20	1.6 - 1.1 (p=0.009)
3-6 mo	11	1.3 - 1.2 (n.s.)
6-12 mo	4	2.0 - 1.4 (!n<6)

both normalised, whereas clinical symptoms persisted. In SPECT0- patients (n = 3): all 3 patients with a positive initial CT but a normal concomitant SPECT, were CLIN- and had a normal control CT at T3mo.

Subgroup of mild trauma (MilTr) (n = 59)

An overview of the results obtained in the MilTr subgroup is given in Figure 3.

Initial SPECT. The initial SPECT (SPECT0) was positive in 32/59 (54%) of patients, with a mean score of abnormality of 1.5 (s.d. 0.5), which is significantly (p = 0.04) smaller than the SPECT0+ score in the ModTr subgroup. SPECT0 was normal in 27/59 (46%) patients. The NPV of SPECT0, given as P (CLIN3mo-/SPECT0-), was 25/27 (93%). Of the remaining 2 patients (CLIN3mo+/SPECT0-), both were CLIN- at T6mo. The PPV, given as P (CLIN3mo+/SPECT0+), was 17/32 (53%); a significantly (p = 0.02) larger SPECT0+ score was found in the CLIN3mo+ group (mean SPECT0 score = 1.6), compared with the CLIN3mo- group (mean SPECT0 score = 1.1).

Follow-up. A gradual and similar decrease in the fraction of SPECT+ and CLIN+ patients was observed at subsequent times of evaluation (Table 3). Of all patients with a positive initial SPECT, 10/32 (31%) had completely negative clinical as well as SPECT findings at 3 months post injury. No patient presenting with the combination SPECT+CLIN- at T3mo, had to be catagorised as SPECT+CLIN+ at T6mo. The 'false negative fraction' (SPECT-CLIN+) at T3mo was 2/32 (6%). Afterwards this combination did not occur anymore.

The 'false positive fraction' (SPECT+CLIN-) decreased from 5/32 (16%) at T3mo over 2/20 (10%) at T6mo to 0/11 (0%) at 12 months months post injury. The number of patients showing the combination of SPECT+ and CLIN+ decreased from 15/32 (47%) at T3mo to 4/11 (36%) at T12mo. Concerning the severity of SPECT lesions, only for the time interval T0-T3mo

a significant (p = 0.009) decrease in SPECT score was found in patients with a persistently positive SPECT at subsequent times of evaluation (Table 4). For the time interval T3mo - T6mo the difference in score was statistically not significant and for the interval T6mo - T12mo the sample size was too small for statistical analysis.

Discussion

In the assessment of the significance of SPECT lesions, two approaches could be followed, theoretically. A first potential approach consists of trying to correlate SPECT findings with parameters reflecting known pathophysiological changes that occur during and after a minor trauma. A second possibility consists of analysing the SPECT result in relation to clincal parameters. Elson[15] gives an excellent overview of the mechanisms and pathophysiology of mild head injury. Knowledge on the pathophysiological substrate in the acute and chronic stages of mild trauma has increased, e.g. from biomechanical analysis of trauma. In particular concerning the localisation of damage, it could be shown that focal changes primarily involve antero-inferior aspects of frontotemporal regions, whereas diffuse axonal injury represents white matter lesions of corpus callosum and frontotemporal lobes with possible cortical hypoperfusion by deafferentiation. However, the formulation of an adequate pathophysiological model and the design of hypothesis-orientated clinical tests are difficult, because even on classification of trauma severity no concensus is found in trauma literature and many pathophysiological aspects still remain unclear, especially concerning the post-concussive syndrome.

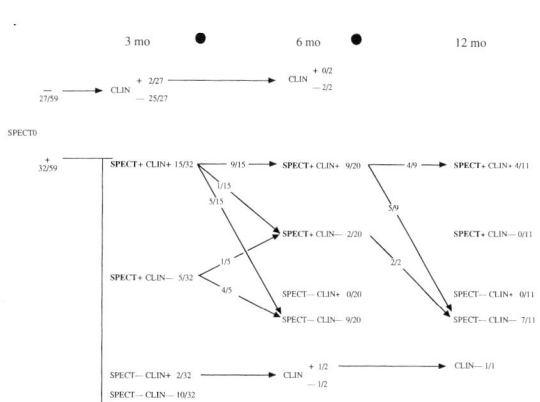

Figure 3 Subgroup of mild trauma. Overview of SPECT and CLIN results at the early post-traumatic stage (SPECT0) and during follow-up at 3 mo, 6 mo and 12 mo post injury

From a practical point of view, an approach based on evaluating the SPECT result in relation to clinical parameters seems therefore to be the most appropriate in estimating whether the rCBF SPECT result accounts for the patient's clinical findings. Comparison of currently available SPECT results from clinical studies is hampered due to differences in patient characteristics (mainly severity of the trauma) and differences in timing of the SPECT study (acute or later stages, varying from some weeks to several years after the trauma).

Criteria for classifying a trauma as being mild range broadly and evenly on the necessity of having a loss of consciousness. No agreement is found in trauma literature. Furthermore, Glasgow Coma Scale scores vary from only 15 to a range of 8 - 15. The same remark applies to other, currently used additional parameters of severity, like amnesia (post-traumatic or retrograde), CT and/or MRI findings and need for and duration of hospital admission[1]. In our study, the patient population was divided into two subgroups (mild or moderate trauma), according to the clinical appearance of the patient at the moment of and shortly after the trauma. The criteria that were used (presence or absence of coma (Glasgow Coma Scale ≥ 11) and/or retrograde amnesia and/or CT lesions) allow a simple, practical approach for patient classification.

The severity of the trauma served as a clinical indicator for evaluating the early post-traumatic SPECT. Although the fraction of positive SPECT cases in ModTr and MilTr subgroups was comparable (57 and 54%, respectively), a significantly smaller degree of abnormality was found in the MilTr subgroup. This observation suggests that, according to our classification criteria, the probability of finding a SPECT lesion is comparable after a ModTr or a MilTr, but that the SPECT abnormality itself corresponds to the severity of the trauma.

In both patient groups, it was confirmed that a negative initial SPECT is a reliable predictor of favourable clinical outcome at 3 months (negative predictive value of >90%), which is an important finding in the evaluation of the patient's ability to return to work.

In contrast to the high negative predictive value of the initial SPECT, its positive predictive value for the clinical outcome at 3 months was low in both patient groups (39% in ModTr and 53% in MilTr). However, a higher score of SPECT abnormality was coupled to an increased probability for the persistence of symptoms at 3 months.

Our data are in accordance with previous findings that SPECT can depict more lesions than CT and confirm the poor predictive capacity of CT in mild and moderate head injury: the absence of CT abnormalities does not guarantee a good outcome, nor does the presence of CT lesions appropriately predict a long-term impairment[8].

In both study groups a gradual decrease in the fraction of patients with persistent clinical signs or symptoms was observed during the 1-year follow-up. At 12 months post injury, less than 10% of patients kept presenting clinical abnormalities. The fraction of patients with a persistently positive SPECT during follow-up also gradually decreased. However, concerning this decrease in relation to the evolution of the frequency of clinical abnormalities, a difference is observed between the ModTr and MilTr group. Whereas in both groups the fractions of CLIN+ and SPECT+ patients are comparable at 12 months post injury, at 3 and 6 months the fraction of SPECT+ patients is considerably larger than the CLIN+ fraction in the ModTr group; this is in contrast with the MilTr group showing comparable fractions of CLIN+ and SPECT+ at all considered times of evaluation. In the ModTr group, a significant decrease of the SPECT abnormality score was observed over the different time intervals during follow-up; in the MilTr group the same trend was found. These data indicate that, during the 1-year follow-up, not only the fraction of patients showing SPECT lesions decreases but also the severity of SPECT disturbances gradually diminishes.

Of all patients with a positive initial SPECT, 20/51 (39%) in the ModTr group and 10/32 (31%) in the MilTr group had completely negative clinical as well as SPECT findings at 3 months post injury and were not re-evaluated afterwards. During the entire follow-up period, a very small or even absent false negative fraction (SPECT- CLIN+) was observed in both groups of patients. This finding suggests that rCBF SPECT can reliably be used in the exclusion of significant clinical sequelae.

On the other hand, the evolution of the false positive fraction (SPECT+ combined with CLIN-) was different for the MilTr compared with the ModTr subgroup. More precisely, at 6 months post injury this fraction was markedly larger (40%) in the ModTr compared to the MilTr group (10%). At 12 months, no false positives were observed in the MilTr group; in the ModTr group the false positive fraction had decreased to 10%. Consequently, the disappearance of subclinical SPECT changes seems to be slower in the ModTr compared with the MilTr group.

In conclusion, our study confirms that SPECT is more sensitive than CT in the detection of post-traumatic cerebral abnormalities in moderate head injury. SPECT lesions detected with the early post injury

SPECT in moderate trauma are more severe than in mild trauma cases. A normal SPECT, at the early post-traumatic stage as well as during a 1-year follow-up of mild and moderate head injury, reliably excludes significant clinical sequelae. In judging the clinical importance of a positive SPECT result, caution is warranted because subclinical SPECT alterations are frequently observed during the early stages ($\leq$6 months post injury) of moderate trauma.

References

1   Kraus, J.F., McArthur, D.L. and Silberman, T.A. Epidemiology of mild brain injury. *Semin. Neurol.* 1994, 14, 1

2   Kraus, J.F. and Nourjah, P. The epidemiology of mild head injury in 'Mild head injury', (Eds. H.S. Levin, H.M. Eisenberg, A.L. Benton), Oxford University Press, New York, USA, 1989, p.8

3   Dacey, R.G. Jr., Alves, W.M., Rimel, R.W. *et al.* Neurosurgical complications after apparently minor head injuries: assessment of risk in a series of 610 patients. *J. Neurosurg.* 1986, 65, 203

4   Bohnen, N and Jolles, J. Neurobehavioural aspects of postconcussive symptoms after mild head injury. *J. Nerv. Mental. Dis.* 1992, 180, 683

5   Englander, J., Hall, K., Stimpson, T. and Chaffin, S. Mild traumatic brain injury in an insured population: subjective complaints and return to employment. *Brain Inj.* 1992, 2, 161

6   Rimel, R.W., Giordani, B., Barth, J.T. *et al.* Disability caused by minor head injury. *Neurosurgery* 1981, 9, 221

7   Mohanty, S.K., Thompson, W. and Rakower, S. Are CT scans for head injury patients always necessary? *J. Trauma* 1991, 31, 801

8   Kido, D.K., Cox, C., Hamill, R.W. *et al.* Traumatic brain injuries: predictive usefulness of CT. *Radiology* 1992, 182, 777

9   Gray, B.C., Ichise, M., Chung, D.-G. *et al.* Technetium-99m-HMPAO SPECT in the evaluation of patients with a remote history traumatic brain injury: a comparison with X-ray computed tomography. *J. Nucl. Med.* 1992, 33, 52

10 Abdel-Dayem, H.M., Sadek, S.A., Kouris, K. *et al.* Changes in cerebral perfusion after acute head injury: Comparison of CT with Tc-99m HMPAO SPECT. *Radiology* 1987, 165, 221

11 Roper, S.N., Mena, I., King, W.A. *et al.* An analysis of cerebral blood flow in acute closed-head injury using Technetium-99m-HMPAO SPECT and computed tomography. *J. Nucl. Med.* 1991, 32, 1684

12 Ichise, M., Chung, D.-G., Wang, P. *et al.* Technetium-99m-HMPAO SPECT, CT and MRI in the evaluation of patients with chronic traumatic brain injury: a correlation with neuropsychological performance. *J. Nucl. Med.* 1994, 35, 217

13 Jacobs, A., Put, E., Ingels, M. and Bossuyt, A. Prospective evaluation of Technetium-99m-HMPAO SPECT in mild and moderate traumatic brain injury. *J. Nucl. Med.* 1994, 35, 942

14 Rutherford, W.H., Merrett, J.D. and McDonald, J.R. Sequelae of concussion caused by minor head injuries. *Lancet* 1977, 1, 1

15 Elson, L.M. and Ward, C.C. Mechanisms and pathophysiology of mild head injury. *Semin. Neurol.* 1994, 14, 8

SPECT in Neurology and Psychiatry, edited by P.P. De Deyn, R.A. Dierckx, A. Alavi and B.A. Pickut
© 1997 John Libbey & Company Ltd, pp. 423–430

SPECT and MR in Focal and Diffuse Head Injury

Chapter
51

J.T.L. Wilson, D.J. Wyper[*], D.M. Hadley[*], J. Patterson[*] and
G.M. Teasdale[*]

Introduction

Fully identifying brain damage in head injury survivors is an unresolved problem. CT is relatively insensitive to many of the lesions in head injury[1,2]; MR is more sensitive than CT but still does not reveal the full spectrum of abnormalities present. Early experience with HMPAO SPECT has shown that it detects abnormalities after traumatic brain injury not revealed by CT[3] or MR CT[4].

We have been studying head injury in Glasgow using SPECT and MR. The design of the study calls for both acute and follow-up SPECT and MR, together with an extensive neuropsychological assessment at follow-up. One hundred and three patients have been recruited to the study, of whom 102 have had SPECT imaging. The aim of this chapter is to discuss some of the major issues surrounding SPECT in head injury, and illustrate points raised with examples drawn from the study.

Focal head injury

The extent of correspondence between functional and structural abnormalities

Initial SPECT studies in acute head injury showed regions of low blood flow, some of which agreed with the locations of lesions on CT and some of which did not[3]. A first question is whether SPECT can reliably detect abnormalities corresponding to the haemorrhagic lesions typically seen on CT after traumatic injury. Choksey *et al.*[5] studied 8 patients with traumatic intracranial haematomas identified by CT: in these patients SPECT clearly demonstrated perfusion defects that corresponded to the location of the haematomas seen on CT. Bullock *et al.*[6] found that all patients with a focal lesion on CT greater than 1.5 cm diameter had a corresponding region of low blood flow. Thus, it appears that there is typically a region of reduced blood flow associated with significant haematoma demonstrated by CT.

The early studies also showed that the region of reduced CBF is often larger than the lesion seen on CT. Abdel-Dayem *et al.*[3] report that the low density areas seen on CT scans were much smaller than corresponding SPECT perfusion deficits. Choksey *et al.*[5] suggest that the degree of mismatch between haematoma size seen on CT and the deficit on SPECT may predict late deterioration.

University of Stirling, Stirling, Scotland
[*]Institute of Neurological Sciences, Southern General Hospital, Glasgow, Scotland

Although SPECT abnormalities may be larger than lesions shown on CT, they are probably similar in size to focal lesions shown by MR. MR studies show the haemorrhagic contusions visualised by CT are usually surrounded by a more extensive area of increased signal on T_2 weighted images[1,2]. This region of hyperintensity is assumed to correspond to oedema associated with the contusion. Bullock et al.[6] found that SPECT perfusion deficits corresponded to the area of hyperintensity on T_2 weighted images associated with contusions seen on CT, but the region of low blood flow was not larger than this increased signal area. In these circumstances, low blood flow on SPECT seems to represent haematoma together with surrounding oedema.

Although SPECT usually shows a region of low blood flow corresponding to haemorrhagic contusions observed on CT, this is not found in every case. Roper et al.[7] compared CT and SPECT findings in 15 patients with acute head injury. Out of a total of 44 abnormalities, 12 were seen on CT only. As might be expected, SPECT failed to detect abnormalities corresponding to thin subdural haematoma, and subarachnoid haemorrhage. SPECT will also fail to detect flow abnormalities corresponding to small contusions below the level of resolution of the technique. However, the study by Roper et al.[7]

indicates that in some relatively large contusions demonstrated on CT, blood flow on SPECT was equal to surrounding tissue. This implies a relative hyperaemia in these areas (i.e. blood flow in excess of metabolic demand), which effectively masks the abnormality. Hyperaemia is discussed in more detail below.

Functional abnormalities without corresponding structural lesions

Perhaps the most exciting finding in SPECT studies of head injury is the presence of a range of abnormalities not shown by structural imaging. Roper et al.[7] found that 39% of focal abnormalities occurred only on SPECT and not on CT. Abnormalities can take the form of focal regions of low or high flow that may be adjacent or distant to abnormalities demonstrated by structural imaging. More global abnormalities in flow such as frontal occipital slope reversal[7], and asymmetric hemispheric perfusion[8] have also been documented. A classification and review of these abnormalities is given elsewhere[9].

An interesting example of a blood flow abnormality without a corresponding MR lesion is shown in Figure 1. In this patient, there is a zone of compromised perfusion below an extradural haematoma (EDH). On

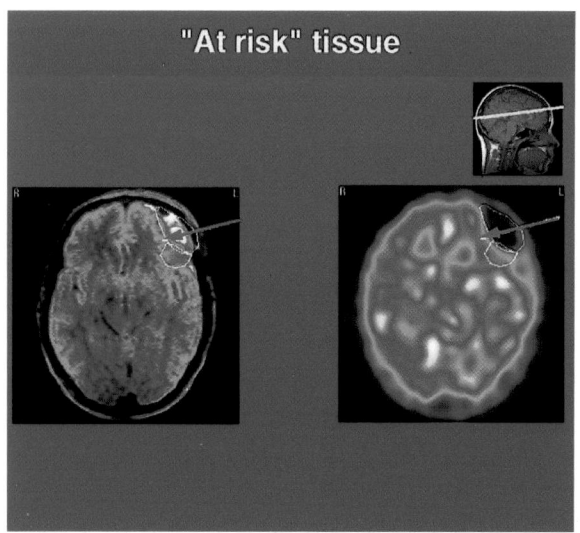 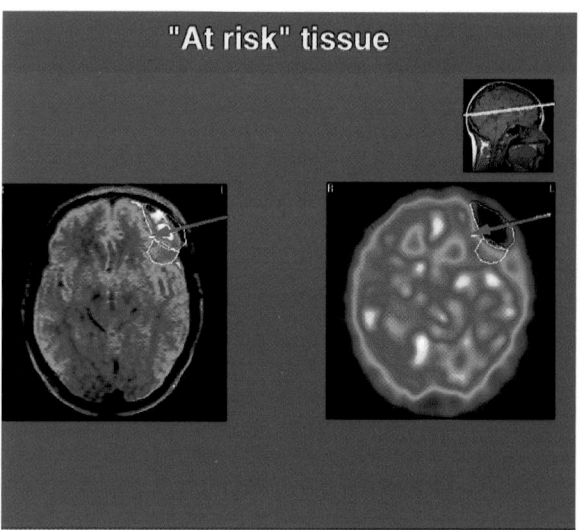

Figure 1 A male aged 49 who fell from a ladder, and was only briefly unconscious. Glasgow Coma Scale (GCS) score on admission was 15. The figure shows: left, MR and HMPAO-SPECT imaging at 4 days post injury; right, at 6 months post injury. Regions of interest (ROIs) have been drawn around extradural and intradural haematomas on acute MR imaging. The ROIs have been transferred to the acute SPECT image and the follow-up MR and SPECT images. A region of reduced perfusion (arrowed) is evident on acute SPECT in a region that is normal on MR; blood flow remains low in this region at 6 months, and there is now a corresponding area of cerebromalacia on MR. At six months, this patient was moderately disabled. On cognitive testing he had poor memory, and showed slow reaction times

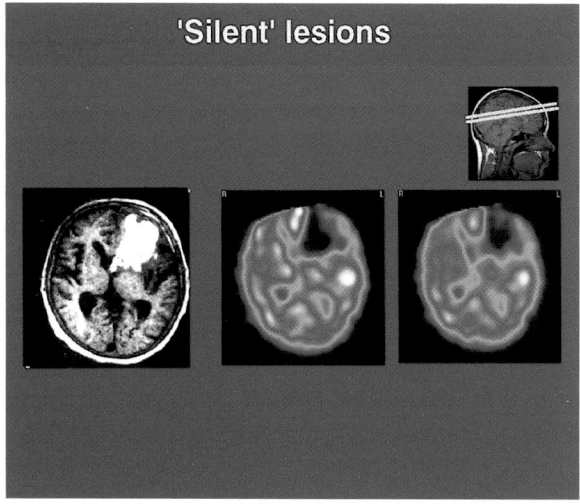
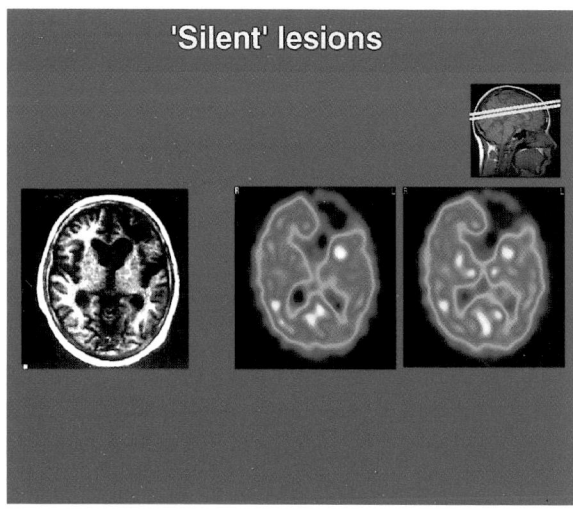

Figure 2 A male aged 48 who fell at work, and was conscious on admission to hospital (GCS=13). The patient was in a state of post-traumatic confusion for a period after injury. However, at follow-up, he had little if any cognitive impairment on neuropsychological testing. He did not report any significant continuing problems associated with his injury, and was back at work. Left, SPECT and MR at 3 days post injury show a large left-frontal abnormality; right, six months post injury, the abnormality is smaller but is still very extensive

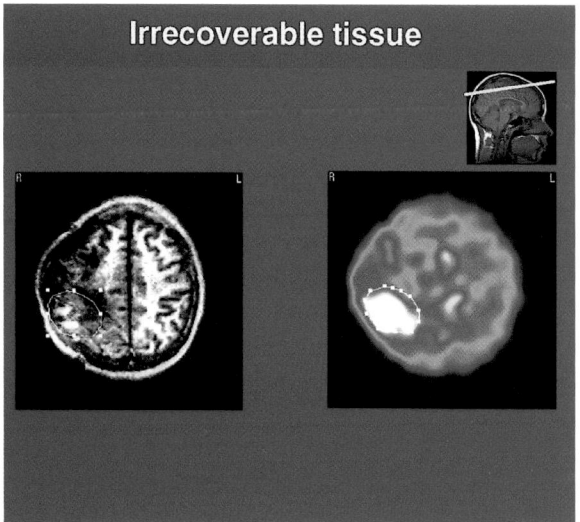
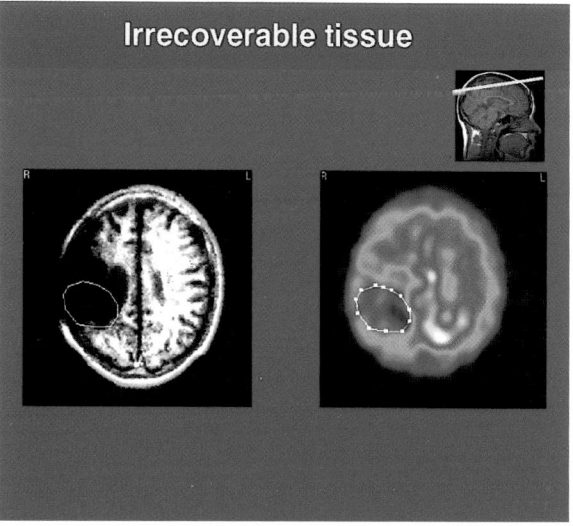

Figure 3 A male aged 24 who fell 30 metres from scaffolding. The patient was in coma on admission (GCS=7). After raised ICP he had a right temporo parietal craniotomy with excision of contused brain and evacuation of intracerebral haematoma. Swelling and further haemorrhage were unresponsive to medical treatment. At six months he was moderately disabled. He had left hemi-paresis, was dysarthric, and had moderate cognitive impairment. Left, SPECT imaging at 5 days post injury shows a zone of hyperaemia associated with the contusion evident on MR; right, at 6 month follow-up there is cerebromalacia in this region

acute MR this region is compressed by EDH and is apparently normal, but by follow-up there is cerebromalacia. The initial region of low blood flow thus appears to represent tissue which is at risk, and which might benefit from neuroprotective intervention.

Changes in focal abnormality and prediction of outcome

An important issue in head injury is the extent to which imaging in the acute stage after injury relates to later outcome. We assessed recovery from focal injury in 23 patients who fulfilled Glasgow Coma Scale (GCS) criteria for minor head injury[10]. All patients had an admission GCS of 13-15 and a positive finding on MR. The MR lesion at 6 month follow-up was on average 31% of the initial size, but there was considerable variation in the extent to which lesions resolved in individual patients. At follow-up the group as a whole showed neuro-psychological impairment in comparison to matched controls. There were no convincing relationships between MR lesions in particular locations and specific cognitive tests, but patients with bilateral lesions performed more poorly than those with unilateral lesions. The findings indicated that the relationship between acute MR findings and 6 month neuropsychological outcome was weak.

Jacobs et al.[11] describe a SPECT study of recovery from mild and moderate head injury suggesting that there is a strong relationship between acute SPECT and later outcome. They studied 42 patients with moderate trauma, and 25 with mild trauma. All patients had HMPAO SPECT in the acute stage; patients with positive findings on acute SPECT had a repeat scan at 3 months. In 32 out of 33 patients with initially negative SPECT findings, clinical symptoms had resolved at follow-up. Positive initial findings were associated with continuing symptoms in 20/34 patients. The results reported[11] thus indicate that a negative initial scan is a reliable predictor of favourable outcome from mild and moderate head injury. This is a potentially important finding that deserves further investigation. In future studies of this kind, it is important that personnel who are performing the follow-up clinical examination are blind to the results of acute imaging.

Our experience suggests that predicting outcome from MR and SPECT findings is problematic. The issue goes beyond simply the question of the sensitivity of the modalities, but also concerns the variable response of the brain to injury. A case illustrating recovery from focal injury is shown in Figure 2. This case made a clinically excellent recovery despite his large left frontal lobe abnormality. The recovery made by this patient indicates the extent of plasticity of the brain in response to focal injury. In this example it appears that the functions previously accomplished by the left frontal lobe have been taken over by other structures, presumably the intact right frontal region. The existence of patients with unexpected patterns of recovery must set limits on reliable prediction of outcome from initial imaging.

Focal hyperaemia

Blood flow studies using the ^{133}Xe method have shown that global cerebral blood flow after head injury may show both abnormally low flow or abnormally high flow[12]. Global hyperaemia is associated with raised intracranial pressure, and is a key part of intracranial dynamics in acute head injury[13]. However, the significance of hyperaemia for later outcome in survivors is not clear; some studies have reported poorer outcome in patients with hyperaemia[12,14], while others have not.

Focal hyperaemia on SPECT in acute head injury has been described by several authors[6,8,15,16]. Hyperaemia is usually associated with focal contusions, but the precise relationship to haemorrhagic areas shown on CT and MR is a matter of controversy. Fumeya et al.[15] suggest that hyperaemic lesions may appear as areas of high intensity in T_2 weighted MR imaging. On the other hand, Sakas et al.[16], extending earlier work[6], report that hyperaemia does not occur in areas which are abnormal on CT or MR, but only affects surrounding tissue. Zones of focal hyperaemia were demonstrated[16] in 38% of patients scanned within two weeks of injury. Those zones occurred adjacent to SPECT perfusion deficits, in tissue that appeared normal on CT and MR. Furthermore they present evidence that when focal hyperaemia occurs it is benign, leaving no abnormality on follow-up MR and having no demonstrable effect on outcome.

Two cases from the present series illustrating acute hyperaemia are shown in Figures 3 and 4. These cases appear to conflict with the idea of benign focal hyperaemia[6,16]. Figure 3 illustrates marked acute hyperperfusion in an area that is abnormal on MR. At six month follow-up, MR shows that the previously hyperaemic area has become a cerebromalacic CSF-filled space. The patient was moderately disabled and had left hemiparesis. In this case the early marked focal hyperperfusion appears to be indicative of tissue which is irrecoverably damaged, and which is associated with impairment at outcome. The case shown in Figure 4 is a moderate head injury with mild focal hyperperfusion. It is consistent with the previous study[16] in that the hyperperfusion is in structurally normal tissue, but there is evidence of subsequent reduced perfusion and impairment at outcome. In this example, there is a right-sided hyperaemia underlying a thin subdural haematoma in the acute stage. At follow-up there is a mild hypoperfusion in the same regions, and some residual neuropsychological impairment. This case shows that even mild hyperaemia can be associated with lasting dysfunction. These cases indicate that the significance of hyperaemia is unclear. In some cases hyperaemia appears to be a benign phenomenon, which leaves little or no sequelae, while in others it is associated with continuing impairment. The conflicting evidence concerning focal hyperperfusion may be influenced by the outcome measures used. In some cases coarse clinical outcome scales may not be sufficiently sensitive to detect a significant effect. In others, brain plasticity as demonstrated in case 2 may compensate for the focal tissue damage which may remain undetected unless SPECT is used as a follow-up.

Diffuse head injury

Funtional abnormalities in diffuse injury

SPECT appears to show promise in assessing brain dysfunction in diffuse head injury. Diffuse brain injury may arise in a number of ways, but diffuse axonal injury (DAI) is one of the distinctive and characteristic lesions after traumatic injury[17]. Many head injuries with severe DAI show no evidence of brain lesions on acute CT. MR is often able to detect small focal lesions in the brainstem, corpus callosum, and at grey-white matter interfaces which are associated with diffuse damage[1,18]. However, such signs are indirect, and do not indicate the precise spatial extent of the injury. Furthermore, these lesions may resolve quite quickly after injury and become undetectable. Diffuse axonal damage can also occur without any macrosopic focal lesions[17]. Experience with SPECT shows that it can visualise regions of brain dysfunction in diffusely injured patients.

Prayer et al.[19] studied 18 patients with severe closed head injury who were normal on CT examination. On MR they found patterns of lesions consistent with diffuse axonal injury in half of the patients, and DAI was associated with poorer outcome. On SPECT imaging, patients with DAI had low blood flow over large areas of cortex (primarily frontal, temporal and parietal lobes) and in the thalamus. Prayer et al.[19] argue that low blood flow in these patients is a consequence of multiple disconnection of cortical regions due to DAI.

A patient showing blood flow patterns after severe diffuse axonal injury is shown in Figure 5. It is not usually possible to assert categorically that a head injured patient has DAI, since this necessitates microscopic level examination of the brain. However, this patient died shortly after the follow-up imaging, and autopsy confirmed DAI as the main pathology. As can be clearly seen, frontal blood flow is low initially and remains low at follow-up. His clinical state was very poor at follow-up: he remained very severely disabled. The extensive abnormality visualised by SPECT contrasts with the appearance on MR. Acute MR demonstrated small lesions typical of DAI, but did not indicate the extent of this injury. On follow-up there was moderate ventricular enlargement, but again there was no indication of the severity of injury in this case.

Recovery after diffuse injury

Wiedmann et al.[4] contrasted 8 patients with focal head injury and 12 patients with diffuse injuries. Patients with focal mass lesions had, proportionally, a greater number of abnormal regions of interest than patients with diffuse injuries. However, the patients with focal lesions were less severely injured by GCS or post traumatic amnesia (PTA) criteria, and showed less evidence of neuropsychological impairment than the diffuse group. This finding underscores the importance of distinguishing different subtypes of head injury when relating imaging findings to outcome. A small abnormality after a diffuse injury may be associated with poorer outcome than an extensive abnormality due to a focal mass[20]. Wiedmann et al.[4] investigated relationships between blood flow deficits and neuropsychological test performance in each subgroup separately. There were few significant associations in the focal group; however, in the diffuse group, 9 of the 12 neuropsychological measures were related to blood flow abnormalities.

Ichise et al.[21] studied a group of 29 patients with SPECT, CT and MR. The majority of patients had been involved in road traffic accidents, and diffuse shearing lesions were implicated in all cases. SPECT abnormalities were found predominantly in frontal and temporal regions. Ichise et al.[21] found that the anterior/posterior ratio on SPECT was related to injury severity and later neuropsychological test performance. The APR was more strongly related to outcome than the ventricle/brain ratio measured from MR. These findings suggest that the degree of frontal blood flow abnormality may be a sensitive index of the extent of diffuse injury. Frontal blood flow has been related to cognitive deficits and psychosocial problems after head injury[22,23].

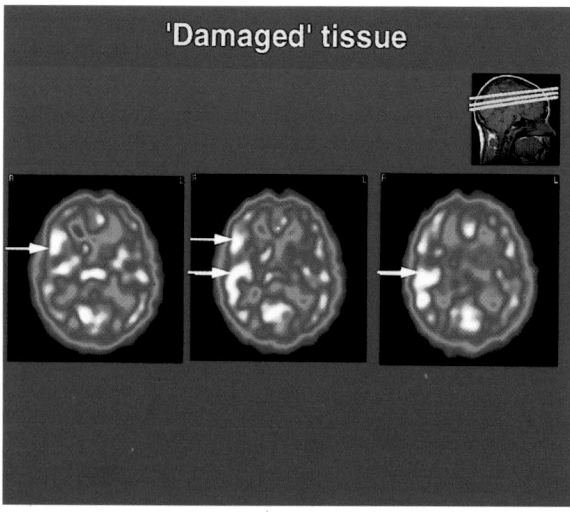 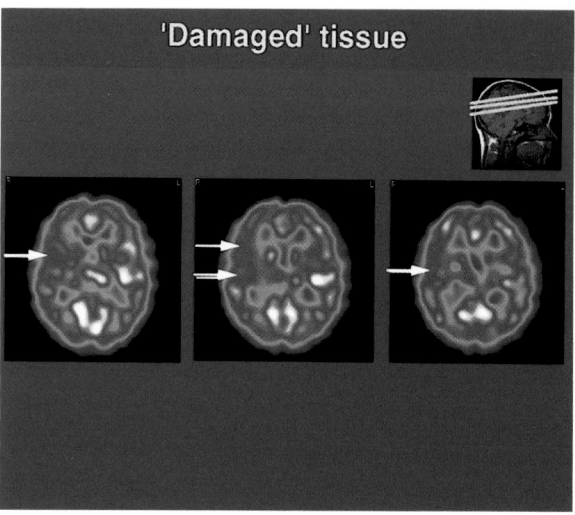

Figure 4 A male aged 23 who was assaulted, and was conscious on admission to hospital (GCS=14). Acute MR demonstrated a thin right frontal subdural haematoma. Left, SPECT imaging at 8 days post injury shows regions of mild hyperaemia (arrowed) underlying the haematoma; right, at six months post injury, the region that was previously hyperaemic has become mildly hypoperfused (arrowed). Although the patient had made a good recovery, he still complained of tiredness and had moderate impairment on visuo-spatial measures (block design and object assembly)

Change over time in a patient with a diffuse injury is shown in Figure 6. This patient was a young man who was assaulted and was in coma on admission to hospital. Acute MR imaging in this patient was normal, thus strongly suggesting that the underlying pathology was diffuse axonal injury. As can be seen, there was low blood flow in frontal regions at 2 weeks post injury; this blood deficit persisted at 3 months post injury. It is particularly interesting that the recovery in this case was delayed, and that there was major change

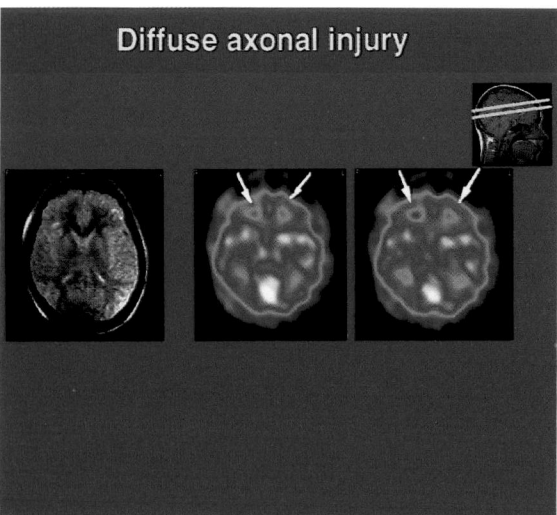 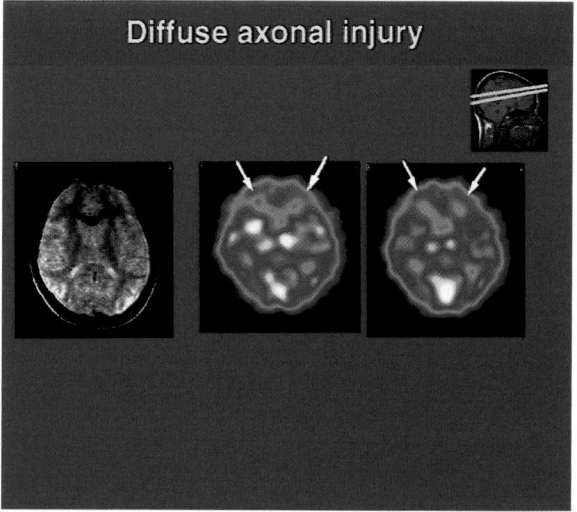

Figure 5 A male aged 36 who was assaulted and who was unconscious on admission. The patient remained in coma for 9 weeks after injury. MR at 5 days post injury shows small lesions in the frontal lobes. Left, SPECT shows marked hypoperfusion in frontal regions (arrowed). The patient was conscious, but severely disabled at follow-up at 5 months. He was unable to walk, was very confused, and had periods of agitation. Right, SPECT imaging at 5 months again demonstrated low blood flow in frontal regions (arrowed). The patient died at 7 months post injury and autopsy showed that diffuse axonal injury was the main pathology

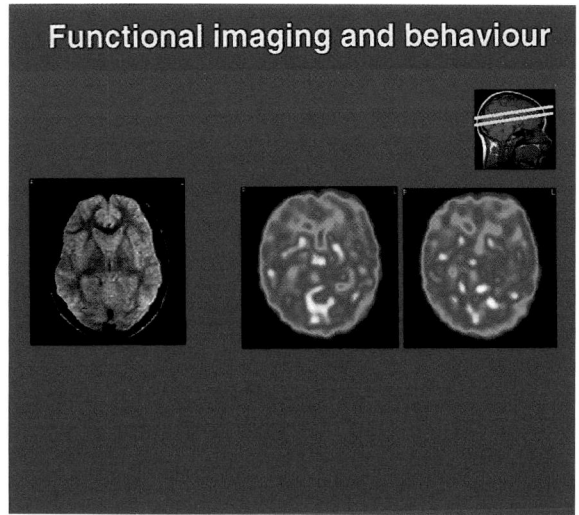
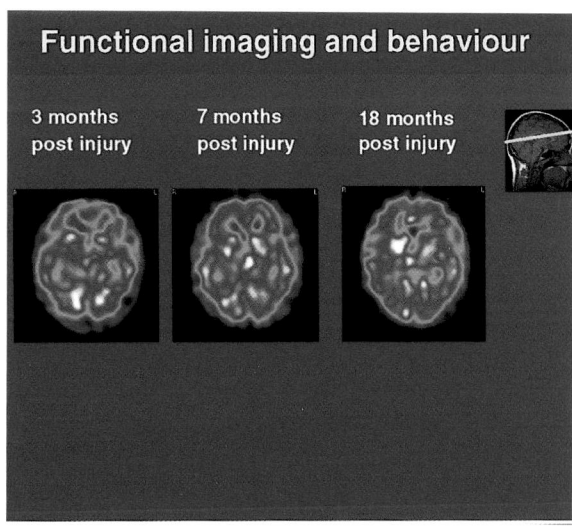

Figure 6 A male aged 19 who was assaulted and was unconscious on admission (GCS=6). MR imaging was normal. Serial SPECT images are shown at 2 weeks (left), 3 months, 7 months and 18 months (right) after injury. At two weeks post injury, low blood flow is particularly apparent in frontal regions. The blood flow pattern at 3 months post injury is quite similar to the acute image. At this time the patient was conscious, but severely disabled; he had periods of agitation and hostility. By 7 months, blood flow in frontal regions is substantially restored, although there is still a blood flow abnormality in the right medial frontal region. There was a corresponding improvement in his clinical state between 3 and 7 months. At 7 months it was reported by relatives that his personality had changed, but he showed little cognitive impairment apart from mental slowing. Follow-up at 18 months indicated a deteriorating clinical picture: the patient has been involved in a series of delinquent acts, and required 24 h supervision. SPECT imaging at 18 months is similar to imaging at 7 months

between 3 and 7 months. We interpret this as evidence that in diffuse axonal injury there are processes underlying brain recovery that can restore input to cortical regions late after injury.

Acknowledgement

This work was supported by the Wellcome Trust.

References

1   Hadley, D.M., Teasdale, G.M., Jenkins, A. *et al.* Magnetic resonance imaging in acute head injury. *Clin. Radiol.* 1988, 39, 131

2   Snow, R.B., Zimmerman, R.D., Gandy, S.E. and Deck, M.D.F. Comparison of magnetic resonance imaging and computed tomography in the evaluation of head injury. *Neurosurgery* 1986, 18, 45

3   Abdel-Dayem, H.M., Sadek, S.A., Kouris, K. *et al.* Changes in cerebral perfusion after acute head injury: Comparison of CT with Tc-99m HMPAO SPECT. *Radiology* 1987, 165, 221

4   Wiedmann, K.D., Wilson, J.T.L., Wyper, D. *et al.* SPECT cerebral blood flow, MR imaging and neuropsychological findings in traumatic head injury. *Neuropsychology* 1989, 3, 267

5   Choksey, M.S., Costa, D.C., Iannotti, F. *et al.* 99TCm-HMPAO SPECT studies in traumatic intracerebral haematoma. *J. Neurol. Neurosurg. Psychiatry* 1991, 54, 6

6   Bullock, R., Sakas, D., Patterson, J. *et al.* Early post-traumatic cerebral blood flow mapping: Correlation with structural damage after focal injury. *Acta Neurochirurgica (Wien)* 1992, 55, 14

7   Roper, S.N., Mena, I., King, W.A. *et al.* An analysis of cerebral blood flow in acute closed head injury using technetium-99m-HMPAO-SPECT and computed tomography. *J. Nucl. Med.* 1991, 32, 1684

8   Nedd, K., Sfakiankis, G., Ganz, W. *et al.* 99mTc-HMPAO SPECT of the brain in mild to moderate traumatic brain injury patients: compared with CT - a prospective study. *Brain Injury* 1993, 7, 469

9   Wilson, J.T.L. and Mathew, P. SPECT in head injury in 'SPECT imaging of the brain', (Ed. R. Duncan), Kluwer Academic, Dordrecht, 1997, p.69

10 Wilson, J.T.L., Hadley, D.M., Scott, L.C. and Harper, A. The neuropsychological significance of contusional lesions indentified by MR imaging in 'Recovery after traumatic brain injury', (Eds. B.P. Uzzell, H.H. Stonnington), Lawrence Erlbaum, Hillsdale, NJ, USA, 1996, p.29

11 Jacobs, A., Put, E., Ingels, M. and Bossuyt, A. Prospective evaluation of technetium-99m-HMPAO SPECT in mild and moderate traumatic brain injury. *J. Nucl. Med.* 1994, 35, 942

12 Overgaard, J. and Tweed, W.A.. Cerebral circulation after head injury. Part 1: Cerebral blood flow and its regulation after closed head injury with emphasis on clinical correlations. *J. Neurosurg.* 1974, 41, 531

13 Obrist, W.D., Marion, D.W., Aggarwal, S. and Darby, J.M. Time course of cerebral blood flow and metabolism in comatose patients with acute head injury. *J. Cereb. Blood Flow Metab.* 1993, 13(1), 5571

14 Uzzell, B.P., Obrist, W.D., Dolinskas, C.A. and Langfitt, T.W. Relationship of acute CBF and ICP findings to neuropsychological outcome in severe head injury. *J. Neurosurg.* 1986, 65, 630

15 Fumeya, H., Ito, K., Yamigawa, O. *et al.* Analysis of MRI and SPECT in patients with acute head injury. *Acta Neurochirurgica (Wien)* 1990, 51, 283

16 Sakas, D.E., Bullock, M.R., Patterson, J., Hadley, D. *et al.* Focal cerebral hyperaemia after focal head injury in humans: a benign phenomenon? *J. Neurosurg.* 1995, 83, 277

17 Adams, J.H., Doyle, D., Ford, I. *et al.* Diffuse axonal injury in head injury: definition, diagnosis and grading. *Histopathology* 1989, 15, 49

18 Gentry, L.R., Godersky, J.C. and Thompson, B. MR imaging of head trauma: Review of the distribution and radiopathologic features of traumatic lesions. *Am. J. Neuroradio.* 1988, 9, 101

19 Prayer, L., Wimberger, D., Oder, W. *et al.* Cranial MR imaging and cerebral ^{99m}Tc HMPAO-SPECT in patients with subacute or chronic severe closed head injury and normal CT examinations. *Acta Radiologica* 1993, 34, 593

20 Wilson, J.T.L. and Wyper, D. Neuroimaging and neuropsychological functioning following closed head injury: CT, MR and SPECT. *Head Trauma Rehab.* 1992 7, 29

21 Ichise, M., Chung, D.G., Wang, P. *et al.* Technetium-99m-HMPAO SPECT, CT and MRI in the evaluation of patients with chronic traumatic brain injury - A correlation with neuropsychological performance. *J. Nucl. Med.* 1994, 35(2), 217

22 Goldenberg, G., Oder, W., Spatt, J. and Podreka, I. Cerebral correlates of disturbed executive function and memory in survivors of severe closed head injury: A SPECT study. *J. Neuro. Neurosurg. Psychiatry* 1992, 55, 362

23 Oder, W., Goldenberg, G., Spatt, J. *et al.* Behavioural and psychosocial sequelae of severe closed head injury and regional cerebral blood flow: A SPECT study. *J. Neurol. Neurosurg. Psychiatry* 1992, 55, 475

Section

10

Specific Applications

SPECT in Neurology and Psychiatry, edited by P.P. De Deyn, R.A. Dierckx, A. Alavi and B.A. Pickut
© 1997 John Libbey & Company Ltd, pp. 433–446

Functional Neuroimaging and Chronic Fatigue Syndrome

Chapter

52

K. Audenaert, L. Lambrecht*, C. Van de Wiele,
K. Osmanagaoglu, P.P. De Deyn** and R.A. Dierckx

Introduction

Chronic fatigue syndrome (CFS) is defined as a chronic disabling illness with both somatic and neuropsychological symptoms in the absence of other known medical conditions that may cause chronic fatigue states[1]. Descriptions of syndromes combining severe chronic fatigue, fever, diffuse pain and other complaints, often preceded by an infectious disease and worsened by physical and emotional influences, appeared in the literature more than two centuries ago[2]. Beard[3] introduced the name 'neurasthenia' in 1880. A possible aetiological agent was proposed by Isaacs[4] in 1948 in reporting on a subset of patients recovering from mononucleosis infectiosa having fatigue and exhaustion for a period of three months to four years. In the UK, after an epidemic of unknown origin in the Royal Free Hospital in London in 1955, patients with symptoms of muscle pain and fatigue were described as suffering from 'benign myalgic encephalomyelitis', later abbreviated as 'myalgic encephalomyelitis'[5,6]. A series of names was introduced in the literature, some of them referring to an epidemiological clue, e.g. Iceland disease[7,8] or Yuppie Flu[9], others referring to a possible aetiopathogenesis, e.g. post-viral fatigue syndrome[10], chronic active Epstein-Barr virus infection syndrome[11] or chronic fatigue and immune dysfunction syndrome[4].

Being confronted with an entangling constellation of symptoms and a lack of objective case definition and even a lack of uniform denomination, the Centres of Disease Control (CDC) in Atlanta formulated a working case definition of CFS for research purposes, without making assumptions about its aetiology[1]. The definition relied entirely on a combination of symptoms and signs, not on laboratory data, and on the exclusion of chronic active organic or psychiatric illness that can produce chronic fatigue (Table 1). In 1991, the National Institutes of Health refined the generalising diagnostic criteria of CFS. Instead of excluding all psychiatric conditions, it was recommended to exclude only schizophrenia, bipolar disorder, psychotic depression and substance abuse, and to include other affective and anxiety disorders as well as somatisation disorder. The major and minor inclusion criteria remained essentially unchanged[12]. In 1994, a new set of criteria from the Centres of Disease Control was published. Recommendations for the clinical evaluation of fatigued persons (Table 2) and a revised case definition of the chronic fatigue syndrome (Table 3) were presented. Changes in definition included the disappearance of the '50%' reduction in activity in the major criteria and the elimination of some somatic symptoms in the minor criteria of chronic fatigue syndrome and the introduction of an 'idiopathic chronic fatigue' as a separate diagnostic class. A strategy for subgrouping fatigued persons in formal investigations was presented. Research

Division of Nuclear Medicine, University Hospital of Ghent, Belgium
*Outpatient Internal Medicine Clinic, Ghent, Belgium
**Department of Neurology, Middelheim Hospital and University of Antwerp and Born-Bunge Foundation, UIA, Antwerp, Belgium

Table 1 Diagnostic criteria for chronic fatigue syndrome

Major criteria (both required for diagnosis)

1. New onset of persisted or relapsing, debilitating fatigue or easy fatigability in a person who has no previous history of similar symptoms, which do not resolve with bedrest and which are severe enough to reduce or impair average daily activity below 50% of the patient's premorbid activity level for a period of at least six months
2. Exclusion of other illnesses that cause fatigue

Minor criteria

Presence of 8 of 11 symptoms listed or 6 of 11 symptoms and 2 of the 3 signs listed

Symptoms

1. Mild fever - oral temperature between 37.5°C and 38.6°C, if measured by the patient - or chills
2. Sore throat
3. Painful lymph nodes in the cervical or axillary distribution
4. Unexplained generalised muscle weakness
5. Muscle discomfort or myalgia
6. Prolonged fatigue (24 h or greater) after previously easily tolerated exercise
7. Generalised headaches (of a type, severity, or pattern that is different from headaches in the premorbid state)
8. Migratory arthralgia without joint swelling or redness
9. Neuropsychological complaints (one or more of the following: photophobia, transient visual scotoma, forgetfulness, excessive irritability, confusion, difficulty thinking, inability to concentrate, depression)
10. Sleep disturbances (hypersomnia or insomnia)

Description of the main symptom complex as initially developing over a few hours to a few days

Physical criteria (must be documented by a physician on at least two occasions, at least one month apart)

1. Low grade fever
2. Non-exsudative pharyngitis
3. Palpable or tender cervical or axillary lymph nodes

(Adapted from reference 1)

cases can be subgrouped by the presence or absence of the following essential parameters: 1) co-morbid conditions, 2) current level of fatigue, 3) duration of fatigue and 4) current level of physical function[13]. In 1996, Komaroff *et al.*[14] analysed the experience from a large centre to examine the adequacy of the CDC case definition. It was concluded that patients meeting the major criteria of the current CDC working case definition of CFS reported symptoms that were clearly distinguishable from the experience of healthy control subjects and from disease comparison groups with multiple sclerosis and depression. Eliminating three symptoms (i.e. muscle weakness, arthralgias and sleep disturbance) and adding two others (i.e. anorexia and

Table 2 Initial clinical evaluation of prolonged or chronic fatigue

A. History and physical examination

B. Mental status examination (abnormalities require appropriate psychiatric, psychological, or neurological examination)

C. Tests

1. Screening lab tests: complete blood count, erythrocyte sedimentation rate, alanine aminotransferase, total protein, albumin, globulin, alkaline phosphatase, calcium, phosphorus, glucose, blood urea nitrogen, electrolytes, creatinine, thyroid stimulating hormone and urinalysis

2. Additional tests as clinically indicated to exclude other diagnoses

Table 3 Diagnostic criteria for chronic fatigue syndrome or idiopathic chronic fatigue

Classify case as either chronic fatigue syndrome or idiopathic chronic fatigue if fatigue persists or relapses for ≥6 months

A. Classify as chronic fatigue syndrome if:

a.   there is a clinically evaluated, unexplained, persistent or relapsing fatigue that is of new or definite onset (has not been lifelong); is not the result of ongoing exertion; is not substantially alleviated by rest; and results in substantial reduction in previous levels of occupational, educational, social, or personal activities, and

b.   four or more of the following symptoms are concurrently present for ≥6 months:

1.   impaired memory or concentration
2.   sore throat
3.   tender cervical or axillary lymph nodes
4.   muscle pain
5.   multi - joint pain
6.   new headaches
7.   unrefreshing sleep
8.   post-exertion malaise

B. Classify as idiopathic chronic fatigue if fatigue severity or symptom criteria for chronic fatigue syndrome are not met

---

nausea) would appear to strengthen the CDC case definition of CFS.

Other case definitions for the syndrome have been developed by British[15] and Australian[16] investigators. There are a number of similarities with the CDC definition, such as the requirement of substantial functional impairment in addition to the complaint of fatigue. On the other hand, differences are apparent as well. For example, the American criteria attach particular significance to somatic symptoms, reflecting the idea that an infectious and/or immune process underlies CFS. In contrast, the British definition does not emphasise somatic symptoms, but insists instead on both physical and mental fatigue and fatigability[17].

Epidemiological data

Fatigue as a symptom is considered to be a common complaint in developed countries, as shown in both community surveys and in general practice reports. In a large community survey, 20% of men and 25% of women 'always feel tired'[18]. Buchwald[19] found 20% of patients in general practice reporting suffering from fatigue. Lane[20] found 30% of people with the complaint of chronic fatigue to satisfy the CDC-criteria[20]. The point prevalence of patients with CFS in primary care or community surveys ranges from 2 to 560 per 100000 population[21,22]. A possible explanation for these discrepancies is the fact that many subjects who fulfil operational criteria are not labelled as such by themselves or by their general practitioners[22].

Chronic fatigue syndrome can affect both men and women of all ages, races and socio-economic classes. Some studies[23-25], found a female predominance, others found an equal gender ratio[16,21]. Recently, Levine[26] reported a peak age incidence of 40-49 years. However, diagnosis of CFS in children and adolescents has been reported and seems even to be underestimated as the CDC criteria do not specifically fit for children[27]. Most studies showed that CFS patients visiting specialists are more likely to come from upper socio-economic strata, although there is no evidence of any excess of higher socio-economic status with fatigue, chronic fatigue or CFS in the community or in primary care settings[17]. Also, systematic surveys do not provide support for the idea that health care workers are more vulnerable to chronic fatigue or CFS[17]. No consistent explanation for the above stated epidemiological variables can be given.

Chronic fatigue has a substantial impact, at both individual and socio-economic levels. Twenty-six per cent of patients who were admitted for tiredness said it forced them to restrict their normal activities[28]; 28% of patients with chronic fatigue have been completely bedridden at some stage[29]. Patients may become bedridden, housebound, unable to work and alienated from their families, friends and colleagues. On the socio-economic level, these patients consume vast resources from both the health care and social security systems[30,31]. The mean number of visits to a doctor in one year is 14 to 19 visits[32]. Fifty to sixty per cent of CFS patients were unemployed and 23 to 38% received

Table 4 Excluding other illnesses

Malignancies

Auto-immune diseases

Localised infections

Chronic or subacute bacterial infections (such as endocarditis, Lyme, tuberculosis)

Fungal diseases (such as histoplasmosis, blastomycosis, coccidiodomycosis)

Parasitic infections (such as toxoplasmosis, amoebiasis, giardiasis)

HIV-related diseases

Chronic inflammatory diseases (such as sarcoidosis, Wegener's granulomatosis, chronic hepatitis)

Neuromuscular diseases (such as myasthenia gravis, multiple sclerosis)

Endocrinal diseases (such as hypothyreosis, Addison's disease, Cushing's syndrome, diabetes mellitus)

Chronic medication or toxic products (such as beta-adrenergic receptor antagonists, interferon, pesticides, solvents)

Chronic psychiatric diseases (such as major depression, anxiety disorders, schizophrenia)

Addictions to alcohol and drugs

---

disability benefits[32]. One main reason for the high costs is the poor prognosis since most CFS patients remain functionally impaired for several years[33]. Hickie *et al.*[32] found a mean duration of illness of six to eight years[32].

Symptoms

Everyone has experienced acute fatigue and probably everyone has had periods of fatigue which are not explained by recent mental and physical challenges[18]. From that point of view, the first major criterion of the CDC strictly requires reduction in activity for at least six months. Many of the physical symptoms of chronic fatigue resemble classical physical symptoms of other diseases. For that purpose, the second of the required major criteria in diagnosing CFS is the exclusion of other illnesses that can cause fatigue. A list is presented in Table 4. Of the minor symptoms, between 90 and 100% of patients report loss of concentration and headache, at least 80 to 89% of patients report disturbed sleep and needing to sleep for long periods, muscle pain with activity and memory loss, at least 70 to 79% report muscle pain at rest, sore throat without common cold and 60 to 69% report joint pain and tender glands in neck. Percentages on post-exertion malaise were not available[32].

Aetiology

At one end of the continuum are those who believe the illness is a purely physical condition, most likely due to infection with a novel infectious agent. At the other end are those who believe that all the symptoms of the illness are due to an unrecognised and untreated underlying primary psychiatric disorder.

Viral infection

A viral aetiopathogenesis can be hypothesised because onset of CFS may follow initial infection or illness, often of a respiratory or gastrointestinal nature[34]. A number of infectious agents were proposed as aetiological agents of CFS, including Epstein-Barr virus[1,35], cytomegalovirus, human herpesvirus 6[36], enterovirus, in particular Coksackie B[37], and retrovirus, in particular human T lymphotropic virus-II[38]. Epstein-Barr virus was strongly suggested as the cause of CFS until it was demonstrated that the incidence of positive serological antibody tests to the Epstein-Barr virus in patients with CFS could not be distinguished from age and gender matched controls[1,35]. In summary, although controlled studies of seroepidemiology have not demonstrated that viral infection is a tenable explanation for most cases of the syndrome, a role for persistent viral infection in the pathogenesis of the disorder has not been excluded definitively[18].

Immune dysfunction

Various abnormalities of immunological parameters in CFS patients have been published, but the reported abnormalities have been generally modest and inconsistent[22]. Abnormalities of both humoral and cellular immunity have been demonstrated[39]. Reduced natural killer cell function is perhaps the most consistently reproducible immunological abnormality, and is similar to findings reported in patients with major depression[40]. However, these abnormalities have not been shown to bear any relationship to the clinical severity of the chronic fatigue syndrome[18].

Neuromuscular pathophysiology

A review of neuromuscular histopathology and function concluded that accumulated evidence revealed normal muscle function, supporting the view 'that the fatigue reported in CFS is central in origin, reflecting abnormal drive rather than peripheral failure of force generation'[41]. Plyoplys et al.[42] performed an electron-microscopic investigation of muscle mitochondria and found no difference between CFS patients and controls.

Neuroendocrine pathophysiology

The prominence of sleep, energy, mood and appetite symptoms in chronic fatigue points to the hypothalamus, which has a controlling function over these states, as a possible pathway to explain symptom generation in chronic fatigue syndrome. Laboratory studies have shown definite hypothalamic dysfunction governing water metabolism with abnormal excretion of a water load[43]. Research also indicates that patients with CFS may have reduced cortisol levels perhaps due to a deficiency in corticotrophin releasing factor[44]. Finally, serotonin pathways are known to be involved in the regulation of a number of hypothalamic functions and central 5 HT receptors were found to be upregulated in chronic fatigue syndrome patients[45].

Psychiatric hypothesis

In a population of patients, consulting for chronic fatigue, Manu[46] found 39/100 of cases to be depressed. High prevalence rates of lifetime major depression in CFS patients were reported. For instance, Gold et al.[47] found that CFS patients in 73% of cases had periods of depression compared with 22% in healthy controls. Hickie et al.[48] diagnosed depression in patients with CFS in 22/48 (46%) of the cases and found a depression preceding the CFS episode in 6/48 (13%) cases. Also, high prevalence rates of panic disorder, ranging between 41%[49] and 82%[20], and somatisation disorder[20], were reported in CFS. Fischler[22] found a significant difference between the prevalence of generalised anxiety disorder (p<0.001) and somatisation disorder (p=0.002) in CFS population compared with medical controls. The psychiatric hypothesis consists of denying the mere existence of CFS as a separate condition and in considering these patients to suffer from major depression, panic disorder or somatisation disorder[22]. Although there is evidence for certain overlap, there are some clear distinctions between major depression and CFS. Hypotheses that depression represents merely a normal reaction to illness burden was criticised on the grounds that three controlled studies of CFS using chronic medical illnesses with similar illness burden (multiple sclerosis, neuromuscular disorder, rheumatoid arthritis) found a higher level of depression in CFS[22,49-51]. Evidence is emerging that psychiatric illness often predates, or is concurrent with, the development of chronic fatigue syndrome[52,53].

Limbic hypothesis

Goldstein[54] introduces the hypothesis that CFS is a consequence of a 'limbic encephalopathy'. The limbic system should be viewed as a higher order, sophisticated regulatory system responding to a wide variety of inputs. Diffuse projection systems can be modulated rapidly in this manner. Goldstein explains all symptoms of CFS by a dysfunction of the limbic system.

Diagnosis

The discrepancy between patients' symptoms and objective findings on physical and neuropsychiatric examination has given rise to long debates in the literature[9,25,55]. Up to now the diagnosis of CFS is based on the recognition of a constellation of symptoms and signs, along with the exclusion of other illnesses [15,16,56]. At present, the diagnosis of CFS is made predominantly on clinical grounds, although serological and immunological correlates of the disease continue to be investigated. However, the non-specific and subjective nature of the symptoms, as well as the absence of a proved causal agent or characteristic pathological abnormality, makes the condition difficult to diagnose[57].

Laboratory tests

Laboratory tests are performed for exclusion of other illnesses and in order to find elements to substantiate the diagnosis of CFS. A list can be proposed, see Table 5.

Table 5 Laboratory test for patients with suspected chronic fatigue syndrome

Full blood cell count

Routine biochemistry analysis

Blood glucose

Erythrocyte sedimentation rate/plasma viscosity

Thyroid function tests

Chest X-ray

Antibody titres:

   antinuclear factor

   rheumatoid factor

Lyme disease

hepatitis A and B

cytomegalovirus

toxoplasma gondii

influenza virus A and B

adenovirus

Coxsackie B virus

Pituitary-adrenal axis dysfunction (cortisol, ACTH, aldosterone)

Immunological status (C3, C4, IL-1, IL-2, CD4%, CD8%, NK%)

(Adapted from reference 18)

Neuropsychological assessment

Neuropsychological assessments have demonstrated marked disturbance of cognitive function, but these have been inconsistent and contradictory. Joyce *et al.* recruited 20 patients with CFS and 20 normal controls to test for neuropsychological functioning. Patients with CFS were impaired, predominantly in the domain of memory, on tests of spatial span, on spatial working memory and a selective reminding condition of the pattern-location association learning test. They performed normally on tests of spatial and pattern recognition memory, simultaneous and delayed matching to sample and pattern-location association learning test. Psychomotor performance is known to be impaired in depression and the effects of depression on neuropsychological functioning may be responsible for at least part of the deficits seen in CFS[59]. Grafman[60]

found that the neuropsychological deficits in CFS were strongly correlated with the severity of mood disturbance.

Neurophysiology and neuroimaging

Polysomnographic findings in a group of patients with CFS were compared with those found in healthy controls. Sleep initiation and sleep maintenance disturbances were observed in the CFS group. The percentage of stage 4 was significantly lower in the CFS group (p=0.001). Sleep onset latency contributed significantly to the discriminating function (p<0.001). Fischler stated that it is unknown whether polysomnographic disturbances in CFS are merely the expression of co-existent conditions or whether they are specific for CFS[22]. Twenty-one ambulatory patients with prominent sleep disorders underwent both HMPAO SPECT and polysomnography. Results were compared with 20 age-matched, healthy volunteers. The series presented suggested the absence of a correlation between polysomnography data and SPECT scan findings in ambulatory patients suffering from CFS[61]. Discrepancies have been found in multi-modal sensory evoked potentials and auditory event related cognitive potentials[62,63]. In conclusion, no pathognomonic signs or diagnostic tests for this condition have been identified.

Neuroimaging

Based on the symptom complex, hypothetically, the brain may be the major seal of disease involvement. Hence, an organic component in the pathogenesis of CFS can be suspected, providing evidence for functional impairment of the brain in CFS. Single photon emission computed tomography allows sensitive exploration of functional brain changes. CT findings are generally normal, but MR abnormalities have been reported. These are discussed below and compared with SPECT imaging.

SPECT imaging studies aimed at identifying: a (differential) diagnostic tool; an instrument for possible therapeutic follow-up; and a tool in pathophysiological research.

SPECT as a possible diagnostic tool

Assessing global and regional cerebral blood flow

Several authors have assessed global cerebral blood flow. Ichise *et al.*[56] studied 60 CFS patients (CDC criteria), compared with 14 normal control subjects. A significantly lower global regional cerebral blood flow (p<0.04) was found in CFS patients[56]. This finding could be confirmed by Costa *et al.*[64] who demonstrated a general reduction in the brain perfusion ratios in all 24 patients of a pilot study (CDC criteria and British criteria)[64]. However Fischler[22], in a study of 16 CFS outpatients (modified CDC criteria) versus 19 major depressed inpatients and 20 healthy controls, did not find a global brain hypoperfusion. A possible explanation could be the large ROIs measured with a single-head camera as compared with more discrete areas assessed with three-head cameras. Some researchers assessed regional cerebral blood flow. The percentage of CFS patients with one or more regional perfusion defects were investigated. It is of great importance to give a correct definition of a defect when comparing studies. Ichise *et al.*[56] found that 48 of 60 (80%) subjects with CFS showed at least one or more regional CBF ratios two standard deviations below normal mean. Defects were described as mild in degree (80-90% of normal controls). Schwartz *et al.*[57], in a study of 16 CFS patients (CDC criteria, British and/or Australian criteria), reported SPECT abnormalities in 13 of 16 (81 %) cases versus 3 of 14 (21%) controls (p<0.01). SPECT defects were defined according to stringent criteria as a region of less than 60% of the maximum activity, greater than 1 cm in diameter, and spanning the full thickness of the cortex. Lambrecht *et al.*, in a study of 113 CFS outpatients found perfusion defects in 26/113 (23%) patients. The lower incidence of SPECT abnormalities in this series presented as compared with the 80%, found in Schwartz *et al.*[57] and Ichise *et al.*[56], may be explained by the bias of an ambulatory patient group, suggesting less severe disease activity. No definition of defect was given (Lambrecht *et al.* unpublished data). Fischler[22] did not find regional hypoperfusion compared with normals. Wyper[65] stated that SPECT did not show a consistent regional abnormality, but did show a greater inhomogeneity in cerebral blood flow in CFS patients compared with normals and non-CFS patients. In summary, some studies report on global cerebral hypoperfusion and most studies report one or more regional hypoperfusion areas, although this phenomenon is not specific for CFS.

The number of defects per patient

Schwartz *et al.* found 7.31±6.49 defects per patient versus 0.43±0.94 defects per control patient (p<0.001) in a smaller study of 16 CFS patients versus 15 controls[57] and 6.53±4.94 regional defects in CFS patients compared with 1.66±2.60 defects in controls (p<0.005) in a larger study of 45 CFS patients versus 38 healthy controls[66]. Lambrecht *et al.* found a mean of 1.5 defects per patient. The difference between Schwartz *et al.* and Lambrecht *et al.* is possibly attributable to the less severe disabled patients in the outpatient population of Lambrecht *et al.* (Lambrecht, unpublished data).

Left to right asymmetry in regional cerebral blood flow

Fischler[22] reported on a statistically significant right greater than left parietotemporal perfusion index asymmetry in CFS compared with major depression and healthy controls, both normalised to mean total ROI perfusion (p=0.001) and to maximum cerebellar activity (p=0.002).

Localisation of regional cerebral perfusion defects

Frontal cortex. Costa[64] reported on hypoperfusion in the frontal cortex (right and left, both p<0.0001). Ichise *et al.* found the left superomedial frontal lobe (p<0.001, 21/60), left superoposterior frontal lobe (p−0.006, 21/60), right superomedial frontal lobe (p<0.001, 19/60) and right infero-anterior frontal lobe (p=0.049, 19/60) to be among the most frequently affected regions. At least one or more abnormal regional CBF ratios were seen in the frontal cortex in 38/60 of the cases[56]. Schwartz *et al.* described

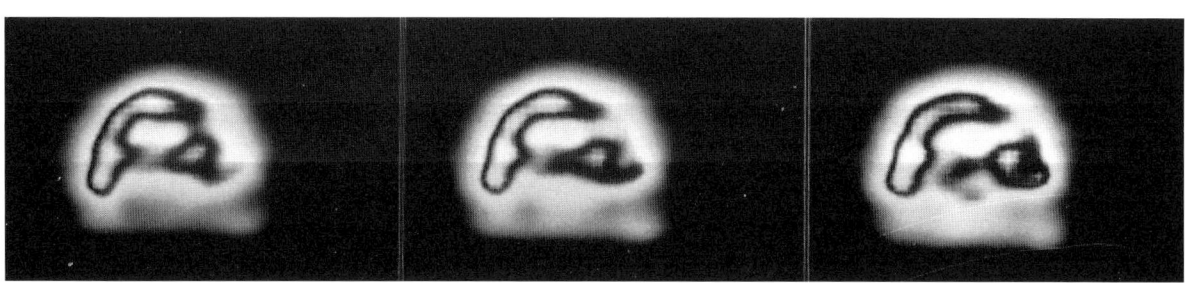

Figure 1 Transverse and coronal SPECT images of a 44 year old female CFS patient presenting with a Karnofsky Index between 50 and 60 (subgroup E) showing left temporoparietal hypoperfusion grade III (decreased activity between 40 and 100%)

significantly more defects than control subjects in the lateral frontal lobe (1.71±1.75 versus 0.21±0.66)[66] and found the hypoperfusion of the lateral frontal cortex to be significantly different from this one in control subjects (p<0.0005)[57]. Lambrecht et al. reported that the frontal lobe was affected in 6/113 of the cases (Lambrecht et al., unpublished data). Fischler[22] reported on a positive correlation between CFS and frontal regional cerebral blood flow.

Temporal cortex. Costa[64] reported on hypoperfusion in temporal lobes (right lateral p=0.009; right mesial p=0.0001; left lateral p=0.007; left mesial p=0.03). Ichise et al.[56] found that at least one or more abnormal regional CBF ratios were seen in the temporal cortex in 21/60 of cases. Schwartz et al. described significantly more defects in CFS in the lateral temporal lobe (1.67±1.73 versus 0.39±0.79) and medial temporal lobe (1.11±0.93 versus 0.42±0.64)[66] and found the hypoperfusion of the lateral temporal cortex to be significantly different from this one in control subjects (p<0.01)[57]. Lambrecht et al. reported that the left and right temporal lobes were affected in 15/113 and 6/113 of the cases, respectively (Lambrecht et al., unpublished data).

Parietal cortex. Costa[64] reported hypoperfusion in the parietal cortex (right p=0.001, left p=0.008). Ichise et al.[56] found that at least one or more abnormal regional CBF ratios were seen in the parietal cortex in 32/60 of cases. Lambrecht et al. reported that the parietal lobe was affected in 7/113 of the cases (Lambrecht et al., unpublished data).

Occipital cortex. Ichise et al.[56] found that at least one or more abnormal regional CBF ratios were seen in the occipital cortex in 23/60 of the cases. Lambrecht et al. reported that the occipital lobe was affected in only 4/113 of the cases (Lambrecht et al., unpublished data).

Deep nuclei. Costa et al.[64] reported on hypoperfusion in the thalamus (right p=0.001; left p=0.002) and in the nucleus caudatus (right p<0.0001; left p=0.001). Ichise et al.[56] found the basal ganglia (p<0.001, 20 cases) to be among the most frequently involved brain regions. They found at least one or more abnormal regional CBF ratios in the basal ganglia in 24/60 of cases. Schwartz et al.[57] found the hypoperfusion of the basal ganglia to be significantly different from the one in control subjects (p<0.02).

Brainstem. Costa et al.[64] was the only one to study and report hypoperfusion in brainstem. This finding is criticised by other research groups because the brainstem lies at the spatial resolution limit of SPECT[67]. Defining a brainstem region of interest involves the risk of incorporating the surrounding CFS spaces, which would lower the apparent count

density[68]. In conclusion, the greater part of the authors report on frontal hypoperfusion, although no specific findings for CFS can be shown. The brainstem hypoperfusion as a marker for CFS, suggested by Costa et al., is criticised by other authors.

Regional cerebral blood flow and clinical functioning

Fischler reported a significant positive correlation between CFS and frontal blood flow. In a group of 13 patients with both CFS and the exclusion of major depressive disorder, a significant positive correlation between Hamilton Depression Rating Scale[69] and right and left superofrontal perfusion index (both p=0.001) and left inferofrontal perfusion index (p=0.002) when normalising to maximal cerebellar perfusion was found. Fischler hypothesised that since the Hamilton Depression Rating Scale includes many somatic symptoms overlapping with CFS symptomatology, it is not proven that only depression is measured with Hamilton Depression Rating Scale; Hamilton total score can represent a composite of CFS intensity and depression. There is also a significant positive correlation between the self-rated items 'impairment in physical activities (CIS-2)' and the right superofrontal perfusion index (p=0.002) and between 'neuropsychological functioning (CIS-4)' and right superofrontal (p=0.004), right mediofrontal and left inferofrontal (p=0.001) perfusion index. Both CIS-2 and CIS-4 are subscales from the CIS Fatigue Scale[70]. Again it must be stated that this was found when normalising to maximal cerebellar perfusion. However, when normalising to total ROI, there were no significant data found for both the correlation between Hamilton and frontal regional perfusion index and CIS Fatigue Scale and frontal regional perfusion index. This can be explained by the fact that in the total ROI perfusion normalisation, the frontal activity is divided by the mean value including several regional perfusion indices which are moderately to highly correlated to Hamilton or CIS so that the correlations between frontal regional perfusion indices and these rating scales become weaker. Fischler found correlations between neuropsychological variables and left superofrontal perfusion index in a group of CFS patients without major depression. Significant correlations were found for the 'Memory for location test, fourth trial' and left superofrontal perfusion index (p=0.003) and for both the 'Buschke's selective reminding test, trial 8' and 'delayed recall' and the left superofrontal perfusion index (respectively, p=0.002 and p=0.001). These tests are indicators of attentional functions, immediate recall, visual and verbal memory. The direction of the association means higher frontal tracer uptake being related to greater neuropsychological impairment[22]. Lambrecht *et al.* showed that most pathological studies were found in the Karnofsky score C (14/26) and D (10/26)-subgroup. The Karnofsky scale can be interpreted as a clinical parameter reflecting disability, in which patients classified as 'B' are less affected than patients classified as 'D'. The concordance, in the group of patients presenting lesions, between number and severity of SPECT lesions and Karnofsky index suggests a possible clinical utility of brain SPECT. SPECT can reflect clinical disability, as scored on the Karnofsky scale[71]. Van De Wiele[61] reported on 21 ambulatory patients with prominent sleep disorders who underwent both HMPAO SPECT and polysomnography. Results were compared with 20 age-matched, healthy volunteers. The series presented suggested the absence of a correlation between polysomnography data and SPECT scan findings in ambulatory patients suffering from CFS.

Differential diagnostics

The most important differential clue is CFS versus depression, since for other diseases presenting with apparent CFS symptomatology, laboratory tests and paraclinical investigations do exist to differentiate.

Schwartz *et al.* performed SPECT scanning for distinguishing patients with CFS from patients with a virus-induced encephalitis (early AIDS dementia complex) and patients with unipolar major depression. Forty-five patients with CFS, 27 patients with AIDS dementia complex, 14 patients with unipolar major depression and 38 healthy controls were included. It should be noted that patients were not matched for age and gender in a way that the patients with unipolar major depression and the controls were significantly older (p<0.001) and that there were significantly more male patients (p<0.001) in the group with AIDS dementia complex. A defect was defined as a region of less than 60% of the maximum activity, greater than 1 cm in diameter, and spanning the full thickness of the cortex. The midcerebral uptake index (MCUI), an objective measurement reflecting radionuclide uptake in the brain, was a 1.5 cm slab centred at the thalamus; this slab included portions of the frontal, temporal, parietal, and occipital lobes, as well as the caudate nucleus and putamen. CFS was found to share some similarities on SPECT imaging with both AIDS dementia complex and unipolar major depression. The number of regional defects was significantly lower in controls (1.66±2.60) compared with patients with CFS (6.53±4.94; p<0.005) or unipolar major depression (6.43±5.61; p<0.005). The number of defects was significantly higher in patients with AIDS dementia complex (9.15±6.43; p<0.05) compared with patients

with CFS. Compared with normal subjects, all three groups had significantly more defects than control subjects in the lateral frontal, lateral temporal and medial temporal lobes. The major unipolar depression population also had significantly more defects in the occipital lobe and the AIDS dementia complex population also had significantly more defects in the medial frontal lobe, both compared with healthy controls. No comparison of number of localised defects was made between CFS population and, respectively, AIDS dementia complex population and unipolar major depression population. Defects may account for various cognitive and affective symptoms (depression, irritability and decreased memory and mental capacities) common to the patients in the three groups. The Midcerebral Uptake Index was significantly lower in CFS (0.667±0.06) and AIDS dementia complex (0.650±0.05) compared with the major unipolar depression (0.731±0.16) and healthy control (0.716±0.09) groups (p<0.002). There were significant differences in the Midcerebral Uptake Index between patients with CFS and control subjects (p<0.005) and depressed patients (p<0.025), but not between patients with CFS and AIDS dementia complex patients (p<0.8). The average counts per pixel in each midcerebral slab were similar in patients with CFS and AIDS dementia complex, and these values were both significantly reduced compared with those of control subjects (p<0.005). The difference between patients with CFS and depression did not reach significance (p<0.075). There was a significant negative correlation between the Midcerebral Uptake Index and the total number of regional defects in the CFS group (p<0.005) and the AIDS dementia complex group (p<0.025)[66]. Fischler found that the major depression group showed a significantly lower left superofrontal regional perfusion index compared with the CFS and the healthy controls group (p=0.001)[22]. This is in accordance with previous reports of superofrontal hypoperfusion in major depression[72,73]. This finding adds further evidence to the existence of biological differences reported between major depression and CFS[22]. Fischler reported on a statistically significant right greater than left parietotemporal perfusion index asymmetry in CFS compared with healthy control and major depression patients (p=0.001). In major depression, both the absence[74] and the presence of temporal asymmetry with iofetamine SPECT[6] were reported. Fischler[22] concluded that the asymmetry in the parietotemporal perfusion is not specific for CFS. Costa[64] found a strongly significant hypoperfusion in the brainstem in CFS patients when compared with normal volunteers (p<0.0001). He divided the total CFS population into a category of CFS patients without major depression or other psychiatric diseases, a category of CFS patients with major depression and a category of CFS patients with an other psychiatric disease. He compared these groups with both normal volunteers and depressed patients with respect to brainstem perfusion. He found statistically significant differences between all CFS patients of the three categories (p<0.0001; p=0.0002 and p=0.03, respectively) and normal controls, and found only statistical significance when comparing the CFS group without depression or other psychiatric disease and the group with depressed people (p<0.0001). There were no significant differences between the CFS group with depression and the CFS group with another psychiatric disease. There also appeared to be a slight significant brainstem hypoperfusion when comparing the depressed group with normals (p=0.04).

An important finding was that brainstem hypoperfusion appears to be the differentiating factor between CFS patients without and CFS patients with depression or other psychiatric disease.

Follow-up

Schwartz et al.[57] performed serial SPECT scans and MR imaging within a six month period in four patients. The second SPECT scan showed far fewer perfusion defects than did the first. The majority of the defects on the second scan were present on the initial study. No changes were noted over time on any of the MR images. Although the group of patients with repeated SPECT scans was very small, these findings may indicate that SPECT abnormalities are reproducible and appear to correlate more closely with overall clinical status.

SPECT compared with MRI

Schwartz compared MR imaging and SPECT on the detection of intracranial abnormalities in patients with CFS. Sixteen patients who fulfilled the criteria for CFS (CDC, British and/or Australian criteria) had MR and SPECT examinations within a 10 week period. Sixteen CFS patients and 15 age-matched controls were included for comparing, respectively, MR images and SPECT findings. MR abnormalities were considered only if they were of increased signal on both proton density and T_2 weighted images. SPECT defects were defined according to stringent criteria as a region of less than 60% of the maximum activity, greater than 1 cm in diameter, and spanning the full thickness of the cortex. The most frequent abnormal findings on MR examination in patients with CFS consisted of small foci of increased T_2 signal in the white matter, involving the centrum semiovale, the corona radiata, the internal capsule, the periventricular region, or the subcortical white matter (U fibres); occasionally, the

white matter near the basal ganglia was also involved. The cortex was of normal intensity in all cases. MR abnormalities were present in eight of 16 subjects, compared with three of 15 control subjects (p>0.1) The number of abnormal foci per patient, 2.06±2.54 in CFS patients versus 0.80±1.74 in control subjects, did not reach statistical significance (p>0.1). Patients with CFS had multiple perfusion defects throughout the cerebral cortex and basal ganglia. SPECT abnormalities were present in 13 of 16 patients versus three of 14 control patients (p<0.01). CFS patients had 7.31±6.49 defects per patient versus 0.43±0.94 defects per control patient (p<0.001). It can be concluded that SPECT scans showed more abnormalities than MRI scans did in patients with CFS. The location of abnormalities on the MR image did not correlate with the location of uptake defects on SPECT scans. On SPECT examination, more than 10 times as many defects as control subjects and defects were present in the vast majority (81%) of patients. These data indicate that SPECT may be more useful than MR in evaluating neurological abnormalities in CFS[66]. Lambrecht et al. found in a group of 30 CFS patients who underwent MRI that 3 patients showed a solitary focus of demyelinisation, respectively hippocampally, in the corona radiata and right frontally, whereas 2 patients showed multiple foci of demyelinisation. In the remaining 25 patients no abnormalities were found (Lambrecht et al., unpublished data). When comparing SPECT to MRI findings, Lambrecht et al. found 3 patients with a solitary focus on MRI whereas SPECT findings were normal. In 6 patients MRI was normal, whereas SPECT showed regions of hypoperfusion. In 2 patients, in whom both MRI and SPECT were abnormal, findings were discordant as to the localisation of the visualised lesions. This may suggest that both imaging techniques may reflect separate processes[75].

Aetiopathophysiological issues

Generally, cortical defects measured with SPECT may result from direct infection of neuroglial elements, from cellular dysfunction due to circulating cytokines, or from decreased flow through cortical arterioles owing to vasculitis[57]. The white matter abnormalities seen on MR images may represent foci of gliosis or chronic demyelinisation, which appear to be irreversible, whereas the cortical abnormalities on SPECT scans may reflect foci of neuronal dysfunction or transient regional hypoperfusion that may correlate with the changing clinical status of the patient[57]. As with any chronic inflammatory condition affecting the CNS, the T_2 bright foci on MR in CFS may represent a perivascular cellular infiltrate and/or reactive demyelinisation of the surrounding white matter[19]. Alternatively, these abnormalities may reflect the results of a vasculopathy specifically involving the small vessels of the cerebral white matter; indeed the distribution of lesions of MR in CFS is similar to that observed in occlusive arteriolar disease of any origin[57].

SPECT imaging resulted in testing some of the above stated aetiologic hypotheses

Viral hypothesis. By comparing SPECT imaging of CFS patients with AIDS related dementia complex and with major unipolar depression, both the viral and the psychiatric hypotheses could be tested. Schwartz et al.[66] hypothesised a direct viral infection in CFS comparable with the one in AIDS dementia complex, hereby supporting the viral hypothesis. This was hypothesised because the pathophysiological process in the central nervous system of patients with CFS would seem more similar to that in patients with AIDS dementia complex than that in patients with unipolar major depression. The Midcerebral Uptake Index values correlated with the regional defect count in the CFS and the AIDS dementia complex groups, but not in the depressed patients or control subjects. The similarity in the location and number of defects in patients with major unipolar depression and CFS may pertain to the clinical similarity of patients with these disorders; however the differences in Midcerebral Uptake Index between these conditions implies a qualitative difference in the pathophysiology of the CNS defects in the two conditions. The normal Midcerebral Uptake Index values in depressed patients militates against the presence of a diffuse inflammatory or vasculitis process. Focal abnormalities throughout the cortex in these patients may reflect decreased cortical activity in subcortical projection sites owing to reduced neurotransmitter release[76] without intrinsic cellular dysfunction[66]. The similarity in Midcerebral Uptake Index data between patients with AIDS dementia complex and CFS suggests a similar origin for the neurological dysfunction in these conditions. SPECT abnormalities in AIDS dementia complex are believed to be due to direct central nervous system infection by the HIV virus. Pathological studies have shown that HIV infection results in a subacute encephalitis characterised by demyelinisation and the presence of the virus in multinucleated giant cells, as well as in the endothelial cells, astrocytes and neurones distributed throughout the brain[77]. Although neuro-pathological data in CFS patients are unavailable, the above stated findings in CFS are consistent with the hypothesis that CFS also results from viral infection of neurones, glia or vasculature. Moreover, previous studies have suggested that EBV, enteroviruses, retroviruses or human herpesvirus 6 alone or in concert, may play a role in CFS. Viral infection can produce neuroglial dysfunction by interfering with intracellular mechanisms or membrane transport systems, by producing focal demyelinisation in association with circulating immune complexes or by cerebral hypoperfusion due to vasculitis[10].

Limbic hypothesis. Fischler reported the possible involvement of the frontal lobe in the pathogenesis of CFS. He hypothesised that as frontal areas are interconnected to the limbic system, limbic dysfunction could be involved in the association between frontal blood flow, neuropsychological functions and physical activities in CFS[22]. Limbic dysfunction has already been hypothesised to be of pathophysiological significance in CFS[54]. Lambrecht et al. hypothesised that the frequent involvement of the left temporal lobe is in agreement with previous reports on the location of regional cerebral perfusion abnormalities in CFS patients using both SPECT and PET (Lambrecht et al., unpublished data). The possible predominant involvement of the left temporal lobe in patients suffering from CFS may be further supported by the results obtained from visual and from auditory evoked brain mapping and neuropsychological evidence[54].

Mena et al.[78] reported on SPECT findings measuring rCBF using ^{133}Xe inhalation method and using HMPAO. They compared late life chronic fatigue syndrome with late life depression. CFS cortical abnormalities were found to be extensive in the right frontotemporal lobes in the projection of the limbic system, preferentially the hippocampus.

Resuming neuroimaging issues in SPECT, one can quote Fukuda and the CDC that there is no uniform modality in neuroimaging studies, including MRI and radionuclide scans (such as PET and SPECT) that can confirm or exclude the diagnosis of CFS[13].

Future neuroimaging research issues

From the above summarised literature, we became aware of some methodological problems that could be tackled in the future. One should: give a clear definition of 'perfusional defect'[56,57]; be cautious when using the cerebellum as a reference since PET studies in CFS patients have shown hypometabolism in the anterior cerebellum[54]; exclude major depressed patients when selecting the reference population since frontal hypoperfusion has been found in major depressive illness patients[68]; take into account whether the studied CFS population is an outpatient or an inpatient one since the gravity of the illness is correlated to neuroimaging issues (Lambrecht et al., unpublished data); clearly state whether or not the patient is taking medication.

Possible further efforts include: comparative studies of subjects who fulfil CFS criteria versus subjects with chronic fatigue secondary to other medical conditions since these can help in differentiating whether hypoperfusion is a result of a primary injury or whether hypoperfusion is a consequence of fatigue; neuropsychological testing and detailed assessment of symptoms on the day of MR or SPECT scanning in order to search for correlation between focal radiographic findings and specific clinical abnormalities[57]; longitudinal studies of patients with CFS to confirm the efficacy of SPECT in follow-up of the course of the illness since it was suggested by this group that SPECT defects could be replicated[57]; the use of FDG-PET to examine cerebral perfusion/metabolism in patients with CFS and those with major depression since glucose hypometabolism measured with PET and ^{18}F-FDG has been reported in CFS patients compared to normal and other patients with depression[64]; the use of receptor ligand studies since possible neurotransmitter deficiencies, e.g. the serotonin system are supposed[45]; activation studies using cognitively demanding tasks since performance deficits in CFS emerge on tasks requiring sustained mental effort[68].

References

1 Holmes, G.P., Kaplan, J.E., Gantz, N.M. *et al.* Chronic fatigue syndrome: a working case definition. *Ann. Intern. Med.* 1988, 108, 387

2 Manningham, R. in 'The symptoms, nature, causes, and cure of the febricula, or little fever', Robinson, London, 1750

3 Beard, G. in 'A practical treatise on nervous exhaustion (neurasthenia): its symptoms nature, sequences, treatment', William Wood, 1880

4 Dekker, M.J., Romkes, J.A. and Haveman, L.M. Het chronisch vermoeheidssyndroom/myalgische encefalomyelitis. Groningen: Wetenschapswinkel Geneeskunde en Volksgezondheid Groningen, 1994

5 The Medical Staff of the Royal Free Hospital. An outbreak of encephalomyelitis in the Royal Free Hospital Group, London, in 1955. *B.M.J.* 1957, 2, 895

6 Acheson, E. The clinical syndrome variously called benign myalgic encephalomyelitis, Iceland disease and epidemic neuromyasthenia. *Am. J. Med.* 1959, 4, 569

7 Levine, P.H., Jacobson, S. and Pocinki, A.G. *et al.* Clinical, epidemiologic, and virologic studies in four clusters of the chronic fatigue syndrome [see comments]. *Arch. Intern. Med.* 1992, 152, 1611

8 Sigurdsson, B., Sigurdsson, J. and Sigurdsson, H. A disease in Iceland simulating poliomyelitis. *Am. J. Hygiene* 1950, 52, 222

9 Palca, J. On the track of an elusive disease [news] [see comments]. *Science* 1991, 254, 1726

10 Behan, P., Behan, W. and Bell, E. The postviral fatigue syndrome-an analysis of the findings in 50 cases. *J. Infect.* 1985, 10, 211

11 Vereker, M.I. Chronic fatigue syndrome: a joint paediatric-psychiatric approach [see comments]. *Arch. Dis. Child.* 1992, 67, 550

12 Schluederberg, A., Straus, S.E., Peterson, P. *et al.* Chronic fatigue syndrome research, definition and medical outcome assessment. *Ann. Intern. Med.* 1992, 117, 325

13 Fukuda, K., Straus, S., Hickie, I. *et al.* The Chronic Fatigue Syndrome: a comprehensive approach to its definition and study. *Ann. Intern. Med.* 1994, 121, 953

14 Komaroff, A., Fagioli, L., Geiger, A. *et al.* An examination of the working case definition of CFS. *Am. J. Med.* 1996, 100, 56

15 Sharpe, M.C., Archard, L.C., Banatvala, J.E. *et al.* A report - chronic fatigue syndrome: guidelines for research. *J. R. Soc. Med.* 1991, 84, 118

16 Lloyd, A.R., Hickie, I., Boughton,C.R. *et al.* Prevalence of chronic fatigue syndrome in an Australian population. *Med. J. Aust.* 1990, 153, 522

17 Wessely, S. The epidemiology of Chronic Fatigue Syndrome. *Epidemiol. Rev.* 1995, 17, 139

18 Lane, R.M. Aetiology, diagnosis and treatment of chronic fatigue syndrome. *J. Serotonin Res.* 1994, 1, 47

19 Buchwald, D., Cheney, P.R., Peterson, D.L. *et al.* A chronic illness characterized by fatigue, neurologic and immunologic disorders, and active human herpesvirus type 6 infection [see comments]. *Ann. Intern. Med.* 1992, 116, 103

20 Lane, T.J., Manu, P. and Matthews, D.A. Depression and somatisation in the chronic fatigue syndrome [see comments]. *Am. J. Med.* 1991, 91, 335

21 Lawrie, S. and Pelosi, A. Chronic Fatigue Syndrome in the community. Prevalence and associations. *Br. J. Psychiatry* 1995, 166, 793

22 Fischler, B. Contribution to the study of the psychopathology and psychobiology of the chronic fatigue syndrome. Brussels: Brussels Free University, 1995

23 Behan, P. and Behan, W. Postviral fatigue syndrome. *Crit. Rev. Neurobiol.* 1988, 4, 157

24 Bates, D., Schmitt, W. and Buchwald, D. Prevalence of fatigue and chronic fatigue syndrome in a primary care practice. *Arch. Intern. Med.* 1993, 153, 2759

25 Gunn, W., Connel, D, and Randall, B. Epidemiology of chronic fatigue syndrome: the Centre for Disease Control Study in 'Chronic fatigue syndrome', (Eds. G.Bock and J.Whelan), John Wiley, Chichester, 1993, p.83

26 Levine, P. Section IX: Review of Research Conference. Epidemiology. *J. Chronic Fatigue Synd.* 1995, 1, 177

27 Bell, D. Diagnosis of Chronic Fatigue Syndrome in Children and Adolescents: Special Considerations. *J. Chronic Fatigue Synd.* 1995, 1, 29

28 Morrell, D. and Wale, C. Symptoms percieved and recorded by patients. *J. R. Coll. Gen. Pract.* 1976, 26, 398

29 Buchwald, D., Sullivan, J. and Komaroff, A. Frequency of 'chronic active Epstein-Barr virus infection' in a general medical practice. *J.A.M.A.* 1987, 257, 2303

30 David, A.S., Wessely, S. and Pelosi, A.J. Postviral fatigue syndrome: time for a new approach. *Br. Med. J. Clin. Res. Ed.* 1988, 296, 696

31 David, A.S., Wessely, S. and Pelosi, A.J. Chronic fatigue syndrome: signs of a new approach [see comments]. *Br. J. Hosp. Med.* 1991, 45, 158

32 Hickie, I., Lloyd, A., Hadzi-Pavlovic, D. *et al.* Can the chronic fatigue syndrome be defined by distinct clinical features? *Psychol. Med.* 1995, 25, 925

33 Wilson, A., Hickie, I., Lloyd, A. *et al.* Longitudinal study of outcome of chronic fatigue syndrome. *B.M.J.* 1994, 308, 756

34 Straus, S.E., Tosato, G. and Armstrong, G. Persisting illness and fatigue in adults with evidence of Epstein-Barr virus infection. *Ann. Intern. Med.* 1985, 102, 7

35 Hellinger, W.C., Smith, T.F., Van Scoy, R.E. *et al.* Chronic fatigue syndrome and the diagnostic utility of antibody to Epstein-Barr virus early antigen [see comments]. *J.A.M.A.* 1988, 260, 971

36 Mendelson, W. and Friedman, R. An overview of chronic fatigue syndrome. *J. Clin. Psychiatr.* 1991, 52, 403

37 Muir, P., Nicholson, F., Banatvala, J. and Bingsley, P. Coxsackie B virus and post viral fatigue syndrome. *B.M.J.* 1991, 302, 658

38 Khan, A., Heneine, W. and Chapman, L. *et al.* Assessment of a Retrovirus Sequence and other possible risk factors for the chronic fatigue syndrome. *Ann. Intern. Med.* 1993, 118, 241

39 Lloyd, A., Wakefield, D. and Hickie, I. Immunity and the pathophysiology of chronic fatigue syndrome in 'Chronic fatigue syndrome', (Eds. G.Bock and J.Whelan), John Wiley, Chichester, 1993

40 Stein, M., Miller, A.H. and Trestman, R.L. Depression, the immune system, and health and illness. Findings in search of meaning. *Arch. Gen. Psychiatry* 1991, 48, 171

41 Edwards, R., Gibson, H., Clague, J. and Helliwell, T. Muscle histopathology and physiology in chronic fatigue syndrome in 'Chronic fatigue syndrome', (Eds. G. Bock and J. Whelan), John Wiley, Chichester, 1993, p.102

42 Plyoplys, A. and Plyoplys, V. Electron-microscopic investigation of muscle mitochondria in chronic fatigue syndrome. *Neuropsychobiology* 1995, 32, 175

43 Bakheit, A.M., Behan, P.O., Watson, W.S. and Morton, J.J. Abnormal arginine-vasopressin secretion and water metabolism in patients with postviral fatigue syndrome. *Acta Neurol. Scand.* 1993, 87, 234

44 Demitrack, M.A., Dale, J.K., Straus, S.E. *et al.* Evidence for impaired activation of the hypothalamic-pituitary-adrenal axis in patients with chronic fatigue syndrome. *J. Clin. Endocrinol. Metab.* 1991, 73, 1224

45 Bakheit, A.M., Behan, P.O., Dinan, T.G. *et al.* Possible upregulation of hypothalamic 5-hydroxytryptamine receptors in patients with postviral fatigue syndrome [see comments]. *B.M.J.* 1992, 304, 1010

46 Manu, P., Matthews, D. and Lane, T. The mental health of patients with a chief complaint of chronic fatigue: a prospective evaluation and follow-up. *Arch. Intern. Med.* 1988, 148, 2213

47 Gold, D., Bowden, R., Sixbey, J. *et al.* Chronic fatigue: a prospective clinical and virologic study. *J.A.M.A.* 1990, 264, 48

48 Hickie, I., Lloyd, A., Wakefield, D. and Parker, G. The psychiatric status of patients with the chronic fatigue syndrome [see comments]. *Br. J. Psychiatry* 1990, 156, 534

49 Wood, G., Bentall, R., Gopfer, M. and Edwards, R. A comparative assessment of patients with chronic fatigue syndrome and muscle disease. *Psychol. Med.* 1991, 21, 619

50 Katon, W.J., Buchwald, D.S., Simon, G.E. *et al.* Psychiatric illness in patients with chronic fatigue and those with rheumatoid arthritis [see comments]. *J. Gen. Intern. Med.* 1991, 6, 277

51 Wessely, S., Butler, S., Chalder, T. and David, A. The cognitive behavioural management of the post-viral fatigue syndrome in 'Post-viral fatigue syndrome', (Eds. R.Jenkins and J.Mowbray) John Wiley, London, 1991

52 Manu, P., Matthews, D. and Lane, T. Depression among patients with a primary complaint of chronic fatigue. *J. Affect. Dis.* 1989, 17, 165

53 Taerk, G.S., Toner, B.B., Salit, I.E. *et al.* Depression in patients with neuromyasthenia (benign myalgic encephalomyelitis). *Int. J. Psychiatry Med* 1987, 17, 49

54 Goldstein, J. in 'Chronic fatigue syndromes, the limbic hypothesis', Haworth Medical Press, New York, 1993

55 Ray, C. Chronic fatigue syndrome and depression: conceptual and methodological ambiguities [editorial]. *Psychol. Med.* 1991, 21, 1

56 Ichise, M., Salit, I., Abbey, S. *et al* Assessment of regional cerebral perfusion by 99m Tc HMPAO SPECT in CFS. *Nucl. Med. Comm.* 1992, 13, 767

57 Schwartz, R., Komaroff, A., Garada, B. *et al.* SPECT Imaging of the brain: Comparison of findings in patients with chronic fatigue syndrome, AIDS Dementia Complex, and Major Unipolar Depression. *Am. J. Roent.* 1994, 162, 943

57 Schwartz, R., Garada, B., Komaroff, A. *et al.* Detection of intracranial abnormalities in patients with chronic fatigue syndrome: comparison of MR Imaging and SPECT. *Am. J. Roent.* 1994, 162, 935

58 Joyce, E., Blumenthal, S. and Wessely, S. Memory, attention, and executive function in chronic fatigue syndrome. *J. Neurol. Neurosurg. Psychiatr.* 1996, 60, 495

59 Robbins, T., Joyce, E. and Sahakian, B. Neuropsychology and imaging in 'Handbook of affective disorders', (Ed. E. Paykel), Churchill Livingstone, Edinburgh, 1992, p.298

60 Grafman, J., Schwartz, V., Dale, J.K. *et al.* Analysis of neuropsychological functioning in patients with chronic fatigue syndrome. *J. Neurol. Neurosurg. Psychiatry* 1993, 56, 684

61 Van De Wiele, C., Lambrecht, L., Osmanagaoglu, K. *et al.* Tc-99m HMPAO SPECT and polysomnography in 21 ambulatory patients suffering from chronic fatigue syndrome. *Acta Neurol. Belgica* 1995, 95, 86

62 Prasher, D., Smith, A. and Findley, L. Sensory and cognitive event related potentials in Myalgic Encephalomyelitis. *J. Neurol. Neurosurg. Psychiatr.* 1990, 53, 253

63 Scheffers, A. Attention and short term memory in chronic fatigue syndrome patients: an event related potential analysis. *Neurolog.* 1992, 42, 1667

64 Costa, D.C., Tannock, C. and Brostoff, J. Brainstem perfusion is impaired in chronic fatigue syndrome. *Q.J.M.* 1995, 88, 767

65 Wyper, D., Patterson, J., Aitchison, F. *et al.* SPECT imaging of the brain with chronic fatigue syndrome. *Acta Neurol. Belgica* 1995, 95, 85

66 Schwartz, R., Garada, B., Komaroff, A. *et al.* Detection of intracranial abnormalities in patients with chronic fatigue syndrome, AIDS Dementia Complex, and Major Unipolar Depression. *Am. J. Roent.* 1994, 162, 943

67 Patterson, J., Aitchison, F. and Wyper, D. SPECT brain imaging in chronic fatigue syndrome. *J. Immunol. Immunopharmacol.* 1995, 15, 53

68 Cope, H. and David, A. Neuroimaging in chronic fatigue syndrome. *J. Neurol. Neurosurg. Psychiatr.* 1996, 60, 471

69 Hamilton, M. Development of a rating scale for primary depressive illness. *Br. J. Soc. Clin. Psychol.* 1967, 6, 278

70 Vercoulen, J., Swaninck, C., Fennis, J. *et al.* Dimensional assessment of Chronic Fatigue Syndrome. *J. Psychosom. Res.* 1994, 5, 383

71 Troch, M., Lambrecht, L., Van De Wiele, C. *et al.* Brain perfusion SPECT findings and Karnofsky performance scale scores in 113 patients suffering from chronic fatigue syndrome. *Acta Neurol. Belgica* 1995, 95, 85

72 Mayberg, H., Lewis, P., Regenold, W. and Wagner, H. Paralimbic hypoperfusion in unipolar depression. *J. Nucl. Med. Comm.* 1994, 9, 397

73 Morinobu, S., Sagawa, K., Kawakatsu, S. *et al.* Regional cerebral blood flow in refractory depression. *Adv. Neuropsychiat. Psychopharmacol.* 1991, 2, 65

74 Maes, M., Dierckx, R. and Meltzer, H. *et al.* Regional cerebral blood flow in unipolar depression measured with 99m Tc HMPAO single photon computed tomography: negative findings. *Psychiat. Res. Neuroimag.* 1993, 50, 77

75 Osmanagaoglu, K., Lambrecht, L., Van De Wiele, C. *et al.* Tc 99m HMPAO SPECT and magnetic resonance imaging in 30 patients suffering from chronic fatigue syndrome. *Acta Neurol. Belgica* 1995, 95, 86

76 Coffey, C.E., Wilkinson, W.E., Weiner, R.D. *et al.* Quantitative cerebral anatomy in depression. A controlled magnetic resonance imaging study. *Arch. Gen. Psychiatry* 1993, 50, 7

77 Gray, F., Gherardi, R. and Scaravilli, F. The neuropathology of the acquired immune deficiency syndrome (AIDS). A review. *Brain* 1988, 111, 245

78 Mena, I., Goldstein, J., Jouane, E. and Lesser, I. Cerebral hypoperfusion in late life chronic fatigue syndrome and late life depression. *J. Nucl. Med.* 1993, 34, 210

SPECT in Neurology and Psychiatry, edited by P.P. De Deyn, R.A. Dierckx, A. Alavi and B.A. Pickut
© 1997 John Libbey & Company Ltd, pp. 447–453

SPECT and Central Nervous System Infectious Diseases

Chapter
53

R. Crols, J. Goeman, B.A. Pickut, R.A. Dierckx[*] and P.P. De Deyn[**]

Human immunodeficiency virus (HIV) infection

The central nervous system frequently becomes involved during the course of HIV infection and AIDS. The reasons for this involvement are multiple and they include opportunistic infections and opportunistic neoplasms as well as primary degenerative processes such as those encountered in AIDS dementia complex (ADC). Among the opportunistic infections, Toxoplasma gondii (toxoplasmosis) is the most common cause of focal encephalitis in patients with AIDS. Other infectious causes of focal encephalitis include bacterial, fungal, and viral infections (progressive multifocal leuko-encephalopathy).

AIDS dementia complex - HIV encephalitis

Diagnosis and staging of ADC

ADC, or HIV encephalitis, is a degenerative disease of the brain in HIV-infected subjects. It is characterised by a progressive cognitive deterioration accompanied later by motor dysfunction. The symptoms become predominant only late in the course of the disease, although subtle deterioration may preceed the full blown complex for a considerable period.

In 1985, months after the presentation of regional cerebral blood flow mapping with ^{99m}Tc-HMPAO, Ell *et al.*[1] published the first images of ^{99m}Tc-HMPAO SPECT scans of two HIV-1 infected individuals with cognitive disturbances. In both patients, this functional imaging technique provided more and earlier evidence of brain dysfunction than did CT scans. Figure 1 illustrates a ^{99m}Tc-HMPAO SPECT in a patient with ADC.

In a study by Pohl *et al.*[2], 12 patients with AIDS dementia complex varying in degree from mild to moderate, underwent ^{123}I-IMP SPECT and 4 of these also HMPAO SPECT. SPECT showed pathological findings in all patients, while computed tomographic (CT) scans were normal in four patients. Five patients had MRI of which two showed leukencephalopathy, which was not apparent on CT images. IMP SPECT showed multiple focal lesions in the cerebral cortex of six patients, while six other patients had isolated unilateral lesions. Additional HMPAO SPECT images showed HMPAO uptake defects in identical regions as IMP uptake defects in two patients and additional areas of reduced HMPAO uptake in two affected individuals. The authors concluded that, although the findings of IMP and HMPAO SPECT were not specific for AIDS encephalopathy, SPECT was a very sensitive method to show pathophysiological changes at an early stage.

Department of Neurology, General Hospital Middelheim, Lindendreef 1, B-2020 Antwerp, Belgium
[*]Department of Nuclear Medicine, University Hospital of Ghent, 9000 Ghent, Belgium
[**]Laboratory of Neurochemistry and Behaviour, Born-Bunge Foundation, University of Antwerp, Universiteitsplein 1, B-2610 Wilrijk, Belgium

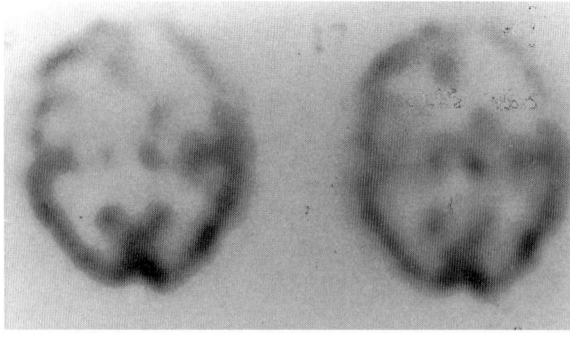

Figure 1 ^{99m}Tc-HMPAO SPECT in a patient with AIDS dementia complex. Oblique ^{99m}Tc-HMPAO SPECT slices showing multiple cortical and subcortical defects. Hypoperfusion of the frontal lobes, the left being more affected; hypoperfusion of the right temporal lobe; focal perfusion deficits of the right and left occipital lobes; hypoperfusion of the right thalamus

Kuni et al.[3] examined 7 patients with AIDS and 7 HIV-negative subjects with ^{123}I-IMP SPECT brain imaging. To quantitate regions of decreased ^{123}I-IMP uptake, pixel intensity histograms of normalised SPECT images of the basal ganglia level were analysed for the fraction of pixels in the lowest quartile of the intensity range. This fraction was significantly higher in AIDS patients than in HIV-negative subjects. Furthermore, a correlation existed between the neuropsychological performance, studied in 4 patients, and the pixel intensity distribution.

Tran Dinh et al.[4] demonstrated with ^{133}Xe-SPECT that cerebral locations of perfusion deficits varied greatly between individuals. Further, Maini et al.[5] demonstrated a cerebellar hypoperfusion in a patient with HIV infection.

Harris et al.[6] used ^{123}I-IMP SPECT to create a quantitative measure of inhomogeneity in HIV-seropositive subjects through estimation of variance frequencies in cortical profiles. The 8 seronegative controls were characterised by strong middle frequency and week high-frequency power. HIV-1-infected subjects with and also without dementia (9 and 10, respectively) showed a significant power shift from middle to high frequencies, indicating diffuse cortical perfusion changes compared with HIV-seronegative individuals.

Masdue et al.[7] studied the contribution of SPECT in differentiating between psychogenic mechanisms and HIV-encephalopathy in HIV-positive subjects with depression or psychosis. In most such cases, CT and MRI are unrevealing. They compared ^{123}I-IMP SPECT

scan results of 32 HIV positive patients, 15 non-AIDS patients with psychosis and 6 normal controls in a retrospective study. The degree of SPECT abnormalities (cortical and subcortical defects) correlated well with the degree of both cognitive and motor impairment.

[99m]Tc hexametazine brain SPECTs of five patients with different stages of AIDS dementia complex, ranging from mild to severe, revealed uptake defects , even in the early stages. The blood flow defects were more pronounced in the later stages. CT scans remained negative except in patients with the most advanced stages of dementia[8]. Fourteen of 20 HIV-infected patients without signs of dementia or severe neurological dysfunction proved to have pathological patterns of ^{99m}Tc-HMPAO uptake on their brain perfusion SPECT[9], suggesting that subtle changes in cerebral perfusion seem to arise early in the course of HIV infection.

Holman et al.[10] compared ^{99m}Tc-HMPAO SPECT scan results of 20 patients with ADC with SPECT scan images of 20 cocaine polydrug users and 20 normal control subjects. They observed very similar results among ADC patients and drug users, with 100 and 90%, respectively, showing cortical defects. Cortical defects were most frequent in the frontal, temporal and parietal lobes and no defects at all were observed in the primary visual cortex and the cerebellum. The mean number of cortical defects was also similar in AIDS dementia patients (10.0) and drug users (10.1), and was significantly greater than among the control subjects (0.7). Background activity was also similar among AIDS dementia patients (65%) and drug users (60%), and was significantly higher than among normal subjects (5%). Finally, AIDS dementia patients and drug users showed equal involvement of the basal ganglia: 40 and 65%, respectively. The authors concluded that brain perfusion SPECT from patients with ADC and from chronic drug users can not be distinguished from each other. Since intravenous drug use is a major risk factor for HIV-1 infection, such subjects may also be scanned for diagnosis of AIDS dementia complex. Caution should therefore be applied before making a specific diagnosis.

Sacktor et al.[11] compared ^{99m}Tc-exametazime SPECT scans of 20 HIV-positive patients, non-intravenous drug users (12 without cognitive deterioration and 8 with mild cognitive impairment) with similarly obtained SPECT scans from 10 HIV-negative subjects. An abnormal SPECT scan result was defined as the presence of two or more focal defects. Sixty-seven per cent of the HIV-positive individuals without cognitive impairment, and 80% of HIV-positive subjects with mild cognitive deterioration had abnormal SPECT scan results. The proportion of abnormal scans was higher in both groups of HIV-positive patients as compared with the proportion of abnormal results among HIV-negative controls, which accounted for 20%. The authors stressed that semiquantitative analysis using cortical region-of-interest/subcortical or cerebellar activity ratios could not be used because of the presence of focal defects within the subcortical structures and cerebellum. In a second study, the same authors[12] demonstrated that cerebral SPECT abnormalities correlated with impaired motor speed performance, which is often an early sign of ADC.

Physiopathology of focal SPECT abnormalities in ADC

The cause of the focal defects remains unclear. They may result from direct neuronal damage by HIV or toxic effects of enzymes and cytokines that are secreted by infected cells[4,13]. The SPECT abnormalities could also represent a neuroimaging marker of vascular inflammation such as cerebral vasculitis, which was demonstrated by Gray et al.[14,15] in asymptomatic HIV-positive patients.

Rubbert et al.[16] studied the correlation of the presence of antibodies to cardiolipin (ACA) with cerebral perfusion defects as demonstrated on ^{99m}Tc-HMPAO SPECT in HIV-1-infected subjects. Only 23.5% of patients with ACA had a normal brain perfusion pattern as compared with 82.4% of patients without ACA.

Geier et al.[17] proved a close association between severity of HIV-1 related ocular microangiopathic syndrome and severity of hypoperfusion in 28 HIV-1 infected patients, suggesting that intracerebral microvascular alterations might contribute to the pathogenesis of neurological symptoms.

Improvement with therapy

CNS infection is characterised histologically by the presence of multinucleated giant cells, reactive astrocytosis, microglial nodules, vacuolar myelopathy and vascular infarcts[18]. As antiretroviral treatment may ameliorate cognitive deterioration in HIV encephalopathy and may reduce the incidence of multinucleated cells (Vago et al.[19]), early diagnosis of CNS involvement may become very important.

Masdeu et al.[7] studied retrospectively the evolution of ^{123}I-IMP SPECT findings in four HIV-positive patients treated with zidovudine (AZT) who had serial SPECT examinations. Clinical amelioration following 6 to 8 weeks of AZT treatment was reflected by an improvement in the SPECT pattern as scored visually by two blinded nuclear medicine physicians. When therapeutic choices become available, SPECT might play an important role as a predictable and early test indicative of the brain's response to therapy[10].

Focal encephalitis in patients with AIDS

The majority of cases of focal encephalitis is caused by cerebral toxoplasmosis. CNS lymphoma is found with increasing frequency and is the second leading cause of focal CNS disease[20]. Other opportunistic bacterial, fungal, and viral infections make up the majority of cases. The differential diagnosis is particularly difficult, especially because lymphoma and toxoplasma encephalitis may have similar characteristics on CT and/or MRI.

SPECT contributes to the differentiation between toxoplasmosis and intracranial lymphoma, since MR imaging alone is not reliable for differentiation. Ganz et al.[21] and Vanarthos et al.[22] postulated the value of ^{201}Tl-SPECT for differentiating lymphoma from infectious processes in AIDS patients. Uptake of ^{201}Tl has been demonstrated in a number of tumours, including cerebral lymphomas[23,24]. O'Malley et al.[25] investigated 13 patients with AIDS and intracranial masses on MR imaging with ^{201}Tl-SPECT to find out whether SPECT could discriminate between neoplasm and opportunistic infection. Seven of these patients had marked increased uptake of ^{201}Tl in the region of the lesion seen on MRI and were interpreted as consistent with lymphoma. At biopsy, six were found to have lymphoma. The seventh patient, who showed increased uptake in one of three brain lesions, had a toxoplasmosis abcess surrounded by cytomegalovirus meningitis as well as scattered foci of Mycobacterium tuberculosis throughout the brain, as revealed on autopsy. The six patients without increased ^{201}Tl uptake were found to have a non-malignant cause for their lesions (four had toxoplasmosis, one PML and one had a venous angioma). Retrospective quantification of the uptake ratios showed a significantly higher uptake ratio in patients with a tumour, suggesting that the addition of quantification of the subjective image interpretation might improve the overall accuracy of diagnosis.

In the same year, Ruiz et al.[26] published the results of a prospective study on the use of ^{201}Tl brain SPECT to differentiate cerebral lymphoma from cerebral toxoplasmosis in 37 AIDS patients with CNS mass lesions on CT and/or MRI. In 12 patients the brain SPECT showed a positive ^{201}Tl uptake. The biopsies and results of autopsy were positive for primary brain lymphoma in each case. Twenty-five patients had no ^{201}Tl uptake. Twenty-four of these cases had positive serial serum antitoxoplasmosis antibodies and improved following introduction of antitoxoplasmosis treatment. One patient had a positive culture for Mycobacterium tuberculosis.

Acute viral encephalitis

Herpes simplex virus (HSV) infection

The diagnosis of herpes simplex virus encephalitis (HSVE) is based upon clinical symptoms and signs indicating temporal lobe dysfunction and the demonstration of a herpes virus infection. However, the clinical picture may be misleading and even brain biopsy may give a falsely negative result[27]. Because treatment is most effective when started early, a sensitive and specific method for early diagnosis is required. At this moment, the diagnosis of HSVE is based on demonstrating herpes virus in cerebrospinal fluid by means of a polymerase chain reaction[28]. However, it takes two to three days in a normal clinical setting to obtain the results. So there is still a need for techniques that indicate immediately a viral encephalitis.

Launes et al.[29] examined 14 patients with encephalitis (6 with HSVE and 8 with non-HSVE), using either ^{123}I-IMP or ^{99m}Tc-HMPAO SPECT. Initial CT scans were normal in all patients. The 6 patients with HSVE had an area of abnormally high tracer accumulation in the affected temporal lobe (4 to 13 days after onset of symptoms, and evident in the first SPECT scan). This initial hyperperfusion was followed by progressive hypoperfusion in the corresponding area, 37 to 165 days after onset of symptoms. Of the 8 patients with non-HSVE, none had focal hyperperfusion during the first two weeks and no hypoperfusion was demonstrated in the two patients who had a follow-up scan. Although the authors reported that focal unilateral hyperperfusion also exists in the ictal phase of focal epilepsy and the luxury perfusion phase of stroke, they concluded that their findings may be specific because of the very prominent intensity of the hyperperfusion in patients with HSVE. They considered the image to be most likely to be caused by hyperperfusion, while the subsequent appearance of hypoperfusion in the same area was attributed to decreased metabolism following neuronal death. Duncan et al.[30], however, demonstrated that increased uptake can also be seen in non-HSVE. Figure 2 illustrates a focal right temporal hyperperfusion on ^{99m}Tc-HMPAO SPECT in a patient with HSVE.

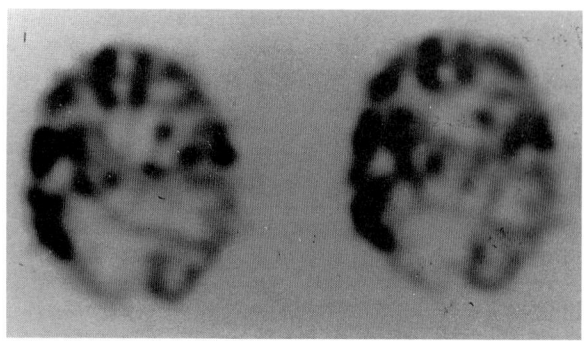

Figure 2 ^{99m}Tc-HMPAO SPECT in a patient with acute herpes simplex encephalitis. Oblique ^{99m}Tc-HMPAO SPECT slices illustrating a marked hyperperfusion in the right temporal lobe. In addition there is a less pronounced increased tracer uptake bifrontally and in the region of the left gyrus postcentralis. The right occipital lobe shows a relative hypoperfusion

Kao et al.[31] also reported increased regional blood flow in a case of HSVE but also in a case of Epstein-Barr virus encephalitis. The follow-up SPECT of the patient with HSVE showed decreased regional cerebral blood flow in the corresponding area, while the follow-up scan of the other patient tended towards normality. In a second publication of the same authors[32] on 18 children with viral encephalitis, of which there were four with HSVE, 17 had increased regional cerebral blood flow on ^{99m}Tc HMPAO brain SPECT during the acute episode. The follow-up SPECT was normal in 12 of these children. In five there was a decreased regional blood flow in those regions showing an increased blood flow on the first SPECT scan. The patients with a normal SPECT during follow-up had a better outcome.

Le Scao et al.[23] recorded similar findings on ^{99m}Tc-HMPAO brain SPECT in a patient with HSVE with localised frontal hyperperfusion in the acute stage and hypoperfusion in the same area six months after onset of symptoms. Again, the CT scan showed no specific abnormalities in the acute stage, while it showed frontal atrophy in the chronic stage.

Park et al.[34] documented reversed crossed cerebellar diaschisis in a ^{99m}Tc-HMPAO SPECT in a patient with intractable epilepsy following successful acyclovir treatment of biopsy-proven HSVE. The SPECT scan showed an area of hyperperfusion in the right temporal lobe and in the contralateral cerebellum.

Encephalitis caused by other viruses

As mentioned before, Launes et al.[29] could not demonstrate the regional hyperperfusion pattern they discovered during the onset period of HSVE, during the acute episode of non-HSVE. However, Duncan et al.[30] also demonstrated regional hyperperfusion on the SPECT scans of patients with non-HSVE.

Kao et al.[31] demonstrated increased regional cerebral blood flow in the right temporal occipital area in a 9-year-old child suffering from an acute episode of Epstein-Barr virus encephalitis. In their second publication[32], the ^{99m}Tc-HMPAO brain SPECTs of 17 of 18 patients with viral encephalitis (12 Epstein-Barr virus, 4 HSV, 2 Japanese B virus) revealed areas of hyperperfusion.

Follow-up scans of non-HSVE seem to yield different results as compared with follow-up scans obtained in patients with HSVE. Non-HSVE does not result in areas of remaining hypoperfusion as is described in HSVE[29,31]. Kao et al.[32] revealed that children with a normal follow-up brain SPECT had a better outcome than children with regional hypoperfusion on the follow-up scan.

Subacute sclerosing panencephalitis (SSPE)

SSPE is a rare subacute measles encephalitis of children and adolescents, characterised by the development of a progressive dementia, myoclonia, epilepsy and ataxia, leading towards spasticity and decortication. Survival is less than 3 years in the vast majority of cases. About 10% evolve in a prolonged course. Diagnosis is based on abnormalities on the EEG and on increased measles antibody titres in serum and CSF.

Few reports have appeared in the literature. Crols et al.[35] described ^{99m}Tc-HMPAO SPECT findings in two cases, one at the very beginning of the disease and one with chronic, stabilised SSPE. In the case of recent onset, a brain perfusion SPECT scan showed a relative hypoperfusion of the right temporo occipital region. This correlated well with the hyperintense signal of the right parieto occipital white matter on MRI and with the findings of the neuropsychological examination, which showed a pronounced involvement of the right hemisphere functions (Figure 3). In stabilised SSPE, SPECT showed only a small zone of cortical activity, consistent with severe atrophy as demonstrated upon CT and MRI. The authors concluded that SPECT became abnormal early in the course of SSPE and that it proved useful in determining the extent and severity of the disease.

In another report, Yagi et al.[36] performed subsequent brain SPECTs on an 8-year old girl with SSPE. In

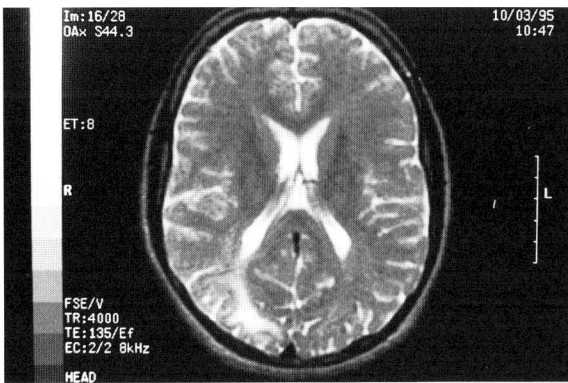

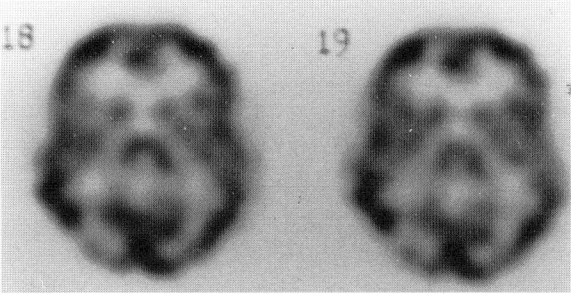

Figure 3 a, T_2-weighted MRI and b, ^{99m}Tc-HMPAO SPECT in a 18 year old patient with SSPE; in MRI there is a hyperintense signal in the right temporo occipital region; in SPECT there is an hypoperfusion in the same region

clinical stage I of the disease, ^{99m}Tc-HMPAO and ^{123}I-IMP-SPECTs showed hypoperfusion in the bilateral occipital areas and part of the cerebellum. At the same time, CT and MRI showed no abnormalities. Subsequently, MRI showed abnormal signal intensity predominantly in the area with hypoperfusion on the SPECT scan. After the introduction of therapy with inosiplex and alpha interferon, the hypoperfusion improved and the abnormal signal intensity on MRI decreased.

Creutzfeldt-Jakob disease

Shih et al.[37] found decreased perfusion of the left frontal and left temporo parietal cortex on the brain perfusion ^{123}I-IMP SPECT scan of a patient with neuropathologically proven Creutzfeldt-Jakob disease (CJD) and proposed the development of SPECT into a useful tool for pre mortem diagnosis of CJD, guiding or avoiding brain biopsy.

Cohen et al.[38] found perfusion defects in the left frontal and right temporo parietal areas on a ^{99m}Tc-HMPAO brain SPECT study of a patient with biopsy-proven CJD. The brain CT scan was normal. Kao et al.[39]

described decreased perfusion in the right frontal and temporal areas on a [99mTc]-HMPAO brain SPECT study of a patient with CJD. This patient also had a normal CT. In a patient with probable Heidenhain type of CJD, which was characterised by the initial onset of visual symptoms, [123I]-IMP brain SPECT showed focal hypoperfusion in the occipital lobes, before CT or MRI revealed any abnormalities[40].

One case of CJD in a recipient of human growth hormone had a [99mTc]-HMPAO SPECT performed. It showed marked impairment of tracer uptake in the basal ganglia and cerebral cortex at a time when the clinical picture was predominantly cerebellar[41].

Bacterial abcesses

In the differential diagnosis between brain tumours and bacterial abcesses, labelled leucocytes may be the first choice rather than perfusion SPECT. With this regard, the contribution of [201Tl]-SPECT remains uncertain since two case studies of positive thallium accumulation in abcedations have been reported.

[201Tl] does not always perform well in differentiating cerebral abscesses from neoplastic lesions, as demonstrated in a patient with a prior history of renal malignancy who developed a solitary brain lesion which had been felt to represent either a primary or metastatic neoplasm on MRI and [201Tl]-SPECT. Upon operation, this lesion was discovered to be a bacterial abscess[42]. False positive [201Tl] accumulation could be due to breakdown of the blood brain barrier[24].

Conclusion

Many different applications of SPECT were examined in several infections of the CNS. The results can be roughly divided into two groups, namely those in which SPECT abnormalities are an important tool for making a diagnosis, and those in which SPECT supports the diagnosis or parallels the clinical evolution.

The first group is the most interesting since SPECT can help in starting treatment at an earlier stage. In this category, the results of perfusion SPECT in encephalitis are very important. Although not limited to this diagnosis, a focal hyperfusion in the context of an infectious CNS disease offers a sensitive instrument, improving an early diagnosis of in particular herpes simplex encephalitis which is essential for good outcome after therapy with acyclovir. SPECT is also an important tool in neurological complications of AIDS. Perfusion SPECT abnormalities correlate not only with the diseased state in ADC, they seem also to predict preclinical HIV-encephalopathy in asymptomatic

patients. Since zidovudine is curative in ADC when used for primary prevention, perfusion SPECT can help in selecting those HIV-infected patients, which should be treated preventively. Finally, [201Tl] SPECT can help in the differential diagnosis of CNS lymphoma versus toxoplasma encephalitis in AIDS patients.

In the second group, perfusion SPECT abnormalities correlate with CNS damage caused by several infections such as opportunistic infections in AIDS, subacute sclerosing panencephalitis or prion diseases. In most patients there is a good correlation between the clinical symptoms and the localization and/or the severity of the disease. Also in the late stages of viral encephalitis, the clinical outcome correlates well with the absence or extent of perfusion SPECT deficits.

References

1   Ell, P.J., Costa, D.C. and Harrison, M. Imaging cerebral damage in HIV infection. *Lancet* 1987, 2, 569

2   Pohl, P., Vogl, G., Fill, H. *et al.* Single photon emission computed tomography in AIDS dementia complex. *J. Nucl. Med.* 1988, 29, 1382

3   Kuni, C.C., Rhame, F.S, Meier, M.J. *et al.* Quantitative I-123-IMP brain SPECT and neuropsychological testing in AIDS dementia. *Clin. Nucl. Med.* 1991, 16, 174

4   Tran Dinh, Y., Mamo, H., Cervoni, J. *et al.* Disturbances in the cerebral perfusion of human immune deficiency virus-1 seropositive asymptomatic subjects: a quantitative tomography study of 18 cases. *J. Nucl. Med.* 1990, 31, 1601

5   Maini, C., Pigorini, F., Pau, F. *et al.* Cortical cerebral blood flow in HIV-1-related dementia complex. *Nucl. Med. Commun.* 1990, 11, 639

6   Harris, G.J., Pearlson, G.D., McArthur, J.C. *et al.* Altered cortical blood flow in HIV-seropositive individuals with and without dementia: a single photon emission computed tomography study. *AIDS* 1994, 8, 495

7   Masdeu, J.C., Yudd, A., Van Heertum, R.L. *et al.* Single-photon emission computed tomography in human immunodeficiency virus encephalopathy: a preliminary report. *J. Nucl. Med.* 1991, 32, 1471

8   Ajmani, A., Habte-Gabr, E., Zarr, M. *et al.* Cerebral blood flow SPECT with [99mTc] exametazine correlates in AIDS dementia complex stages. *Clin. Nucl. Med.* 1991, 16, 656

9   Schielke, E., Tatsch, K., Pfister, H.W. *et al.* Reduced cerebral blood flow in early stages of human immunodeficiency virus infection. *Arch. Neurol.* 1990, 47, 1342

10 Holman, B.L., Garada, B., Johnson, K.A. *et al.* A comparison of brain perfusion SPECT in cocaine abuse and AIDS dementia complex. *J. Nucl. Med.* 1992, 33, 1312

11 Sacktor, N., Prohovnik, I, Van Heertum, R.L. *et al.* Cerebral single-photon emission computed tomography abnormalities in human immunodeficiency virus type 1-infected gay men without cognitive impairment. *Arch. Neurol.* 1995, 52, 607

12 Sacktor, N., Van Heertum, R., Dooneief, G. *et al.* A comparison of cerebral SPECT abnormalities in HIV-positive homosexual men with and without cognitive impairment. *Arch. Neurol.* 1995, 52, 1170

13 Koenig, S., Gendelman, H., Orenstein, J.M. *et al.* Detection of AIDS virus in macrophages in brain tissue from AIDS patients with encephalopathy. *Science* 1986, 233, 1089

14 Gray, F., Lescs, M-C. and Paraire, F. Early brain changes in HIV infection : neuropathological study of 11 HIV seropositive, non-AIDS cases. *J. Neuropathol. Exp. Neurol.* 1992, 51, 177

15 Gray, F., Hurtrel, M. and Hurtrel, B. Early central nervous system changes in human immunodeficiency virus (HIV)-infection. *Neuropathol. Appl. Neurobiol.* 1993, 19, 3

16 Rubbert, A., Bock, E., Schwab, J. *et al.* Anticardiolipin antibodies in HIV infection:association with cerebral perfusion defects as detected by 99mTc-HMPAO SPECT. *Clin. Exp. Immunol.* 1994, 98, 361

17 Geier, A., Schielke, E., Tatsch, K. *et al.* Brain HMPAO-SPECT and ocular microangiopathic syndrome in HIV-1 infected patients. *AIDS* 1993, 7, 1589

18 Weis, S., Bise, K., Lenos, I.C. and Mehraein, P. Neuropathologic features of the brain in HIV-1 infection in 'HIV-1 infection of the central nervous system', (Eds. S. Weis, H. Hippius), Hogrefe & Huber, Gottingen, 1992, p.159

19 Vago, L., Castagna, A., Lazzarin, A. *et al.* Reduced fequency of HIV-induced brain lesions in AIDS patients treated with zidovudine. *J. Acquir. Immune Defic. Syndr.* 1993, 6, 42

20 Rosenblum, M.L., Levy, R.M. and Bredesen, D.R. Neurosurgical implications of the acquired immuno-deficiency syndrome (AIDS). *Clin. Neurosurg.* 1988, 34, 419

21 Ganz, W.I. and Serafini, A. The diagnostic role of nuclear medicine in the acquired immunodeficiency syndrome. *J. Nucl. Med.* 1989, 30, 1935

22 Vanarthos, W.J., Ganz, W.I., Vanarthos, J.C. *et al.* Diagnostic uses of nuclear medicine in AIDS. *Radiographics* 1992, 12, 731

23 Borggreve, F., Dierckx, R.A., Crols, R. *et al.* Repeat Thallium-201 SPECT in cerebral lymphoma. *Functional Neurol.* 1993, 8, 95

24 Dierckx, R.A., Martin, J.J., Dobbeleir, A. *et al.* Sensitivity and specificity of thallium-201 single photon emission tomography in the functional detection and differential diagnosis of brain tumors. *Eur. J. Nucl. Med.* 1994, 21, 621

25 O'Malley J.P., Ziessman, H.A., Kumar, P.N. *et al.* Diagnosis of intracranial lymphoma in patients with AIDS: value of 201Tl single-photon emission computed tomography. *A.J.R.* 1994, 163, 417

26 Ruiz, A., Ganz, W.I., Post, M.J.D. *et al.* Use of thallium-201 brain SPECT to differentiate cerebral lymphoma from Toxoplasma encephalitis in AIDS patients. *Am. J Neuroradiol.* 1994, 15, 1885

27 Landry, M.L., Booss, J. and Hsiung, G.D. Duration of vidarabine therapy in biopsy-negative herpes simplex encephalitis. *J.A.M.A.* 1982, 247, 332

28 Lakeman, F.D. and Whitley, R.J. Diagnosis of herpes simplex virus encephalitis : application of polymerase chain reaction to cerebrospinal fluid from brain-biopsied patients and correlation with disease. National Institute of Allergy and Infectious Diseases Colloborative Study Group. *J. Infect. Dis.* 1995, 171, 857

29 Launes, J., Nikkinen, P., Lindroth, L. *et al.* Diagnosis of acute Herpes simplex encephalitis by brain perfusion single photon emission computed tomography. *Lancet* 1988, 1, 1188

30 Duncan, R., Patterson, J., Bone, I. and Kennedy, P.G. Single photon emission computed tomography in diagnosis of herpes simplex encephalitis. *Lancet* 1988, 2, 516

31 Kao, C-H., Wang, S-J., Mak, S-C. *et al.* [99mTc] HMPAO brain SPECT findings in pediatric viral encephalitis. *Clin. Nucl. Med.* 1994, 19, 590

32 Kao, C-H., Wang, S-J., Mak, S-C. *et al.* Viral encephalitis in children: detection with [99mTc] HMPAO brain single photon emission CT and its value in prediction of outcome. *Am. J. Neuroradiol.* 1994, 15, 1369

33 Le Scao, Y., Turzo, A., Guias, M. *et al.* Changes of [99mTc] HMPAO brain distribution in herpes encephalitis. *Clin. Nucl. Med.* 1993, 18, 452-453

34 Park, C.H., Kim, S.M., Streletz, L.J. *et al.* Reverse crossed cerebellar diaschisis in partial complex seizures related to Herpes simplex encephalitis. *Clin. Nucl. Med.* 1992, 17, 732

35 Crols, R., Pickut, B.A., Mariën, P. and De Deyn, P.P. [99mTc]-HMPAO-SPECT in two patients with subacute sclerosing panencephalitis (SSPE). NeuroSPECT Symposium, Antwerp, Belgium, 1995. *Acta Neurol. Belg.* 1995, 95, 24

36 Yagi, S., Miura, Y., Mizuta, S. *et al.* Chronological SPECT studies of a patient with subacute sclerosing panencephalitis. *Brain Dev.* 1993, 1, 141

37 Shih, W.J., Markesbery, W.R., Clark, D.B. *et al.* Iodine-123 HIPDM brain imaging findings in subacute spongiform encephalopathy (Creutzfeldt-Jakob disease). *J. Nucl. Med.* 1987, 28, 1484

38 Cohen, D., Krausz, Y., Lossos, A. *et al.* Brain SPECT imaging with [99mTc] HMPAO in Creutzfeldt-Jakob disease. *Clin. Nucl. Med.* 1989, 14, 808

39 Kao, C-H., Wang, S-J., Liao, S-Q. and Yeh, S-H. [99mTc] HMPAO brain SPECT findings in Creutzfeldt-Jakob disease. *Clin. Nucl. Med.* 1993, 18, 234

40 Jibiki, I., Fukushima, T., Kobayashi, K. *et al.* Utility of 123I-IMP brain scans for the early detection of site-specific abnormalities in Creutzfeldt-Jakob disease (Heidenhain type): a case study. *Neuropsychobiology* 1994, 29, 117

41 Markus, H.S., Duchen, L.W., Parkin, E.M. *et al.* Creutzfeldt-Jakob disease in recipients of human growth hormone in the United Kingdom: a clinical and radiographic study. *Q. J. Med.* 1992, 82, 43

42 Krishna, L., Slizofski, W.J., Katsetos, C.D. *et al.* Abnormal intracerebral thallium localization in a bacterial brain abscess. *J. Nucl. Med.* 1992, 33, 1017

SPECT in Neurology and Psychiatry, edited by P.P. De Deyn, R.A. Dierckx, A. Alavi and B.A. Pickut
© 1997 John Libbey & Company Ltd, pp. 455–466

SPECT in Headache with Special Reference to Migraine

Chapter
54

P.P. De Deyn, G. Nagels, B.A. Pickut, M. Schwartz[*],
V. Saxena, R.A. Dierckx[**]

SPECT image analysis and scoring in headache studies

The information obtained during a SPECT examination can be scored in several ways. Two methods can be distinguished: visual and quantitative analysis. In visual analysis, symmetry of perfusion, and inhomogeneity of regional perfusion can be used. Interhemispheric comparisons using ROIs lead to semi-quantitative scoring[1]. ROIs can also be compared with reference areas, e.g. cerebellum and frontal cortex[2]. Friberg[3] evaluated the presence of regional perfusion asymmetries in symmetrically located regions in the two hemispheres. Each picture was scored from 1 (normal) to 4 (clearly abnormal). Scores for four observers were added. A value of 4-8 was normal while a value of 9-16 was asymmetrical.

In his quantitative analysis, Friberg[3] scored interhemispheric side to side differences by summing counts in predefined ROIs (anterior, middle and posterior cerebral artery and three other territories). An asymmetry index was calculated, after normalisation to an internal reference (cerebellum = 100%), using the formula (ROIright - ROIleft) / ROIright. Deviations exceeding 2.5 s.d. of the values obtained in the control population were considered abnormal. Intrasubject comparisons can be made to determine which values are abnormal Batistella[4] considered any asymmetry beyond 10% observed in at least two perpendicular planes and two adjacent sections abnormal.

In our study considering interictal SPECT in patients suffering from migraine and tension headache, a systematic visual analysis system was used, considering hypoperfusion severity in 10 sections indicated on a series of transaxial slices. Using our above mentioned formula, this scoring system yields a number indicating the hypoperfusion by giving a total hypoperfusion severity score (SeS).

SPECT in migraine

A large number of SPECT studies have been performed in patients with migraine. The studies related to migraine can be differentiated according to several criteria: the clinical types of migraine which were studied; the ictal or interictal timing of the recordings; the tracers and acquisition techniques which were used; the age of the population studied; and the presence or absence of anti-migraine medication. A number of studies lead to interesting conclusions regarding the pathophysiological mechanisms underlying migraine.

Department of Neurology A.Z.
Middelheim and University of
Antwerp and Born-Bunge
Foundation, Lindendreef 1,
2020 Antwerp, Belgium
[*]Department of Neurology,
Bnai-Zion Hospital, Technion
University, Haifa, Israel
[**]Division of Nuclear Medicine,
University Hospital Ghent

Migraine types

According to the International Headache Society[5], migraine is a clinical condition in which the patient typically suffers from attacks of moderate or severe, unilateral, pulsating headache, lasting 4 to 72 h, which are aggravated by routine physical activity and are accompanied by nausea or vomiting, photophobia and phonophobia. Not all of these criteria have to be present to reach the diagnosis. The diagnosis of migraine with aura can be made when all or some of the attacks are preceded by the gradual occurrence of one or more fully reversible symptoms indicating focal cerebral cortical or brainstem dysfunction, not lasting more than 60 min per symptom, and followed by headache with a free interval of less than 60 min. Again, not all of these criteria have to be fulfilled to reach the diagnosis.

Several types of aura may occur: visual aura (classical migraine or migraine with typical aura) (CLM), sensorimotor involvement (hemiplegic migraine) (HM), basilar artery migraine (Bickerstaff migraine) (BAM), migraine aura without headache. Migraine without aura is sometimes referred to as common migraine or hemicrania simplex (CM).

Interictal SPECT in migraine

Scintigraphic studies in migraine patients under interictal conditions have demonstrated both normal and abnormal flow patterns. Interictal abnormalities in cerebral blood flow have been demonstrated by rCBF studies[6-12]. These conventional methods using ^{133}Xe did not allow precise assessment of the localisation of the CBF changes. Some authors report that interictal SPECT in an adult population usually shows hypoperfusions only in patients with aura[13,14] while others demonstrate abnormalities in both patients with and without aura.

Friberg demonstrated moderate flow asymmetries on interictal SPECT examination in migraine patients. He investigated migraine patients with (n=60) and without (n=32) aura under interictal conditions (at least five days after their last migraine attack) and a healthy control group (n=42) using quantitated and visual methods. SPECT was performed using either ^{133}Xe or HMPAO. Patients with aura showed abnormalities in 63% of cases using a quantitated analysis (30% of HMPAO scans, 70% of xenon scans). Patients without aura showed abnormalities in 20/32 cases using a quantitated analysis (30% in HMPAO scans, 77% in xenon scans). This means that asymmetries were depicted with the same frequency in both patient groups. In the visual evaluation, interrator variability was high. Interrator variability in the normal control

group, however, was low. Visual scoring was 50% less sensitive than the quantification method for identification of asymmetries. Both visual and quantitated scores were correlated to age, duration and attack frequency in the two patient groups. No significant correlations were found[3].

Several other studies demonstrated flow abnormalities under interictal conditions; Robertson[10] found interictal asymmetries in 60% (n=20) of patients with aura, and 69% (n=29) of patients without aura using a stationary probe and xenon. Cavestri et al.[15] studied 39 controls and 20 migraine patients in interictal phase (10 with and 10 without aura) using the ^{133}Xe inhalation method, and showed significant reductions of CBF in the migraine population. Lagrèze[6] described interictal abnormalities in 50% (n=8) of patients with aura. Schlake[16] reported interictal abnormalities in 79% (n=24) of patients without aura and in 60% (n=22) of patients with aura using one-observer visual analysis of HMPAO images. Suess[17] found interictal distribution abnormalities of the same size in 28 migraine patients examined with HMPAO. Colamussi et al.[18], using interictal HMPAO SPECT in 28 patients with migraine with aura, showed a slight hypoperfusion in 79% of cases and a correlation between hypoperfusion areas and the neurological symptoms of aura in 55% of individuals.

Schlake investigated, according to his description, 5 patients with classical migraine and 18 with migraine accompagnée (headache associated with transient neurological symptoms) using ^{123}I IMP SPECT, and found interictally decreased cerebral blood flow in all patients suffering from migraine accompagnée (16 hemiplegic migraine, 2 BAM), often corresponding to the site of the headache as well as to the topography of transient neurological symptoms. The hypoperfusion was most obvious in patients with persisting neurological symptoms. Most patients suffering from classical migraine did not show hypoperfusions (4/5)[14]. Interictal SPECT in 14 patients with classical migraine showed hypoperfusions in 13 cases, 6 patients showing a hypoperfusion in the frontal lobe, 1 in the temporal, 11 in the parietal and 5 in the occipital lobe. Right parietal regions were involved more often than left. Only three patients showed involvement in only one lobe. The parieto-occipital cortex appeared to be the site most commonly involved with a right side predominance[19]. Other authors also reported a high number of interictal CBF abnormalities in migraine[8,20].

Alterations of regional hypoperfusion do appear to be more more pronounced in migraine with aura and frequently correlate to ictal neurological abnormalities[14,17,21-24]. Batistella located hypoperfusions on interictal HMPAO SPECT in 5 out of 19 migraine patients aged 8 to 16 years (ten affected with common migraine, 6 with classical migraine and 3 with hemiplegic migraine) in the temporo occipital and parietal regions[4]. Podreka[25] examined eleven patients suffering from headache with HMPAO SPECT, and found abnormalities in seven of them. These were located in the parietal and frontal cortex in one hemisphere.

Several other studies failed to demonstrate any abnormalities of cerebral blood flow in migraine patients under interictal conditions[7,9,26-32]. In a recent study, we evaluated ^{99m}Tc-HMPAO perfusion SPECT in two patient populations, one suffering from migraine with or without aura and one suffering from tension headache. Interictal ^{99m}Tc-HMPAO SPECT images were obtained using a three-head SPECT system (Triad 88, Trionix) equipped with Fan Beam Collimators (FWHM 7.3mm). A 20 miCi dose of ^{99m}Tc-HMPAO was administered intravenously in a quiet and light dimmed room. Acquisition was started after 20 min; accumulation performed in a 128x64 matrix, pixel size 3.5mm, 40s per angle, 40 angles per detector (3 steps, 120° rotation); reconstruction in a 64x64 matrix using Butterworth-filtered backprojection. A total of 51 patients was studied. The group suffering from migraine (n = 38) was composed of individuals suffering from migraine with aura (n = 22) and patients

with migraine without aura (n = 16). This group consisted of 27 women and 11 men aged 39 ± 2.4 yrs (M±s.d.). The group of 13 patients suffering from tension headache was aged 49 ± 3.4 yrs (M ± s.d.) and consisted of 9 women and 4 men. Age and sex distribution was not significantly different for the two patient groups.

Visual scoring of hypoperfusion severity (SeS) was performed on the transaxial ^{99m}Tc-HMPAO SPECT slices. Each transaxial slice was divided into 10 sectors as indicated in Figure 1. The absence or presence and severity of hypoperfusion was scored for each sector and for all slices. Scores were given for each sector (Se$_i$) as follows: 0: absent (or no hypoperfusion), 1: mild hypoperfusion, 2 : moderate, 3 : severe: breaching. Hypoperfusion was scored by 3 independent raters blinded for diagnosis. A total hypoperfusion severity score was obtained using the following formula:

$$SeS = \frac{32}{TNS} \sum_{i=1}^{10} NS_I \times Se_I$$

in which: NSi is the number of slices showing hypoperfusion in sector i; TNS is the total number of slices. In cases of severe hypoperfusion in all sectors on all slices, one would obtain a hypothetical SeS of 960.

The perfusion SPECT deficit scores for the different patient populations (total migraine population,

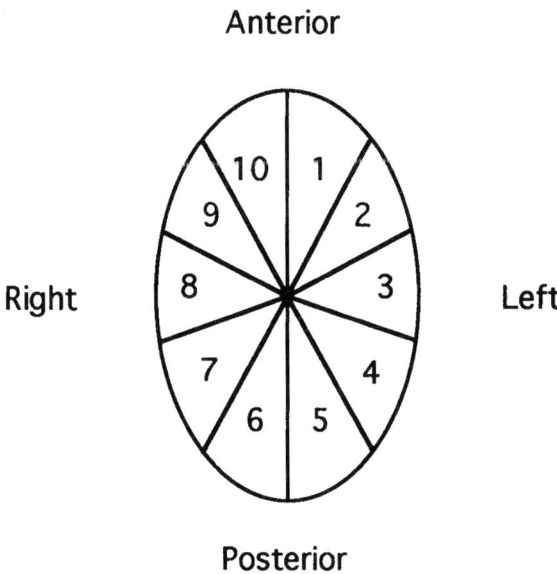

Anterior

Right / **Left**

Posterior

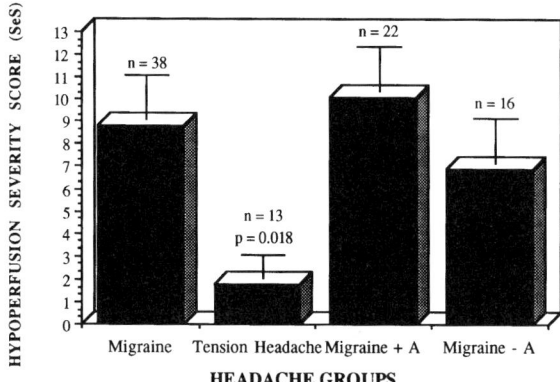

Figure 1 Visual scoring on transaxial ^{99m}Tc-HMPAO SPECT slices. The absence or presence and severity of hypoperfusion was scored for each sector and for all slices. From these scores, a total hypoperfusion severity score (SeS) was calculated according to the formula represented in the text

Figure 2 Perfusion SPECT deficit score (SeS) in migraine and tension headache. The ordinate indicates the hypoperfusion total severity score (SeS) values while the abscissa represents the different patient groups. Migraine + A = migraine with aura. Migraine - A = migraine without aura

migraine without aura, migraine with aura and tension headache group) are represented in Figure 2. The SeS was 8.8 ± 1.6 (n=38, M ± SEM) in the total migraine population and significantly lower in the tension headache group namely 1.8 ± 0.9 (n=13, M ± SEM)(p=0.018). The SeS in the migraine group with aura was 10.1 ± 2.5 (n=22, M ± SEM) and not significantly different from the hypoperfusion in the migraine group without aura where the SeS was somewhat lower with a value of 6.9 ± 1.9 (n=16, M ± SEM) (p=0.339). In the migraine group with sensori-motor aura, the SeS was 9.7 ± 2.3 (n=17, M ± SEM). No significant lateralisation of the perfusion deficits was observed in the migraine group; the SeS Left being 5.4 ± 1.5 (n = 38,M ± SEM) while the SeS Right was 3.4 ± 0.9 (n = 38, M ± SEM) (p=0.243).

In addition, we attempted to investigate a possible correlation between interictal hypoperfusion localisation and lateralisation of headache and/or aura. In the group of individuals with exclusively lateralised headache (n = 21), an ipsilateral deficit was observed in 14/21. A contralateral deficit was seen in 2/21, while no deficit was observed in 5/21 and a bilateral deficit in 5/21. Subjects with migraine with lateralised sensorimotor aura (n=15) displayed the following hypoperfusion pattern: ipsilateral deficit in 5/15; contralateral deficit in 7/15; no deficit in 5/15 and finally, a bilateral deficit in 2/15. From our study, we concluded that interictal hypoperfusion SeS was significantly higher in individuals suffering from migraine than in patients presenting with tension headache. Interictal hypoperfusion SeS was not significantly higher in migraine with aura than in migraine without aura. SeS values of the left and right hemispheres were not statistically significantly different. Lateralisation of interictal hypoperfusion and headache seemed to correlate quite well, while this was not the case for the topographical lateralisation of sensorimotor disturbances in the migraine with aura subgroup.

Ictal SPECT in migraine

Ictal migraine studies in adults usually evidence a focal hypoperfusion in patients with aura and no hypoperfusions in patients without aura[13]. Figures 3-5 illustrate ictal ^{99m}Tc-HMPAO SPECTs in some of our migraine patients with aura. Figure 3 is obtained in a woman with typical right sensorimotor aura, aphasia and right hemianopsia. Figure 4 shows the ictal SPECT findings in a man with a migraine aura consisting of right hemiparesis. Finally, Figure 5 illustrates the findings in a woman with visual aura consisting of right-sided hemianopsia.

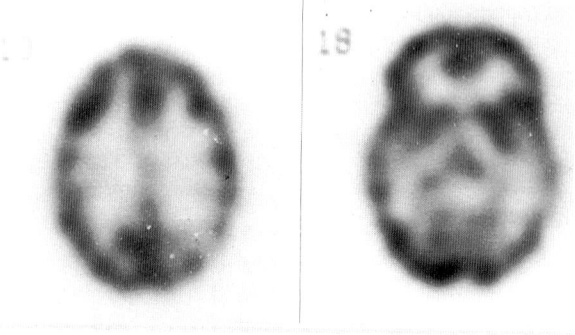

Figure 3 Patient GE. Ictal ^{99m}Tc-HMPAO SPECT in migraine with typical right sensorimotor aura in a 22 year old woman presenting since the age of 13. The patient presented with paroxystic episodes of lateralised pulsating headache preceded by paraesthesias followed by paresis of the right arm and face accompanied by aphasia and right-sided hemianopsia. All complementary diagnostic tests (including arteriography) remained negative. SPECT demonstrated a hypoperfusion left parieto-occipitally with extension to the temporal lobe

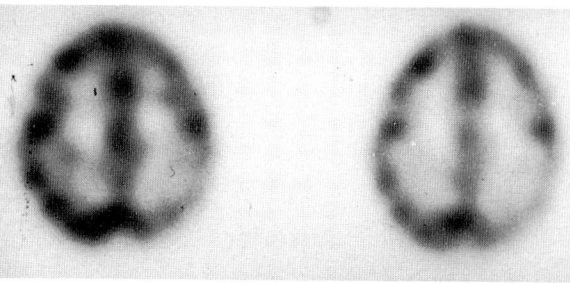

Figure 4 Patient DBF. Migraine with typical aura consisting of right sided hemiparesis in a 43 year old man with paroxystic episodes of pulsating headache on the left preceded by paresis of the right hemicorpus. ^{99m}Tc-HMPAO SPECT shows focal left fronto parietal hypoperfusion

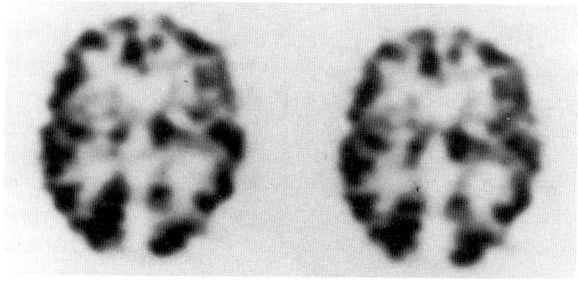

Figure 5 Patient VC. Migraine with typical aura consisting of right hemianopsia in a 23 year old woman presenting with paroxystic pulsating headache localised left occipitally preceded and accompanied by right-sided hemianopsia. ^{99m}Tc-HMPAO SPECT showed hypoperfusion in the left occipital region involving the optic radiation and visual cortex

Nature of the perfusion changes

During migraine attacks with aura, marked focal changes in brain tissue perfusion have been described[7,28,33,34]. Sakai and Meyer[11] and Juge and Gauthier[35] described a global blood flow increase during attacks with aura. Decreased CBF in adults during migraine attacks was seen in the classic and in the common type[26,28,36]. During the aura phase of the attack, rCBF can reach ischaemic levels[33,37].

Timing and localisation of the perfusion changes

Most SPECT studies show reduction of CBF during the prodromal stage of migraine headache[9,26-32]. Ictal SPECT using ^{133}Xe in migraine with aura has shown both global hyperperfusion throughout the attack[11,38] and focal initial hypoperfusion followed by delayed hyperaemia[21,34,39]. Focal hypoperfusion in spontaneous attacks of classical migraine persisted for several hours in some patients studied using xenon inhalation SPECT[7].

During the visual or sensorimotor prodromi of CLM, CBF is decreased in the cortical area corresponding to the focal neurologic symptoms when studied using xenon SPECT[7]. The hypoperfusion is on the side of the headache. The hypoperfusion is sometimes followed by a transient hyperaemia 12-24 h after the attack. Andersen[39] performed ^{133}Xe inhalation SPECT in seven patients during and repeatedly after spontaneous classic migraine attacks. CBF was reduced in the first three hours, in the hemisphere corresponding to the neurological deficit, followed by hyperperfusion in the same region, often persisting after the headache. After one week no asymmetries were found. All patients developed headache while hypoperfusion was still present. Some authors remark on the common occurrence of regional flow changes in the 'migraine ROI', which covers the watershed area between posterior and middle cerebral artery during the attack[7,34,39].

A number of SPECT studies performed during migraine attacks without aura showed no focal changes[7,13,28,30,40,41]. Ferrari[2] performed ictal and interictal HMPAO SPECT in 20 patients without aura and found no significant asymmetries outside or during the attack. The rCBF ratios did not differ significantly when comparing ictal and interictal SPECT per patient. A smaller number of studies suggests a 25% to 35% global increase[11,38]. No asymmetric or focal rCBF changes have been reported[2].

Enhancemnet of SPECT alterations in migraine

Pharmacological activation

Administration of some compounds may lead to enhanced detection of abnormalities. In a paediatric population, 5% CO_2 inhalation showed a focal reduction of blood flow surge on xenon inhalation in only those patients suffering from migraine[42]. CO_2 inhalation was proven to increase blood velocity as measured by intracranial doppler, leading to changes in the level of physiological activation[43]. Both 5% CO_2 and 100% O_2 inhalation were shown to lead to increase in blood flow in migraine patients[44,45].

Administration of acetazolamide, a carbonic anhydrase inhibitor, resolved hypoperfusions on HMPAO SPECT in 14/20 migraine patients. Of the remaining patients, three showed less pronounced hypoperfusions compared with baseline. Three older patients showed no difference in regional hypoperfusion compared with baseline. In these patients, the loss of vasodilatatory capacity could be due to age or cerebrovascular disease. In patients with cerebrovascular ischaemia, acetazolamide usually enhances low-flow regions. The acetazolamide test might thus be useful in the differential diagnosis of migraine with aura from transient cerebrovascular ischaemia[1].

Pathophysiology of migraine

SPECT studies have been proven to be an important tool for clarifying the pathophysiology of migraine. One case report states that the increase in cerebral perfusion recorded in a patient suffering from chronic paroxysmal hemicrania might be caused by a non-specific pain-induced activation of rCBF[22]. Most authors, however, do not adhere to this view and the proposed mechanism has not been proven in other kinds of pain syndrome. Wolff[46] suggests a cerebrovascular hypothesis. According to this hypothesis, transient cerebral arterial constriction causes focal ischaemia, leading to aura symptoms. The hypoperfusion is followed by intra and/or extracranial vasodilatation, which in turn causes headache.

A number of authors made observations supporting this mechanism. Skinhoj[12,32] described increased rCBF in the headache phase of classic and common migraine attacks. Enhanced vasoconstrictor activity might predispose to a more marked vascular instability and focal hypoperfusion resulting in a migraine attack with aura[7,28,33]. During the visual or sensorimotor prodromi of CLM, CBF is decreased in the cortical area corresponding to the focal neurological symptoms when studied by xenon SPECT. The hypoperfusion is on the side of the headache. The hypoperfusion is sometimes followed by a transient hyperaemia 12-24 h after the attack. No interictal hypoperfusions were noticed. According to Lauritzen[7], migraine without aura showed no ictal or interictal hypoperfusions.

Later studies yielded data in contradiction with this important hypothesis. Andersen[39] showed that headache occurred sooner than the transition from vasoconstriction to hyperaemia. Some patients with classical migraine were found to develop headache before the hyperaemic phase, i.e. during hypoperfusions. This suggests that cerebral hyperaemia is not the cause of the headache in migraine[7,39].

In addition, Lauritzen showed that the reduction of rCBF lasts longer than the aura symptoms. Late hyperaemia does not occur in classic migraine until hours after the aura symptoms have resolved. Hyperaemia can last from about 1 h to more than 24 h after aura symptoms. Hyperaemia is focal and limited to the area previously hypoperfused. There are indications that the severity of the aura symptoms relates to the severity and duration of the hypoperfusion, which in turn determines the severity and duration of the hyperaemia. There were no neurological deficits during hyperperfusion[7]. Sakai[11] described persistence of hyperaemia up to 48 h after headache resolved in both common and classic migraine. Friberg[37] described cerebrovascular tone instability (fluctuating washout rates in low-flow regions, indicating that short episodes of severe ischaemia alternate with periods of normal or slightly reduced flow) in patients with classic migraine and during TIAs. In 1907, Gowers[47] stated that a primary disturbance of the brain parenchyma elicits the migraine attack and that the vascular abnormalities are only secondary phenomena. In this view, migraine attacks are initiated by a cortical spreading depression inducing posterior oligemia which progresses anteriorly[33,48,49]. PET studies support this hypothesis by pointing to cerebral glucose hypometabolism as the initial event of the migraine attack[50]. The hypoperfusion observed by SPECT may be a manifestation of spreading cortical depression and leads to moderate ischaemia[41]. Also interictal SPECT abnormalities yield data allowing us to obtain a better understanding of the pathophysiology of migraine. Friberg[21] suggests a common involvement of the larger intracranial arteries in the painful phase in both migraine with and without aura. Indeed, the fact that interictal studies show the same percentage of abnormalities in patients with and without aura suggests a common pathophysiological basis[3]. This is supported by the similar intracranial haemodynamic changes observed during both types of attack[21] and by the effectiveness of 5HT agonists on both types of

migraine attacks[3]. Friberg presumes that the cause of abnormal CBF asymmetries arises from desynchronised vascular tone regulation and cites evidence of marked rapid oscillations in CBF during a migraine attack with aura suggesting an instability of cerebrovascular tone[13,37].

Spina[51] published data that were in agreement with similar reports in the paediatric population and could be explained by both the vascular pathogenesis of migraine[52,53], directed or intermediated by other haemodynamic transmitters[54] or by the neuronal theory causing perhaps a spreading depression, coinciding with a short period of decreased cortical blood flow, following or producing hypometabolism in the cortex combined with a diminished vascular reactivity. Olesen[28] states that oligemia is followed by focal signs which precede the classic migraine attack, while in common migraine this phenomenon has rarely been observed. Oligemia persists when neurological signs have disappeared, which suggests the existence of a different relation between variations of cerebral flow, distorted neuronal activity and neurotransmitters[55].

Sakai and Meyer[11] suggest interictal dysregulation in response to physiological stimuli such as CO_2, O_2 and functional activation[11,43,44,56]. MRI studies suggest discrete (subcortical) white matter lesions in migraine[57,58].

[123]I IMP SPECT data presented by Schlake[14] suggest that migraine, and in particular migraine accompagnée, is characterised by a permanent alteration of cerebral perfusion and perhaps of neuronal activity, which also exists in symptom free intervals. Friberg[3] noted moderate asymmetries in the interictal phase of migraine, both with and without aura which did not resemble the massive changes seen in ischaemic stroke. There was no clear pattern in the distribution of the asymmetries. They were not restricted to one vascular territory and their appearance was described as being 'patchy'.

Batistella[4] confirms the hypothesis that in patients suffering from migraine, the clinical attack may occur concomitantly with an exacerbation of pre-existing modifications of cerebral vascular autoregulation which are detectable even during headache free periods.

In summary, during the aura, ictal perfusion SPECT tends to show regional hypoperfusion, followed by hyperperfusion in the ensuing headache phase. These data support the vascular hypothesis. In migraine with sensorimotor accompanying symptomatology, there is a tendency towards correlation between the hypoperfusion area and the focal neurological symptoms. Early studies failed to show these perfusion changes in common migraine, but later observations demonstrated ictal hyperaemia ipsilateral to the headache, or in some cases, more generalised. These data lead to the conclusion that the same pathophysiological mechanisms are causing both migraine with and without aura, and that the aura surfaces only when a certain threshold of hypoperfusion is reached. Vascular mechanisms appear to be important in the development of aura symptoms and headache, but do not appear to be the initial mechanism of migraine. Evidence supports the neural theory in which a spreading cortical depression induces anteriorly progressing oligemia.

BAM

Schlake[14] described two BAM patients. Both showed interictal ^{123}I IMP SPECT perfusion deficits with marked correlations to the site of headache but with no correlations to the neurological symptoms. Spina[51] presented six paediatric patients suffering from BAM, aged 11 to 14. He measured a decreased CBF in five out of six, mostly in the posterior regions in the interictal phase.

Migrainous stroke

Vascular disturbances accompanying the migraine attack can cause local cerebral ischaemia[33,59-61]. CT and MRI studies have shown that migraine can be associated with structural brain changes, which are probably related to vascular derangements[62-66]. Migraine-induced strokes most commonly occur in the posterior circulation or in the posterior branches of the middle cerebral artery, which is consistent with the prominence of visual symptoms in migraine[1]. Several causative mechanisms leading to migrainous stroke have been proposed: cerebral oedema, increased platelet aggregation and ensuing ischaemia[33,67,68]. Migrainous stroke may occur in pre-existing low-flow regions[59,69]. Migraine could play an aetiological role in about 5% of strokes in young patients[70]. Strokes occur more frequently in migraine patients who have an aura[71-73]. SPECT with acetazolamide may be used for the estimation of cerebrovascular risk in migraine patients[1].

Migraine in childhood

Feggi[74] performed ictal and interictal HMPAO SPECT in a paediatric population (26 patients between 8 and 16 years, 9 with typical aura, 8 with prolonged aura, 6 BAM, 3 had aura without headache). Nine patients only had interictal SPECT, while 10 had only ictal

SPECT. Interictal SPECT showed a significant hypoperfusion in 1/16 whereas ictal SPECT was positive in 13/24.

Spina[51] investigated 19 migraine patients aged from 10 to 16 years within five days after the last migrainous episode using HMPAO, and compared them with a control group of 9 subjects. He found decreased CBF in 15/19 patients (3/4 HM, 5/6 BAM, 5/5 CLM, 2/4 CM). Five cases showed hypoperfusion in the left hemisphere, 3 in the right and 7 in both hemispheres. In BAM, most hypoperfusions were noticed in the posterior regions.

Batistella[4] described 19 paediatric patients with decreased uptake of HMPAO in classic and hemiplegic forms. All 10 patients with CM showed negative interictal SPECT. Three out of 6 CLM cases and 1 out of 3 HM cases showed hypoperfusions in the temporo occipital regions (2 cases) and parietal regions (2 cases), leading to the conclusion that cerebrovascular autoregulation can be impaired even in the headache free period in migraine with aura.

Cluster headache

Involvement of cerebral haemodynamics in cluster headache have been described by several authors[22,75-77]. Gawel[78] presents evidence for a sympathetic defect of vasomotor control of the anterior cerebral artery on the side of the headache during cluster periods by measuring CO_2 reactivity of the major intracranial vessels using transcranial doppler. During the cluster period, reactivity was significantly lower, but only in the anterior cerebral artery on the side of the headache. Gallium SPECT performed in six patients, showed a lesion in the region of the cavernous sinus (which faded when the patient moved out of the cluster) in three of them. This abnormality had not been seen in any other condition. CT was normal in the three patients. The lesion might be the cavernous sinus plexus, which has been postulated by Moskowitz[79] to be the pathophysiological focus in cluster, since it can explain the parasympathetic symptoms of lacrimation, rhinorroe and nasal congestion, the Horner's syndrome, the facial and forehead sweating and the peri- and retro-orbital pain.

SPECT applicability in differential diagnosis and therapy of headache

Differential diagnosis

In addition to the valuable contribution SPECT has made to the research on pathophysiology of migraine, several authors report on the potential clinical value of

SPECT in migraine. The relative benign nature of migraine was put to question by reports on migrainous stroke[19]. Patients with classic migraine should be monitored for possible ischaemic complications. In patients showing interictal hypoperfusions, vasoconstricting drugs are contraindicated and instead, calcium antagonists should be used[6]. Andersen[39] states that a laboratory procedure is needed to distinguish between different types of migraine attacks to evaluate the time course and severity of the attacks in the individual patient. SPECT is valuable in the diagnosis of migraine, since an exact CBF time profile has been demonstrated: initial focal decrease followed by an increase in the same region and final normalisation.

NeuroSPECT depicts blood flow abnormalities in acute aphasic disorders, either due to ischaemia, or due to hyperaemia secondary to migraine or epilepsy. Since the treatment of these conditions differs, SPECT plays a role in patient management. Receptive aphasia is a neurological syndrome frequently associated with an ischaemic event that neuroSPECT detects before a CT abnormality is present[80-82]. Lewis[83] describes two patients in whom the unexpected appearance of hyperaemia in Wernicke's area shown on HMPAO SPECT had implications for the patients' further diagnostic testing and treatment. Migraine and epilepsy are paroxysmal disorders that can be difficult to distinguish[84]. Migraine prevalence is between 1 and 25%[83] while that of epilepsy is below 1%. Differential diagnosis of hyperaemia is between seizure activity and the vasodilatory phase of migraine. The latter is less likely because usually the oligemic phase is associated with neurological signs and symptoms[25,26,83,85].

BAM patients are the most frequently misdiagnosed headache patients[86,87]. The differential diagnosis includes cerebrovascular disease, brain tumour, mental disorder, temporal lobe epilepsy, hysteria and complications of drug abuse. The diagnosis requires the presence of reversible ischaemia in the territory of the basilar artery combined with a clinical tableau of dysfunction of the brain stem, cerebellum and occipital cortex[86]. Seto describes a 33 year old woman suffering from basilar artery migraine who was initially misdiagnosed as having a cerebrovascular or mental disorder. An emergency HMPAO scan showed significant hypoperfusions in right temporo occipital and cerebellar regions during an attack. During a symptom free period these changes had normalised, allowing a diagnosis of BAM. IMP SPECT, however, failed to show rCBF changes in the basilar territory in two cases.

Schlake[22] published on a chronic paroxysmal hemicrania in a 69 year old woman (first described by Sjaastad[88]). This condition is similar to cluster headache but is characterised by shorter attack duration and higher frequency of attacks. The patient underwent HMPAO SPECT which showed a regional reduction (as compared with cerebellum) of tracer uptake bilaterally in the fronto parietal region in the pain free state and an absence of significant hypoperfusions during a typical attack. HMPAO SPECT in an attack free period under verapamil monotherapy again showed bilateral fronto parietal hypoperfusions.

Our findings in migraine and tension headache showed significantly different hypoperfusion scores in these two headache populations. Although the clinical presentation of migraine and tension headache may be quite typical, our findings might be helpful in making a more precise diagnosis in individual patients. Moreover, our findings further indicate the differences in pathophysiology of these two headache syndromes.

Therapy

The effect of several compounds used in the prophylaxis and acute treatment of migraine has been evaluated using SPECT. Spina[51] repeated HMPAO SPECT in four children suffering from migraine after six months of treatment with pizotifen and/or flunarizine, and found a normalisation of flow in previously hypoperfused areas which corresponded with subjective improvement. In one case, however, CBF worsened in spite of a decrease of the migrainous attacks.

Schlake[22] found no marked differences in the distribution and severity of hypoperfusions in a patient with chronic paroxysmal hemicrania who underwent an interictal SPECT before and during treatment with verapamil. When comparing SPECT images before and after administration of acetazolamide, he found resolution of interictal hypoperfusions in migraine patients with and without aura in 14/20 cases, which may suggest that acetazolamide should be investigated for therapeutic effect in migraine[1].

The influence of flunarizine on D_2 receptors was studied in vivo using interictal ^{123}I-iodobenzamide SPECT, a ligand with high affinity and specificity for D_2 receptors, in 11 migraine patients treated with 10 mg flunarizine per day. Striatal activity was expressed as a relative number using frontal cortex as an internal reference. A reduction of the dopamine receptor binding potential was noticed in all patients compared with age-matched controls. No extrapyramidal signs were observed. Flunarizine at clinically used doses blocks D_2 receptors. The degree of dopamine D_2 receptor blockade did not correlate with the efficacy of flunarizine in the prophylaxis of migraine. Therefore the antimigraine action of flunarizine is propably not mediated by an antidopaminergic mechanism[89].

Flunarizine has an inhibitory effect on transmembrane calcium influx, inhibiting calcium related contraction of smooth muscle. There is also evidence of an antidopaminergic mechanism[90,91]. Antidopaminergic drugs improve nausea and vomiting during migraine attacks and prevent migraine[92]. The antimigraine action of flunarizine may therefore be mediated by the dopaminergic system. This lack of correlation between the antidopaminergic mechanism and the antimigraine action of flunarizine contradicts other reports[93].

Ergotamine was shown to have no influence on central dopamine D_2 receptor binding potential. Since the affinity of ergotamine for dopamine receptors is well known, it was concluded that ergotamine does not cross the blood brain barrier, and that a central action of ergotamine is unlikely to explain its therapeutic benefit[94]. Two migraine patients were studied during ergotamine abusus and after withdrawal and compared with 15 normal controls. Striatum/cerebellum and striatum/occipital cortex ratios did not differ between normal controls and patients who were taking or not taking ergotamine[94]. In a recent paper, Friberg[95] discussed the need for additional *in vivo* neuroreceptor imaging studies in migraine. This would be of importance for the study of the pathophysiology of migraine, as well as for the study of pharmacological agents.

Ferrari[2] performed HMPAO SPECT interictally, ictally and after treatment of an attack with 6 mg of subcutaneous sumatriptan in 20 patients suffering from migraine without aura and found no significant changes when comparing ictal SPECT before and after treatment. Sumatriptan is believed to act via vascular and neuronal 5HT receptors[96-98]. Scott performed HMPAO SPECT in six volunteers treated with 2 mg iv sumatriptan, compared with treatment with placebo in the same volunteer and found no detectable effect[99]. Similarly, no effect of sumatriptan on rCBF was found using xenon SPECT during a migraine attack, but a substantial correction of the reduction in blood velocity in the middle cerebral arteries was demonstrated, suggesting a vasoconstrictor effect on the dilated large arteries but not on normal vessels[21].

Dormehl[100], using HMPAO SPECT, demonstrated in the baboon model that sumatriptan attenuated the blood flow increasing effect of nimodipine by 47%, while it did not influence the acetazolamide or halothane induced alterations of blood flow. This type of study contributes to a better understanding of the mechanisms of action of neuroactive drugs.

Conclusions

Interictal SPECT in migraine often reveals hypoperfusion. Hypoperfusion was observed in several studies in 50%-80% of patients suffering from migraine with and without aura[3,8,10,16,17,20,25,51]. Our interictal findings in a mixed population of individuals with migraine with and without aura, are in agreement with these papers. Indeed, we found interictal hypoperfusions in 63% of cases. Some authors report a lower incidence of hypoperfusion in 'classical migraine' (visual aura) than in 'migraine accompagnée'. This is also consistent with our findings, interictal SPECT being positive in 73% of patients with migraine with aura and in 50% of patients presenting migraine without aura. Side of headache and topography of neurological symptoms tend to correlate according to some authors[4,14]. On interictal SPECT in patients with exclusively lateralised headache, we found an ipsilateral deficit in 67% of individuals. Localisation of interictal hypoperfusion and neurological lateralisation of clinical symptomatology in our group of patients with sensorimotor aura did not correspond that well (47%).

Most reports dealing with ictal SPECT in migraine, indicate regional hypoperfusion during migraine aura[7,34,36,39]. Ictal SPECT seems to be more sensitive than interictal[74]. Negative ictal SPECTs were reported in patients without aura[2]. In migraine without aura, there is either normal perfusion or hyperperfusion during the attacks[7,38,40]. The hypoperfusion area tended to correspond to the topography of the neurological symptomatology and the side of the headache[7]. Some reports indicate a transient hyperaemia following the initial hypoperfusion[39,41].

Data related to flunarizine, ergotamine and sumatriptan are scanty, often involving small patient populations or isolated case reports. Ferrari *et al.*[2] did not demonstrate significant changes on HMPAO SPECT interictally, ictally and after treatment of an attack with sumatriptan.

Besides the contribution of SPECT to our further understanding of the pathophysiology of migraine and other headache types, the possible implications of SPECT findings in clinical neurology are considerable. SPECT may contribute to the diagnosis of basilar artery migraine, differential diagnosis epilepsy versus migraine and migraine versus tension headache. Furthermore, SPECT observations may contribute to optimalisation of patient management e.g. concerning treatment strategies where vasoconstricting agents should perhaps be avoided in patients with interictal hypoperfusion(s). Finally, SPECT may be applied as a scientific tool in the further identification and mechanistic study of anti-migraine agents.

Acknowledgements

This work was supported by the Flemish Ministry of Education, the Baron Bogaert-Scheid Fund, Born-Bunge Foundation, Medical Research Foundation OCMW Antwerp, University of Antwerp, Neurosearch Antwerp, and NFWO grants numbers 3.0044.92 and 3.0064.93.

References

1　Schlake, H.P., Böttger, I.G., Grotemeyer, K.H. *et al.* The influence of acetazolamide on cerebral low-flow regions in migraine - an interictal ^{99m}Tc-HMPAO SPECT study. *Cephalalgia* 1992, 12, 284

2　Ferrari, M., Haan, J., Blokland, J.A.K. *et al.* Cerebral blood flow during migraine attacks without aura and effect of sumatriptan. *Arch. Neurol.* 1995, 52, 135

3　Friberg, L., Olesen, J., Iversen, H. *et al.* Interictal "patchy" regional cerebral blood flow patterns in migraine patients. A single photon emission computerized tomographic study. *Eur. J. Neurol.* 1994, 1, 35

4　Battistella, P.A., Ruffilli, R., Dalla Pozza, F. *et al.* [99m]Tc HMPAO SPECT in pediatric migraine. *Headache* 1990, 30, 646

5　Olesen, J. and Lipton, R.B. Migraine classification and diagnosis. *Neurology* 1994, 44, 6

6　Lagrèze, H.L., Tsuda, Y., Hartman, A. and Bulan, P. Effect of flunarizine on regional cerebral blood flow in common and complicated migraine. *Eur. Neurol.* 1986, 25S1, 122

7　Lauritzen, M. and Olesen, J. Regional cerebral blood flow during migraine attacks by xenon-133 inhalation and emission tomography. *Brain* 1984, 107, 447

8　Levine, S.R., Welch, K.M.A., Ewing, J.R. and Robertson, W.M. Asymmetric cerebral blood flow patterns in migraine. *Cephalalgia* 1987, 7, 245

9　Norris, J.W., Hachinski, V.C. and Cooper, P.W. Changes in cerebral blood flow during a migraine attack. *Br. Med. J.* 1975, 3, 676

10　Robertson, M.W., Welch, K.M.A., Levine, S.R. and Shultz, L.R. Age-related changes in cerebral blood flow in patients with migraine in 'Migraine and other headaches: the vascular mechanisms', (Ed. J.Olesen), Raven Press, New York, 1991

11　Sakai, F. and Meyer, J.S. Regional cerebral hemodynamics during migraine and cluster headache measured by the Xenon inhalation method. *Headache* 1978, 18, 122

12　Skinhoj, E. Hemodynamic studies within the brain during migraine. *Arch. Neurol.* 1973, 29, 95

13　Friberg, L., Olesen, J. and Iversen, H.K. Regional cerebral blood flow during attacks and whenfree of symptoms in a large group of migraine patients. *Cephalalgia* 1989, 9S10, 29

14　Schlake, H.P., Grotemeyer, K.H., Böttger, I. *et al.* ^{123}I-amphetamine-SPECT in classical migraine and migraine accompagnée. *Neurosurg. Rev.* 1987, 10, 191

15　Cavestri, R., Arreghini, M., Longhini, M. *et al.* Interictal abnormalities of regional cerebral blood flow in migraine with and without aura. *Minerva Med.* 1995, 86, 257

16　Schlake, H.P., Böttger, I.G., Grotemeyer, K.H. *et al.* Brain imaging with 99mTc-HMPAO and SPECT in migraine with aura: an interictal study in 'Migraine and other headaches: the vascular mechanism', (Ed. J.Olesen), Raven Press, New York, USA, 1991, p.209

17　Suess, E., Wessely, P., Koch, G. and Podreka, I. 99mTc-d, 1-HMPAO SPECT in migraine with aura in the headache-free interval in 'Migraine and other headaches: the vascular mechanisms', (Ed. J.Olesen), Raven Press, New York, 1991, p.65

18　Colamussi, P., Giganti, M., Cittanti, C. *et al.* Significato ed utilità della SPECT con 99mTc HMPAO nella diagnostica dell'emicrania con aura. *Radiol. Med.* 1995, 89, 324

19　Maini, C.L., Turco, G.L., Castellano, G. *et al.* Cerebral blood flow and volume in symptom-free migraineurs: a SPECT study. *Nuklearmedizin* 1990, 29, 210

20　Lagrèze, H.L., Dettmers, C. and Hartmann, A. Abnormalities of interictal perfusion in classic but not common migraine. *Stroke* 1988, 19, 1108

21　Friberg, L., Olesen, J., Iversen, H.K. and Serling, B. Migraine pain associated with middle cerebral artery dilatation: reversal by sumatriptan. *Lancet* 1991, 1, 13

22　Schlake, H.P., Böttger, I.G., Grotemeyer, K.H. *et al.* Single photon emission computed tomography (SPECT) with 99mTc-HMPAO (hexamethyl propylenamino oxime) in chronic paroxysmal hemicrania - a case report. *Cephalalgia* 1990, 10, 311

23　Schlake, H.P., Böttger, I.G., Grotermeyer, K.H. and Husstedt, I.W. Brain imaging with I-IMP-SPECT in migraine between attacks. *Headache* 1989, 29, 344

24　Wesseley, P., Suess, E., Koch, C. and Podreka, I. 99 Tc-d, 1-HMPAO SPECT in migraine without aura in 'Migraine and other headaches: the vascular mechanisms', (Ed. J.Olesen), Raven Press, New York, 1991, p.203

25　Podreka, I., Suess, E., Goldenberg, G. *et al.* Initial experience with technetium-99m HMPAO brain SPECT. *J. Nucl. Med.* 1987, 28, 1657

26　Lauritzen, M., Skyhoj-Olsen, T., Lassen, N.A. and Paulson, O.B. Changes in regional cerebral blood flow during the course of classic migraine attacks. *Ann. Neurol.* 1983, 13, 633

27　O'Brien, M.D. Cerebral blood flow changes in migraine. *Headache* 1971, 10, 139

28　Olesen, J. The common migraine attack may not be initiated by cerebral ischaemia. *Lancet* 1981, 29, 438

29　Olesen, J. Migraine and regional cerebral blood flow. *Trends in Neurosci.* 1985, 8, 318

30　Olesen, J., Tfelt-Hansen, P., Henriksen, L.M. and Larsen, B. The common migraine attack may not be initiated by cerebral ischemia. *Lancet* 1982, 45, 438

31　Simard, D. and Paulson, O.B. Cerebral paralysis during migraine attack. *Arch. Neurol.* 1973, 29, 207

32 Skinhoj, E. and Paulson, O.B. Regional cerebral blood flow in internal carotid distribution during migraine attack. *Br. Med. J.* 1969, 3, 569

33 Olesen, J. The ischemic hypothesis of migraine. *Arch. Neurol.* 1987, 44, 321

34 Olesen, J., Friberg, L., Olsen, T.S. *et al.* Timing and topography of cerebral blood flow, aura, and headache during migraine attacks. *Ann. Neurol.* 1990, 28, 791

35 Juge, D. and Gauthier, G. Mésures de debit sanguin cérébral régional (DSCR) par inhalation de Xenon 133, applications cliniques. *Bulletin der Schweiserishn Akademie der Medizinischen Wissenschaften* 1980, 36, 101

36 Nappi, G. and Savoldi, F. in 'Headache: diagnostic system and taxonomic criteria', Eurotext, London, 1985

37 Friberg, L., Olesen, T.S. and Lassen, N.A. Cerebrovascular tone instability causing focal ischemia in 'Neuronal messengers in vascular function', (Eds. H. Nobin, C. Ouman, B. Arnekho-Nobin), Elsevier Science, Amsterdam, 1987, p.549

38 Kobari, M., Meyer, J.S., Ichijo, M. *et al.* Hyperperfusion of cerebral cortex, thalamus and basal ganglia during spontaneously occuring migraine headaches. *Headache* 1989, 29, 282

39 Andersen, A.B., Friberg, L., Olsen, T.S. and Olesen, J. Delayed hyperaemia following hypoperfusion in classic migraine. *Arch. Neurol.* 1988, 45, 154

40 Juge, O. Regional cerebral blood flow in different clinical types of migraine. *Headache* 1988, 28, 537

41 Lassen, N.A. Cerebral blood flow tomography with Xenon-133. *Seminars in Nuclear Medicine* 1985, 15, 347

42 Roach, E.S. and Stump, D.A. Regional cerebral blood flow in childhood headache. *Headache* 1989, 29, 379

43 Thie, A., Fuhlendorf, A., Spitzer, K. and Kunze, K. Transcranial doppler evaluation of common and classic migraine. Part 1. Ultrasonic features during the headache-free period. *Headache* 1990, 30, 201

44 Meyer, J.S., Zetusky, W., Jonsdottir, M. and Mortel, K. Cephalic hyperaemia during migraine headaches. A prospective study. *Headache* 1986, 26, 388

45 Sakai, F. and Meyer, J.S. Abnormal cerebrovascular reactivity in patients with migraine and cluster headache. *Headache* 1979, 19, 257

46 Wolff, H.G. in 'Headache and other head pain', Oxford University Press, New York, USA, 1963

47 Gowers, W.R. in 'The borderland of epilepsy', J&A Churchill, London, 1907

48 Lauritzen, M. Cerebral blood flow in migraine and cortical spreading depression. *Acta Neurol. Scand.* 1987, 76S113, 1540

49 Leao, A.P.P. and Morrison, R.S. Propagation of cortical spreading depression. *J. Neurophysiol.* 1945, 8, 33

50 Sachs, H., Russell, J.A.G., Christman, D.R. *et al.* Positron emission tomographic studies on induced migraine. *Lancet* 1984, 1, 465

51 Spina, A., Damato, V., Losito, R. *et al.* Brain SPECT and migraine in childhood. *Acta Neurol. Napoli* 1992, 14, 10

52 Olesen, J. and Lauritzen, M. The role of vasoconstriction in the pathogenesis of migraine in 'The pharmacological basis of migraine therapy', (Ed. W.K. Amery), Blackwell Scientific, Oxford, UK, 1984

53 Prencipe, M. Focal cerebral ischemia and migraine. *Cephalalgia* 1985, 5, 21

54 Raskin, N.H. Pharmacology of migraine. *Ann. Rev. Pharmacol.* 1981, 21, 463

55 Covelli, V., Achille, P. and De Marinis, M. I preside psicofarmacologici nelle terapie delle cefacee. *Giorn. Neuropsicofarmac.* 1990, 12, 99

56 Thomas, T.D., Harpold, G.J. and Troost, B.T. Cerebrovascular reactivity in migraineurs as measured by transcranial doppler. *Cephalalgia* 1990, 10, 95

57 Ferbert, A., Busse, D. and Thron, A. Microinfarction in classic migraine? A study with magnetic resonance imaging findings. *Stroke* 1991, 22, 1010

58 Igarishi, H., Sakai, F., Kan, S. *et al.* Magnetic resonance imaging of the brain in patients with migraine. *Cephalalgia* 1991, 11, 69

59 Broderick, J.P. and Swanson, J.W. Migraine related strokes, clinical profile and prognosis in 20 patients. *Arch. Neurol.* 1987, 44, 868

60 Featherstone, H.J. Clinical features of stroke in migraine: a review. *Headache* 1986, 26, 128

61 Rothrock, J.F., Walicke, P., Svenson, M.R. *et al.* Migrainous stroke. *Arch. Neurol.* 1988, 45, 63

62 du Boulay, C.H., Ruiz, J.S., Rose, F.C. *et al.* CT changes associated with migraine. *Am. J. Neuroradiol.* 1983, 4, 472

63 Kaplan, R.D., Solomon, C.D., Diamond, S. and Freitag, F.G. The role of MRI in the evaluation of a migraine population: preliminary data. *Headache* 1987, 27, 315

64 Mathew, N.T., Meyer, J.S., Welch, K.M.A. and Nebhett, C.R. Abnormal CT scan in migraine. *Headache* 1977, 16, 272

65 Sargent, J.D., Lawson, R.C., Solbach, P. and Coyne, L. Use of CT scan in an outpatient headache population: an evaluation. *Headache* 1979, 19, 388

66 Soges, L.J., Cacayorin, E.D., Petro, C.R. and Ramachandran, T.S. Migraine: an evaluation by MR. *Am. J. Neuroradiol.* 1988, 9, 425

67 Shah, A.B., Coull, B.M. and Beamer, N.B. In vivo platelet activation and strokes in young adults with migraine. *Neurology* 1983, 33, 206

68 Peatfield, P.C. Can transient ischemic attacks and classical migraine always be distinguished? *Headache* 1987, 27, 240

69 Nichtweiss, M. Hirninfarkte als migränekomplikation. *Nervenartz* 1986, 57, 408

70 Hart, G.H. and Miller, V.T. Cerebral infarction in young adults: a practical approach. *Stroke* 1983, 14, 110

71 Castaldo, J.E., Anderson, M. and Reeves, A. Middle cerebral artery occlusion with migraine. *Stroke* 1982, 13, 308

72 Cohen, R.J. and Taylor, J.R. Persistent neurologic sequelae of migraine: a case report. *Neurology* 1979, 29, 1175

73 Dorfman L.J., Marshall W.H. and Enzmann, D.R. Cerebral infarction and migraine: clinical and radiologic correlations. *Neurology* 1979, 29, 317

74 Feggi, L., Soriani, S., Arnaldi, C. *et al.* Interictal and ictal phase study with 99mTc-HMPAO brain SPECT in childhood migraine with aura. *Neurology* 1995, 1, 47

75 Gawel, M.J. and Krajewski, A. Intracranial hemodynamics in cluster headache. *Headache* 1988, 28, 484

76 Schlake, H.P., Böttger, I.G., Grotemeyer, K.H. and Husstedt, I.W. Brain imaging with 123I-IMP-SPECT in migraine between attacks. *Headache* 1989, 29, 344

77 Wesseley, P., Suess, E., Koch, G. *et al.* Tc HMPAO findings in acute headache and during symptom-free interval. *Cephalalgia* 1989, 9, 62

78 Gawel, M.J., Krajewski, A., Luo, Y.M. and Ichise, M. The cluster diathesis. *Headache* 1990, 30, 652

79 Moskowitz, M.A. Cluster headache: evidence for a pathophysiologic focus in the superior pericarotid cavernous sinus plexus. *Headache* 1988, 28, 584

80 Dierckx, R., Dobbeleir, A., Pickut, B.A. *et al.* [99m]Tc HMPAO SPECT in acute supratentorial ischaemic infarction, expressing deficits as milliliter zeroperfusion. *Eur. J. Nucl. Med.* 1995, 22, 427

81 Neirinckx, R., Canning, L. and Piper, I Technetium-99md, 1-HMPAO: a new radiopharmaceutical for SPECT imaging of regional cerebral blood flow. *J. Nucl. Med.* 1987, 28, 191

82 O'Leary, D.H., Hill, T.C. and Lee, R.G. The use of 123-iodoamphetamines and single photon emission computed tomography to assess local cerebral blood flow. *A. J. N. R.* 1983, 4, 547

83 Lewis, D.H., Longstreth, W.T., Wilkus, R. and Copass, M. Hyperemic receptive aphasia on neuroSPECT. *Clinical Nuclear Medicine* 1993, 18, 409

84 Pedley, T.A. Differential diagnosis of episodic symptoms. *Epilepsia* 1983, 24S1, S31

85 Leao, A.P.P. Spreading depression of activity in cerebral cortex. *J. Neurophysiol.* 1944, 7, 359

86 Diamond, S. Basilar artery migraine, a commonly misdiagnosed disorder. *Postgraduate Med.* 1987, 81, 45

87 Seto, H., Shimizu, M., Futatsuya, R. *et al.* Basilar artery migraine reversible ischemia demonstrated by ^{99m}Tc HMPAO brain SPECT. *Clinical Nuclear Medicine* 1994, 19, 215

88 Sjaastad, O. and Dale, I. Evidence for a new treatable headache entity. A preliminary report. *Headache* 1974, 14, 105

89 Wöber, C., Brücke, T., Wöber-Bingöl, C. *et al.* Relation of dopamine D_2 receptor blockade and therapeutic efficacy in migraine prophylaxis with flunarizine. *Cephalalgia* 1993, 13, 248

90 Ambrosio, C. and Stefani, E. Interaction of flunarizine with dopamine D_2 and D1 receptors. *Eur. J. Pharmacol.* 1991, 197, 221

91 Holmes, B., Brogden, R.N., Heel, R.C. *et al.* Flunarizine: a review of its pharmacodynamic and pharmacokinetic properties and therapeutic use. *Drugs* 1984, 27, 6

92 Mitchelson, F. Pharmacological agents affecting emesis. A review (part II). *Drugs* 1992, 43, 443

93 Piccini, P., Nuti, A., Paoletti, A.M. *et al.* Possible involvement of dopaminergic mechanisms in the antimigraine action of flunarizine. *Cephalalgia* 1990, 10, 3

94 Verhoeff, N.P.L.G., Visser, W.H., Ferrari, M.D. *et al.* Dopamine D_2-receptor imaging with ^{123}I-iodobenzamide SPECT in migraine patients abusing ergotamine: does ergotamine cross the blood brain barrier? *Cephalalgia* 1993, 13, 325

95 Friberg, L. In vivo neuroreceptor imaging by SPECT in migraine. *Cephalalgia* 1995, 15, 310

96 Humphrey, P.P.A., Feniuk W., Motevalian, M. *et al.* The vasoconstrictor action of sumatriptan on human isolated dura mater in 'Serotonin, molecular biology, receptors and functional effects', (Eds. J.R.Fozard, P.R.Saxena), Birkhauser Verlag, Basel, 1991

97 Ferrari, M.D. and Saxena, P.R.S. Clinical and experimental effects of sumatriptan in humans. *Trends Pharmacol. Sci.* 1993, 14, 129

98 Moskowitz, M.A. Interpreting vessel diameter changes in vascular headaches. *Cephalalgia* 1992, 12, 5

99 Scott, A.K., Grimes, S., Ng, K. *et al.* Sumatriptan and cerebral perfusion in healthy volunteers. *Br. J. Clin. Pharmacol.* 1992, 33, 401

100 Dormehl, I.C., Oliver, D.W. and Hugo, N. Cerebral blood flow effects of sumatriptan in drug combinations in the baboon model. *Arzneim.-Forsch./Drug Res.* 1995, 45, 952

SPECT in Neurology and Psychiatry, edited by P.P. De Deyn, R.A. Dierckx, A. Alavi and B.A. Pickut

⁵⁷Cobalt: a SPECT Tracer for Local Brain Damage

Chapter
55

H.M.L. Jansen, H. Stevens, A.A.J. Joosten,
S. Knollema, D.A. Piers, A.E.J. de Jager,
J.M. Minderhoud and J. Korf

Introduction

Cobalt (Co), atomic number 27, takes its name either from the German 'kobold' (evil spirit) or from the Greek 'cobalos' (mine)[1]. In the past, Co-isotopes have been used among others for radiotherapy (^{60}Co) and radiodiagnostic purposes (bleomycine-^{57}Co)[1-5]. At present, the isotopes ^{55}Co and ^{57}Co are evaluated for, respectively, PET- and SPECT-imaging in several diseases, including stroke, multiple sclerosis and traumatic brain injury[6-11]. Because of the limited availability of PET-centres and the complexity and costs of the PET methodology, we have studied the clinical applicability of both ^{55}Co (PET isotope; $T_{1/2}$=17.5 h) and ^{57}Co (SPECT isotope; $T_{1/2}$=270 days). ^{55}Co PET has the advantage of high spatial resolution, absolute quantitation and a relatively low radiation dose (7 mSv/mCi)[10]. The disadvantage is low availability for clinical routine application and logistical problems concerning the relatively short half-life of ^{55}Co. In contrast, ^{57}Co SPECT has the disadvantage of a lower spatial resolution (although the resolution gap is narrowing), a lack of quantitative representation (although SPECT can be considered as semi-quantitative) and a relatively high radiation dose (12 mSv/mCi)[10]. The advantage of ^{57}Co, however, is its wider availability and simple logistics due to a much longer half-life. According to WHO recommendments for class II studies, 22 MBq (0.6 mCi) ^{55}Co (excluding any radionuclide contamination) and 15 MBq (0.4 mCi) ^{57}Co can be used in human studies annually following intravenous bolus administration[10].

In stroke, computed tomography (CT) has most often been used to confirm diagnosis and to exclude other brain pathology[9,12,13]. Predictive parameters measured at admission correlating with neurological outcome and recovery following stroke include rCBF, metabolism, site and size of the infarction together with clinical scores of stroke severity[6,12,13]. After stroke, the brain pathology progresses in steps from ischaemia (potential viability) to infarction (brain cell death) and inflammation (concomitant with the activation of astro- and microglia cells and leukocyte-infiltration)[6,9,12,13]. In all these calcium (Ca) plays an important role. As there is no Ca isotope with suitable radiation characteristics for *in vivo* imaging, we have proposed Co as a Ca tracer to visualise the infarction[6,8]. *In vitro* experiments have demonstrated cellular Co accumulation through non-NMDA Ca channels[6,9,14-19]. A recent Co PET study in 6 stroke patients affirmed the clinical applicability of Co to visualise stroke[6,9].

In multiple sclerosis (MS), the subsequent histopathological events are disruption of the blood brain barrier (BBB) followed by perivascular infiltration of leukocytes, inflammation, demyelinisation, glia-proliferation (gliosis) and

Groningen University Hospital,
PO Box 30.001, 9700 RB
Groningen, Netherlands

eventually axonal and neuronal loss[11,20-22]. Since Ca influx occurs in both cell-death and T-lymphocyte activation in MS, it is reasonable to suppose that visualisation of this Ca accumulation may allow detection of MS lesions. The potential role of Co as a Ca analogue for PET in 7 relapsing progressive MS patients has already been investigated[7,10]. A significant correlation between the mean number of lesions per plain in the MS brain and the progression rate (PR) of the disease was demonstrated in this Co PET study[7]. Here we report the results of a SPECT study with ^{57}Co[11].

Methods

Stroke study

Five patients with a middle cerebral artery (mca) territory infarction admitted to the Neurological Department of Groningen University Hospital, Netherlands, were selected for this Co SPECT study. Inclusion criteria were: stable clinical signs of mca infarction; age over 18 years old; and written informed consent. Patients with disabling previous stroke, serious other disorders or deterioration in the course of mca stroke were excluded. These 5 patients (2 men; 3 women) age 23 to 75 (mean of 53) years formed a homogeneous group with respect to the diagnosis of completed mca infarction, but differed regarding the time interval between stroke onset and Co SPECT examination (6-13 days). All patients had suffered their first ischaemic stroke (thrombo-embolic type) and demonstrated a distinct neurological deficit appropriate to mca infarction ranging from mild paresis to hemiplegia. The mca stroke scale according to Orgogozo was used to assess neurological deficits[9,12]. This mca scale evaluates the level of consciousness, verbal communication, eye movement, power in arm, hand, leg and foot, and facial paresis on a score from 0 (death) to 100 (complete recovery). It was made on admission and discharge (at least 60 days after stroke onset), when patients were clinically stable, and had demonstrated no further improvement for at least 14 days.

SPECT examination was performed 24 h after iv adminstration of 0.4 mCi ^{57}CoCl$_2$ (Amersham, UK) using a double-headed rotating gamma camera (MultiSpect 2, Siemens) equipped with high resolution low energy collimator[23]. Sixty-four 60 s images were acquired on a 64x64 pixel matrix. A Butterworth filter with a cut-off frequency of 0.45 f_{Ny} was used. No attenuation correction was applied.

For each mca stroke patient, we analysed 12 sequential transaxial slices that were located in a 8 cm thick brain section displaying the actual infarction. In each slice, a region of interest (ROI) was defined using an arbitrarily chosen threshold value, thus outlining the infarction area. For each ROI in the infarcted area, an identical contralateral ROI was defined (mirror ROI). The average Co uptake in all ROIs was assessed. Data were combined to obtain the area and Co content of each ROI. The cobalt enhancement ratio (CER) was defined as the quotient of Co uptake in the ROI versus mirror ROI. The cobalt infarction load (CIL) was defined as the product of CER and infarction volume.

MS study

Five relapsing progressive MS patients (4 men; 1 woman) had clinically definite disease according to the Poser criteria[7,22]. The scores on the expanded disability status scale (EDSS) varied between 1.5 and 8.0[24]. The duration of disease (DUR) varied between 78 and 332 months. The EDSS and PR (quotient of EDSS and DUR) were obtained for the five patients as indicators of clinical disease activity i.e. motor handicap[7,21]. All patients gave written informed consent.

SPECT examination was performed 24 h after intravenous injection of 0.4 mCi ^{57}CoCl$_2$ (Amersham, UK) using a single-headed rotating gamma camera (Siemens, Diacam) equipped with a low energy all purpose collimator. Sixty-four 60 second images were collected on a 128x128 pixel matrix. A Butterworth filter with a cut-off frequency of 0.3 f_{Ny} was used.

For each patient we analysed 5 sequential transaxial slices that were located in a 4 cm thick brain section, 3.5 cm above the orbito-meatal line, to ensure the presence of sites of predilection of MS in the brain (peri-ventricular region). In each plane an elliptical ROI was defined to exclude all anatomical structures outside the brain. Inside this elliptical ROI, lesions were recognised as areas of increased signal intensity, indicating local increased uptake of ^{57}Co. In accordance with previous work, these lesions were taken to be MS lesions, based on their localisation[7]. Non-specific areas of high intensity due to vessels in the midline area and choroïd plexus, were disregarded.

The number of pixels and the Co uptake in the brain were determined. The lesion borders were outlined as ROIs using an empirical relative contour level (CL) determined by visual assessment (40% of the average Co uptake per plane per patient). The plaque area (PA: total number of pixels appearing in MS plaques in all ^{57}Co SPECT slices) and the Co enhancement ratio (CER: mean of ratios of the total Co uptake in the MS plaque versus in the non-affected brain) were assessed, resulting in the Co plaque load (CPL) for each patient according to the algorithm CPL=PAxCER.

Results

Stroke study

Table 1 summarises the clinical and Co SPECT data. In all patients, Co SPECT displayed relative Co accumulation in the affected appropriate hemisphere. There was no significant correlation between Co SPECT and clinical parameters (Figure 1).

MS study

Table 2 shows both clinical and Co SPECT data. The mean number of lesions per patient was found to be 3.8 (± 1.3). The mean number of counts within an individual lesion was 24.3 (± 8.6) counts per acquisition per slice. A relationship was found between EDSS and CPL (correlation coefficient of 0.90; p<0.05, using the Spearman-Rank test for non-parametric analysis, Figure 2).

Discussion

Stroke study

Our accumulation indices of Co (CER values in Table 1) are in the same order of magnitude as values reported for ^{201}Tl in stroke patients, although Tl SPECT demonstrated equivocal findings[25]. The use of

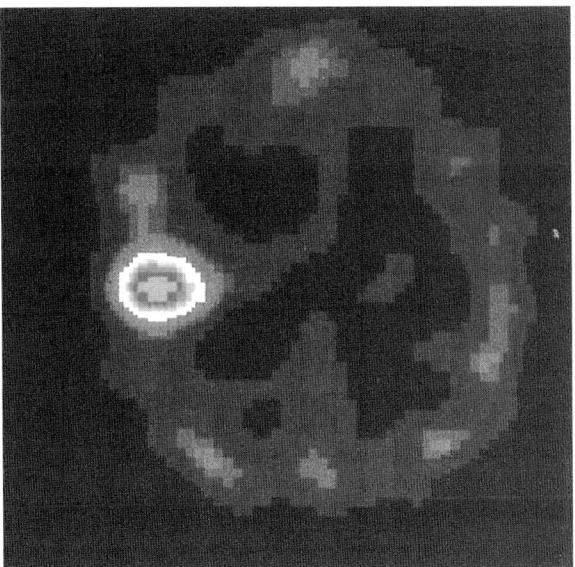

Figure 1 Co SPECT scan of patient 5 performed 9 days after stroke onset, revealing evident Co accumulation in the right mca vascular territory which was 2.7 times the activity in the contralateral region. These findings were affirmed with CT and were in good accordance with the neurological deficit, i.e. mild left-sided hemiparesis and hemihypaesthesia

Tl is based in part on the idea that this monovalent cation may reflect enhanced metabolism, in particular Na/K-ATpase pump activity. In contrast to the present Co study, Tl did not accumulate shortly after the infarction, but only in the subacute phase characterised by hyperperfusion inflammatory processes and BBB breakdown. Thus, Co uptake may therefore have more potential than Tl to detect early damage.

The lack of correlation between Co SPECT and clinical parameters may be explained by the small number of patients in our pilot series. Moreover, other explanations for this discrepancy may be inaccuracy in quantitating clinical parameters, the limited spatial resolution of (double-headed) SPECT and the presence of brain oedema, which cannot be detected on Co SPECT but may well determine the neurological deficit. This pilot study was confined to patients with mca infarction because of its relatively homogeneous clinical presentation and high prevalence[9,12]. All patients demonstrated clinical improvement, which is in good agreement with the general pattern of mca stroke, i.e: moderate recovery accompanied by some degree of permanent clinical deficit. We used the mca scale according to Orgogozo to quantify neurological deficits because of its efficacy in the assessment of mca infarction[9]. An increase in this score is likely to reflect

Table 1 Clinical and Co SPECT data of 5 stroke patients with an acute ischaemic mca infarction

Patient	Interval (days)[a]	Scores at admission mca.adm[b]	Scores at discharge mca.dis[c]	Improvement scores mca.imp[d]	CER
1	12	85	100	15	1.0
2	13	40	45	5	3.6
3	11	20	35	15	2.2
4	6	95	100	5	1.0
5	9	75	100	25	2.7

[a], Time between onset of infarction and acquisition of Co SPECT; [b], neurological status as measured by a mca scale (0-100) on admission; [c], neurological status as measured by a mca-scale (0-100) on discharge;[d], clinical improvement defined as the (positive) difference between the mca score on admission and discharge

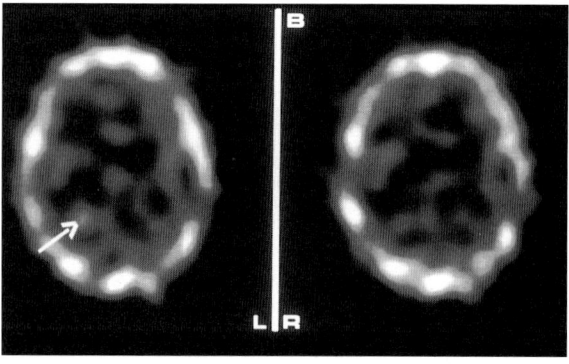

Figure 2 Two sequential SPECT images of patient C showing evident Co uptake in the MS plaque delineated as a ROI (arrow). Co accumulation at the convexity and in the midline area of the brain is due to Co in blood vessels

Table 2 Clinical and [57]Co SPECT data of 5 relapsing progressive MS patients (A-E)

	Clinical data		SPECT data			
	DUR[a]	EDSS[b]	PR[c]	PA[d]	CER[e]	CPL[f]
A	260	7.5	0.029	877	0.032	28.064
B	108	7.0	0.065	655	0.009	5.895
C	332	8.0	0.024	1466	0.027	39.582
D	224	1.5	0.007	356	0.010	3.560
E	78	2.5	0.032	960	0.023	22.080

[a], Duration of the disease (months);[b], expanded disability status scale;[c], progression rate (quotient of EDSS and DUR);[d], plaque area, total number of pixels appearing in MS plaques in all five [57]Co SPECT slices;[e], cobalt enhancement ratio, mean of ratios of the total [57]Co uptake in the MS plaque versus the non-affected brain;[f], cobalt plaque load (product of PA and CER)

neurological improvement. It avoids more unspecific symptoms or signs (cognitive and sensory dysfunction) and disability.

MS study

Our results indicate that Co SPECT using a single-headed camera, readily detects an inhomogeneous Co distribution in the MS brain, displaying multiple sites of increased focal Co uptake[11]. Our preliminary findings suggest a relationship between CPL and EDSS. The poor count rate and signal-to-noise ratio did not allow any statistical analysis. The low spatial resolution of the single-headed SPECT camera in comparison to the PET camera, leads to confluency of multiple MS lesions into one single plaque. For this reason we did not determine the number of MS lesions but instead determined PA and CER, resulting in the CPL parameter[11].

Although we realise that T_2-weighted MRI is considered to be the gold standard in MS, we did not apply this imaging modality. The aim of our study was only to verify the potential of [57]Co as a SPECT nuclide in MS, and not to assess the specificity and/or sensitivity of SPECT versus MRI in MS.

The basic mechanism of detection in [57]Co SPECT may be extravasation of vascular Co and Co labelled T-lymphocytes into the MS lesion irrespective of BBB integrity[10,11,20-22,26]. The character of the MS lesion may vary from one extreme, being predominantly cellular with marked gliosis to the other extreme, inflammation, oedema and demyelination[7,11,21,26].

Hypothetically, [57]Co SPECT may visualise both features of the MS lesion, i.e. axonal and neuronal loss and cell infiltration, inflammation and demyelination[7,11,21,26].

Although we conclude that single-headed Co SPECT is not an appropriate imaging modality in MS, the encouraging results of the present pilot study justify extension by using multi-headed SPECT and longer scan times to improve both qualitative and quantitative interpretations of Co accumulation in both the healthy and the MS brain. The use of a T_2-weighted MRI as a gold standard, is required for further evaluation of the usefulness of Co as a tracer[7,11].

Conclusion

So far, we have studied 5 mca stroke patients and 5 relapsing progressive MS patients with [57]Co SPECT. We are aware of both the potential of our approach and the preliminary nature of our data, which support Co to be a possible marker for cellular decay and/or cellular-mediated infiltration in MS lesions. The actual mechanism of Co uptake poses the hardest question, in which the pharmacology of Co seems to play a pivotal role[6,7,10]. After intravenous administration, Co can be detected for at least 24 h in plasma and the blood-cell fraction (mainly leukocytes)[10]. Plasma Co is recovered both in free unbound and in (ir)reversibly protein-bound form[10]. In MS, immunologically activated T-lymphocytes demonstrate increased Ca influx and may thus accumulate Co in the same manner[7,10,23,27]. In this way, Co may label immune stimulated

T-lymphocytes[23,27]. Thus, Co SPECT may visualise the combination of two features, i.e. axonal and neuronal loss (free Co through non-NMDA Ca channels) and leukocyte infiltration and inflammation (Co labelled T-lymphocytes)[7,10,11]. At this point, our Co SPECT study involves only a few patients, which does not allow assessment of sensitivity and specificity of Co SPECT. Any additional diagnostic or prognostic value and an appropriate time window (i.e. interval stroke onset and Co SPECT) needs further study in larger patient series. In comparison to Tl SPECT (stroke patients) and MRI (MS patients), Co SPECT may have interesting clinical applications.

Acknowledgement

This work was supported by a grant (GGN 22.2741) from the Dutch Technology Foundation (STW).

References

1   Schroeder, H.A., Nason, A.P. and Tipton, I.H. Essential trace metals in man: Cobalt. *J. Chron. Dis.* 1967, 20, 869

2   IARC Working Group on the evaluation of carcinogenic risks to humans. Cobalt and cobalt compounds, Lyon, France, 1991, 52, 363

3   Paans, A.M.J., Wiegman, T., de Graaf, E.J. and Kuilman, T. The production and imaging of [55]Co-labeled bleomycin. Gendreau G. Ninth international conference on cyclotrons and their applications, Caen, France, Les Ulis, Les editions physique, 1981, p.699

4   Rosenberg, D.W. Pharmacokinetics of cobalt chloride and cobalt-protoporphyrin. *Drug Metabolism and Disposition* 1993, 21, 846

5   Lagunas-Solar, M.C. and Jungerman, J,A, Cyclotron production of carrier-free Cobalt-55, a new positron emitting label for bleomycin. *Int. J. Appl. Rad. Isotopes* 1979, 30, 25

6   Jansen, H.M.L., Pruim, J., van der Vliet, A.M. *et al.* Visualization of damaged brain tissue after ischemic stroke with cobalt-55 positron emission tomography. *J. Nucl. Med.* 1994, 35, 456

7   Jansen, H.M.L., Willemsen, A.T.M., Sinnige, L.G.F. *et al.* Cobalt-55 positron emission tomography in relapsing-progressive multiple sclerosis. *J. Neurol. Sci.* 1995, 132, 139

8   Jansen, H.M.L., van der Naalt, J., Van Zomeren, A.H. *et al.* Cobalt-55 positron emission tomography in traumatic brain injury: a pilot study. *J. Neurol. Neurosurg. Psych.* 1996, in press

9   Jansen H.M.L., Paans A.M., van der Vliet, A.M. *et al.* Cobalt-55 positron emission tomography in ischemic stroke: relation to clinical outcome. *J. Cereb. Blood Flow Metab.* 1995, 15, S674

10 Jansen, H.M.L., Knollema, S., Veenma van der Duin, L. *et al.* Pharmacokinetics and dosimetry of 55- and 57-Cobalt chloride. *J. Nucl. Med.* 1996, in press

11 Joosten, A.A.J., Jansen, H.M.L., Piers, A. *et al.* 57-Cobalt SPECT in relapsing-progressive multiple sclerosis: a pilot-study. *Nucl. Med. Comm.* 1995, 16, 703

12 Baron, J.C. Neuroimaging procedures in acute ischemic stroke. *Curr. Opin. Neurol.* 1993, 6, 900

13 Marchal, G., Serrati, C., Rioux, P. *et al.* PET imaging of cerebral perfusion and oxygen consumption in acute ischaemic stroke: relation to outcome. *Lancet* 1993, 341, 925

14 Dienel, G.A. and Pulsinelli, W.A. Uptake of radiolabeled ions in normal and ischemia-damaged brain. *Ann. Neurol.* 1986, 19, 465

15 Dubinsky, J.M. Examination of the role of calcium in neuronal death. *Ann. NY Acad. Sci.* 1993, 679, 34

16 Gibbons, S.J., Brorson, J.R., Bleakman, D. *et al.* Calcium influx and neurodegeneration. *Ann. NY Acad. Sci.* 1993, 679, 22

17 Gramsbergen, J.B.P., Veenma van der Duin, L., Loopuijt, L. *et al.* Imaging of the degeneration of neurons and their processes in rat or cat brain by [45]CaCl2 autoradiography or [55]CoCl2 positron emission tomography. *J. Neurochem.* 1988, 50, 1798

18 Pruss, R.M., Akeson, R.L., Racke, M.M. and Wilburn, J.L. Agonist-activated cobalt uptake identifies divalent cation-permeable kainate receptors on neurons and glial cells. *Neuron* 1991, 7, 509

19 Williams, L.R., Pregenzer, J.F. and Oostveen, J.A. Induction of cobalt accumulation by excitatory amino acids within neurons of the hippocampal slice. *Brain. Res.* 1992, 581, 181

20 Ffrench-Constant, C. Pathogenesis of multiple sclerosis. *Lancet* 1994, 343, 271

21 McDonald, W.I., Miller, D.H. and Thompson, A.J. Are magnetic resonance findings predictive of clinical outcome in therapeutic trials in multiple sclerosis? The dilemma of interferon . *Ann. Neurol.* 1994, 36, 14

22 Poser, C.M., Paty, D.W., Schelnberg, L. *et al.* New diagnostic criteria for multiple sclerosis: guidelines for research protocols. *Ann. Neurol.* 1983, 13, 227

23 Clementi, E., Martino, G., Grimaldi, L.M.E. *et al.* Intracellular Ca^{2+} stores of T lymphocytes: changes induced by in vitro and in vivo activation. *Eur. J. Immunol.* 1994, 24, 1365

24 Kurtzke, J. Rating neurological impairment in multiple sclerosis: an expanded disability status scale (EDSS). *Neurology* 1983, 33, 1444

25 Bernat, I., Toth, G. and Kovacs, L. Tumour-like thallium-201 accumulation in brain infarcts, an unexpected finding on single photon emission tomography. *Eur. J. Nucl. Med.* 1994, 21,191

26 Minderhoud, J.M., Mooyaart, E.L., Kamman, R.L. *et al.* In vivo phosphorus magnetic resonance spectroscopy in multiple sclerosis. *Arch. Neurol.* 1992, 49, 161

27 Martino, G., Clementi, E., Brambilla, E. *et al.* Interferon activates a previously undescribed Ca2+ influx in T-lymphocytes from patients with multiple sclerosis. *Proc. Natl. Acad. Sci. USA* 1994, 91, 4825

SPECT in Neurology and Psychiatry, edited by P.P. De Deyn, R.A. Dierckx, A. Alavi and B.A. Pickut
© 1997 John Libbey & Company Ltd, pp. 473–475

Regional Cerebral Blood Flow in Patients with Ergotamine Misuse: a SPECT study using ^{99m}Tc-HMPAO

Chapter
56

F. Ahmed, K.S. Nijran, R. Hering, B.E. Jones and
T.J Steiner

Introduction

Between 5 and 10% of patients presenting to headache clinics fulfil the criteria for medication misuse headache. Although ergotamine is of undoubted benefit in the treatment of migraine attacks, its mode of action is unclear. It has both partial agonist activity at alpha-receptors and powerful vasoconstrictor effects possibly due to stimulation of vessel wall serotonin receptors[1,2]. The vasoconstrictor effects are prolonged for at least 24 h[3] and regular use may induce a continuous vasoconstriction. The effects of peripheral vasospasm are well known. Whether there are any such effects in the intracranial vasculature is uncertain. We are unaware of any regional cerebral blood flow (rCBF) studies in ergotamine misuse, but regular use of ergotamine clinically produces cumulative effects[4] and a chronic dull occipital pain with nausea which is relieved by a further dose and worsens on withdrawal[3].

Study design

Patients and controls

Patients aged 18-65 years were recruited from The Princess Margaret Migraine Clinic at Charing Cross Hospital, London (UK). Patients in the experimental group were using ergotamine twice or more weekly on a regular basis for longer than 3 months. The control group had tension type headache. Neurological illness other than migraine and other vascular disorders were excluded from the study.

SPECT scanning

HMPAO (Coreteo, Amersham) was mixed with freshly eluted technetium and 7-10 MBq/kg injected intravenously within 30 min. Injections were given under standardised conditions of ambient light and noise levels.

SPECT scans were performed using an SME 810 high resolution dedicated brain scanner with twelve detectors and focussed collimators scanning the axial plane one slice at a time. Multiple 3 or 5 min slices were acquired in sequence at 6 or 10 mm intervals, respectively, from the base to the top of the brain, and the data were corrected for decay of ^{99m}Tc before tomographic reconstruction.

Reconstruction was perfomed using SMB Neuro 900 (version 2.91) 3-slice reconstruction software with a low resolution filter. Attenuation of the 140 keV gamma emission from ^{99m}Tc was corrected using a 99 mm attenuation path length and edge detection to locate the boundary of the head. The 3D data were

Charing Cross and Westminster
Medical School, London (UK),
St. Dunstan's Road, London, UK

reorientated if necessary and interpolated to produce 43 slices, giving a voxel of 1.61 x 1.61 x 2 mm, for transfer to the SPM software.

Analysis

The data were analysed using software from the Wellcome Department of Cognitive Neurology, London UK, implemented in Matlab (Mathworks Inc., Sherborn MA, USA), previously used for PET data. Statistical parametric maps are spatially extended statistical processes which are used to characterise regionally specific effects in imaging data. Statistical parametric mapping combines the general linear model (to create the statistical map or SPM) and the theory of Gaussian fields to make statistical inferences about regional effects[6].

All images (43 slices) studied were normalised by transforming into a standard stereotactic space as defined by the Talairach atlas[7]. A group comparison was made and SPM projections were obtained to look for areas of perfusion which were significantly different between the two groups.

Results

Twenty-seven patients were studied in the experimental group (11M, 16F; mean age 46.6 years, range 30-62). The average weekly consumption of ergotamine was 9 mg (range 4-14 mg) and the mean duration of ergotamine consumption was 68.4 months (range 7 months-27 years). None of the patients were taking any treatment for migraine prophylaxis at the time of assessment. Twenty patients (7M, 13F; mean age 36.1 years, range 25-62) with episodic tension type headache were used as controls, 15 on amitriptyline (tricyclic antidepressant), 3 on fluoxetine (serotonin reuptake inhibitor) and 2 on no treatment.

On visual assessment, most individual scans appeared normal, with only 2 scans showing obvious areas of reduced perfusion (Figure 1). SPM analysis revealed significant areas of both reduced and increased perfusion in patients with ergotamine misuse. The areas of increased perfusion were more marked in the left occipital and both temporal cortices while areas of reduced perfusion were more pronounced in the fronto-parietal cortex, in the cingulate gyrus around the corpus collosum (Figure 2).

Discussion

The mechanism of ergotamine misuse headache is unknown. Reduced serotonin vascular sensitivity in

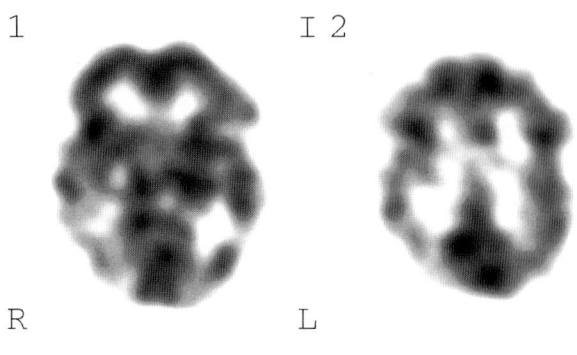

Figure 1 SPECT scan of a patient with ergotamine misuse showing areas of patchy perfusion

ergotamine abusers has been suggested[8]. Our study demonstrates areas of altered perfusion throughout much of the cerebral cortex. Areas of reduced perfusion suggest risk to the cortex from this iatrogenic condition, and it is possible that hyperperfused areas may steal further blood from already hypoperfused areas. We need to know whether the extent of hypoperfusion reaches the level of critical ischaemia.

Withdrawal of ergotamine produces severe headache for up to 7 days in almost all patients[2]. Subsequent relief is excellent and the relapse rate is less than 25%[9]. It would be interesting to see whether the rCBF changes found in our study are reversible after medication withdrawal. If so, a combination of reduced perfusion and rebound vasodilation may be contributory to the cause of headache during ergotamine misuse.

References

1   Fozare, J.R. The animal pharmacology of drugs used in the treatment of migraine. *J. Pharm. Pharmacol.* 1975, 27, 297

2   Muller-Schweinitzer, E. and Fanchamps, A. Effects on arterial receptors of ergot derivatives used in migraine. *Adv. Neurol.* 1982, 33, 343

3   Tfelt-Hansen, P., Eickhoff, J.H., and Olesen, J. The effect of single dose ergotamine tartrate on peripheral arteries in migraine patients, methodological aspects and time effect curve. *Acta Pharmacol. Toxicol.* 1980, 47, 151

4   Ala-Hurula, V., Myllyla, V. and Kokkanen, E. Ergotamine abuse: results of ergotamine discontinuation with special reference to plasma concentration. *Cephalalgia* 1982, 2, 189

5   Tfelt-Hansen, P. and Krabbe, A.A. Ergotamine abuse do patients benefit from withdrawal? *Cephalalgia* 1981, 1, 29

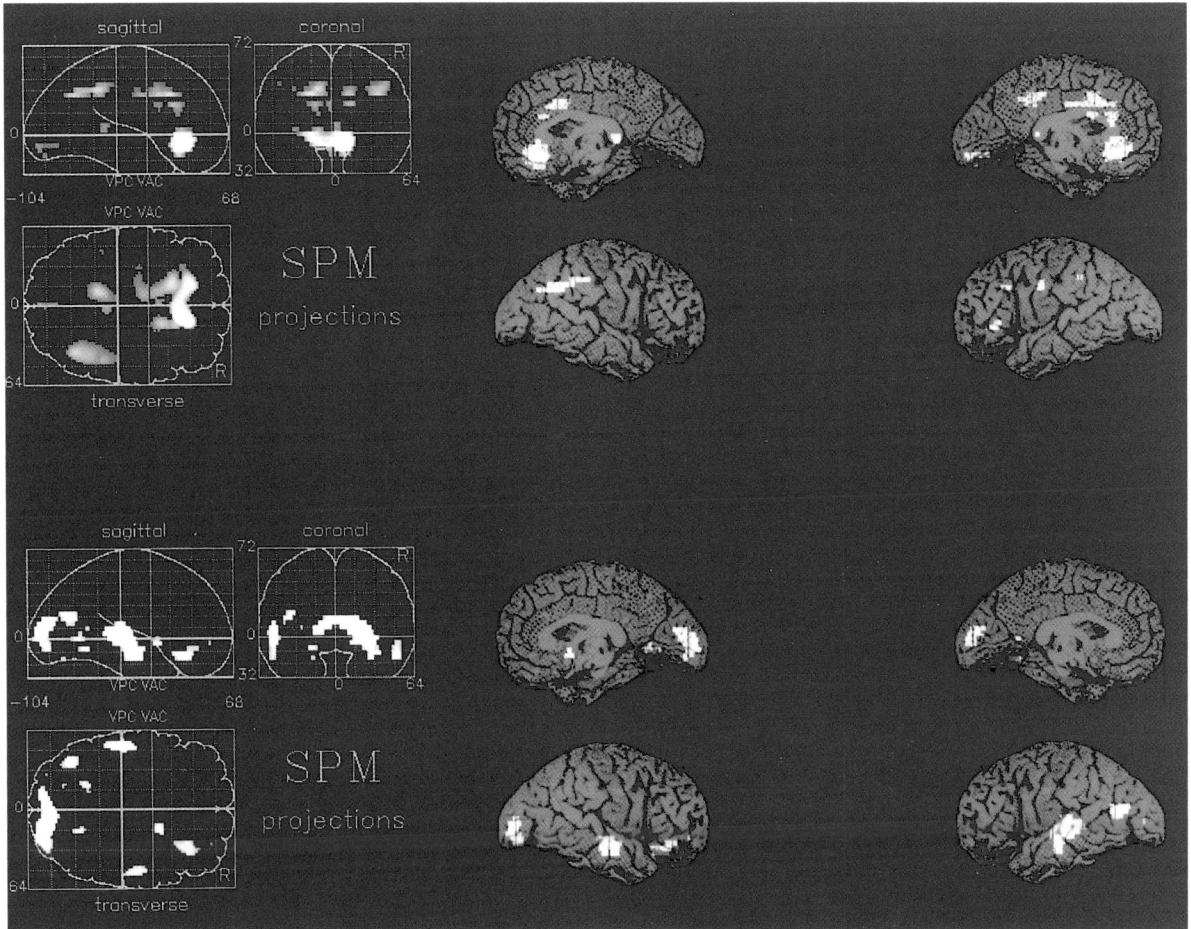

Figure 2 SPM projections and brain maps showing: above, areas of reduced perfusion; and, below, increased perfusion

6   Friston, K.I., Passingham, R.E., Nutt, J.G. *et al.* Localisation in PET image: direct fitting of the intercommisural (AC-PC) line. *J. Cereb. Blood Flow Metab.* 1989, 9, 690

7   Talairach, J., Zilkha, G., Tournoux, P. *et al.* Atlas d'Anatomie Stereotaxique au Telencephale, Masson, Paris, 1988

8   Panconesi, A., Franchi, G., Del-Bianco, P.L. *et al.* Reduced serotinin vascular sensitivity in ergotamine abusers. *Cephalalgia* 1989, 9, 259

9   Pearce, J. Hazards of ergotamine tartrate. *B. M. J.* 1976, 1, 834

Techniques

SPECT in Neurology and Psychiatry, edited by P.P. De Deyn, R.A. Dierckx, A. Alavi and B.A. Pickut
© 1997 John Libbey & Company Ltd, pp. 479-494

Brain SPECT Instrumentation: State-of-the-Art and Future Direction

Chapter

57

J. Vandevivere[*], H. Ham[**], A. Dobbeleir[*], J. Naudts[†] and P.P. De Deyn[*†]

Introduction

Brain single photon emission computed tomography (SPECT) camera provides the clinician with a three-dimensional distribution of the radiopharmaceutical used. The tomographic images are reconstructed from multiple images acquired by the detector around the patient's head. Modern tomographic principles of single photon emission tomography (SPECT) and X-ray computed tomography (CT) are based on quantitative projection data obtained with the detection system placed or rotated around the object.

The mathematical principles underlying the axial tomographic reconstruction were first published by Radon[1] in 1917. In 1956 the first practical application was implemented in radioastronomy by Bracewell[2]. Although the most widely known medical application of tomographic reconstruction is in radiology, it is in nuclear medicine that the first tomographic scanner was build by Kuhl[3] in 1963. The practical application of the principles of tomographic imaging in medicine was initiated by Hounsfield[4] and Ambrose[5] in 1973, with the introduction of X-ray transmission computed tomography (CT) (Table 1). This modern three-dimensional reconstruction algorithm developed for X-ray CT was introduced by Budinger[6] a year later in nuclear medicine. The first SPECT camera using the scintillation camera was designed by Jaszczak *et al,*[7] in 1977

Most SPECT imaging as well as all the other nuclear medicine procedures are performed with a single-head SPECT camera. The detector is mounted on a gantry allowing rotation of the detector around the patient's head and body. The trimmed head geometry of the detector, combined with the ability to magnify the acquisition matrix anywhere across the detector at any desirable factor, ensures an excellent detector-to-patient head proximity and optimal sampling resolution (Figure 1).

The advances in brain SPECT imaging are due to the convergence of developments in the radiopharmaceuticals, the detector[8], the computer, and the reconstruction algorithm used in other imaging modalities (Table 2). Brain SPECT resurged in the beginning of the eighties with the introduction by Winchell[9] of the first regional cerebral blood flow tracers, iodine-labelled amphetamines, followed by [99mTc]-labelled tracers ([99mTc]-HMPAO[10]; [99mTc]-ECD[11]). In the mid eighties the clinical practical multi-headed camera was developed by Lim[12], providing good quality brain SPECT images. He introduced the single ring gantry and radial-motion-only detector travel that guarantees the centre-of-rotation accuracy to 0.1 mm precision. This patented system overcomes the failure of the commercial multiple-detector SPECT system of the early eighties. Gantry instability and detector misalignment of the

[*]Department of Nuclear Medicine and Neurology, Middelheim Hospital Antwerp, Belgium
[**]St Peter's Hospital Brussels, Belgium
[†]Department of Neurochemistry and Behaviour, University of Antwerp, Antwerp, Belgium

Table 1 Time-line SPECT reconstruction

1917	Radon	mathematical principles
1956	Bracewell	astronomy
1963	Kuhl	tomographic scanner
1973	Hounsfield	X-ray CT
1974	Budinger	gamma camera

Table 2 NeuroSPECT advances

Year	Instrumentation: SPECT	Radiopharmaceutical
63	Mark 4 scanner (Kuhl)	
73	Scanner (Meyers)	^{99m}Tc ^{133}Xe
77	Single-head camera(Jaszczak)	
80		^{123}I amphetamines
85	Triple-headed camera(Lim)	
87		^{99m}Tc HMPAO
88		^{99m}Tc ECD

first systems were mainly due to pivoting detectors. The triple-headed gamma camera has the advantage to collect three times more data during the same imaging time in contrast to the single-head detector. The triple-headed gamma camera together with the fan-beam collimator, which magnifies the images on the detector, provides images with a spatial resolution on a phantom of 7.3 mm full width at half maximum (FWHM)[13]. The FWHM is a useful measurement to compare the spatial resolution or the ability to produce the least blurred images of different gamma cameras. It is clear that the current state-of-the-art for neuro-SPECT cameras is the triple-headed system[14,15](Figure 2). The dual-headed SPECT camera is now becoming the 'workhorse' of a nuclear medicine department, by providing maximum clinical versatility (Figure 3).

The triple-headed systems of Picker™ and Trionix™ have the capability to satisfy the unique requirements for xenon regional cerebral blood flow (rCBF) imaging. The multiple detector heads and high speed

capability rotation (a 360° study in 10 s), allow the xenon study to be easily acquired. SPECT studies of the transit of ^{133}Xe, when combined with a measure of the input function, can be fitted to a mathematical model yielding quantitative estimates of the brain flow[16-19].

The gamma camera

Over the past 35 years, the basic technology of the gamma camera, invented by Anger[20], has hardly changed. The actual gamma camera works pretty much as the first commercial PHO gamma camera of Nuclear Chicago™, which was built in 1964. The basic principles of image formation are very simple. The radiopharmaceutical distribution is projected by the collimator onto a NaI (Tl) detector crystal, creating a pattern of scintillations in the crystal that outlines the distribution of radioactivity in front of the collimator. The collimator is usually a large plate of lead with thousands of small holes placed in front of the crystal. Only gamma rays travelling through the collimator holes may contribute to the image formation. The NaI (Tl) scintillation crystal acts as a transducer and produces a light pulse when hit by a photon. These light pulses are collected by photomultiplier tubes, which generate a measurable electric current by multiplication. The array of photomultiplier tubes fixed on the crystal, and connected to electronic position logic circuits, determines the 'x' and 'y' coordinates of the photon interaction.

Each scintillation event is also analysed for its energy 'E' by a pulse-height analyser. When the source radioactivity is distributed in the body of a patient, scattering of the emitted photons may take place. During scattering, the photon trajectory changes and a fraction of the photon's energy is lost. During the imaging most scattered photons are removed because they are not useful, as they do not correspond to the original distribution of the radiopharmaceutical in the

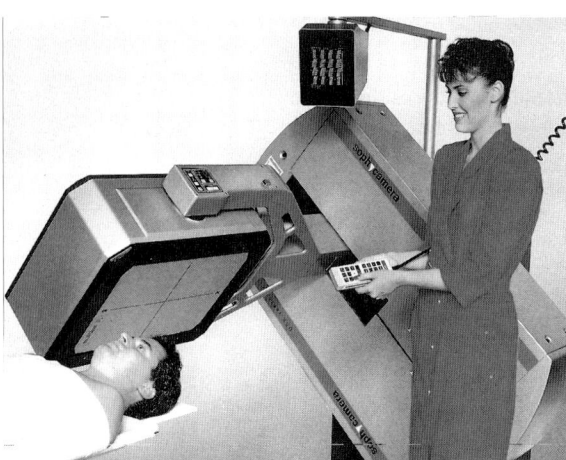

Figure 1 Single-head gamma camera. The detector is mounted on a gantry allowing rotation of the detector around the patient's head and body. The trimmed head geometry, combined with the ability to magnify the acquisition matrix anywhere across the detector at any desirable factor, ensures an excellent detector-to-patient head proximity and optimal sampling

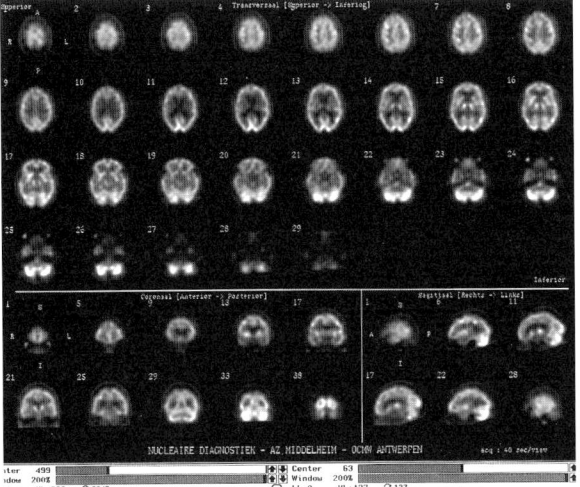

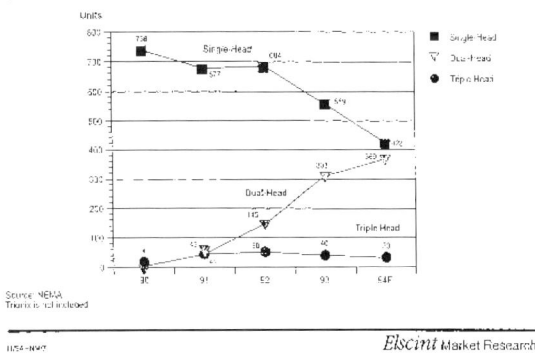

Rotating Cameras in the U.S.

Figure 3 The amount of single-, dual-, and triple headed SPECT cameras sold in the US between 1990 and 1993

Figure 2 ^{99m}Tc-HMPAO brain study with a triple-headed SPECT camera equipped with lead superfine fan-beam collimators, with a sensitivity at 10 cm of 106 counts/ Ci min, and with a system resolution of 7.3 mm FWHM (rotating radius 13 cm). Clinical history: 23 year-old healthy male volunteer. Injected dose: acquisition started 20 min after injection of 20 mCi ^{99m}Tc-HMPAO (Ceretec, Amersham^{TM}). SPECT parameters: Trionix TRIAD 88^{TM}; acquisition: 30 min, 40 s/stop, 3.5 mm pixel, projection images were rebinned to parallel images and reconstructed in 64x64 matrix using a Butterworth filter 0.7 cycles/cm, roll-off 5

body. The scattered photons are removed by the pulse-height analyser, which selects only those photons falling within a predefined selected window energy range.

It is not easy to determine exactly the 'x' and 'y' coordinates and the 'E' energy of the photon interaction in the detector. This is due to the main disadvantage of the Anger design and its inherent non-uniformity across the field of view, which arises from the non-uniformity of the collimator and the NaI (Tl) crystal itself, defects in optical coupling between the crystal and the photomultipliers, variations in the performance of the photomultipliers and the non-linearity in the processing circuitry. Engineering of the gamma camera to correct these distortions has progressed considerably.

The fundamental limitation of the Anger algorithm is that the determination of the spatial 'x' and 'y' coordinates of the photon interacting within the scintillation crystal and the energy 'E' deposit in the crystal are interdependent. This is due to the fact that the sum of the outputs of all

photomultiplier tubes is computed to calculate the 'E'. This interdependence is fundamental to Anger methodology and limits the performance specification of the Anger camera whether partially digital or analogue.

With the development of the cheaper microprocessor, manufacturers are digitising the output of each photomultiplier tube. This so-called totally 'digital camera' permits a better determination of 'x' and 'y' coordinates and the energy 'E' of the photon which interacts with the scintillation crystal. ADAC^{TM} and Park Medical Systems^{TM} propose a 'Non Anger' digital detector. Here, a cluster of photomultipliers around the interacting photon is used, to compute in real time 'x' and 'y' positions and the energy (E) deposit in the crystal by the incident photon.

With regard to scatter and attenuation correction, today's state-of-art camera should be able to produce non-spatial distorted images in a wide energy range. The energy dependent spatial distortions are primarily the result of the different penetration/absorption depths within the scintillation crystal for photons of different energies. The varying interaction depth results in different solid angles with respect to the photomultiplier tubes. Since the depth of interaction has a direct impact on the spectral response of the photomultiplier tubes, the values for 'x', 'y' and 'E' are directly impacted. Several manufacturers are providing digital processors correcting for energy dependent spatial resolution.

A summary of the NEMA performance of the recent gamma cameras is presented in Table 3.

Table 3 Comparison chart NEMA specification

	ISR[a]	SIP[b]		CR[c]	IER[d]
		ESR[e]	SS[f]		
ADAC (vertex epic)	3.5	8.8	285	200	10
Elscint(Helix-HR)	3.3	9.0	540	180	9.8
GE (Maxxus)	3.8	10.2	330	180	9.8
Park	2.7	8.8	325	250	9.2
Picker (3000XP)	3.3	7.7	230	110	10
Siemens (Multispect 3)	3.9	7.6	210	190	10.1
SMV (DST-XL)	3.1	8.7	317	220	9.5
Toshiba	3.8	10.2	295	200	10
Trionix (Triad XLT)	3.8	9.6	320	65	9.8

All measurements performed per ' NEMA standards publication for performance measurements of scintillation cameras, NEMA NU-1986'

[a] ISR (intrinsic spatial resolution): in mm; FWHM UFOV (full width at half maximum; useful field of view); [b] SIP (system imaging performance): ESR (extrinsic spatial resolution): in mm; FWHM with LEAP (low energy all purpose) collimator in air and at 10 cm distance; [c] CR (count rate) : in kcps (kilocounts per s); observed with 20% loss, without scatter and 20% energy window; [d] IER (intrinsic energy resolution): in%; ratio of FWHM to photopeak energy,140 keV, 20 Kcps; [e] ESR (extrinsic spatial resolution): in mm; FWHM with LEAP (low energy all purpose) (system sensitivity): in counts/min/μCi; LEAP collimator; [f] SS (system sensitivity): in counts/min/μCi; LEAP collimator

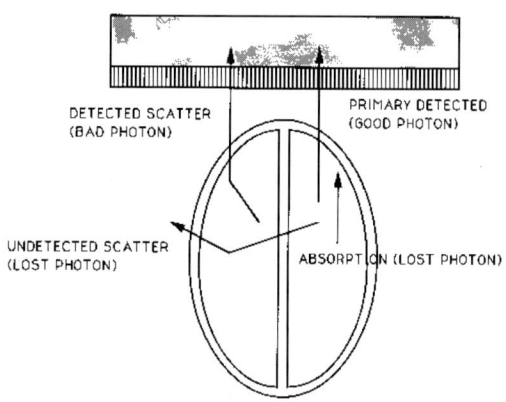

Figure 4 Potential path of the emitted photon in the brain. The 'good' unscattered primary photons follow a straight-line trajectory through a collimator hole and contain the correct information. The 'bad' Compton scattered photons that reach the detector are backprojected along lines from which they did not originate and contain incorrect positional information. Consequently their inclusion in the SPECT images decreases the contrast and the spatial resolution and affects the quantitation. The 'lost' photons cause attenuation. This is due to the loss of useful photons in the body tissues, either by photoelectric absorption or by scatter through an angle sufficiently large that they can no longer be detected

Towards SPECT quantification

Although the image quality of the SPECT images has improved tremendously, we are actually not able to quantify studies in mCi of radioactive tracer per g tissue, except for those studies based on xenon washout curves. Combining good scatter, attenuation compensation and resolution recovery would have the potential to move SPECT imaging from its mostly qualitative role into a fully quantitative clinical diagnostic imaging modality. During the past years, a great amount of experimental work has been published to correct for attenuation, scatter and resolution recovery, the essential limiting factors that affect the quantitative aspects of SPECT images. In the near future, the growing capabilities in electronics and computer technology may offer a cost effective solution for this correction. It is encouraging to see much progress in this area. Since the mid-nineties, some manufacturers are proposing scatter and attenuation compensation and resolution recovery[21].

It is important to remember some basic physics to understand scatter and attenuation. According to the potential path of the emitted photon in brain tissue we can divide the photons into the 'good', the 'bad' and the 'lost'[22], (Figure 4). The 'good' unscattered primary photons follow a straight-line trajectory through a collimator hole, and deposit their full energy in the crystal. Those photons contain the correct information.

The 'bad' scattered photons are deflected and lose a fraction of their original energy. The scattered photons contain incorrect positional information. Consequently their inclusion in the SPECT images decreases the contrast and the spatial resolution and affects the quantitation.

The 'lost' photons cause attenuation. This is due to the loss of useful photons in the body tissues, either by photoelectric absorption or by scatter through a sufficiently large angle so that they can no longer be detected.

Scatter

Excellent reviews have been written by Buvat[23,24] and Rosenthal[25]. The 'good' and the 'bad' photons are selected at a system level on the basis of the energy deposited in the crystal. The determination of the energy of a photon with the system is far from ideal. In case of a source emitting monoenergic photons in front of a detector, the pulse height analyser will register a spread of the energy response instead of a narrow line as ideally would be expected at the location corresponding with the energy of the photon. The parameter to measure the energy spread is the FWHM. The FWHM is expressed as a percentage of the photopeak energy 'E'. The energy resolution for ^{99m}Tc of the actual systems varies between 10 and 9.2%, which is practically the theoretical limit of 8.5% that can be achieved. The theoretical limit is the energy resolution measured with a single crystal coupled to the specific photomultiplier tube. The poor energy resolution is due to the fluctuations in the crystal's light output by each 'good' photon interacting in the NaI (Tl) crystal and, ultimately, by the variability of the electrons produced by the photomultiplier tube. Moreover, the physics of the Compton interaction tells us that the energy loss slowly changes with increasing angle. The so-called 'small-angle' scatter is the most abundant in the photopeak for the common radionuclides. A 140 keV photon scattered through an angle of 52° produces a photon of 126 keV, which is within a 20% energy window[25]. Since the energy resolution of the system is 9-9.5% for ^{99m}Tc, a wide (20-15%) pulse-height discriminator is usually chosen to include the 'good' photons. Unfortunately many 'bad' photons will also be recorded in the photopeak window of the camera's pulse-height analyser. For a ^{99m}Tc-planar acquisition of a normal-sized patient, about 30% of the photons detected within the 20% window are scattered photons[23]. Total scatter rejection at system level is insufficient and further analysis of the Compton scatter is necessary. It should be noted, however, that an analytical study of the relative proportion of the detected photons with different pathways is not feasible, since these pathways cannot be retraced. Therefore scatter correction methods constitute approximations based on various assumptions.

Elimination of scatter events

The common goal of the energy-based scatter elimination methods is to estimate the spatial distribution of the scattered photons in order to remove them from the acquired image. If one window is placed on the photopeak of the radionuclide's spectrum and another is placed in another region to estimate the Compton fraction, and if an appropriate relationship

Table 4 Scatter correction methods commercially implemented

ADAC	work in progress
Elscint	scatter free image (SFI^{TM})
GE	work in progress
Park	Holospectral^{TM} imaging
Picker	dual photopeak window
Siemens	weighted window scatter substraction
SMV	work in progress
Toshiba	triple energy window (TEW^{TM})
Trionix	work in progress

between the counts in the two windows can be determined, the scatter correction can be scaled and subtracted from the photopeak image. Multiple finer windows covering a wider range of the energy spectrum could allow a better discrimination between different scattering environments. This yields an image with reduced scatter and better contrast. This scatter free image appears more noisy and unpleasant to interpret, even if its contents are more reliable.

More scatter correction methods are implemented on the gamma camera by the manufacturers. Those currently available in clinical practice are discussed briefly in Table 4. Other techniques that do not require particular hardware or software, such as the dual energy window method, can also be implemented clinically. The currently available clinical methods can be divided into 2 groups. First, relatively simple methods, such as the dual photopeak window and the triple energy window. The data are acquired in the photopeak and the estimation of the scatter component is based on a few parameters.

The dual-photopeak window method of King[26] is based on the hypothesis that the lower part of the photopeak will contain a large amount of scatter, while the upper energy portion of the photopeak will be practically scatter free. Furthermore this method assumes that there is an existing relationship between the scatter fraction within the photopeak for the pixel i and the ratio of the number of counts detected in two equal wide non-overlapping subwindows splitting the photopeak window. The dual photopeak window, according to a simulation study of Buvat[24], tends to overestimate the amount of unscattered photons in pixels with low counts and to underestimate it when it is high so that relative quantification performance is expected to be poor. For absolute quantification, the method may be a good compromise. In the triple energy window (TEW™) method of Ichihara[27], the number of scattered photons is estimated in each pixel from the events acquired within two narrow (2 keV) subwindows located on each side of the photopeak window. The scatter component in the photopeak is estimated by the trapezoidal area located under the linear fit determined between the 2 subwindows. Practically, the images are acquired simultaneously in the three windows. In SPECT the substraction is performed on each projection before the reconstruction. The low number of photons recorded within the two narrow subwindows in each pixel, in particular the upper one, may make correction particularly sensitive to statistical fluctuation which hinders accurate local quantification. The triple energy window method globally overestimates the number of scattered photons in the photopeak window according to the simulation studies of Buvat[24]. It may be a valuable alternative to the dual photopeak window method, in particular for relative quantification.

The more sophisticated methods, such as scatter free image (SFI™) proposed by Berlad *et al.*[28], Holospectral™ imaging of Gagnon[29,30] and factor analysis of medical image sequences, initiated by Di Paola[31] and elaborated by Mas[32], using theoretically more comprehensive analysis of the data, are potentially more reliable in terms of quantification, and are confirmed by the simulation studies of Buvat[23]. The Holospectral™ imaging of Park Medical Systems proposes scatter correction at the data acquisition stage. This is one of the most advanced approaches for scatter correction available in clinical practice. From each photon interaction the 'E' energy and the 'x' and 'y' position is digitised and stored in 16 adjacent energy bins covering an energy range from 53 to 165 keV. Each energy bin is 7 keV wide. The mathematical algorithm later purges the scattered photons. This yields an image with reduced scatter, better contrast and less counts (Figure 5).

The methods relying on both wide spectral range analysis far from the photopeak and fine sampling will be more sensitive to camera non-uniformity. The superiority of these sophisticated methods over those which are less demanding will have to be proved clinically to justify the additional storage and computational investment that they require.

Weighting of the detected events

This approach intends to take into account all photons detected within a wide energy window. Indeed, it uses the energy information of the photons in order to weight their contribution and statistically relocate them by spreading the weights around their detection

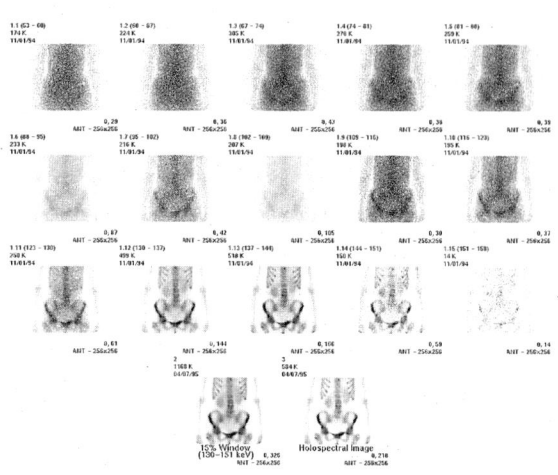

Figure 5 The 'Holospectral™' acquisition of a bone scan. Upper 3 rows The raw data stored in 16 adjacent energy bins covering an energy range from 53 to 165 keV. Each energy bin is 7 keV wide. The frames outside the photopeak contain a significant number of 'good' photons that can contribute to the final image. Last row: left side: represents the conventional bone scan 15per cent window. Right side: represents the bone scan processed by the Holospectral algorithm. This yields an image with reduced scatter, better contrast and less counts (images provided courtesey of Park Medical System)

location. This basic idea was first suggested by Beck[33] in 1972. It was not until 1988 that Halama[34] brought about the practical application. Each photon detected at a position 'x', 'y' with an energy 'E' is distributed by the weighted acquisition module (WAM™) over a 21-pixel matrix centred on 'x','y' and selected as a function of 'E'. The major drawbacks are that the weighting matrices are predetermined and do not adapt themselves to the patient's size and the geometry during acquisition; and the smoothing effect of the correction algorithm on the obtained images. Siemens™, which commercialised the system, does not promote it anymore.

Attenuation

The accuracy of SPECT images is hampered by attenuation of the emitted photons inside the body. The physical importance of photon attenuation can be appreciated from the fact that the half-value layer for 140 keV photons through soft tissue is about 4.5 cm for narrow beam geometry. The simplest and most well known method for correcting attenuation was described by Chang[35]. The measured projection data are first reconstructed without attenuation correction. A correction factor is calculated at each point as the average attenuation factor. A more sophisticated and theoretically more accurate compensation for photon attenuation requires knowledge of the geometry and composition of the attenuation coefficient for brain tissues and the surrounding bone structures. This problem can be solved with a measured attenuation map. The well known X-ray CT image is such a map. It would be ideally reconstructed from transmission data obtained simultaneously with the emission data. Nuclear manufacturers are developing two different methods:

1. The dual-head systems use the dual-scanning line-source, a moving line-source which scans the patient's body during each step in the SPECT acquisition[36].
2. In the triple head system[37,38], one detector head is dedicated to acquire the transmission scan and for this purpose a line-source is mounted at the focal line of a fan-beam collimator, (Figure 6).

In the brain one generally assumes the attenuation is uniform. Several problems remain and clinical validation is necessary: the cross-talk between transmission and emission energy windows when both transmission and emission images are acquired simultaneously; the attenuation compensation algorithm used which varies from vendor to vendor from a single iteration of pre-reconstruction correction, to single and multiple iterations with attenuation compensation; and the transmission data truncation artefact when fan-beam collimators are used.

Variable spatial resolution

A third important aspect of SPECT is the non-uniformity of resolution with depth for parallel-hole collimation. A promising method for dealing with this collimator problem is to incorporate correction factors from measured or theoretical spread function in an iterative reconstruction algorithm[39].

Scatter, attenuation and variable spatial resolution compensation: inseparable issues

It is fundamental that the three main causes for SPECT artefacts are corrected. Compensation for one parameter creates other artefacts. The images obtained, after eliminating the root causes for SPECT artefacts, will improve in contrast, signal-to-noise, enhance in detail and increase activity quantification accuracy. The complexity in the distribution of the 'good', the 'bad' and the 'lost' photons makes it almost impossible to compensate for all the variables associated with photon scatter and attenuation. Accurate quantification therefore remains impossible at this time. Furthermore the image noise will increase as 30 to 40% of the detected counts will be rejected. A clinical system will become available in the near future. The actual number-crunching computer is easily accessible and can handle sophisticated correction algorithm image sets at an incredible speed.

Computers, towards standardisation and connectivity

Standardisation of the hardware

There is a trend to move towards standardisation of the hardware. Practically all the manufacturers are abandoning the concept of building their own computer. This trend has fuelled an explosion of systems in nuclear medicine called workstations, which are small powerful computers, that run an open industry operating system (UNIX) (Table 5). The graphical user interface (X window with OSF/Motif or Open Look) provides easy control for non-computer orientated physicians.

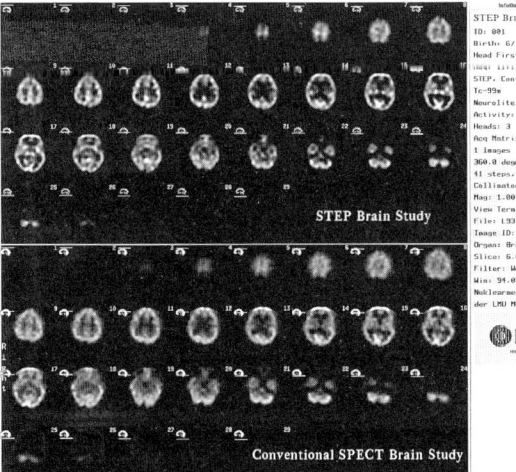

Figure 6 ^{99m}Tc-ECD perfusion brain study acquired on PRISM 3000 and corrected for attenuation by STEPTM (simultaneous transmission emission protocol). The STEPTM of the triple-headed gamma camera of Picker involves a collimated line source ^{153}Gd and fan-beam collimation on all three heads

Imaging software from third parties

Several gamma camera manufacturers are moving to license (or adapt) imaging software from third parties. These companies develop software library toolboxes

Table 5 Workstation

ADAC	SUN SPARC 20
Elscint	Xpert (pentium)
Toshiba	SUN SPARC 20
Park Medical	SUN SPARC 20
Siemens	Mac PowerPC 601/110 MHz
GE	HP-715
Trionix	SUN SPARC 20
SMV	IBM Power 6000
Picker	DEC AXP 175

Table 6 Third party software toolbox

Nuclear manufacturers	Software companies
Adac	AVS
Siemens	IDL
GE	ISG
SMV	PV Wave

that are operating mostly outside of nuclear medicine, in CT and MRI. Examples of cooperation are ADAC-AVS, Siemens-IDL, GE-ISG and SMV-PV wave (Table 6). Developing new software is expensive and is not the core business of nuclear manufacturers. Some manufacturers have practical objections because nuclear medicine images have a considerable number of specific features.

Connectivity

Although the concept of image communication on a multi-vendor, multimodality network of image acquisition, storage and display devices is desirable from the physician's point of view, the reality is that it can be very difficult for vendors to implement it until now. Local area networks interconnect multi-vendor equipment to the propriety networks, either directly, or via bridges, routers or gateways. There is a chance, in the near future, that computers from different modalities will actually talk to each other.

Limited connectivity between the systems is now available through Interfile 3.3 as standard[40,41]. It seems likely that a step further will be taken with the recently published, completely documented, DICOM 3.0, US standard. The goal of the redesigned standard DICOM, introduced by Bigwood[42], is to promote communication between imaging devices. The DICOM standard is maintained by the Working group VI of the MED-PACS section of the Diagnostic Imaging and Therapy Systems Division of the National Electrical Manufacturers Association (NEMA[43]). The Nuclear Medecine Ad Hoc Med-PACS committee proposed a 'supplement 7'[44] to version 3 of DICOM . This committee is in contact with the members of the European Standards Committee (CEN). The new

nuclear medicine Image Object Definition (IOD) redefines a DICOM image to be a multi-dimensional, multi-frame image set. DICOM 'supplement 7' meets the specific requirements of nuclear medicine image data and a 'static image' becomes a special case of the general multi-dimensional image.

The DICOM 3.0 'send' and 'receive' capabilities will permit : standardisation of the nuclear procedures; multimodality image fusion and compensation for partial volume effect; and information management.

Standardisation of the nuclear procedures

The referring physician expects that nuclear medicine is able to produce the same and reproducible results within a defined margin of error, wherever the test is performed.

Until now, this is not the case as every manufacturer, or even nuclear centre, has its own software packages and standards.

A minimum of standardisation and rigorous quality assurance are needed to ensure that all results have the same significance. Efforts need to be made by manufacturers and centres of nuclear medicine to allow the routine exchange of tomography data. A large scale distribution of data, to build the statistical distribution of the parameters of interest to help define normal conditions and decision thresholds is necessary. DICOM may be the potential software toolbox to achieve this goal.

Multimodality image fusion and compensation for partial volume effect

Multimodality image fusion is very important for nuclear medicine. It allows combination of the functional character of nuclear medicine studies with the anatomical detail available in CT or MRI. Appropriate correlation of both can be a big aid for nuclear medicine.

The co-registration of functional images with CT or MRI may provide a solution to the partial volume effect[45]. It refers to the inaccuracy in the determination of the activity in anatomically small structures, because of the influence on the adjacent structures. The phenomenon is due to the mismatch between system resolution and object size. This effect will decrease the apparent mean activity within small structures surrounded by lower activity region and vice versa[46,47]. Partial volume effects are important in comparing the relative activity in small brain structures of different sizes. It may be even more important when comparing activities in small structures across individuals whose structures volume may differ. Examples of situations where the effect of partial volume effect is important include Alzheimer disease and temporal lobe epilepsy[48]. In these diseases, CT and MRI have reported atrophy in the tissue volume in the corresponding SPECT regions where the relative uptake of the regional blood flow tracer is low. Today, correction methods remain experimental. They depend either on measuring or calculating a recovery coefficient as a function of the object size. The object size can be estimated independently by CT or MRI.

Information management

The organisation of clinical practices will evolve further. A new generation of Picture Archiving and Communication Systems (PACS) is underway and, this time, it is likely to affect the majority of nuclear medicine installations. Its characteristics are: decentralised systems, the era of mainframes is over, data remain distributed over a large number of small but powerful computers interconnected by local and wide area networks; open environment with multivendor equipment based on industry standards; departmental information systems (NMIS) in which automatisation of work flow is the key to quality improvement and cost reduction, acquisition and viewing stations, PACS, NMIS, all of these cooperate in the same manner; integration of text and image reports together with additional features such as oral or hand written annotations (multimedia).

There is hope that the failures of the past can be avoided by progressing in an incremental way, reducing the complexity to small manageable pieces[49]. The evolution of computer systems will certainly influence the technical solutions available for carrying on the automatisation of information flow. Clearly, under the pressure of video applications, communication bandwidth will become available at low prices, in quantities sufficient for fast transport of medical images. Of more concern are the developments in the area of software engineering. Due to mass market effects, only a few software houses worldwide have the means to commercialise powerful tools. Medical software developers will prefer to use these tools even if as a consequence the resulting product

does not comply to the standards of the medical world. In other words, the medical standards will have to be supersets of the *de facto* standards established in mass consumer markets. Finally, the Internet has gained such an impetus that it cannot remain without effect. Already, the first applications of using the Internet for training of nuclear medicine specialists have been reported in the literature. One can expect further applications to follow[50].

PET imaging with SPECT camera

There is a trend for performing one of the most useful clinical applications of positron emission tomography (PET) imaging with a conventional SPECT gamma camera[51-54]. ^{18}F-fluorodeoxyglucose ([18]FDG) gives an image that is related to regional glucose metabolism and until now has been restricted essentially to PET imaging[55-57]. The initial application of [18]FDG was for the evaluation of seizure disorders, brain tumours, and dementia, where PET imaging is usually more sensitive and specific than other imaging modalities[58-63]. The technique was then applied to the heart where myocardial viability is virtually assured by significant [18]FDG activity measured within a myocardial region, demonstrating diminished coronary blood flow[64]. Recently, [18]FDG has been shown to be a promising radiopharmaceutical for oncology, where malignant tumours succesfully accumulate [18]FDG in proportion to their high proliferation. Extracranial tumours succesfully imaged with [18]FDG PET include colon[65], lung[66], breast[67], pancreas[68], various sarcomas[69], and squamous cell carcinoma of head and neck[70].

The easiest and cheapest way to perform [18]FDG images with the SPECT camera is to treat 511 keV annihilation photons resulting from positron decay as single photons. This method is used by most manufacturers[51-53]. Two easy modifications in the SPECT camera are required for 511 keV imaging, namely an ultra high energy collimator in front of the crystal and modification of the standard 70-360 keV energy range. To constrain 511 keV photons in the lead channels of the collimator, very thick septa of at least 2.5 mm are required resulting in a very heavy collimator [142 kg (APEX Helix, Elscint[TM]) 215 kg (TRIAD XLT, Trionix[TM])]. The SPECT camera needs a stable gantry to support the collimator(s) and to maintain an acceptable centre of rotation. The low sensitivity of the 3/8" thick NaI (Tl) crystal for 511 keV can be enhanced with 36% by providing a 1/2" thick crystal. The intrinsic spatial resolution for [99mTc] maintains good NEMA measurements when selecting a 3/8" or a 1/2" crystal, the FWHM is, respectively, 3.8 and 4.3 mm for crystal[52]. Both thicker crystal and

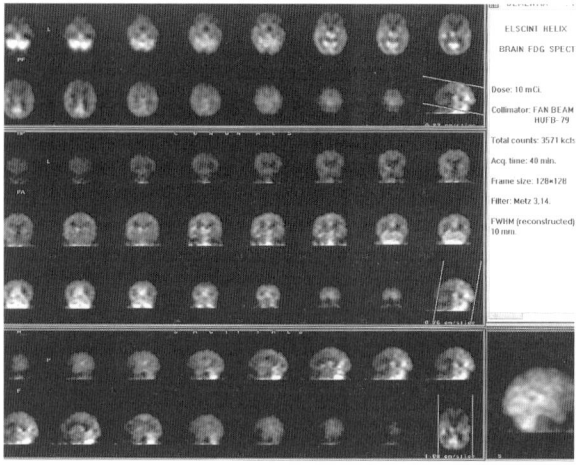

Figure 7 [18]FDG brain study with dual-headed SPECT camera fitted with a dedicated fan-beam collimator. Clinical history: patient with Alzheimer dementia. Injected dose: 10 mCi [18]FDG. SPECT parameters: Elscint Helix; acquisition: 40 min, Frame size 128x128; Filter: Metz 3,14; FWHM (reconstructed transaxial slice): 10 mm (Courtesy of Sandler MP, MD, Vanderbilt University)

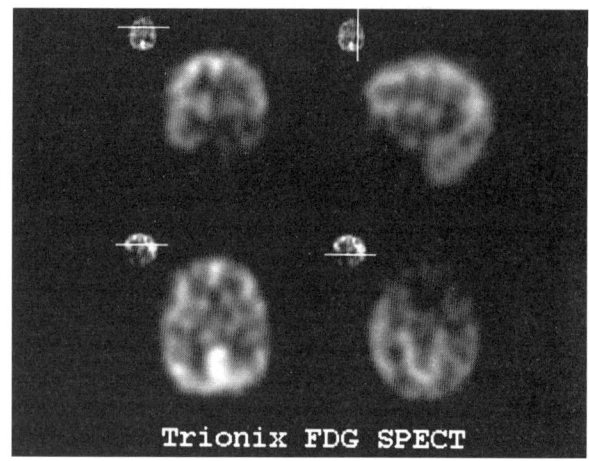

Figure 8 [18]FDG brain study with triple-headed SPECT camera fitted with a dedicated parallel-hole collimator. Clinical history: 27 year-old female with history of seizure disorder. Injected dose: 10 mCi 18FDG; SPECT study performed subsequent to PET study (time from injection to PET study unknown). Both studies interictal. SPECT parameters: Trionix TRIAD XLT[TM]; acquisition: 40 min, 60 s/stop, 3.56 mm pixel, Butterworth pre-filter 0.5 cycle/ cm, 5 roll-off.(Courtesy of Cleveland Clinic Foundation)

specially designed high energy collimators enhance 511 keV imaging quality and increase sensitivity[71]. Elscint[TM] and Trionix[TM] use a multiple-headed gamma camera, fitted with an optimised high energy collimator, to obtain brain SPECT images with a spatial resolution of about 10 mm in the reconstructed slice (Figures 7 and 8). The advantage of the concept is that the supplementary costs to upgrade the SPECT camera are low and limited to the purchase of a dedicated collimator. It is available to every nuclear practice without cyclotron, if there is a production site within 2 h shipping distance.

Muehllehner[54] showed for the first time in 1995, at the annual meeting of the Society of Nuclear Medicine, [18]FDG coincidence imaging with a two-headed SPECT system in collaboration with the ADAC[TM] laboratories. The resulting reconstructed images have a spatial resolution of 4.7 mm FWHM, which is comparable to a typical PET camera (Figure 9). The spatial resolution of the coincidence images is twice as good as those obtained from a multi-headed SPECT system fitted with dedicated high resolution 511 keV collimators. The difference in spatial resolution is due to the acquisition method. In coincidence detection, there is no collimator and imaging spatial resolution equals the detector's intrinsic spatial resolution.

The collimator in front of the detector is the major limitation in nuclear imaging. Practically all the photons are absorbed by the septa of the collimator and only those in front of, and parallel to the septa are projected onto the detector. This limits the accepted solid angle so that typically one out of the 10 000 emitted photons reaches the detector. This 'projection by absorption' technique is an inherently inefficient method, and therefore SPECT images have poor statistics. Additionally, the spatial resolution is limited because the diameter of the holes must be relatively large to obtain a reasonable count rate[22].

The fundamental physical difference between PET and SPECT systems is the use of annihilation coincidence detection in the detection process[55]. The annihilation coincidence detection is based on the fact that two 511 keV photons are emitted in opposite directions following annihilation of a positron and an ordinary electron. The annihilation photons are detected by two detectors, orientated at 180° to each other, and only those pairs that are in coincidence are recorded. In coincidence imaging, the projection line is determined by two points. In collimated SPECT one is limited to one point, and the direction of the projection line is determined by the orientation of the septa of the collimator. It should be noted that electronic collimation by coincidence detection dates back to

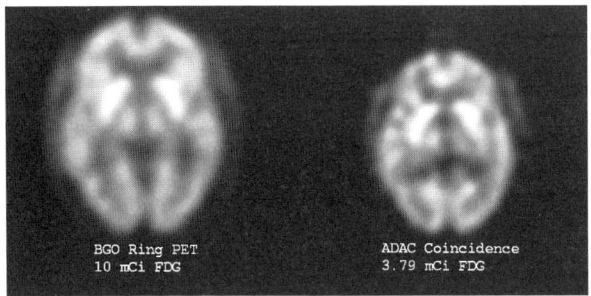

Figure 9 Left side: brain study after injection of 10 mCi [18]FDG acquired with a state-of-the-art ring PET scanner with Bismuth germanato detector. Right side: the brain images obtained from the same individual half an hour later (3.79 mCi) with dual-SPECT camera in coincidence (ADAC[TM]). Muehlehner not only used the photopeak-photopeak events, but also photopeak-Compton events. This image represents 4 slices out of a total of 90. The normal slice spacing was 4 mm. (Courtesy of ADAC[TM] laboratories)

Anger [20], the inventor of the gamma camera, and a considerable amount of fundamental work was performed in the early seventies[72]. Until now coincidence detection was not implemented in clinical practice using conventional Anger detectors, because of a fundamental limiting factor, the low count rate capability of the detector. At the time of Anger[73] 50-100 mCi was enough to flood the electronics of the analogue camera.

Before we continue with coincidence imaging we should review the limiting factors of the gamma camera at high count rate. Gamma cameras, like other radiation detectors, suffer from the effects of dead time and pulse pileup at high count rate studies. The absorption of a gamma ray in the scintillation camera gives rise to the emission of light photons, which in turn are converted into electronic pulses. During the time the system converts the scintillation event into electronic pulses and analyses and records it, the imager is incapable of handling other events correctly. This time is known as the system dead time. If a second pulse occurs before the first has disappeared, the two pulses will overlap to form a single distorted output pulse. The pulse pileup phenomenon simulates an event with a higher energy than that of either of the two individual photons, and it takes place somewhere midway between the two true events. The system thus ignores two true events, artificially creating another with false energy and location figures. Furthermore the gamma camera detector is a paralysable system. It is a system that introduces a dead time for each event, whether or not that event is actually counted. Thus an event occurring during the dead time of a preceding event would not be counted, but would still introduce its own dead time during which subsequent events could not be recorded. Therefore the paralysable gamma camera has at high count rate an extendable dead time. The physical limit is the finite scintillation decay time of the NaI (Tl) crystal. The relative time constant is approximately 0.250 ms [22]. Ideally, accurate collection of light photons requires light pulse integration of 4x time constant (approximately 1 ms) in order to obtain 98% information[74]. Taking into account all the preceding considerations, it is obvious that the image quality deteriorates at high count rates, because the counts are misplaced or lost. The images have lesser spatial and energy resolution and less uniformity.

A continuing aim of the gamma camera designers is to reduce the dead time in order to produce acceptable images at high count rate. The gamma camera count rate has improved substantially over the years. Fast digital pipe-line processing makes the electronics contribution to the dead time negligible as compared with the finite duration of the scintillation. Further improvement in gamma camera count rate is hampered by the extended scintillation time of NaI (Tl) (> 800 ns), causing overlap of the events and the inability to image extremely high count rates. Several methods have been proposed to avoid this pulse pileup phenomenon. The first methods were pulse pileup reduction methods. They are based on an integrator that processes the first part of the pulse and truncates the tail electronically[22,75-78]. This strategy diminishes the effects of pulse pileup, but degrades energy and spatial resolution. In 1989, Lewellen[79] evaluated a pulse tail extrapolation method that allows the separation of individual pulses involved in pulse pileup events at high event rate. Lewellen was able to achieve a high count rate with the adapted a GE Maxxus[TM] camera. In 1995, Tournier[80] proposed an anti pileup system by signal deconvolution that would be implemented in the Sopha Medical Vision[TM] cameras. According to their specifications, the gamma count-rate would improve to more than 1 million counts per s. This patented digital deconvolution detection (DDD[TM]) technique allows restoration of the original incident pulses by deconvolution of the signal. Theoretically, there should be less degradation of the spatial resolution at high count rate with both systems separating the events. The original incident pulses are theoretically restored and the 'x' and 'y' coordinates the 'E' can be calculated more accurately. This fully digital detector technology to maximise counting efficiency is ultimately limited by the physics of NaI (Tl) scintillation.

Only 1% of the detector photons is in coincidence with a dual-headed SPECT. It is due to a number of factors including attenuation in the patient, low interaction probability with the scintillation material, limited solid angle for coincidence detection and activity outside the coincidence field of view, but not outside the single detection aperture. It is easy to calculate that operating at a count rate of 500 000 counts per s, the useful count rate expected is 5000 counts per s.

NaI (Tl) as a scintillator is not ideal for positron imaging due to its inherent low efficiency for stopping 511 keV photons. The vast majority of 511 keV photons pass through a typical 3/8" thickness of NaI (Tl) without interacting with the crystal. Until now the manufacturers optimised the imaging performances of the camera for low and very low energy emitting tracers, namely ^{99m}Tc and [201]Tl. The importance of ^{201}Tl is declining and is substituted progressively by ^{99m}Tc-labelled myocardial radiopharmaceuticals. The biological tracer [18]FDG has been succesfully applied with the PET scanner in brain, cardiac and tumour studies. Since [18]FDG can be performed with a SPECT camera, manufacturers should optimise the SPECT camera in the future for low, medium and high energy emitting tracers. A good compromise might be to use 1/2" thick NaI (Tl) crystal and optimise the count rate capability of the detector.

When the collimator is removed, photons from multiple angles can interact with the detector. In coincidence imaging, the only constraint is that both of the accepted photons must interact with the two detectors within a narrow timing window of 15 ns. This short integration time requires that the SPECT camera can operate in two separate modes to achieve high performance in each mode. In the SPECT mode, longer integration times are requested to collect the low light levels in order to improve spatial and energy resolution. Digital electronics with software control enabled the design of a single system that can operate in both SPECT and coincidence modes.

To handle such high count rate, Muehllehner[54,78] uses three main techniques already developed for the UGM 500H/GE Quest[TM] NaI (Tl) PET scanner. The Anger algorithm, where all the photomultiplier tubes are involved to calculate the position and the energy of the event, is abandoned. Instead, when the two detectors are hit simultaneously by an event the photomultiplier collecting the maximal signal is localised on both detectors. To calculate the position, only the photomultiplier tube with the maximal signal and the six photomultiplier tubes around it are used. Muehllehner calls it the multicentroid position calculation. By limiting the amount of photomultiplier tubes for the calculation of the position and the energy

you allow the system to handle events, on other places, 20 ns later, without interference.

The long decay time of a scintillation event in NaI (Tl) crystal is shortened by clipping the pulse electronically after 150 ns so that after the smoothing effect another event can occur 200 ns later. Instead of having one set of electronics on the crystal, multiple overlapping triple channels are used to avoid the dead time effects. Twenty-five per cent of the photomultipliers producing a pulse of 200 ns, which is relatively long, is put in a discriminator to shape the pulse to a 5 ns signal. Combining the four sections of the crystal, the electronics are able to handle the events at a maximum count rate of 1 million counts per s instead of 250K per s.

There are significant computional problems with the reconstruction of the image since the number of coincidence lines exceeds the total number of events typically collected. Assuming a 256x256 matrix size (needed for the 4 mm resolution), counts are integrated for each of the possible 256x256x256x256 coincidence pairs. The size of a typical acquisition of 32 views amounts to about 100 MBytes.

The characteristics of [18]FDG SPECT imaging with and without collimator are summarised in Table 7. Compared with the conventional PET scanner, both methods are hampered by the low efficiency of the

Table 7 FDG imaging performances with SPECT and PET

	SRT[a]	CR[b]
Collimated SPECT (3/8" thick crystal)	10-20	1000/detector
Collimated SPECT (1/2" thick crystal)	10-20	1400/detector
Coincidence SPECT (3/8" thick crystal)	3.5-4.7	3 000-7 000[c]
PET	3.5-6.8	40 000-90 000

[99m]Tc and ^{201}Tl performances with SPECT

Thallium SPECT (single- head)	>17	2 500
Sestamibi SPECT (single-head)	>15	10 000
HMPAO SPECT (3-headed, fan-beam)	7.3	6 000

[a], SRT (spatial resolution transaxial) : in mm ; FWHM (full width at half maximum); [b], CR (count rate) : in cps (counts per s); [c], depending on windowing technique and reconstruction algorithm

NaI (Tl) crystal for high energy photons. With collimated SPECT you put a low resolution high energy collimator in front of a high resolution detector, the worst combination from a physical point of view. This results in images with a reconstructed transversal spatial resolution of 10 and 20 mm depending on the collimator performances. The current count rate per detector is 1000-1400 counts per s depending on the crystal thickness. In coincidence imaging, the reconstructed spatial resolution is about 5 mm FMHM, thus excellent, and the maximum count rate is 3000 to 7000 counts per s depending on the energy windowing and acquisition technique. An increase in count rate of 40% can be expected using 1/2" thick crystal. The irradiation dose in coincidence studies is low because the count rate capability of the detector is limited. It should be noted that the count rate observed with a SPECT camera in coincidence mode is similar to those obtained with a SPECT system operating for [99mTc] single photon emitters SPECT studies.

The performance of the SPECT/PET scanner will increase by optimising the crystal thickness and the so called three-dimensional coincidence acquisition, where coincidences, from large axial angles are accepted. The bottleneck for further progress is essentially due to the physical characteristics of the NaI (Tl) crystal. Ideally, to perform PET with SPECT equipment we should have a detector with the following characteristics : a sufficient large pulse output allowing good energy resolution; a short scintillation decay time reducing image quality deterioration at high count rate due to the effects of dead time, pulse pileup and random coincidence events; a greater stopping power for efficient detection of 511 keV annihilation photons.

The search for new alternatives includes a material called LSO (lutetium orthosilicate)[81]. LSO has excellent efficiency at 511 keV and good overall light output, making it a promising alternative to NaI (Tl). Further areas of exploration include the forging of multiple scintillation materials to combine high stopping power with high light output.

Cost benefit

In the years ahead, the development of the equipment will not only be determined by the clinical efficacy but also by cost reduction.

The choice of the instrument and the tracer will be determined by clinical outcome. In brain tumour evaluation, contrast resolution is the critical issue and not spatial resolution. The detection of a hot spot is easier with the metabolic tracer [201Tl], which has a more

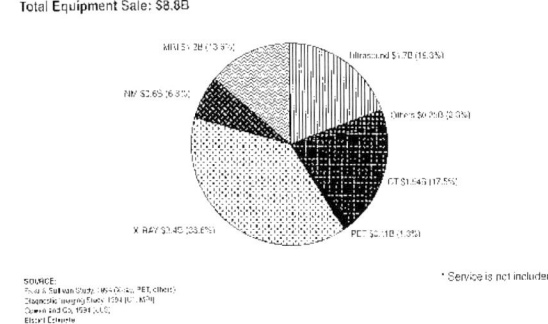

Figure 10 World Diagnostic Imaging Market by modality expected in 1994

favourable target/non-target ratio, than with [18]FDG. The [201Tl] SPECT is the most cost-effective and first choice examination to perform to distinguish radiation necrosis from recurrent tumour, as well as to grade tumours[58,59,82-84]. Although the dedicated collimated SPECT is the worst combination for [18]FDG imaging, their efficiency for myocardial viability detection seems equal with the state-of-the-art PET scanner[85]. If these first results are confirmed, it offers the opportunity to apply this powerful [18]FDG imaging method to smaller community hospitals at a lower fee. The possibility to perform [18]FDG images with a SPECT camera does not change the fundamental economical problem of PET imaging. Although we avoid the purchase of a PET scanner ($1 million), the high costs of establishing a full-scale PET centre ($5-7 million) are due to the cyclotron, its maintenance and the production of ultrashort PET radiopharmaceuticals ($ 1.5-2 million)[86]. It is different if the nuclear department is within 2 h of a medical cyclotron/radio-pharmaceutical establishment, where [18]FDG can be purchased and shipped to the remote site at the expense of $250-$500 per dose[87]. Furthermore, FDG imaging may cut the total cost in the evaluation of a patient with occult metastasis by reducing the amount of multiple expensive, time consuming examinations. Indeed, a single [18]FDG SPECT examination can depict the regional abnormal metabolic sites and focus the complementary examinations to those abnormal sites. The reading time of CT or MRI images can also be shortened as the attention of the radiologist is focussed essentially to the abnormal FDG sites.

The sale of nuclear medicine equipment represents only 7% of the medical imaging worldwide and is made by at least 10 different equipment manufacturers. The world imaging market including service grew from 1.5 billion US$ in 1970 to 14 billion US$ in 1994 (Figure 10). The prospect is a flat or declining market.

Conclusion

Basic gamma camera technology has not changed, but the engineering involved has progressed considerably. From the new generation SPECT cameras, better quantification can be expected by scatter and attenuation compensation and resolution recovery in depth into the SPECT reconstruction method. Ideally, it is always desirable to correct images for all errors to produce quantitative results. Realistically, absolute quantification is not possible at this time. All computer systems in nuclear medicine are now based on standard hardware and operating systems. Nevertheless some vendors still use dedicated display boards.

The DICOM 3.0 'send' and 'receive' capabilities will provide connectivity of proprietary images from vendors in nuclear medicine and even other imaging modalities such as CT and MRI. Until now, nuclear procedures vary from centre to centre and DICOM 3.0 may be the key tool for standardisation. The multimodality image fusion is a new powerful clinical tool where appropriate correlation of function and anatomy can be performed. It gives prospects to make corrections for partial volume effect.

Combining SPECT/PET imaging in one system may expand the capability of many nuclear medicine departments by adding [18]FDG imaging. It would be unrealistic to expect the same high performance to be achieved with a dedicated PET, however, the performance of the SPECT imager in coincidence mode has at least the same sensitivity as a SPECT system operating for imaging single photon emitters and a resolution of a dedicated PET system.

The bottleneck for further progress in the SPECT/PET scanner is essentially due to the physical characteristics of the Na I (Tl) crystal. LSO has excellent efficiency at 511 keV and good light output at 140 keV making it a promising alternative to NaI (Tl).

Acknowledgements

The authors would like to acknowledge the discussions during the SNM and the EANM meetings in Brussels about the scintillation camera with the management teams of the different manufacturers, as well as their advising physicists.

References

1   Radon, J. Uber die bestimmung von functionen durch ihre integralwerte langs gewisser manningfaltigkeiten. *Berichte Sacchsische Akad. Wiss Leipzig Math. Phys. K* 1917, 69, 262

2   Bracewell, R.N. Strip integration in radioastronomy. *Aust. J. Phys.* 1956, 9, 198

3   Kuhl, D.E., Eduards, R.Q., Ricci, A.B. *et al.* The Mark IV system for radionuclide computed tomography of the brain. *Radiology* 1976, 80, 405

4   Hounsfield, G.N. Computerized transverse axial scanning (tomography): Description of system. *Br. J. Radiol.* 1973, 46, 1023

5   Ambrose, J. Computerized transverse axial scanning (tomography): Part 2 Clinical application. *Br. J. Radiol.* 1973, 46, 1023

6   Budinger, T.F. and Gullberg, G.T. Three-dimensional reconstruction in nuclear medicine emission imaging. *EEE Trans. Nucl. Sci.* 1974, 21, 2

7   Jaszczak, R.J., Murphy, P.H., Huard, D. and Burdine, J.A. Radionuclide emission tomography of the head with Tc-99m and a scintillation camera. *J. Nucl. Med.* 1977, 18, 373

8   Jaszczak, R.J., Coleman, R.E. and Lim, C.B. SPECT : Single emission computed tomography. *IEEE Trans. Nucl. Sci.* 1980, NS-27, 1137

9   Winchell, H.S., Baldwin, R.M. and Lin, T.H. Development of I-123 labeled amines for brain studies: localization of I-123 iodophenylalkylamines in rat brain. *J. Nucl. Med.* 1980, 21, 940

10 Neirinckx, R.D., Canning, L.R., Piper, I.M. *et al.* Tc-99m d,l-HMPAO: a new radiopharmaceutical for SPECT imaging of regional cerebral blood perfusion. *J. Nucl. Med.* 1987, 28, 191

11 Walovitch, R.C., Hall, K.M., O'Toole, J.J. and Williams, S.J. Metabolism of Tc-99m ECD in normal volunteers. *J. Nucl. Med.* 1988, 29, 747

12 Lim, C.B., Gottschalk, S., Walker, R. *et al.* Triangular SPECT system for 3-D total organ volume imaging: Design-concept and preliminary imaging results. *IEEE Trans. Nucl. Sci.* 1985, NS-32, 741

13 Dobbeleir, A., Dierckx, R. and Vandevivere, J. High resolution SPECT using a three-head rotating camera and super fine lead fan-beam collimators. *Eur. J. Nucl. Med.* 1991, 18, 600

14 Dierckx, R.A., Dobbeleir, A. and Martin, J.J. Tc-99m HMPAO tomography using a three-headed SPECT system equipped with lead fan-beam collimator. *Clin. Nucl. Med.* 1993, 18, 532

15 Dierckx, R., Dobbeleir, A., Vandevivere, J. *et al.* Visualisation of brainstem perfusion using a high spatial resolution SPECT system. *Clin. Nucl. Med.* 1992, 17, 378

16 Devous, M.D., Stokely, E.M. and Bonte, F.J. Quantitative imaging of regional cerebral blood flow in man by dynamic single photon tomography in 'Radionuclide imaging of the brain', (Ed. B.L. Holman), Churchill Livingstone, New York, 1985, p.135

17 Glas, H.I. and Harper, A.M. Measurement of the regional blood flow in cerebral cortex of man through intact skull. *Br. Med. J.* 1963, 2, 1611

18 Mallett, B.L. and Veall, N. The measurement of regional cerebral clearance rate in man using ^{133}Xe inhalation and extracranial recording. *Clin. Sci.* 1965, 29, 179

19 Kano, I. and Lassen, N.A. Two methods for calculating regional cerebral blood flow from emission computed tomography of inert gas concentrations. *J. Comput. Assist. Tomogr.* 1979, 371

20 Anger, H.O. Scintillation camera. *Rev. Sci. Instr.* 1958, 29, 27

21 Slomka, P. and Swerhone, D. SNM camera and computer system report. Postscript copy: nuc.vichosp.london.on.ca filepub/snm92-snm95.ps.

22 Sorenson, J.A. and Phelps, M.E. in 'Physics in nuclear medicine', W.B. Saunders, Philadelphia, 1987

23 Buvat, I., Benali, H., Todd-Pokoprek, A. *et al.* Scatter correction in scintigraphy: the-state-of-the-art. *Eur. J. Nucl. Med.* 1994, 21, 675

24 Buvat, I., Rodriguez-Villafuerte, M., Todd-Pokropek, A. *et al.* Comparative assessment of nine scatter correction methods based on spectral analysis using Monte Carlo simulations. *J. Nucl. Med.* 1995, 36, 1476

25 Rosenthal, M.S., Cullom, J., Hawkins, W., *et al.* Quantitative SPECT imaging: a review and recommendations by the focus committee of the society of nuclear medicine computer and instrumentation council.

26 King, M.A., Hademenos, G.L. and Glick, S.J. A dual-photopeak window method for scatter correction. *J. Nucl. Med.* 1992, 33, 605

27 Ichihara, T., Ogawa, K., Motomura, N. *et al.* Compton scatter compensation using a triple-energy window method for single and dual-isotope SPECT. *J. Nucl. Med.* 1993, 2216

28 Maor, D., Berlad, G., Chrem, Y. *et al.* A Klein-Nishina based energy factors for Compton free imaging (CFI) [abstract] *J. Nucl. Med.* 1991, 32, 1000

29 Gagnon, D., Pouliot, N. and Laperriere, L. Statistical and physical content on low photons in Holospectral imaging. *IEEE Trans. Med. Imaging* 1991, 10, 284

30 Gagnon, D., Todd-Pokropek, A., Arsenault, A. *et al.* Introduction to Holospectral imaging in nuclear medicine for scatter substraction. *IEEE Trans. Med. Imaging*, 1989, 8, 245

31 Di Paola, R., Bazin, J.P., Aubry, F. *et al.* Handling of dynamic sequences in nuclear medicine. *IEEE Trans. Nucl. Sci.* 1982, 29, 1310

32 Mas, J., Hannequin, P., Ben Younes, R. *et al.* Correction de la diffusion Compton en Imagerie isotopique par analyse factorielle sous contraintes. *Innov. Tech. Biol. Med.* 1990, 11, 641

33 Beck, R.N., Zimmer, L.T., Charleston, D.B. and Hoffer, P.B. Aspects of imaging and counting in nuclear medicine using scintillation and semi conductors detectors. *IEEE Trans. Nucl. Sci.* 1972, 19, 173

34 Halama, J.R., Henkin, R.E. and Friend, L.E. Gamma camera radionuclide images: improved contrast with energy-weighted acquisition. *Radiology* 1988, 19, 533

35 Chang, L.T. A method for attenuation correction in radionuclide computed tomography. *IEEE Trans. Nucl. Sci.* 1978, NS-25, 638

36 Tan, P. and Bailey, D.L. *et al.* A scanning line source for simultaneous emission and transmission measurements in SPECT. *J. Nucl. Med.* 1993, 30, 1752

37 Tung, C.H., Gulberg, G.T., Zeng, G.L. *et al.* Non uniform attenuation correction using simultaneous transmission converging tomography. *IEEE Trans. Nucl. Sci.* 1992, 39, 1134

38 Bourguignon, M.H., Berrahm H., Berdriem, B. *et al.* Correction of attenuation in SPECT with an attenuation coefficient map: *J. Nucl. Biol. Med.*1993, 37, 26

39 Formiconi, A.R., Pupi, A. and Passeri, A. Compensation of spatial system response in SPECT with conjugate gradient reconstruction technique. *Phys. Med. Biol.* 1989, 34, 69

40 Cradduck, T.D., Bialey, D.L., Hutton, B.F. *et al.* A standard protocol for the exchange of nuclear medicine image files. *Nucl. Med. Commun.* 1989, 10, 703

41 Todd-Prokropek, A. Interfile conformance claim. *Nucl. Med. Commun.* 1994, 15, 659

42 Bigwood, W.D. and Horii, S. Introduction to the ACR NEMA DICOM Standard. *Radiographics* 1993, 12, 345

43 NEMA. Digital imaging and communications. ACR-NEMA Standard publication, 1988

44 'Supplement 7' The nuclear medicine component of the DICOM standard. Postscript copy: /dicom_docs /drafts/nm_iod.ps.

45 Pelizzari, C.A., Chen, G.T.Y., Spelbring, D.R. *et al.* Accurate three-dimensional registration of CT, PET and/or MR images of the brain. *J. Comput. Assist. Tomogr.* 1989, 13, 20

46 Hoffman, E.J., Huang, S.C., Phelps, M.E. *et al.* Quantification in positron emission computed tomography: Effect of object size. *J. Comput. Assist. Tomogr.* 1979, 3, 299

47 Kojima, A., Matsumoto, M., Takahashi, M. *et al.* Effect of spatial resolution on SPECT quantification values. *J. Nucl. Med.* 1989, 30, 508

48 Videen, T.O., Perlmutter, J.S., Mintun, M.A. *et al.* Regional correction of the positron emission tomography data for the effect of cerebral atrophy. *J. Cereb. Blood Flow Metab.* 1988, 8, 662

49 Van de velde, R. in 'Hospital information systems: the next generation', Springer-Verlag, Berlin, 1992

50 Wallis, J.M., Miller, M.M., Miller, T.R. and Vreeland, T.H. An Internet based Nuclear Medecine Teaching File. *J. Nucl. Med.* 1995, 35, 1520

51 Drane, W.E., Abbott, F.D., Nicole, M.W. *et al.* Technology for FDG SPECT with a relative inexpensive gamma camera. *Radiology* 1994, 191, 461

52 Martin, W.H. *et al.* FDG SPECT: Correlation with FDG-PET. *J. Nucl. Med.* 1995, 36, 988

53 Noelpp, U.B., Roesler, H., Ritter, E.P. *et al.* Myocardial ^{18}F-FDG tomography using conventional gamma camera and a seven pinhole collimator. *J. Comput. Assist. Tomogr.* 1994, 18, 102

54 Muehlehner, G., Geagan, M. and Countryman, P. SPECT scanner with PET coincidence capability. *J. Nucl. Med.* 1995, 36, 70P

55 Phelps, M.E., Hoffman, E.J., Mullani, N.A. *et al.* Applications of annihilation coincidence detection to transaxial reconstruction tomography. *J. Nucl. Med.* 1975, 16, 210

56 Phelps, M.E., Maziotta, J.C. and Huang, S.C. Study of cerebral function with positron emission tomography. *J. Cereb. Blood Flow Metab.* 1982, 2, 113

57 Phelps, M.E., Maziotta, J.C. and Schelbert, H.R. (Eds.) in 'Positron emission tomography and autoradiography: Principles and applications in the brain and heart', Raven Press, New York, 1986

58 Alavi, A. and Hirsch, L.J. Studies of central nervous system disorders with single photon emission computed tomography and positron emission tomography : evolution over the past 2 decades. *Semin. Nucl. Med.* 1991, 21, 58

59 Brooks, D.J., Beaney, R.P. and Thomas, D.G. The role of positron emission tomography in the study of cerebral tumors. *Semin. Oncol.* 1986, 13, 83

60 Coubes, P., Awad, I.A., Antar, M. *et al.* Comparison and spatial correlation of interictal HMPAO-SPECT and FDG-SPECT in intractable temporal lobe epilepsy. *Neurol. Res.* 1993, 15, 160

61 Di Chiro, G. Positron emission tomography using [18F] fluoro-deoxyglucose in brain tumors: a powerful diagnostic and prognostic tool. *Invest. Radiol.* 1986, 22, 360

62 Heiss, W.D. and Phelps, M.E. (Eds.) in 'Positron Emission tomography of the brain', Spinger-Verlag, New York, 1983

63 Weinstein, H.C., Scheltens, P. and Hijdra, W. *et al.* Neuroimaging in the diagnosis of Alzheimer disease. II. Positron and single photon emisssion tomography. *Clin. Neurosurg.* 1993, 314, 884

64 Tillisch, J., Brunken, R., Marshall, R. *et al.* Reversibility of cardiac wall motion abnormalities predicted by positron tomography. *N. Engl. J. Med.* 1986, 314, 884

65 Strauss, L.G., Clorius, J.H., Schlag, P. *et al.* Recurrence of colorectal tumors: PET evaluation. *Radiology* 1989, 170, 329

66 Kubuto, K., Matsuzawa, T., Fujiwara, T. *et al.* Differential diagnosis of lung tumor with positron emission tomography: a prospective study. *J. Nucl. Med.* 1990, 31, 1927

67 Wahl, R.L., Cody, R.L., Hutchins, G.D. *et al.* Primary and metastatic breast carcinoma: initial clinical evaluation with PET with the radiolabeled glucose analogue 2-[F-18]-fluoro-2-deoxy-D-glucose. *Radiology* 1991, 179, 765

68 Bares, R., Klever, P., Hellwig, D. *et al.* Pancreatic cancer detected by positron emission tomography with 18F-labeled deoxyglucose: method and first results. *Nucl. Med. Commun.* 1993, 14, 596

69 Adler, L.P., Blair, H.F., Makley, J.T. *et al.* Noninvasive grading of musculoskeletal tumor using PET. *J. Nucl. Med.* 1991, 32, 1508

70 Reisser, C., Haberkorn, U. and Strauss, L.G. PET scan in tumor diagnosis in the head and neck. *Laryngorhinootologie* 1991, 70, 214

71 Rappoport, V., Chen, E.Q. and Jiang, J. SPECT imaging by 511 keV photons. *J. Nucl. Med.* 1995, 36, XXP

72 Muehllehner, G., Buchin, M.P. and Dudek, J.H. Performance parameters of positron imaging camera. *IEEE Trans. Nucl. Sci.* 1976, 23, 528

73 Anger, H.O. Radioisotope cameras in 'Instrumentation in Nuclear Medecine', (Ed. G.L. Hine), The Academic Press, New York, 1967, 496

74 Bollinger, L.M. and Thomas, G.E. Measurements of time dependence of scintillation intensity by delayed-coincidence method. *Rev. Sci. Instr.* 1961, 32, 1044

75 Elscint, The Apex family, a product profile, 1982

76 Imbar, D. Fast gamma camera US patent 4,455,616, 1984

77 Dirkse, F.J. and Kulberg, G.H. A method and a circuit for processing pulses of a pulse train. European patent 121703

78 Muehllehner, G. and Karp, J.S. A positron camera using positive-sensitive detectors. PENN-PET. *J. Nucl. Med.* 1986, 27, 9098

79 Lewellen, T.K., Bice, A.N., Pollard, K.R. *et al.* Evaluation of a clinical scintillation camera with pulse tail extrapolation electronics. *J. Nucl. Med.* 1989, 30, 1554

80 Tournier, E., Chaillout, J.J., Janin, C. *et al.* An antipileup system by signal deconvolution: A feasability study to improve gamma camera count rate without loss of spatial resolution (personal communication)

81 Melcher, C.L., Lutetium orthosilicate single crystal scintillator detector, US Patent Numbers 4,958,080, 1990, and 5,025,151, 1991

82 Biersack, H.J., Grunwald, F. and Kropp, J. Single photon emission computed tomography imaging of brain tumors. *Semin. Nucl. Med.* 1991, 21, 2

83 Dierckx, R.A., Martin, J.J. and Dobbeleir, A. Sensitivity and specificity of Thallium-201 single-emission tomography in the functional detection and differential diagnosis of brain tumours. *Eur. J. Nucl. Med.* 1994, 21, 621

84 Ell, P.J. and Costa, D.C. The role of nuclear medicine in neurology and psychiatry. *Curr. Opin. Neurol. Psychiatry* 1992, 5, 863

85 Burt, R.W., Perkins, O.W. and Oppenhiem, B.E. *et al.* Direct comparison of fluorine-18-FDG Spect, Fluorine-18-FDG PET and rest Thallium-201 SPECT for detection of myocardial viability. *J. Nucl. Med.* 1995, 36, 176

86 Conti, P.S., Keppler, J.S. and Halls, J.M. Positron emission tomography: a financial and operation analysis. *A.J.R.* 1994, 162, 1270

87 Drane, W. Is PET worth its cost? *Administrators in Radiology* 1994, 27

SPECT in Neurology and Psychiatry, edited by P.P. De Deyn, R.A. Dierckx, A. Alavi and B.A. Pickut
© 1997 John Libbey & Company Ltd, pp. 495-499

Quantification in SPECT using Non-Invasive Methods

Chapter

58

A. Dobbeleir, R.A. Dierckx[*], J. Vandevivere and P.P. De Deyn

Introduction

Many neurological disorders are associated with a decrease of perfusion. For many years, attempts at quantification of brain function have been made. In 1945, Kety and Schmidt[1] measured absolute cerebral blood flow, using inhalation of nitrous oxide in low concentrations. As shown by the Fick[2] equation, arterial and venous blood samples are needed:

$$Q_{brain}(T) = Flow \times (A_C - V_C) \, dt$$

in which Q_{brain} = amount of substance delivered to the brain, A_C = arterial concentration and V_C = venous concentration.

Several models, especially for PET studies, have been derived from this equation. For absolute quantification, several asssumptions are made in the kinetic blood flow models. In SPECT, absolute quantification is mainly used to validate semi-quantification methods for specific patient groups.

Cerebral blood flow

Due to the introduction of ^{123}I-amphetamine and ^{99m}Tc-HMPAO at the end of the 1980s, and the use of high resolution tomographic scanners, the interest in regional distribution of the brain perfusion increased tremendously. The first pass extraction of HMPAO was explained by Nickel[3] in a simple circulation model:

$$A_{brain} = A_{inject} \times (1 - R_{lung}) \times (CBF/CO) \times R_{brain}$$

in which A_{brain} = activity trapped in the brain, A_{inject} = total injected activity, R_{lung} = retention factor of the lung, CBF = cerebral blood flow, CO = cardiac output and R_{brain} = retention factor of the brain.

After intravenous injection of a known activity of ^{99m}Tc-HMPAO the tracer flows through the right heart chamber, the lung and the left heart chamber. Within the lung a small part of the radioactivity is trapped due to diffusion to the lung tissue. This fraction is indicated as the retention factor of the lung.

Departments of Nuclear Medicine and Neurology, Middelheim Hospital Antwerp and University of Antwerp
[*]Department of Nuclear Medicine, University Hospital Ghent, Belgium

Afterwards, in the aorta the blood flow splits into the brain circulation and the systemic circulation. Therefore, only the fraction of activity given by the ratio of cerebral blood flow on cardiac output reaches the brain. The amount of radioactivity retained in the brain depends on the extraction and retention fraction of the brain.

To quantitate the retention fraction in the brain, arterial and venous blood samples are needed. A technique that avoids these blood samples is necessary for clinical applications. Generally, for practical reasons, it is also considered that the retention fraction is constant over the brain and that the HMPAO SPECT image mainly represents a distribution of blood flow.

Absolute quantification

The first non-invasive absolute quantification method was proposed by Lassen and Kanno[4], and Celsis et al.[5]

Their method is based on the inhalation and expiration of the ^{133}Xe. Four 1 min sequential tomographic images of the cross-section of the brain were obtained using a dedicated tomograph. The shape of the arterial input function was recorded using a separate detector placed over the right lung. This was the only non-invasive method until recently. The technical disadvantages are the need for a dedicated expensive fast rotating single photon tomograph and the poor resolution of the low energetic xenon isotope.

Besides arterial sampling methods, compartmental models have been developed by predicting the blood flow from a linear relationship with a calculated index, such as the absolute quantification method of Matsuda[6]. This method uses the brain input and aortic arch curves to calculate a brain perfusion index which is correlated to blood flow. A detailed explanation is given in another chapter.

Visual and semi-quantitative analysis

Quantification remains difficult in routine practice. Therefore most physicians evaluate the distribution of blood flow in the brain by visual interpretation. In an attempt to be more sensitive and reducing the variation coefficient by referring to a stable region, many semi-quantitative methods using ^{99m}Tc-HMPAO have been described over the past few years[7]. Operator defined or automatic left to right ratios have been used. The activity in functional regions has been studied. In order to delineate more precisely the anatomical structures, SPECT images have been matched to CT or NMR images. The volume of the defect has been calculated by comparison to the contralateral healthy structures.

Significant improvement in image resolution has been achieved by using multidetector systems and high resolution fanbeam collimators[8]. When comparing images made with a single detector to a multidetector system, physicians had to adapt their visual interpretation due to a dramatic improvement in reconstructed resolution, from about 15 mm to about 8 mm, providing functional details never observed before. The images were close to those observed with PET systems.

Matsuda et al.[9] at Kanazawa University in Japan presented the first high resolution functional brain atlas. Major topographical reference points could be defined and a comparison was made with the MRI data[10].

Meanwhile, progress was also made in computer speed, permitting reconstruction or reprojection methods which were too time consuming a few years ago[11]. Three-dimensional display utilising volume rendering facilitates understanding of spatial relationships and anatomical-functional correlation[12].

In smaller structures, a relative hypoperfusion is observed. This is not necessarily a physiological phenomenon, but is associated with the tomographical resolution of the gamma camera, and is well known as a partial volume effect. For this reason, visual or quantitative structures of the left hemisphere are compared with the same structures in the right hemisphere.

In Figure 1, a Hofmann brain phantom is presented. The first and third row represents planar images of slices through the phantom. The second and fourth row are tomographic reconstructions of the phantom. Due to poor resolution, the images of the tomographic reconstruction are less sharp and a drop in activity is observed in smaller structures[13].

In Figure 2 a circumferential profile of the phantom in a basal ganglia slice is presented. Although the same radioactivity is present everywhere, different activities of the cortex are observed. Frontal cortical activity is higher then in the other cortical regions. This corresponds to the region in the phantom where the cortex has the largest diameter. This means also that normal distribution of the tracer in the brain depends on the resolution of the acquisition system. A mental picture of normality and pictures of different disease states are therefore mandatory. Gender differences in brain uptake were described by Podreka in a large group of normal subjects[14]. This is why some research establishments try to develop a normal database of regional cerebral uptake[15]. Sectorial regions of interest were drawn on brain slices of normal volunteers in order to obtain strict reference values to be used in interindividual and intergroup clinical comparisons.

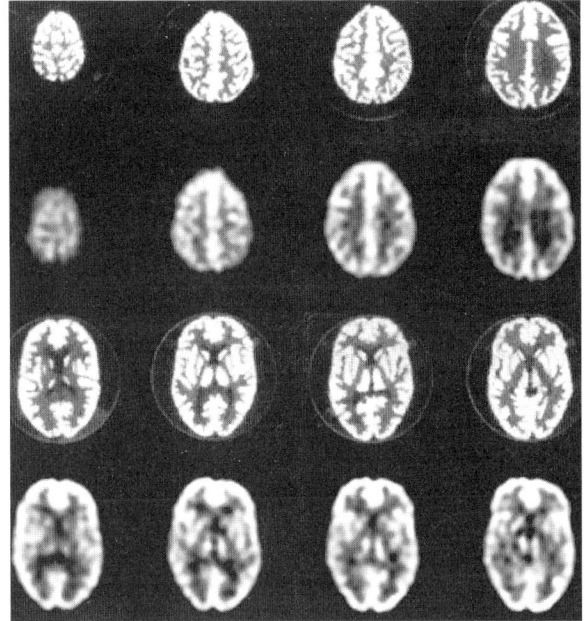

Figure 1 Hofmann brain phantom. First and third row represent planar images of slices through the phantom. Second and fourth row are tomographic reconstructions

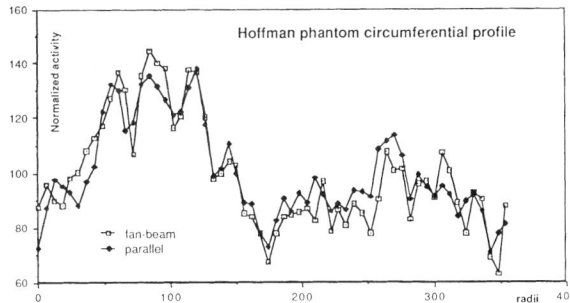

Figure 2 Circumferential maximum value profile of a Hoffman phantom in a basal ganglia slice normalised to the mean activity. 90° corresponds to frontal activity.

The activity in each region is generally compared with contralateral activity and cerebellar activity. A mean and s.d. value can be obtained for each region. Most of the cortical normal values are situated at a level of about 80 to 85% of the cerebellar activity. The spread was in general around 5% except in the fronto orbital region, where it was about 10%. In all similar studies, for example in Alzheimer patients, the assumption has to be made on clinical grounds that the cerebellar activity is normal, since the cerebellum is needed as reference region. In the same way, the mean activity in the whole slice or even in the whole brain is used as reference. Automatic transformation of 3D images into a stereotaxic Talairach atlas for establishing a normal database and patient comparison has been achieved [16].

Effective volume determination

Defect volumes can be calculated. ROIs have to be drawn over the lesion on all slices involved. These ROIs are mirrored to the contralateral homologous region. The total functional volume loss, expressed as an imaginary volume of zero perfusion can then be calculated. This method, first used by Mountz [17], takes into account the pixel volumes, number of slices and the activity difference at each slice between the normal and in our case ischaemic hemisphere.

We used this method in patients suffering from unilateral acute ischaemic infarction [18]. By expressing the infarction as milllitre zeroperfusion, this semi-quantification method simultaneously takes into account the extent and degree of hypoperfusion. SPECT defects may be measured in an accurate and reproducible way. Moreover, this study showed a significant correlation between the volume zeroperfusion and the neurological deficit on admittance as scored on the Orgogozo scale.

Brain uptake quantification

We have developed an absolute quantification method [19], not to quantify blood flow, but to quantify exactly what is seen in the images: the regional brain uptake of ^{99m}Tc-HMPAO, which is the product of blood flow and retention of the brain. We studied the influence of individual body surface, brain volume and heart rate fluctuation on brain uptake [20]. The influence of these factors were investigated in 33 healthy volunteers. Afterwards, they were applied to 13 patients suffering from probable dementia of the Alzheimer type, in order to correct for interindividual variation [21]. An equation has been tested to calculate from known point source activities a factor K. Multiplying SPECT slices on pixel by pixel base by this factor provides image values expressed as 10^6 of the injected lipophilic dose per ml brain tissue.

This allows intra or interindividual comparison between different ^{99m}Tc-HMPAO studies. In healthy volunteers with similar heart rate at injection in the two studies, a mean deviation of 7.2% in cerebellar uptake was observed between repeated acquisitions [19]. On the contrary, testing the reproducibility of the method on healthy volunteers, we noted a significant influence of the heart rate at injection time. This could be expected since brain uptake is inversely proportional to cardiac output.

Table 1 Cerebellar uptake (mean and standard deviation) in health volunteers and DAT patients at rest heart rate, corrected for a body surface factor of BS/1.73 and corrected for body surface and a brain volume factor of BV/1350

	rBU at rest HR	rBU BS Corrected	rBU BS+BV Corrected
Volunteers (33)	48.4 ± 9.7	52.1 ± 7.7	52.0 ± 7.3
Men Vol (18)	43.1 ± 7.6	49.9 ±8.4	51.6 ±8.7
Women Vol (15)	54.8 ± 8.1	54.7 ± 6.2	52.5 ± 5.5
DAT (13)	75.2 ± 18.3	66.2 ± 10.9	53.9 ±7.4

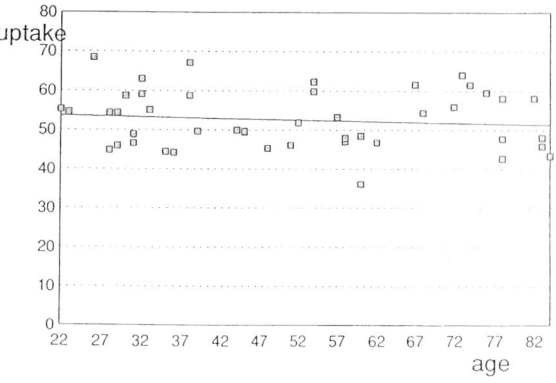

Figure 3 Regional brain uptake rBU in healthy volunteers and DAT patients, after cumulative corrections for heart rate, body surface and brain volume, plotted versus age. The decline of the cerebellar uptake with age becomes negligible rBU = age (54.7 - 0.04)

Table 1 shows the cerebellar uptake of the total group of 33 healthy volunteers, 18 men, 15 women and 13 Alzheimer patients. The mean uptake at basal heart rate indicated in the first column varies from 43.1 for men to 75.2 for Alzheimer patients. The second column shows the brain uptake corrected for the body surface. The value 49.9 for men becomes closer to the uptake value of 66.2 for the Alzheimer patients, who had a much smaller body weight. The third column shows the results after the correction for body surface and brain volume index. In each of these groups, the cerebellar uptake nears 52×10^{-6} of the injected dose per ml brain tissue, with a similar standard deviation of about 7.

In Figure 3 the cerebellar uptakes of 33 healthy volunteers and 13 Alzheimer patients, after cumulative corrections for heart rate, body surface and brain volume are plotted versus age. As seen on this graph the decline of the cerebellar uptake with age becomes negligible.

Normalised brain uptake values allow extension of the application of the quantification method from longitudinal studies to group comparisons. This study proved that the cerebellum is a practical and reliable region to choose as a reference in patients with Alzheimer's dementia.

Discussion

The aim of quantification is to provide a reliable and reproducible numerical measure of brain perfusion in different regions and time windows. Since absolute quantification is difficult and time consuming in daily practise, absolute quantification is certainly important for identifying stable regions in different disease states, regions which afterwards can be used in semi-quantitation as control or reference regions. In these cases, semi-quantitation is advisable since possible

measurement errors are smaller. However, in cases where an overall change in blood flow can be expected, like carotid obstruction or in stimulation studies, the absolute quantification method is mandatory.

References

1 Kety, S.S. and Schmidt, C.F. The determination of cerebral blood flow in man by use of nitrous oxide in low concentrations. *Am. J. Physiol.* 1945, 143, 53

2 Fick, A. Uber die Messung des Blutquantums in den Herzventrikeln. Verhandl Phys Med Ges Wurzburg. (Transl. H.E. Hoff, H.J.Scott), *N. Engl. J. Med.* 1948, 239, 476

3 Nickel, O., Nagele-Wohrle, B., Ulrich, P. *et al.* RCBF-quantification with 99mTc HMPAO-SPECT: Theory and first results. *Eur. J. Nucl. Med.* 1989, 15,1

4 Kanno, I. and Lassen, N.A.Two methods for calculating regional cerebral blood flow from emission computed tomography of inert gas concentrations. *J. Comput. Assist. Tomogr.* 1979, 3, 71

5 Celsis, P., Goldman, T., Henriksen, L. and Lassen, N.A. A method for calculating regional cerebral blood flow from emission computed tomography of inert gas concentrations. *J. Comput. Assist. Tomogr.* 1981, 5, 641

6 Matsuda, H., Tsuji, S., Shuke, N. *et al.* A quantitative approach to technetium-99m hexamethylpropylene amine oxime. *Eur. J. Nucl. Med.* 1992, 19, 195

7 Mountz, J. Quantification of the SPECT Brain Scan in 'Nuclear Medicine Annual', Raven Press, New York, 1991, p. 67

8 Dobbeleir, A., Dierckx, R. and Vandevivere, J. High spatial resolution SPECT using a three-head rotating gamma camera and super fine lead fanbeam collimators. *Eur. J. Nucl. Med.* 1991, 18, 600

9   Matsuda, H., Oskoie, S.D., Kinuya, K. *et al.* Tc-99m HMPAO brain perfusion tomography atlas using high resolution SPECT system. *Clin. Nucl. Med.* 1990, 15, 428

10 Dierckx, R., Dobbeleir, A., Martin, J.J. and De Deyn, P.P. Tc-99m HMPAO tomography using a three-headed SPECT system equipped with lead fan-beam collimators. *Clin. Nucl. Med.* 1993, 18, 532

11 Wallis, J. and Miller, T. Volume rendering in three-dimensional display of SPECT images. *J. Nucl. Med.* 1990, 31, 1421

12 Dierckx, R., Dobbeleir, A., Borggreve, F. *et al.* Three-dimension reconstruction of brain perfusion. *Eur. J. Nucl. Med.* 1991, 18, 597

13 Kim, H., Zeeberg, B., Fahey, F. *et al.* Three-dimensional SPECT simulations of a complex three-dimensional mathematical brain model and measurements of the three-dimensional physical brain phantom. *J. Nucl. Med.* 1991, 32, 1923

14 Podreka, I., Goldenberg, G., Baumgartner, C. *et al.* HMPA0 brain uptake in young normal subjects: gender differences and hemispheric asymmetries. *J. Cereb. Blood Flow Metab.* 1989, 9, 202

15 De Sadeleer, C., de Metz, K., Somers, G. and Bossuyt, A. Relative quantification of Tc99m HMPAO SPECT based on sectorial regions of interest in normal volunteers. *Eur. J. Nucl. Med.* 1989, 21, 781

16 Vanhove, C., Monte, C., Colaert, H. and Demonceau, G.Standardised atlas for brain studies. *Eur. J. Nucl. Med.* 1994, 21, 773

17 Mountz, J. A method of analysis of SPECT blood flow image data for comparison with computed tomography. *Clin. Nucl. Med.* 1989, 14, 192

18 Dierckx, R., Dobbeleir, A., Pickut, B. *et al.* Technetium-99m HMPAO SPET in acute supratentorial ischaemic infarction, expressing deficits as millilitre of zero perfusion. *Eur. J. Nucl. Med.*1995, 22, 427

19 Dobbeleir, A. and Dierckx, R. Quantification of Tc-99m HMPAO brain uptake in routine clinical practice using calibrated point sources as an external standard: phantom and human studies. *Eur. J. Nucl. Med.*1993, 20, 684

20 Dierckx, R., Dobbeleir, A., Maes, M. *et al.* Parameters influencing SPET regional brain uptake of Tc-99m HMPAO measured by calibrated point sources as an external standard. *Eur. J. Nucl. Med.*1994, 21, 514

21 Dobbeleir, A., De Deyn, P.P. and Dierckx, R. The cerebellum as reference region: comparison of absolute cerebellar uptake of Tc-99m HMPAO in 33 healthy volunteers and 13 DAT patients. *Eur. J. Nucl. Med.*1994, 21, S5

SPECT in Neurology and Psychiatry, edited by P.P. De Deyn, R.A. Dierckx, A. Alavi and B.A. Pickut
© 1997 John Libbey & Company Ltd, pp. 501-505

A Non-Invasive Quantitative Approach to ^{99m}Tc-Ethyl Cysteinate Dimer

Chapter

59

H. Matsuda and A. Yagishita[*]

Introduction

^{99m}Tc-ethyl cysteinate dimer (^{99m}Tc-ECD)[1-4] is a new brain perfusion imaging agent for single photon emission computed tomography (SPECT). This agent has some advantages over a ^{99m}Tc-labelled compound for brain perfusion imaging, ^{99m}Tc hexamethylpropylene amine oxime (^{99m}Tc-HMPAO). It has excellent radiochemical stability after it is reconstituted[4], and it is superior to ^{99m}Tc-HMPAO in its sensivity to lesion detection and lesion contrast[5]. Both tracers possess many of the same characteristics in their kinetics in the brain[6]. Therefore, the same quantitative method as has been previously reported using ^{99m}Tc-HMPAO[7,8] may also be applicable to ^{99m}Tc-ECD. We describe here a non-invasive approach to measure regional cerebral blood flow (rCBF) using ^{99m}Tc-ECD without any blood sampling.

Materials and methods

Eleven subjects, 5 women and 6 men, aged 42-87 years (mean 64 years), gave informed consent to participation in the study. Three of these subjects had brain infarction in the chronic phase, 4 Parkinson's disease, 2 spinocerebellar degeneration, 1 amyotrophic lateral sclerosis and 1 Alzheimer's disease. They underwent two types of radionuclide angiography and SPECT using ^{99m}Tc-ECD and ^{99m}Tc-HMPAO within 2 to 8 days (mean 5 days). The ^{99m}Tc-HMPAO and the ^{99m}Tc-ECD each used 555 MBq. The passage of the tracer from the aortic arch to the brain was monitored in a 128 x 128 format for 100 s at 1 s intervals using a rectangular gamma camera of the three-head SPECT system (Siemens, Multispect3). Regions of interest (ROIs) were hand-drawn over the aortic arch (ROI_{aorta}) and bilateral brain hemispheres (ROI_{brain}). A hemispheric brain perfusion index (BPI) was determined using the same method as has been described previously[7]. Ten minutes after injection of ^{99m}Tc-HMPAO or ^{99m}Tc-ECD, brain SPECT imaging was carried out using the SPECT system equipped with high-resolution parallel-hole collimators. The projection data were obtained in a 128 x 128 format for 24 angles in a 120° arc for each camera with 50 s per angle. A Shepp and Logan filter was used for SPECT image reconstruction. Attenuation correction was performed using Chang's method.

In the current study, the initial distribution volume for the tracer (Vn) [7] was corrected for ROI sizes (Corr. Vn) for standardisation as follows

Division of Radiology, National Center Hospital for Mental, Nervous, and Muscular disorders, NCNP, 4-1-1, Ogawahigashi, Kodaira, Tokyo 187, Japan
*Department of Neuroradiology, Tokyo Metropolitan Hospital for Nervous Diseases, Tokyo, Japan

$$\text{Corr. Vn} = 100 \text{ Vn} \; \frac{\text{ROI}_{\text{aorta}}\text{size}}{\text{ROI}_{\text{brain}}\text{size}}$$

In rCBF quantification using ^{99m}Tc-HMPAO, the linearisation factor α in Lassen's correction algorithm[9] was adapted to cerebral blood flow (CBF) values in the referential cerebral hemisphere, as described previously[8]. This correction algorithm was also applied to ^{99m}Tc-ECD. In this application, the linearisation factor α was set to: 1.5, a value proposed by Lassen *et al.*[9] in a ^{99m}Tc-HMPAO study; 2.6, a proposed value by Friberg *et al.*[6] in a ^{99m}Tc-ECD study; and infinite, no linearisation correction. Using this algorithm, both ^{99m}Tc-HMPAO and ^{99m}Tc-ECD transaxial SPECT images were converted to rCBF maps. Thirty-six regions of interest (ROIs) were drawn in bilateral hemispheres in slice 2, slice 6, and slice 10 according to Figure 3 of a previous report[8] in both ^{99m}Tc-HMPAO and ^{99m}Tc-ECD rCBF maps. The rCBF values for these 36 ROIs for each patient (396 ROIs in total) were compared between ^{99m}Tc-HMPAO and ^{99m}Tc-ECD.

Results

The mean ± s.d. of the hemispherical BPI for ^{99m}Tc-ECD was 5.7 ± 1.8, which was signficantly lower than that for ^{99m}Tc-HMPAO, 6.1 ± 1.8 (paired t-test, p=0.0046). Hemispherical BPI values for both tracers showed a highly significant correlation (Figure 1, n=22, r=0.935, p<0.0001). The linear regression line

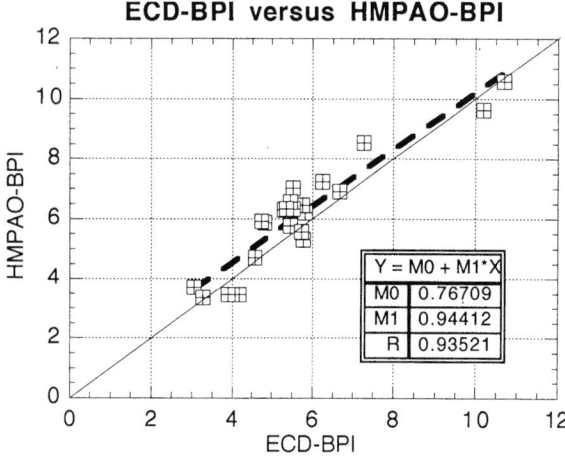

Figure 1 Hemispherical brain perfusion indices (BPI) for ^{99m}Tc-ECD compared with BPI for ^{99m}Tc-HMPAO in 11 patients. They showed a highly significant correlation (n=22, r=0.935, p<0.0001). The linear regression line equation was y=0.944x + 0.767

equation was y=0.944x + 0.767. Using both linear regression line equations between ^{99m}Tc-ECD BPI and ^{99m}Tc-HMPAO BPI, and between ^{99m}Tc-HMPAO BPI and mean CBF values obtained from a ^{133}Xe inhalation SPECT method in a previous study (y=2.75x+17.7)[7], ^{99m}Tc-ECD BPI was converted to ^{133}Xe-CBF values (y=2.60x+19.8). The mean ± s.d. of the hemispherical corr. Vn for ^{99m}Tc-ECD was 3.6 ± 1.5, which was also significantly lower than that for HMPAO, 4.8 ± 2.1 (paired t-test, p=0.0278). The relationships of rCBF values between ^{99m}Tc-HMPAO and ^{99m}Tc-ECD are shown in Figure 2. The mean ± s.d. of the rCBF values for ^{99m}Tc-HMPAO was 49.9 ± 17.3 ml/100 g/min. However, the mean ± s.d. of the rCBF values for ^{99m}Tc-ECD was 43.2 ± 12.5, 58.8 ± 23.8, and 50.1 ± 16.9 ml/100 g/min when the α value was set to infinite, 1.5, and 2.6, respectively. There were no significant differences in rCBF values between ^{99m}Tc-HMPAO and ^{99m}Tc-ECD when α was set to 2.6 (paired t-test, p=0.4661). On the other hand, rCBF values for ^{99m}Tc-ECD were significantly higher and lower (paired t-test, p<0.0001) than those for ^{99m}Tc-HMPAO when α was set to 1.5 and infinite, respectively. Comparative rCBF images for ^{99m}Tc-HMPAO and ^{99m}Tc-ECD are represented in Figure 3.

Discussion

In the present study, BPI values for ^{99m}Tc-ECD were slightly lower than those for ^{99m}Tc-HMPAO. This might be due to low first-pass brain extraction for ^{99m}Tc-ECD as compared with that for ^{99m}Tc-HMPAO. Friberg *et al.*[6] reported a first-pass extraction ratio of 0.60 on the average for ^{99m}Tc-ECD when CBF was 46 ml/100 g/min. Whereas Andersen *et al.*[10] reported a higher first-pass extraction ratio of 0.72 on the average for ^{99m}Tc-HMPAO when CBF was 59 ml/ 100 g/ min. BPI represents the unidirectional influx rate from blood to brain, and it is proportional to a product of CBF and the first-pass extraction ratio. Therefore BPI depends on the first-pass extraction ratio for the used tracer under constant CBF. However, differences between ^{99m}Tc-ECD BPI and ^{99m}Tc-HMPAO BPI were smaller than those expected from this difference in the first-pass extraction ratios. This might be attributed to a difference in the radiochemical purity (RCP) between two tracers. The RCP of ^{99m}Tc-HMPAO is somewhat lower than that of ^{99m}Tc-ECD[4]. The lower the RCP becomes, the smaller BPI becomes. Although this slight difference is present, BPI values for the two tracers showed a highly significant correlation. Therefore, ^{99m}Tc-ECD BPI can be converted to ^{133}Xe-CBF values using two linear

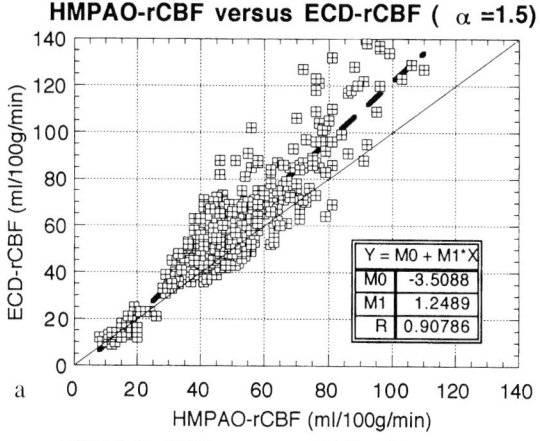

HMPAO-rCBF versus ECD-rCBF (α =1.5)

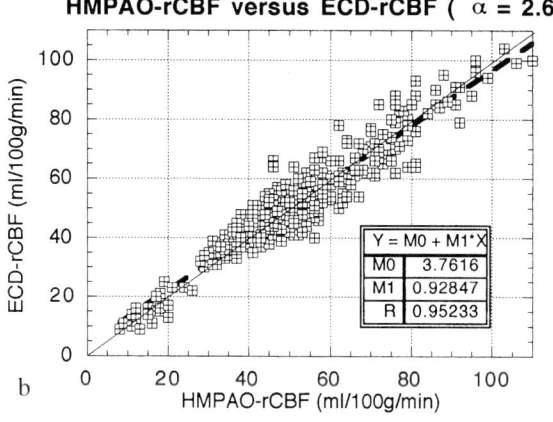

HMPAO-rCBF versus ECD-rCBF (α = 2.6)

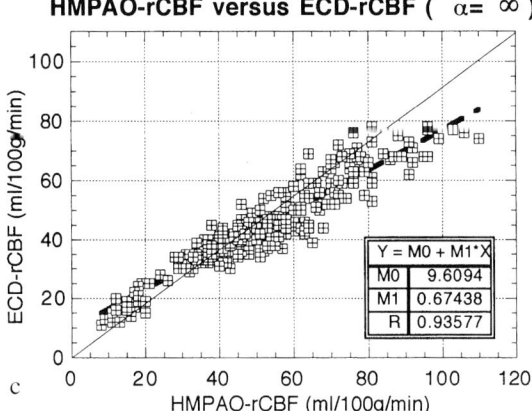

HMPAO-rCBF versus ECD-rCBF (α= ∞)

Figure 2 a-c Correlation of regional cerebral blood flow (rCBF) values calcuated from Lassen's correction algorithm between ^{99m}Tc-HMPAO and ^{99m}Tc-ECD in 35 regions of interest (ROIs) for each patient (396 ROIs in total). For ^{99m}Tc-HMPAO, the linearisation factor α in the algorithm was adapted to cerebral blood flow (CBF) values in the referential cerebral hemisphere. For ^{99m}Tc-ECD the linearisation factor α was fixed to: a, 1.5; b, 2.6; c, infinite. The fixed α value of 2.6 for ^{99m}Tc-ECD gave the linear regression line (dashed line) very close to the line of identity (solid line)

regression line equations between ^{99m}Tc-ECD BPI and ^{99m}Tc-HMPAO BPI, and between ^{99m}Tc-HMPAO BPI and ^{133}Xe-CBF.

The corr. Vn value represents the initial distribution volume for the tracer that may be related to the plasma space[11]. The low corr. Vn values for ^{99m}Tc-ECD may result from lack of significant protein binding in the blood in comparison with substantial protein binding of ^{99m}Tc-HMPAO[10,12]. This result agrees with higher blood activity for ^{99m}Tc-HMPAO than for ^{99m}Tc-ECD[4].

Friberg et al.[6] reported a lower k_2 value for ^{99m}Tc-ECD kinetics, which is the rate constant of the back-diffusion from the brain to the blood, than that for ^{99m}Tc-HMPAO kinetics. This low level of back-diffusion leads to a higher λ value for ^{99m}Tc-ECD, which is the brain-blood partition coefficient, than that for ^{99m}Tc-HMPAO. In Lassen's linearisation algorithm of a curve-linear relationship between brain activity and blood flow, the correction factor α was determined by the ratio of k_3, which is the conversion rate constant from lipophilic to hydrophilic tracer in the brain, to k_2 in a reference region[9]. Although the reported mean k_3 value of 0.57 for ^{99m}Tc-ECD was lower than that of 0.80 for ^{99m}Tc-HMPAO[9], an almost three-fold smaller k_2 value for ^{99m}Tc-ECD[6] than for ^{99m}Tc-HMPAO[9] results in a higher α value of 2.6 in the linearisation

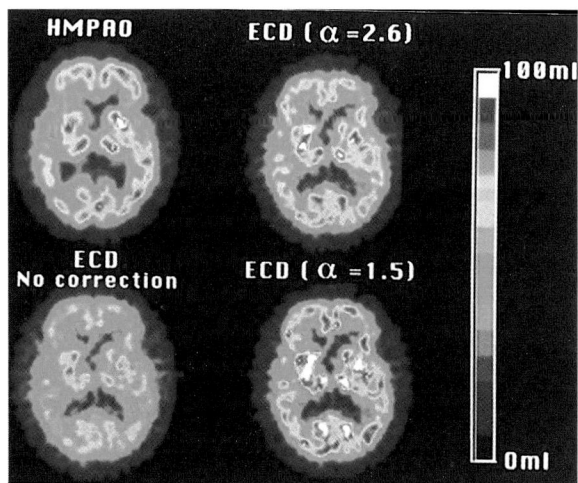

Figure 3 Representative rCBF maps for ^{99m}Tc-ECD and ^{99m}Tc-HMPAO in a 71 year-old woman with Parkinson's disease. The whole-brain CBF was 44 ml/100 g/min. The fixed α value of 2.6 for ^{99m}Tc-ECD gave an almost identical rCBF map to ^{99m}Tc-HMPAO. However, the fixed α value of 1.5 and infinite (no correction) caused higher and lower rCBF values for ^{99m}Tc-ECD than those for ^{99m}Tc-HMPAO, respectively

algorithm of ^{99m}Tc-ECD than ^{99m}Tc-HMPAO as described by Friberg *et al.*[6]. When CBF in the reference region ranged from 20 to 60 ml/100 g/min, optimised α values can be estimated using equations 5 and 6 from a previous report[8] and ranged from 3.2 to 1.2 for ^{99m}Tc-HMPAO and from 6.3 to 2.1 for ^{99m}Tc-ECD. The use of the fixed α value in the linearisation algorithm gives rise to deviation of the obtained rCBF values from true rCBF values when using optimised α values that vary with CBF in a referential region. However, much lower deviation of obtained rCBF values from true values was observed in a simulation study (Figure 4) for ^{99m}Tc-ECD than for ^{99m}Tc-HMPAO. This was supported by the present comparative study in rCBF values between ^{99m}Tc-ECD and ^{99m}Tc-HMPAO. The use of the fixed α value of 2.6 gave the nearly same rCBF for ^{99m}Tc-ECD as those for ^{99m}Tc-HMPAO through whole flow levels, and may be practically appropriate to acquire rCBF values in a ^{99m}Tc-ECD study.

In conclusion, non-invasive rCBF measurements using graphical analysis were applicable to ^{99m}Tc-ECD as well as ^{99m}Tc-HMPAO without any blood sampling. This quantitative approach may be quite useful for routine clinical studies, and may exert several advantages of ^{99m}Tc-ECD over ^{99m}Tc-HMPAO.

References

1 Vallabhajosula, S., Zimmerman, R.E., Picard, M. *et al.* Technetium-99m ECD: a new brain imaging agent: in vivo kinetics and biodistribution studies in normal human subjects. *J. Nucl. Med.* 1989, 30, 599

2 Walovitch, R.C., Hill, T.C., Garrity, S.T. *et al.* Characterization of technetium-99m-L,L-ECD for brain perfusion imaging, part 1: pharmacology of technetium-99m-ECD in non-human primates. *J. Nucl. Med.* 1991, 30, 1892

3 Léveillé, J., Demonceau, G., De Roo, M. *et al.* Characterization of technetium-99m-L,L-ECD for brain perfusion imaging, part 2; biodistribution and brain imaging in humans. *J. Nucl. Med.* 1989, 30, 1902

4 Léveillé, J., Demonceau, G. and Walovitch, R.C. Intrasubject comparison between technetium-99m-ECCD and technetium-99m-HMPAO in healthy human subjects. *J. Nucl. Med.* 1992, 33, 480

5 Matsuda, H., Li, Y.M., Higashi, S. *et al.* Comparative SPECT study of stroke using Tc-99m ECD,I-123 IMP, and Tc-99m HMPAO. *Clin. Nucl. Med.* 1993, 18, 75

6 Friberg, L., Andersen, A.R., Lassen, N.A. *et al.* Retention of ^{99m}Tc-bicisate in the human brain after intracarotid injection.

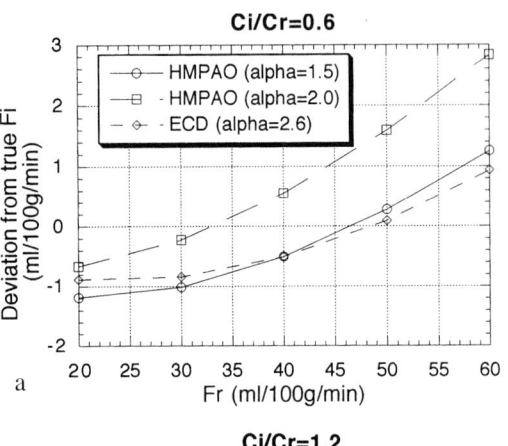

a

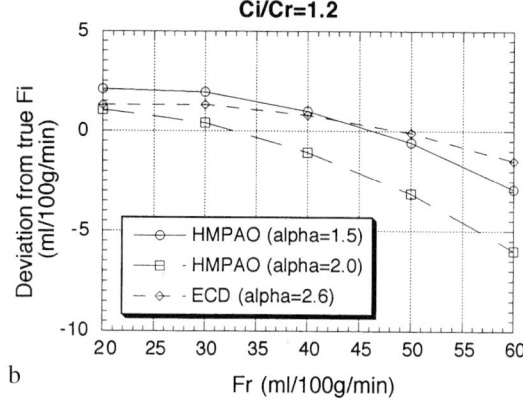

b

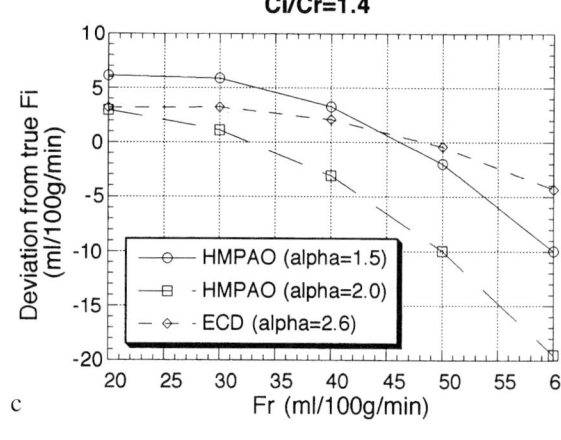

c

Figure 4 a-c Simulated graphs of the influence of the fixation of the linearisation factor α value on resulting rCBF values in the Lassen's correction algorithm. Ordinate denotes deviation of calcuated rCBF values from true values in a region (Fi) when the fixed α value (1.5 and 2.0 for ^{99m}Tc-HMPAO, and 2.6 for ^{99m}Tc-ECD) is used in the algorithm instead of optimised α values that vary with CBF in the referential hemisphere (Fr, abcissa). Simulation was performed in conditions that SPECT count ratio of a region (Ci) to a referential hemisphere (Cr) was set to: a, 0.6; b, 1.2 and c, 1.4. Much less deviation within 5 ml/100 g/min was observed for ^{99m}Tc-ECD than for ^{99m}Tc-HMPAO in all conditions

7   Matsuda, H., Tsuji, S., Schuke, N. *et al.* A quantitative approach to technetium-99m hexamethylpropylene amine oxime. *Eur. J. Nucl. Med.* 1992, 19, 195

8   Matsuda, H., Tsuji, S., Shuke, N. *et al.* Noninvasive measurements of regional cerebral blood flow using technetium-99m-hexamethylproplene amine oxime. *Eur. J. Nucl. Med.* 1993, 20, 391

9   Lassen, N.A., Andersen, A.R., Freiberg, L. and Paulson, O.B. The retention of [^{99m}Tc]-D,L-HMPAO in the human brain áfter intracarotid bolus injection: a kinetic analysis. *J. Cereb. Blood Flow Metab.* 1988, 8(1), S44

10 Andersen, A.R., Friberg, H., Knudsen, K.B.M. *et al.* Extraction of [^{99m}Tc]-d,l-HMPAO across the blood-brain barrier. *J. Cereb. Blood Flow Metab.* 1988, 8(1), S44

11 Peters, A.M. Graphical analysis of dynamic data: the Patlak- and Rutland plot. *Nucl. Med. Commun.* 1994, 15, 669

12 Knudsen, G.M., Andersen, A.R., Somnier, F.E. *et al.* Brain extraction and distribution of ^{99m}Tc-bicisate in humans and rats. *J. Cereb. Blood Flow Metab.* 1994, 14(1), S12

SPECT in Neurology and Psychiatry, edited by P.P. De Deyn, R.A. Dierckx, A. Alavi and B.A. Pickut
© 1997 John Libbey & Company Ltd, pp. 507-512

Automated Template-Based Quantification of Brain SPECT

Chapter
60

P.J. Slomka, J. Stephenson, R. Reid and G.A. Hurwitz

Introduction

Reliable and objective assessment of images in single photon emission computed tomography (SPECT) of the brain can reduce the variability and subjectivity of the test. One method of objective assessment of the abnormalities is relative quantification of counts. In order to be able to interpret the results of such quantification, there is a need for the reference and limit values obtained from normal images. Several existing brain SPECT quantification schemes are based on such principles[1,2]; however, they require some form of user interaction during placement and definition of ROIs, or during the alignment stage. This interaction can introduce subjectivity to the final results. Full automatisation of these procedures should result in overall improved reproducibility of the image interpretation. Several investigators have been pursuing development of methods for the inter-subject registration of brain images in order to develop a standardised brain atlas for PET and MRI images[3-6].

Previously, we have developed a fully automated quantification scheme for the inter-subject registration and relative quantification of myocardial perfusion SPECT images based on the normal and variation templates[7,8]. In this study, we test the possibility of applying the previously developed algorithms for myocardial perfusion quantification to perform fully automated quantification of brain SPECT. The technique is based on the concept of three-dimensional (3D) and automated image registration[9-12]. We apply image registration techniques to normalise images of different subjects, to a common orientation and size using anisotropic scaling, which subsequently allows for voxel by voxel image quantification.

Methods

For the creation of the normal database, images from 10 normal patients (8 men, 2 women, aged 25-53) were used. In addition, 6 scans with perfusion abnormalities have been used for the qualitative assessment of the registration and quantification procedure. ^{99m}Tc-ECD SPECT brain images were collected by on a Multispect-2 dual headed Siemens (Hoffman Estates, IL) camera with matrix size 64x64, zoom 1.78, 32 stops and 360° rotation. The time per stop was individually determined from the first projection frame for which the count limit was set at 80,000; this time ranged from 50 to 60 s. Images have been reconstructed using uniform Chang attenuation correction and 3D Butterworth Fourier filter with a cut-off 0.4 of Nyquist frequency applied to post-filter the reconstructed data volume. The pixel size of the acquisition data was 5.38 mm. The reconstruction, and all image processing was performed on the Nuclear

Department of Diagnostic Radiology and Nuclear Medicine, University of Western Ontario and Victoria Hospital, 375 South Street, London, Ontario, Canada, N6A 4G5

Diagnostics (Stockholm, Sweden) Hermes workstation. The pixel size of zoomed, reconstructed slices was 3.59 mm.

The registration algorithms were implemented in the C programming language using the Solaris operating environment on a Sun Microsystems Inc. (Mountain View, CA) Sparc 10/512 workstation. Reconstructed transverse studies were correlated to each other in 3D by means of an automated image registration algorithm, which was identical to the previously described method applied to cardiac images[7,8]. Briefly, in the first step, an approximate image alignment was accomplished using a technique based on the principal axes transformation[10,13] and subsequently a simplex minimisation technique[14] was applied to improve the fit. The simplex-downhill minimisation algorithm was applied to iteratively improve upon the initial principal axes image fit by independently adjusting nine transformation parameters. The x, y, and z scaling parameters were included in the search for the best fit as separate parameters, therefore allowing for anisotropic compensation for size variations between brains of different subjects. The sum of absolute count differences[12] between 2 image volumes represented the function value. Each evaluation of function value involved a full reorientation of one dataset (64 slices 64x64) using trilinear (3D) interpolation analogous to the bilinear method[15]. The reorientation was applied to the raw transverse data, thus avoiding the accumulation of linear interpolation errors.

Based on the results in our previous assessment of various convergence methods[7] the absolute count-difference method was chosen for the amalgamation of templates and the test-patient registration. The result of each automated alignment was carefully assessed by an experienced nuclear medicine technologist by overlaying of the template image and aligned patient image, a roving window display technique[7] and a subtracted display. The quality of the fit was examined on all image slices in transverse, coronal and sagittal orientations.

The mean and variation templates were built according to the scheme previously described for cardiac images[7,8]. In the first stage, patients were sequentially registered to the first patient, which was centred in the image matrix and manually reorientated. It should be noted that currently this initial orientation has been chosen arbitrarily, but it would possible to align the initial image to standardised 3D coordinates, such as Talaraich space[16]. The images were then added voxel-by-voxel, creating the mean image. Subsequently, original images of normal patients were re-registered to this mean image and normalised using the ratio of the total counts. This approach ensured that the

registration did not depend on the selection of the first patient. The 3D mean (Figure 1) and variation templates (Figure 2a) were obtained by calculating the mean and coefficient of variation (standard deviation divided by the mean) of the count distribution at each voxel. The asymmetry variation template has been created by calculating the mean of left-to-right differences at each voxel and for each subject (Figure 2b). The asymmetry template has been mirrored and replicated around the y-axis for display purposes.

To assess quantitatively the robustness of the fitting algorithm and its performance in case of abnormal brain scans, we analysed the effect of simulated defects and the effect of the initial alignment on registration accuracy. Ten different simulated defects were generated on images of one normal patient. The simulated defects were introduced at various locations in the brain; their size varied between 5% to 20% of the brain volume. Voxels belonging to the simulated defects were set to 0. Images with simulated defects were then arbitrarily misaligned (angles and shifts) by up to 10 pixels and up to 15 degrees, and subsequently re-registered to the normal templates. Registration parameters from the original study without defects provided an absolute reference to which the registrations of images with simulated defects were compared. The registration error for each transformation parameter was defined as the absolute change in the registration parameters related to the introduction of the defect.

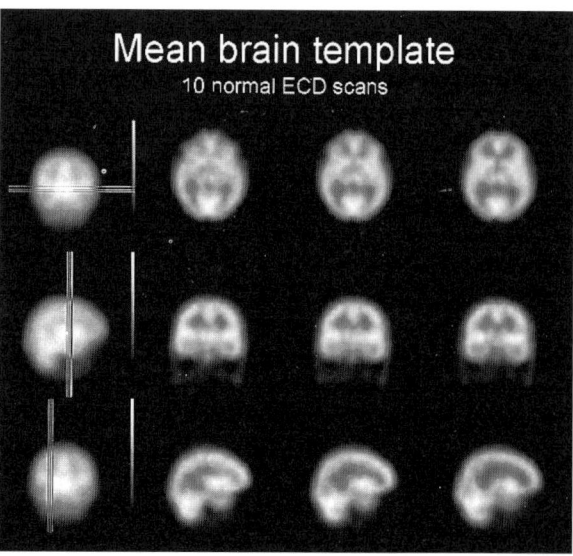

Figure 1 Mean brain template accumulated from 10 normal patients

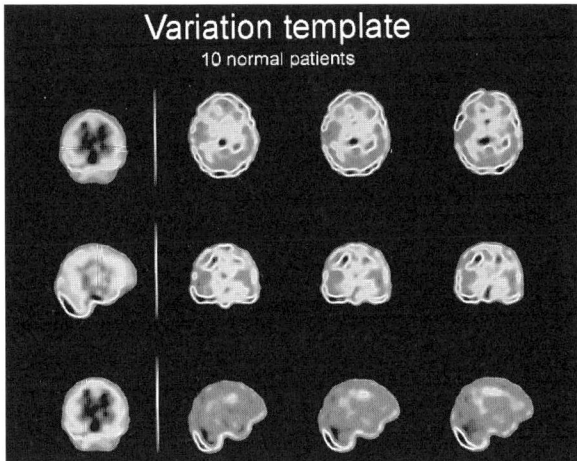

Figure 2a Variation template

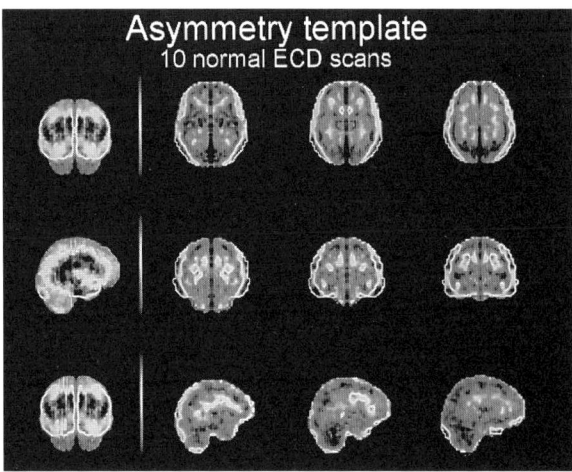

Figure 2b Asymmetry template

To estimate size and location of perfusion abnormalities we used a 3D recursive region-growing scheme, as described previously[8]. The algorithm used the variation and mean templates to mark contiguous voxels in the patient image that were below normal limits (Figure 3). The counts in test-patients' images were normalised using the ratio of total counts in the template and the individual images. The region growing was initiated from the point where the difference between voxel values of the test-patient image and the mean template image divided by the coefficient of variation at that location was maximal. The region-growing marked all contiguous voxels (belonging to one 3D cluster) if their value was smaller than the mean minus a predefined s.d. threshold. The region-growing procedure was repeated 5 times, avoiding the already marked voxels. Therefore, it was possible to derive up to 5 separate defects on the patient data. In addition to the above scheme, we also devised an asymmetry-based region growing scheme. The asymmetry-based region growing did not use the mean template map, but the left-to-right voxel difference has been evaluated at each voxel and compared with the corresponding asymmetry range at that location (Figure 2b). Voxels with asymmetry values higher than the range obtained from the asymmetry map were then marked as abnormal. The display of the original tomographic images and defects was integrated by overlaying the bitmap images representing the abnormal voxels outlined by the region- growing and the original patient images (Figure 4). To estimate the effect of increasing the number of patients included in the template we have also built the mean template from n=4 images (Figure 5).

Results

The mean number of iterations required by the simplex-downhill algorithm for each patient registration was 327. The total time for finding the minimum ranged from 3 to 10 min. All results of fitting algorithms have been evaluated visually by an experienced technologist in all orientations (transverse, coronal, sagittal). In all cases (10 normal studies, 10 simulated studies and 6 abnormal patients) no visual discrepancies has been observed. In addition, the results of the quantitative assessment of the influence of the presence of the defect on the registration are presented in Table 1.

In the population of normal subjects, the coefficient of variation was higher on edges, around the major fissures and in the periventricular areas (Figure 2a).

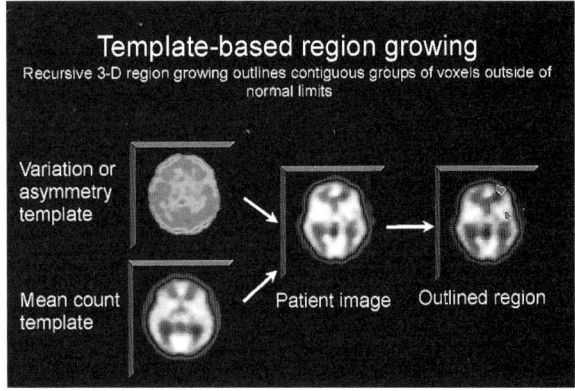

Figure 3 Principle of the template-based region-growing

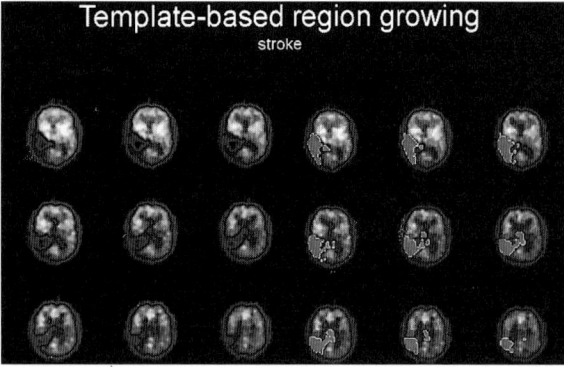

Figure 4 An example of the template region-growing applied to the abnormal brain scan. Original images (left) and the results of the region-growing procedure overlaid on the images (right)

Table 1 Registration errors in the simulated defect experiment

Parameter	Mean ±s.d.	Maximum
x shift (pixels)[a]	0.8±0.3	1.6
y shift (pixels)	0.5±0.4	1.8
z shift (pixels)	0.5±0.3	1.2
x scale (%)	1.3±0.8	4.9
y scale (%)	1.0±0.8	3.6
z scale (%)	1.1±0.7	2.3
xy angle (deg)	1.4±0.6	3.1
xz angle (deg)	1.4±1.0	4.6
yz angle (deg)	0.9±0.5	1.9

[a] pixel size is 3.59 mm

The highest values were around 50% at the posterior edge of the cerebellum. The lowest values of the coefficient of variation and were in the range of 7-8%. The region-growing procedure was evaluated visually and the derived regions were generally consistent with visual observation of the defects.

Discussion

Anisotropic, linear scaling parameters play an important role because the dimensions and shape of the brain vary between patients. It is possible, however, to apply non-linear scaling, or 'warping' techniques that adjust more than nine parameters to compensate for different shapes[4]. For example, one such method was recently proposed for the registration of HMPAO SPECT brain studies[6] and PET studies[4,5]. It seems, however, that warping methods can distort relative count distribution in the brain. The implications of warping schemes for 3D MRI brain mapping are discussed by Collins *et al.*[17], suggesting that the amount of allowed warping should be variable across the brain volume and defined by 'stiffness coefficient'. Current warping schemes do not use such constraints[4] and it seems that a careful analysis of warping effects in a variety of abnormal conditions is needed. Another method for dealing with non-linear differences could be the normalised surface projection approach proposed recently for evaluating PET images[5]. It has to be stressed, however, that SPECT images are generally of low resolution (8-10 mm) and warping may not be as important as it is in the case of PET. Nevertheless, the anisotropic scaling methods may be limited in the quantification of voxels on the edges of the brain.

Despite amalgamating a number of patients using anisotropic but linear transformations, the composite images retain the essential characteristics of brain image, and there does not appear to be a significant loss of resolution when the number of patients is increased in the template (Figure 5). The most noticeable characteristics of the composite templates were the low level of noise and the slightly smoothed and 'blurred' appearance of the edges The smooth appearance could be attributed to a much higher number of counts in the templates than in single-patient images. Blurred edges were caused by differences in brain shapes still remaining after the anizotropic scaling. Due to the low resolution of the original images, however, these differences do not seem to affect significantly the resolution of the composite images (Figure 1 and Figure 5). The relatively good quality of template images can be explained by the lack of fine details in the original images, which are of relatively low resolution.

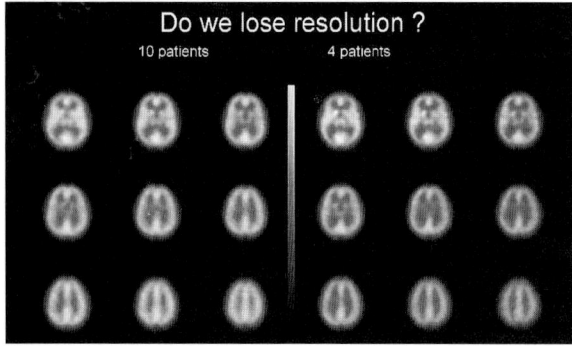

Figure 5 Mean template formed from the images of 10 patients (left) and 4 patients (right)

An important advantage of the method is fully automated fitting, which may allow better and more reproducible selection of angles. By automated reorientating to standardised 3D orientation, the subjectivity of interpretation should be reduced. Perhaps especially important is the accurate determination of the rotation angle in the coronal plane, which will play a significant role in evaluating subtle side-to-side differences. The use of the normal limits of asymmetry from the asymmetry map may further enhance the reliability of estimating the side-to-side differences. The software adjustment of the angles is simpler to implement and reported to be more accurate than using customised head moulds[18] for the determination of the angles.

The accuracy of the automated registration (Table 1) compared with the resolution of the scan (generally 8-10 mm) is encouraging. An objective measure of the anticipated algorithm performance with abnormal data was provided by the simulated-defect registration (Table 1). The results showed that alignment was accurate even when a considerable part of the brain was missing. The method is robust despite the presence of defects because the algorithm searches for the relative minimum of the count-difference. Although the simulated-defects resulted in overall higher count-difference between patient image and the template, the relative minimum was found for transformation parameters similar to those in the original data registration. The results imply that fitting of the brain studies will not be affected by the presence of perfusion defects. This confirms our earlier findings when using this method for heart studies[7,8].

Although increasing the number of patients does not seem to change the appearance of the normal mean template, the number used in this study (n=10) may not be sufficient to represent standard variation and the asymmetry map. Therefore, these maps should be treated as preliminary results. We are currently investigating possibilities for building the normal models from a larger group of patients. Ideally, these groups should be age matched.

Conclusions

The concept of automated inter-subject registration and creating of 3D normal distribution templates can be applied to brain SPECT images. Despite amalgamating several images, we did not observe a significant loss of resolution in the mean template. We were able to use such 3D normal maps for the relative quantification of counts in test-patients. The registration technique is insensitive to the abnormalities in the tracer distribution. The region-growing procedure provides an appealing and natural presentation of the defects. Such visualisation and regional quantification may enable more objective image interpretation. The technique developed promises to be an uncomplicated and reliable technique for computer-aided interpretation of brain SPECT images.

References

1 Hooper, R.H., McEwan, A.J., Lentel, B.C.*et al.* Interactive three-dimensional region of interest analysis of HMPAO SPECT Brain Studies. *J. Nucl. Med.*1990, 31, 2046

2 Johnson, K.A., Kijewski, M.F., Becker, A.*et al.* Quantitative Brain SPECT in Alzheimer's disease and normal ageing. *J. Nucl. Med.*1993, 34, 2044

3 Fox, P.T. and Perlmutter, M.A. Enhanced detection of focal brain responses using inter-subject averaging and change distribution analysis of subtracted PET images. *J. Cereb. Blood Flow Metab.*1988, 8, 642

4 Minoshima, S., Koeppe, R.A. *et al.* Anatomic Standarization: Linear Scaling and Nonlinear warping of functional brain images. *J. Nucl. Med.*1994, 35, 1528

5 Minoshima, S., Frey, K.A., Koeppe, R.A.*et al.* A diagnostic approach in Alzheimer's disease using three-dimensional stereotactic surface projections of fluorine-18-FDG-PET. *J. Nucl. Med.*1995, 36, 1238

6 Houston, A.S., Kemp, P.M. and Macleod, M.A. A method for assessing the significance of abnormalities in HMPAO brain SPECT images. *J. Nucl. Med.*1994, 35, 239

7 Slomka, P.J., Hurwitz, G., Stephenson, J.A. and Cradduck, T.D. Automated alignment and sizing of myocardial stress and rest scans to three-dimensional normal templates using an image registration algorithm. *J. Nucl. Med.* 1995, 36, 1115

8 Slomka, P.J., Hurwitz, G., St. Clement, G. and Stephenson, J.A. Three dimensional demarcation of perfusion zones corresponding to specific coronary arteries : application for automated interpretation of myocardial SPECT. *J. Nucl. Med.* 1995, 36, 2120

9 Pelizzari, C.A., Chen, G.T.Y., Spelbring, D.R. *et al.* Accurate three-dimensional registration of CT, PET, and/or MR images of the brain. *J. Comput. Assist. Tomogr.* 1989, 13, 20

10 Alpert, N.M., Bradshaw, J.F., Kennedy, D. and Correia, J.A. The principal axes transformation - a method for image registration. *J. Nucl. Med.* 1990, 31, 626

11 Junck, L., Moen, J.G., Hutchins, G.D.*et al.* Correlation methods for the centering, rotation and alignment of functional brain images. *J. Nucl. Med.* 1990, 31, 1220

12 Hoh, C.K., Dahlbom, M., Harris, G. *et al.* Automated iterative three-dimensional registration of positron emission tomography images. *J. Nucl. Med.* 1993, 34, 2009

13 Faber, T.L. and Stokely, E.M. Orientation of 3-D structures in medical images. *IEEE Trans. Pattern Anal. Machine Intell.* 1988, 10, 376

14 Press, W.H., Teukolsky, S.A., Vetterling, W.T. and Flannery, B.P. in 'Numerical recipes in C', 2nd edition, Cambridge University Press, New York, 1992, p.123

15 Press, W.H., Teukolsky, S.A., Vetterling, W.T. and Flannery, B.P. in 'Numerical recipes in C', 2nd edition, Cambridge University Press, New York, 1992, p.408

16 Talaraich, J. and Tournoux, P. in 'Co-planar stereotaxic atlas of the human brain', Thieme, New York, 1988

17 Collins, D.L., Neelin, P., Peters, T.M. and Evans, A.C. Automatic 3D intersubject registration of MR volumetric data in standarized Talaraich space. *J. Comput. Assist. Tomogr.* 1994, 18, 192

18 Strother, S.C., Anderson, J.R., Xu, X.L. *et al.* Quantitative comparisons of image registration techniques based on high-resolution MRI of the brain. *J. Comput. Assist. Tomogr.* 1994, 8, 95

SPECT in Neurology and Psychiatry, edited by P.P. De Deyn, R.A. Dierckx, A. Alavi and B.A. Pickut
© 1997 John Libbey & Company Ltd, pp. 513-519

Biological Basis of Cerebral Perfusion SPECT

Chapter
61

D.O. Slosman and P. Magistretti[*]

Introduction

The introduction of [99mTc]-labelled brain-retained tracers for cerebral perfusion SPECT imaging has stimulated their widespread use in clinical settings and has initiated enthusiastic developments concerning methodological issues such as the quantification of regional cerebral blood flow (rCBF) or functional neuroimaging. Nevertheless, the biological mechanisms that enable the cellular retention of these new tracers reflect only indirectly rCBF. In this chapter, our aims are: to summarise the acquired knowledge for identifying the cellular target(s) of [99mTc]-tracers in the brain; to demonstrate the limits of the cellular mechanisms involved in the brain tissue's retention of these tracers as well as their potential value, in understanding physiopathological issue's; and to discuss their potential impact in a clinical setting.

Brain imaging and tissue target

Since the original article by Roy and Sherrington[1], written more than a century ago, it has been understood that brain activity, cerebral perfusion and brain tissue metabolism itself (glucose consumption) are closely related. In the late 1970s, Sokoloff's model[2] and the development of a quantitative technique for measuring glucose consumption in regional brain tissue such as FDG PET as a marker of neuronal activity[3], opened a new era of functional brain imaging. Only recently, however, has the cellular site of FDG retention during activation been identified. Thus *in vitro* evidence strongly suggests that astrocytes are the targets of fluorodeoxyglucose cellular retention and not neurons, as was thought previously[4,5]. In addition, glutamate appears to be a candidate for providing the coupling between neuronal activity and activation-linked glucose consumption[4,5]. Therefore, one might wonder which population of cells retains the SPECT brain imaging agents that are administered intravenously. In particular, is there any cellular specificity (e.g., in endothelial cells, astrocytes or neurons)?

Similar to other brain SPECT markers (IMP: isopropyl-iodoamphetamine, HIPDM: trimethyl-propanediamine, HMPAO: hexamethyl-propanediamine oxime, or ECD: ethyl cysteinate dimer), [133Xe] crosses the blood-brain barrier (BBB). But unlike the others, xenon is not trapped in the brain, and regional cerebral blood flow (rCBF) measurement is obtained by modelling its brain dynamic transit[6,7]. Therefore, cell specificity is less likely to be of any importance when [133Xe] is used, while it becomes an important issue when the other SPECT brain imaging agents are concerned. These radio-labelled 'chemical microspheres' are trapped in brain tissue, and their total amount

Division of Nuclear medicine, Geneva University Hospital, 1211 Geneva 14, Switzerland
[*]Neurological Research Laboratory, Institute of Physiology and Department of Neurology, Lausanne University Medical School, 1005 Lausanne, Switzerland

retained is considered to reflect the magnitude of rCBF. However, the cell type involved, its metabolic activities and its behaviour in brain diseases are among other factors which will determine retention. Indirect evidence suggests that the basic lipophilic amines IMP and HIPDM are retained in endothelial cells. It has already been demonstrated that biogenic amines (such as serotonin) and basic lipophilic amines (such as amphetamine) are largely taken up by pulmonary endothelial cells and, for nearly two decades now, their lung extraction has been measured as an index of pulmonary endothelial cell function[8]. We have previously studied the nature and extent of the pulmonary extraction of these markers in isolated-perfused lung models[9,10]. In particular, we observed that the extent of IMP lung extraction is linearly dependent on the pulmonary vascular surface available for blood flow[10]. Therefore, at the brain tissue level, the endothelial cell appears to be a good candidate for the cellular retention of IMP or HIPDM. This could also explain the importance of back-diffusion/redistribution over time and the importance of early imaging with IMP[11,12]. No other specific binding system could be proposed to explain

pulmonary retention of ECD or HMPAO, and there are no relevant observations to suggest that endothelial cells could be the cellular target. Based on the observations made with FDG, one also could consider astrocytes as a cellular target for ECD and HMPAO retention.

Brain imaging and cellular uptake mechanism

Despite the wide clinical and research use of functional brain imaging, the cellular and molecular mechanisms that underlie the signal that is detected with PET/SPECT techniques are still poorly understood. Recently, the uptake of glutamate into astrocytes has been identified as playing a role, during activation, in providing the signal for FDG PET[4,5]. The evidence can be summarised as follows: when a given cerebral area is physiologically activated, glutamate, the principal excitatory neurotransmitter, is released from afferent pathways; in other words, glutamate release is a concomitant of local activation, implying that glutamate is a likely candidate for providing the

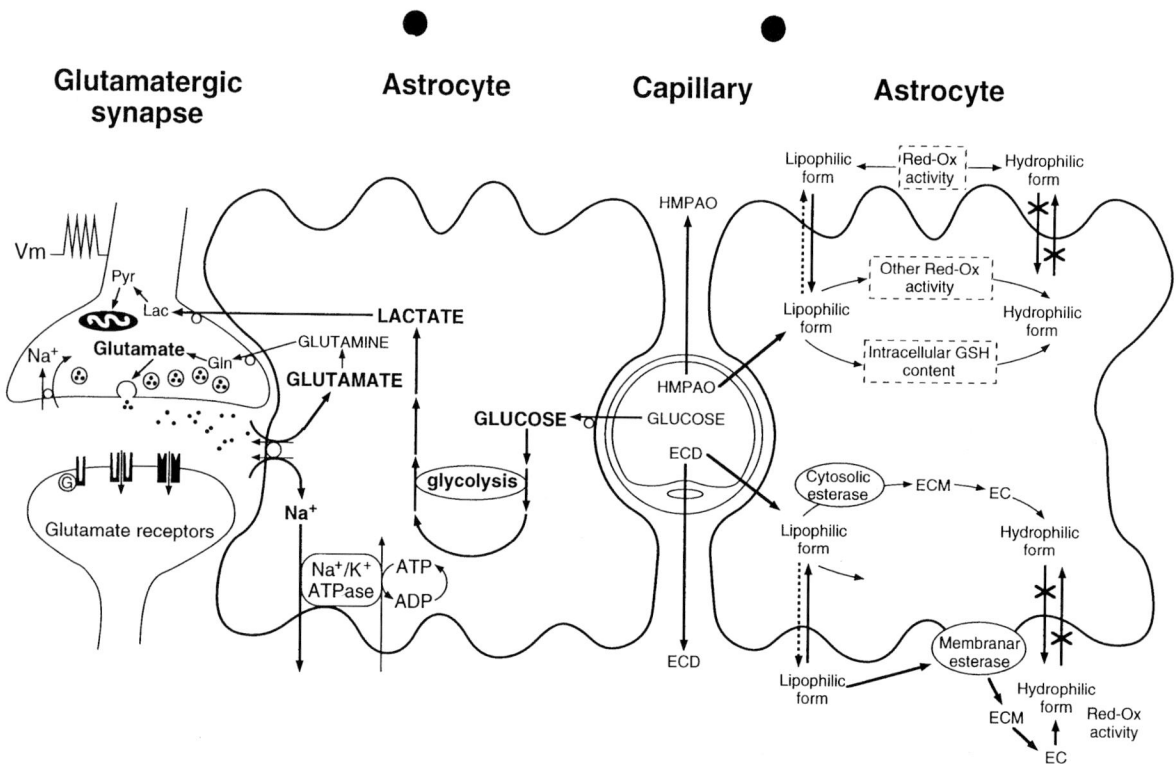

Figure 1 Schematic of the mechanism for glutamate-induced glycolysis, HMPAO and ECD uptake in astrocytes during physiological activiation

coupling between neuronal activity and activation-linked glucose utilisation. Moreover, glutamate that is released from excitatory afferents is avidly taken up by astrocytes that ensheath synaptic contacts[13]. Other astrocyte processes, the end-feet, surround intraparenchymal capillaries, which are the source of glucose[14]. This feature implies that astrocytes form the first cellular barrier which the glucose encounters when entering the brain parenchyma, and it makes them a likely site for prevalent glucose uptake (Figure 1). This cytoarchitectural arrangement along with the capacity of astrocytes to sense synaptic activity (through the reuptake of glutamate), provide suggestive evidence of the key role that astrocytes play in coupling neuronal activity to glucose utilisation. Indeed, it has been demonstrated recently using the well-established 2-deoxyglucose (2-DG) technique[4,5] that glutamate stimulates glucose uptake and phosphorylation by astrocytes. This effect is not mediated by specific glutamate receptors known to be present on astrocytes[15], since it is not inhibited by any of the specific antagonists tested, nor is it mimicked by agonists specific to each receptor subtype. Rather, a detailed pharmacological analysis indicates a tight coupling between Na^+-dependent glutamate uptake and

glucose utilisation by astrocytes (Figure 1)[4,16]. These observations have recently been replicated in the laboratory of Louis Sokoloff[5], who originally developed the use of 2-DG as a way to image, by autoradiography and PET, activity-linked glucose utilisation[2]. In addition, activation-dependent glucose uptake into glial cells has been demonstrated clearly using simple and well-compartmentalised neural preparation, such as the retina[17]. Thus, a consensus is now emerging that supports the view that uptake of the labelled glucose into astrocytes contributes significantly, particularly, during activation, to the signal observed with FDG PET[4,5]. In addition, according to this model, the impairment of glutamate uptake by astrocytes is likely to be reflected in a decreased FDG PET signal.

The cellular locus of the signals originating from HMPAO or ECD SPECT is still largely unknown. Given their high degree of lipophilicity, HMPAO and ECD readily cross membranes; they are converted to hydrophilic forms which are retained inside cells[18-23]. Based on these physicochemical properties, the uptake of HMPAO or ECD by the brain is taken to reflect rCBF[7,24-32].

Table 1 Review of the literature reporting cases of increased uptake of cerebral SPECT imaging agents

Authors	Agents	Cases	Authors' conclusion
Non-malignant diseases			
Moretti et al.[12]	HMPAO/IMP	2/10	'Luxury perfusion' only seen on HMPAO SPECT
Meyer et al.[54]	HMPAO	1/ 1	Limbic encephalitis
Tamgac et al.[37]	IMP / ECD	7/52	Reflow hyperaemia only seen on IMP SPECT
Lassen et al.[38]	^{133}Xe / ECD	1/ 1	Hyperaemia in subacute stroke only seen on ^{133}Xe SPECT
Tsuchida et al.[55]	HMPAO/IMP/ECD	2/10	'Luxury perfusion' only seen on HMPAO or IMP SPECT
Malignant diseases			
Babich et al.[39]	HMPAO	2/12	Hyperaemia associated with high-grade glioma
Lindegaard et al.[41]	HMPAO	1/12	Hyperaemia associated with glioma
Rodriguez et al.[42]	HMPAO/Thallium	8/21	Glioma uptake and indicator of therapy response
Schwartz et al.[40]	HMPAO/Thallium	4/15	Hyperaemia associated with high-grade glioma

However, experimental evidence has suggested that the intracellular conversion to the hydrophilic form of HMPAO is related to the glutathione content of cells[18]. Reduced glutathione is an essential component of the cell's armamentarium and its capacity to scavenge oxygen free radicals, which has been widely implicated in neuronal death[33]. The amount of reduced glutathione is directly related to the redox state of a cell, particularly to its NADP/NADPH ratio. Thus, changes in the levels of NADPH, which are produced notably as a by-product of glucose metabolism through the pentose phosphate pathway, will result in an abnormal redox state of a cell, a 'condition' that will have an impact on the uptake of HMPAO. Indeed, very recent observations indicate that the cellular retention of HMPAO is determined by the redox state in a variety of cell types, including a human astrocyte-derived cell line (Figure 1)[34]. These observations in particular may provide a useful tool to elucidate certain pathophysiological mechanisms involved in neurodegeneration. Thus, in addition to being a valuable indicator of rCBF, HMPAO may provide unique information on the specific energy metabolism processes of a given cortical region.

If the intracellular conversion of ECD to the hydrophilic forms has been related to an intracellular process (activity of esterases) similar to that of HMPAO (glutathione and related activities), recent experimental evidence also suggests that the membrane-bound esterasic activity represents a limiting step in the regulation of total ECD cellular retention[35] (Figure 1). Minimal or no membranar esterasic activity will favour intracellular ECD uptake, while an important membranar esterasic activity will largely reduce the lipophilic form of ECD available to cross the cell membrane. A large variation in the regulation of membrane-bound esterase is less likely to occur than is a variation in the redox state. Therefore, contrary to HMPAO, these observations support ECD as a more accurate indicator of rCBF, which is unlikely to be altered by abnormal metabolic processes.

Relationship between *in vivo* brain imaging and the cellular behaviour of tracers

HMPAO and ECD SPECT have been performed in numerous clinical conditions, particularly in patients with brain tumours, with epilepsy or after strokes. As shown in Table 1, the discordant results between ECD and other rCBF agents have been identified in several conditions[7,36-38].

Babich *et al.*[39] have reported two patients out of 12 with intracranial tumours and focal hyperperfusion. Schwartz *et al.*[40] brought additional evidence when they reported four out of 15 patients with brain tumours and increased HMPAO uptake. Among them, three patients had a local recurrence of irradiated tumours, while one was free of recurrent disease. These observations were related to tumour hyperperfusion; the falsely positive case was associated with a possible transient hyperperfusion due to irradiation. In another series of 12 patients, one presented a focal hyperperfusion that was associated with a brain infarction of the contralateral hemisphere[41]. More recently, Rodriguez *et al.*[42] studied 21 patients with histologically proven astrocytoma and reported that six out of seven patients, prior to therapy, had increased HMPAO uptake and did not show neurological improvement after therapy. In contrast, only two out of nine patients with increased HMPAO uptake before therapy showed neurological improvement after therapy. These observations enabled the authors to support the previously stated hypothesis of the relationship between hyperperfusion and the increased uptake of HMPAO, and they suggested the use of HMPAO SPECT as a predictor of a tumour's response to therapy. The presence of hyperperfusion, *per se*, could not explain our discrepant observations of increased HMPAO uptake compared with normal ECD uptake. Although both HMPAO and ECD have been shown to reflect rCBF in normal subjects, these observations suggest that metabolic abormalities are responsible for the increased HMPAO retention. In a tumoral process, a necrotic centre is surrounded by intact tumour cells but separated from them by a ring of dying cells in relation to the regional anoxo-ischaemic state. In this condition, the production of proinflammatory cytokines, in particular tumour necrosis factor alpha (α-TNF), stimulates the activation of inflammatory cells, resulting in oxidative stress and causing intracellular xanthine dehydrogenase to convert into xanthine oxidase. During the metabolisation of xanthine or hypoxanthine in uric acid mediated by xanthine oxidase, there is a generation of free radicals, such as superoxide radicals and hydrogen peroxide, which alter the intracellular glutathione content as well as the redox equilibrium. Therefore, one can hypothesise that the focal increase of free radicals around the central necrotic tumour area will enhance (or even trigger) the cellular retention of HMPAO in a manner independent of rCBF, while ECD uptake will be unaffected by these inflammation-promoted metabolic changes. Results obtained in clinical settings may be related to the determination of predictive factors associated with the increased uptake of HMPAO (particularly in the presence of stroke, tumours or inflammatory processes) or in the field of epileptical functional imaging (i.e., falsely positive readings may occur in ictal SPECT when tumours or other structural abnormalities are present and responsible, *per se*, for the increased focal uptake).

As discussed previously, the abnormal redox state of a cell will alter the cellular retention of HMPAO. This biological behaviour may be useful for testing *in vivo* the role of oxygen free radicals in neurodegeneration, or for identifying early non-invasive alterations related to neurodegeneration, particularly for Alzheimer's disease (AD). The definitive diagnosis of AD depends upon post mortem histological verification. Diagnosis can be supported during the course of the disease by neuropsychological testing and by neuroimaging using CT or MRI[43]. Thus, pre mortem neuroimaging findings (CT and MRI) can be correlated with post mortem temporal lobe neuropathological changes (atrophy)[44]. In addition to the structural findings revealed with CAT and MRI imaging, functional imaging procedures have revealed a decrease in energy metabolism in selected brain areas in those patients who present clinical symptoms corresponding to the diagnosis of probable AD[43,45]. The three parameters of brain energy metabolism, namely blood flow, oxygen consumption (CMRO$_2$) and glucose utilisation (CMRglu), are affected to varying degrees. These observations have been obtained essentially with two imaging techniques, PET and SPECT[46,47]. In particular, decreases in CMRglu, visualised with FDG PET, and reductions in rCBF, monitored with HMPAO SPECT, are maximal in the temporal and parietal cortices of patients with probable AD[46,47]. This hypometabolism has generally been interpreted as reflecting the degree of cortical atrophy, which is manifested by the clinical symptoms of dementia, and is supported by structural imaging acquisitions (CT and MRI). However, a few studies have indicated that cortical hypometabolism is present at the very early stages of the disease, when cortical atrophy is absent and neuropsychological deficits are circumscribed by a moderate and isolated age-associated memory impairment that shows normal, neocortically mediated language and cognitive function[48-50]. The longitudinal nature of these studies, in which metabolic imaging and neuropsychological tests were performed on the same patients over a 48 month period, provided the initial evidence that cortical hypometabolism could precede cognitive impairment and not merely be the result of cortical atrophy. In addition, correlations between cognitive impairment, middle cerebral artery-flow velocity and cortical glucose metabolism in the early phase of AD has recently been reported[51]. These observations hint at the possible predictive value of metabolic reductions monitored by PET or SPECT in dementias of the Alzheimer type[48-50]. Two recent studies in asymptomatic at risk individuals have further strengthened this view[52,53].

In this chapter, we have attempted to integrate recent experimental results and clinical observations concerning HMPAO and ECD, and to correlate them to FDG PET imaging. The data highlight the discrepancies between HMPAO and ECD behaviours existing *in vitro* at the cellular level, as well as clinically[56]. In addition, it suggests that HMPAO cerebral uptake does not solely represent rCBF but also reveals some specific metabolic activities and that, in the future, HMPAO could be used in some pathological states, as a metabolic tracer similar to FDG, while ECD would remain a more specific rCBF tracer.

References

1   Roy, C.S. and Sherrington, C.S. On the regulation of the blood-supply of the brain, 1889

2   Sokoloff, L., Reivich, M., Kennedy, C. *et al.* The (14C)deoxyglucose method for the measurement of local cerebral glucose utilization: theory, procedure and normal values in the conscious and anesthetized albino rat. *J. Neurochem.* 1977, 28, 897

3   Phelps, M.E., Huang, S.C., Hoffman, E.J. *et al.* Tomographic measurement of local cerebral glucose metabolic rate in humans with F-18 2-fluoro-2-deoxy-D-glucose : validation of method. *Ann. Neurol.* 1979, 6, 371

4   Pellerin, L. and Magistretti, P.J. Glutamate uptake into astrocytes stimulates aerobic glycolysis : a mechanism coupling neuronal activity to glucose utilization. *Proc. Natl. Acad. Sci. USA* 1994, 91, 10625

5   Takahashi, S., Driscoll, B.F., Law, M.J. and Sokoloff, L. Role of sodium and potassium ions in regulation of glucose metabolism in cultured astroglia. *Proc. Natl. Acad. Sci. USA* 1995, 92, 4616

6   Lassen, N.A., Henriksen, S., Holm, S. *et al.* Cerebral blood-flow tomography: Xenon-133 compared with isopropyl-amphetamine-iodine-123. *J. Nucl. Med.* 1983, 24, 17

7   Devous, M.D., Payne, J.K., Lowe, J.L. and Leroy, R.F. Comparison of technetium-99m- ECD to Xenon-133 SPECT in normal controls and in patients with mild to moderate regional cerebral blood flow abnormalities. *J. Nucl. Med.* 1993, 34, 754

8   Junod, A.F. 5-Hydroxytryptamine and other amines in the lungs in 'Handbook of Physiology: section 3 - The respiratory system', (Ed. A.P. Society), The Williams and Witkins Company, Bethesda, 1985, p.337

9   Slosman, D.O., Brill, A.B., Polla, B.S. and Alderson, P.O. Evaluation of [Iodine-125] N,N,N'-trimethyl-N'-[2-Hydroxy-3-methyl-5-iodobenzyl]-propanediamine lung uptake using an isolated-perfused lung model. *J. Nucl. Med.* 1987, 28, 203

10 Slosman, D.O., Donath, A. and Alderson, P.O. 131I-metaiodobenzyl-guanidine and 125I-iodoamphetamine lung extraction in rat: parameters of lung endothelial cell function and pulmonary vascular area. *Eur. J. Nucl. Med.* 1989, 15, 207

11 Yonekura, Y., Nishizawa, S., Mukai, T. *et al.* Functional mapping of flow and back-diffusion rate of N-isopropyl-p-idoamphetamine in human brain. *J. Nucl. Med.* 1993, 34, 839

12 Moretti, J.L., Caglar, M. and Weinmann, P. Cerebral perfusion imaging tracers for SPECT: which one to choose ? *J. Nucl. Med.* 1995, 36, 359

13 Barres, B.A. New roles for glia. *J. Neuroscience* 1991, 11, 3685

14 Peters, A., Palay, S.L. and Webster de, H.F. in 'The fine structure of the nervous system: neurons and their supporting cells', W.B. Saunders, Philadelphia, 1991

15 Pearce, B. Amino acid receptors in 'Astrocytes: pharmacology and function', (Ed. S. Murphy), Academic Press, San Diego, 1993, p. 47

16 Kanner, B.I. Glutamate transporters from brain: a novel neurotransmitter transporter family. *FEBS Lett.* 1993, 325, 95

17 Tsacopoulos, M. and Magistretti, P.J. Metabolic coupling between glia and neurons. *The Journal of Neuroscience* 1996, 16, 877

18 Neirinckx, R., Burke, J.F., Harrison, R.C. *et al.* The retention mechanism of technetium-99m-HM-PAO: intracellular reaction with glutathione. *J. Cereb. Blood Flow Metab.* 1988, 8, S4

19 Andersen, A.R. 99mTc-D,L-Hexamethylene-propyleneamine oxime (99mTc-HMPAO): basic kinetic studies of a tracer of cerebral blood flow. *Cerebrovascular and Brain Metabolism Reviews* 1989, 1, 288

20 Léveillé, J., Demonceau, G., De Roo, M. *et al.* Characterization of technetium-99m-L,L-ECD for brain perfusion imaging, part 2 : biodistribution and brain imaging in humans. *J. Nucl. Med.* 1989, 30, 1902

21 Walovitch, R.C., Hill, T.C., Garrity, S.T. *et al.* Characterization of technetium-99m- L,L-ECD for brain perfusion imaging, part 1: pharmacology of technetium-99m ECD in nonhuman primates. *J. Nucl. Med.* 1989, 30, 1892

22 Walovitch, R.C., Franceschi, M., Picard, M. *et al.* Metabolism of 99mTc-L,L-Ethyl cysteinate dimer in healthy volunteers. *Neuropharmacology* 1991, 30, 283

23 Walovitch, R.C., Cheesman, E.H., Maheu, L.J. and Hall, K.M. Studies of the retention mechanism of the brain perfusion imaging agent 99mTc-bicisate (99mTc-ECD). *J. Cereb. Blood Flow Metab.* 1994, 14, S4

24 Yonekura, Y., Nishizawa, S., Mukai, T. *et al.* SPECT with (99mTc)-d,l-hexamethyl-propylene amine oxime (HM-PAO) compared with regional cerebral blood flow measured by PET: effect of linearization. *J. Cereb. Blood Flow Metab.* 1988, 8, S82

25 Andersen, A.R., Friberg, H., Lassen, N.A. *et al.* Assessment of the arterial input curve for 99mTc-d,I-HMPAO by rapid octanol extraction. *J. Cereb. Blood Flow Metab.* 1988, 8, S23

26 Lassen, N.A., Andersen, A.R., Friberg, L. and Paulson, O.B. The retention of 99mTc-d,l-HMPAO in the human brain after intracarotid bolus injection : a kinetic analysis. *J. Cereb. Blood Flow Metab.* 1988, 8, S13

27 Orlandi, C., Crane, P.D., Platts, S.H. and Walovitch, R.C. Regional cerebral blood flow and distribution of 99mTc ethyl cysteinate dimer in nonhuman primates. *Stroke* 1990, 21, 1059

28 Gemmell, H.G., Evans, N.T. S., Besson, J.A.O. *et al.* Regional cerebral blood flow imaging : a quantitative comparison of technetium-99m-HMPAO SPECT with C-15 O2 PET. *J. Nucl. Med.* 1990, 31, 1595

29 Pupi, A., deCristofaro, T.R., Bacciottini, L. *et al.* An analysis of the arterial input curve for technetium-99mHMPAO : quantification of rCBF using single-photon emission computed tomogtraphy. *J. Nucl. Med.* 1991, 32, 1501

30 Murase, K., Tanada, S., Fujita, H. *et al.* Kinetic behavior of technetium-99m-HMPAO in the human brain and quantification of cerebral blood flow using dynamic SPECT. *J. Nucl. Med.* 1992, 33, 135

31 Greenberg, J.H., Araki, N. and Karp, A. Correlation between Tc99m-bicisate and regional CBF measured with iodo-[C-14] antipyrine in a primate focal ischemia model. *J. Cereb. Blood Flow Metab.* 1994, 14, S36

32 Pupi, A., Castagnoli, A., De Cristofaro, M.T.R. *et al.* Quantitative comparison between 99m Tc-HMPAO and 99m Tc-ECD: measurement of arterial input and brain retention. *Eur. J. Nucl. Med.* 1994, 21, 124

33 Coyle, J.T. and Puttfarcken, P. Oxidative stress, glutamate, and neurodegenerative disorders. *Science* 1993, 262, 689

34 Jacquier-Sarlin, M., Polla, A. and Slosman, D.O. Oxido-reductive state: the major determinant for cellular retention of HMPAO-Tc99m. *J. Nucl. Med.* 1996, 37, 1413

35 Jacquier-Sarlin, M., Polla, A. and Slosman, D.O. The cellular basis of ECD brain retention. *J. Nucl. Med.* 1996, 37, 1694

36 Tsuchida, T., Nishizawa, S., Yonekura, Y. *et al.* SPECT Images of technetium-99m ethyl cysteinate dimer in cerebrovascular diseases : comparison with other cerebral perfusion tracers and PET. *J. Nucl. Med.* 1993, 35, 27

37 Tamgac, F., Moretti, J.-L., Defer, G. *et al.* Non-matched images with I-123 IMP and Tc-99m bicisate single-photon emission tomography in the demonstration of focal hyperaemia during the subacute phase of an ischemic stroke. *Eur. J. Nucl. Med.* 1994, 21, 254

38 Lassen, N.A. and Sperling, B. 99mTc-bicisate reliably images CBF in chronic brain diseases but fails to show reflow hyperemia in subacute stroke: report of a multicenter trial of 105 cases comparing 133-Xe and 99mTc-bicisate (ECD, Neurolite) measured by SPECT on the same day. *J. Cereb. Blood Flow Metab.*1994, 14, S44

39 Babich, J.W., Keeling, F., Flower, M.A. *et al.* Initial experience with Tc99m-HMPAO in the study of brain tumors. *Eur. J. Nucl. Med.* 1988, 14, 39

40 Schwartz, R.B., Carvalho, P.A., Ill, E.A. *et al.* Radiation necrosis vs High-Grade recurrent glioma : differentiation by using dual-isotope SPECT with 201 TI and 99m Tc-HMPAO. *A. J. N. R.* 1992, 12, 1187

41 Lindegaard, M.W., Skretting, A., Hager, B. *et al.* Cerebral and cerebellar uptake of Tc99m-d,l-hexamethyl-propyleneamine oxime (HMPAO) in patients with brain tumor studied by single photon emission computerized tomography. *Eur. J. Nucl. Med.* 1986, 12, 417

42 Rodriguez, M., Fonseca, A.T., Salgado, D. and Vieira, M.R. Tc99m-HMPAO brain SPECT in the evaluation of prognosis after surgical resection of astrocytoma. Comparison with other noninvasive imaging techniques (CT, MRI and Tl201 SPECT). *Nucl. Med. Com.* 1993, 14, 1050

43 Corey-Bloom, J., Thal, L.J., Galasko, D. *et al.* Diagnosis and evaluation of dementia. *Neurology* 1995, 45, 211

44 Davis, P.C., Gearing, M., Gray, L. *et al.* The CERAD Experience, part VIII: neuroimaging -neuropathology correlates of temporal lobe changes in Alzheimer's disease. *Neurology* 1995, 45, 178

45 Herholz, K. FDG PET and differential diagnosis of dementia. *Alzheimer Dis. Assoc. Disord.* 1995, 9, 6

46 Frackowiak, R.S.J., Pozzilli, C., Legg, N.J. *et al.* Regional oxygen supply and utilization in dementia : a clinical and physiological study with oxygen-15 and positron tomography. *Brain* 1981, 104, 753

47 Messa, C., Perani, D., Lucignani, G. *et al.* High-resolution technetium-99m-HMPAO SPECT in patients with probable Alzheimer's disease : comparison with fluorine-18-FDG PET. *J. Nucl. Med.* 1994, 35, 210

48 Wolfe, N., Reed, B.R., Eberling, J.L. and Jagust, W.J. Temporal lobe perfusion on single photon emission computed tomography predicts the rate of cognitive decline in Alzheimer disease. *Arch. Neurol.* 1995, 52, 257

49 Haxby, J.V., Grady, C.L., Duara, R. *et al.* Neocortical metabolic abnormalities precede nonmemory cognitive defects in early Alzheimer's-type dementia. *Arch. Neurol.* 1986, 43, 882

50 Haxby, J.V., Grady, C.L., Koss, E. *et al.* Longitudinal study of cerebral metabolic asymmetries and associated neuro-psychological patterns in early dementia of the Alzheimer type. *Arch. Neurol.* 1990, 47, 753

51 Franceschi, M., Alberoni, M., Bressi, S. *et al.* Correlations between cognitive impairment, middle cerebral artery velocity and cortical glucose metabolism in the early phase of Alzheimer's disease. *Dementia* 1995, 6, 32

52 Kennedy, A.M., Frackowiak, R.S.J., Newman, S.K. *et al.* Deficits in cerebral glucose metabolism demonstrated by positron emission tomography in individuals at risk of familial Alzheimer's disease. *Neurosci. Lett.* 1995, 18, 17

53 Small, G.W., Mazziotta, J.C., Collins, M.T. *et al.* Apolipoprotein E Type 4 Allele and cerebral glucose metabolism in relatives at risk for familial Alzheimer disease. *J. A. M. A.* 1995, 273, 942

54 Meyer, M. and Wahner, H.W. Focal high uptake of HMPAO in brain perfusion studies : a clue in the diagnosis of encephalitis. *J. Nucl. Med.* 1990, 31, 1094

55 Tsuchida, T., Nishizawa, S., Yonekura, Y. *et al.* SPECT images of technetium-99m-ethyl cysteinate dimer in cerebrovascular diseases: comparison with other cerebral perfusion tracers and PET. *J. Nucl. Med.* 1994, 35, 27

56 Papazyan, J.-P., Delavelle, P., Burkhard, P. *et al.* Discrepancies between HMPAO and ECD SPECT imaging in brain tumor. *J. Nucl. Med.* 1997, 38, 592

SPECT in Neurology and Psychiatry, edited by P.P. De Deyn, R.A. Dierckx, A. Alavi and B.A. Pickut

The Primate Model in Neuropharmacology for Cerebral Blood Flow Determinations with HMPAO SPECT

Chapter

62

I.C. Dormehl, D.W. Oliver* and N. Hugo

Animal models in medical research

Early man obtained information by observing his environment. Animals, as an integral part of the environment, contributed to stimulate the understanding and creativity of reasoning man to improve his way of life.

Early recordings of serious investigations on human biology and anatomy point towards initial dissections on human corpses and cadavers, until these fell into disfavour and were banned in the Middle Ages. The emphasis for research in the medical sciences then reverted to the deliberate use of a variety of animals. Richard Lower successfully performed blood transfusions on dogs in the middle of the 17th century. In June 1667, the first blood transfusion on a human was carried out in France by Jean Baptiste Denis who transfused sheep's blood into two boys, both of whom subsequently died. It was much later that the research activities of Nobel Prize winner, Karl Landsteiner (1868-1943) eventually provided blood transfusions with sound scientific basis, and thus confirmed the impact of early animal research on the shaping of civilisation.

In the 1800s, David Ferrier stimulated animal cortex to localise brain functions, and around 1892 animal seizure models were demonstrated using a variety of techniques. Such animal research, made with circumspection, with care to avoid suffering, with respect for life, and upholding scientific merit, is still justifiable, and continuing even if under the watchful eye of concerned animal protection groups. Among others, animal models have been useful in pharmacology for evaluating drug efficacy, and for supplying information on the toxicity of a wide variety of pharmaceutical agents, including those active on the central nervous system (CNS) and influencing cerebral blood flow (CBF) patterns.

The use of non-human primates for medical research has been documented already in the early years of this century, when Robert Koch used monkeys to study the pattern of infection with human trypanosomiasis. Non-human primates are morphologically and often functionally similar to man. The morphological and functional superiority of the non-human primate is represented by its human-like brain, hands and uterus. The kidney of the non-human primate is also unique among animals, because only man and the non-human primate have kidneys with a multi-papillar structure, and microscopic examination of nephritis in rhesus monkeys confirmed identical results to those in man. Also the ECG of the non-human primate has been identified to be similar to that of man[1].

AEC Institute for Life Sciences, Faculty of Medicine, University of Pretoria, Box 2034 Pretoria 0001, South Africa
*Department of Pharmacology, Potchefstroom University for CHE, Private Bag X6001, Potchefstroom 2520, South Africa

The susceptibility of the non-human primate to pharmacological and toxicological effects of drugs frequently resembles that of man, and many examples exist where drugs were relatively toxic to the rat and dog in comparison to the non-human primate and man. The importance of the non-human primate in dependence studies is well recognised[2,3]. Withdrawal syndrome, manifested in morphine or barbiturate dependent rhesus monkeys, closely resembles that in human addicts. It shows a similar attitude to that of man in his drug-seeking behaviour and psychological susceptibility to the principal drugs of abuse, such as morphine, codeine, pentobarbital and alcohol. Even if hypnotics or alcohol are freely available, the rat will not self-administer drugs up to the point that it is severely depressed or anaesthetised, but the rhesus monkey loves to self-anaesthetise. There is a limitation, however, in the use of the monkey for drug assessment: it does not take hallucinogens and THC.

The relatively large size of the Cape baboon Papio ursinus with a weight of 27-30 kg for a large male, makes this animal especially suitable for *in vivo* studies, using nuclear medical instrumentation and techniques. It becomes an almost ideal model for *in vivo* rCBF investigations with SPECT imaging and a perfusion tracer such as ^{99m}Tc-HMPAO. The brain of the baboon is relatively large when compared with its body weight. The relative sizes of the cerebral hemispheres, pons, cerebellum and medulla are similar to the values for man[4] (Figure 1). The cerebral hemispheres are incompletely separated from each other by the longitudual fissure. The cerebral cortex spreads over the surface of the hemisphere, and its area is increased by the presence of gyri, separated by sulci. It is demarcated by several important sulci into frontal, parietal, temporal and occipital lobes. The configuration of the convolutions shows a general increase in complexity with man. There is a relation between the degree of fissuration and the size of the brain, and these factors are related to body weight[5]. The major difference from baboon to man is the development of secondary and tertiary sulci, which adds greater detail of fissuration. The cerebellum of the baboon is, as with man, divisible into three main lobes; the floccular lobes are comparatively large and the petrosal lobe projects from the anterolateral margin of the paraflocculus. According to most authorities the anatomical differences between baboon and human brain appear to be quantitative, e.g. cell densities, rather than qualitative. 'There is no known neomorphic element' that distinguishes the one from the other[6]. It is therefore with some confidence that the baboon is being used for neuroSPECT purposes.

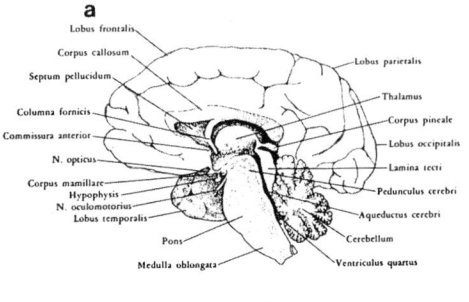

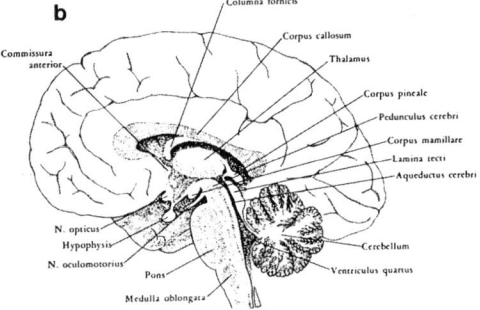

Figure 1 The brain of a, Papio and b, Homo (from An Atlas of Primate Gross Anatomy, Doris R Swindler and Charles D Wood, 1982)

Cerebral blood flow as disease indicator in neurophysiology and neuropsychiatry

SPECT brain studies with ^{99m}Tc-HMPAO have been used for the assessment of cerebral perfusion in many neurological and psychiatric diseases, demonstrating that abnormalities of cerebral perfusion may be present in both neurological as well as psychiatric pathology. ^{133}Xe-inhalation investigations with scintillation multiprobe systems were performed by several teams[7-9] to measure rCBF, and it was noted under many circumstances that it could be equated with local brain physiology.

The assessment of rCBF therefore could and usually does provide useful diagnostic information, and/or information for a better understanding of the complex clinical presentations in patients with such neurological and psychiatric manifestations.

Mean normal CBF is kept relatively constant by autoregulation. It varies between 50 and 60ml/min/ 100 g brain substance and is higher in grey matter than in white matter. Normal cerebral function is still possible with mean CBF values as low as 20 ml/min/100 g, the brain compensating with an increase in oxygen extraction from the circulation. Values below this lead to abnormalities of brain functioning detectable by electroencephalography. Task-related variations in rCBF in healthy brains, and in patients with functional psychiatric disease are of smaller magnitude, 2 - 35% of resting flow[10]. In the normal brain as well as in neuropsychiatric pathology, rCBF is coupled to metabolic demand and changes in CBF could reflect on neuronal metabolism.

Local reductions in CBF in Alzheimer's Disease (AD) may point to reductions in neuronal activity in relevant areas due to cell loss through atrophy and loss of synapses. In the early phase of AD, abnormal patterns of perfusion, i.e. hypoperfusion have been established in the temporo parietal cortex. The predictive value of this observation is high in AD patients with memory and cognitive impairment[11].

Using HMPAO SPECT, it was found that increasing age (range 21-80 years) was associated with both an increase in side-to-side asymmetry and a preferential decline of rCBF in the frontal cortex[12,13].

CBF evaluations with HMPAO SPECT of patients with schizophrenia indicated a physiological dysfunction of the prefrontal cortex and sometimes the temporal lobe, at the onset of the illness prior to neuroleptic treatment[14] (Figure 2).

Paralimbic hypoperfusion was detected in unipolar depression from HMPAO SPECT studies, although the psychiatric rating scales correlated poorly with CBF (Figure 3). Major differences in functional images are found in cases of epilepsy, depending on whether the patient is in the interictal, ictal or postictal state (Figure 4). Hyperfusion at the focus during the ictal state is to 95% positively predictive, but the study is logistically difficult to perform, especially with HMPAO. ^{99m}Tc-ECD with its longer *in vitro* consistency appears to be a better proposition for use in patients with epilepsy[15,16].

Cerebral toxoplasmosis is a common opportunistic CNS infection in AIDS patients. Neuropathological findings include inflammatory infiltrates with polymorphonuclear leukocytes, in addition to lymphocytes, plasma cells and histocytes. In the later stages, cysts and areas of necrosis are present. Initially no abnormalities may be observed on a CT scan. AIDS patients present with abnormal HMPAO SPECT indicating the early stage of a CNS toxoplasma lesion[17].

Patients with AIDS dementia complex (ADC - an AIDS-related dementia) were found, using HMPAO SPECT, to have exclusive cortical CBF derangements and maximum hypoperfusion in the frontal and parietal lobes. The degree of hypoperfusion significantly correlated with the severity of the dementia complex[18]. Cocaine-induced seizures occur due to the local

anaesthetic actions of this compound. Severe vasospasm is caused by the brain catecholamines leading to reduced CBF[19]. Various resting patterns of disruption of rCBF and metabolism as observed in functional imaging are associated with Parkinsonian disorders. Temporal frontal lobe perfusion seems to be affected.

There is increasing evidence that HMPAO SPECT for rCBF determinations is a viable technique for detecting cortical lesions following traumatic brain injury (TBI) (moderate and mild), revealing a greater number of lesions than CT or MRI[20], especially during the first hours following an ictus (Figure 5). In a study on patients with chronic traumatic brain injury, brain SPECT was found to correlate with performance on a number of neurophysiological tests[21].

A combination of HMPAO SPECT and carotid angiography increased the reliability of the Matas test as a means of determining the effect of carotid artery ligation[22]. CBF changes relating to neurotoxicity from various industrial substances, e.g. Cd, Mn, were detected with SPECT and correlated to behavioural abnormalities[23]. It is also true that confirmed normal CBF coupled to changed receptor distributions for e.g. D_2-distribution, measured in the basal ganglia by IBZM, contributes to the diagnostic result[24].

The evidence is, therefore, that SPECT has obvious diagnostic potential, and with pharmacological interventions and computer analysis, is a new tool in the assessment of brain disease. Although the literature clearly abounds with applications of SPECT in neuropathology, only small numbers of patients are being scanned in nuclear medicine facilities compared with the large numbers treated for neurological disorders. Clinicians are still sceptical about the diagnostic sensitivity and specificity of brain SPECT.

Cerebral blood flow from HMPAO SPECT data

Fundamentally, all medical imaging involves visual comparisons. When used for diagnosis, images are frequently compared with mental pictures, which in any event are the interpreter's concepts of normality and different diseased states. For prognosis or treatment, monitoring comparisons often focus on changes in serial studies in the same patient, and depend on patterns seen in the images.

In nuclear medicine, these patterns represent spatial and temporal arrangements and rearrangements of the physiological and biochemical processes under investigation. The imaging techniques, should have

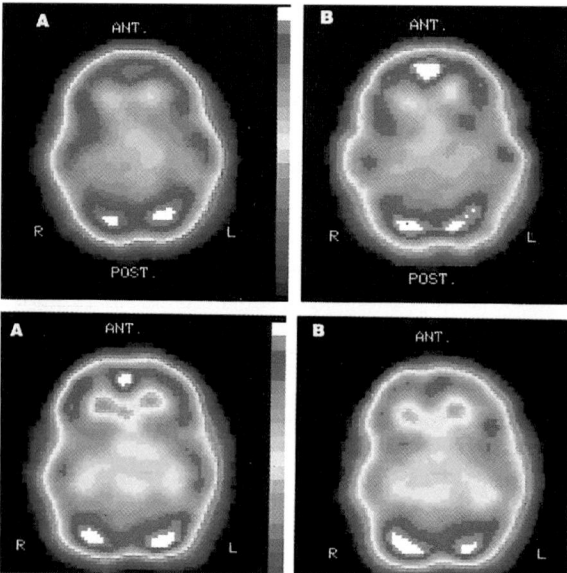

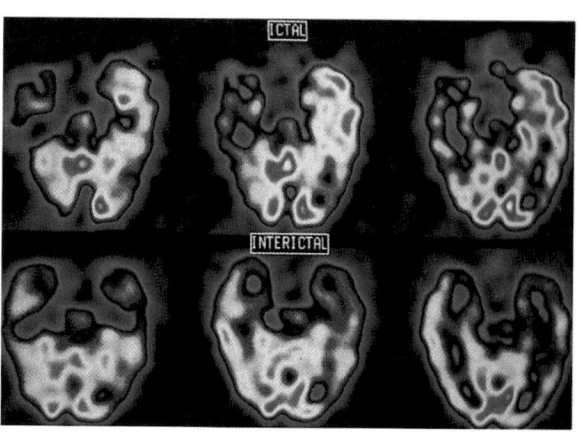

Figure 2 HMPAO SPECT slices at 36 mm above the frontocerebellar line in (top) a representative control subject, and (bottom) a representative schizophrenic patient. a, Resting scan; b, Wisconsin Card Sorting Test (WCST). An increase in prefrontal rCBF is noticed in the control during WCST. For the patient prefrontal hyperperfusion is present at rest, and a decrease in rCBF for this region follows during WCST (reference 14)

Figure 4 Ictal and interictal perfusion patterns in a 38-year-old woman with bilateral EEG foci and suspected left temporal sclerosis. ^{99m}Tc-HMPAO SPECT shows decreased perfusion in the left temporal lobe interictally and markedly increased perfusion in the left temporolateral and temporopolar region, and slightly increased perfusion in the mesial structures during the seizure (taken from Grünwald *et al. J. Nucl. Med.* 1994)

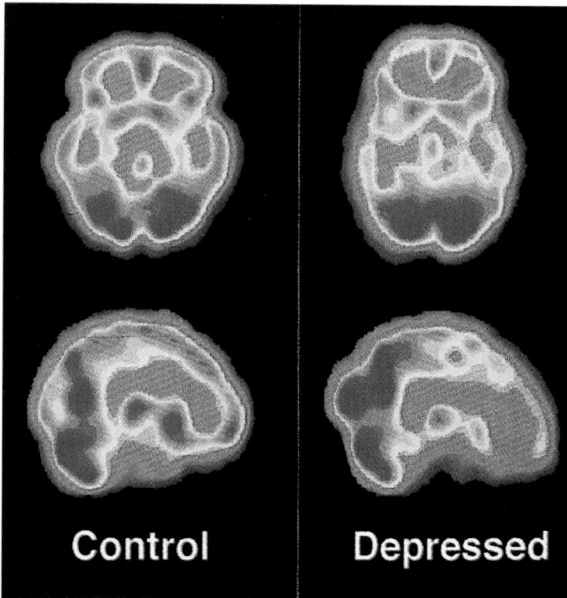

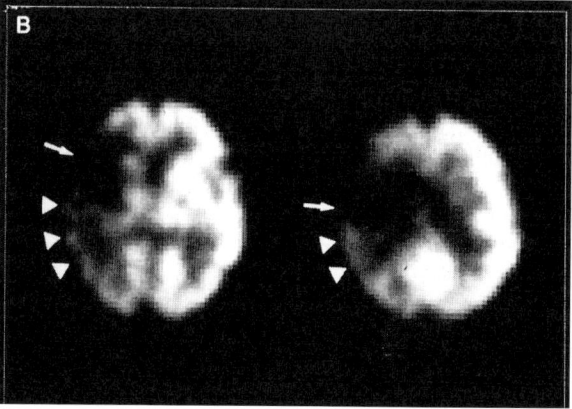

Figure 3 Transaxial (upper) and sagittal (lower) views of HMPAO SPECT images from a depressed patient and an age-matched, sex-matched, non-depressed control (taken from Mayberg *et al. J. Nucl. Med.* 1994)

Figure 5 A 65-year-old woman with sudden onset of total aphasia: transaxial SPECT images obtained at 1.8 h after onset demonstrate an area of severe low perfusion (arrows) enclosed by a large area of mild hypoperfusion (arrowheads) which is consistent with the territory of the right middle cerebral artery (taken from Shimosegawa *et al. J. Nucl. Med.* 1994)

adequate spatial and time resolution to capture the available information in as much detail as possible.

A methodology for brain SPECT has been defined for establishing consensus among experts - a kind of modified Delphi-technique for tracer preparation and optimal imaging[25], but still no formal guidelines or recommendations exist whereby the diagnostic efficacy could be universally validated.

A key test of computer-based techniques for qualitative as well as quantitative image information will be their ability to detect lesions at low thresholds without loss of specificity. Image manipulation, such as filtering and smoothing should be standardised, as should be slice orientation. Computer-assisted image interpretation follows three routes: comparing activity in one part of the image with another, looking for ratios; comparing activity in the regions of interest (ROI) with a normal data base; and generating kinetic data. These procedures introduce a degree of quantitation into the SPECT technique. Quantitation is desirable above visual-only interpretation for better differentiation, e.g. between AD and other possible treatable dementia-related diseases, and also for sensitive monitoring of therapy.

Although it is known that counts/pixel in regions of the brain are related to blood flow in the region[26,27], absolute blood flow non-invasively with radiopharmaceuticals such as HMPAO is not easily attainable. The approach of calculating ratios could vary: the ratio of counts in a particular ROI to the counts in an identical contralateral region as in unilateral TBI, or to the counts in the unaffected hemisphere[26], even to counts in the cerebellum which could be corrected for early diffusion of tracer[27,28]. The last ratio depends on the assumption that the cerebellum is itself not activated by the test procedure. In AD, the basal ganglia can be the reference structure as it is in this case usually spared. A lesion is identified if the ratio is below a certain threshold value. This threshold is chosen by defining a range of values from 'normal' volunteers.

Normals, especially where age-matching is needed, are not always adequately available. Furthermore, what is normal? A clear and unequivocal knowledge of normal brain perfusion is an absolute prerequisite to objective interpretation of scans and assessment of the accuracy of such interpretations. Normal perfusion and the acceptable limits at each region must be mapped and recognised. The appreciation of normal patterns and variability is the accumulated result of a large number of normal observations.

With respect to the analysis of SPECT images, the limited anatomical information derived from blood flow images renders it difficult to localise the anatomical site of interest. Hence the ability of the technique to give information about small areas of brain is limited not only by intrinsic properties such as spatial resolution and the partial volume effect, but also by the reliable identification of precisely the brain regions observed. The extent of anatomic variability must be recognised and accounted for.

To aid interpretation of normals, an atlas of normal structures was defined and correlated with the widely recognised Talairach Tournoux stereotactic neurosurgical atlas[29,30]. Hereby the brain image is mathematically resized into a defined stereotactic space, following which the use of the corresponding coordinate system allows identification of specific areas (Figure 6). All normals are, however, not alike, not only anatomically, but also there are age-related changes in cortical perfusion, and gender differences[31]. A brain SPECT database from different participating institutions is needed. Important advances at various centres have been made in defining normal brain

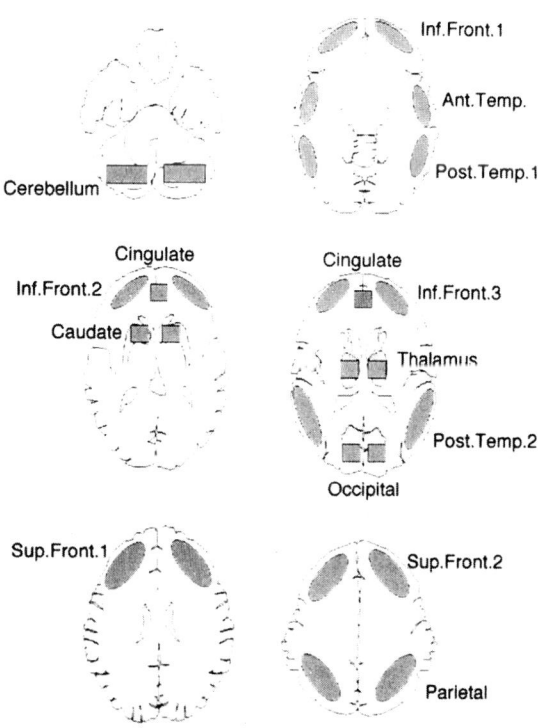

Figure 6 SPECT region of interest template: transaxial views at six standardised brain levels. The rCBF was measured in standardised brain regions by using generalised template modifications from the Matsui and Hirano brain atlas (taken from Matsui *et al. Igaku-Shoin (New York)*1978. The regions of interest were defined in cortical and subcortical regions (taken from Mayberg *et al. J. Nucl. Med.* 1994)

perfusion and condensing such descriptions into usable digital formats - also identifying the perfusion patterns associated with various disease entities and correlating these patterns with clinical outcome. A multicentre interobserver agreement on dementia studied with HMPAO SPECT was published[32], with encouraging discrimination of subtypes of dementia. More imaging centres are developing the resources necessary to superimpose functional images onto similarly orient-ated cranial MR images of the same subject. This technique currently represents the best way to obtain precise anatomical localisation in functional brain images.

Shapes of ROIs are also not consistent. Sometimes predetermined and regular shapes are used, in other cases irregular shapes designed to enclose a specific structure. The placement of regions can likewise vary, i.e. either individually and manually, or with the aid of a standardised computer algorithm. Region placement is normally planned before results become available for objectivity (Figure 6).

The reality, however, remains that threshold values of ratios are observer-dependent and also display-dependent. Work is in progress on the accuracy of various methods of image display and colour scale mapping[33]. However, one has to recognise a high level of complexity and normal variability in brain structure and functional interrelationships which make brain SPECT difficult to interpret with the unaided eye, and the techniques for analysis are not yet adequately standardised.

Automated computer pattern recognition could be the alternative. Given one set of images from a normal population and another from patients (e.g. with AD), the artificial neural network (ANN) will find the best means of differentiating these two image patterns with no interference from pathophysiological knowledge of the disease process. A neural network algorithm[34] proved effective at recognising the pattern of AD - more than just a measure of parietal uptake or an asymmetry index. An image is reviewed for patterns, not a single finding but a constellation of findings, individually non-specific but diagnostic when taken together. This is also the way the human mind works. However it provides neither a quantitative measure of distinguishing between groups for comparisons nor kinetic data, and therefore does not yet fully tap the diagnostic potential of SPECT. Nor could more than two different groups be handled successfully.

The sensitivity and specificity of diagnostic brain SPECT is therefore still an unknown, and a reason why clinicians do not in general involve this modality in their diagnostic procedures. Interpretation and techniques applied to that effect are also not simple.

Measurement and interpretation of CBF changes following interventions

Although tracer uptake in the brain is influenced by various parameters such as cardiac output[35], retention fraction[36], and lipophilic and hydrophilic fractions[37], a numerical value that could monitor brain uptake of HMPAO would be useful for follow-up, activation and pharmacological studies. Quantification of absolute CBF or uptake has been pointed out to be problematic and not yet a routine diagnostic clinical practice. Various methods have been suggested to convert brain counts into brain uptake, such as using calibrated point sources as external standard[38], but these have not yet found easy application.

Follow-up studies, however, measuring changes in CBF and HMPAO uptake in the same patient after an intervention do not demand absolute values, e.g. relative rCBF increases could be measured after shunt surgery in patients with normal pressure hydrocephalus, and some of these regional improvements correlated with improvement in psychiatric symptomatology. Successful follow-up CBF-measurements after vascular reconstructive surgery in moyamoya disease have also been reported.

Measures of pharmacological modulation of rCBF have been used to learn about cerebral activity of the administered drug. It provides the ideal scenario of the follow-up study to assess pharmacological effect and treatment efficacy in neurological and psychiatric pathologies. Another example would be to involve activation paradigms whereby the magnitude of CBF change could be monitored after a pharmacological challenge[39]. This could show how reversible the deficits are and how treatable a patient might be. Acetazolamide is a drug often used to determine cerebral reserve before and after a surgical intervention[40].

Alignment of multiple studies for comparison is a major problem. Pelizzari[41] looks at surface contours, others at the anterior commissure - posterior commissure line for reference[42]. Alternatively, external fiducial markers can be used[43]. To avoid subjectivity, alignment of scans can be performed by an automated computer algorithm. However, with each patient as his own control, the trained human observer is still very good at compensating for artefacts and recognising anatomical variability and functional changes.

Semiquantification of CBF changes, induced pharmacologically or otherwise, becomes comparat-ively easy and still reliable, using the split-dose method[44,45]. It is an ideal method to use in drug development where acute effects of the drug need to be monitored, as is the case with cerebral infarction. An advantage is that often the patient can stay in position for the before-and-after intervention measurement, taking care of alignment by devising a proper stable head rest.

According to the split-dose method of HMPAO SPECT, two consecutive i.v. injections of ^{99m}Tc-HMPAO will be administered before and after an expected CBF change could have taken place. The second injection has two to three times the dosage of the first to allow better manipulation of the background remaining from the first injection. Each HMPAO administration is followed by a SPECT acquisition, the data of which will represent rCBF during conditions at the injection time. The effect of a drug intervention performed after completion of the first SPECT can be measured by the second SPECT, following on the second HMPAO-injection, which was so administered to reflect appropriately (e.g. at the required response time) on the drug interaction. The result is expressed as a ratio of count rate data obtained during SPECT-2 with respect to SPECT-1, after subtraction of the decay corrected background from SPECT-1.

$$R = \frac{(\text{SPECT-2}) - (\text{SPECT-1})^*}{\text{SPECT-1}}$$

[*] decay corrected

^{99m}Tc-HMPAO appears to be the best commercially available tracer-ligand for this type of procedure due to its rapid deposition in the active brain ($\approx$ 4 min).

Wyper[46], who studied 10 patients at rest on two occasions, showed that this method was more accurate than test-retest with a week interval. When compared with delayed SPECT studies, the advantages of the split-dose method are that the total amount of radioactivity administered to the patient can be kept lower and that the same vial of HMPAO can often be used for both injections. When a pharmacological effect requires a long time response, e.g. longer than 10 min after drug administration, the two HMPAO doses should be prepared individually from two different vials, because of the rapid *in vitro* degradation of the tracer after reconstitution[45,47,48]. Single head gamma cameras usually take 20-30 min to acquire statistically meaningful data during a 360° arc of rotation. Often because of poor structural detail these devices yield only slice-related information. With properly chosen positioning, individual tomographic slices can relate predominantly to a specific structure(s), which is only

rough regional information. With multiple head detectors (e.g. three in the IGE Neurocam Triad, or the Trionix, built in a triangular shape around a space for the patient's head) the sensitivity and efficiency of photon detection increases significantly, and a 360° arc of rotation will take a shorter period of time to acquire the same total counts per study as a single detector head gamma camera would.

Structural information on the brain can be obtained from the first and second scans using more sophisticated equipment despite the low dose ($\approx$ 8 mCi) of the first HMPAO injection and ROIs across interesting structures can readily be chosen for comparison. CBF increases of 10% have been shown to be significant[44] using this method.

The split-dose method is based on the chemical properties of the tracer that crosses the blood-brain barrier and is trapped in brain cells. Since the intracellular conversion of the tracer to non-diffusible complexes is dominated by glutathione, which is present in excess[49], the trapping process may be considered as not saturable. Therefore if ^{99m}Tc-HMPAO is injected, the tracer distribution will be proportional to the regional CBF in both scans. Results show that mean brain activity recorded in the second scan is proportional to the total injected dose. Therefore, the tracer uptake is not limited by the first dose injection.

Cerebropharmacodynamics of psychotropic drugs acting in major psychiatric illnesses could ideally be developed and investigated by HMPAO SPECT. An investigation into cholinergic involvement in the memory deficits of AD utilised the cholinomimetic properties of L-acetylcarnitine to observe the effects of increasing cholinergic activity on regional, particularly parietal, CBF in AD patients[50]. The effect of physostigmine on patterns of rCBF was investigated[51]. In this study, it was observed that the pharmacological challenge was associated with focal increases in tracer uptake in posterior parietal temporal regions in the patients but not in the controls.

The response to nitroglycerin in dilating cerebral vasculature was investigated to assess its therapeutic actions[52]. Other substances, e.g. 7% CO_2 inhaled, having similar effects, have also been used in activation paradigms[53]. Acetazolamide has, in this respect, been thoroughly studied. It is a powerful vasodilator that exerts its effects within 10 min following i.v. injection[54,55], increasing CBF by approximately 35%. It has been used to study CBF reactivity in patients with transient ischaemic attacks[56], significantly increasing the sensitivity of SPECT for detecting regions of pathological blood flow (Figure 7).

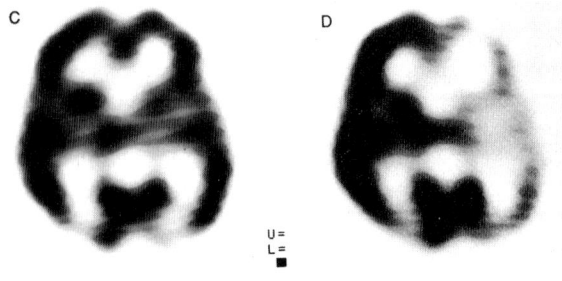

Figure 7 Patient with narrowing of the right carotid-fork IMP SPECT image before acetazolamide (C). Activity slightly decreased in the entire left cerebral hemisphere. (D) IMP SPECT image after acetazolamide. Markedly decreased activity in the entire left cerebral hemisphere (taken from Hoshi *et al.* *J. Nucl. Med.* 1994)

Acetazolamide stress testing has also been used to assess cerebrovascular reserve in patients with epilepsy and dementia[57]. In these instances the purpose of the test is to determine whether alterations in resting rCBF are of neuronal or vascular origin. Primary neuronal dysfunction (such as AD), produces rCBF abnormalities only as an epiphenomenon, through autoregulation. Such areas have a normal acetazolamide response.

CBF changes measured after pharmacological intervention can be assessed for their therapeutic significance in various diseases, e.g. the use of calcium channel blockers in stroke patients, where the drug might only be effective prior to induced or spontaneous reperfusion. If given acutely, some antidepressants administered to patients with affective disorders inhibit the re-uptake of noradrenaline and/or serotonin in the synapse, while others block inactivation[58]. Possible CBF changes induced in this manner and their significance could be studied by the split-dose method of HMPAO SPECT. Research has also demonstrated that many antidepressants exhibit effects on receptor sensitivity after chronic administration. A decrease in beta-adrenergic receptor sensitivity and enhanced responsiveness to serotonergic and alpha-adrenergic stimulation has been noted. Monoamine oxidase inhibitors block the inactivation of biogenic amines and thus increase the concentration of those neurotransmitters[59]. Therefore monitoring changes of rCBF in patients with mood disorders may be useful to direct therapy. It could also be applied in the development of appropriate pharmacological agents, and for better understanding of the pathophysiology of depression, the latter especially when correlated to cognitive behavioural changes. A clear correlation between pathological HMPAO SPECT findings and an

increasing Hamilton depression rating scale (HDRS) was reported[60], which was not the case in patients with normal brain SPECT.

It appears that deranged CBF and cerebral metabolism are present in schizophrenia[61], and subsyndromes could be regionally correlated in the brain. It has been hypothesised that in schizophrenia there is an overactivity of the dopaminergic system, with higher D_2 receptor densities in the left than right putamen, not found in controls[62]. This agrees with the work showing increased perfusion and metabolism in the basal ganglia on the left side. The phenomenon will find application in the field of pharmacology, i.e. studying receptor systems and cerebral metabolism and the perfusion response to pharmacological interaction by agonists and antagonists[63]. This research provides exciting opportunities to test hypotheses relating to antipsychotic pharmacodynamics and clinical response in living humans.

Preliminary results from a group of normal ageing patients under extended therapy with oral piracetam, or alternatively a combination of nicotinic acid with pentifylline, point towards improved rCBF and corresponding improvement in memory. Drugs may increase blood flow without altering cerebral metabolism. A significant increase in glucose metabolism was found with PET after piracetam treatment in an AD group of patients[64]. The small number of patients, however, prohibits a conclusion on the therapeutic relevance of metabolic effects in this case.

Although neurotransmitter and receptor interactions with drugs can be effectively monitored *in vivo* with SPECT and PET, leading to dose determinations and investigations of the impact of pharmacological manipulations on receptor systems, the arrival of both the tracer and the drug is blood flow and brain perfusion dependent, and this must be taken into consideration, if not also measured.

The split-dose method with HMPAO lends itself ideally to neuro-activation studies[65,66]. In order to observe the pattern of CBF associated with a task, it is necessary to perform that task only during the relatively short fixation period of the tracer, starting shortly before administration of HMPAO and continuing for approximately 4 min. This minimises problems such as initial learning effects in cognitive tasks and the time needed for the development of a physiological response after the HMPAO injection.

The verbal fluency task was found to be associated with a small but significant increase in rCBF in the left dorsolateral prefrontal cortex, which did not always prove to be the case with the Wisconsin Card Sorting Test[66], despite it being considered equally robust in testing this cerebral region. A SPECT study of schizophrenic patients performing a verbal fluency task showed that compared with a control group, the schizophrenic sample had decreased HMPAO uptake in left frontal cortical and left posterior cortical regions[67].

Two tests were also performed during the CBF-imaging of 20 medication-free schizophrenics and 25 normals, viz the Wisconsin Card Sorting Test, and a simple number matching test. In the controls, the flow to the dorsolateral prefrontal cortex was clearly increased during the card test, not so in the patients. Number matching did not affect flow to this area for either group[68].

A split-dose subtraction HMPAO SPECT study was performed on schizophrenic patients in collaboration with a verbal memory activation test to look for deficiencies in temporal lobe function (Busatto, un-published results). Despite low frontal lobe flow and significantly poorer performance on the memory task, the degree of medial temporal activation measured in the schizophrenic group was not significantly different from that of the control group. Grossly, the brain is only subtly abnormal in schizophrenia. It is instructive in this regard to note that the frontal lobe, which has the more subtle pathology, tends to be more disordered functionally.

Based upon the premise that increased neuronal (synaptic) activity leads to an increase in regional cerebral blood flow, activation studies for Parkinson's disease patients have been developed in which subjects are scanned under two or more differing conditions e.g. at rest and while moving a limb in order to identify brain regions whose blood flow differs between the conditions. From this, it is inferred that localised changes in neuronal activation are responsible for, or at least involved in, the human activity under study.

Interactions between cognitive and pharmacological manipulations (i.e. neuro-modulation) and measured by SPECT and PET can also be very informative. Certain drugs were found to augment task-induced increases in rCBF e.g. buspirone and apomorphine acting on memory-induced rCBF increases in the retrospinal region and dorsolateral prefrontal cortex respectively[69]. The particular experimental model can be chosen for pharmacological reasons, i.e. to find the effect of a drug on cognition, or for neuropsychological purposes where a task will be selected if it is known to implicate a particular neurotransmitter system. Methodological problems are matching the time-course of drug activity with that of tracer uptake and washout[63], and analysing data to distinguish between global and regional drug effects on blood flow/metabolism.

A recent example of this strategy is the reaction of akinetic Parkinson's patients before and after a subcutaneous injection of apomorphine (a dopamine agonist), during a finger opposition task[70]. The akinetic patients, unlike normal controls, failed to increase rCBF to contralateral primary sensory areas and the supplementary motor cortex during the task. Following apomorphine, akinesia resolved and rCBF to motor regions in patients resembled that of controls. This was the evidence for functional differentiation of motor areas in akinetic patients, which was shown to be reversible by a dopaminergic drug.

It was also found that schizophrenic patients did not activate frontal regions following apomorphine - unlike controls. Schizophrenic patients are known to perform poorly on the Wisconsin Card Sorting Test, which is a measure of prefrontal function and have relatively low flow to frontal regions[68]. These data provide support for the hypothesis of a relative frontal cortical dopamine deficiency in schizophrenia (Pedro, unpublished results).

The importance of the methods of neuropharmacology outlined above is clear. In future brain SPECT and PET studies will have a necessary role to play in the development and evaluation of novel and classical psychotropic drugs, and some of this of necessity involves animal experimentation.

The non-human primate and split-dose HMPAO SPECT

Although it is now possible to relate the basic molecular structure of a receptor to its cellular, biochemical and biophysical responses and pharmacological specificity in the test-tube, animals have a major use to enable understanding drug action on neurophysiology. Behavioural responses of animals to psychotropic drugs provide some indication of neuroreceptor function *in vivo* but extrapolation to human neuropsychology, even from the non-human primate, has limitations. For one there are no appropriate animal models for schizophrenia, but models of traumatic brain injury and seizures have been used, as were primates which were rendered parkinsonian by administration of MPTP (1-methyl-4-phenyl-1,2,3,6-tetrahydropyridine)[71].

The baboon model has found frequent application in receptor imaging with SPECT.

In developing a baboon model for CBF determinations with SPECT imaging and ^{99m}Tc-HMPAO, it was found to be meaningfully sensitive to the effects of anaesthesia on CBF[72].

Anaesthesia is necessary for restraining the animal during scintigraphy, and it becomes critical when the procedure becomes prolonged. The split-dose method used with the model compares rCBF before and after a drug intervention, (i.e. from two sets of SPECT data, viz SPECT-1 and SPECT-2), and the result is given as a ratio (R) of the two determinations once the background contribution from SPECT-1 to the SPECT-2 data had been subtracted. To assess and understand the results from this model, i.e. the R values, a control representation for each investigation is required which describes through R values, rCBF changes taking place during an anaesthesia-only experimental run, and choosing a corresponding point in time for the second HMPAO injection to match the intervention response in the subsequent drug-intervention study. Anaesthesia is chosen to least disturb normal CBF, and to be easy to maintain and monitor. A useful form of anaesthesia would be ketamine-barbiturate combinations. The ketamine (10 mg/kg of ketamine hydrochloride) is necessary for induction, but not useful for maintenance because of the possibility of convulsions during longer studies. Thiopentone sodium can be used for maintenance (70 ml/h of a 0.5% solution) for shorter studies (1 h), and pentobarbitone for studies of 2 h and longer. The baseline study will then have the first HMPAO injection with the baboon still under the influence of ketamine from darting, and the second double dose of HMPAO after SPECT-1, (performed under barbiturate maintenance), and injected to match the intervention of the experimental protocol.

Table 1 gives R values from various anaesthesia combinations for tomographic slices as acquired in the transaxial, sagittal and coronal views, and for the global brain[72]. The ratio R is an indication of the level change of rCBF at a chosen time during the second anaesthesia with respect to the first. Curves plotted of R versus slice number (Figure 8) display some regional information from the various slices as they pertain predominantly to anatomical structures.

If no changes in CBF occur during the switch to a second anaesthesia (e.g. ketamine-thiopentone), or during prolonged anaesthesia, (e.g. thiopentone-thiopentone) (Table 1), a value of R = 2 would be expected because of the double dose of HMPAO for the second injection. The mean value of R= 1.79 ± 0.03 for ketamine-thiopentone from many studies is statistically meaningfully less than two (R<2). Ketamine hydrochloride is known, and has been shown in correlation studies, to increase blood pressure and heart rate, leading to augmented CBF which is not maintained during the barbiturate phase, and this will reduce the R values.

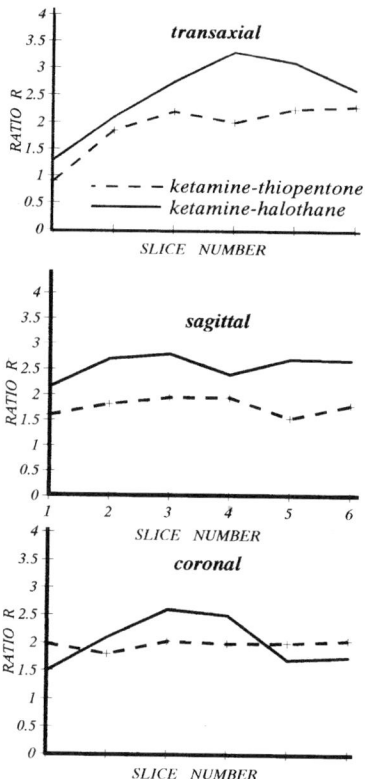

Figure 8 A set of typical curves of ratio (R) versus slice number, starting at a, the occipital lobes transaxially, b, from right to left of the brain sagitally and c, from the cerebellum to the dorsal slice of the cerebrum coronally. Dotted lines represent ketamine-thiopentone data; solid lines ketamine-halothane data

The model under halothane anaesthesia (ketamine-halothane; 1.5% halothane in oxygen) renders R values significantly > 2. Halothane reduces blood pressure and heart rate. Inhibition of the autoregulation of CBF in response to blood pressure changes leads to the vasodilatory effects of halothane, and changed blood flow distribution to various organs, with specifically decreased cerebral vascular resistance, which explains the increased CBF measured in this case.

With the cerebrovascular effects of the anaesthesia known, the model has found application for assessing acute responses from drug intervention. A study with acetazolamide (500 mg) produced a similar increase in CBF after 10 min, i.e. 32% as has been shown in humans[73]. An infusion of the calcium channel blocker nimodipine increased CBF globally after 10 min by approximately 35%, also known for humans; in addition it has a distinct regional effect with a near to 90% increase of rCBF in the cerebellum. These two

Table 1 Mean ($\pm$ s.d.) ratios from transaxial, sagittal and coronal views of four equal cerebral regions and from the total brain regions

	Region 1	Region 2		Region 3	Region 4	Total Brain
Procedure A	2.27 ± 0.62	2.17 ± 0.36	Transaxial	2.16 ± 0.33	2.13 ± 0.22	2.18 ± 0.06
Procedure B	1.73 ± 0.87	1.88 ± 0.19		1.86 ± 0.37	1.95 ± 0.36	1.86 ± 0.09
Procedure C	1.82 ± 0.52	2.06 ± 0.35		1.92 ± 0.29	2.18 ± 0.36	2.00 ± 0.16
Procedure D	2.21 ± 0.50	3.04 ± 0.18		2.82 ± 0.28	2.74 ± 0.31	2.70 ± 0.35
			Sagittal			
Procedure A	2.35 ± 0.83	2.25 ± 0.36		2.30 ± 0.29	2.56 ± 0.67	2.37 ± 0.14
Procedure B	1.84 ± 0.29	2.10 ± 0.18		1.97 ± 0.39	1.83 ± 0.54	1.94 ± 0.13
Procedure C	2.06 ± 0.49	2.06 ± 0.42		1.82 ± 0.55	1.62 ± 0.38	1.89 ± 0.21
Procedure D	2.43 ± 0.70	2.90 ± 0.22		2.99 ± 0.19	2.86 ± 0.32	2.80 ± 0.25
			Coronal			
Procedure A	2.18 ± 0.48	2.08 ± 0.27		2.71 ± 0.90	2.47 ± 0.48	2.36 ± 0.29
Procedure B	1.91 ± 0.32	1.93 ± 0.23		1.92 ± 0.28	1.73 ± 0.59	1.87 ± 0.10
Procedure C	1.96 ± 0.24	2.04 ± 0.35		2.09 ± 0.45	2.30 ± 0.52	2.10 ± 0.15
Procedure D	2.20 ± 0.37	2.99 ± 0.34		2.99 ± 0.22	2.66 ± 0.51	2.71 ± 0.37

A, Prolonged thiopentone (1.79 ± 0.03 {n = 48}); B, ketamine-thiopentone; C, ketamine-pentobarbitone; D, ketamine-halothane

results help to validate the baboon model for HMPAO SPECT and the split-dose method. In addition it was observed that, although acetazolamide is known to produce metabolic acidosis due to its carbonic anhydrase activity, the increase in CBF did not correlate with an increase in $PaCO_2$, but rather with an increase in PaO_2 (35%). The increased CBF from nimodipine was achieved without influence on blood pressure and arterial blood gases. It is known that cerebrovascular autoregulation is resistant to nimodipine.

An investigation of the combined effect of acetazolamide and nimodipine on the CBF in the baboon model showed a suppression of CBF with respect to the individual responses; also the increase in PaO_2 due to acetazolamide, was reduced to 23%, suggesting that nimodipine attenuates the effect of acetazolamide, and that acetazolamide may have an effect on the local cerebral metabolic rate for oxygen. This observation was substantiated in a subsequent study where dose and time responses of acetazolamide were investigated with this model[74].

The antimigraine drug sumatriptan, a 5-HT serotonergic agonist, yielded with this model no or an insignificant effect (slight increase) on CBF, 10 min after being administered intramuscularly[75]. However, after 25 min, a significant decrease (20%) was observed in the CBF, when compared with an anaesthesia-only baseline study which showed a marked increase in CBF during the prolonged anaesthesia. It was proposed that sumatriptan only had an effect when an abnormal increased CBF existed. Still using the split-dose HMPAO SPECT method, a combination study of sumatriptan (at 25 min) with nimodipine showed a significant decrease in the nimodipine-induced high CBF, but no effect on the increased CBF due to acetazolamide. There was also no effect on increases found under halothane anaesthesia. There is therefore a specificity in the action of sumatriptan, which implicates Ca^{2+}, and an indication that the serotonin receptors are likely to be involved in the normalisation of CBF (Dormehl, unpublished results).

The baboon model was modified to investigate the effect of various forms of local anaesthesia on CBF in the acute phase. It allowed for control of $PaCO_2$ by ventilation under general anaesthesia. This model describes the functional dependence of ΔCBF versus $\Delta PaCO_2$ using SPECT HMPAO and the split-dose method together with induced $PaCO_2$ changes between the two HMPAO injections. Normal reactivity to

PaCO$_2$ changes were validated (Figure 9). The model with thiopentone anaesthesia and controlled ventilation was used to investigate the mechanisms of CBF increase known to follow on the local anaesthetic lidocaine (6 mg/kg). The baboons were maintained at constant respiratory rate and volume. The results indicate that the correlation between ΔCBF and the corresponding change in PaCO$_2$ deviated from the baseline pattern of the model, and had only a slight dependence on ΔPaCO$_2$ confirming a cerebrovascular contribution by the lidocaine. The increase in CBF (24%) at around 2 min after lidocaine administration, agrees with known information[76]. The increased slope of the CO$_2$ reactivity curve might indicate an increased sensitivity to CO$_2$ after administration of lidocaine[77].

The use of ^{123}I-iodoamphetamine (IMP) with the split-dose technique was explored. The question was whether it provides the same information as does HMPAO - can the two agents be interchanged at will? Comparing R values (i.e. rCBF changes) as measured by the HMPAO, and by the IMP split-dose method during prolonged thiopentone anaesthesia, produced 13% higher values as determined by IMP, which were not statistically significant, but could relate to the i.v. IMP needing 20 min to reach a steady state. However, doing the same comparison but with an acetazolamide intervention, increased CBF as measured with IMP by 52%, with respect to the IMP anaesthesia-only study, compared with the 37% from the HMPAO measurement to its own control. This could have positive diagnostic implications identifying IMP as the more sensitive drug to check CBF changes in a test of cerebrovascular reserve. The induced metabolic acidosis and alkaline urine from acetazolamide had

Table 2 Percentage changes[a] in total brain uptake of HMPAO and IMP due to various procedures

Procedures	Percentage change	Statistical significance p-values
A to C	+ 13 ± 1	p>0.05
A to B	+ 37 ± 8	p<0.01
C to D	+ 52 ± 3	p<0.01
B to D	+ 26 ± 8	p>0.05
A to D	+ 74 ± 4	p<0.01
C to B	+ 21 ± 6	p<0.05, p>0.01

[a]Percentage changes are expressed with respect to the procedure mentioned first; A , thiopentone anaesthesia and ^{99m}Tc-HMPAO for both tracer injections; B, thiopentone anaesthesia ^{99m}Tc-HMPAO for both tracer injections and acetazolamide (500 mg and 10 min response time); C, thiopentone anaesthesia, ^{123}I(IMP) for both tracer injections; D, as above with C, but with acetazolamide (500 mg, 10 min response time)

apparently altered biodistribution of the two radiopharmaceuticals to different degrees. A dual-isotope study, split-dose with the two tracers combined for whichever reason will, according to this study, give incorrect values (Table 2)[78].

Conclusion

The diagnostic and investigative importance of cerebral blood flow measurements, using SPECT techniques with lipophilic tracers such as HMPAO has been shown here. It is also apparent that both diagnosis and investigation benefit tremendously when pharmacological modulation of rCBF is applied. Semiquantitative data on cerebral function can be gained from the split-dose method. This method is also ideal to assess the therapeutic significance and directions of pharmacological interventions in neuropathology and psychiatric disease. It is especially here, in drug research and development, that the baboon model as described can find wide application.

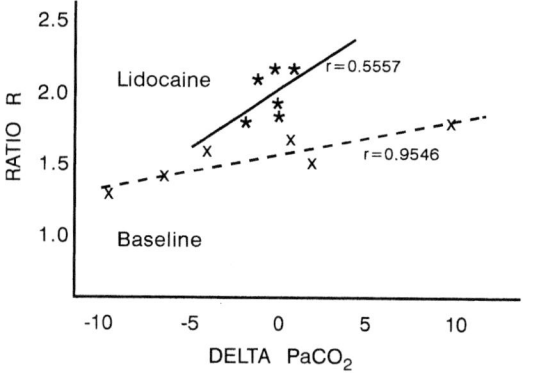

Figure 9 Linear regression lines to fit the raw data of CBF changes (R) versus PaCO$_2$ changes for the baseline study (r = 0.9546, p<0.00001) and the lidocaine study (r = 0.5557, p=0.0001)

References

1   Cheetam, R.W.S. Premature artificial systoles in the baboon. *S. Afr. Med. J.* 1934, 8, 739

2   Wagenen, G. Proceedings conference on nonhuman primate toxicology, U.S. Gov. Print Office, 1966, p. 103

3   Wilson, J.G. Proceedings conference on nonhuman primate toxicology, U.S. Gov. Print Office, 1966, p. 114

4   Hill, W.C.O. in Primates: comparative anatomy and taxonomy, volume 8: cynopithecinae, Wiley Interscience, New York, 1970, p. 5

5   Connolly, C.J. in 'External morphology of the primate brain', Charles C. Thomas Co., Springfield, USA, 1950, p. 3

6   Le Gros Clark, W.E. in 'The antecedents of man: an introduction to the evolution of the primates', Quadrangle Books, Chicago, USA, 1960, p. 262

7   Lassen, N. and Ingvar, D. Regional cerebral blood flow measurement in man: a review. *Arch. Neurol.* 1963, 9, 615

8   Veall, N. and Mallett, B.L. The two-compartment model using ^{133}Xe inhalation and external counting. *Acta Neurol. Scand.* 1965, 14, 83

9   Warkentin, S., Nilsson, A., Risberg, J. *et al.* Regional cerebral blood flow in schizophrenia: repeated studies during a psychotic episode. *Psychiatr. Res. Neuroimaging* 1990, 35, 27

10 Fox, P.T. Functional brain mapping with positron emission tomography. *Semin. Neurol.* 1989, 9, 323

11 Holman, B.L., Johnson, K.A., Gerada, B. *et al.* The scintigraphic appearance of Alzheimer's disease: a prospective study using technetium-99m-HMPAO SPECT *J. Nucl. Med.* 1992, 33, 181

12 Markus, H.S., Costa, D.C., Lennox, G. *et al.* ^{99m}Tc-HMPAO rCBF SPECT in corticobasal degeneration. Abstract of 20th Annual Meeting of the British Nuclear Medicine Society. *Nucl. Med. Commun.* 1992, 13

13 Waldemar, G., Hasselbach, S.G., Anderson, A.R. *et al.* ^{99m}Tc-d,l-HMPAO and SPECT of the brain in normal ageing. *J. Cereb. Blood Flow Metab.* 1991, 11, 508

14 Catafau, A.M., Parellada, E., Lomena, F.J. *et al.* Prefrontal and temporal blood flow in schizophrenia: resting and activation technetium-99m-HMPAO SPECT patterns in young neuroleptic-naive patients with acute disease. *J. Nucl. Med.* 1994, 35, 935

15 Kuikka, J.T. and Berkovic, S.F. Localization of epileptic foci by single-photon emission tomography with new radiotracers. *J. Nucl. Med.* 1994, 21, 1173

16 Menzel, C., Grünwald, F., Pavics, L. *et al.* Brain single-photon emission tomography using technetium-99m bicisate (ECD) in a case of complex partial seizure. *J. Nucl. Med.* 1994, 21, 1243

17 Catafau, A.M., Sol, M., Lomena, F.J. *et al.* Hyperfusion and early technetium-99m-HMPAO SPECT appearance of central nervous system toxoplasmosis. *J. Nucl. Med.* 1994, 35, 1041

18 Maini, C.L., Pigorini, F., Pau, F.M. *et al.* Technetium-99m-HMPAO brain SPECT in acquired immune deficiency syndrome (AIDS). *Eur. J. Nucl. Med.* 1989, 15, 417

19 Miller, B.L., Mena, I., Giombetti, R. *et al.* Neuropsychiatric effects of cocaine: SPECT measurements. *J. Addict. Dis. (US)* 1992, 11, 47

20 Jacobs, A., Put, E., Ingels, M. and Bassuyt, A. Prospective evaluation of technetium-99m-HMPAO SPECT in mild and moderate traumatic brain injury. *J. Nucl. Med.* 1994, 35, 942

21 Ichise, M., Chung, D.-G., Wang, P. *et al.* Technetium-99m-HMPAO SPECT, CT and MRI in the evaluation of patients with chronic traumatic brain injury: a correlation with neuropsychological performance. *J. Nucl. Med.* 1994, 35, 217

22 Matsuda, H., Higashi, S., Neshandar, I. *et al.* Evaluation of cerebral collateral circulation by technetium 99m-HMPAO brain SPECT during Matas test: report of three cases. *J. Nucl. Med.* 1988, 29, 1724

23 Lill, D.W., Mountz, J.M. and Darji, J.T. Technetium-99m-HMPAO brain SPECT evaluation of neurotoxicity due to manganese toxicity. *J. Nucl. Med.* 1994, 35, 863

24 Ichise, M., Toyama, H., Fornazzari, L. *et al.* Iodine-123-IBZM dopamine D2 receptor and technetium-99m-HMPAO brain perfusion SPECT in the evaluation of patients with and subjects at risk for Huntington's disease. *J. Nucl. Med.* 1993, 34, 1274

25 Fletcher, J.W., Woolf, S.H. and Royal, H.D. A consensus-development method for producing diagnostic procedure guidelines: SPECT brain perfusion imaging with Tc-99m-HMPAO. *J. Nucl. Med.* 1994, 35, 2003

26 Andersen, A.R., Friberg, H.H., Schmidt, J.F. and Hasselbalch, S.G. Quantitative measurements of cerebral blood flow using SPECT amd 99mTc-d,l-HMPAO compared to xenon-133. *J. Cereb. Blood Flow Metab.* 1988, 8, 569

27 Lassen, N., Andersen, A., Friberg, L. and Paulson, O. The retention of 99Tcm-d,l-HMPAO in the human brain after intracarotid bolus injection: a kinetic analysis. *J. Cereb. Blood Flow Metab.* 1988, 8, 513

28 Matsuda, H., Tsuji, S., Shuke, N. *et al.* A quantitive approach to technetium-99m-hexamethylpropylene amine oxime. *Eur. J. Nucl. Med.* 1992, 19, 195

29 Minoshima, S., Koeppe, R.A., Fray, K.A. *et al.* Stereotactic PET atlas of the human brain: aid for visual interpretation of functional brain images. *J. Nucl. Med.* 1994, 35, 949

30 Talairach, J. and Tournoux, P. in 'Co-planar stereotaxic atlas of the human brain', Thieme, New York, USA, 1988

31 Levin, J.M., Holman, B.L., Mendelson, J.H. *et al.* Gender differences in cerebral perfusion in cocaine abuse: ^{99m}Tc-HMPAO SPECT study of drug abusing women. *J. Nucl. Med.* 1994, 35, 1902

32 Hellman, R.S., Tikofsky, R.S., Van Heertum, R. *et al.* A multi-institutional study of interobserver agreement in the evaluation of dementia with rCBF/SPET technetium-99m exametazime (HMPAO). *Eur. J. Nucl. Med.* 1994, 21, 306

33 Stapleton, S.J., Caldwell, C.B., Leonhardt, C.L. *et al.* Determination of thresholds for detection of cerebellar blood flow deficits in brain SPECT images. *J. Nucl. Med.* 1994, 35, 1547

34 Kippenhan, J.S., Barker, W.W., Nagel, J. *et al.* Neural network classification of normal and Alzheimer's disease subjects using high-resolution and low-resolution PET cameras. *J. Nucl. Med.* 1994, 35, 7

35 Nickel, O., Nägele-Wöhrle, B., Ulrich, P. *et al.* rCBF-quantification with [99mTc]-HMPAO SPECT: theory and first results. *Eur. J. Nucl. Metab.* 1989, 32, 1501

36 Szabo, Z., Seki, C., Rhine, J. *et al.* Effect of spatial resolution on absolute quantification with high resolution SPECT (Abstract). *Eur. J. Nucl. Med.* 1991, 18, 604

37 Nakamura, K., Tukatani, Y., Kubo, A. *et al.* The behaviour of [99mTc]-hexamethylpropylene amine oxime ([99mTc]-HMPAO) in blood and brain. *Eur. J. Nucl. Med.* 1989, 15, 100

38 Dobbeleir, A. and Dierckx, R. Quantification of technetium-99m hexamethylpropylene amine oxime brain uptake in routine clinical practice using calibrated point sources as an external standard: phantom and human studies. *Eur. J. Nucl. Med.* 1993, 20, 684

39 Cohen, M.B. *et al.* SPECT brain imaging in Alzheimer's disease with oral tetrahydroaminoacridine and lecithin. *Clin. Nucl. Med.* 1992, 17, 312

40 Vorstrup, S., Brun, B. and Lassen, N.A. Evaluation of the cerebral vasodilatory capacity by the acetazolamide test before EC-IC bypass surgery in patients with occlusion of the internal carotid artery. *Stroke* 1986, 17, 1291

41 Pelizzari, C.A., Chen, G.T., Spelbring, D.R. *et al.* Accurate three-dimensional registration of CT, PET, and/or MR images of the brain. *J. Comput. Assist. Tomogr.* 1989, 13, 20

42 Friston, K.J., Passingham, R.E., Nutt, J.G. *et al.* Localization in PET images: direct fitting of the intercommissural (AC-PC) line. *J. Cereb. Blood Flow Metab.* 1989, 9, 690

43 Crosson, B., Williamson, D.J.G., Shukla, S.S. *et al.* A technique to localize activation in the human brain with technetium-99m-HMPAO SPECT: a validation study using visual stimulation. *J. Nucl. Med.* 1994, 35, 755

44 Pantano, P., De Piero, V., Ricci, M. *et al.* Motor stimulation response by technetium-99m hexamethylpropylene amine oxime split-dose method and single photon emission tomography. *Eur. J. Nucl. Med.* 1992, 19, 939

45 Sharp, P.F., Smith, F.W., Gemmell, H.G. *et al.* Technetium-99m HMPAO stereoisomers as potential agents for imaging regional cerebral blood flow: human volunteer studies. *J. Nucl. Med.* 1986, 27, 171

46 Wyper, D.J., Hunter, R., Patterson, J. *et al.* A split-dose technique for measuring changes in cerebral blood flow patterns. *J. Cereb. Blood Flow Metab.* 1991, 11, S449

47 Hung, J.C. Corlija, M. Volkert, W.A. *et al.* Kinetic analysis of technetium-99m d,l-HMPAO decomposition in aqueous media. *J. Nucl. Med.* 1988, 29, 1568

48 Lucignani, G., Rosetti, C., Ferrario, P. *et al.* In vivo metabolism and kinetics of [99mTc]-HMPAO. *Eur. J. Nucl. Med.* 1990, 16, 249

49 Neirinckx, R.D., Canning, L.K., Burke, J.F. *et al.* The retention mechanism of [99mTc]-HMPAO: intracellular reaction with glutathione. *J. Cereb. Blood Flow Metab.* 1988, 8, S4

50 Battistin, L., Pizzolato, G., Dam, M. *et al.* Regional cerebral blood flow study with 99mTc-hexamethylpropylene amine oxime single photon emission tomography in Alzheimer's and multi-infarct dementia. *Eur. Neurol.* 1990, 30, 296

51 Geany, D.P., Soper, N., Shepstone, B.J. *et al.* Effect of central cholinergic stimulation on regional cerebral blood flow in Alzheimer's disease. *Lancet* 1990, 335, 1484

52 Dahl, A., Russel, D., Nyberg-Hansen, R. *et al.* Effect of nitroglycerin on cerebral circulation measured by transcranial doppler and SPECT. *Stroke* 1989, 20, 1733

53 Ringelstein, E.B., Eyck, S.V. and Mertens, I. Evaluation of cerebral vasomotor reactivity by various vasodilating stimuli: a comparison of CO_2 to acetazolamide. *J. Cereb. Blood Flow Metab.* 1992, 12, 162

54 Bonte, F., Devous, M. and Reisch, J. The effect of acetazolamide on regional blood flow in normal subjects as measured by single photon emission tomography. *Invest. Radiol.* 1988, 23, 564

55 Matsuda, H., Higashi, S., Kinuya, K. *et al.* SPECT evaluation of brain perfusion reserve by the acetazolamide test using Tc-99m-HMPAO. *Clin. Nucl. Med.* 1991, 16, 572

56 Chollet, F., Celsis, P., Clanet, M. *et al.* SPECT study of cerebral blood flow reactivity after acetazolamide in patients with transient ischemic attacks. *Stroke* 1989, 20, 458

57 Bonte, F.J., Devous, M.D., Reisch, J.S. *et al.* The effect of acetazolamide on regional cerebral blood flow in patients with Alzheimer's disease or stroke as measured by single-photon emission computed tomography. *Invest. Radiol.* 1989, 24, 99

58 Goodman, W.K. and Charney, D. Therapeutic applications in mechanism of action of monoamine oxidase inhibitor and heterocyclic anti-depressant drugs. *J. Clin. Psychiatry* 1985, 46, 6

59 Tollefson, G.D. Monoamine oxidase inhibitors: a review. *J. Clin. Psychiatr.* 1983, 44, 280

60 Klemm, E., Grunwuäld, F., Overbeck, B. *et al.* HMPAO SPECT in depression and schizophrenia. *Eur. J. Nucl. Med.* 1992, 19, 616

61 Liddle, P.F., Friston, K.J., Frith, C.D. *et al.* Patterns of cerebral blood flow in schizophrenia. *Br. J. Psychiatr.* 1992, 160, 179

62 Farde, L., Wiesel, F.A., Halklin, C. *et al.* Central D2 dopamine receptor in patients treated with antipsychotic drugs. *Arch. Gen. Psychiatr.* 1988, 45, 71

63 Dolan, R., Bench, C. and Friston, K. Positron emission tomography in psychopharmacology. *Int. Rev. Psychiatry* 1990, 2, 427

64 Mielke, R., Pietrzyk, U., Jacobs, A. *et al.* HMPAO, SPET and FDG PET in Alzheimer's disease vascular dementia comparison of perfusion and metabolic pattern. *Eur. J. Nucl. Med.* 1994, 21, 1052

65 George, M.S., Ring, H.A., Costa, D.C. *et al.* Demonstration of human motor cortex activation using SPECT. *J. Neural Trans.* 1992, 87, 231

66 Holm, S., Madsen, P.L., Rubin, P. *et al.* [99mTc] HMPAO activation studies: validation of the split-dose, image subtraction approach. *J. Cereb. Blood Flow Metab.* 1991, 11, S766

67 Lewis, S.H., Ford, R.A., Syed, G.M. *et al.* A controlled study of ^{99m}Tc-HMPAO single photon emission imaging in chronic schizophrenia. *Psychol. Med.* 1992, 22, 27

68 Weinberger, D.R., Berman, K.F., Zec, R.F. *et al.* Physiologic dysfunction of dorsolateral prefrontal cortex in schizophrenia I. Regional cerebral blood flow evidence. *Arch. Gen. Psychiatr.* 1986, 43, 114

69 Friston, K.J., Frith, D.C., Liddle, P.F. *et al.* Comparing functional (PET) images: the assessment of significant change. *J. Cereb. Blood Flow Metab.* 1991, 11, 690

70 Rascol, O., Sabatini, U., Chollett, F. *et al.* Supplementary and primary sensory motor area activity in Parkinson's disease. *Arch. Neurol.* 1992, 32, 749

71 Hantraye, P., Brownwel, A.L., Elmalch, D. *et al.* Dopamine fibre detection by [11C]-CFT and PET in a primate model of parkinsonism. *Neuro Report* 1992, 3, 265

72 Dormehl, I.C, Redelinghuys. F., Hugo, N. *et al.* The baboon model under anaesthesia for in vivo cerebral blood flow studies using SPECT techniques. *J. Med. Prim.* 1992, 21, 270

73 Oliver, D., Dormehl, I., Redelinghuys, F. *et al.* Drug effects on cerebral blood flow in the baboon model - Acetazolamide. *Nucl. Med.* 1993, 32, 292

74 Dormehl, I.C., Oliver, D.W. and Hugo, N. Dose response from pharmacological interventions for CBF determinations in a baboon model using ^{99m}Tc-HMPAO and SPECT *Nucl. Med. Comm.* 1993, 14, 573

75 Oliver, D., Dormehl, I. and Hugo, N. Effects of sumatriptan on CBF in the baboon model. *Arzeneimittel Forschung/Drug Research* 1994, 8, 925

76 Dutka, A.J., Mink, R., McDermot, J. *et al.* Effect of lidocaine on somatosensory evoked response and cerebral blood flow after canine cerebral embolism. *Stroke* 1992, 23, 1515

77 Dormehl, I.C., Lipp, M.D.W., Hugo, N. *et al.* Influence of intravenously administered lidocaine on cerebral blood flow in a baboon model standardized under controlled general anaesthesia using single photon emission tomography and technetium-99m hexamethylpropylene amine oxime. *Eur. J. Nucl. Med.* 1993, 20, 1095

78 Dormehl, I.C., Oliver, D.W., Hugo, N. and Rossouw, D. A comparative cerebral blood flow study in a baboon model with acetazolamide provocation: ^{99m}Tc-HMPAO versus [123]I(IMP). *Nucl. Med. Biol.* 1995, 22, 373

SPECT in Neurology and Psychiatry, edited by P.P. De Deyn, R.A. Dierckx, A. Alavi and B.A. Pickut
© 1997 John Libbey & Company Ltd, pp. 537-546

Functional Magnetic Resonance Imaging of the Brain

Chapter
63

F. Aichner, C. Kremser, M. Wagner and S. Felber

Introduction

Brain activation is reflected by changes in the electromagnetic fields as produced by changes in the membrane potential of the neuronal cellular membranes. These changes can be directly observed by electroencephalography and nowadays by means of magnetencephalography. However, both methods allow only limited spatial resolution. The topographical distribution of activation in certain brain structures has been obtained by direct stimulation of the cortex in animal experiments and during open brain surgery in humans.

A tremendous step towards the non-invasive mapping of brain activation was the observation that brain activation is accompanied by an increase in regional blood flow using positron emission tomography (PET). PET requires the administration of radionuclides, which means this method is not employed on a routine basis.

At the beginning of the 1990s, it was shown that activation coupled changes in cerebral blood flow and blood volume could also be observed using magnetic resonance imaging techniques. In 1991, Belliveau[1] demonstrated an increase in blood volume of the primary visual cortex as a direct response to visual stimulation using Gd-DTPA enhanced MRI. Based on the results of Ogawa *et al.*[2,3] and Turner *et al.*[4], Kwong et al.[5] could demonstrate that changes in regional brain perfusion can also be observed by MRI, using the inherent magnetic properties of oxygenated and deoxygenated blood as a contrast agent. With this approach, now referred to as blood oxygenation level dependent (BOLD) MRI, it became possible to map brain activation non-invasively.

The main advantage of BOLD MRI is that activation tasks can be observed repeatedly without any harm to the patient. This has interested neuroscientists, clinical neurologists, neurosurgeons, psychiatrists and psychologists, and drawn them into the use of functional magnetic resonance imaging (fMRI). At present, the method is still in its infancy and the scope of this article is to outline some of its potentials and limitations that have to be taken under consideration while planning fMRI experiments.

The basic principles of fMRI

In general, the signal intensities of tissues on MRI depend on a number of tissue specific and equipment specific parameters[6]. The tissue specific parameters include the total number of contributing protons and their microenvironment properties T_1 and T_2. The T_2 relaxation of protons depends on spin-spin

Department of Magnetic Resonance
Medical School, University of Innsbruck
Anichstrasse 35, A-6020
Innsbruck, Austria

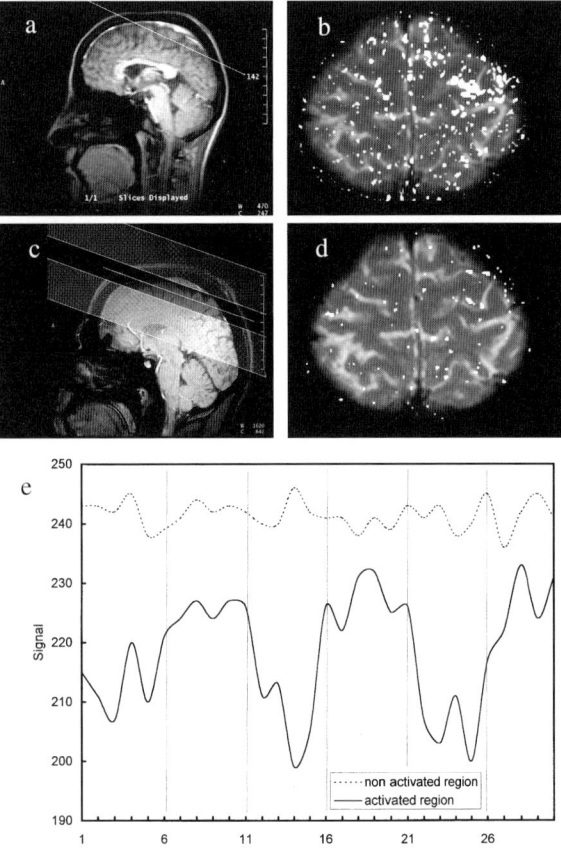

Figure 1 a, b, Motor stimulation study within the basal ganglia involving a hand movement task obtained with a coronary orientation. The same pulse sequence as used for Figure 3 was employed without parallel presaturation pulses. Finger tapping of the right hand was performed by the subject. c, Functional activation map through the basal ganglia obtained with a subtraction based z-score analysis. For the image acquisition a flip angle of 30° was used. Activation found in the left hemisphere. d, The same activation map with an excitation flip angle of 12°. The activation within the basal ganglia is unchanged whereas activation in the cortex region is reduced. Reduced excitation flip angles lead to a suppression of inflow effects and thus to a reduction in the influence of blood flow changes on the activation maps

interactions within the observed molecule and on the magnetic susceptibility of the environment (T_{2*}). T_{2*} effects increase with the field strength of the scanner employed and since brain activation effects are strongly correlated to T_{2*} effects, fMRI studies require magnets with field strengths >1T. In addition, the excitable protons may macroscopically (blood flow) and microscopically (diffusion and perfusion) move

between excitation and signal collection, which further influence their signal intensity on the MR image[7]. Since, fMRI depends on the changes in regional blood flow and changes in the magnetic properties of blood or the administered contrast agent, T_1 and T_2 and other effects have to be encountered for interpreting results of fMRI studies. Signal changes can also be observed on T_1 weighted MR images[8].

FMRI using paramagnetic contrast agents

Gd-DTPA, which is routinely applied for diagnostic MRI, has been used for fMRI studies[1]. In contrast to diagnostic MRI, which takes advantage of T_1 changes induced by Gd-DTPA, fMRI depends on the T_{2*} effect of Gd-DTPA that is present during the first pass of the contrast agent through the brain. The first bolus of contrast agent that passes through the capillary network has concentrations of Gd-DTPA high enough to cause a T_{2*} shortening within the parenchyma surrounding the capillaries. This T_{2*} shortening leads to a decrease in signal intensity on the MR images, which is more prominent in regions with augmented regional blood flow during brain activation. In order to monitor this effect, T_{2*} susceptible images have to be acquired within short time frames[7]. Usually, gradient echo images with short repetition times and longer echo times are employed to meet these requirements. Since the initial T_{2*} effect of Gd-DTPA compensates for T_1 changes due to inflow effects, higher excitation angles around 60° can be used to maximise signal to noise ratios. Up to 10% signal differences between activated and non-activated regions can be observed at 1.5 T[9].

FMRI using the BOLD effect

As shown by Kwong, brain activation maps can also be created using the different magnetic properties of haemoglobin as an inherent contrast agent[10]. When blood passes through the capillary bed, the tissue parenchyma removes oxygen from oxyhaemoglobin, which is thereby transformed to deoxyhaemoglobin. Deoxyhaemoglobin has a stronger T_{2*} effect as compared with oxyhaemoglobin on the adjacent parenchyma and causes signal void around the postcapillary venoles. PET studies have shown that the increase in the regional blood flow to the activated brain area exceeds the increase of the tissue oxygen extraction fraction. This difference leads to a net decrease of deoxyhaemoglobin in activated brain structure and consequently to an increase in signal intensity on the final fMR image. The effect yields a 2 - 5% signal difference between activated and non-activated brain on T_{2*} weighted images at a field strength of 1.5 T.

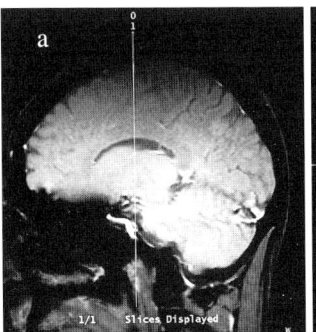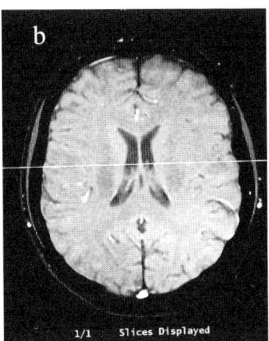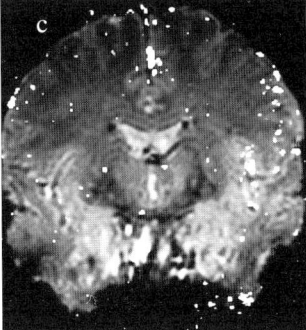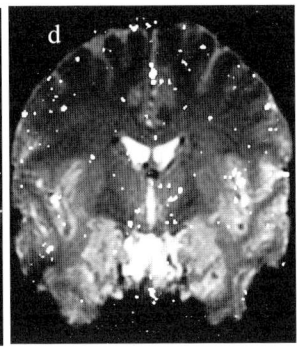

Figure 2 a,c,e Motor stimulation study involving a hand movement task, obtained with different slice positions. Finger tapping of the right hand was performed by the subject. For the image acquisition a 2D FLASH sequence with centric reordered phase encoding and parallel presaturation pulses was used for a complete reduction of flow effects. b,d,f Corresponding activation maps obtained with a subtraction based z-score analysis. A strong dependence of the activation pattern on the respective slice position is found indicating that for reproducible fMRI results imaging sequences enabling the simultaneous acquisition of several slices would be preferred. Such imaging strategies are mainly based on EPI making special MR scanner hardware necessary which is not yet widely available

The sequences that have been employed to detect the BOLD effect, are also gradient echo images (2D Flash, Echo Planar Imaging EPI) with a short TR and a rather long TE[11-13]. Inflow effects that modulate T_1 of blood can increase the signal intensity in the pre- and post-capillary vascular bed, thus influencing the signal intensity parallel to the BOLD effect, and may thereby lead to incorrect activation patterns. The use of low flip angles can reduce this effect, however, it also diminishes the overall signal to noise ratio (Figure 1).

FMRI study protocols

FMRI examinations

FMRI examinations are usually performed by repeated image acquisition at the same slice position during activated and non-activated periods. Using 2D flash techniques only a single slice position can be imaged, whereas with EPI up to 20 slice positions can be acquired simultaneously. The single slice approach (2D flash) reduces the reproducibility of fMRI studies due to the dependency of activation patterns on the slice position and orientation (Figure 2)[14]. Typically, the image acquisition is repeated 30 to 60 times. For motor cortex stimulation, the subject is asked to perform the respective motor task paradigm in a periodic sequence. During an examination with 30 images, five rest images alternate with five activation images (Figure 3). The acquired images are then subjected to some sort of statistical or correlation analysis in order to identify activated brain regions. It should be noted that fMRI can also be performed with non-periodic tasks requiring modified statistical methods.

Paradigm

Functionality is defined by the following approaches: imaging of architectonics, imaging of connectivity, topography mapping, imaging of physiological function and behavioural studies and imaging. PET and fMRI attempt to localise information processing within the brain at the four mentioned levels. A further consideration of fMRI is the correct application of standardised paradigm protocols because the paradigm design is essential for the interpretation and comparison of fMRI findings. The signal changes are determined by the stimulus repetition rate, the stimulus duration, by the stimulus feature density and the spatial extent of stimulus[15]. Simple and complex motor tasks, auditory stimulation, visual imagery, cognitive tasks in the form of word finding, word and language processing, word generation have been added successfully to the repertoire of fMRI observable brain activations.

Rest is defined behaviourally, but even during rest subjects can think, recall events from memory, or dream. Even a person asleep and without external stimuli has an intrinsic brain activity in the brain in the form of metabolic activity (PET) as well as action- and post-synaptic potentials (EEG). The purpose of a rigorous rest definition is a state in which the subject is awake but has a minimum of brain activity. It is known that the eyes closed and ears plugged condition is the best baseline state for measuring activations[16]. This is easily achieved in the PET facilities, but represents a problem due to the noise produced by the gradients within the magnet.

There are several other factors that can influence the CBF during rest and activation. They include age, sex, medication, alcohol, fatigueness, drowsiness, sleep, handedness, hemispheric differences, learning effects, fear, uneasiness, and other psychological factors.

Postprocessing

For the data postprocessing of fMRI, different strategies are available and in use. All postprocessing strategies are sensitive to minimal movements of the head leading to severe errors in the final activation map (Figure 4). Therefore, fMRI results can be improved using co-registration techniques to minimise the influence of patient movements. The simplest fMRI postprocessing technique is the so-called subtraction method, where the difference between all averaged activated images and all averaged non-activated images is calculated. Non-zero regions in the obtained subtraction image should correspond to activated brain regions. The subtraction method can be further refined if a threshold (standard signal fluctuation of all rest images, z-scan analysis) image is applied to the subtraction.

More sophisticated postprocessing strategies such as cross-correlation and auto-correlation techniques have been proposed. These account not only for calculated signal differences but also for the time course of the applied paradigm in cases of periodic stimulation. These methods reduce signal changes that are not correlated to the stimulation on the calculated activation maps (e.g. large signal fluctuations at large vessels such as sagittal sinus).

Application of fMRI in brain activation studies

The emergence of sophisticated modalities such as PET and MRI with their activation studies has led to an explosion of experimental data and made the brain accessible to modern science. Tables 1 - 4 show a brief list of some of this work in functional brain mapping.

Somatotopic mapping (Tables 1 and 2)

Knowledge of the somatotopic organisation of the primary motor cortex in human is derived from electrophysiological stimulation studies and positron

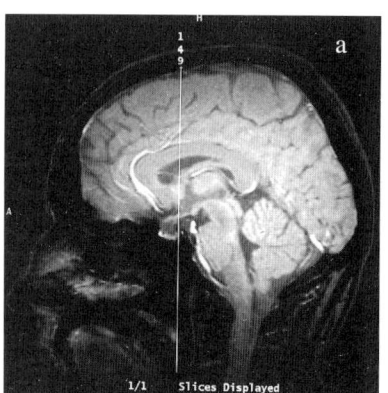 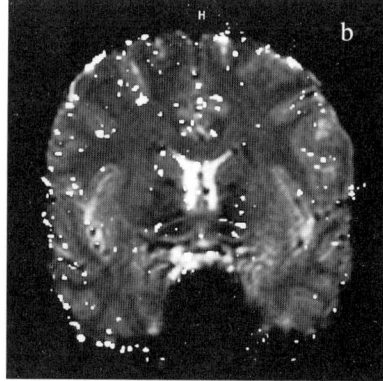 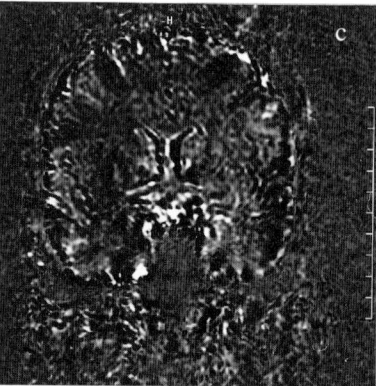

Figure 3 a, Motor stimulation study involving a hand movement task, obtained with a slice orientation. For the image acquisition a 2D FLASH sequence with TR = 102ms, TE = 56ms, a = 20° and a slice thickness of 3 mm were used with a scan matrix of 128 x 128. b, Functional activation map obtained with a subtraction based z-score analysis. No parallel presaturation pulses were used for the image acquisition. Activation is observed, as expected, in the left hemisphere. c, To suppress the contribution of blood flow changes to the observed activation the image acquisition was also performed with parallel presaturation pulses. All 30 consecutive image acquisitions were performed with a time delay of 2 s. The whole fMRI acquisition was organised in 6 blocks of 5 images each, representing 3 periods where the subject was at rest and 3 periods where the subject was asked to perform finger tapping of the right hand. d, Functional activation map obtained with a subtraction based z-score analysis. Parallel presaturation pulses were used for the image acquisition to suppress the influence of activation related blood flow changes. The striking activation pattern seen in b is strongly reduced due to the flow suppression indicating the strong influence of blood flow effects on fMRI. e, Signal time course obtained from ROI measurement in activated (solid line) and non-activated (dotted line) brain regions. The periodic signal enhancement due to the performed motor task is clearly seen for the activated brain region, whereas no signal changes take place in non-activated regions

Table 1 Functional brain mapping: motor system

Paradigm/anatomic structure	Method	Reference
Motor cortex	fMRI	17
	fMRI	18
	fMRI	19
	fMRI	20, 21
Arm and hand movements	fMRI	22
	PET	23
	fMRI	24
	fMRI	25
Complex movements	fMRI	26
Finger movements	fMRI	25
Willed action	PET	27
Handedness and hemispheric		
asymmetry	fMRI	28
basal ganglia	fMRI	29
cerebellar cortex	fMRI	30
saccadic eye movements	PET	31
Musical sight reading and	PET	32
keyboard performance	PET	33

Table 2 Functional brain mapping: sensory system

Paradigm	Method	Reference
Vibration	PET	34
Shape	PET	35
Pain	PET	36
	PET	37
Sensory stimulation	fMRI	38
	fMRI	5
	fMRI	39
	fMRI	40

Table 3 Functional brain mapping: vision

Paradigm	Method	Reference
Retinotopy	PET	41
Stimulus rate	PET	15
Visual stimulation	fMRI	10
	fMRI	42
	fMRI	1
	fMRI	43
	fMRI	44
	fMRI	45
	fMRI	46
	fMRI	47
Colour	PET	48
Face and object process	PET	49
	fMRI	1
Functional specialisation	PET	50
	fMRI	51
Visual recall	fMRI	52

emission tomographical investigations. A replication of this work with fMRI is needed because somatotopic organisation of the motor cortex is defined and can serve as a validation of the technique. FMRI has sufficient functional spatial resolution to demonstrate somatotopic organisation of the primary motor cortex. FMRI is able to distinguish arm from finger movements. The cortical areas activated by voluntary movements appear larger than those described from electrical stimulation. Studies that have correlated fMRI results with electrical stimulation findings derived from patients undergoing intraoperative cortical mapping have only shown a correspondence within several millimetres.

In addition to the by now familiar activation of primary and supplementary motor cortex, cerebellar activation has been demonstrated. Preliminary data have shown activation at the basal ganglia. Presurgical planning work using motor stimulation may assist neurosurgeons to identify motor-sensory areas from tumours to be resected.

Mapping the representation of the visual field (Table 3)

The data collected in the last years have demonstrated that fMRI maps of the visual cortex correlate well with known retinotopic organisation. Higher order visual processing areas can be discerned using fMRI, if appropriately designed discrimination tasks are used. Successful studies have been carried out at higher

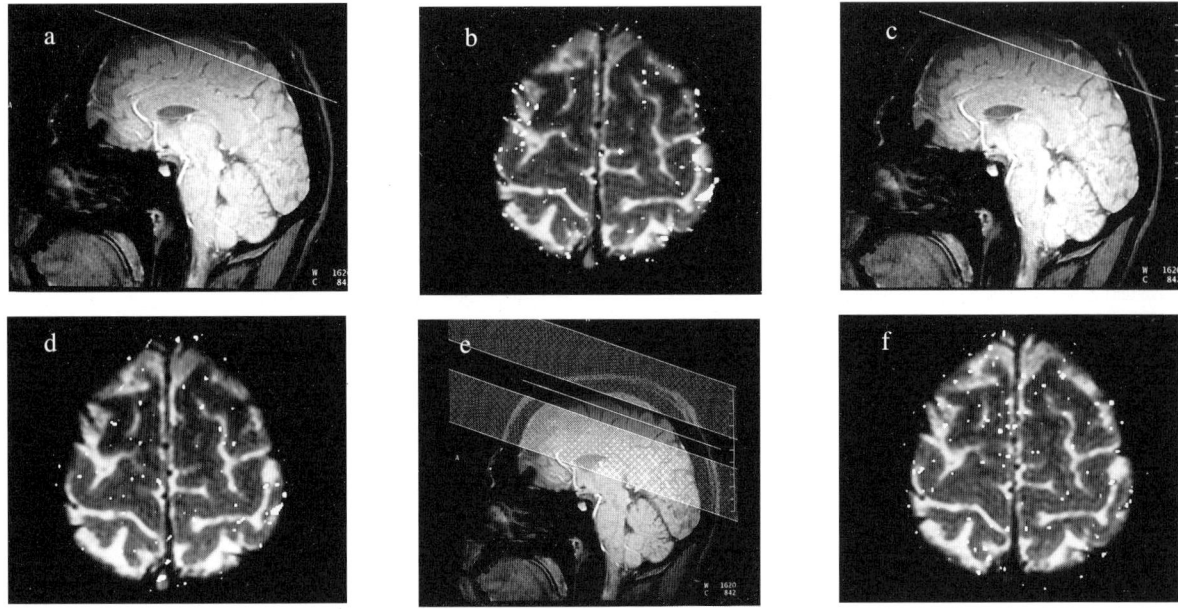

Figure 4 a, Motor stimulation study within the basal ganglia involving a hand movement task obtained with a slice orientation. The same pulse sequence as used for Figure 3 was employed without parallel presaturation pulses. Finger tapping of the right hand was performed by the subject. b, Functional activation map obtained with a subtraction based z-score analysis. Contrary to expectation, the main activation is found in the cortex region of the right hemisphere. c, Subtraction image between the first and last image corresponding to non-activated periods. Without the occurrence of patient movements, no image structures should be visible in the subtraction image. Patient movement, which especially for motor stimulation studies is very often correlated to the activation task, represents a major problem for fMRI examinations resulting in wrong activation patterns

visual regions such as motion sensitive area V_5/MT and the face/object recognition area V_4. Visual imagery has been explored.

Mapping of human auditory cortex

The published fMRI data from the human auditory cortex are in agreement with findings from other functional maps indicating that both left and right temporal regions are involved with processing and auditory speech stimuli. The processing of speech stimuli requires the activity of more wide spread brain areas than does processing of simpler non-speech sounds.

Mapping of cognitive functions (Table 4)

For higher cognitive functions, several fMRI language-associated regions have been demonstrated. With either auditory or visual stimuli, language lateralisation has been demonstrated, matching results obtained by the standard, yet extremely invasive WADA test. For memory studies, prefrontal cortex regions have been implicated in working memory tasks. For picture encoding, fMRI also revealed significant signal

intensity increases bilaterally in hippocampal and parahippocampal regions and at the temporal occipital junction.

Epilepsy

In studies of epilepsy, simultaneous fMRI and electrophysiological recording has been achieved. In a recent study, the spatial localisation of fMRI was more accurate than electroencephalography recorded from a subdural grid in predicting the site of successful surgical therapy[63].

Present problems in fMRI

During fMRI of the brain, several problems arise, e.g. low contrast noise ratio, low contrast artefact ratio, intra- and interimage artefacts, difficulties of brain-vein, separation and inflow artefacts. Intense studies of possible artefacts and errors are under way. The most serious practical problem arises by virtue of fMRI's excellent spatial resolution. Even a tiny, 0.5 mm movement of the head can change the intensity of a boundary pixel by as much as 40%. Head motion

Table 4 Functional brain mapping: language

Paradigm/anatomical structure	Method	Reference
Covert word production	fMRI	53
Word finding	PET	54
Single word processing	PET	55
Visual words	PET	56
Letter and object processing	PET	49
Word generation	PET	57
	fMRI	58
	fMRI	59
Phonetic and pitch discrimination	PET	60
Broca area	fMRI	61
Auditory cortex	fMRI	62

between conditions results in confusing structures in the difference image. This registration can be corrected by comparing the image details, especially if volume information is provided at each scan.

Experimentally at 1.5 T systems, one observes an MR signal change upon brain activation to be in the order of 2 - 5% from base line conditions. The optimum signal change predicted by theoretical models is normally not larger than 2%[5].

Conventional fMRI gradient echo sequences have serious problems of intraimage and interimage motion artefacts. Navigator echo-based motion correction schemes are used to minimise the phase in consistency among k-space lines. For functional MRI, interimage motion artefacts are still a serious problem. The utilisation of a bite bar made from a dental mould is useful in reducing the up and down inclination head motion problem. The better the head is restrained during the image acquisition, the less one has to rely on any postprocessing reregistration scheme[64].

One of the most basic problems of fMRI is to differentiate the BOLD effect from macroscopical flow. Three different mechanisms account for the signal alterations: deoxyhaemoglobin dependent susceptibility changes; stimulus related flow changes; and signal fluctuations not related to the actual stimulation protocol ('vascular noise').

Some authors suggest that exact differentiation of flow from BOLD effects may not be necessary in fMRI, because the nett difference in signal intensity may even be augmented if arterioles and venoles may be allowed

to contribute signal. While, this may hold true for neuropsychological activation studies, others have reasonable concern that the resulting loss of topographical accuracy may be critical for surgical planning[65].

Several approaches have been evaluated to differentiate the signal response of postcapillary veins from larger draining veins, including presaturation regimens (Figure 5) and 3D slab acquisitions. The simplest way to diminish inflow and outflow effects is the reduction of the excitation angle (Figure 1), which however has the penalty of overall signal to noise reduction.

Furthermore, present interpretation of fMRI studies are hampered by our incomplete understanding of the physiological correlation between parenchymal activation and augmentation of regional perfusion. There is still much work ahead to elucidate the influence of the frequency and type of stimuli on blood flow increase. In addition, repetitive experiments in the same person may lead to adaptive changes in the processing of stimuli and eventually to adaptive changes in the degree of blood flow changes. It is still not known whether different brain structures have different blood flow responses to activation. In addition, most of the published studies were carried out in healthy young volunteers and the response of elderly subjects with decreased autoregulation capabilities of the cerebral vasculature remains to be evaluated.

Conclusion

FMRI using BOLD contrast is a new method for observing brain activation. Regions activated in the motor cortex by movement of fingers, elbows and toes have been mapped. Regions involved with performance and mental rehearsal of complex motor tasks have been imaged. The primary visual cortex has been retinotopically mapped and retinotopic organisation of some of the higher levels of the visual pathways have been observed. Differences have been observed in the temporal lobes during passive listening to white noise as opposed to speech sounds. Regions activated by the tasks of reading and listening to spoken words have been observed. Much additional work will contribute to the complete understanding of the precise nature of the BOLD contrast.

FMRI has a sufficient spatial and temporal resolution, no radiation hazard and the opportunity to study single subjects as often as required. It can be performed using a routine 1.5 T MR scanner. There are many important areas related to fMRI that may become integrated into clinical applications. FMRI is helpful for identification of critical gyri or sulci before neurosurgical or

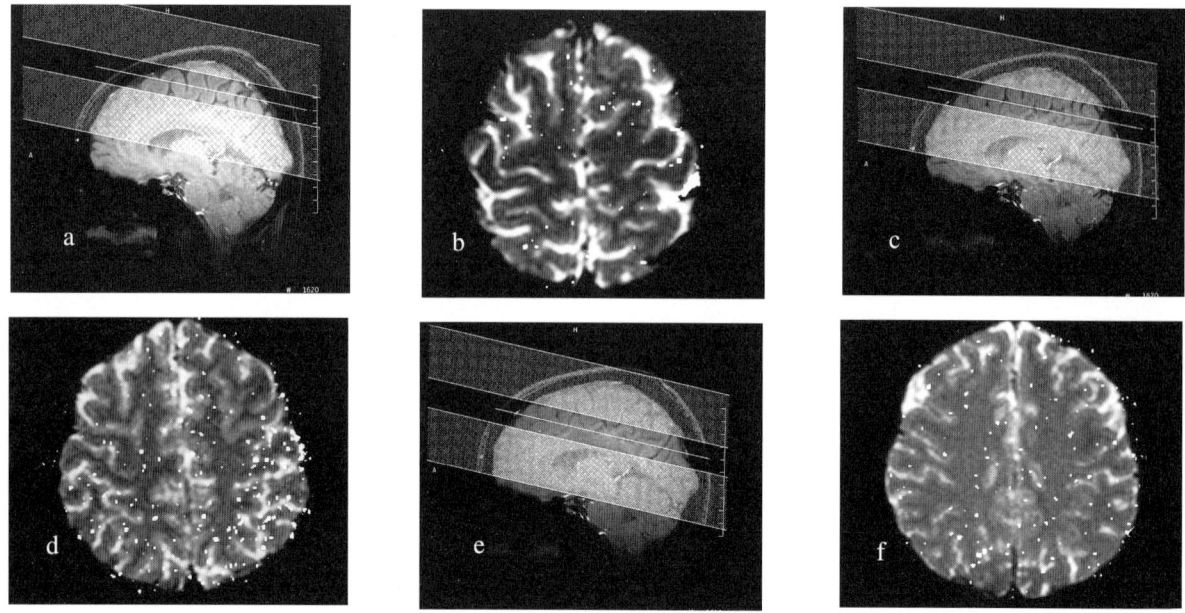

Figure 5 a,c,e Motor stimulation study involving a hand movement task, obtained with slice orientations. Finger tapping of the right hand was performed by the subject. b, Activation map obtained with the same pulse sequence as used for Figure 3 without parallel presaturation pulses. Activation patterns are as expected found in the left hemisphere. Inspection of the activation maps gives evidence that the major contributions to the found patterns are from brain vessels. d, Reduction of blood flow effect by using a 2D FLASH sequence with a centric reordered phase encoding without parallel presaturation pulses. The use of centric reordered phase encoding leads to a reduction of the inflow effect eliminating the contribution of slow blood flow on the activation maps. f, Almost complete reduction of blood flow effects due to the additional usage of parallel presaturation pulses. The small activation patterns seen in the image correspond to calculation errors due to the rather simple subtraction based z-score analysis. Employing more sophisticated cross correlation analysis would eliminate these erroneous signals

neuroradiological procedures including epileptic surgery, and hopefully fMRI will replace the invasive WADA test. Functional human neuroanatomy and pharmaceutical studies will have a new and completely non-invasive armamentarium. When used with care, fMRI has a bright future in basic research, in surgical planning for tumour excision and epilepsy, in studies of cognitive development and in investigations of neuropsychiatric disorders including monitoring effects of drug therapy and brain function.

References

1 Belliveau, J.W., Kennedy, D.N., Mc Kinstry, R.C. *et al.* Functional mapping of the human visual cortex by magnetic resonance imaging. *Science* 1991, 254, 716

2 Ogawa, S., Lee, T.M., Kay, A.R. and Tank, D.W. Brain magnetic resonance imaging with contrast dependent on blood oxygenation. *Proc. Natl. Acad. Sci. USA* 1990, 187, 9868

3 Ogawa, S., Lee, T.M., Nayak, A.S. and Glynn, P. Oxygenation-sensitive contrast in magnetic resonance image of rodent brain at high magnetic fields. *Magn. Reson. Med.* 1990, 14, 68

4 Turner, R., Le Bihan, D., Moonen, C.T.W. *et al.* Echo-planar time course MRI of rat brain deoxygenation changes. *Magn. Reson. Med.* 1991, 22, 159

5 Kwong, K.K., Belliveau, J.W., Chesler, D.A. *et al.* Dynamic magnetic resonance imaging of human brain activity during primary sensory stimulation. *Proc. Natl. Acad. Sci. USA* 1992, 89, 5675

6 Aichner, F.T., Felber, S.R., Muller, R.N. and Rinck, P.A. in 'Three-dimensional magnetic resonance imaging', Blackwell Scientific Publications, London, 1994

7 Le Bihan, D. in 'Diffusion and perfusion magnetic resonance imaging. Applications to functional MRI', Raven Press, New York

8 Detre, J.A., Leigh, J., Williams, D. and Koretsky, A. Perfusion imaging. *Magn. Reson. Med.* 1992, 23, 37

9   Bandettini, P.A., Wong, E.C., Hinks, R.S. *et al.* Time course EPI of human brain function during activation. *Magn. Reson. Med.* 1992, 25, 390

10 Kwong, K.K. Functional magnetic resonance imaging with echo planar imaging. *Magn. Reson. Quarterly* 1995, 11, 1

11 Bandettini, P.A., Binder, J.R., De Yoe, E.A. *et al.* Functional MR Imaging using the BOLD approach, in 'Diffusion and Perfusion Magnetic Resonance Imaging', (Ed. D. Le Bihan), Raven Press, New York, 1994, p. 351

12 Edelman, R.R., Siewert, B., Darby, D.G. *et al.* Qualitative mapping of cerebral blood flow and functional localization with echo-planar MR imaging and signal targeting with alternating radio frequency. *Radiology* 1994, 192, 513

13 Edelman, R.R., Wielopolski, P. and Schmitt, F. Echo-planar MR Imaging. *Radiology* 1994, 192, 600

14 Cox, R.W., Binder, J.R., De Yoe, E.A. and Rao, S.M. Analysis of Inter-trial and Inter-subject repeatability in whole brain functional magnetic resonance imaging. *Proc. Soc. Magn. Reson.* 1995, 2, 833

15 Fox, P.T. and Raichle, M.E. Stimulus rate determines local brain blood flow in striate cortex. *Ann. Neurol.* 1985, 17, 303

16 Roland, P.E. in 'Brain activation', Wiley - Liss, New York, 1993

17 Yousry, T.A., Schmid, U.D. and Jassoy, A.G. Topography of the cortical motor hand area: prospective study with fMRI and direct motor mapping. *Radiology* 1995, 195, 23

18 Kim, S.G., Ashe, J., Georgopouplos, A.P. *et al.* Functional imaging of human motor cortex at high magnetic field. *J. Neurophysiol.* 1993, 69, 297

19 Schad, L.R., Trost, U., Knopp, M.V. *et al.* Motor cortex stimulation measured by magnetic resonance imaging on a standard 1.5 T clinical scanner. *Magn. Reson. Imaging* 1994, 11, 461

20 Cao, Y., Towle, V.L., Levin, D.N. and Balter, J.M. Functional mapping of human motor cortical activation by conventional MRI at 1.5 T. *J. Magn. Reson. Imaging* 1993, 3, 869

21 Cao, Y., Vikingstad, E.M., Huttenlocher, P.R. *et al.* Functional magnetic resonance studies of the reorganization of the human hand sensorimotor area after unilateral brain injury in the perinatal period. *Proc. Natl. Acad. Sci. USA* 1994, 91, 9612

22 Rumeau, C., Tzourio, N., Murayama, N. *et al.* Location of hand function in the sensorimotor cortex: MR and functional correlation. *Am J. Neuroradiol.* 1994, 15, 567

23 Colebatch, J.G., Deiber, M.P., Passingham, R.E. *et al.* Regional cerebral blood-flow during voluntary arm and hand movements in human subjects. *J. Neurophysiol.* 1991, 65, 1392

24 Cao, Y., Towle, V.L., Levin, D.N. *et al.* Conventional 1.5 T functional MRI localization of human hand sensorimotor cortex with intraoperative electrophysiologic validation. Proceedings 12th of SMRM, 1993, p. 1417

25 Connelly, A., Jackson, G.D., Frackowiak, R.S.J. *et al.* Functional mapping of activated human primary cortex with a clinical MR imaging system. *Radiology* 1993, 188, 125

26 Rao, S.M., Binder, J.R., Bandettini, P.A. *et al.* Functional magnetic resonance imaging of complex human movements. *Neurology* 1993, 43, 2311

27 Frith, C.D., Friston, K., Liddle, P.F. and Frackowiak, R.S.J. Willed action and the prefrontal cortex in man: a study with PET. *Proc. R. Soc. Lond. B. Biol. Sci.* 1991, 244, 241

28 Kim, S.G., Ashe, J., Hendrich, K. *et al.* Functional magnetic resonance imaging of motor cortex: hemispheric asymmetry and handedness. *Science* 1993, 261, 615

29 Bucher, S.F., Seelos, K.C., Stehling, M. *et al.* High resolution activation mapping of basal ganglia with functional magnetic resonance imaging. *Neurology* 1995, 45, 180

30 Kim, S.G., Ugurbil, K. and Strick, P. Activation of a cerebellar output nucleus during cognitive processing. *Science* 1994, 265, 949

31 Fox, P.T., Fox, J.M., Raichle, M.E. and Burde, R.M. The role of cerebral cortex in the generation of saccadic eye movements: a positron emission tomographic study. *J. Neurophysiol.* 1985, 552, 348

32 Sergent, J., Zuck, E., Terrians, S. and MacDonald, B. Distributed neural network underlying musical sight-reading and key board performance. *Science* 1992, 257, 106

33 Grafton, S.T., Woods, R.P., Mazziotta, J.C. and Phelps, M.E. Somatotopic mapping of the primary motor cortex in humans: Activation studies with cerebral blood flow and positron emission tomography. *J. Neurophysiol.* 1991, 66, 735

34 Fox, P.T., Burton, H. and Raichle, M.E. Mapping human somatosensory cortex with positron emission tomography. *J. Neurosurg.* 1987, 67, 34

35 Seitz, R.J., Roland, P.E., Bohm, C. *et al.* Somatosensory discrimination of shape: tactile exploration and cerebral activation. *Eur. J. Neurosci.* 1991, 3, 481

36 Jones, A.K.P., Brown, W.D., Friston, K.J. *et al.* Cortical and subcortical localization of response to pain in man using positron emission tomography. *Proc. R. Soc. Lond. B. Biol. Sci.* 1991, 244, 39

37 Talbot, J.D., Marrett, S., Evans, A.C. *et al.* Multiple representations of pain in human cerebral cortex. *Science* 1991, 251, 1355

38 Jack, C.R., Thompson, R.M., Butts, R.K. *et al.* Sensory motor cortex: correlation of presurgical mapping with functional MR imaging and invasive cortical mapping. *Radiology* 1994, 190, 85

39 Hammeke, T.A., Yetkin, F.Z., Mueller, W.M. *et al.* Functional magnetic resonance imaging of somatosensory stimulation. *J. Neurosurg.* 1994, 35, 677

40 Yetkin, F.Z., Papke, R.A., Mark, L.P. *et al.* Location of the sensorimotor cortex: functional and conventional MR compared. *Am. J. Neuroradiol.* 1995, 16, 2109

41 Fox, P.T., Miezin, F.M., Allman, J.M. *et al.* Retinotopic organization of human visual cortex mapped with positron-emission tomography. *J. Neurosci.* 1987, 7, 913

42 Frahm, J., Bruhn, H., Merbolt, K. and Hanicke, W. Dynamic MR imaging of human brain oxygenation during rest and photic stimulation. *J. Magn. Reson. Imaging* 1992, 2, 501

43 Eddy, W.F., Behrmann, M., Carpenter, P.A. *et al.* Test-Retest reproducibility during fMRI studies: Primary visual and cognitive paradigms. *Proc. Soc. Magn. Reson.* 1995, 2, 843

44 Turner, R., Jezzard, P., Wen, H. *et al.* Functional mapping of the human visual cortex at 4 Tesla and 1.5 Tesla using deoxygenation contrast EPI. *Magn. Reson. Med.* 1993, 29, 277

45 Blamire, A., Ogawa, S., Ugurbil, K. *et al.* Dynamic mapping of human visual cortex by high-speed magnetic resonance imaging. *Proc. Natl. Acad. Sci. USA* 1992, 89, 11069

46 Menon, R., Ogawa, S., Tank, D. and Ugurbil, K. 4-Tesla gradient recalled echo characteristics of photic stimulation-induced signal changes in the human primary visual cortex. *Magn. Reson. Med.* 1993, 30, 380

47 Merboldt, K.D., Bruhn, H., Hanicke, W. *et al.* Decrease of glucose in the human visual cortex during visual stimulation. *Magn. Reson. Med.* 1992, 22, 68

48 Lueck, C.J., Zeki, S., Friston, K.J. *et al.* The colour centre in the cerebral cortex of man. *Nature* 1989, 340, 386

49 Sergent, J., Zuck, E., Leversque, M. and MacDonald, B. Positron emission tomography study of letter and object processing: empirical findings and methodological considerations. *Cerebral Cortex* 1992, 2, 68

50 Zeki, S., Watson, J.D.G., Lueck, C.J. *et al.* A direct demonstration of functional spezialisation in human visual cortex. *J. Neurosci.* 1991, 11, 641

51 Ogawa, S., Tank, D.W., Menon, R. *et al.* Intensic signal changes accompanying sensory stimulation - functional brain mapping with magnetic resonance imaging. *Proc. Natl. Acad. Sci. USA* 1992, 89, 5951

52 Le Bihan, D., Turner, R., Zeffiro, T. *et al.* Activation of human primary visual cortex during visual recall: an MRI study. *Proc. Natl. Acad. Sci. USA* 1993, 90, 11802

53 Rueckert, L., Appolonio, I., Grafman, J. *et al.* Magnetic resonance imaging functional activation of left frontal cortex during covert word production. *J. Neuroimag.* 1994, 4, 67

54 Frith, C.D., Friston, K.J., Liddle, P.E. and Frackowiak, R.S.J. A Pet study of word finding. *Neuropsychologia* 1991, 29, 1137

55 Petersen, S.E., Fox, P.T., Posner, M.I. *et al.* Positron emission tomographic studies of the cortical anatomy of single word processing. *Nature* 1988, 331, 585

56 Petersen, S.E., Fox, P.T., Snyder, A.Z. and Raichle, M.E. Activation of extrastriate and frontal cortical areas by visual words and word like stimuli. *Science* 1990, 249, 1041

57 Friston, K.J., Frith, C.D., Liddle, P.E. and Frackowiak, R.S.J. Investigating a network model of word generation with positron emission tomography. *Proc. R. Soc. Lond. B. Biol. Sci.* 1991, 244, 101

58 McCarthy, G., Blamire, A.M., Rothman, D.L. *et al.* Echo-planar MRI studies of frontal cortex activation during word generation in humans. *Proc. Natl. Acad. Sci. USA* 1993, 90, 4952

59 Cuenod, C.A., Bookheimer, S.Y., Hertz-Pannier, L. *et al.* Functional MRI during word generations, using conventional equipment. A potential trial for language localization in the clinical environment. *Neurology* 1995, 45, 1821

60 Zatorre, R.J., Evans, A.C., Mayer, E. and Gjedde, A. Lateralization of phonetic and pitch discrimination in speech processing. *Science* 1992, 256, 846

61 Hinke, R.M., Hu, X, Stillman, A.E. *et al.* Magnetic resonance functional imaging of Broca's area during internal speech. *Neuroreport* 1993, 4, 675

62 Binder, J.R., Rao, S.M., Hammeke, T.A. *et al.* Functional magnetic resonance imaging of human auditory cortex. *Am. Neurol.* 1994, 35, 662

63 Detre, J.A., Sirven, J., Alsop, D.C. *et al.* Localization of subclinical ictal activity by functional magnetic resonance imaging: correlation with invasive monitoring. *Am. Neurol.* 1995, 38, 618

64 Woods, R., Mazziota, J. and Cherry, S. Automated algorithm for aligning tomographic images. II Cross-modality MRI-PET registration. *J. Comput. Assist. Tomogr.* 1992 16, 620

65 Frahm, J., Merboldt, K.D., Hänicke, W. *et al.* Brain or vein - Oxygenation or flow? On Signal Physiology in functional MRI of human brain activation. *NMR in biomedicine* 1994, 7, 45

SPECT in Neurology and Psychiatry, edited by P.P. De Deyn, R.A. Dierckx, A. Alavi and B.A. Pickut
© 1997 John Libbey & Company Ltd, pp. 547-560

Integration of Brain Imaging Techniques

Chapter
64

G. Lucignani, G. Rizzo, C. Messa, M.C. Gilardi and F. Fazio

Introduction

The combined use of several biomedical imaging techniques (BITs), including X-ray computed tomography (X-ray CT), magnetic resonance imaging (MRI), single photon emission tomography (SPECT), and positron emission tomography (PET), represents a powerful strategy to probe cerebral functions for research and clinical purposes, since the integration of multi-modal information allows us to overcome intrinsic limitations and to enhance the specific potential of each BIT. The analysis of information obtained by several BITs is required to achieve a more complete comprehension of pathophysiological mechanisms, and to generate a more accurate definition of the clinical picture. This strategy is based first on the sequential and chronologically ordered acquisition of information by different BITs, and second on the use of registration techniques to integrate the data. Different information is represented in a customised spatial reference system that is specific for each subject being examined, to obtain a point by point correspondence of each anatomical structure present in the different images.

This paper will review: a) the technical possibilities offered by each MRI, X-ray CT, SPECT, PET; b) the registration techniques currently used for the integration of multimodal cerebral images; c) the main reasons for pursuing the integration of multi-modal information. Some of the clinical applications of the integrated use of the various BITs will be discussed.

Imaging techniques

Emission tomography

Emission tomography requires the administration of a radiopharmaceutical to the subject examined, either intravenously or by inhalation, followed by the measurement of the radioactivity distributed in the body by external detection of the emitted gamma rays. Radionuclides that decay emitting gamma rays (e.g. ^{123}I, ^{99m}Tc) are used for single photon emission tomography (SPECT), while those that decay emitting positrons (^{11}C, ^{15}O, ^{13}N, ^{18}F) are used for positron emission tomography (PET). The detection of 511keV gamma rays, originated by the positron annihilation events detected by PET, permits quantitation of radioactivity concentration. PET instrumentation, based on coincidence detection circuitry, is more complex and costly than SPECT equipment. The availability of radiotracers for the *in vivo* assessment of biochemical, physiological, and pharmacological processes, is another major advantage of

INB-CNR, University of Milan, Scientific Institute H. San Raffaele, Via Olgettina 60, I 20132, Milan, Italy

PET over SPECT, but the short half-life of the positron emitters (of the order of seconds or minutes) makes the presence of a cyclotron mandatory in the proximity of the PET scanner, thus increasing the cost and limiting the diffusion of PET, as compared with SPECT.

PET allows the quantitative assessment of cerebral haemodynamics (regional blood flow, blood volume, cerebral oxygen extraction and consumption) by use of ^{15}O-labelled tracers. Cerebral perfusion can be assessed also by SPECT using ^{99m}Tc or ^{123}I labelled tracers, which cross the blood-brain barrier and are retained in the brain tissue in proportion to regional blood flow.

The tracer most commonly used for PET studies of cerebral metabolism is $[^{18}F]$-fluorodeoxyglucose $([^{18}F]FDG)$, for quantification of regional glucose metabolism. Cerebral protein synthesis can also be assessed with PET and ^{13}N or ^{11}C labelled amino acids. Both these variables cannot be assessed with SPECT. Several PET and SPECT tracers are also available for the examination of various neurotransmitter systems.

Image quality in PET and SPECT results from a compromise between spatial resolution, affecting the ability of the technique to discriminate small structures, and count density, which depends on the system detection efficiency and regulates the levels of noise in the image. PET scanners consist of multiple rings of detectors, to provide multiple image slices of the organ under examination. Improvement in spatial resolution is the result of reducing the size and increasing the number of detectors in a ring. In most of the presently available commercial scanners, the detection system consists of high density bismuth germanate scintillators. These are organised in blocks of small detectors (e.g. a matrix of 8x8 crystals, 4x4x30mm each), allowing a good balance between crystal size, crystal/photomultipliers ratio, energy spectroscopic characteristics to be achieved. Spatial resolution of the order of 4 mm is achieved in current generation PET systems, very close to the intrinsic limits of the technique, imposed by the finite range of the positrons' path in matter and by the gamma rays deviation from 180° opposite paths following the annihilation event.

Current generation PET tomographs consist of up to 24 adjacent detector rings, covering an axial field of view of 15 cm or more. This multi-slice configuration allows the study of a whole organ in a single acquisition and the three-dimensional assessment of the radioactivity distribution. Furthermore, the axial extension of these tomographs has allowed a significant increase in detection efficiency, by the development of three-dimensional (3D) acquisition methods, made possible by increasing the axial acceptance angle. This increase

of sensitivity by a factor of 5 or more, allows a reduction of noise in the image, a reduction in the amount of radioactivity administered to the patient, or alternatively a reduction in the acquisition time.

Temporal resolution in PET, defined as the minimum acquisition time, notwithstanding the increase of detection efficiency, remains of the order of seconds/minutes to obtain acceptable noise levels in the image.

Rotating gamma-camera systems, consisting of a large crystal of NaI(Tl), mounted on a gantry to allow 360° rotation around the patient, continue to be the instrument of choice for SPECT. This is because of the relatively affordable costs and universal use to image all organs of the body either in planar or tomographic mode. The axial extension of the detector allows coverage of the whole organ under study in a single acquisition. Using this device, spatial resolution of approximately 1 cm is obtained with a radius of rotation of 10 cm, which means making the gamma camera rotate very close to the head. Improvement in detection efficiency is obtained by multidetector SPECT systems, which increase the detection volume around the patient. Three-headed gamma camera systems are nowadays widely available, representing a more versatile device than other dedicated brain tomographic scanners, with an increase in detection efficiency by a factor of 3 when compared with single-headed cameras. A slight improvement in spatial resolution is also obtained.

It should be noted that detection efficiency in PET is orders of magnitude higher than in SPECT, because collimation systems, filtering the radiations reaching the detectors, are not required. PET is more powerful, complex, and expensive than SPECT, but recent technological improvements make SPECT more and more competitive and more widely available than PET[1-3]. Notwithstanding the increasing interest for the clinical use of PET, the main field of application of PET is research. SPECT, which is nowadays widely used for clinical purposes, will offer further opportunities for research.

Magnetic resonance imaging

Magnetic resonance imaging is one of the most powerful BIT, and permits the production of tomographic images in any plane of the organ under examination. Various atomic nuclei, particularly the proton nucleus of the hydrogen atoms (^{1}H), which when placed in a strong and homogeneous magnetic field, align themselves with this field and reach a thermal equilibrium. The proton nuclei precess about the applied magnetic field at a characteristic frequency, but at a random phase (or orientation) with respect to each other. The application of a brief radio frequency (RF) electromagnetic pulse disturbs the equilibrium and introduces a transient phase coherence to the nuclear magnetisation that can, in turn, be detected as a radio signal (MR signal). By forming a magnetic field that varies spatially, it is possible to separate the signal from different locations according to frequency. The use of Fourier transform allows us to separate the different frequencies of the MR signals to produce an image.

Besides the density of nuclei, in particular the proton density in the case of ^1H, two fundamental temporal parameters are used to describe the MR signal: the longitudinal relaxation rate, T_1, and the transversal relaxation rate, T_{2*}. T_1 is the rate at which the nuclei placed in a magnetic field exponentially approach thermal equilibrium, after the pulse. In biological tissues, the proton T_1 is quite long: from tens of milliseconds to seconds. Differences in the T_1s of tissues are one of the primary methods used in clinical MRI. T_{2*} describes the rate at which the MR signal decays due to a loss of the phase coherence of the proton nuclei. The observed signal decay rate, T_{2*}, generally ranges from a few milliseconds to tens of milliseconds and also the T_{2*} signal decay rates differ among body tissues.

These two relaxation rates vary with the strength of the applied magnetic field, changing the contrast of different tissues in the MR images. In particular this contrast increases with the strength of the field, and proportionally increases the frequency of the RF pulse. This leads to an upper limit of the field strength for human studies, imposed by radio-frequency penetration. Commercial scanners available today for clinical use range from 0.5 Tesla to 3 Tesla, while there are only a few 4 Tesla machines for research studies on humans.

Within these limits, the major advantage of MRI over conventional radiological techniques is that MRI does not imply the use of ionising radiation and no biological hazard is known. MRI spatial resolution is very high, of the order of submillimetres and allows very detailed structural images to be obtained. The anatomical resolution of MRI images in terms of contrast of tissues with different characteristics (as for example in pathological conditions) can be further improved by using proper sequences of image acquisition. Moreover, due to recent hardware and software developments, it has been possible to implement fast and ultra-fast MRI sequences. Fast sequences allow the implementation of three-dimensional acquisition techniques, providing detailed volumetric visualisation of the body district under

study within a time frame of the order of few minutes. Ultra-fast MRI sequences, such as the Echo-Planar Imaging (EPI) technique, allow a very high temporal resolution (of the order of tens of milliseconds). It has been shown how MRI can be used to map, together with the brain anatomy, human brain activity[4-6].

MRI developments, particularly those involving ultra-fast imaging, have made possible the implementation of techniques by which activity in the human brain can be observed non-invasively with a spatial resolution of a few millimetres and temporal resolution of less than a second. These new techniques, generally termed as functional MRI (fMRI), have already led to the assessment of processes related to neuronal function.

The increases in the signal detected seem to exceed increases in oxygen consumption, and depend largely on blood volume and oxygen concentration in blood. Since the oxygen content of venous blood increases during brain activation, there is an increase in the MR signal, due to the paramagnetic effect of deoxyhaemoglobin as compared with the diamagnetic properties of oxyhaemoglobin. Thus, with fMRI it is possible to examine the locus of the brain activity while a subject was performing a specific task in a completely non-invasive way with a high degree of reliability. Furthermore, the very high temporal resolution of EPI technique can be coupled with the high spatial resolution of conventional MRI to locate precisely the locus of activation, giving fMRI an expanding role in the understanding of brain function.

X-ray computed tomography

X-ray computed tomography (X-ray CT) is a widely available BIT, which provides highly detailed diagnostic information. X-ray CT instrumentation has gone through a fast technological evolution since the appearance of the first generation X-ray CT scanner in 1973. In the X-ray CT imaging devices of first generation, a narrow beam of X-rays was used to scan a patient while a radiation detector on the opposite side of the patient's body was used to detect the transmitted X-rays. By a combination of translations and rotation movements of the X-rays tube-detector system, these 'transmission' measurements were repeated at different positions and orientations and a linear/angular sampling of the attenuation of the beam across the patient was obtained. X-ray CT data are processed by a computer based reconstruction algorithm to generate images of attenuation coefficients across the anatomical plane defined by the scanning X-ray beam.

Subsequently, fan-shaped X-ray beams were introduced instead of pencil beams, so that multiple measurements of X-ray transmission across the tomographic section could be made simultaneously (second generation X-ray CT scanners). A reduction in scanning time to 20-60 s was possible. Third and fourth generation scanners are based on pure rotational movements of the X-ray tube and detectors array, and of the X-ray tube within a stationary circular array of hundreds of detectors, respectively. Scanning time has been further reduced to times as short as 1 s. Short scanning time diminishes the probability of motion artefacts, thus improving image quality.

More recently, continuous rotation of the gantry has become possible by the use of slip ring technology (connection of the tube voltage cables through sliding contact). Using this technology, the X-ray tube can rotate while the patient's table moves without stopping through the X-ray CT gantry, resulting in a spiral acquisition trajectory. The spiral X-ray CT technique presents several potential advantages over the conventional slice-by-slice acquisition mode. A large volume of the patient's body can be axially examined without gaps between contiguous slices, in very short time (e. g. up to 50 cm in less than 1 min); the continuous axial sampling improves the accuracy in the detection of small lesions and the quality of three dimensional reconstruction; this further reduction in acquisition time reduces artefacts due to patient motion and increases patient throughput. Current generation CT scanners are characterised by spatial resolution values as low as 0.25 mm.

Comparative considerations

In the evaluation of the potentials of each imaging modality, whether for scientific research or in the process of defining an optimal diagnostic protocol, one must consider some essential physical features of the instruments available including: 1) spatial resolution; 2) contrast resolution; 3) temporal resolution; 4) short term repeatability of the examination.

At the present time, the highest spatial resolution is provided by X-ray CT and MRI. This feature is of obvious importance in the examination of any organ, but in the examination of brain morphology and function it becomes essential for differentiating contiguous yet distinct anatomo-functional structures. Furthermore, poor spatial resolution results in loss of quantitative accuracy due to partial volume effect in emission tomography, and the assessment of tracer kinetics in regions of interest containing mixtures of different tissues may result in gross errors if functional heterogeneity is overlooked[7,8].

The contrast resolution of MRI is superior to that of X-ray CT and can be further enhanced, both in MRI and X-ray CT by use of contrast agents and in MRI by use

of different acquisition sequences[5]. In nuclear medicine, an improvement in signal-to-noise ratio can be achieved by optimising the instrumentation performance, the choice of the tracer and the time of acquisition, by allowing enough time for the uptake of the tracer in the target organ and for its systemic clearance, i.e. by taking advantage of the kinetics and biodistribution of the tracers used. Temporal resolution may be irrelevant when studying non-dynamic processes, such as brain morphology, when the subject examined is collaborative, whereas it becomes crucial in the examination of dynamic processes such as during brain activation studies and when the subjects examined cannot remain motionless.

The time necessary for SPECT and PET studies is dependent upon the dose of tracer administered, in order to achieve sufficient counting statistics in the images. In SPECT, time resolution is of the order of minutes, and it is shorter for acquisitions carried out with dedicated instruments than with general purpose rotating gamma cameras[1,2,9]. In PET the increase in detection efficiency by the 3D acquisition modality allows a reduction in the acquisition time, which remains of the order of seconds.

Spiral X-ray CT technology has improved temporal resolution (less than 1sec/tomographic slice), significantly reducing motion artefacts in volumetric images. The temporal resolution of MRI is achieved both with hardware and software development, and time required for scanning ranges from the few minutes of conventional spin-echo sequences, to the 30-100 ms of echo-planar imaging (EPI) techniques[4].

While X-ray CT and nuclear medicine studies are limited by radiation exposure, and in nuclear medicine also by the time necessary for decay of the tracers employed, fundamental studies on the dosimetry of MRI are still very limited, however, the results of the studies available so far do not indicate any limitation in the repeatability of the MRI examination[10].

Registration techniques
Several registration techniques have been implemented for the integration of multi-modal biomedical images relative to the same subject. In fact, in each tomographic scanner, the organ under examination is represented as a volume in a spatial coordinate system which is specific for that particular acquisition device. Registration of biomedical images obtained with different tomographic instruments is achieved when a point by point correspondence of the same anatomical functional structures in the different multi-modal studies is established. For this, the different image

volumes must be remapped into the same spatial reference system. Registration techniques are used for the estimation of the geometric transformation parameters among the various studies: a 3x3 rotation matrix, a 3x1 translation vector, and a scaling factor.

Fiducial markers

A very common strategy for image registration is based on the use of fiducial markers, whose coordinates in the two tomographic studies allow the determination of the registration parameters. The markers are in general point or line sources made of selected radioactive or contrast agents, visible in the different imaging modalities. They are either located directly on the patient's skin[11] or fixed to a device used for patient positioning[12]. The coordinates of the markers in the two studies to be registered are used as input in a minimisation algorithm, which estimates the best geometric transformation to overlap the markers and achieve the spatial correspondence of the two image volumes[13].

Registration methods based on such external markers have a widespread application, being independent of the imaging modalities to be matched and the alteration in the image pattern, induced by the pathology. Registration accuracy is strictly related to the precision by which markers are repositioned in the different tomographic studies. The main limitation of this approach is the need for a predefined acquisition protocol, requiring special care in the fixation and filling of the markers.

Image feature matching

A different approach to the registration problem relies on the consideration that in two multi-modal studies of the same organ, it is possible to extract homologous geometrical features, relative to the anatomical district under examination. If these features contain the spatial information needed for correctly identifying the spatial reference systems in which the tomographic images are represented, matching of the equivalent features results in matching the multimodal image volumes.

Based on this principle, several methods have been proposed, differing from each other principally in the class of homologous features chosen for extraction and/or for the registration algorithm, by which the features themselves are overlapped. Thus, these different methods present different performances in terms of registration accuracy, computer time, suitability for clinical use, dependence on the image alterations induced by pathology.

A method, assuming anatomical point markers as matching features, has been proposed by Evans et al.[14] to correlate PET and MRI cerebral images in normal subjects. In the images to be correlated, few homologous cortical and subcortical landmarks are recognised in order to identify two sets of corresponding 3D points.

A strategy that allows a retrospective registration of MRI, X-rays CT and PET cerebral images has been developed by Pelizzari et al.[15]. In this method, equivalent surfaces corresponding to the external surface of the head are identified in each of the two studies. One surface, named 'head' and represented as a set of contours, is used as reference, the second one, named 'hat' and represented by a set of points, is fitted to the first one. For each hat point, the intersection with the head surface of a ray from the transformed hat point to the centroid of the head model is evaluated. A non-linear least squares algorithm is used, which minimises the mean square of such 'hat-head' distances. The allowed class of transformations includes rigid body rotation and translation, and linear scaling along three orthogonal axes, which accounts for uncertainty in the scan pixel sizes and for possible linear distortion in MRI.

However, in general, these techniques are based on image processing methods that can be performed off-line and they do not present constraints during acquisitions. For this reason, they have the common advantage, with respect to the use of external markers, of allowing retrospective registrations, which is a relevant feature for a wide clinical use. On the other hand, a limitation of this approach to image registration is that these methods can be applied only to those imaging modalities in which several homologous anatomical structures can consistently be identified in the studies to be correlated.

Pixel by pixel analysis

Fully automated registration techniques that are based on the pixel-by-pixel analysis of the image characteristics have also been proposed. These techniques rely on the hypothesis that the organ under examination shows similar information characteristics in two independent tomographic scans. This means that pixel values in the two studies to be matched are strongly correlated. For this reason, these methods seem to be very powerful in particular for the registration of studies acquired with the same acquisition modality (i.e. in PET follow-up, test-retest and activation studies)[16,17].

An extension of this approach to the registration of multi-modal studies, in particular MRI and PET, has been also implemented in Woods *et al.*[18]. The hypothesis of pixel value similarity is not verified in this case and some modifications have to be introduced. In particular, the MRI study has to be preprocessed by deleting the structures which are not imaged by PET (e.g. scalp, skull and meninges) and by segmenting MRI data into separate components on a thresholding basis. The algorithm minimises the uniformity of the PET pixel values within each of this partition, by iteratively minimising a weighted average of the standard deviation of the PET pixels. The computation time is quite variable and depends on a wide number of parameters, such as pixel size, number of slices, counting statistics and others. Usually a time of 30-40 min is required for PET/MRI registration, with a standard setting of the parameters. An extra time must be considered in the manual editing of the MRI study to eliminate the structure external to the brain.

The procedure described above allows us to register MRI and PET studies with a residual error estimated to be less than 3 mm. However, in the presence of pathology resulting in altered image pattern, a careful use of this method has to be carried out, by verifying that the presence of a structural lesion does not cause residual misalignment after registration of the two studies.

Integration and joined analysis of multi-modal images

The information acquired with the various imaging modalities is often complementary; therefore, it is a current procedure to exploit the potential of two or more imaging modalities in order to obtain more accurate information and new insight on the status and function of an organ. The collation of the information obtained with different modalities is usually the clinician's task. However, due to developments in the area of biomedical imaging technologies, a new strategy aimed at the synergistic use of the different technologies is evolving. There are at least three main reasons for pursuing the integration of multi-modal information: one is originated by the need to relate radioactive tracers distribution to morphological districts; another is the achievement of tissue characterisation by use of different BITs, the third is in relation to the possibility to improve the informative content of functional studies by use of morphology-based information.

The interpretation of functional images such as those obtained by PET and SPECT can be difficult or even impossible in some cases if the anatomical information provided by X-ray CT or MRI is not available. PET and SPECT functional images are in fact representing physiological and biochemical processes, and they do not intrinsically show the underlying morphology. Extreme situations are found in neuroreceptor studies and in tumour detection, i.e. in those cases in which the radioactivity is distributed in discrete areas without apparent relation to an indentifiable anatomical structure. The point by point correspondence of anatomical and functional images, as obtained by a registration technique, allows the unambiguous association of functional measurements to morphological districts. An immediate benefit of this approach is in assisting the quantitative and semiquantitative analysis of nuclear medicine images, carried out by the definition of regions of interest corresponding to actual anatomical functional structures.

The distribution of contrast media and tracers is determined by a number of variables intrinsic to the organ, structure, and tissue examined, either normal or pathological. The integrity of the structure itself and of the blood-brain barrier, along with the rate of blood flow, of metabolism of different substrates, the expression of receptors, as well as the alterations of all the above, contribute to image formation. By combining the information obtained with the different methods and tracer substances, as well as biochemical information obtained with MRS, it is possible not only to distinguish the structural components of the nervous system, but also to characterise pathological tissues based on the assessment of a unique combination of several biochemical features.

Furthermore an anatomical functional correlation can be applied for a more accurate quantification of functional parameters. Morphological data can be included within the tomographic reconstruction process to improve signal/noise ratio and spatial resolution. Underestimation of radioactivity concentration, resulting from partial volume effect, can be compensated by knowledge of shape and size of the particular anatomical region under examination. Quantification of functional images is affected by the presence of etherogeneous tissues, characterised by different metabolic or flow rate (e.g. grey matter, white matter, cerebrospinal fluid in cerebral images). Quantification accuracy can thus be improved by knowledge of the regional tissue composition. This information is achieved by segmentation into homogeneous tissue components of anatomical images, such as MRI, characterised by high spatial definition and contrast. As an example, the measurement of the degree of cerebral atrophy assessed by MRI could be used for correcting the related apparent reduction of functional activity (blood flow, metabolism) assessed by PET or SPECT.

Matching radioactive tracers distribution and morphological districts

Under several circumstances the pattern of distribution of radioactive tracers does not resemble any known morphological structure. This is, for example, the case of the distribution of a tracer either following alterations of the blood-brain barrier permeability, or within a lesion containing different tissue components. This is often the case encountered in the examination of patients with brain tumours. Several SPECT and PET methods, based on the use of ^{201}Tl, [^{18}F]FDG, [^{11}C]methionine and monoclonal antibodies, as well as numerous other radioisotopic methods, are currently used for the localisation and characterisation of tumours. Some of the tracers used do not cross the blood-brain barrier and can therefore distribute only in areas of altered permeability, as in the case of ^{201}Tl[9] and monoclonal antibodies[19], whereas other substances undergo a differential uptake in normal and pathological tissues, as in the case of [^{18}F]FDG[20,21]. These patterns of distribution may generate either 'hot spots' or 'cold spots', or a mixture of the two. In any case there is the need to match a specific pattern of distribution with a specific tissue component, in most cases without a dependable anatomical reference as provided by SPECT and PET.

A correct spatial relation between radioactive tracer distribution and underlying anatomical structure may be difficult even within a normal region. This may occur when within one structure there are morphologically indistinguishable components that are different among each other with respect to the behaviour of the tracer used, because of distinct neurochemical features. This is a problem encountered when assessing the distribution of tracers used to probe the neurotransmitter systems.

One particular case is represented by the localisation of functions in the human brain. This task has been based for a long time on the correlation between the *in vivo* observation of neurological and neuropsychological deficits, and the detection at autopsy of cerebral lesions. While destructive lesions can cause a functional deficit, irritative lesions are at the basis of pathologically enhanced functions. Both types of lesion have become more identifiable non-invasively *in vivo* by the advent of X-ray CT, MRI and emission tomography. Although the visualisation of lesions with X-ray CT or MRI has represented a major event for the *in vivo* explanation of neurological deficits, these systems cannot always be adequate for the full understanding of cerebral function, i.e. processes that require the integrity of neuronal circuits. Thus, the relationship between neuronal activity and cerebral metabolism and haemodynamics has become the basis for studies with PET and SPECT of neuronal circuits under resting conditions.

Methods for the measurement of blood flow and metabolism during the execution of defined tasks have increased the number of tools available for the assessment of cerebral functional activity. These methods have made possible the definition of neural circuits and pathways involved in sensory-motor activity, attention, memory, word processing, visual recognition, as well as the examination of the recovery of brain functional activity after focal damage. The use of tracers labelled with short-lived isotopes allows us to perform a complete activation study, i.e. baseline and activation, within the same study session by use of PET, e.g. with ^{15}O labelled water or carbon dioxide[22], or with radioactive xenon and SPECT[23]. The complexity of these techniques and their cost has triggered the development of alternative techniques based on the use of SPECT and chemical microspheres labelled with ^{99m}Tc, and on the performance of the baseline and activation studies at least 24 h apart for the decay of the isotope. A method has recently been validated for motor activation studies that requires the administration of two doses of the tracer, in proportion 1:3, for the baseline and activation study, respectively[24].

Activation studies have also been performed by acquiring MR images of the brain in rapid succession[25]. These studies show variations of MR signal intensity in positions corresponding to focal areas of activation, related to the localised increase in blood flow in these areas, as shown by PET or SPECT. One area that appears particularly amenable for neuroimaging studies is epilepsy. For the routine clinical evaluation of patients with epilepsy, the combination of interictal and ictal studies of perfusion provide the most complete information[26-30]. For this purpose, the use of SPECT with chemical microspheres is very convenient since it allows us to obtain an image of the perfusion at the time of the tracer injection, i.e. during seizures, by performing the SPECT study at the end of the seizures. Assessment of perfusion and metabolism is used by some surgeons in the presurgical evaluation of patients with refractory partial epilepsy to confirm the uniqueness of the focus and its location[31]. This practice, however, has not yet gained widespread acceptance and is considered in many cases insufficient for surgical intervention without stereo-EEG with depth electrodes. A high sensitivity of proton-MRS and proton-MRS imaging (chemical shift imaging) in the detection of both the location and extension of the epileptic focus in patients with intractable temporal lobe epilepsy has been demonstrated[32].

Tissue characterisation

Tissue characterisation is substantially based on the assessment of the chemical features intrinsic to the system under examination. The distribution of contrast agents to be used with X-ray CT in the extracellular fluid space is relatively non-specific, and the search for agents targeted to specific systems or to disease has not made substantial progress as yet. On the other hand excellent results for tissue characterisation can be obtained with emission tomography and MR spectroscopy (MRS)[33,34]. Emission tomography and MRS allow the *in vivo* assessment of biochemical variables directly in the organ under examination. By use of these techniques, it is possible to overcome the limitations due to the indirect assessment of metabolic processes by measurements of the concentrations of metabolites and drugs in the body fluids. Emission tomography and MRS provide different yet complementary information. By using emission tomography, it is possible to quantify the concentration of radioactively labelled substances present in the organ examined in nanomolar amounts. However, emission tomography allows only the measurement of the total concentration of radioactive molecules, and it does not distinguish among the various chemical species that may be labelled, i.e. neither the precursor nor any of the possible labelled products. Therefore strategies must be developed that ensure that the radioactivity measured at the time of the study is contained exclusively in the precursor and/or in the products specific to the chemical reaction to be assayed. The labelled precursor must be so selected that its chemical transformations are limited only to the pathway under study[35,36]. Additional problems are encountered with SPECT, as compared with PET, due to the use of tracers labeled with radioactive isotopes that are not naturally occurring in the body.

In contrast with emission tomography, MRS permit us to distinguish the different metabolites formed following the administration of a molecule, although the accurate quantitation of metabolites concentration is not feasible directly with conventional acquisition sequences and the exact localisation of the signal source may be difficult[34]. Moreover, the relatively low sensitivity of MRS is the crucial limiting factor and non-physiological amounts of exogenous tracer substance must be used, in some cases, to obtain a detectable signal[37]. Three brain metabolites can currently be identified with proton-MRS: N-acetyl-aspartate, creatine, and choline. It appears, therefore, that MRS is most suitable for the evaluation of biochemical processes occurring in the brain[33], at different steps along the metabolic pathway, that lead to the formation of relatively large amounts of product,

even without the administration of exogenous tracer substances.

Emission tomography is amenable instead for the assessment of biochemical processes by use of exogenous substances in tracer amounts, when the system studied cannot be perturbed during the study, and when the process examined does not lead to the accumulation of sufficient amounts of product to be measured by MRS. The use of MRS and emission tomography for *in vivo* studies of neurochemistry also appears to be limited by the poor resolution of both techniques. With respect to the clinical use of these techniques, emission tomography has been widely used for over a decade for the assessment of neurochemical variables useful in the diagnostic work-up of patients with cerebral tumours, cerebrovascular diseases, epilepsy and numerous other pathological states[38]. The potentials of MRS in the examination of the neurological diseases are still largely unexploited[33].

With respect to the clinical application of the principle of tissue characterisation, this is a fundamental requirement in the diagnostic work-up of brain tumours. For the past two decades it has been based on morphological imaging, first with X-ray CT and more recently also with MRI, which is becoming the primary diagnostic method for its lower negative rate when compared with X-ray CT[39-41]. However, X-ray CT and MRI remain largely complementary modalities. In the presence of clinical symptoms leading to the suspicion of tumour, however, negative X-ray CT should be promptly followed by MRI for the detection of possible tumours. X-ray CT remains superior to MRI for the evaluation of bone lesions in proximity of the tumour and calcificacion within the tumour. The *in vivo* biochemical imaging of tumours is best achieved by emission tomography. The usefulness of [^{18}F]FDG in the differentiation between tumour recurrence and radionecrosis has been demonstrated and is widely accepted[21,42,43]. The possibility of assessing, in sequence, one or more different biochemical and physiological variables of the tumour, including blood flow, oxygen and glucose consumption, protein synthesis, pH, and receptor density, is unique to PET, and this feature may become extremely useful when these measurements are part of defined diagnostic protocols. In the meantime other imaging modalities with SPECT and monoclonal antibodies are attracting increasing interest, in particular those aimed at the signal amplification by tumour pre-targeting techniques[19].

By use of MRS, in particular proton-MRS, biochemical variables have been assessed in cerebral tumours in man. This technique is very sensitive for the detection of derangements from normal metabolism that are typical of neoplasms. A decrease in the concentration of N-acetyl-aspartate is a common finding in cerebral gliomas due to the neuronal concentration of this metabolite exclusively in neurons. Also, the presence of a relative increase of choline and lactate characterises tumours with high metabolic activity. However, despite its high sensitivity, the specificity of proton-MRS in the differentiation of other types of cerebral tumours is relatively poor.

The non-invasive evaluation of patients presenting with cerebrovascular disorders (CVD) by imaging techniques relies mainly on X-ray CT[44]. Other modalities include MRI, SPECT perfusion scintigraphy and PET based studies of local haemodynamics and energy metabolism. It has been shown that MRI is superior to X-ray CT for localisation of lesions in CVD. One advantage of MRI is that it allows non-invasive angiography[45], useful in the assessment of the cerebral circulation in stroke patients. X-ray CT is used, starting at the time of the stroke onset, for the differential diagnosis between cerebral ischaemia and haemorrhage, and for defining the location and size of the lesion. In most cases, however, X-ray CT becomes positive only after several hours of ischaemic stroke. Following the initial diagnostic phase, the sequential examination of stroke patients with X-ray CT or MRI allows the staging of the lesion and helps in the therapeutical planning and follow-up. In the case of transient ischaemic attacks (TIA), the observation of morphological damage is infrequent, yet possible, as a result of previous ischaemic episodes. During a TIA the defect of perfusion can be demonstrated by a SPECT examination. The perfusion defect may persist also after the functional recovery indicating a condition of critical perfusion[46,47].

The concurrent assessment of blood flow, oxygen extraction fraction and metabolism, key variables in stroke patients, is only possible with PET. However, PET studies of cerebral haemodynamics and energy metabolism in the acute phase of stroke are not practical in large populations and, for this reason PET cannot be considered a diagnostic tool in these patients[48]. At the time of the stroke onset, therefore, the determination of perfusion by SPECT with technetium-labelled tracers may be the only useful measurable variable. The predictive value of SPECT perfusion studies on patient outcome and the relation between the results of SPECT perfusion studies, X-ray CT, and cerebral angiography has been demonstrated[49]. This observation can have a direct impact on therapeutical planning, one of the most relevant issues in acute stroke patients. The treatment must begin as early as possible, when signs of parenchymal damage are not yet visible with X-ray CT and difficult to interpret

using MRI. At this stage of the stroke, the assessment by SPECT of the extent and severity of the perfusion deficit may be crucial to carry out proper therapy, including therapy with thrombolytic drugs that requires a very careful planning due to the attendant risks. The effects of the thrombolytic therapy can be monitored, if necessary, by repeated SPECT perfusion studies. The definition of the anatomically versus the functionally impaired area in the early phases of stroke is very useful to determine the patient's prognosis[50]. This is in agreement with the fact that by combining X-ray CT and SPECT blood flow it is possible to determine the area of penumbra, in view of therapeutic protocols. The evaluation of vascular reserve in patients with chronic ischaemia[51] also requires an intra and intermodality registration technique. In fact, SPECT data obtained with different tracers (i.e. blood flow and blood volume tracers) or in different condition (i.e. before and after acetazolimide) have to be registered to correctly identify the area of abnormal perfusion. The tissue characterisation of the functionally impaired area is also possible by comparing SPECT data with MRS to achieve information on tissue viability.

The development of new MRI acquisition procedures and sequences with high temporal resolution, in particular EPI, has made possible the imaging with MRI of physiological processes such as blood microcirculation, i.e. perfusion, and the evaluation of molecular mobility, i.e. molecular diffusion[4,6]. One area that is specific to MRI is that aimed at the evaluation of molecular diffusion; this area may become of relevance in the future for tissue characterisation in pathological processes[52-54].

Also the assessment of pharmacological features is of particular relevance for the characterisation of structural and functional components of the nervous system. The assessment of neuropharmacological variables can be based on two different strategies. The first is the administration of pharmacological doses of drugs under investigation and the measurement by imaging techniques, most frequently by emission tomography, of variations of local blood flow or metabolism to define the pattern of functional changes induced by the drug[55]. A second strategy is the administration of drugs labelled with radioactive isotopes and the *in vivo* monitoring of the distribution and pharmacokinetics of these tracers[56,57]. In essence, this second strategy allows the *in vivo* definition of the distribution pattern of tracers utilised as specific neuronal markers. This has originated a new form of anatomical imaging and has allowed the visualisation in the brain of specific populations of neurons that express a specific protein on their surface, and thus made it possible to visualise *in vivo* neuronal pathways and projections. Emission tomography-based neuropharmacology has subsequently evolved into a methodology based on experimental procedures and kinetic models used in basic biochemical and pharmacological research[58-61]. This methodology is now being applied to measure neuropharmacological variables, such as regional receptor densities, alterations in receptor occupancy from endogenous neurotransmitters and exogenous drugs, and receptor plasticity[62-64].

Because of the very low concentration of receptors in the brain, their imaging requires the use of tracer substances that, once administered in very low amounts to avoid pharmacological effects, can still bind in a concentration that is sufficient to provide an externally detectable signal. This goal can be achieved with emission tomography by the use of tracers with high specific activity, but it is virtually impossible, at the present time, with MR. The number of radioactively labelled compounds produced for the assessment of several neuropharmacological variables has increased continuously over the past decade since images of brain receptors were produced with SPECT and with PET[35,58-66]. Significant advances in this area have occurred leading to interesting progress in the development of SPECT based pharmacology. The tracers developed for SPECT include substances for the assay of D_1 and D_2 dopaminergic receptors, central and peripheral benzodiazepine receptors, S_1 and S_2 serotoninergic, muscarinic and opiate receptors. Only some of the tracers have also been tested in man. However, it is really in the area of PET, rather than SPECT, that most of the efforts of the neuropharmacological research with emission tomography have been concentrated. Not only have many of the tracers developed for PET been tested, but they have also been used for the evaluation of patients with neurological and psychiatric disorders. Indeed correct design and application of experimental procedures and kinetic analyses are needed not only to understand basic issues in neuropharmacology, but also to use emission tomography for clinical purposes. Some physiological and pathological processes can be studied in living human subjects only by PET, since quantitation of dynamic processes of uptake and release of tracer can be measured only with PET. However, even with the limited number of tracers available, the potentials of SPECT as a tool for the *in vivo* visualisation of neuronal pathways and projections have not been exploited yet for the examination of large populations, a goal that appears more suitable for SPECT than for PET.

Improvement of functional data analysis by using morphology-based information

This is a relatively new area of research and is aimed at the correlation of anatomical and functional information, to improve the accuracy of the measures of functional variables. For this purpose morphological data can be included within the tomographic reconstruction process of SPECT and PET, to improve the signal/noise ratio and the spatial resolution. Underestimation of radioactivity concentration, resulting from partial volume effect can be offset with knowledge of the shape and size of the anatomical region under examination[7].

The presence of functional tissue heterogeneity, due to relative differences of blood flow, metabolism, receptor density etc., can affect the quantification of such variables[8]. Thus, the accuracy of quantitative measures can be improved by the knowledge of the number and type of tissue components within the anatomical region object of the analysis. This information can be pursued by segmentation into homogeneous tissue components, of images with high anatomical contrast, such as MRI images[67].

For example, the measurement of the degree of cerebral atrophy assessed by MRI could be used for correcting the related apparent reduction of metabolic activity and perfusion in PET and SPECT studies, and not only to rule out the presence of a cerebral lesions (e.g. cerebrovascular disorders, hydrocephalus, subdural haematoma or tumours) that may in some cases determine the occurrence of cognitive impairment similar to that observed in dementia.

In a number of cases of dementia associated disorders the diagnosis based on clinical evaluation is questionable, in particular in the early stages of Alzheimer's disease (AD), and additional information is often sought from neuroimaging techniques. X-ray CT and MRI may contribute to the definition of the presence and degree of cerebral atrophy or cerebral lesions that may in some cases determine the occurrence of cognitive impairment similar to that observed in dementia[68]. However, the use of methods of morphological imaging may often be inconclusive for the diagnosis of dementia, since the atrophy that can be observed is not specific to the disease; the assessment of cerebral metabolism and blood flow with emission tomography has been shown to be useful in the evaluation of demented patients, particularly in the early phase of probable Alzheimer's disease[67,69-77].

Considerations

The ultimate goal of diagnostic imaging procedures performed in patients with neurological symptoms is the identification of the abnormal morphological and functional patterns that correlate with the symptoms. Thus, methods are evaluated on the basis of their diagnostic sensitivity and specificity. The ideal diagnostic method is rapid, inexpensive, non-invasive and accurate. Currently X-ray CT and MRI are the diagnostic methods of first choice in all neurological diseases. X-ray CT is the technique of first choice for the evaluation of patients in the acute stage following trauma, ischaemic and haemorrhagic stroke, and subarachnoid haemorrhage. MRI is the technique of choice in the subacute and chronic stage of neurological diseases. Both X-ray CT and MRI are very sensitive techniques, however, in numerous cases signs and symptoms cannot be completely explained by methods of morphological imaging. Functional disturbances can, in fact, precede a detectable morphological damage; therefore, only functional imaging may permit the early assessment of the biochemical damage that precedes the morphological damage, the correlation of functional alterations and clinical symptoms in the absence of a detectable morphological damage, and eventually the explanation of symptoms due to functional abnormalities that occur in areas proximal and remote from the site of the primary lesion, due to neuronal deafferentation. Thus, in several cases it is only with the integration of morphological and functional information that it is possible to achieve a full appreciation of the nature and extent of the damage that produces the clinical symptoms. Depending on the disease under examination, its stage, and the question addressed at the time of the observation, the choice of method(s) may vary. Indeed, the integration of the information specific to each imaging modality might bring a more complete comprehension of pathophysiological mechanisms and generate a more accurate definition of the clinical picture. Although the choice of specific methods to be used in the investigation of patients with neurological diseases must remain, in principle, selective and sequential, new information can be obtained without any further patient involvement at the little additional cost necessary for the fusion of individual images, by correlating and integrating information obtained with different imaging devices and methods. Inasmuch as the synergistic strategy allows us to gain a more complete understanding of any given physiological, pharmacological or pathological process, it could represent the basis for the modification of current diagnostic procedures. The synergistic use of the available biomedical technologies is also crucial for an effective diagnostic process and economic use of the available technology; therefore, this is an issue that can have a relevant economical and social impact and that should be considered by the medical equipment manufacturers in targeting and optimising their products.

References

1   Budinger, T.J. Advances in Emission Tomography. *J. Nucl. Med.* 1990, 31, 628

2   Genna, S. and Smith, A.P. The development of ASPECT, an anular single crystal brain camera for high efficiency SPECT. *IEEE Trans. Nucl. Sci.* 1988, NS-35, 654

3   Kouris, K., Jarritt, P.H., Costa, D.C. and Ell, P.J. Physical assessment of the GE/CGR Neurocam and comparison with a single rotating gamma-camera *Eur. J. Nucl. Med.* 1992, 19, 236

4   Stehling, M.K., Turner, R. and Mansfield, P. Echo-planar imaging: magnetic resonance imaging in a fraction of a second. *Science* 1991, 254, 43

5   Gore, J.C. Contrast agents and relaxation effects in 'Magnetic Resonance Imaging of the Brain and Spine', (Ed. S. W. Atlas), Raven Press, New York, USA, 1991, p. 69

6   Turner, R., Le Bihan, D. Moonen, C.T. *et al.* Echo-Planar Time course of MRI cat brain oxygenation changes. *Magn. Res. Med.* 1991, 22, 159

7   Hoffman, E.J. and Phelps, M.E. Positron emission tomography principles and quantitation in 'Positron emission tomography and autoradiography: principles and application for the brain and heart', (Eds. M. Phelps, J. Mazziotta, H. Schelbert), Raven Press, New York, USA, 1986, p. 237

8   Schmidt, K., Lucignani, G., Moresco, R.M. *et al.* Errors introduced by tissue heterogeneity in estimation of local cerebral glucose utilization with current kinetic models of the [^{18}F] fluorodeoxyglucose method. *J. Cereb. Blood Flow Metab.* 1992, 12, 823

9   Kim, K.T, Black, K.L, Marciano, D. *et al.* Thallium-201 SPECT imaging of brain tumours: methods and results. *J. Nucl. Med.* 1990, 31, 965

10 Shellock, F.G. Bioeffects and safety considerations in 'Magnetic Resonance Imaging of the Brain and Spine', (Ed. S. W. Atlas), Raven Press, New York, 1991, p. 87

11 Hawkes, D.J., Hill, D.L.G., Lehmann, E.D. *et al.* in 'Preliminary work on the interpretation of SPECT images with the aid of registered MR images and an MR derived 3D neuro-anatomical atlas', NATO ASI series, SpringerVerlag, 1990, F60, p. 241

12 Bettinardi, V., Scardaoni, R., Gilardi, M.C. *et al.* A new head-holder for patient positioning repositioning and fixation in PET, MR and CT devices. *J. Comput. Assist. Tomogr.* 1991, 15, 886

13 Arun, K.S., Huang T.S. and Blostein, S.D. Least-squares fitting of two 3D point sets. *IEEE Trans. PAMI* 1987, 9, 698

14 Evans, A.C., Marrett, S., Collins, L. and Peters, T.M. Anatomical-functional correlative analysis of the human brain using three dimensional imaging system in 'Medical Imaging III: Image processing', SPEI Press 1989, 1092, p.264.

15 Pelizzari, C.A., Chen, G.T.Y., Spelbring, D.R. *et al.* Accurate Three-Dimensional Registration of CT, PET and/or MR Images of the Brain *J. Comput. Assist. Tomogr.* 1989, 13, 20

16 Hoh, C.K., Dahlbom, M., Harris, G. *et al.* Automated iterative three-dimensional registration of positron emission tomography images. *J. Nucl. Med.* 1993, 34, 2009

17 Woods, R. P., Cherry, S.R. and Mazziotta, J.C. Rapid automated algorithm for aligning and reslicing PET Images *J. Comput. Assist. Tomogr.* 1992, 16, 620

18 Woods, R.P., Mazziotta, J.C. and Cherry, S.R. MRI-PET Registration with automated algorithm *J. Comput. Assist. Tomogr.* 1993, 17, 536

19 Paganelli, G., Magnani, P., Zito, F. *et al.* Pre-targeting immunodetection in glioma patients: tumour localization and single photon emission tomography imaging of [99mTc]PnAO-biotin. *Eur. J. Nucl. Med.* 1994, 21, 314

20 Alavi, A., Dann, R., Chawluk, J. *et al.* Positron emission tomography imaging of regional cerebral glucose metabolism. *Semin. Nucl. Med.* 1986, 16, 2

21 Di Chiro, G., De LaPaz, R.L., Brooks, R.A. *et al.* Glucose utilization of cerebral gliomas measured by [^{18}F] fluorodeoxyglucose and positron emission tomography. *Neurology* 1982, 32, 1323

22 Roland, P.E. and Friberg, L. Localization of cortical areas activated by thinking. *J. Neurophysiol.* 1985, 53, 1219

23 Lassen, N.A, Ingvar, D.H. and Skinoj, E. Brain function and blood flow. *Sci. Am.* 1978, 239, 62

24 Pantano, P., Di Piero, V., Ricci, M. *et al.* Motor stimulation response by technetium-99m hexamethylpropylene amine oxime split-dose method and single photon emission tomography *Eur. J. Nucl. Med.* 1992, 19, 939

25 Belliveau, J.W., Kennedy, D.N., McKinstry, R.C. *et al.* Functional mapping of the human visual cortex by magnetic resonance imaging. *Science* 1991, 254, 716

26 Baldy-Moulinier, M., Lassen, N.A., Engel, J. and Askienazy, S. in 'Focal epilepsy; clinical use of emission tomography', John Libbey & Co. Ltd, London, 1989

27 Duncan, R., Bone, I., Patterson, J. and Hadley, D.M. SPECT in temporal lobe epilepsy: Interictal and postictal studies in 'Current problems in epilepsy (7) Focal Epilepsy; Clinical use of emission tomography', (Ed. M. Baldy-Moulinier, N.A. Lassen, J. Engel Jr, S. Askienazy), John Libbey & Co. Ltd, London, 1989, p.79

28 Habert, M.O., Parietti, L., Lebtahi, R. *et al.* A ^{99m}Tc-HmPAO interictal study in severe partial epilepsies: correlations with anatomical and electrophysiological data in 'Current problems in epilepsy (7) Focal Epilepsy; Clinical use of emission tomography', (Eds. M. Baldy-Moulinier, N.A. Lassen, J. Engel Jr, S. Askienazy), John Libbey & Co. Ltd,

London, UK, 1989, p.197

29 Rowe, C.C, Berkovic, F., Benjamin Sia, S.T. *et al.* Localization of epileptic foci with postictal single photon emission computed tomography. *Ann. Neurol.* 1989, 26, 660

30 Theodore, W H. Epilepsy in 'Clinical Neuroimaging', (Ed. W.H. Theodore), Alan R. Liss Inc., New York, USA, 1988, p. 183

31 Engel, J. The role of neuroimaging in the surgical treatment of epilepsy. *Acta Neurol. Scand.* 1988, 45, 84

32 Matthews, P.M., Andermann, F. and Arnold, D.L. A proton magnetic resonance spectroscopy study of focal epilepsy in humans. *Neurology* 1990, 40, 985

33 Lenkinski, R.E. and Schnall, M.D. MR Spectroscopy and the Biochemical Basis of Neurological Disease in 'Magnetic Resonance Imaging of the Brain and Spine', (Ed. S. W. Atlas), Raven Press, New York, USA, 1991, p.1099

34 Tofts, P. and Wray, S. A critical assessment of methods of measuring metabolite concentrations by NMR spectroscopy. *NMR Biomed.* 1988, 1, 1

35 Huang S.C. and Phelps, M.E. Principles of tracer kinetic modeling in positron emission tomography and autoradiography in 'Positron emission tomography and autoradiography: principles and application for the brain and heart', (Eds. M. Phelps, J. Mazziotta, H. Schelbert), Raven Press, New York, USA, 1986, p. 287

36 Sokoloff, L. Cerebral circulation, energy metabolism, and protein synthesis: general characteristics and principles of measurement in 'Positron emission tomography and autoradiography: principles and application for the brain and heart', (Eds. M. Phelps, J. Mazziotta, H. Schelbert), Raven Press, New York, 1986, p. 1

37 Gadian, D.G. in 'Nuclear Magnetic Resonance and its applications to living systems', Claredon Press, Oxford, UK, 1982

38 Mazziotta, J.C. and Phelps, M.E. Positron emission tomography studies of the brain in 'Positron emission tomography and autoradiography: principles and application for the brain and heart', (Eds. M. Phelps, J. Mazziotta, H. Schelbert), Raven Press, New York, 1986, p. 493

39 Atlas, S.W. Intraaxial brain tumours in 'Magnetic Resonance Imaging of the Brain and Spine', (Ed. S. W. Atlas), Raven Press, New York, USA, 1991, p.379

40 Fishbein, D.S. Neuroradiologic work-up of brain tumours in 'Clinical Neuroimaging', (Ed. W.H. Theodore), Alan R. Liss Inc., New York, USA, 1988, p.111

41 Goldberg, H.I. Extraaxial brain tumours in 'Magnetic Resonance Imaging of the Brain and Spine', (Ed. S. W. Atlas), Raven Press, New York, USA, 1991, p.327

42 Di Chiro, G. and Brooks, R.A. PET-FDG of untreated and treated cerebral gliomas. *J. Nucl. Med.* 1988, 29, 421

43 Di Chiro, G., Oldfield, E., Wright, D.C. *et al.* Cerebral necrosis after radiotherapy and/or intraarterial chemotherapy for brain tumours: PET and neuropathologic studies. *A. J. R.* 1988, 150, 189

44 Jarenwattananon, A., Khandji, A. and Brust, J.C.M. Diagnostic Neuroimaging in Stroke in 'Clinical Neuroimaging', (Ed. W.H. Theodore), Alan R. Liss Inc., New York, USA, 1988. p.11

45 Masaryk, T.J. and Ross, J.S. MR Angiography: clinical applications in 'Magnetic Resonance Imaging of the Brain and Spine', (Ed. S. W. Atlas), Raven Press, New York, USA, 1991, p. 1079

46 Hartmann, A. Prolonged disturbances of regional cerebral blood flow in transient ischemic attacks. *Stroke* 1985, 16, 932

47 Bogousslawsky, J., Delaloye-Bishof, A., Regli, F. and Delaloye, B. Prolonged hypoperfusion and early stroke after transient ischemic attack. *Stroke* 1990, 21, 40

48 Powers, W.J. Positron Emission Tomography in Cerebrovascular Disease: Clinical Applications? in 'Clinical Neuroimaging', (Ed. W.H. Theodore), Alan R. Liss Inc., New York, USA, 1988, p.11

49 Giubilei, F., Lenzi, G.L., Di Piero, V. *et al.* Predictive value of brain perfusion single-photon emission computed tomography in acute ischemic stroke. *Stroke* 1990, 21, 895

50 Mountz, J., Modell, J.G., Foster, N.L. *et al.* Prognostication of Recovery Following Stroke Using the Comparison of CT and Technetium-99m HM-PAO SPECT. *J. Nucl. Med* 1984, 1, 61

51 Vorstrup, S., Brun, B. and Lassen, N.A. Evaluation of the cerebral vasodilatory capacity by the acetazolamide test before EC-IC bypass surgery in patients with occlusions of the internal carotid artery. *Stroke* 1986, 17, 1291

52 Le Bihan, D., Turner, R., Moonen, C.T. and Pekar, J. Imaging of diffusion and microcirculation with gradient sensitization: design, strategy, and significance. *J. Mag. Res. Imag.* 1991, 1, 7

53 Le Bihan, D., Turner, R., Douek, P. and Patronas, N. Diffusion MR imaging: clinical applications. *Am. J. Roentg.* 1991, 159, 591

54 Ogawa, S., Lee, T.M., Nayak, A.S. and Glynn P. Oxygenation-sensitive contrast in magnetic resonance image of rodent brain at high magnetic fields. *Magn. Res. Med.* 1990, 14, 68

55 Kurumaji, A., Dewar, D. and McCulloch, J. Metabolic mapping with deoxyglucose autoradiography as an approach for assessing drug action in the central nervous system in 'Imaging drug action in the brain', (Ed. E.D. London), CRC Press Inc., 1993, p. 207

56 Chen, C., Ouyang, X. and Wong, W.H. Sensor fusion in image reconstruction. *IEEE Trans. Nucl. Science* 1991, NS-38, 687

57 Wagner, H.N., Burns, H.D., Dannals, R.F. *et al.* Imaging dopamine receptors in the human brain by positron tomography. *Science* 1983, 221, 1264

58 Delforge, J., Syrota, A. and Mazoyer, B.M. Identifiability analysis and parameter identification of an in vivo ligand-receptor model from PET data. *IEEE Trans. Biomed. Eng.* 1990, 37, 653

59 Farde, L., Halldin, C., Stone-Elander, S. and Sedvall, G. PET analysis of human dopamine receptor subtypes using ^{11}C-SCH 23390 and ^{11}C-raclopride. *Psychopharmacology* 1987, 92, 278

60 Wong, D.F., Wagner, H.N., Dannals, R.F. *et al.* Effects of age on dopamine and serotonin receptors measured by positron tomography in the living human brain. *Science* 1984, 226, 1393

61 Young, A.B., Frey, K.A. and Agranoff, B.W. Receptor assays in vitro and in vivo in 'Positron emission tomography and autoradiography: principles and application for the brain and heart', (Eds. M. Phelps, J. Mazziotta, H. Schelbert), Raven Press, New York, USA, 1986, p. 73

62 Lucignani, G., Moresco, R.M. and Fazio, F. PET-Based Neuropharmacology: State of the Art. Cerebrovasc. *Brain Metab. Rev.* 1989, 1, 271

63 Maziére, B. and Maziére, M. Where have we got to with neuroreceptor mapping of the human brain? *Eur. J. Nucl. Med.* 1990, 16, 817

64 Maziére, B. and Maziére, M. Positron emission tomography studies of brain receptors. *Fundam. Clin. Pharmacol.* 1991, 5, 61

65 Comar, D., Maziére, M., Godot, J.M. *et al.* Visualization of ^{11}C-flunitrazepam displacement in the brain of the live baboon. *Nature* 1979, 280, 329

66 Stöcklin, G. Tracers for metabolic imaging of brain and heart. *Eur. J. Nucl. Med.* 1992, 19, 527

67 Herscovitch, P., Auchus, A. P., Gado, M.D. *et al.* Correction of Positron Emission Tomography data for cerebral atrophy. *J. Cereb. Blood Flow Metab.* 1986, 6, 120

68 Alavi, A., Newberg, A.B., Sounder, E. and Berlin, J.A. Quantitative analysis of PET and MRI data in normal aging and Alzheimer's disease: atrophy weighted total brain metabolism and absolute whole brain metabolism as reliable discriminators. *J. Nucl. Med.* 1993, 34, 1681

69 Burns, A., Philpot, M.P., Costa, D.C. *et al.* The investigation of Alzheimer's disease with single photon emission tomography. *J. Neurol. Neurosurg. Psych.* 1989, 52, 248

70 Duara, R., Grady, C., Haxby, J. *et al.* Positron emission tomography in Alzheimer's disease. *Neurology* 1986, 36, 879

71 Friedland, R.P. and Luxenberg, J. Neuroimaging and dementia in 'Clinical Neuroimaging', (Ed. W.H. Theodore), Alan R. Liss Inc., New York , USA, 1988, p. 139

72 Gemmel, H.G., Sharp, P.F., Smith, F.W. *et al.* Cerebral blood flow measured by SPECT as a diagnostic tool in the study of dementia. *Psychiatry Res.* 1989 29, 327

73 Haxby, J.V., Grady, C.L., Duara, R. *et al.* Neocortical metabolic abnormalities precede nonmemory cognitive defects in early Alzheimer's type dementia. *Arch. Neurol.* 1986, 43, 882

74 Jagust, A.J., Budinger, T.F. and Reed, B.R. The diagnosis of dementia with single photon emission computed tomography. *Arch. Neurol.* 1987, 44, 258

75 Johnson, K.A., Mueller, S.T., Walsche, T.M. *et al.* Cerebral perfusion imaging in Alzheimer's disease: use of single photon emission computed tomography and Iofetamine Hydrochloride I-123. *Arch. Neurol.* 1987, 44, 165

76 McGeer, P.L., Kamo, H., Harrop., R. *et al.* Positron emission tomography in patients with clinically diagnosed Alzheimer's disease. *Can. Med. Ass. J.* 1986, 134, 597

77 Perani, D., Di Piero, V., Vallar, G. *et al.* Technetium-99m HM-PAO-SPECT study of regional cerebral perfusion in early Alzheimer's disease. *J. Nucl. Med.* 1988, 29,

Author Index

Subject Index